ANTIVIRAL DRUGS

CONTENTS

CONTRIBUTORS ix

PREFACE xiii

PART I HUMAN IMMUNODEFICIENCY VIRUS

Section I HIV Protease Inhibitors

1 Discovery and Development of Atazanavir 3
Awny Farajallah, R. Todd Bunch, and Nicholas A. Meanwell

2 Discovery and Development of PL-100, A Novel HIV-1 Protease Inhibitor 19
Jinzi J. Wu and Joseph Musto

3 Darunavir (Prezista, TMC114): From Bench to Clinic, Improving Treatment Options for HIV-Infected Patients 31
Marie-Pierre de Béthune, Vanitha Sekar, Sabrina Spinosa-Guzman, Marc Vanstockem, Sandra De Meyer, Piet Wigerinck, and Eric Lefebvre

4 Discovery and Development of Tipranavir 47
Karen R. Romines

Section II HIV Non-nucleoside Reverse Transcriptase Inhibitors

5 TMC278 (Rilpivirine): A Next-Generation NNRTI in Phase III Clinical Development for Treatment-Naive Patients 59
Jérôme Guillemont, Katia Boven, Herta Crauwels, and Marie-Pierre de Béthune

6 Etravirine: From TMC125 to Intelence: A Treatment Paradigm Shift for HIV-Infected Patients 71
Koen Andries, Ann Debunne, Thomas N. Kakuda, Michael Kukla, Ruud Leemans, Johan Vingerhoets, Brian Woodfall, and Marie-Pierre de Béthune

Section III HIV Nucleoside Reverse Transcriptase Inhibitors

7 Discovery and Development of Tenofovir Disoproxil Fumarate 85
Erik De Clercq

8 Discovery and Development of Apricitabine 103
Susan Cox, John Deadman, Justine Southby, and Jonathan Coates

Section IV HIV Entry Inhibitors

9 Discovery and Development of Maraviroc and PF-232798: CCR5 Antagonists for the Treatment of HIV-1 Infection 117
Patrick Dorr and Paul Stupple

10 Discovery of the CCR5 Antagonist Vicriviroc (Sch 417690/Sch-D) for the Treatment of HIV-1 Infection 137
Jayaram R. Tagat, Julie M. Strizki, and Lisa M. Dunkle

11 Discovery and Development of HIV-1 Entry Inhibitors That Target gp120 149
John F. Kadow, John Bender, Alicia Regueiro-Ren, Yasutsugu Ueda, Tao Wang, Kap-Sun Yeung, and Nicholas A. Meanwell

Section V HIV Integrase Inhibitors

12 Discovery of MK-0536: A Potential Second-Generation HIV-1 Integrase Strand Transfer Inhibitor with a High Genetic Barrier to Mutation 163
Melissa S. Egbertson, John S. Wai, Mark Cameron, and R. Scott Hoerrner

13 Discovery and Development of HIV Integrase Inhibitor Raltegravir 181
Vincenzo Summa and Paola Pace

14 Elvitegravir: A Novel Monoketo Acid HIV-1 Integrase Strand Transfer Inhibitor 197
Hisashi Shinkai, Masanori Sato, and Yuji Matsuzaki

PART II HEPATITIS C VIRUS

Section VI Protease Inhibitors

15 Discovery and Development of Telaprevir 209
Anne-Laure Grillot, Luc J. Farmer, B. Govinda Rao, William P. Taylor, Ilan S. Weisberg, Ira M. Jacobson, Robert B. Perni, and Ann D. Kwong

16 Discovery and Development of BILN 2061 and Follow-up BI 201335 225
Montse Llinàs-Brunet and Peter W. White

17 Intervention of Hepatitis C Replication Through NS3-4A, the Protease Inhibitor Boceprevir 239
Srikanth Venkatraman and F. George Njoroge

18 Discovery and Development of the HCV NS3/4A Protease Inhibitor Danoprevir (ITMN-191/RG7227) 257
Scott D. Seiwert, Karl Kossen, Lin Pan, Jyanwei Liu, and Brad O. Buckman

19 **Discovery and Development of the HCV Protease Inhibitor TMC435** 273
Pierre Raboisson, Gregory Fanning, Herman de Kock, Åsa Rosenquist, René Verloes, and Kenneth Simmen

Section VII HCV Polymerase Nucleoside Inhibitors

20 **Discovery and Clinical Evaluation of the Nucleoside Analog Balapiravir (R1626) for the Treatment of HCV Infection** 287
Klaus Klumpp and David B. Smith

21 **Discovery and Development of PSI-6130/RG7128** 305
Phillip A. Furman, Michael J. Otto, and Michael J. Sofia

Section VIII Other HCV Inhibitors

22 **Discovery of Cyclophilin Inhibitor NIM811 as a Novel Therapeutic Agent for HCV** 317
Kai Lin

23 **HCV Viral Entry Inhibitors** 329
Flossie Wong-Staal, Guohong Liu, and Jeffrey McKelvy

PART III RESPIRATORY SYNCYTIAL VIRUS INHIBITORS

24 **Discovery of the RSV Inhibitor TMC353121** 341
Jean-François Bonfanti, Gabriela Ispas, Frans Van Velsen, Wieslawa Olszewska, Tom Gevers, and Dirk Roymans

25 **Discovery and Development of Orally Active RSV Fusion Inhibitors** 353
Nicholas A. Meanwell, Christopher W. Cianci, and Mark R. Krystal

26 **Discovery and Development of RSV604** 367
Joanna Chapman and G. Stuart Cockerill

PART IV INFLUENZA, HEPATITIS B, AND CYTOMEGALOVIRUS INHIBITORS

27 **Discovery and Development of Influenza Virus Sialidase Inhibitor Relenza** 385
Robin Thomson and Mark von Itzstein

28 **Discovery and Development of Entecavir** 401
Richard Wilber, Bruce Kreter, Marc Bifano, Stephanie Danetz, Lois Lehman-McKeeman, Daniel J. Tenney, Nicholas Meanwell, Robert Zahler, and Helena Brett-Smith

29 **Benzimidazole Ribonucleosides: Novel Drug Candidates for the Prevention and Treatment of Cytomegalovirus Diseases** 417
Karen K. Biron, Kristjan S. Gudmundsson, and John C. Drach

INDEX 435

CONTRIBUTORS

Koen Andries, Johnson & Johnson Pharmaceutical Research and Development, Beerse, Belgium

John Bender, Bristol-Myers Squibb Company Research and Development, Wallingford, Connecticut

Marc Bifano, Bristol-Myers Squibb Company Research and Development, Wallingford, Connecticut

Karen K. Biron, Pathfinder Pharmaceuticals, Inc., Durham, North Carolina

Jean-François Bonfanti, Janssen R&D, Janssen-Cilag, Johnson & Johnson, Val de Reuil, France

Katia Boven, Tibotec, Inc., Titusville, New Jersey

Helena Brett-Smith, Bristol-Myers Squibb Company Research and Development, Wallingford, Connecticut

Brad O. Buckman, InterMune, Inc., Brisbane, California

R. Todd Bunch, Bristol-Myers Squibb Company, Evansville, Indiana

Mark Cameron, Merck Research Laboratories, West Point, Pennsylvania

Joanna Chapman, Arrow Therapeutics, Ltd., London, UK

Christopher W. Cianci, Bristol-Myers Squibb Company Research and Development, Wallingford, Connecticut

Jonathan Coates, Avexa Ltd., Richmond, Victoria, Australia

G. Stuart Cockerill, Arrow Therapeutics, Ltd., London, UK

Susan Cox, Avexa Ltd., Richmond, Victoria, Australia

Herta Crauwels, Tibotec BVBA, Beerse, Belgium

Stephanie Danetz, Bristol-Myers Squibb Company Research and Development, Wallingford, Connecticut

John Deadman, Avexa Ltd., Richmond, Victoria, Australia

Marie-Pierre de Béthune, Tibotec BVBA, Beerse, Belgium

Ann Debunne, Johnson & Johnson Pharmaceutical Research and Development, Beerse, Belgium

Erik De Clercq, Rega Institute for Medical Research, Leuven, Belgium

Herman de Kock, Tibotec BVBA, Beerse, Belgium

Sandra De Meyer, Tibotec BVBA, Beerse, Belgium

Patrick Dorr, Abbott Laboratories, Berkshire, UK

John C. Drach, School of Dentistry, University of Michigan, Ann Arbor, Michigan

Lisa M. Dunkle, Merck Research Laboratories, Kenilworth, New Jersey

Melissa S. Egbertson, Merck Research Laboratories, West Point, Pennsylvania

Gregory Fanning, Tibotec BVBA, Beerse, Belgium

Awny Farajallah, Bristol-Myers Squibb Company, Plainsboro, New Jersey

Luc J. Farmer, Vertex Pharmaceuticals, Inc., Cambridge, Massachusetts

Phillip A. Furman, Pharmasset, Inc., Princeton, New Jersey

Tom Gevers, Tibotec BVBA, Beerse, Belgium

Anne-Laure Grillot, Vertex Pharmaceuticals, Inc., Cambridge, Massachusetts

Kristjan S. Gudmundsson, University of Iceland, Reykjavik, Iceland

Jérôme Guillemont, Johnson & Johnson Pharmaceutical Research and Development, Val de Reuil, France

R. Scott Hoerrner, Merck Process Chemistry, Rahway, New Jersey

Gabriela Ispas, Tibotec BVBA, Beerse, Belgium

Ira M. Jacobson, Joan and Sanford I. Weill Medical College of Cornell University, New York, New York

John F. Kadow, Bristol-Myers Squibb Company Research and Development, Wallingford, Connecticut

Thomas N. Kakuda, Tibotec, Inc., Titusville, New Jersey

Klaus Klumpp, Roche Palo Alto LLC, Palo Alto, California

Karl Kossen, InterMune, Inc., Brisbane, California

Bruce Kreter, Bristol-Myers Squibb Company Research and Development, Wallingford, Connecticut

Mark R. Krystal, Bristol-Myers Squibb Research and Development, Wallingford, Connecticut

Michael Kukla, Johnson & Johnson Research and Development, Spring House, Pennsylvania

Ann D. Kwong, Vertex Pharmaceuticals, Inc., Cambridge, Massachusetts

Ruud Leemans, Johnson & Johnson Pharmaceuticals Research and Development, Beerse, Belgium

Eric Lefebvre, Janssen-Cilag BV, Amsterdam, The Netherlands

Lois Lehman-McKeeman, Bristol-Myers Squibb Company Research and Development, Wallingford, Connecticut

Kai Lin, Novartis Institutes for BioMedical Research, Inc., Cambridge, Massachusetts

Guohong Liu, iTherX Pharmaceuticals, Inc., San Diego, California

Jyanwei Liu, InterMune, Inc., Brisbane, California

Montse Llinàs-Brunet, Boehringer Ingelheim (Canada), Ltd., Laval, Quebec, Canada

Yuji Matsuzaki, Central Pharmaceutical Research Institute, JT, Inc., Osaka, Japan

Jeffrey McKelvy, iTherX Pharmaceuticals, Inc., San Diego, California

Nicholas A. Meanwell, Bristol-Myers Squibb Company Research and Development, Wallingford, Connecticut

Joseph Musto, GlaxoSmithKline, Research Triangle Park, North Carolina

F. George Njoroge, Schering Plough Research Institute, Kenilworth, New Jersey

Wieslawa Olszewska, Imperial College, London, UK

Michael J. Otto, Pharmasset, Inc., Princeton, New Jersey

Paola Pace, Merck Research Laboratories, Rome, Italy

Lin Pan, InterMune, Inc., Brisbane, California

Robert B. Perni, Sirtris, Cambridge, Massachusetts

Pierre Raboisson, Tibotec BVBA, Beerse, Belgium

B. Govinda Rao, Vertex Pharmaceuticals, Inc., Cambridge, Massachusetts

Alicia Regueiro-Ren, Bristol-Myers Squibb Company Research and Development, Wallingford, Connecticut

Karen R. Romines, Pathfinder Pharmaceuticals, Inc., Durham, North Carolina

Åsa Rosenquist, Tibotec BVBA, Beerse, Belgium

Dirk Roymans, Tibotec BVBA, Beerse, Belgium

Masanori Sato, Pharmaceutical Division, JT, Inc., Tokyo, Japan

Scott D. Seiwert, InterMune, Inc., Brisbane, California

Vanitha Sekar, Tibotec, Inc., Titusville, New Jersey

Hisashi Shinkai, Central Pharmaceutical Research Institute, JT, Inc., Osaka, Japan

Kenneth Simmen, Tibotec BVBA, Beerse, Belgium

David B. Smith, Roche Palo Alto LLC, Palo Alto, California (currently at Alios BioPharma)

Michael J. Sofia, Pharmasset, Inc., Princeton, New Jersey

Justine Southby, Avexa Ltd., Richmond, Victoria, Australia

Sabrina Spinosa-Guzman, Tibotec BVBA, Beerse, Belgium

Julie M. Strizki, Merck Research Laboratories, Kenilworth, New Jersey

Paul Stupple, Pfizer Global R&D, Kent, UK

Vincenzo Summa, Merck Research Laboratories, Rome, Italy

Jayaram R. Tagat, Merck Research Laboratories, Kenilworth, New Jersey

William P. Taylor, Vertex Pharmaceuticals, Inc., Cambridge, Massachusetts

Daniel J. Tenney, Bristol-Myers Squibb Company Research and Development, Wallingford, Connecticut

Robin Thomson, Institute for Glycomics, Griffith University, Queensland, Australia

Yasutsugu Ueda, Bristol-Myers Squibb Research and Development, Wallingford, Connecticut

Marc Vanstockem, Tibotec BVBA, Beerse, Belgium

Frans Van Velsen, Tibotec BVBA, Beerse, Belgium

Srikanth Venkatraman, Schering Plough Research Institute, Kenilworth, New Jersey

René Verloes, Tibotec BVBA, Beerse, Belgium

Johan Vingerhoets, Tibotec BVBA, Beerse, Belgium

Mark von Itzstein, Institute for Glycomics, Griffith University, Queensland, Australia

John S. Wai, Merck Research Laboratories, West Point, Pennsylvania

Tao Wang, Bristol-Myers Squibb Company Research and Development, Wallingford, Connecticut

Ilan S. Weisberg, Joan and Sanford I. Weill Medical College of Cornell University, New York, New York

Peter W. White, Boehringer Ingelheim (Canada), Ltd., Laval, Quebec, Canada

Piet Wigerinck, Galapagos NV, Mechelen, Belgium

Richard Wilber, Bristol-Myers Squibb Company Research and Development, Wallingford, Connecticut

Flossie Wong-Staal, iTherX Pharmaceuticals, Inc., San Diego, California

Brian Woodfall, Tibotec BVBA, Beerse, Belgium

Jinzi J. Wu, GlaxoSmithKline, Research Triangle Park, North Carolina

Kap-Sun Yeung, Bristol-Myers Squibb Company Research and Development, Wallingford, Connecticut

Robert Zahler, Bristol-Myers Squibb Company Research and Development, Wallingford, Connecticut

PREFACE

We live in an unprecedented era in the antiviral drug discovery. The first antiviral therapies became available about 50 years ago with the introduction of drugs such as idoxuridinefor the treatment of herpetic keratitis and methisazone for the treatment and prophylaxis of smallpox and variola infection. Almost two decades later, the discovery of ACV (acyclovir) ushered in a new era of antivirals. One of the subsequent big milestones was heralded by the discovery of AZT (zidovudine), approved in 1987 for use against HIV, followed by more than two decades of an intense antiretroviral drug discovery effort, which resulted in more than 20 new U.S. Food and Drug Administration (FDA)-approved anti-HIV drugs. Along with drugs discovered and registered for use against hepatitis C virus (HCV), hepatitis B virus (HBV), influenza, and herpes simplex virus (HSV), there are now more than 50 FDA-approved small-molecule antiviral drugs. The pace of viral drug discovery continues unabated as new viral and host targets as well as new drug discovery paradigms emerge.

This book is organized by virus class, such as HIV, HCV, respiratory syncytial virus (RSV), influenza, HBV, and cytomegalovirus (CMV). In turn, the most intensely researched viruses, such as HIV and HCV, are organized further by the inhibitory mechanism (polymerase, entry, integrase, etc.). The book was not intended to be a comprehensive listing of all antiviral drugs and molecules, although it covers many of them. Described is the science of design, discovery, and development of drugs, from bench through the clinic. These compounds include relatively recently approved antiviral drugs as well as molecules in advanced clinical development at the time of writing. Issues encountered and strategies toward their successful resolution are described by top academic and industrial authorities in the field. What strategy was used to discover the initial molecules used in lead optimization? What obstacles had to be overcome in the lead optimization process to yield molecules of clinical value? What were the drug development, pharmacokinetics and viral resistance hurdles, and how were these addressed? Topics showcase challenges and solutions of problems encountered, and it is hoped that the tremendous experience accumulated over many years of research will be particularly useful to basic and bench scientists as well as clinicians as they continue discovering and developing new drugs and therapies. It is hoped that this holistic approach to describing the drug discovery process from bench to clinic will allow the reader to better appreciate the interconnectedness of discovery and development, and will accelerate discovery of new drugs that address unmet patient needs.

This editor would like to thank all the authors for their outstanding contributions, and to dedicate his part of this effort to his sons.

Wieslaw M. Kazmierski

Raleigh, North Carolina

PART I

HUMAN IMMUNODEFICIENCY VIRUS

1

DISCOVERY AND DEVELOPMENT OF ATAZANAVIR

AWNY FARAJALLAH
Bristol-Myers Squibb Company, Plainsboro, New Jersey

R. TODD BUNCH
Bristol-Myers Squibb Company, Evansville, Indiana

NICHOLAS A. MEANWELL
Bristol-Myers Squibb Company Research and Development, Wallingford, Connecticut

INTRODUCTION

Atazanavir is an azapeptide inhibitor of HIV-1 protease that prevents the formation of mature virions in HIV-1-infected cells by inhibiting the cleavage of gag and gag-pol polyproteins. Atazanavir was developed to address a number of concerns with existing protease inhibitors: high pill burden, high frequency of dosing, and metabolic side effects such as hyperlipidemia. The development program focused initially on dosing atazanavir without coadministering a pharmacokinetic enhancer such as ritonavir. Ritonavir inhibits hepatic CYP3A4 and the metabolism of drugs (such as atazanavir) utilizing this pathway, thereby increasing the blood levels of these drugs. The emerging practice of "boosting" with low-dose ritonavir led to the evaluation of this alternative dosing strategy, initially in treatment-experienced subjects who had previously received and failed multiple antiretroviral regimens, then in antiretroviral-naive patients.

DISCOVERY

Atazanavir (BMS-262362, Scheme 1) was identified from studies of a series of pseudosymmetric azapeptide substrate analogs of HIV-1 protease in which fundamental inhibitory activity relies on replacement of the hydrolyzable amide bond by a hydroxyethylene isostere [1–3]. Although the initial examples of this chemotype demonstrated favorable in vitro and in vivo properties [1,2], further optimization for in vitro HIV-1 inhibitory potency and in vivo exposure was required to identify atazanavir [3,4]. As shown in Scheme 1, the two closely related lead compounds **1** and **2** demonstrated disparate properties: The isoamyl derivative (**1**) is a potent HIV-1 protease inhibitor, $IC_{50} = 16$ nM, with good antiviral activity in cell culture, $EC_{50} = 2.7$ nM, but exhibits poor oral bioavailability, while the cyclohexylmethyl analog (**2**) is a 10-fold weaker protease inhibitor, $IC_{50} = 177$ nM, and antiviral agent, $EC_{50} = 55$ nM, that demonstrates good bioavailability following oral administration to mice [3]. Based on x-ray crystallographic information of the early lead CGP-53820 (**3**) cocrystallized with HIV-1 protease [5], the potential of introducing larger P1′ substituents was examined, with the anticipation that potency would be enhanced while preserving the physicochemical properties conferring good absorption. From a drug design perspective, the effort sought to establish additional favorable contacts between the inhibitor and protease residues Arg8, Phe153, Gly148, and Gly149 located at the periphery of the S1′ pocket [4]. The synthesis and evaluation of a derivative in which the cyclohexylmethyl substituent of **2** was replaced by a biphenyl moiety established the validity of the hypothesis since the new compound potently inhibited HIV-1 protease, $IC_{50} = 35$ nM, demonstrating tolerance for a large P1′ element, while expressing excellent antiviral activity in cell culture, $EC_{50} = 1.8$ nM. Replacing the two valine residues with *tert*-Leu resulted in CGP-75355 (**4**), which showed

Antiviral Drugs: From Basic Discovery Through Clinical Trials, First Edition. Edited by Wieslaw M. Kazmierski.

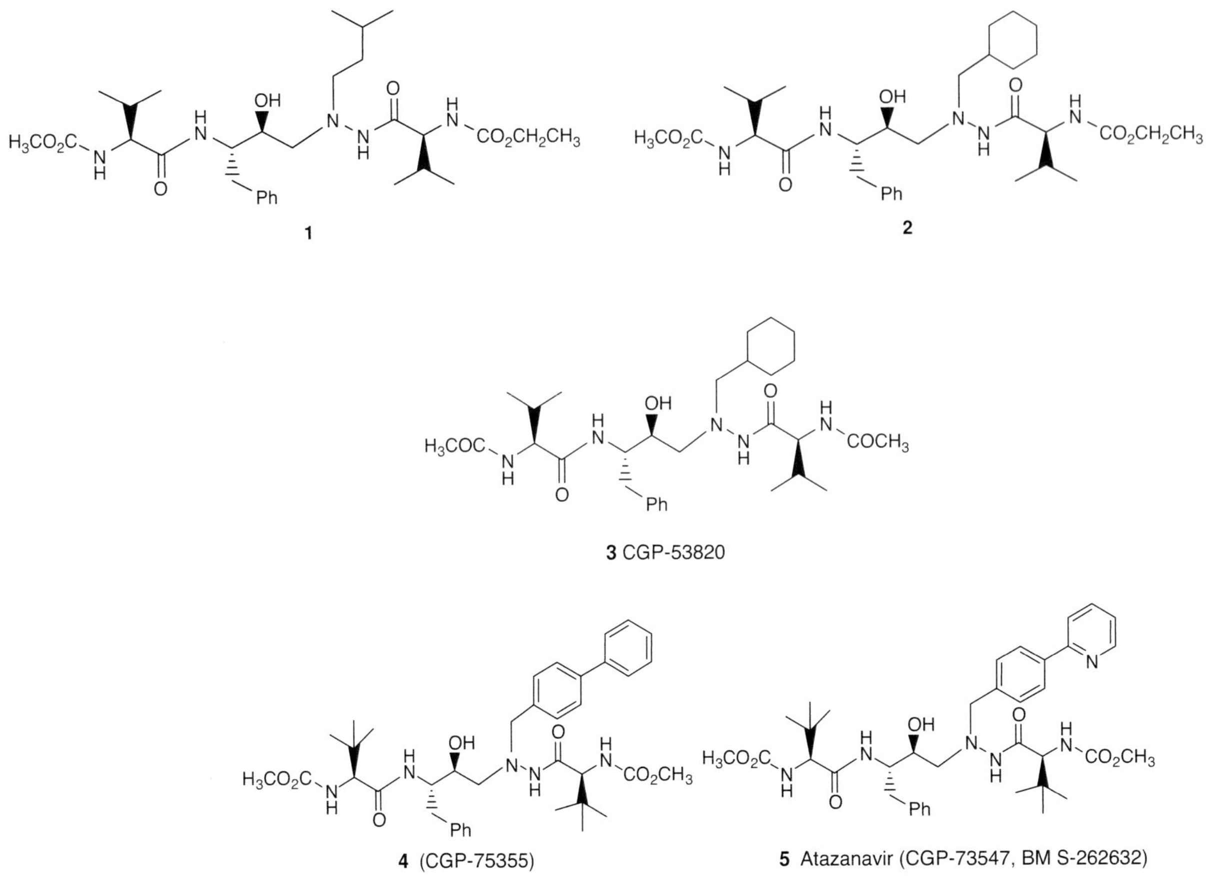

SCHEME 1 Discovery of atazanavir.

a further improvement in cell culture potency, $EC_{50} = 0.7$ nM. More important, protease inhibitors that incorporated *tert*-Leu residues were generally well absorbed in mice following oral administration.

With the structural elements critical for potent antiviral activity established, attention was directed toward improving pharmaceutical properties, with a focus on increasing solubility [4]. To this end, heterocycles designed to increase hydrophilicity were introduced to replace the distal phenyl of the biphenyl moiety. This exercise identified the 2-pyridyl as the optimal element, providing atazanavir (**5**, BMS-262632, CGP-73547) as a potent HIV-1 protease inhibitor, $IC_{50} =$ 26 nM, that retained potency toward HIV-1 protease resistant to saquinavir. Atazanavir (**5**) exhibits excellent antiviral properties in cell culture, $EC_{50} = 1.4$ nM and $EC_{90} = 3$ nM, with a good therapeutic index, $CC_{30} = 21.8$ μM and $CC_{90} =$ 31.8 μM. Following oral administration to mice and dogs, atazanavir (**5**) showed good plasma bioavailability, establishing blood levels in excess of the EC_{90} [4].

SYNTHESIS

The strategic approach to the preparation of atazanavir developed by the discovery chemistry team, summarized in Scheme 2, has largely been followed by the process synthesis depicted in Scheme 3 [4], with several modifications designed to facilitate the preparation of multikilogram quantities of the active pharmaceutical ingredient [6]. The discovery synthesis was satisfactory for the preparation of material for preliminary toxicological evaluation but was deemed to be less than optimal for the synthesis of the significantly larger quantities of drug required for longer-term toxicological studies and clinical trials. The process chemistry strategy was focused on improving the synthesis of the two key intermediates, hydrazine (**9**) and epoxide (**11**), that were used in the discovery synthesis. With access to these molecules in hand, optimization of the reagents and conditions used for their coupling, followed by improvements in the final elaboration to the product, were completed.

In the discovery synthesis (Scheme 2), a nickel-catalyzed cross-coupling reaction between 2-bromopyridine and the Grignard reagent (**7**) derived from a protected form of 4-bromobenzaldehyde (**6**) was used to prepare the aldehyde (**8**) [4]. This procedure required the use of diisobutylaluminum hydride, a problematic reagent when used in large-scale reactions. Access to (**9**) was improved considerably by coupling 2-bromopyridine with commercially available 4-formylbenzeneboronic acid (**13**) under Suzuki conditions (Scheme 3), a process mild enough to obviate the

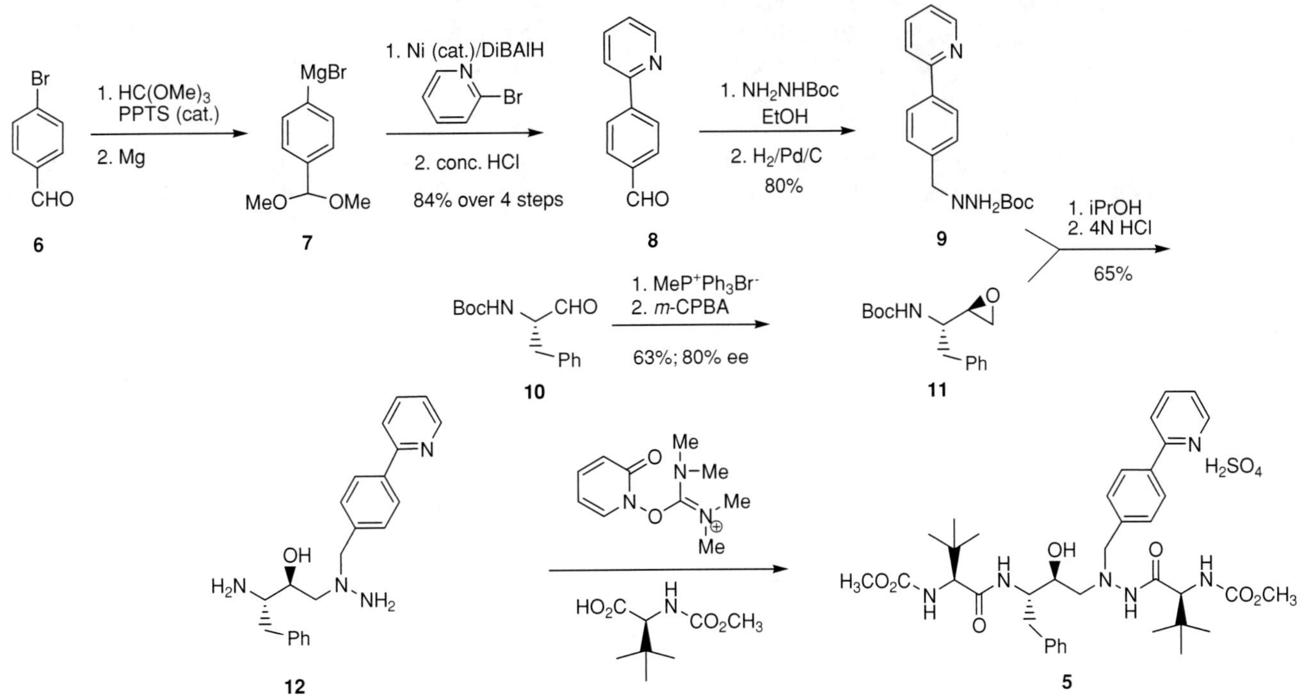

SCHEME 2 Discovery synthesis of atazanavir.

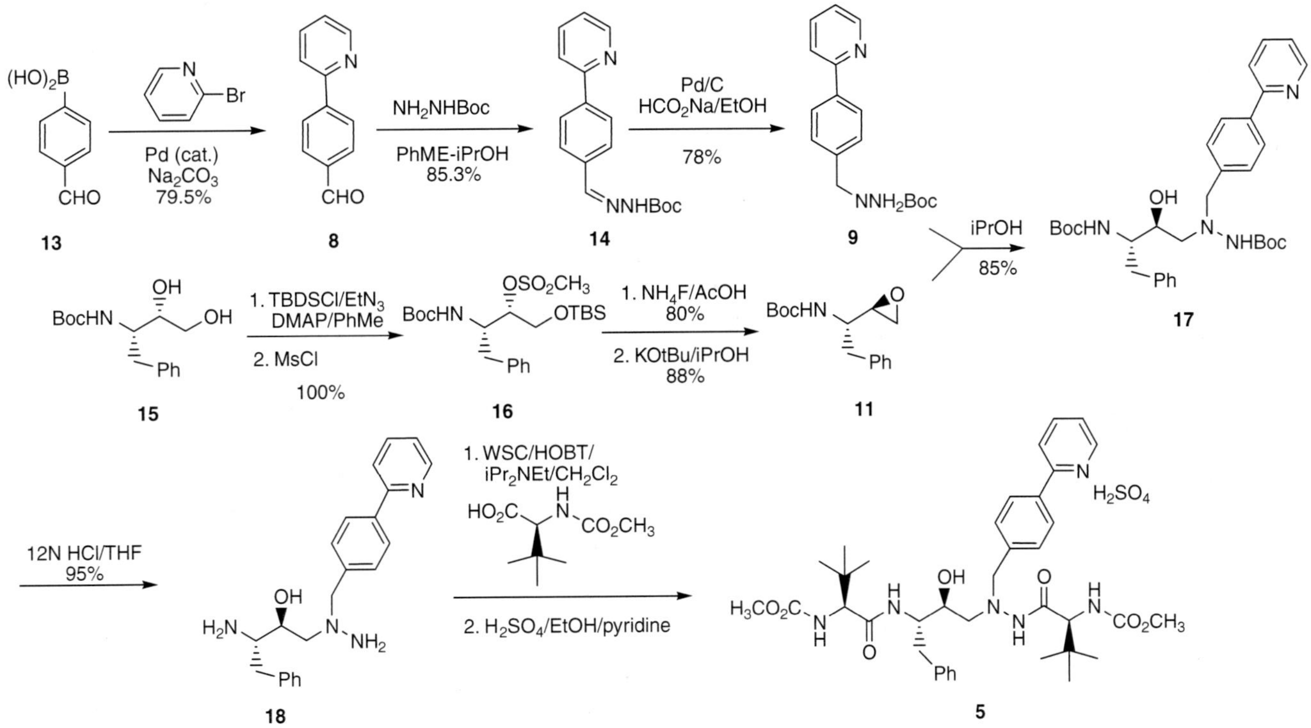

SCHEME 3 Optimized process for the large-scale preparation of atazanavir.

inefficiencies associated with the tandem protection/ deprotection of the formyl group used by the discovery group. Condensation of (**8**) with *tert*-butyl carbazate followed by Pd-catalyzed hydrogenation then afforded the *tert*-butoxycarbonyl (Boc)-protected hydrazine (**9**) in high yield.

An optimized approach to the preparation of epoxide (**11**) relied upon ring closure of a vicinal diol, a process that avoided the racemization-prone L-Boc-phenylalaninal as an intermediate. The secondary mesylate (**16**) was prepared in quantitative yield in a one-pot process comprising silyl protection of the primary alcohol of (**15**) followed by mesylation with methanesulfonyl chloride. Desilylation occurred upon exposure of the product to ammonium fluoride in acetic acid, a much less expensive reagent than the more commonly used tetrabutylammonium fluoride. Epoxide formation was completed by treating the liberated alcohol with potassium *tert*-butoxide in isopropanol, determined to be the optimal base after screening several candidates, to provide (**11**) in good overall yield. The coupling of the two key structural elements (**9**) and (**11**) was effected by heating equimolar quantities in isopropanol at reflux for 24 h. Isolation of (**17**) was straightforward, accomplished by precipitation upon diluting the reaction mixture with water and recrystallization from a mixture of acetonitrile and water which removes small quantities of by-products. The two Boc moieties of (**17**) were removed under acidic conditions and the exposed amines coupled simultaneously with *N*-methoxycarbonyl-L-*tert*-leucine using a water-soluble carbodiimide [6].

A more recent approach to the synthesis of atazanavir (**5**), depicted in Scheme 4, relies upon a diastereoselective reduction of the ketone precursor (**22**) to install the tertiary alcohol with the correct absolute configuration, allowing a different retrosynthetic disconnection [7]. Reduction of ketone (**22**) with lithium tri-*tert*-butoxyaluminum hydride provided the *syn*-1,2-amino alcohol moiety found in atazanavir (**5**), with the high (28 : 1) Felkin–Anh type of diastereoselectivity controlled by the chirality of the proximal *N*-(methoxycarbonyl)-L-*tert*-leucinyl moiety.

The final issue to resolve with atazanavir was the bioavailability of the free base, which is poorly soluble in water, <1 μg/mL, leading to poor bioavailability due to dissolution-limited absorption. The bisulfate salt was identified as the optimal form of atazanavir for development after an extensive survey which identified this salt as possessing excellent aqueous solubility, 4 to 5 mg/mL. The bisulfate salt was found to exist as two crystalline forms with form 1, formed with good reproducibility in acetone, acetonitrile, or ethanol, displaying good crystallinity [8]. Comparison of the ^{1}H-NMR spectra of the free base and bisulfate salt indicated that protonation had occurred on the pyridine ring, as might be anticipated.

PRECLINICAL PHARMACOKINETICS

The nonclinical safety profile of atazanavir has been evaluated extensively in pharmacokinetic/absorption, distribution, metabolism, and excretion (ADME), and toxicology studies. Sensitive and specific bioanalytical methods, high-performance liquid chromatography/ultraviolet, and liquid chromatography/mass spectrometry were used to determine the plasma and urine concentrations of atazanavir, respectively. The concentrations of radioactivity in plasma and urine samples from radiolabeled studies were determined by

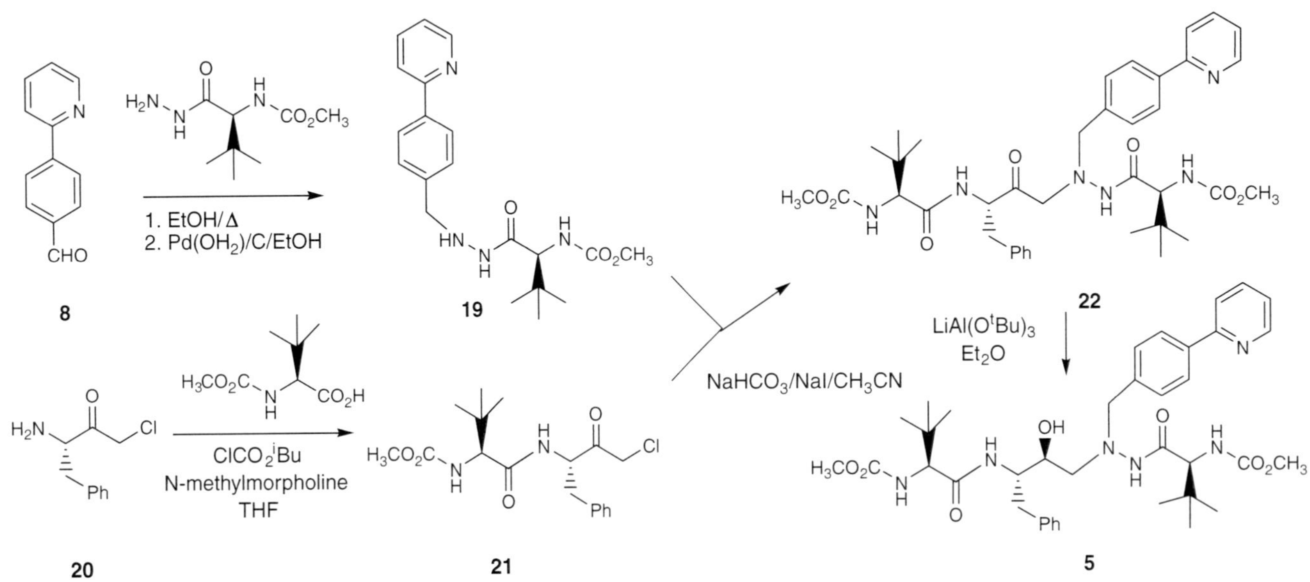

SCHEME 4 Alternative synthesis of atazanavir.

direct liquid scintillation counting (LSC) of the samples mixed with the scintillation cocktail. The samples of blood and the homogenates of feces and various organs/tissues were either bleached, solubilized, or combusted prior to analysis by LSC.

Absorption

Atazanavir exhibited modest absolute oral bioavailability in rats (15.2% from a PEG-400 suspension) and dogs (36.3% from a capsule). The recovery of a significant amount of unchanged drug in rat (39%) and dog (79%) after oral administration suggested incomplete absorption and/or biliary elimination of atazanavir in both species. When compared to the decline in plasma concentrations after intravenous dosing, the slow decline in plasma levels after achieving peak plasma levels (at 2 h) in nonfasted rats and dogs following oral administration suggested prolonged oral absorption [9].

Distribution

The steady-state volume of distribution of atazanavir in rats (1.62 L/kg) and dogs (0.76 to 2.45 L/kg) is greater than the total body water (0.67 L/kg in the rat and 0.60 L/kg in the dog), indicating extravascular distribution and/or tissue protein binding. Accordingly, drug-related radioactivity was distributed extensively into and decayed from all tissues in rats following oral administration of a 100-mg/kg dose of [^{14}C]atazanavir, with no sequestration in any particular tissue. The highest levels of radioactivity were associated with the dosing/absorption site(s) along the gastrointestinal tract and liver. Appreciable levels of radioactivity were noted in tissues known to be reservoirs of HIV, such as lymph nodes and testes. Atazanavir-derived radioactivity was secreted in milk and distributed to fetal tissues of the rat, suggesting placental transfer of the drug. The in vitro binding of atazanavir to mouse, rat, dog, and human serum proteins was comparable, ranging from 86.5 to 92.8%. Tissue and plasma levels of radioactivity were generally higher in female than in male rats following [^{14}C]atazanavir.

Biotransformation

The metabolic pathways of atazanavir in rats, dogs, and humans are similar and involve monooxygenation, dioxygenation, glucuronidation, N-dealkylation, hydrolysis, and oxygenation with dehydrogenation. The multiple monohydroxylated, dihydroxylated, and trihydroxylated metabolites demonstrated that the oxygenation of atazanavir can occur on the phenylmethyl ring, the pyridinylphenylmethyl ring system, and at different positions on the pentaazatetradecanedioic acid dimethyl ester part of the molecule. The major elimination pathway appeared to be CYP3A4-mediated conversion to these oxygenated metabolites and excretion in the bile as either free or glucuronidated metabolites. Additional minor metabolic pathways observed consisted of N-dealkylation metabolites and hydrolytic cleavage of the carbamate moieties. In rat and dog plasma, the major circulating components were atazanavir and 4-(2-pyridyl)benzoic acid (M2), along with small amounts of an unidentified keto metabolite. In addition, traces of an N-dealkylated metabolite, M14, were observed in dog plasma. These metabolites were also identified in humans and are depicted in Scheme 5 [9,10].

Elimination

Atazanavir is an intermediate- to high-extraction drug in animals; the elimination half-life in the rat and dog is 0.94 and 0.45 h, respectively. The minimal recovery of radioactivity in urine (<7%) and substantial recovery in feces (>67%) after intravenous administration in rats and dogs suggested that the major route of excretion of atazanavir and its metabolite(s) is via the bile.

TOXICOLOGY

The ADME profiles of atazanavir in rats and dogs indicated that these species were appropriate for the toxicity evaluation of atazanavir. The oral toxicity of atazanavir was well characterized in a comprehensive nonclinical toxicology program that included single- and repeat-dose toxicity, reproductive and developmental toxicity, in vitro and in vivo genotoxicity, carcinogenicity, and immunotoxicity studies. The safety assessment included comparisons of plasma exposures to atazanavir in animals to those in humans following the recommended clinical dosing regimens of 400 mg/day atazanavir without ritonavir, or 300 mg/day atazanavir and 100 mg/day ritonavir.

Single-Dose Toxicity

Single-dose oral toxicity studies were conducted in mice and rats at doses of 200 to 1600 mg/kg. Atazanavir demonstrated a low order of acute toxicity in both species. In mice, the minimal lethal doses were 1600 and 800 mg/kg in males and females, respectively. Deaths occurred from 1 to 5 days after dosing and were not associated with any drug-related gross or histopathologic changes. Clinical signs, considered to be agonal, were present just prior to or concomitant with death. Nonspecific clinical signs were also observed after dosing in surviving animals at high doses. Atazanavir was well tolerated in mice up to 400 mg/kg. In rats, the minimal lethal dose was greater than 1600 mg/kg. The greater sensitivity of mice to the acute effects of atazanavir compared to rats may be related to higher systemic exposure to atazanavir, as demonstrated in subsequent toxicity studies [9].

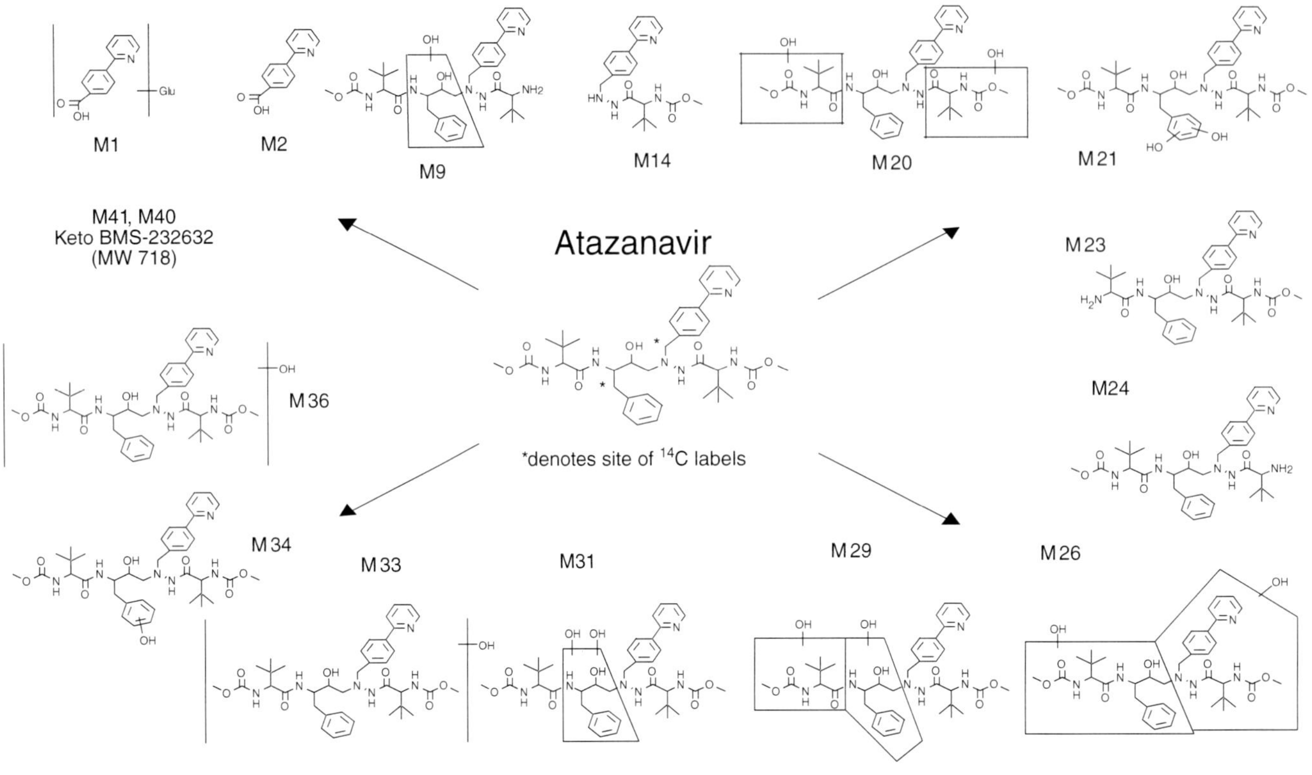

SCHEME 5 Proposed metabolic pathways of atazanavir in humans.

Repeat-Dose Toxicity

Repeat-dose toxicity of atazanavir was evaluated in studies in rats, dogs, and mice of up to 9 months' duration. Atazanavir-related findings in all three species were generally confined to the liver. In rats, the toxicity of atazanavir was evaluated at doses up to 1200 mg/kg per day in the 2-week study and up to 900 mg/kg per day in the 6-month study with a 3-month interim evaluation and a 2-month postdose recovery period. Atazanavir was generally well tolerated. Liver changes consisted of increased serum total bilirubin at $\geq$300 mg/kg per day; increased liver weights and associated minimal to mild hepatocellular hypertrophy at $\geq$ 100 mg/kg per day, that were considered an adaptive response consistent with hepatic enzyme induction; pale livers at 900 mg/kg per day; and minimal to moderate hepatocellular cytoplasmic lipid vacuolation at 100 mg/kg per day. None of the hepatic changes were accompanied by elevations in serum transaminases or microscopic evidence of cholestasis or degenerative liver changes. The hepatic alterations generally did not progress between 3 and 6 months of dosing and, with the exception of increased liver weights at 900 mg/kg per day, were reversible. Systemic AUC exposures at the well-tolerated dose of 900 mg/kg per day for 6 months were 1.2 to 4.0 times the exposure at the recommended clinical dose of 400 mg/day atazanavir or 0.5 to 1.8 times the exposure at the recommended clinical dose of 300 mg/day atazanavir with ritonavir.

In dogs, the toxicity of atazanavir was evaluated at doses up to 360 mg/kg per day in 2-week studies and up to 180 mg/kg per day in the 9-month study. Because of clinical toxicity at 90 to 360 mg/kg per day in the initial 2-week dog study, a second 2-week study was conducted at lower doses (10 to 75 mg/kg per day). In the 9-month study in dogs, the low dose (10 mg/kg per day) was increased to 180 mg/kg per day after 3 months due to the absence of drug-related findings at 10 mg/kg per day. In the initial 2-week study, hepatic changes consisted of minimal to moderate increases in serum total bilirubin, liver enzymes (alanine and aspartate aminotransferases, γ-glutamyltransferase, and alkaline phosphatase), total cholesterol, and triglycerides, and decreases in protein and/or albumin at all doses. In the second 2-week study, there were no drug-related changes. In the 9-month study, hepatic changes were limited to minimally increased serum total bilirubin and γ-glutamyltransferase at $\geq$ 30 mg/kg per day, minimally to moderately increased serum alkaline phosphatase at $\geq$ 90 mg/kg per day in individual animals, and minimally increased liver weights at $\geq$ 90 mg/kg per day. No drug-related gross or microscopic liver changes or evidence of cholestasis were observed in any of the studies in dogs. Additional findings of minimally altered water balance (increased water consumption at 180 mg/kg per day) and minimally decreased heart weights at 30 and 90 mg/kg per day at 3 months only were not associated with any functional impairment or gross or microscopic organ changes, and were considered to be toxicologically insignificant. At the well-tolerated dose of 180 mg/kg per day for 6 months, systemic AUC exposures were 1.7 to 7.9 times the human exposures at 400 mg/day atazanavir or 0.8 to 3.1 times the human exposure at 300 mg/day atazanavir with ritonavir.

In mice, doses of 40 mg/kg per day in males and 160 mg/kg per day in females were generally well tolerated after 3 months with no effects seen at the lower doses of 20 and 40 mg/kg per day in males (M) and females (F), respectively. Similar to the liver changes noted in rats and/or dogs, mild increases in serum total bilirubin at 80 (M) and 640 (F) mg/kg per day; minimal-to-marked increases in liver weights, hepatocellular hypertrophy, and lipid vacuolation at $\geq$ 40 (M) and 160 (F) mg/kg per day; and pale livers at 80 (M) and $\geq$ 160 (F) mg/kg per day were also observed in mice. In addition, clinical and microscopic evidence of hepatotoxicity at 80 (M) and 640 (F) mg/kg per day was present and was characterized by minimal-to-moderate elevations in serum transaminases (M and F) and a low incidence of minimal hepatocellular single-cell necrosis (F only). Increased cellular glycogen [80 (M) and 640 (F) mg/kg per day] was also noted only in mice. Systemic AUC (area under the plasma concentration–time curve) exposures at the well-tolerated doses 40 (M) and 160 (F) mg/kg per day] were 0.4 and 4.1 times the exposure in humans given 400 mg/day atazanavir or 0.2 to 1.8 times the exposure in humans given 300 mg/day atazanavir with ritonavir. Other drug-related findings in female mice included mild-to-moderate decreases in platelet counts at $\geq$ 160 mg/kg per day; minimal-to-mild increases in leukocytes, neutrophils, and lymphocytes at 640 mg/kg per day; and morphological changes in erythrocytes (i.e., poikilocytosis, anisocytosis, polychromasia) at 640 mg/kg/day. Increased spleen weight and size and histological evidence of increased splenic and hepatic extramedullary hematopoiesis in females $\geq$ 160 mg/kg per day were interpreted as secondary effects related to the reduced platelet counts rather than direct drug effects. However, a clinical or morphological basis for the reduction in platelets was not determined. All of these changes, which were limited to female mice, were considered to have no established clinical relevance, as systemic exposures at doses producing these alterations were relatively high (1.8 to 12 times human exposure at the recommended doses), and similar consistent changes were not observed in rats and dogs treated chronically with atazanavir. Importantly, there have been no reports of thrombocytopenia in clinical trials of patients treated with atazanavir.

Reproductive and Developmental Toxicity

A complete battery of reproductive toxicity studies was conducted with atazanavir to assess potential effects on fertility, reproductive function, gestation, parturition, and lactation of the parental generation in rats; on embryonic and fetal development in rats and rabbits; and on growth, development, and reproductive performance of progeny in rats. Systemic exposures supporting the reproductive studies were established in the interim 3-month toxicity study in rats and supportive 7-day toxicokinetic studies in pregnant rats and rabbits. High doses of atazanavir in the reproductive studies in rats were based on a maximum feasible dose (atazanavir concentration and PEG-400 dose volume limitations based on study duration) or results of previous reproductive or repeat-dose toxicity studies. The high dose in the embryo–fetal development study in rabbits was based on toxicity in a range-finding study.

In the study of fertility and reproductive performance in rats (100, 375, and 1400 mg/kg per day), drug-related effects were limited to prolonged diestrus with abbreviated estrus and metestrus in females at all doses. Minimally lower fertility was seen in female rats at 1400 mg/kg per day; however, fertility was only marginally below that observed historically in control rats. This finding was not duplicated in a second fertility study at 1400 mg/kg per day; and therefore, the reduced fertility was considered not to be drug related. There were no effects of atazanavir on early embryonic development or reproductive performance, including mating, at doses up to and including 1400 mg/kg per day. In the absence of any adverse effects on mating, fertility, or reproductive performance or microscopic changes in the ovaries and female reproductive tract in toxicity studies, the perturbation of estrous cyclicity in female rats was considered to be of limited toxicological significance. Systemic AUC exposures in male and female rats at 1400 mg/kg per day, which had no effect on fertility, were at least 1.4 (M) and 3.4 (F) times human exposure at 400 mg/day atazanavir or 0.6 (M) and 1.5 (F) times the human exposure with 300 mg/day atazanavir with ritonavir. Systemic AUC exposure in pregnant rats at 1400 mg/kg per day, which produced no effects on reproductive performance or early embryonic development, was 0.9 or 1.9 times the human exposure with 300 mg/day atazanavir with ritonavir, or 400 mg/day atazanavir dose, respectively.

In the embryo–fetal development studies, atazanavir produced no adverse embryonic or fetal effects at maternally toxic doses (up to 1920 mg/kg per day in rats and 60 mg/kg per day in rabbits). Maternal AUC exposures at the fetal no-effect doses were in rats 0.8 or 1.8 times and 0.4 or 1.0 times the human exposure at 300 mg/day atazanavir with ritonavir or 400 mg/day atazanavir, respectively.

In a study of pre- and postnatal development in rats exposed to atazanavir (50, 220, and 1000 mg/kg per day), findings were limited to mean body weight gain suppression in the F_1 generation from 4 days of age through the early postweaning growth period at the maternally toxic dose of 1000 mg/kg per day. This finding was considered likely to be secondary to the maternal body weight reductions rather than a direct effect of atazanavir. At the highest no-effect dose

(220 mg/kg per day), systemic AUC exposure to atazanavir was 0.5 times the human exposure at the recommended daily dose of atazanavir with ritonavir and 1.1 times the human exposure at the recommended daily dose of atazanavir alone. Atazanavir had no effect on the reproductive performance in the F_1 generation.

In summary, atazanavir demonstrated no selective developmental toxicity and no effects on reproductive function or fertility at exposures generally equivalent to that in humans at the recommended daily dose of atazanavir or ritonavir.

Genetic Toxicity

The genotoxic potential of atazanavir was evaluated in a battery of in vitro and in vivo test systems. All in vitro assays were conducted with and without metabolic activation (rat liver S9 fraction). Atazanavir was not mutagenic in either the bacterial mutagenicity screening assay or in the definitive Ames reverse-mutation study. In the definitive Ames assay, cytotoxicity was observed in each of the *Salmonella* and *Escherichia coli* strains at the highest concentration evaluated (2500 μg/plate), both with and without metabolic activation. In the in vitro chromosomal aberration test in primary human lymphocytes, atazanavir was clastogenic at cytotoxic concentrations of 30 μg/mL in the absence of metabolic activation and of 240 μg/mL in the presence of metabolic activation. In contrast, atazanavir was not clastogenic in the in vivo micronucleus test in rats at doses up to 2000 mg/kg for 3 days. As positive in vitro results and a negative bone marrow micronucleus test were obtained, it was necessary to perform a second in vivo test based on the International Conference on Harmonization guidelines. In vivo/in vitro unscheduled DNA synthesis (UDS) assays in both male and female rats were conducted with single oral doses up to 2000 mg/kg, and atazanavir did not induce UDS in the liver. Since the UDS endpoint may not have been sensitive for detection of any clastogenic effect, as such damage is not readily repaired by UDS mechanisms, an alternative assay, the single-cell gel electrophoresis (Comet) assay, with a more appropriate endpoint, was conducted with assessments of liver and duodenum. Although no valid data could be obtained from livers of atazanavir-treated rats (assay failure due to lack of positive control response), clear negative results for DNA damage were obtained in the duodenum at single oral doses up to 2000 mg/kg.

Carcinogenicity

The carcinogenic potential of atazanavir was evaluated in mice and rats by oral gavage administration for two years. In mice administered atazanavir at doses of 20, 40, or 80 mg/kg per day in males and 40, 120, or 360 mg/kg per day in females, an increased incidence of benign hepatocellular adenomas was observed in females given the highest dose of atazanavir. Systemic exposure at the high dose in females was three times the exposure in humans given 300 mg/day atazanavir with 100 mg/day ritonavir and seven times the exposure in humans given 400 mg/day atazanavir. No increased incidence of tumors was observed in females at lower doses or in males at any dose. Exposures at the nontumorigenic doses in males and females ranged from 1.8 to 4.2 times the human exposure with the two clinical dosing regimens. Based on the nonneoplastic liver findings and the overall lack of genotoxicity, the hepatocarcinogenic effect in high-dose female mice was considered secondary to atazanavir-related cytotoxicity and lacking in clinical relevance because of the relatively high dose and exposure associated with this finding.

In rats administered atazanavir at doses of 100, 350, or 1200 mg/kg per day for two years, there were no statistically significant positive trends in the incidence of neoplasms at any dose. Exposures in rats at the high dose of 1200 mg/kg per day were 0.7 (males) and 2.5 (females) times the exposure in humans at the recommended dose of atazanavir with ritonavir and 1.6 (males) and 5.7 (females) times the human exposure at the recommended dose of atazanavir without ritonavir.

Based on the results of the mouse carcinogenicity study, additional investigative studies were conducted in mice which strongly supported the hypothesis that the female mouse-specific increased incidence in hepatocellular tumors was due to increased hepatocellular proliferation secondary to cytotoxicity, based on 5-bromo-2′-deoxyuridine (BrdU) staining and terminal deoxynucleotidyl transferase-mediated dUTP-X nick end labeling (TUNEL), respectively. Increased cell proliferation secondary to drug-related cytotoxic changes is a well-recognized nongenotoxic (epigenetic) mechanism of tumor development in rodents [11–14].

In addition, the absence of a carcinogenic effect of atazanavir in other tissues or organs in the mouse carcinogenicity study and the absence of any carcinogenic effect in the companion rat carcinogenicity study further support the nongenotoxic nature of the hepatocellular tumorigenic effect since mutagens are more likely than nonmutagens to induce tumors in multiple organs in a single study and in more than one animal species [15]. Moreover, the collective results of the genotoxicity and carcinogenicity studies and of the investigation of atazanavir-induced hepatic effects support a threshold nongenotoxic, cytolethal-proliferative mechanism of tumor development that does not occur at clinically relevant exposures in mice. Together, the result from the genotoxicity and carcinogenicity studies support that atazanavir is not a genotoxic carcinogen and does not pose a carcinogenic risk to humans at therapeutic doses and exposures.

In conclusion, the toxicity of atazanavir was adequately evaluated in a comprehensive battery of GLP (good laboratory practices)–compliant nonclinical toxicology studies. Based on the results of these studies, only the liver was identified as a potential target organ, with microscopic evidence of hepatotoxicity observed only in female mice. Atazanavir demonstrated no selective developmental toxicity, no effects on reproductive function or fertility, and no evidence of immunotoxicity. The results of the genotoxicity, carcinogenicity, and investigative studies support the fact that atazanavir is not a genotoxic carcinogen and does not pose a carcinogenic risk to humans. Therefore, there were no nonclinical findings that precluded the safe administration of atazanavir for treatment of HIV infection in humans.

MICROBIOLOGY AND RESISTANCE

Atazanavir exhibits anti-HIV-1 activity with a mean 50% effective concentration (EC_{50}) in the absence of human serum of 2 to 5 nM against a variety of laboratory and clinical HIV-1 isolates grown in peripheral blood mononuclear cells, macrophages, CEM-SS cells, and MT-2 cells. Atazanavir has activity against HIV-1 group M subtype viruses A, B, C, D, AE, AG, F, G, and J isolates in cell culture. Atazanavir has variable activity against HIV-2 isolates [9].

In vitro studies were conducted to assess the development of resistance in three strains (RF, LAI, and NL4-3) of HIV-1 virus in cell culture in the presence of increasing concentrations of atazanavir for up to 4.8 months. Genotypic and phenotypic analysis indicated that an N88S substitution in protease appeared first during passage of the RF and LAI viruses. The LAI virus exhibiting a 93-fold reduced susceptibility to atazanavir contained five amino acid changes in protease (L10Y/F, I50L, L63P, A71V, and N88S), while the NL4-3 virus showing a 96-fold decrease in susceptibility contained four amino substitutions (V32I, M46I, I84V, L89M). The NL4-3 variant has a well-documented resistance substitution (protease I84V) located near the active site, whereas the resistance phenotype of LAI is attributed to the appearance of I50L and N88S substitutions, in combination with other secondary substitutions at residues 10, 63, and 71. Atazanavir-resistant virus remained susceptible to saquinavir while showing varying levels (0.06- to 71-fold change) of cross-resistance to nelfinavir, indinavir, ritonavir, and amprenavir. Atazanavir-resistant LAI viruses (harboring the unique protease I50L substitution) exhibited increased susceptibility to ritonavir and amprenavir.

Analysis of the genotypic profiles of 943 of the 950 protease inhibitor susceptible and resistant clinical isolates from atazanavir clinical trials identified a strong correlation between the presence of the specific protease amino acid changes at 10I/V/F, 20R/M/I, 24I, 33I/F/V, 36I/L/V, 46I/L, 48V, 54V/L, 63P, 71V/T/I, 73C/S/T/A, 82A/F/S/T, 84V, and 90M and decreased susceptibility to atazanavir. Although no single substitution or combination of substitutions is predictive of atazanavir resistance, the presence of at least five of these substitutions correlated strongly with loss of atazanavir susceptibility [16].

PRECLINICAL SAFETY ASSESSMENTS

Electrophysiology and Cardiac Conduction Studies

The ECG effects of atazanavir were assessed in rabbit Purkinje fibers. Atazanavir minimally increased action potential duration (13% at 30 μM). This concentration is approximately four times the mean C_{max} and 17 times the mean C_{ss} in humans given atazanavir 400 mg/day. Weak inhibition of sodium currents ($IC_{50} > 30$ μM) and moderate inhibition of calcium currents (IC_{50} of 10.4 μM) were also identified in vitro. Atazanavir was also evaluated in the in vitro IKr (hERG) and IKs potassium channels, where it produced weak inhibition of IKr current and no significant inhibition of the IKs current. The clinical significance of these weak inhibitory effects on several ion channels, including hERG, and modest prolongations of the action potential duration is not clear. In in vivo studies, no direct drug-related effects on cardiac function were noted in dogs treated with atazanavir for up to 9 months. Plasma concentrations of atazanavir at the high dose of 180 mg/kg per day in the 9-month toxicity study, which produced no ECG changes, were up to three times the C_{max} and seven times the AUC in humans given atazanavir 400 mg/day.

Metabolic Effects

Preclinical findings showed that atazanavir exhibited markedly less interference with lipid metabolism in cell culture models of hepatocytes and adipocytes than did other protease inhibitors. Atazanavir exhibited lesser effects on expression of lipogenic genes in hepatocyte and adipocyte models. Direct assays of human 20S proteasome in vitro showed that atazanavir is a weak inhibitor of proteasome activity with IC_{50} values several times higher than typical plasma C_{max}, while several other protease inhibitors inhibited proteasome activity with IC_{50} values below reported plasma C_{max} values.

Additionally, data from in vitro studies demonstrated that atazanavir has little or no effect on GLUT-4 or GLUT-1 glucose transporters in cell culture models of adipocytes and myocytes. These glucose transporters are critical for glucose uptake in fat and muscle tissues. Because of the role of glucose metabolism in lipid biosynthesis and its regulation, the lack of inhibition of GLUT-4 or GLUT-1 activity by atazanavir may contribute to its neutral lipid profile.

Hyperbilirubinemia

Elevation in bilirubin is the most frequent laboratory abnormality observed in atazanavir clinical trials. In a heterologously expressed human UGT 1A1 in vitro system, atazanavir—at clinically relevant concentration—inhibits the glucuronidation of bilirubin. This has also been observed in human liver microsomes. The majority of elevations in total bilirubin are indirect (unconjugated) and not associated with liver function test elevations. Bilirubin elevations are reversible upon discontinuation or interruption of atazanavir.

PHASE I–III SAFETY AND EFFICACY

Atazanavir clinical safety and efficacy were demonstrated through a clinical development program in antiretroviral therapy naive and experienced patients. Two randomized controlled dose-ranging phase II studies compared unboosted atazanavir at doses of 200 to 600 mg against nelfinavir [17,18], and two comparative phase III studies compared unboosted atazanavir at a dose of 400 mg against efavirenz [19] in treatment-naive patients and lopinavir/ritonavir in treatment-experienced patients [20]. Atazanavir 300 mg with ritonavir 100 mg used as a pharmacokinetic enhancer was compared to unboosted atazanavir in treatment-naive patients [21] and studied against lopinavir/ritonavir in both treatment-naive [22] and treatment-experienced patients [23]. The clinical development program of atazanavir has resulted in its approval in combination with other antiretroviral drugs for treatment-naive patients with either boosted or unboosted dosing of atazanavir, and for treatment-experienced with boosted atazanavir dosing.

CLINICAL PHARMACOLOGY

Pharmacokinetics

Most atazanavir pharmacokinetic studies were conducted in HIV-uninfected subjects. Atazanavir is rapidly absorbed after oral administration, reaching peak plasma concentrations after 2 to 3 h. Steady state is reached by around day 6 with once-daily dosing. Nonlinear pharmacokinetics were demonstrated, resulting in greater than dose-proportional increases in bioavailability over a dose range of 200 to 800 mg daily in HIV-uninfected subjects [24].

Administration of atazanavir with food enhances its bioavailability and reduces pharmacokinetic variability [25, 26]. The absolute oral bioavailability of atazanavir was not determined in humans; however, the bioavailability of atazanavir capsules relative to a solution was 68% in humans. Peak concentrations of atazanavir in humans were achieved in 1.5 h after a single oral capsule dose in the fed state, with no evidence of a plateau effect after peak levels, indicating that the absorption is rapid. Consistent with the findings in animals, approximately 79% of the administered radioactivity was recovered in the feces of humans, suggesting biliary elimination and/or incomplete absorption. Renal elimination was a minor pathway in humans, since only 13% of the radioactivity administered was recovered in the urine after a single 400-mg oral dose, with unchanged drug accounting for approximately half of that radioactivity. In humans, females have modestly higher exposures to atazanavir compared to males, but the difference (< 25%) is considered not to be of clinical relevance. Scheme 5 shows the chemical structures of the proposed human metabolites. Atazanavir was the major circulating component in human plasma. Additionally, M2, M14, and the unidentified keto metabolite, each constituting approximately 10% of the plasma radioactivity, were present in human plasma. M2 and M14 possess no anti-HIV activity.

Atazanavir is $\geq$ 86% protein bound in human plasma (86% to albumin and 89% to α_1-acid glycoprotein). Atazanavir is a substrate of human cytochrome P450 3A4 (CYP3A4) in vitro. Consistent with these in vitro data, ritonavir (a potent CYP3A4 inhibitor) increases [27] and efavirenz (a potent CYP3A4 inducer) decreases the exposure to atazanavir [28] following concomitant administration in humans. The inhibitory effect of low-dose ritonavir on CYP3A4 substantially increases atazanavir concentrations. Compared to the atazanavir 400 mg once daily at steady state, atazanavir AUC and $C_{\min}$ for atazanavir/ritonavir 300/100 mg once daily is 4- and 12-fold greater, respectively [29]. Atazanavir inhibits, but does not induce, human CYP3A4 in vitro, and is a moderate inhibitor of uridine diphosphate glucuronosyl transferase 1A1 (UGT1A1) in vitro. In clinical studies, elevations in endogenous serum bilirubin, a UGT1A1 substrate, are observed but rarely result in treatment discontinuation.

Atazanavir requires acidic pH for dissolution. Therefore, concomitant use of medications that raise gastric pH, such as antacids, histamine (H_2) blockers, and proton pump inhibitors, reduce atazanavir bioavailability. Atazanavir boosting with ritonavir and concomitant or temporal separation with acid-reducing agents decrease the effect of acid-reducing agents on atazanavir pharmacokinetics [30–32].

Pharmacodynamics

Seven non-placebo-controlled clinical pharmacology studies to evaluate the effect of atazanavir exposure on ECG parameters were completed in healthy subjects. Doses of unboosted atazanavir at 200 through 800 mg once daily were studied. ECG parameters were measured prior to and during study drug administration. Equivocal effects of atazanavir on the QTc interval were observed in these non-placebo-controlled studies. A dose- and concentration-dependent effect on PR interval was seen in these initial non-placebo-controlled studies [9].

A definitive, placebo-controlled double-blind three-treatment three-period crossover study in 72 healthy subjects was designed to determine the effect of unboosted atazanavir (400 and 800 mg) on ECG parameters, specifically the QTcB and PR intervals. While boosted atazanavir (atazanavir 300 with ritonavir 100 mg) was not included in this study, boosted atazanavir results in concentrations intermediate between atazanavir 400 and 800 mg [9]. In this study, atazanavir had neither a clinically significant nor a statistically significant concentration-dependent effect on the QTcB interval. Fourteen percent of patients taking atazanavir 400 mg/day developed PR intervals greater than 200 ms (normal range 120 to 200 ms). The PR prolongations was dose related, and their frequency and magnitude increased with increasing dose of atazanavir. PR prolongations at the 400-mg dose of atazanavir were all mild ($\leq$ 250 ms). All prolongations of the PR interval were asymptomatic and not associated with significant clinical findings. No episodes of 2° or 3° AV block were observed.

Studies with other protease inhibitors demonstrated that C_{min} (trough) concentrations of HIV protease inhibitors correlate with efficacy. Atazanavir trough concentrations and inhibitory quotient using the clinical dosing regimens of atazanavir 400 and 300 mg with ritonavir were determined in patients naive to antiretroviral therapy [33]. The inhibitory quotient was defined as the atazanavir C_{trough}/individual's HIV-1 protein binding-adjusted EC_{90} for atazanavir against HIV and was available from 32% of subjects at baseline. In these antiretroviral-naive subjects, C_{trough} in both regimens was associated with the probability of virologic suppression at 48 weeks; however, even in the lowest C_{trough} quartile, 88% of subjects achieved virologic suppression. Total bilirubin levels and the development of jaundice were positively associated with atazanavir C_{trough}. Higher atazanavir C_{trough} and a regimen of atazanavir 300 mg with ritonavir were associated with greater increases in fasting triglycerides and total cholesterol. Despite a statistically significant regimen effect for fasting triglycerides and total cholesterol elevations, only a weak positive correlation of atazanavir C_{trough} was noted, suggesting a stronger association of these lipid elevations with ritonavir administration rather than atazanavir C_{trough} values. Hepatic transaminase elevation (AST or ALT) and the probability of diarrhea or nausea were not associated with atazanavir C_{trough}. The relationship of atazanavir C_{trough} and total bilirubin, lipid profile, and liver transaminase changes was confirmed further in study AI424-138 (CASTLE) pharmacokinetic/pharmacodynamic analysis [34].

Clinical Trials in Antiretroviral-Naive Patients

Study AI424-007 [17] was a 48-week dose-ranging phase II study comparing the safety and efficacy of atazanavir in doses of 200, 400, and 500 mg once daily to nelfinavir 750 mg three times a day in combination with didanosine and stavudine in 420 antiretroviral naive patients. The study was blinded to atazanavir dose but included an open-label comparison to nelfinavir. Subjects received atazanavir monotherapy for 2 weeks followed by the combination regimen for 46 weeks. After 48 weeks, mean change from baseline in plasma HIV-1 RNA (-2.57 to -2.33 $\log_{10}$ copies/mL), the proportion of subjects with plasma HIV-1 RNA < 400 copies/mL (56 to 64%) and < 50 copies/mL (28 to 42%), and mean increases in $CD4^{+}$ T-cell count (185 to 221 cells/mm^3) were comparable across treatment groups. Diarrhea was two to three times more common in the nelfinavir group (61% of subjects) than in the atazanavir groups (23 to 30% of subjects), and jaundice occurred only in atazanavir-treated subjects (6, 6, and 12% in the 200-, 400-, and 500-mg groups, respectively). There was minimal effect on blood lipids parameters at all atazanavir doses, in contrast to the nelfinavir arm, which experienced an increase from baseline in total cholesterol, triglycerides, and fasting low-density lipoprotein (LDL) cholesterol levels.

Atazanavir 400 and 600 mg once daily were compared to nelfinavir 1250 mg twice a day in combination with lamivudine and stavudine in another phase II study (AI424-008) in 467 antiretroviral-naive patients [18]. At 48 weeks, mean changes in plasma HIV-1 RNA ($\log_{10}$ copies/mL) from baseline to 48 weeks were -2.51, -2.58, -2.31; HIV-1 RNA < 400 copies/mL were 64, 67, and 53%; and HIV-1 RNA < 50 copies/mL were 35, 36, and 34% in atazanavir 400 mg, 600 mg, and nelfinavir arms, respectively. $CD4^{+}$ T-cell count increases were similar across all arms. Adverse events were similar across treatments with the exception of diarrhea (more frequent with nelfinavir) and jaundice (more frequent with atazanavir). Unconjugated hyperbilirubinemia was reported more frequently in the higher-dose atazanavir (600 mg) arm. Similar to study AI424-007, both atazanavir arms had minimal effects on lipids compared to nelfinavir. Based on these data and the risk–benefit profile, atazanavir 400 mg once daily was chosen as the recommended dose of unboosted atazanavir.

Study AI424-044 was a rollover study of patients completing the earlier nelfinavir comparative phase of AI424-008 with plasma HIV-1 RNA fewer than 10,000 copies/mL [35]. Patients were maintained on atazanavir, or (if they received nelfinavir) switched to atazanavir and followed for 24 weeks after completing 48 weeks of study AI424-008. Atazanavir was well tolerated and effective during extended use and also in patients who switched from nelfinavir. In virologically suppressed, nelfinavir-treated patients switched to atazanavir, virologic suppression continued, whereas nelfinavir-induced lipid elevations were reversed within 12 weeks, approaching pretreatment values. Extended atazanavir use in patients who received atazanavir previously resulted in continued viral suppression and lipid changes that were not clinically relevant.

Study AI424-034 [19] was a phase III randomized double-blind double-dummy active-controlled two-arm study in 810 patients comparing the antiviral efficacy and safety of atazanavir 400 mg administered once daily vs. efavirenz 600 mg administered once daily in combination with open-label fixed-dose zidovudine plus lamivudine twice daily in treatment-naive patients. At week 48, plasma HIV-1 RNA levels were lower than 400 copies/mL in 70% of patients receiving atazanavir and 64% of patients receiving efavirenz. Immunological responses were similar in both treatment arms. Atazanavir-treated patients did not demonstrate significant increases in total cholesterol, fasting LDL cholesterol, fasting triglycerides, fasting glucose or insulin levels, and atazanavir-related bilirubin elevations resulted in treatment discontinuation in less than 1% of participants.

Boosted atazanavir (atazanavir 300 mg with ritonavir 100 mg) was compared to atazanavir 400 mg in antiretroviral naive patients in a phase II study, AI424-089, which randomized 200 patients (95 to boosted atazanavir and 105 to unboosted atazanavir). Response rates of plasma HIV-1 RNA < 400 copies at week 48 were 86% and 85% on the boosted atazanavir and unboosted atazanavir regimens. There were 3 and 10 patients with virologic failure in the boosted atazanavir and unboosted atazanavir groups, respectively. Plasma lipid elevations were low with both regimens. At 96 weeks, discontinuation rates were similar in both arms, but the response rates were slightly higher in the boosted atazanavir arm, with fewer virological failures than in the unboosted atazanavir arm. Increases in plasma lipids in both regimens were similar; however, there were higher rates of hyperbilirubinemia on the boosted atazanavir arm [36].

The CASTLE study (AI424-138) was a large, open-label randomized phase III study comparing atazanavir/ritonavir (300/100 mg once daily) to lopinavir/ritonavir (400/100 mg twice daily) in antiretroviral-naive patients. The study randomized 440 and 443 patients to atazanavir/ritonavir and lopinavir/ritonavir arms, respectively. At 48 weeks, 78% of those on atazanavir/ritonavir and 76% of those on lopinavir/ritonavir achieved the primary endpoint of plasma HIV-1 RNA fewer than 50 copies/mL, demonstrating the noninferiority of atazanavir/ritonavir to lopinavir/ ritonavir. Similar increases in $CD4^+$ T-cell count were noted in both arms. The rates of discontinuation were 9 and 13% in the atazanavir/ritonavir- and lopinavir/ritonavir-containing arms, respectively. The atazanavir/ritonavir arm was associated with significantly lower increases in total cholesterol, triglycerides, and non-high-density lipoprotein cholesterol.

Atazanavir/ritonavir demonstrated higher rates of hyperbilirubinemia and lower rates of gastrointestinal events than those of lopinavir/ritonavir [22]. Noninferiority of atazanavir/ritonavir to lopinavir/ritonavir was also confirmed at week 96. Virological failure rates were low with both regimens. Atazanavir/ritonavir had a better lipid profile, such that 2% of subjects on atazanavir/ritonavir vs. 9% of subjects on lopinavir/ritonavir initiated lipid-lowering drugs on study. Additionally, atazanavir/ritonavir had a more favorable gastrointestinal tolerability than lopinavir/ritonavir [37]. Similar results were demonstrated regardless of the patients' race or gender [38,39].

Clinical Trials in Antiretroviral-Experienced Patients

BMS studies AI424-043 and AI424-045 were conducted in treatment-experienced patients. In study AI424-045 [23], 358 patients who had failed two or more prior antiretroviral regimens were randomized to receive atazanavir/ritonavir 300/100 mg once a day, atazanavir/saquinavir 400/1200 mg once a day, or lopinavir/ ritonavir 400/100 mg twice a day, each with tenofovir and another nucleoside reverse transcriptase inhibitor. The primary endpoint of time-averaged reductions in plasma HIV-1 RNA from baseline for atazanavir/ritonavir and lopinavir/ritonavir were comparable at 48 weeks (1.93 and 1.87 $\log_{10}$ copies/mL, respectively). Mean $CD4^+$ T-cell-count increases were 100 and 121 cells/mm^3 for atazanavir/ritonavir and lopinavir/ritonavir, respectively. The efficacy of atazanavir/saquinavir was lower than lopinavir/ritonavir by both these parameters and this arm was discontinued at 24 weeks. Declines in total cholesterol and fasting triglycerides were greater with atazanavir/ritonavir and atazanavir/saquinavir than with lopinavir/ritonavir, with lipid-lowering agents used more frequently in the lopinavir/ritonavir arm than in the atazanavir arms. Hyperbilirubinemia was more common on the atazanavir/ritonavir arm, and diarrhea was more common in lopinavir/ritonavir arm, which also had greater use of antidiarrheal agents. In the extended follow-up period, to 96 weeks, once-daily atazanavir/ritonavir demonstrated durable safety and efficacy and was associated with significant reductions in total cholesterol and fasting triglycerides [40].

In study AI424-043 [20], 300 patients failing protease inhibitor–based antiretroviral therapy were randomized to receive atazanavir 400 mg once a day without ritonavir or lopinavir/ritonavir 400/100 mg twice daily, each with two nucleoside reverse transcriptase inhibitors. Lopinavir/ritonavir resulted in significantly greater reduction in plasma HIV-1 RNA than that of unboosted atazanavir at 48 weeks. However, both regimens were equally effective in patients who had no baseline nucleoside reverse transcriptase inhibitors mutations. Atazanavir resulted in either no change or decreases in fasting LDL cholesterol, total cholesterol, and fasting triglycerides, whereas lopinavir/ritonavir resulted in increases in these lipid parameters. Based on these results, unboosted atazanavir is not recommended for use in treatment-experienced patients.

Clinical Trials in Pediatric Patients

The PACTG 1020A (AI424-020) study was designed as a phase I/II open-label pharmacokinetics and safety study of atazanavir (powder and capsules) in combination regimens in antiretroviral-naive and antiretroviral-experienced HIV-1-infected infants, children, and adolescents. Consistent with the adult experience, the results of AI424-020 support the fact that atazanavir/ritonavir is generally safe and well tolerated in pediatric populations. Compared with adults, no new safety findings related to atazanavir/ritonavir were identified in the pediatric population. The results of this study have led to the approval of pediatric dosing recommendation in adolescents and children above the age of 6 in the United States [41–43].

FUTURE DIRECTIONS

Atazanavir in combination with two nucleosides has been studied extensively in both antiretroviral treatment-naive and experienced patients. However, since nucleoside reverse transcriptase inhibitors may be associated with long-term toxicities or development of extensive nucleoside cross-resistance, studying atazanavir in new treatment regimens without nucleoside reverse transcriptase inhibitors is warranted. With the introduction of new classes of antiretroviral therapy with new mechanism of action, the use of atazanavir with these new compounds is being explored, including ongoing studies with integrase inhibitors (raltegravir [44] and elvitegravir [45]), CCR5 inhibitors (maraviroc [46] and vicriviroc [47]), as well as with new nonritonavir pharmacokinetic enhancers (such as GS 9350) [48].

Studies of boosted atazanavir monotherapy as a potential option for maintenance therapy after initial virological suppression with a full antiretroviral regimen have also been conducted. These studies have shown mixed results regarding the efficacy of boosted atazanavir monotherapy and the value of this strategy [49–51].

CONCLUSIONS

Atazanavir was developed as the first potent once-a-day protease inhibitor. The efficacy, safety, and tolerability of the compound have been demonstrated in both treatment-naive and treatment-experienced patients, and atazanavir is now recommended as part of a preferred regimen in many HIV treatment guidelines [52–54]. Atazanavir is currently approved unboosted for antiretroviral-naive patients who cannot tolerate ritonavir and boosted with ritonavir for both antiretroviral-naive and antiretroviral-experienced patients. Atazanavir is being evaluated in new treatment paradigms as antiretroviral therapy, and patients' medical needs continue to evolve.

REFERENCES

[1] Fässler, A.; Rösel, J.; Grütter, M.; Tintelnot-Blomley, M.; Alteri, E.; Bold, G.; Lang, M. Novel pseudosymmetric inhibitors of HIV-1 protease. *Bioorg. Med. Chem. Lett.* **1993**, *3*, 2837–2842.

[2] Sham, H. L.; Zhao, C.; Marsh, K. C.; Betebenner, D. A.; Lin, S.; McDonald, E.; Vasavanonda, S.; Wideburg, N.; Saldivar, A.; Robbins, T.; et al. Potent inhibitors of the HIV-1 protease with good oral bioavailabilities. *Biochem. Biophys. Res. Commun.* **1995**, *211*, 159–165.

[3] Fässler, A.; Bold, G.; Capraro, H.-G.; Cozens, R.; Mestan, J.; Poncioni, B.; Rösel, J.; Tintelnot-Blomley, M.; Lang, M. Aza-peptide analogs as potent human immunodeficiency virus type-1 protease inhibitors with oral bioavailability. *J. Med. Chem.* **1996**, *39*, 3203–3216.

[4] Bold, G.; Fässler, A.; Capraro, H.-G.; Cozens, R.; Klimkait, T.; Lazdins, J.; Mestan, J.; Poncioni, B.; Rösel, J.; Stover, D.; et al. New aza-dipeptide analogues as potent and orally absorbed HIV-1 protease inhibitors: candidates for clinical development. *J. Med. Chem.* **1998**, *41*, 3387–3401.

[5] Priestle, J. P.; Fässler, A.; Rösel, J.; Tintelnot-Blomley, M.; Strop, P.; Grütter, M. G. Comparative analysis of the x-ray structures of HIV-1 and HIV-2 proteases in complex with CGP-53280, a novel pseudosymmetric inhibitor. *Structure* **1995**, *3*, 381–389.

[6] Xu, Z.; Singh, J.; Schwinden, M. D.; Zheng, B.; Kissick, T. P.; Patel, B.; Humora, M. J.; Quiroz, F.; Dong, L.; Hsieh, D.-M.; et al. Process research and development for an efficient synthesis of the HIV protease inhibitor BMS-232632. *Org. Process Res. Dev.* **2002**, *6*, 323–328.

[7] Fan, X.; Song, Y.-L.; Long, Y.-Q. An efficient and practical synthesis of the HIV protease inhibitor atazanavir via a highly diastereoselective reduction approach. *Org. Process Res. Dev.* **2008**, *12*, 69–75.

[8] Singh, J.; Pudipeddi, M.; Lindrud, D. M. Bisulfate salt of HIV protease inhibitor. World Patent Application, WO 1999036404, 1999.

[9] Bristol-Myers Squibb Company. Atazanavir briefing document BMS-232632, May 2003. Available at http://www.fda.gov/ohrms/dockets/ac/03/briefing/3950B1_01_Bristol MyersSquibbAtazanavir.pdf. Accessed Nov. 19, 2009.

[10] ter Heine, R.; Hillebrand, M. J. X.; Rosing, H. E.; van Gorp, C. M.; Mulder, J. W.; Beijnen, J. H.; Huitema, A. D. R. Identification and profiling of circulating metabolites of atazanavir, a HIV protease inhibitor. *Drug Metab. Dispos.* **2009**, *37*, 1826–1840.

[11] Williams, G. E.; Whysner, J. Epigenetic carcinogens: evaluation and risk assessment. *Exp. Toxicol. Pathol.* **1996**, *48*, 189–195.

[12] Williams, G. E.; Iatropoulos, M. J.; Weisburger, J. H. Chemical carcinogen mechanisms of action and implications for testing methodology. *Exp. Toxicol. Pathol.* **1996**, *48*, 101–111.

[13] Lima, B. S.; Van der Laan, J. W. Mechanisms of nongenotoxic carcinogenesis and assessment of the human hazard. *Regul. Toxicol. Pharmacol.* **2000**, *32*, 135–143.

[14] Butterworth, B. E.; Conolly, R. B.; Morgan, K. T. A strategy for establishing mode of action of chemical carcinogens as a guide for approaches to risk assessments. *Cancer Lett.* **1995**, *93*, 129–146.

[15] Gold, L. S.; Slone, T. H.; Stern, B. R.; Bernstein, L. Comparison of target organs of carcinogenicity for

mutagenic and non-mutagenic chemicals. *Mutat. Res.* **1993**, *286*, 75–100.

[16] Bristol-Myers Squibb Company. Reyataz® (atazanavir sulfate) capsules: US prescribing information. Available at http://packageinserts.bms.com/pi/pi_reyataz.pdf. Accessed Dec. 7, 2009.

[17] Sanne, I.; Piliero, P.; Squires, K.; Thiry, A.; Schnittman, S. Results of a phase 2 clinical trial at 48 weeks (AI424–007): a dose ranging, safety, efficacy and comparative trial of atazanavir at three doses in combination with didanosine and stavudine in antiretroviral-naive subjects. *J. Acquir. Immune Defic. Syndr.* **2003**, *32*, 18–29.

[18] Murphy, R.; Sanne, I.; Cahn, P.; Phanuphak, P.; Percival, L.; Kelleher, T.; Giordano, M. Dose-ranging, randomized, clinical trial of atazanavir with stavudine and lamuvidine in antiretroviral-naive subjects: 48-week results. *AIDS* **2003**, *17*, 2603–2614.

[19] Squires, K.; Lazzarin, A.; Gatell, J.; Powderly, W.; Pokrovskiy, V.; Delfraissy, J. F.; Jemsek, J.; Rivero, A.; Rozenbaum, W.; Schrader, S.; et al. Comparison of once daily atazanavir with efavirenz, each in combination with fixed-dose zidovudine and lamivudine, as initial therapy for patients infected with HIV. *J. Acquir. Immune Defic. Syndr.* **2004**, *36*, 1011–1019.

[20] Cohen, C.; Nieto-Cisneros, L.; Zala, C.; Fessel, W. J.; Gonzalez-Garcia, J.; Gladysz, A.; McGovern, R.; Adler, E.; McLaren, C. Comparison of atazanavir with lopinavir/ritonavir in patients with prior protease inhibitor failure: a randomized multinational trial. *Curr. Med. Res. Opin.* **2005**, *10*, 1683–1692.

[21] Malan, D. R.; Krantz, E.; David, N.; Wirtz, V.; Hammond, J.; McGrath, D. Efficacy and safety of atazanavir, with or without ritonavir, as part of once-daily highly active antiretroviral therapy regimens in antiretroviral-naive patients. *J. Acquir. Immune Defic. Syndr.* **2008**, *47*, 161–167.

[22] Molina, J.-M.; Andrade-Villanueva, J.; Echevarria, J.; Chetchotisakd, P.; Corral, J.; David, N.; Moyle, G.; Mancini, M.; Percival, L.; Yang, R.; et al. Once-daily atazanavir/ritonavir vs. twice-daily lopinavir/ritonavir, each in combination with tenofovir and emtricitabine, for the management of anti-retroviral-naive HIV-1 infected patients. *Lancet* **2008**, *372*, 646–655.

[23] Johnson, M.; Grinsztejn, B.; Rodriguez, C.; Coco, J.; DeJesus, E.; Lazzarin, A.; Lichtenstein, K.; Wirtz, V.; Rightmire, A.; Odeshoo, O.; McLaren, C. Atazanavir plus ritonavir or saquinavir and lopinavir/ritonavir in patients experiencing multiple virological failures. *AIDS* **2005**, *19*, 685–694.

[24] Agarwala, S.; Graesela, D.; Child, M.; Geraldes, M.; Geiger, M.; O'Mara, E. Characterization of the steady-state pharmacokinetic (PK) profile of atazanavir (atazanavir) beyond the 24-hour dosing interval. *Antivir. Ther.* 2003, *8* (Suppl. 1). Abstract 845.

[25] Child, M.; Agarwala, S.; Boffito, M.; Jones, A.; Mahnke, L.; Nettles, R.; Persson, A.; Xu, X.; Bertz, R. Effect of food on the pharmacokinetics of atazanavir when administered with ritonavir in healthy subjects. 8th International Workshop on Clinical Pharmacology of HIV Therapy, Budapest, Hungary, Apr. 16–18, 2007. Abstract 25.

[26] O'Mara, E.; Mummaneni, V.; Randall, D.; Sagali, N.; Olsen, S.; Tanner, T.; Schuster, A.; Raymond, R.; Kaul, S. BMS-232632: a summary of multiple dose pharmacokinetic, food effect and drug interaction studies in healthy subjects. 7th Conference on Retroviruses and Opportunistic Infections, San Francisco, Jan. 30–Feb. 2, 2000. Abstract 504.

[27] Agarwala, S.; Russo, R.; Mummaneni, V.; Randall, D.; Geraldes, M.; O'Mara, E. Steady-state pharmacokinetic (PK) interaction study of atazanavir (atazanavir) with ritonavir (ritonavir) in healthy subjects. 42nd Interscience Conference on Antimicrobial Agents and Chemotherapy, San Diego, CA, 2002. Abstract H-1716.

[28] Tackett, D.; Child, M.; Agarwala, S.; Geiger, M.; Geraldes, M.; Laura, B.; O'Mara, E. Atazanavir: a summary of two pharmacokinetic drug interaction studies in healthy subjects. 10th Conference on Retroviruses and Opportunistic Infections, Boston, 2003. Abstract 543.

[29] Agarwala, S.; Eley, T.; Filoramo, D. Steady-state pharmacokinetics and inhibitory quotient of atazanavir with and without ritonavir in treatment naive HIV-infected patients. 7th International Workshop on Clinical Pharmacology of HIV Therapy, Lisbon, Portugal, 2006. Abstract 85.

[30] Agarwala, S.; Eley, T.; Child, M.; Wang, Y.; Hughes, E.; Chung, E.; Wang, R.; Grasela, D. Pharmacokinetic effect of famotidine on atazanavir with or without ritonavir in healthy subjects. 6th International Workshop on Clinical Pharmacology of HIV Therapy, Québec City, Québec, Canada, Apr. 28–30, 2005. Abstract 11.

[31] Agarwala, S.; Persson, A.; Eley, T.; Child, M.; Filoramo, D.; Sevinsky, H.; Li, T.; Xu, X.; Bertz, R. Effect of famotidine 20 mg and 40 mg dosing regimens on the bioavailability of atazanavir with ritonavir in combination with tenofovir in healthy subjects. 14th Conference on Retroviruses and Opportunistic Infections, Los Angeles, Feb. 25–28, 2007. Poster 568.

[32] Eley, T.; Zhu, L.; Dragone, J.; Persson, A.; Filoramo, D.; Li, T.; Xu, X.; Mahnke, L.; Agarwala, S.; Bertz, R. Effect of omeprazole 20-mg daily on the bioavailability of multiple-dose atazanavir with ritonavir in healthy subjects. 8th International Workshop on Clinical Pharmacology of HIV Therapy, Budapest, Hungary, Apr. 16–18, 2007. Abstract 66.

[33] Bertz, R.; Wang, Y.; Mahnke, L.; Persson, A.; Chung, E.; Mathew, M.; Agarwala, S.; Filoramo, D.; Hammond, J.; Grasela, D., et al. Assessment of pharmacokinetic/pharmacodynamic relationships through 48 weeks from a study of HIV+, ARV-naive subjects receiving antiretroviral therapy containing atazanavir 400 mg or atazanavir/ritonavir 300/100 mg once daily. 14th Conference on Retroviruses and Opportunistic Infections, Los Angeles, Feb. 25–28, 2007. Poster 565.

[34] Zhu, L.; Liao, S.; Absalon, J.; Child, M.; Zhang, J.; Mathew, M.; McGrath, D.; Wang, Y.; Bertz, R.; Molina, J.-M. Exploration of pharamcokinetic/pharamcodynamic relationships of boosted atazanavir and lopinavir over 48 weeks in HIV-infected treatment naive patients: CASTLE study.

10th International Workshop on Clinical Pharmacology of HIV Therapy, Amsterdam, Apr. 15–17, 2009. Poster P19.

[35] Wood, R.; Phanuphak, P.; Cahn, P.; Pokrovskiy, V.; Rozenbaum, W.; Pantaleo, G.; Sension, M.; Murphy, R.; Mancini, M.; Kelleher, T.; Giordano, M. Long-term efficacy and safety of atazanavir with stavudine and lamuvidine in patients previously treated with nelfinavir or atazanavir. *J. Acquir. Immune Defic. Syndr.* **2004**, *36*, 684–692.

[36] Malan, N.; Krantz, E.; David, N.; Mathew, M.; Rightmire, A.; Wirtz, V.; Yang, R.; McGrath, D. Efficacy and safety of atazanavir-based therapy in anti-retroviral naive HIV-1 infected subjects, both with and without ritonavir; 96-week results from AI424089. 4th International AIDS Society Conference on HIV-1 Pathogenesis, Treatment and Prevention, Sydney, Australia, July 22–25, 2007. Abstract WEPEB024.

[37] Molina, J.-M.; Andrade-Villanueva, J.; Echevarria, J., Chetchotisakd, P.; Corral, J.; David, N.; Mancini, M.; Yang, R.; McGrath, D. Atazanavir–ritonavir vs. lopinavir–ritonavir in anti-retroviral naive HIV-1 infected patients: CASTLE 96-week safety and efficacy. 48th Interscience Conference on Antimicrobial Agents and Chemotherapy/Infectious Diseases Society of America 46th Annual Meeting, Washington, DC, Oct. 25–28, 2008. Abstract H-1250d.

[38] McGrath, D.; Uy, J.; Yang, R.; Thiry, A.; Mancini, M.; Absalon, J. Efficacy and safety by racial group in ARV-naive subjects treated with atazanavir/ritonavir or lopinavir/ritonavir: 48-weeks results for the CASTLE study (AI424138). XVII International AIDS Conference, Mexico City, Mexico, Aug. 3–8, 2008. Abstract TUPE0058.

[39] Absalon, J.; Uy, J.; Yang, R.; Mancini, M.; McGrath, D. Gender-based differences in ARV-naive patients treated with boosted protease inhibitors: results from the CASTLE study (AI424138). XVII International AIDS Conference, Mexico City, Mexico, Aug. 3–8, 2008. Abstract TUPE0062.

[40] Johnson, M.; Grinsztejn, B.; Rodriguez, C.; Coco, J.; DeJesus, E.; Lazzarin, A.; Lichtenstein, K.; Wirtz, V.; Rightmire, A.; Odeshoo, L.; McLaren, C. 96-Week comparison of once-daily atazanavir/ritonavir and twice-daily lopinavir/ritonavir in patients with multiple virologic failures. *AIDS* **2006**, *20*, 711–718.

[41] Kiser, J.; Rutstein, R.; Aldrovandi, G.; Samson, P.; Graham, B.; Schnittman, S.; Smith, M.; Fletcher, C.; and the PACTG 1020 Study Team. Pharmacokinetics of atazanavir/ritonavir in HIV-infected infants, children and adolescents: PACTG 1020A. 12th Conference on Retroviruses and Opportunistic Infections, Boston, Feb. 22–25, 2005. Abstract 767.

[42] Rutstein, R.; Samson, P.; Aldrovandi, G.; Graham, B.; Schnittman, S.; Fletcher, C. V.; Kiser, J.; Smith, M. E.; Mofenson, L.; Fenton, T. Effect of atazanavir (ATAZANAVIR) on serum cholesterol (CH) and triglyceride (TG) levels in HIV-infected infants, children, and adolescents: pediatric AIDS Clinical Trials Group (PACTG) 1020A. 12th Conference on Retroviruses and Opportunistic Infections, Boston, Feb. 22–25, 2005. Abstract 774.

[43] Rutstein, R.; Samson, P.; Fenton, T.; Kiser, J.; Fletcher, C.; Schnittman, S.; Mofenson, L.; Smith, E.; Graham, B.; Aldrovandi, G. The NIH PACTG Protocol 1020: atazanavir (ATAZANAVIR), ± ritonavir in HIV-infected infants, children and adolescents. 14th Conference on Retroviruses and Opportunistic Infections, Los Angeles, Feb. 25–28, 2007. Abstract 715.

[44] Phase IIB pilot of atazanavir + raltegravir (SPARTAN). Available at http://clinicaltrials.gov/ct2/show/NCT00768989. Accessed June 25, 2009.

[45] Mathias, A.; Ramanathan, S.; Hinkle, J.; West, S.; Enejosa, J.; Kearney, B. Effect of atazanavir/r on the steady-state pharmacokinetics of elvitegravir. 47th Interscience Conference on Antimicrobial Agents and Chemotherapy, Chicago, Sept. 17–20, 2007. Poster A-1417.

[46] A pilot study of a novel treatment regimen, maraviroc + ritonavir-boosted atazanavir, in treatment naive HIV-infected Patients. Available at http://clinicaltrials.gov/ct2/show/NCT00827112. Accessed June 25, 2009.

[47] Efficacy and safety of vicriviroc in HIV-infected treatment-naive subjects (study P04875AM3). Available at http://clinicaltrials.gov/ct2/show/NCT00551018. Accessed June 25, 2009.

[48] Safety and efficacy of GS-9350-boosted atazanavir compared to ritonavir-boosted atazanavir in combination with emtricitabine/tenofovir disoproxil fumarate in HIV-1 infected, antiretroviral treatment-naive adults. Available at http://clinicaltrials.gov/ct2/show/NCT00892437. Accessed June 25, 2009.

[49] Karlström, O.; Josephson, F.; Sönnerborg, A. Early virologic rebound in a pilot trial of ritonavir-boosted atazanavir as maintenance monotherapy. *J. Acquir. Immune Defic. Syndr.* **2007**, *44*, 417–422.

[50] Vernazza, P.; Daneel, S.; Schiffer, V.; Decosterd, L.; Fierz, W.; Klimkait, T.; Hoffmann, M.; Hirschel, B. The role of compartment penetration in PI-monotherapy: The atazanavir–ritonavir monomaintenance (ATARITMO) trial. *AIDS* **2007**, *21*, 1309–1315.

[51] Wilkin, T.; McKinnon, J.; DiRienzo, A. G.; Mollan, K.; Fletcher, C.; Margolis, D.; Bastow, B.; Thal, G.; Woodward, W.; Godfrey, C.; et al. Regimen simplification to atazanavir–ritonavir alone as maintenance antiretroviral therapy: final 48-week clinical and virologic outcomes. *J. Infect. Dis.* **2009**, *199*, 866–871.

[52] Department of Health and Human Services, Panel on Antiretroviral Guidelines for Adults and Adolescents. Guidelines for the use of antiretroviral agents in HIV-infected adults and adolescents. Available at http://www. aidsinfo.nih.gov/ContentFiles/AdultandAdolescentGL.pdf. Accessed Jan. 11, 2010.

[53] Hammer, S.; Eron, J.; Reiss, P.; Schooley, R.; Thompson, M.; Walmsley, S.; Chan, P.; Fischl, M.; Gatell, J.; Hirsch, M.; et al. Antiretroviral treatment of adult HIV infection. 2008 Recommendations of the International AIDS Society–USA Panel. *JAMA* **2008**, *300*, 555–570.

[54] European AIDS Clinical Society. EACS guidelines. Available at http://www.eacs.eu/guide/index.htm. Accessed Jan. 11, 2010.

2

DISCOVERY AND DEVELOPMENT OF PL-100, A NOVEL HIV-1 PROTEASE INHIBITOR

JINZI J. WU AND JOSEPH MUSTO
GlaxoSmithKline, Research Triangle Park, North Carolina

INTRODUCTION

The introduction of HIV-1 protease inhibitors (PIs) for the treatment of HIV/AIDS patients more than a decade ago hallmarked the era of highly active antiretroviral therapy (HAART). In sharp contrast to earlier treatment modalities, the use of PIs in conjunction with other classes of antiviral drugs, such as nucleoside reverse transcriptase inhibitors (NRTIs), in triple (or simpler) combination therapy regimens resulted in effective suppression of viral replication commensurate with significant reduction of HIV/AIDS-related morbidity and mortality [1–5]. However, as is the case with all current and experimental anti-HIV drugs, the development of resistance to these drugs has been shown to be a major cause of virological failure of combination antiretroviral therapy [6–9]. The majority of HIV patients ultimately experience some form of drug resistance during therapy [10]. In addition, the percentage of patients presenting with viral resistance upon diagnosis has been increasing rapidly [11]. Some PIs are considered to be high-genetic-barrier compounds for the development of drug resistance. Furthermore, cross-resistance between these drugs is frequently observed and has been shown to increase together with an increasing number of mutations in the PR gene, as is usually the case following sequential therapy with regimens that include these drugs [12,13]. Cross-resistance can result in significant erosion of therapeutic options and may be of greater concern in heavily treatment-experienced patients because of the more extensive and complex mutational patterns harbored by their viruses.

PL-100, a lysine-derived novel protease inhibitor (PI) of human immunodeficiency virus type 1 (HIV-1), and its prodrug, PPL-100, were discovered and developed by Ambrilia Biopharma, Inc., a Montreal-based biopharmaceutical company devoted to antiviral drug development. PL-100 was discovered during the period 2002–2004 by scientists at Pharmacor, Inc., a small Montreal-based biotech which was acquired by Procyon Biopharma, Inc., which later became Ambrilia Biopharma, which assumed the responsibility of preclinical and clinical development of PL-100. Preclinical studies showed that PL-100 possessed suboptimal solubility and pharmacokinetic, (PK) properties, possibly hindering further development. Scientists at Ambrilia developed a prodrug approach to further optimize solubility and the PK profile of PL-100, which led to the discovery of a phosphorylated prodrug, PPL-100. Ambrilia successfully completed preclinical and clinical development (phase I in healthy volunteers) of PPL-100 in approximately 18 months and licensed it to Merck in 2006. Scientists at Ambrilia and its precursor companies had the following remits during the discovery and development of PL-100 and its prodrug, PPL-100: (1) a potent and selective next-generation PI with a novel scaffold; (2) a favorable cross-resistance profile compared to approved PIs at that time, mainly lopinavir (LPV) and atazanavir (ATV) (darunavir and tipranavir were not available for comparison then); (3) a high genetic barrier to the development of resistance; and (4) a unique PK profile with the potential of becoming the first unboosted PI. This chapter summarizes the discovery and development of PL-100 and PPL-100 in the context of the foregoing objectives.

Antiviral Drugs: From Basic Discovery Through Clinical Trials, First Edition. Edited by Wieslaw M. Kazmierski.

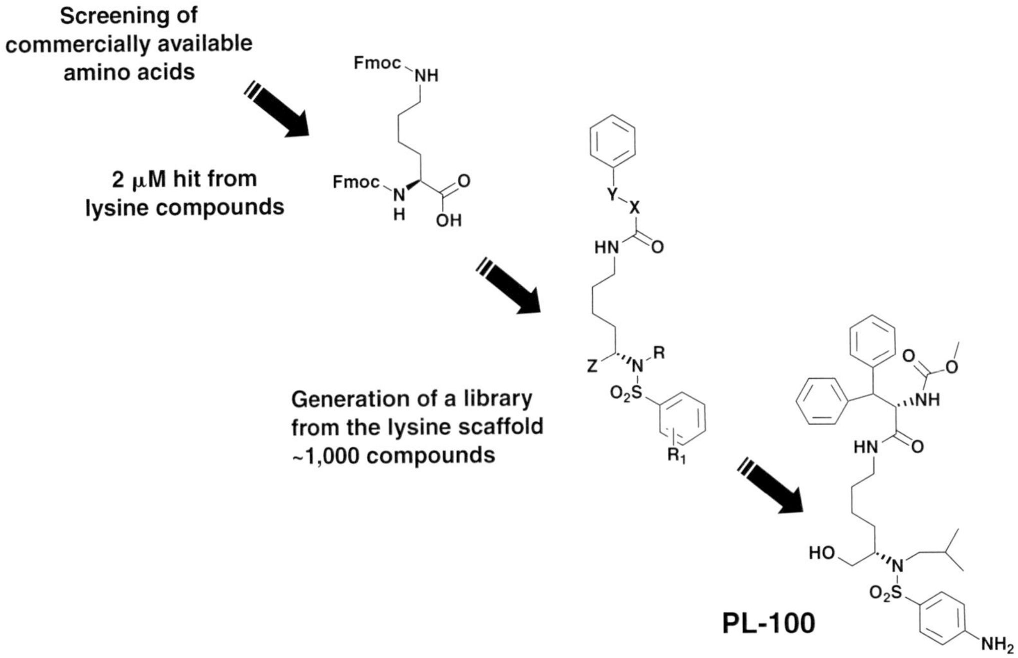

SCHEME 1 Screening and lead optimization.

DISCOVERY

Next-Generation PI with a Novel Lysine Scaffold

A series of HIV-1 PIs with a novel scaffold based on lysine were discovered via the screen of an amino acid library and subsequent rational drug design, as illustrated in Scheme 1. This novel scaffold generated potent lead compounds for both protease enzyme inhibition and antiviral activities [14]. Furthermore, initial cross-resistance studies of one such lead compound suggested that this class of molecules was promising [15]. The lead optimization process giving rise to PL-100 was reported by Stranix et al. [16,17]. The testing results obtained during the optimization work are provided in Tables 1 and 2.

The inhibition of HIV-1 PR, activity against HIV-1 in the cell-based assay, and cellular toxicity were reported by Dandache et al. [18], Stranix et al. [17], and Wu et al. [19]. PL-100, a novel L-lysine derivative HIV PI, inhibited purified HIV-1 PR with a mean K_i value of 36 pM, as determined by a tightly binding inhibitor plot [15]. With the exception of IDV (K_i, ~ 2 nM), all of the PIs tested demonstrated K_i values in the same picomolar range (14 to 306 pM).

The selectivity of PL-100 was evaluated by testing its ability to inhibit the activities of other aspartyl PRs: namely, pepsin and cathepsin D. In these assays, PL-100 showed no inhibitory activity (its IC_{50} values were > 50 μM for both cathepsin D and pepsin), whereas APV's IC_{50} values were 15.2 and 0.28 μM, respectively. These results demonstrate that PL-100 is a potent and selective competitive HIV-1 PI.

To determine whether PL-100 effectively blocks the proteolytic processing of HIV-1 p55 polyprotein, H9 cells chronically infected with HIV-1 IIIB were incubated in the presence of various concentrations of PL-100, and the p55 cleavage product p24 was detected by Western blotting. The results show that PL-100 effectively prevented the processing of the p55 precursor protein, as demonstrated by a dose-dependent decrease in the amount of p24 product [15]. These results confirm that PL-100 is an effective inhibitor of the HIV-1 PR in infected cells.

TABLE 1 Inhibition of HIV-1 Aspartyl Protease (IC_{50}) and Antiviral Activity (EC_{50}) in the Cellular Assay (MT-4)

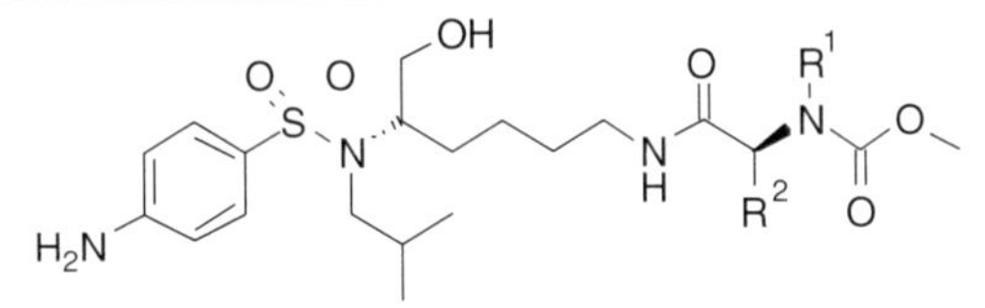

R^1	R^2	IC_{50} (nM)	EC_{50} (nM)
H	$C_6H_5CH_2$	12	2000
H	Ph	>300	N.D.[a]
H	$C_6H_5CH_2CH_2$	40	9000
CH_2	$C_6H_4CH(TIC)$	130	N.D.
CH_3	$C_6H_5CH_2$	6.5	1000
H	Naphthyl-1-CH_2	1.2	120
H	Naphthyl-2-CH_2	1.2	258
H	Biphenyl-2-CH_2	0.521	200
H	$(C_6H_5)_2CH$	0.500	16

[a]N.D., not determined.

TABLE 2 Structure–Activity Relationship[a]

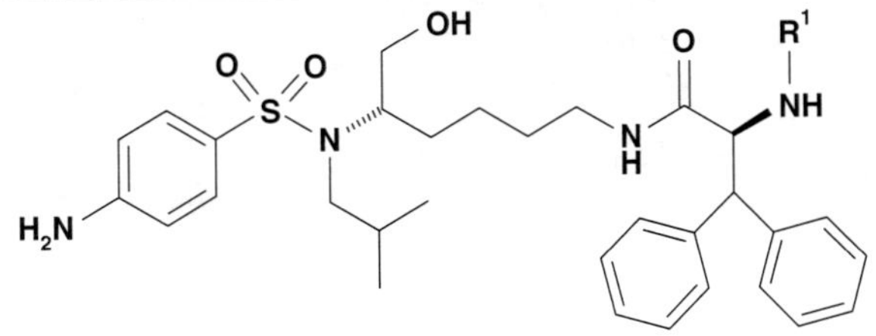

R^1	IC_{50} (nM)	EC_{50} (nM)
H	0.50	44
Ac	1.5	66
Cyclopropyl-CO	0.43	25
CH_3O-CO	0.50	16 (PL-100)
$(CH_3)_3CO$-CO	0.40	41
$(CH_3)_2N$-CO	0.44	62
Pyrazine-CO	0.52	19
2-Pyridyl-CO	0.46	68
3-Pyridyl-CO	0.68	39
4-Pyridyl-CO	0.65	32
2-CH_3-3-pyridyl-CO	0.40	42
6-CH_3-3-pyridyl-CO	0.40	24
3-HO-2-pyridyl-CO	0.90	153
6-H_2N-3-pyridyl-CO	0.40	84
3-Picolyl-CO	0.24	194
2-Picolyl-O-CO	0.12	17
3-Picolyl-O-CO	0.48	18
4-PicolylO-CO	0.39	20
2-HO-phenyl-CO	0.63	64
3-HO-phenyl-CO	0.40	64
4-HO-phenyl-CO	0.53	88
3-HO-4-NO_2-phenyl-CO	0.33	16

[a]IC_{50}, enzyme activity; EC_{50}, antiviral activity.

The in vitro antiviral activity of PL-100 was tested by a standard MTT cytoprotection assay. PL-100 potently suppressed viral replication of the laboratory-adapted strain NL-4.3 in MT-4 cells with an average EC_{50} of 16 nM and an EC_{90} of 23 nM, while the selected FDA-approved PIs gave EC_{50} values that ranged between 4 and 67 nM (Table 3) [17–19]. Furthermore, the cytotoxicity of PL-100, with a CC_{50} value of 37,000 nM and a selectivity index of 2313, was similar to those of commercially available PIs (Table 3) [17–19]. In addition, EC_{50} values of PL-100 against wild-type viruses in other cellular assays have been reported [EC_{50} = 0.006 to 0.011 μM in cord blood mononuclear cells (CBMCs)] [17].

Favorable Cross-Resistance Pattern

The antiviral activity of PL-100 and its backup PL-337 were evaluated in parallel with a series of commercially available PIs at the time of investigation [17–20] using a panel of 63 constructs containing PR and RT gene sequences from PI-experienced patients in a replication-defective reporter-gene-based phenotypic assay (PhenoSense HIV assay; Monogram Biosciences). The selection criteria for the 63 NL-4.3-based constructs included high-level loss of susceptibility to specific PIs and high-level loss of susceptibility to multiple PIs. The following primary PI mutations were considered in the study: D30N, V32I, L33F, M46I/L, I47A/V, G48V, I50L/V, V82A/F/L/S/T, I84V, N88D/S, and L90M, as defined by the International AIDS Society–USA. The numbers of constructs in the panel harboring zero, one, two, three, four, five, or six of these primary PI mutations were 2, 4, 7, 30, 15, 4, and 1, respectively. Hence, the majority of the constructs in this panel harbored three or four primary PI mutations; this emphasizes the strength of the panel. The representation of each primary PI mutation in the panel of 63 constructs tested in the cross-resistance profiling of PL-100 was as follows: 2 constructs with D30N, 3 with V32I, 21 with L33F, 38 with M46I/L, 5 with I47A/V, 6 with G48V, 7 with I50L/V, 33 with V82A/F/L/S/T, 35 with I84V, 11 with N88D/S, and 31 with L90M. Mixed genotypes in the samples were not considered. The mean EC_{50} of PL-100 in this assay was 5.3 nM against the wild-type NL-4.3 reference construct compared to 10.7, 1.5, 7.8, 2.8, 5.8, and 1.8 nM for APV, ATV, IDV, LPV, NFV, and SQV, respectively. The PI susceptibility of each patient-derived resistance test vector was compared to that of the wild-type NL-4.3 reference

TABLE 3 Comparison of Antiviral Activity and Cytotoxicity of PL-100 vs. Approved PIs

Protease Inhibitor	Antiviral Activity, EC_{50} (μM)[a]	Cytotoxicity, CC_{50} (μM)	Selectivity Index, SI[b]
PL-100	0.016 ± 0.003	37 ± 16	2,313
ATV (atazanavir-BMS)	0.004 ± 0.001	71 ± 19	17,750
APV (amprenavir-GSK)	0.051 ± 0.014	>100	>1,961
IDV (indinavir-Merck)	0.067 ± 0.010	>100	>1,493
LPV (lopinavir-Abbott)	0.019 ± 0.001	28 ± 8	1,474
NFV (nelfinavir-Pfizer)	0.031	8 ± 2	258
RTV (ritonavir-Abbott)	0.061 ± 0.003	26 ± 6	426
SQV (saquinavir-Roche)	0.013	19 ± 7	1,462

[a]EC_{50} obtained using the NL4-3 strain and MT-4 cell line, 6 days postinfection.
[b]The selectivity index (SI) = cytotoxic concentration 50 (CC_{50})/antiviral EC_{50}.

TABLE 4 Antiviral Activity of PL-100 and PL-337 vs. Marketed PIs Against 63 Multi-PI-Resistant Strains[a]

	ATV: Atazanavir-BMS	APV: Amprenavir-GSK	IDV Indinavir-Merck	LPV Lopinavir-Abbott	NFV Nelfinavir-Pfizer	SQV Saquinavir-Roche	PL-100	PL-337
Median FC[b]	15.6	9.7	8.1	17.0	15.0	23.2	**3.6**	**4.7**
Mean FC[b]	25.7	18.5	16.5	31.3	31.7	85	**8.7**	**9.3**
%FC < 2.5	16	14	13	10	10	27	**37**	**38**
%FC < 10	38	52	54	37	27	40	**76**	**72**
%FC > 50	22	8	5	19	10	37	**3**	**2**

[a]Tipranavir and darunavir were not available for comparison at the time of this study.
[b]FC, fold change of antiviral activity against resistant strains vs. wild-type virus.

construct; the results were expressed as the fold change in EC_{50} in relation to the reference. Table 4 shows activity of PL-100 and its backup, PL-337, and marketed PIs against 63 multi-PI resistant strains in fold change or (FC) in EC_{50} using the PhenoSense assay compared to wild-type viruses.

As expected from the genotypes in the panel, there was broad cross-resistance among the approved PIs tested, with a range in the median change of 8.1- to 23.2-fold. Between 73 and 91% of the viruses had > 2.5-fold-reduced susceptibility to the approved PIs, and 46 to 73% had changes of > 10-fold. Overall, PL-100 and its backup, PL-337, showed the lowest median change and the lowest mean change. The number of constructs with changes in EC_{50} to PL-100 of < 2.5-fold was also the highest (36% with changes of < 2.5-fold vs. 9 to 27% for the other PIs). It was also observed that only 3% of the strains tested showed a change above 50-fold for PL-100, compared to 5 to 37% for the other PIs. The genotypic analysis was focused on key mutations for approved PIs. The samples from the panel of 63 were selected depending on the presence of only primary/signature mutations for each PI tested, as defined by the International AIDS Society–USA. Thirty-four strains harbored the I50L, I84V, and/or N88S signature mutation associated with resistance to ATV. The median changes were 23.1-fold (range, 3.1- to 81.2-fold) and 3.9-fold (range, 0.4- to 84.0-fold) for ATV and PL-100, respectively. The LPV primary mutations V32I, I47A/V, and/or V82A/F/ S/T were present in 37 of the isolates. The median changes were 20.1-fold (range, 2.9- to 151.8-fold) and 5.3-fold (range, 0.6- to 51.5-fold) for LPV and PL-100, respectively.

In summary, both the median and mean changes observed with PL-100 and PL-337 were the lowest of all PIs in these genotype-based comparisons. Finally, at the time that this cross-resistance study was performed, the recently approved PIs TPV and DRV were not available for direct comparison with PL-100.

High Genetic Barrier to Resistance

Genotypic Analysis PL-100 has a novel lysine-based scaffold with a flexible linker, differentiating itself from approved PIs. With such a flexible linker, one could hope that this novel PI might have a higher barrier to the development of drug resistance than that of many of approved PIs. Although clinical data on the barrier to the resistance are not available, in vitro resistance selection studies were carried out to provide some information on the genetic barrier of PL-100 [21–24]. The genotypic analysis of the HIV-1/IIIb variants growing after 8 weeks of culture in the presence of PL-100 (Table 5) revealed a T80I mutation in PR that was maintained throughout the selection. Increasing the concentration of PL-100 led to the selection of three additional mutations in PR: K45R, M46I, and P81S (Table 5). A genotype that is intermediate between the single mutant T80I and the quadruple mutant K45R/M46I/ T80I/P81S (Table 5: weeks 15 to 25) was not identified. No highly fit variant emerged after 48 weeks in the presence of PL-100, and genotyping of the virus at that time did not show changes in PR from that of week 25 (i.e., K45R/M46I/T80I/P81S). Results obtained with APV (Table 5) were consistent with published findings [25–27]. Two mutations selected by PL-100 affect amino acid residues located in the flaps of HIV PR (K45R and M46I). In addition, PL-100 selected for two novel active-site mutations (T80I and P81S) located in the 80S loop of HIV PR. No mutations were observed in the p7/p1 and p1/p6 protease cleavage sites of Gag [24].

Phenotypic Analysis A standard MTT assay was performed to compare the sensitivity to PL-100 of the site-directed mutant viruses (SDMVs) produced by transfection of COS-7 cells with that of the wild-type laboratory-adapted strain NL-4.3 (Table 6). These assays revealed that each mutation on its own did not confer significant resistance to PL-100. Indeed, only the single-mutant T80I showed an FC value in EC_{50} of 2.25, while both the K45R and the M46I single mutants had FCs in EC_{50} below 2. The P81S mutant as well as the double mutants harboring the P81S mutation could not be tested in this assay, since the virus harboring P81S mutation has a defect in the replication capacity (processing p55Gag precursor into p24). Only when the four mutations coexisted in PR did one observe high enough viral titers to get 100% MT-4 cell killing after 6 days and thus to detect

TABLE 5 PL-100 In Vitro Selected a Novel Mutation Pattern (K45R, M46I, T80I, and P81S)

Virus	Week	PL-100: New Mutations (concentration μM)	APV: New mutations (concentration μM)
IIIb	8	(0.1) T80I	(0.5) Not done
	15	(1.0) T80I	(2.5) L10F, I84V, Q92K
	18	(1.0) T80I	(2.5) Not done
	20	(1.0) T80I	(2.5) Not done
	22	(1.0) T80I	(2.5) Not done
	25	(2.5) K45R, M46I, T80I, P81S	(5.0) L10F, M46I, I84V, Q92K
	34	(5.0) K45R, M46I, T80I, P81S	(5.0) L10F, M46I, I84V, Q92K
	48	(5.0) K45R, M46I, T80I, P81S	(5.0) L10F, M46I, I84V, Q92K

a signal in the MTT assay: The KMTP quadruple mutant showed only a mild resistance to PL-100 with an FC value in $EC_{50} = 10.82$.

The sensitivity of PL-100-selected mutations to several marketed PIs was compared to that of the wild-type virus by MTT assay (Table 7). Data showed that no cross-resistance to other PIs was conferred by the mutants studied. Even with an FC in EC_{50} of 2.7 against atazanavir (ATV), the quadruple mutant did not show significant resistance to any PI tested. Interestingly, the single mutant T80I even showed a marked hypersusceptibility to several PIs tested (Table 6), especially nelfinavir (NFV) and saquinavir (SQV), showing 8- and 10-fold hypersensitivity to T80I.

In summary, the data suggest that PL-100 has a high genetic barrier to drug resistance. It is a promising new PI that may force HIV-1 into a unique mutational pathway that in addition to conferring only low-level resistance, may be detrimental to viral replication capacity. Furthermore, the mutations selected by PL-100 in vitro showed no cross-resistance to other PIs. Interestingly, the mutational pathway may also render HIV-1 more sensitive to several other PIs that could potentially be used in combination with PL-100.

TABLE 6 Site-Directed Mutagenesis Analysis[a]

Mutation	Virus Genotype	Replication Capacity[b]	Average Fold Change in $EC_{50} \pm$ S.D. (n)[c]
N.A.	Wild-type	++++	1 (7)
Single	K45R	N.D.	1.51 ± 0.40 (3)
	M46I	N.D.	0.81 ± 0.18 (2)
	T80I	+++	2.25 ± 0.52 (5)
	P81S	—	N.A.
Double	K45R/M46I	+++/++++	0.98 ± 0.32 (2)
	K45R/P81S	—	N.A.
	M46I/P81S	—	N.A.
	T80I/P81S	—	N.A.
Triple	K45R/M46I/P81S	++	N.A.
	K45R/T80I/P81S	—	N.A.
	M46I/T80I/P81S	+	N.A.
Quadruple	K45R/M46I/T80I/P81S	+++	10.82 ± 2.25 (5)

[a]N.A., not applicable; N.D., not determined.
[b]Antiviral activity of PL-100 against HIV/NL-4.3 site-directed mutants was determined by MTT assay in MT4, 6 days' postinfection.
[c]Determined by standard replication kinetics in MT4 for 7 days.

TABLE 7 Activity of Marketed PIs vs. Viruses with PL-100-Selected Mutations

	Fold Change in EC_{50}	
Marketed PI	Single, Double, and Quadruple Mutations (Except Single T80I Mutation)	T80I
ATV	0.43–2.70	0.48
LPV	0.63–1.62	0.39
APV	0.60–1.48	0.95
SQV	0.45–1.11	0.10
NFV	0.56–1.34	0.13
IDV	0.52–1.46	0.30

Structural Basis for Resistance

Co-crystallization of PL-100 with WT HIV-1 protease and x-ray crystallography were performed [24,28]. Analysis of the enzyme–inhibitor complex reveals that the inhibitor has an extended conformation that provides hydrophobic side chains that fill four of the subpockets of the enzyme proximal to the catalytic dyad spanning from S2 to S4. The primary hydroxyl group present in PL-100 serves to mimic the catalytic water molecule necessary for aspartyl protease functionality. To understand the novel resistance profile inherent in PL-100, as well as the hypersensitivity of T80I to the other PIs, a model was created in the active site of the wild-type protease. A T80I single-point mutation and a M46I/K45R/T80I/P81S quadruple mutation were separately incorporated into the WT crystal structure, and the binding of PL-100 was reexamined in these mutant enzyme models [24]. Thr80 is the only polar residue within the P1 loop, and its hydroxyl group forms highly conserved hydrogen bonds with the backbone of Val82. Both SQV and NFV have a lipophilic decahydroisoquinoline moiety that is proximal to the rigid Thr80 residue. An isoleucine mutation at this position would have a positive effect on the binding affinity, as the inhibitor would benefit from a more favorable hydrophobic contact with the protease as well as having less-restrictive non-hydrogen-bonding interaction between Ile80 and Val82. Calculation of the interaction energy of SQV in models of both the wild-type and T80I mutant enzyme confirms the approximate 10-fold increase in binding affinity that was found experimentally (Table 7, T80I with NFV and SQV). Furthermore, examination of the x-ray crystal structure of the PL-100/wild-type enzyme complex suggests that the aromatic rings of the diphenylalanine group are responsible for the loss in binding affinity. A model of the P81S containing quadruple mutation illustrates that the serine mutant residue is less than 4 Å from both of the phenyl groups of PL-100. This mutation reduces the hydrophobic character of the S1 and S3 subsites and creates a more hydrophilic environment for binding. A calculation of the interaction energy of PL-100 in models of both the wild-type and P81S-containing quadruple mutant enzyme suggests an approximate 10-fold loss in activity. This is consistent with the data from site-directed mutagenesis (Table 6).

A crystal structure of HIV-1 protease and lysine sulfonamide-8 inhibitor, a close analog of PL-100, was reported by Madhavi et al. [29]. The data suggest that lysine sulfonamide-8 inhibitor binds to the HIV-1 protease in a novel fashion. Most of the inhibitors that are on the market are peptidomimetics, where a conserved water molecule mediates hydrogen-bonding interactions between the inhibitors and the flaps of the protease. The lysine sulfonamide-8 inhibitor binds to the active site of HIV-1 protease in a novel manner, displacing the conserved water and making extensive hydrogen bonds with every region of the active site. The authors speculated that the hydrogen-bonding pattern of the PL-100/protease complex is likely to be similar to that of the protease complex of the lysine sulfonamide-8 inhibitor, except for bonds made by the amine group at P2′, where the benzylamine is replaced by a phenylamine in PL-100. In summary, co-crystallization and x-ray crystallography provided the insight of a structural basis for favorable cross-resistance and a high genetic barrier of PL-100.

PRECLINICAL PHARMACOKINETICS AND METABOLISM

PPL-100, a Prodrug of PL-100

Although it has a favorable cross-resistance profile and a high genetic barrier to resistance development in vitro, PL-100 has a low solubility (79 μg/mL). Furthermore, the pharmacokinetic profile of PL-100 is not optimal. A prodrug approach was used to increase aqueous solubility and oral bioavailability [17]. A phosphorylated prodrug (bissodium salt), PPL-100, was selected as a clinical candidate for further development (Scheme 2). The published data [17,19,20,22,23] suggest that PPL-100 (> 145 mg/mL) is 1800-fold more water soluble than is PL-100, and the oral bioavailability of PPL-100 increases two- to threefold compared to the parent compound, PL-100. This prodrug is not active against HIV-1 protease. The studies in cannulated rats demonstrate that PL-100 was the major metabolite found in the portal vein and systemic circulation when prodrug PPL-100 was orally dosed, suggesting that most of the prodrug is converted to the parent drug in the gastrointestinal tract [30].

In Vitro Metabolism

In vitro metabolism of PL-100 in human and rat liver microsomes was compared with amprenavir, lopinavir, saquinavir, indinavir, nelfinavir, and ritonavir [30]. PL-100 was more stable than lopinavir, saquinavir, and indinavir. Metabolism of PL-100 in human liver microsomes was significantly

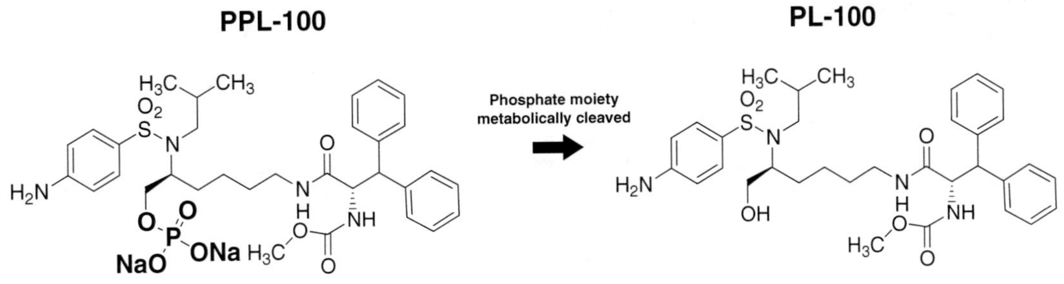

SCHEME 2 PPL-100 and PL-100.

inhibited by ritonavir and other CYP3A4 inhibitors, which was consistent with in vivo data showing that pharmacokinetics of this PI was boosted significantly by ritonavir (Fig. 1). PL-100 did not inhibit CYP2C9 and CYP2D6 but did inhibit CYP3A4/5 in vitro (Table 8). PL-100 did not induce the activity of CYP2C9 and CYP3A4 in the freshly isolated primary human hepatocytes [30].

Pharmacokinetics

PK profiles in rats between PL-100 and PPL-100 were investigated [17,19,20,22,23]. PL-100 or PPL-100 was administered orally at doses indicated in Figure 1. Each time point in the figure represents the average plasma (PL-100; ng/mL) of six female rats at a given dose. Absolute oral bioavailability for PL-100 and PPL-100 at 30 mg/kg was calculated as 8.7 and 23%, respectively. The PK profile of PPL-100 in rats was also investigated when boosted by RTV (Fig. 1). PPL-100 and RTV were coadministered orally at doses indicated in Figure 1. Each time point in the figure represents the average plasma (PL-100; ng/mL) of six female rats at a given dose. In comparison to the cross-resistance profile of the parent drug, PL-100, the data suggest that PPL-100 has potential as a novel unboosted PI for the treatment of PI-naive patients as well as PI-experienced patients infected with drug-resistant HIV strains bearing two or fewer primary PI mutations. Furthermore, when boosted by ritonavir, PPL-100 has potential for the treatment of patients infected with drug-resistant HIV strains bearing three to four primary PI mutations, as defined in the cross-resistance profiling study.

CLINICAL OBSERVATIONS

Study Design

A first-in-man single-dose escalation study was conducted to assess the product's safety and pharmacokinetic profile [17,22,23]. Consenting healthy male volunteers aged 18 to 45 years were enrolled in the study. The study was a double-blind randomized placebo-controlled single-dose escalation trial whose objective was the evaluation of the safety and pharmacokinetics of PPL-100. The study was conducted at a

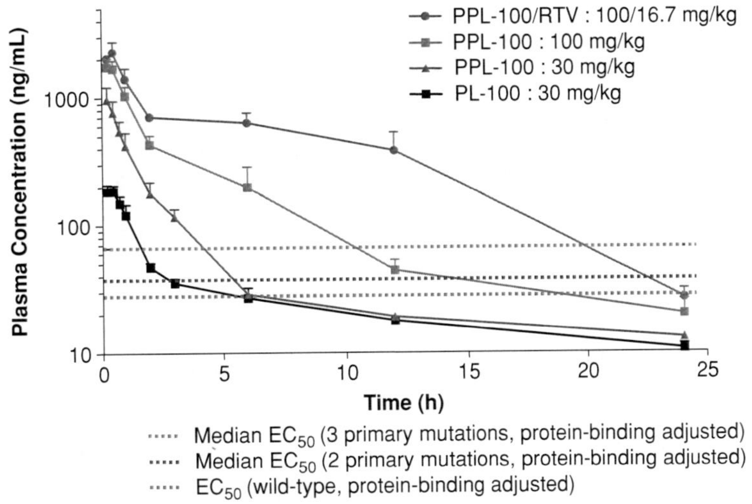

FIGURE 1 Pharmacokinetic profiles of PL-100 and PPL-100 in rats in relation to cross-resistance patterns. (*See insert for color representation of the figure.*)

TABLE 8 In Vitro CYP Inhibition

			K_i (μM)	
Enzyme	Substrate	Metabolic Reaction	PL-100	Ritonavir
CYP2C9	Tolbutamide	Tolbutamide Methyl-hydroxylation	13.3 ± 1.7	13.9 ± 2.0
CYP2D6	Dextromethorphan	Dextromethorphan O-Demethylation	27.8 ± 2.3	2.7 ± 0.3
CYP3A4/5	Testosterone	Testosterone 6β-Hydroxylation	0.445 ± 0.050	0.033 ± 0.005

single Canadian center. Sixty-four subjects were enrolled in a total of eight cohorts, as shown in Table 9. For each cohort, six subjects received a single dose of PPL-100, and two subjects received placebo. Subjects were to be nonsmokers able to provide informed consent and to have discontinued the use of grapefruit juice and foods containing poppy seeds 7 days and 24 h, respectively, prior to a study of drug administration. Subjects were to discontinue the consumption of coffee and alcohol 48 h prior to dosing and while in residence at the study clinic. For cohorts 1 to 5, subjects were dosed after a supervised overnight fast of at least 10 h, whereas in cohorts 6 to 8, subjects also received a light meal.

Sample Collection and Analysis

All subjects had blood samples drawn by dead-volume intravenous catheter or via direct vein puncture 30 min prior to study drug administration or 60 min in cohorts 6 to 8 as well as at 0.25, 0.5, 0.75, 1,1.5, 2, 2.5, 3, 4, 6, 8, 12, 18, and 24 h post-dose. Determination of PL-100, PL-461, and ritonavir in human EDTA K2 plasma was achieved using a high-performance liquid chromatographic method with tandem mass spectrometry detection. Plasma concentrations data for PL-100, PL-461 (the free acid form of PL-100), and ritonavir were used to generate pharmacokinetic parameters using noncompartmental analysis with the WinNonlin Professional version 5.0. Descriptive statistics was performed for: $AUC_{0\text{-}t}$, $AUC_{0\text{-}\infty}$, C_{max}, $AUC_{t/\infty}$, T_{max}, λz, $t_{1/2,el}$, T_{lag}, Cl/F, Vz/F, $AUMC_{0\text{-}\infty}$, and MRT with SAS version 8.02. The time from dosing to the first observable concentration (T_{lag}), the maximum observed concentration (C_{max}), and the time to reach C_{max} were observed directly. $AUC_{0\text{-}t}$ was calculated using the linear trapezoidal rule.

TABLE 9 Treatment per Cohort

Cohort	Dose of PPL-100
1	300 mg
2	600 mg
3	1200 mg
4	1800 mg
5	2400 mg
6	600 mg with a light meal
7	1200 mg with a light meal
8	600 mg with a light meal and 100 mg of ritonavir

Safety Monitoring

Criteria for monitoring safety and tolerability included medical history, vital signs, electrocardiogram, and clinical laboratory tests. Clinical laboratory tests, physical examination, electrocardiogram, and vital signs were performed at screening, post-study procedures, and on day 2 following administration if the study drug. Supine electrocardiograms were also performed within 60 min prior to dosing and at 1, 2, 3, 4, 6, and 8 h after dosing (the 3-h post-dose measurement was taken only with cohorts 7 and 8, whereas the 6- and 8-h post-dose measurements were performed only for cohort 8). Vital signs were also taken within 30 min prior to dosing or 60 min prior to dosing for cohorts 6 to 8 and at 0.5, 1, 1.5, 2, 4, 8, and 12 h post-dose. Throughout the study, subjects were monitored for adverse events. At admission and prior to departure, subjects were asked a standard probe question concerning the onset of any new health problems. All adverse events, including those reported within 7 days following the last drug administration, were recorded.

Pharmacokinetics

In total, 64 male subjects were randomized and received the study drug and were included in the pharmacokinetic, safety, and statistical analyses. The subject population had an age range of 19 to 45 years and ranged from 164.0 to 184.5 cm in height and 63.0 to 96.6 kg in weight. All subjects were Caucasian. Pharmacokinetic parameters are described in Table 10. For the first five cohorts, the mean $AUC_{0\text{-}t}$ varies from 2147 ± 521 for subjects enrolled in cohort 1 treated with 300 mg of PPL-100 to 7096 ± 4406 for subjects enrolled in cohort 5 treated at 2400 mg. The T_{max} is reached after approximately 1 h, and the mean half-life (mean $t_{1/2}$) varies from 29.99 to 37.27 h.

Examination of the results in Table 10 suggest that the $AUC_{0\text{-}t}$ increases linearly with increasing doses but in a less than dose-proportional manner, whereas the C_{max} increases

TABLE 10 Main Pharmacokinetic Parameters[a]

Cohort	$AUC_{0\text{-}t}$ (ng·h/mL) Mean ± S.D.	C_{max} (ng/mL) Mean ± S.D.	T_{max} (h) Mean ± S.D.	$t_{1/2}$ (h) Mean ± S.D.
1	2147.72 ± 521.54	496.03 ± 426.32	1.00 ± 0.758	37.27 ± 7.57
2	2972.66 ± 918.09	940.87 ± 577.15	1.13 ± 0.685	35.74 ± 15.76
3	4805.47 ± 536.27	1998.92 ± 529.89	0.917 ± 0.129	29.99 ± 4.47
4	5673.88 ± 1236.67	2039.46 ± 800.76	1.04 ± 0.252	35.48 ± 9.73
5	7096.42 ± 4406.17	2526.94 ± 1370.53	1.13 ± 0.306	30.41 ± 24.66
6	2784.79 ± 308.73	498.52 ± 205.82	3.08 ± 2.46	50.79 ± 43.35
7	5705.22 ± 2127.1	1406.79 ± 916.85	2.75 ± 0.758	27.54 ± 4.97
8	3988.14 ± 1357.9	667.95 ± 415.20	3.08 ± 1.07	45.83 ± 25.72

[a]Cohorts 1, 2, 3, 4, and 5 received, respectively, 300, 600, 1200, 1800 and 2400 mg of PPL-100 under fasting conditions. Cohorts 6 and 7 received, respectively, 600 and 1200 mg of PPL-100 with a light meal. Cohort 8 received 600 mg of PPL-100 with a light meal and 100 mg of ritonavir. Data are normalized for subject body weight in kilograms.

linearly until 1200 mg, increasing less thereafter. The plasma concentration vs. time curves for the doses used in cohorts 1 through 5 are presented in Figure 2. It is to be noted that plasma concentrations are maintained above the protein binding–adjusted EC_{50} for periods of at least 24 h. An exceptional long half-life of PL-100 in plasma samples was observed, ranging from 30 to 37 h.

A light meal (Fig. 3) does not affect the AUC and elimination half-life significantly but reduces the C_{max}. T_{max} increases from 1 to 3 h with a light meal. Coadministration of PPL-100 (Fig. 4) with a single dose of ritonavir (100 mg) results in a slight increase in both C_{max} and AUC.

Safety and Tolerability

There was a total of 56 treatment-emergent adverse events, of which 21 were reported as treatment related. The severity of the adverse events was graded according to the Division of AIDS Adverse Event Grading Table. The severity was graded as follows: grade 1 (mild), grade 2 (moderate), grade 3 (severe), and grade 4 (life-threatening). All adverse events were graded 1 (mild), except two adverse events that were graded 2 (moderate). The most common drug-related clinical adverse experiences reported were dizziness (six events in six subjects, one receiving placebo), headache (three events in three subjects, one receiving placebo), and nausea (three events in three subjects, one receiving placebo). No clinically meaningful dose–response relationship was observed. In addition, the unblinded data show no clinically meaningful treatment-related effects of PPL-100 upon analysis of chemistry/hematology, laboratory, or vital signs parameters. A summary of the adverse events is presented in Table 11. The tabulation is according to the Medical Dictionary for Regulatory Activities (MedDRA).

DISCUSSION

Although significant progress has been made in HIV/AIDS treatment, a number of key issues remain unresolved. Viral eradication is not achieved with current highly active

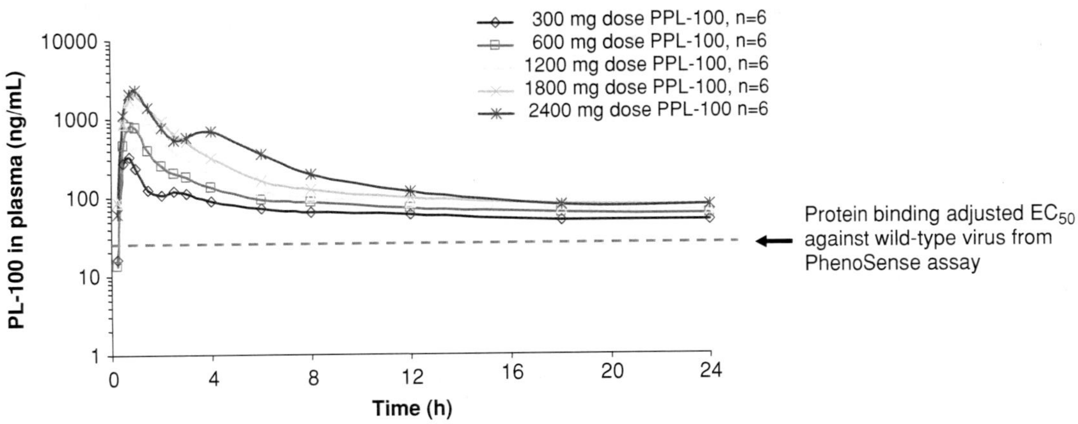

FIGURE 2 Clinical PK profile of PL-100 in single-dose escalation studies in relation to its protein binding–adjusted antiviral activity. (*See insert for color representation of the figure.*)

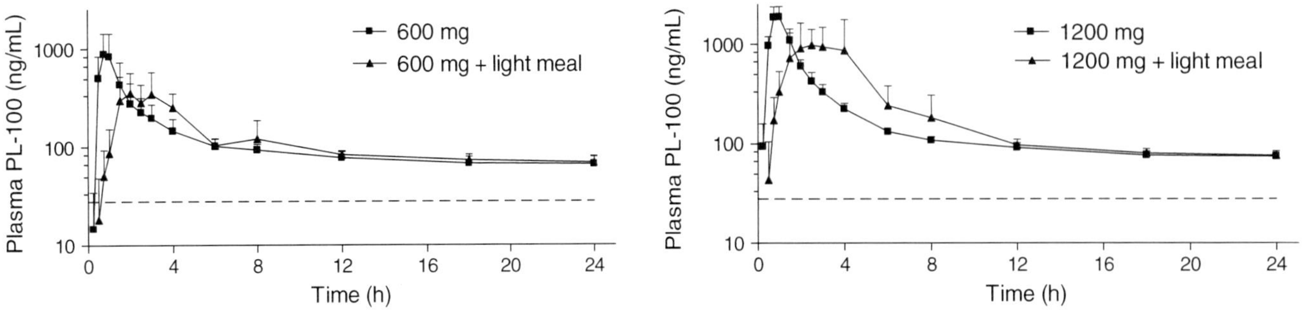

---Protein binding-adjusted EC_{50} against wild-type virus from PhenoSense assay.

*The light meal is two slices of white bread, one pat of butter, one portion of mild cheddar cheese (21 g), two pats of strawberry jam, and one carton (200 mL) of 3.25% M.F. milk.

FIGURE 3 Pharmacokinetics of PPL-100 without RTV boosting in the absence and presence of a light meal in relation to its antiviral activity.

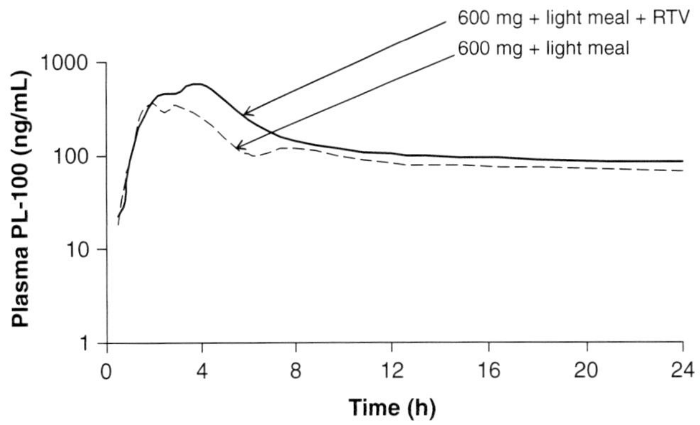

FIGURE 4 Pharmacokinetics of PPL-100 with RTV boosting in the presence of a light meal.

TABLE 11 Number of Adverse Events per Cohort

	PPL-100 Cohort									
Number of Adverse Events	1	2	3	4	5	6	7	8	Placebo	Total
Dizziness				2	2	1			1	6
Protein urine present				2	1		1		1	5
Blood cholesterol increased		1				1	1	1	1	5
Catheter-site pain		2					1			3
Blood uric acid increased		1					1	1	1	4
Nausea				1	1				1	3
Headache				1	1				1	3
Alanine aminotransferase increased		1							1	2
Diarrhea		1					1			2
Blood triglycerides increased		1						1		2
All others	2	3	1	3	3	2	1	2	4	21
Total per cohort	2	10	1	9	8	4	6	5	11	56

antiretroviral therapy (HAART) regimens because of the persistence of a long-lived pool of latently infected memory T-cells. Instead, the treatment of HIV infection involves maintaining patients on suppressive HAART regimens indefinitely. Therefore, there are a number of obstacles in maintaining lifetime suppression of viral replication, such as drug tolerability and convenience, drug–drug interaction, and drug resistance. The protease inhibitors (PIs) were the second class of HIV therapeutics to be launched following the NRTIs and proven to be a class of potent antiviral drugs with a high genetic barrier to the development of drug resistance. As a result, the PI class underwent rapid development, with nine drugs (excluding ritonavir) reaching the market by 2006, when the clinical safety and PK studies of PPL-100 were completed. However, the class is associated with a number of issues, including pharmacokinetic problems, and side effects such as lipodystrophy. Boosting PIs with ritonavir improves pharmacokinetics, increases efficacy, and is now standard practice. All approved PIs, given once or twice daily, require boosting by ritonavir due to their suboptimal pharmacokinetic profiles. Some physicians recommend unboosted ATV twice or once daily, but this is not yet common standard practice, due to its less robust PK and interpatient PK variation. Ritonavir is a significant CYP inhibitor and inducer, giving rise to major drug–drug interaction problems. Therefore, the development of a next-generation PI not requiring ritonavir boosting is an unmet medical need and a very challenging task.

The present studies, evaluating pharmacokinetics, safety, and tolerability of a single escalated dose of PPL-100 suggest that PPL-100 has a pharmacokinetic profile characterized by a long elimination half-life ranging from 30 to 37 h, in contrast to most marketed PIs, which have relatively short terminal half-lives, varying from 2 to 10 h. The long elimination half-lives provide the hope for PPL-100 as the first unboosted PI in the clinical development, yet to be confirmed in further clinical studies. A recent report from Concert Pharmaceutical indicates that deuterated ATV with reduced metabolism by CYPs may potentially be another PI which does not require RTV boosting. Furthermore, pharmacokinetic profiles of PPL-100 were very similar in the presence and absence of food. In the presence of a light meal, C_{max} decreases as expected, while terminal half-lives remain for more then 27 h. In contrast, many PIs, such as ATV, have to be taken with food since their C_{max} and C_{min} values decrease significantly in the absence of food. The coadministration of PPL-100 with ritonavir in humans did not result in a significant increase in drug exposure, suggesting that PPL-100 could be administered without ritonavir boosting. In the presence of 100 mg of ritonavir, drug exposure (AUC) increased by only 60%. These clinical findings are inconsistent with PK studies in animal models where significant boosting of PK by RTV was observed. From the beginning, a novel PI with a favorable cross-resistance profile and a high genetic barrier was central to the discovery of the next generation of PIs at Ambrilia and its precursor companies. The identification of a novel lysine sulfonamide scaffold and subsequent lead optimization has proven to be a winning strategy to answer the challenges described above. Studies from co-crystallization and x-ray crystallography provide a structural basis for the unique and favorable resistance patterns offered by this novel PI.

REFERENCES

[1] Palella, F. J. Jr.; Delaney, K. M.; Moorman, A. C.; Loveless, M. O.; Fuhrer, J.; Satten, G. A.; Aschman, D. J.; Holmberg, S. D. Declining morbidity and mortality among patients with advanced human immunodeficiency virus infection. *N. Engl. J. Med.* **1998**, *338*, 853–860.

[2] Hogg, R. S.; Heath, K. V.; Yip, B.; Craib, K. J.; O'Shaughnessy, M. V.; Schechter, M. T.; Montaner, J. S. Improved survival among HIV-infected individuals following initiation of antiretroviral therapy. *JAMA* **1998**, *279*, 450–454.

[3] Vittinghoff, E.; Scheer, S.; O'Malley, P.; Colfax, G.; Holmberg, S. D.; Buchbinder, S. P. Combination antiretroviral therapy and recent declines in AIDS incidence and mortality. *J. Infect. Dis.* **1999**, *179*, 717–720.

[4] Colman, P. M. New antivirals and drug resistance. *Annu. Rev. Biochem.* **2009**, *78*, 95–118.

[5] Fernández-Montero, J. V.; Barreiro, P.; Soriano, V. HIV protease inhibitors: recent clinical trials and recommendations on use. *Expert Opin. Pharmacother.* **2009** Jul; *10*(10), 1615–1629.

[6] Quiros-Roldan, E.; Signorini, S.; Castelli, F.; Torti, C.; Patroni, A.; Airoldi, M.; Carosi, G. Analysis of HIV-1 mutation patterns in patients failing antiretroviral therapy. *J. Clin. Lab. Anal.* **2001**, *15*, 43–46.

[7] Rousseau, M. N.; Vergne, L.; Montes, B.; Peeters, M.; Reynes, J.; Delaporte, E.; Segondy, M. Patterns of resistance mutations to antiretroviral drugs in extensively treated HIV-1-infected patients with failure of highly active antiretroviral therapy. *J. Acquir. Immune Defic. Syndr.* **2001**, *26*, 36–43.

[8] Winters, M. A.; Baxter, J. D.; Mayers, D. L.; Wentworth, D. N.; Hoover, M. L.; Neaton, J. D.; Merigan, T. C. Frequency of antiretroviral drug resistance mutations in HIV-1 strains from patients failing triple drug regimens. *Antiviral Ther.* **2000**, *5*, 57–63.

[9] Lorenzi, P.; Opravil, M.; Hirschel, B.; Chave, J. P.; Furrer, H. J.; Sax, H.; Perneger, T. V.; Perrin, L.; Kaiser, L.; Yerly, S. Impact of drug resistance mutations on virologic response to salvage therapy. Swiss HIV Cohort Study. *AIDS* **1999**, *13*, F17–F21.

[10] Molla, A.; Korneyeva, M.; Gao, Q.; et al. Ordered accumulation of mutations in HIV protease confers resistance to ritonavir. *Nat. Med.* **1996**, *2*, 760–766.

[11] Condra, J. Virologic and clinical implications of resistance to HIV-1 protease inhibitors. *Drug Resist. Update* **1998**, *1*, 292–299.

[12] Deeks, S. Failure of HIV-1 protease inhibitors to fully suppress viral replication: implications for salvage therapy. *Adv. Exp. Med. Biol.* **1999**, *458*, 175–182.

[13] Yenni, P. G.; Hammer, S. M.; Hirsch, M. S.; et al. Treatment for adult HIV infection: 2004 recommendations of the International AIDS Society–USA Panel. *JAMA* **2004** Jul 14; *292*(2), 266–268.

[14] Stranix, B. R.; Sauvé, G.; Bouzide, A.; Côté, A.; Sévigny, G.; Yelle, J. *Bioorg. Med. Chem. Lett.* **2003**, *13*, 4289.

[15] Sévigny, G.; Stranix, B. R.; Tian, B.; Dubois, A.; Sauvé, G.; Petropoulos, C.; Lie, Y.; Hellmann, N.; Conway, B.; Yelle, J.*Antiviral Res.* **2006**, *70* (2), 17.

[16] Stranix, B. R.; Lavallée, J. F.; Sévigny, G.; Yelle, J.; Perron, P.; LeBerre, N.; Herbart, D.; Wu, J. J. *Bioorg. Med. Chem. Lett.* **2006**, *16*, 3459–3462.

[17] Stranix, B. R.; Dandache, S.; Milot, G.; Wu, J. J. Novel HIV protease inhibitors, containing a lysine backbone. Zing Drug Discovery Conference, 2007.

[18] Dandache, S.; Sévigny, G.; Yelle, Y.; Stranix, B. R.; Parkin, N.; Schapiro, J. M.; Wainberg, M. A.; Wu, J. J. In vitro antiviral activity and cross-resistance profile of PL-100, a novel protease inhibitor of human immunodeficiency virus type 1. *Antimicrob. Agents Chemother.*, **2007**, Nov; 4036–4043.

[19] Wu, J. J.; Sévigny, G.; Stranix, B. R.; et al. Pharmacological and cross-resistance profiling of PL-100 and its pro-drug, PPL-100. 6th Clinical Pharmacology Workshop, 2005.

[20] Wu, J. J.; Sévigny, G.; Stranix, B. R.; et al. PL-100 and its derivatives, a novel class of potent human immunodeficiency virus type 1 protease inhibitors: resistance profile and pharmacokinetics. 14th International HIV Drug Resistance Workshop, 2005.

[21] Wu, J. J.; Dandache, S.; Stranix, B. R.; Panchal, C.; Wainberg, M. A. The HIV-1 protease inhibitor PL-100 has a high genetic barrier and selects a novel pattern of mutations. 15th International HIV Drug Resistance Workshop, 2006.

[22] Dandache, S.; Daigneault, L.; Stranix, B. R.; Ge, M.; Wainberg, M. A.; Panchal, C.; Wu, J. J. PL-100, a novel protease inhibitor with a high genetic barrier. 16th International AIDS Conference, 2006.

[23] Wu, J. J.; Daigneault, L.; Stranix, B. R.; Ge, M.; Milot, G.; Dandache, S.; Wainberg, M. A.; Panchal, C. Preclinical and clinical evaluation of PPL-100, a next generation HIV protease inhibitor. HIV DART, 2006.

[24] Dandache, S.; Coburn, C.; Oliveira, M.; Allison, T. J.; Holloway, M. K.; Wu, J. J.; Stranix, B. R.; Panchal, C.; Wainberg, M. A.; Vacca, J. P. PL-100, a novel HIV-1 protease inhibitor displaying a high genetic barrier to resistance: an in vitro selection study. *J. Med. Virol.* **2008**, *80*, 2053–2063.

[25] Partaledis, J. A.; Yamaguchi, K.; Tisdale, M.; Blair, E. E.; Falcione, C.; Maschera, B.; Myers, R. E.; Pazhanisamy, S.; Futer, O.; Cullinan, A. B. In vitro selection and characterization of human immunodeficiency virus type 1 (HIV-1) isolates with reduced sensitivity to hydroxyethylamino sulfonamide inhibitors of HIV-1 aspartyl protease. *J. Virol.* **1995**, *69*, 5228–5235.

[26] Pazhanisamy, S.; Partaledis, J. A.; Rao, B. G.; Livingston, D. J. In vitro selection and characterization of VX-478 resistant HIV-1 variants. *Adv. Exp. Med. Biol.* **1998**, *436*, 75–83.

[27] Johnson, V. A.; Brun-Vezinet, F.; Clotet, B.; Gunthard, H. F.; Kuritzkes, D. R.; Pillay, D.; Schapiro, J. M.; Richman, D. D. Update of the drug resistance mutations in HIV-1: 2007. *Top. HIV Med.* **2007**, *15*, 119–125

[28] Vacca, J. P.; Holloway, M. K.; Allison, T. J.; Coburn, C. A.; Wu, J. J.; Wainberg, M. A. A structural basis for resistance to PL-100, 16th International HIV Drug Resistance Workshop, 2007.

[29] Madhavi, N. L.; Nalam, A. P.; Tim, H. M.; Jonckers, I. D.; Schiffer, C. A. Crystal structure of lysine sulfonamide inhibitor reveals the displacement of the conserved flap water molecule in human immunodeficiency virus type 1 protease. *J. Virol.* **2007**, *81*, 9512–9518.

[30] Wu, J. J.; Stranix, B. R.; Milhot, G.; Ge, M.; Dandache, S.; Forte, A.; Panchal, C. PL-100, a next generation protease inhibitor against drug-resistant HIV: in vitro and in vivo metabolism. *Interscience Conference on Antimicrobial Agents and Chemotherapy*, 2006.

3

DARUNAVIR (PREZISTA, TMC114): FROM BENCH TO CLINIC, IMPROVING TREATMENT OPTIONS FOR HIV-INFECTED PATIENTS

Marie-Pierre de Béthune

Tibotec BVBA, Beerse, Belgium

Vanitha Sekar

Tibotec, Inc., Titusville, New Jersey

Sabrina Spinosa-Guzman, Marc Vanstockem, and Sandra De Meyer

Tibotec BVBA, Beerse, Belgium

Piet Wigerinck

Galapagos NV, Mechelen, Belgium

Eric Lefebvre

Janssen-Cilag BV, Amsterdam, The Netherlands

INTRODUCTION

From the mid-1990s, new antiretroviral (ARV) drugs and classes and the use of highly active ARV therapy (HAART: at least three ARV agents from a minimum of two classes) have improved the long-term management of human immunodeficiency virus (HIV) infection [1]. However, by the early to mid-2000s, several limitations of HAART had become apparent. Such limitations meant that the treatment goal of achieving full virologic suppression was not possible in almost half of treatment-experienced patients at that time [2]. Instead, the most realistic treatment goals for these patients were the maintenance of viral load and immune status.

Adverse events (AEs) and relatively complex and frequent dosing regimens resulted in suboptimal adherence [3,4] and affected quality of life. In addition, poor adherence contributed to an increased prevalence of multidrug-resistant (MDR) virus. Furthermore, a decade of suboptimal ARV regimens, such as the use of mono/dual therapy and sequential monotherapy, resulted in incomplete viral suppression and persistent low-level viremia, ultimately leading to resistance development [5].

Multidrug resistance has probably been one of the greatest limitations to effective long-term HIV therapy [6]. ARV regimens had a low ability to prevent resistance development and therefore failed to preserve future treatment options [7,8]. Furthermore, despite excellent adherence, some patients failed ARV therapy due to inadequate drug levels as a result of variability in pharmacokinetics [9] or drug–drug interactions (DDIs) [10].

Darunavir (DRV; Prezista, TMC114), a protease inhibitor (PI) with a dual mode of action (inhibition of both HIV-1 protease catalytic activity and subunit dimerization), was developed to address some of these limitations. As a result of a unique profiling process involving a panel of MDR viruses, DRV was selected with very potent activity in drug-resistant

Antiviral Drugs: From Basic Discovery Through Clinical Trials, First Edition. Edited by Wieslaw M. Kazmierski.

virus, high binding properties, and a very slow dissociation rate. Moreover, DRV with low-dose ritonavir (RTV; Norvir, 100 mg; DRV/r) had favorable pharmacokinetic (PK) properties after oral administration and a potential for few DDIs with commonly used medications.

DRV was first tested in highly treatment-experienced patients, with excellent results. Trials in less treatment-experienced then treatment-naive patients quickly followed. In 2006, DRV was approved for use in treatment-experienced adult patients in the United States and then in February 2007 in the European Union (EU), and was licensed for treatment-naive adults with HIV-1 infection in 2008 in the United States [11] and in early 2009 in the EU. In this chapter we review the discovery, chemistry, and pharmacokinetics/pharmacodynamics (PD) of DRV and highlight its clinical development in HIV-infected patients.

DISCOVERY

Although HAART resulted in considerable efficacy benefits, such treatment had several shortcomings. Improvements were required in several areas, including safety, tolerability, and ease of administration. However, as outlined above, an additional unmet medical need was the availability of new drugs that were active against HIV strains resistant to treatment. Thus, DRV was designed and selected to improve on the aforementioned areas, with strong emphasis on high binding affinity to HIV protease and potent activity across a range of both wild-type and resistant HIV strains.

In the late 1990s, Tibotec embarked on a search for a new PI by evaluating the activity of various molecules structurally related to amprenavir (APV) [12,13]. DRV was identified in a unique research and development program [14]. Two steps in this process involved screening the activity of potential candidates against clinical HIV-1-resistant strains. The first screen assessed the antiviral activity of the synthesized compounds against a 19-strain panel of HIV strains. Eighteen of these were derived from patient samples and were therefore active, pathogenic forms of HIV with a variety of resistance mutations, representative of the diversity found in current clinical practice at that time. The second screen utilized Antivirogram (Virco) profiling with thousands of different clinical PI-resistant isolates.

Replacing the tetrahydrofuran (THF) group of APV with a fused bicyclic THF moiety, and the 4-aminobenzenesulfonamide group with a 4-methoxybenzenesulfonamide in the P2′ pocket resulted in TMC126. This compound had a high antiviral activity against wild-type HIV-1 [12,13], but was also active against a selected panel of five PI-resistant mutants. Indeed, this molecule exhibited a very potent broad-spectrum activity, which was higher than that of reference PIs [15]. However, TMC126 was not developed further, since preliminary PK studies in rats and dogs demonstrated low plasma drug levels [14,15].

Using TMC10, a racemate of TMC126 and one of the first PIs to be tested against a set of PI-resistant HIV strains [14], a chemical template was derived. More than 1000 analogs were generated and assessed in the profiling process described above.

To improve the PK profile of TMC126 while maintaining the high potency, a new series of closely related compounds was synthesized [15]. The compounds all shared the bis-THF moiety, which improved interaction with the P2′ pocket of the HIV-1 protease. The benzenesulfonamide substituent and/or the stereochemistry of the bis-THF group were modified. With regard to the P2′ phenyl group, introducing *p*-CN, *p*-CH_3, or *m*-NH_2 substituents had little effect on the antiviral activity against both wild-type and mutant viruses. However, *p*-nitro, *p*-acetyl, and *p*-iodo substituents increased activity against mutant viruses significantly, but not activity against the wild type. Increased activity against both types of virus was achieved when *p*-OCH_3 or 3,4-dioxolane groups were included. The best profile was achieved by the 4-NH_2 substituent (i.e., TMC114 = DRV). Single-oral-dose PK studies in rats and dogs showed rapid absorption of DRV, resulting in high blood levels [15].

A key factor in the selection of DRV was its high genetic barrier in vitro to the development of resistance [16]. Such results suggested that DRV showed potential resilience to the development of resistance in clinical practice, and therefore the potential to help preserve future treatment options for HIV-infected patients [17]. Further details of the in vitro characterization of DRV, which demonstrate the potent activity of this molecule, confirming its choice for further development, are summarized in the "Preclinical Development" section below.

SYNTHESIS

DRV, as DRV ethanolate, has the chemical name [(*1S*,*2R*)-[3]-[[([4]-aminophenyl)sulfonyl](2- methylpropyl)amino]-2-hydroxy-1-(phenylmethyl)propyl]carbamic acid (*3R*,*3aS*,*6aR*)-hexahydrofuro [2,3]-*b*]furan-3-yl ester monoethanolate. Its molecular formula is $C_{27}H_{37}N_3O_7S{\cdot}C_2H_5OH$ with a molecular weight of 593.83 Da. Scheme 1 depicts the structural formula. DRV is a white to off-white hygroscopic powder with slight water solubility (approximately 0.15 mg/mL at 20°C). Its solubility varies widely in organic solvents.

DRV is synthesized in a three-step process (Scheme 1) [18]. The starting material is optically active bis-THF. First, the alcohol group of bis-THF is converted to a mixed carbonate by reaction with *N*,*N*′-disuccinimidyl carbonate in the presence of triethylamine. Next, a sulfonamide scaffold is made by reacting a commercially available epoxide with isobutylamine in 2-propanol to provide

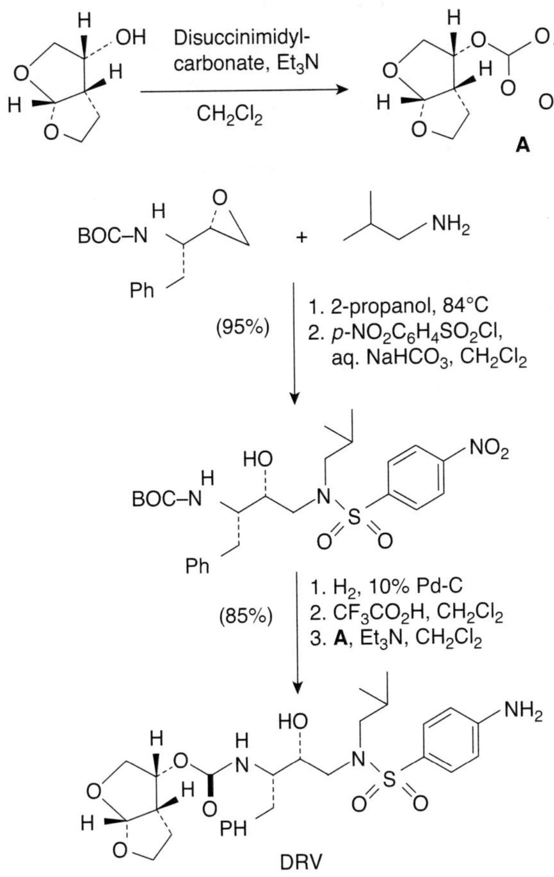

SCHEME 1 Synthetic method for the preparation of DRV. (From [18], copyright © 2009 American Chemical Society.)

the corresponding amino alcohol, which in the presence of *p*-nitrobenzenesulfonyl chloride and sodium bicarbonate produces the sulfonamide scaffold. In the final step, the *p*-nitro group is hydrogenated to the aromatic amine and the protective *tert*-butoxycarbonyl (Boc) group is removed, resulting in the formation of a diamine. When this diamine is exposed to the mixed carbonate in the presence of triethylamine, DRV is formed (Scheme 1) [18].

FORMULATION

For patient use, DRV presents as orange or white (depending on country) oval-shaped film-coated tablets. Currently, three strengths are available, containing DRV ethanolate equivalent to 300, 400, or 600 mg DRV for adult use. Inactive ingredients include microcrystalline cellulose, colloidal anhydrous silicon dioxide, crospovidone, and magnesium stearate. The film coating, Opadry Orange, contains FD&C Yellow No. 6, poly(ethylene glycol) 3350, poly(vinyl alcohol)-partially hydrolyzed talc, and titanium dioxide (E171). Two formulations are available as white caplet-shaped (75 mg) or oval-shaped (150 mg) film-coated (colored with Opadry White) tablets for pediatric use. The 75-, 150-, 400-, and 600-mg tablets are dose proportional and are compressed from a common powder blend.

For adults, the recommended DRV/r doses are 600/100 mg twice daily (b.i.d.; treatment-experienced) and 800/100 mg once daily (q.d.; treatment-naive). For children (6 to $<$ 18 years), DRV/r bid dosing is body weight based: $\geq$ 20 kg to $<$ 30 kg = 375/50 mg; $\geq$ 30 kg to $<$ 40 kg = 450/60 mg; $\geq$ 40 kg = 600/100 mg [11].

PRECLINICAL DEVELOPMENT

In Vitro Characterization of DRV

DRV inhibited the catalytic activity of isolated wild-type HIV-1 protease and of two drug-resistant mutant proteases [19]. For wild-type protease, the DRV binding affinity was >100-fold higher than that of the PIs: lopinavir (LPV), atazanavir (ATV), APV, and tipranavir (TPV) [20]. Binding to MDR proteases showed that all five PIs had lower binding affinities. However, although this lower affinity reduced antiviral activity in vitro for LPV, ATV, APV, and TPV, a 1000-fold reduction in DRV binding affinity did not translate into weaker antiviral activity [20].

High-resolution crystallography studies showed that DRV binds, via strong hydrogen bonds, with main-chain atoms of the HIV-1 protease [19], [21], [22]. DRV has an unusually close fit within the protease active site [23]. The high binding affinity and close fit may explain DRV's potent inhibitory activity against MDR proteases [23].

DRV also inhibits dimerization of the HIV-1 protease enzyme monomers, which is also seen with TPV but not with APV, ATV, indinavir (IDV), LPV, nelfinavir (NFV), RTV, or saquinavir (SQV) [24]. This dual mechanism may explain why DRV is a potent HIV-1 protease inhibitor compared with other PIs. Cell-based assays demonstrated the highly potent antiviral activity of DRV against wild-type and MDR viruses [16], [20], [21]. Median 50% effective concentration (EC_{50}) DRV values were 1 to 5 nM [16]. The DRV CC_{50} (50% cytotoxic concentration) was >100 μM. Thus, the DRV selectivity index (CC_{50}/EC_{50}) was > 20,000 for wild-type HIV, making it a potent and selective HIV inhibitor [16].

DRV also demonstrated equivalent antiviral activity against different HIV-1 subtypes [16], [25]. In 3309 recombinant PI-resistant clinical isolates, DRV was active against a greater proportion of the isolates than were any other PIs tested (Fig. 1) [26].

In vitro selection experiments with wild-type HIV-1 have shown that selecting DRV-resistant viruses is very difficult [16], [27]. Selection of resistant HIV-1 with APV, ATV, LPV, NFV, RTV, SQV, and TPV was more rapid and easier than with DRV, resulting in strains with clinically relevant PI

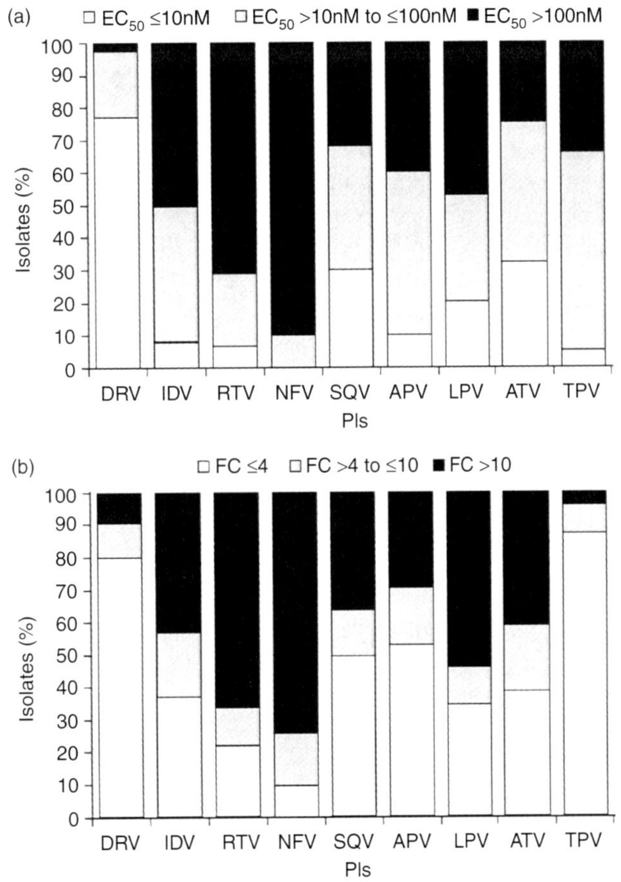

FIGURE 1 Antiviral activity of various PIs against a panel of 3309 recombinant clinical isolates of HIV-1 resistant to at least one PI: clustered by (a) EC_{50} values and (b) fold-change (FC) values. (From [26].)

resistance-associated mutations (RAMs). In contrast, mutations eventually emerging in DRV-exposed strains were not associated with decreased DRV susceptibility [27]. Furthermore, the pathway to DRV resistance in wild-type HIV-1 is different than for other PIs.

Preclinical Toxicology Studies

DRV was evaluated in routine preclinical toxicity studies [11]. DRV was not mutagenic or genotoxic in in vitro and in vivo assays. Two-year oral gavage studies in rats and mice showed an increase in liver and thyroid (male rats only) tumors; such findings in rodents have limited relevance to humans. Repeated DRV administration to rats induced hepatic microsomal enzyme activity and increased thyroid hormone elimination, a mechanism predisposing rats, but not humans, to thyroid neoplasms. DRV did not affect fertility or early embryonic development in rats. DRV has also shown no teratogenic potential in mice (with or without RTV), rats, and rabbits.

Pharmacokinetic Properties

Preclinically, DRV was shown to have favorable PK properties. DRV exhibits high protein binding, being 95% bound to plasma proteins, primarily α_1-acid glycoprotein [28]. The primary metabolic route for DRV is oxidative metabolism mainly by cytochrome P450 (CYP450) enzymes [29]. At least three oxidative metabolites with some anti-HIV activity have been identified in humans, although they are at least 10-fold less active than DRV against wild-type virus [11].

CLINICAL DEVELOPMENT

Clinical Pharmacology Studies

DRV is metabolized by and inhibits CYP3A; thus, as with other PIs, increased DRV concentrations could be achieved by coadministration with a potent CYP3A inhibitor. In a phase I four-way crossover study, HIV-negative healthy male volunteers ($n = 8$) received DRV (one 600-mg dose orally) $\pm$ RTV (100 mg b.i.d.) [30]. The absolute bioavailability of DRV alone was 37%, whereas with RTV (DRV/r), it was 82%. The area under the plasma concentration–time curve (AUC_{last}) for DRV was 14-fold higher following coadministration with RTV vs. administration alone. Systemic exposure to DRV was not increased with higher doses of RTV (200 mg b.i.d.) [29]. As this early study showed that the exposure to DRV was increased by coadministering low-dose RTV as a PK enhancer, the majority of clinical studies have involved the coadministration of DRV and RTV. As fasting decreased plasma levels [31], DRV should also be taken with food [11]. Studies in patients with mild or moderate hepatic impairment had shown that no dose adjustment of DRV is considered necessary for these populations and that routine clinical monitoring is recommended [11], [28]. Dose modification of DRV/r is also not required in patients with renal impairment [11].

An extensive DRV/r drug–drug interactions (DDI) program in > 650 HIV-negative healthy volunteers and HIV-infected patients has been conducted. Consequently, guidance is available on coadministrating DRV/r with many commonly used ARV or non-ARV medications (Table 1) [11], [28]. Generally, the DDI profile of DRV/r is well characterized and manageable. No dose adjustment for DRV/r is recommended for any coadministration.

Phase IIa Proof-of-Concept Study

One proof-of-concept study, TMC114-C207, was a randomized open-label controlled trial in 50 highly treatment-experienced patients infected with MDR HIV-1 [32]. Patients substituted their failing PI for DRV/r at 300/100 mg b.i.d., 900/100 mg q.d. or 600/100 mg b.i.d., or continued

TABLE 1 Summary of Key DRV–Drug Interaction Data*

Drug Class	Guidance re Coadministration with DRV/r: No Dose Adjustment of DRV/r or Coadministered Drug	Guidance re Coadministration with DRV/r: Modify and/or Monitor Dose or Schedule of Coadministered Drug	Guidance re Coadministration with DRV/r: Coadministration Not Recommended
PIs	ATV	IDV[a]	LPV SQV
NRTIs	Tenofovir Didanosine		
NNRTIs	Efavirenz ETR NVP		
Fusion inhibitor	Enfuvirtide		
Integrase inhibitor	Elvitegravir		
CCR5-entry inhibitor	—	MRV[b]	
HMG-CoA reductase inhibitors	—	Atorvastatin[c] Pravastatin[c] Rosuvastatin[c]	
Gastric pH modifiers	Omeprazole Ranitidine		
Narcotic analgesics	Methadone		
Oral contraceptives	—	Ethinyl oestradiol[d] Norethindrone[d]	
PDE-5 inhibitors	—	Sildenafil[e] Vardenafil[e] Tadalafil[e]	
Selective serotonin reuptake inhibitors	—	Paroxetine[f] Sertraline[f]	
Anticonvulsants	—	CBZ[g] Phenobarbital[h] Phenytoin[h]	
Anti-infectives	Clarithromycin[i]	Rfb[j] Ketoconazole[k]	Rifampicin
Cardiac glycosides		Digoxin[c]	

Source: [11,28].
NRTI, nucleoside reverse transcriptase inhibitor; NNRTI, nonnucleoside reverse transcriptase inhibitor; PED-5, phosphodiesterase type 5; ETR, etravirine (Intelence); MRV, maraviroc; CBZ, carbamazepine; Rfb, rifabutin.
[a]In case of intolerance, reduce dose of IDV from 800 mg to 200 mg b.i.d.
[b]Reduce MRV by 50%.
[c]Start at lowest dose and titrate to clinical response.
[d]Plasma levels are reduced; additional/alternative contraception recommended.
[e]Dose adjustment recommended; refer to Prezista PI (2009).
[f]Levels are decreased, so monitor and titrate to clinical effect.
[g]CBZ dose may need to be reduced by 25 to 50%; titrate dose and monitor toxicity.
[h]Monitor levels, as they may be decreased.
[i]May need to reduce dose in patients with renal impairment.
[j]Dose-reduce Rfb by at least 75% and monitor toxicity.
[k]Maximum dose recommended of 200 mg recommended.

with their preentry PI treatment (control). At day 14, 46, 31, and 42% for the DRV/r groups, respectively, vs. 8% (control) of patients had plasma HIV-1 RNA < 400 copies/mL. The AEs with DRV/r were mainly mild to moderate, with no dose–response relationship [32]. These results provided the basis for dose selection and regimens in the phase IIb program.

Phase IIb Development

POWER 1 and 2 Trials DRV/r was first evaluated in highly treatment-experienced patients with MDR HIV. This population represented a high unmet medical need, as these patients are the hardest to treat successfully, due to cross-resistance and the dwindling number of treatment options.

TABLE 2 Baseline Characteristics of Patients in the POWER 1, 2, and 3 and TITAN Trials

	POWER Trials			TITAN Trial	
Parameter	CPIs[a] POWER 1 and 2 ($n = 124$)*	DRV/r 600/100 mg b.i.d. POWER 1 and 2 ($n = 131$)	DRV/r 600/100 mg b.i.d. POWER 3 ($n = 336$)	DRV/r 600/100 mg b.i.d. ($n = 298$)	LPV/r 400/100 mg b.i.d. ($n = 297$)
Demographics					
Male, *n* (%)	109 (88)	117 (89)	292 (87)	229 (77)	241 (81)
Mean age, years (S.D.)[b]	44.4 (7.05)	43.9 (8.57)	43 (20–70)[c]	40.9 (9.0)	40.8 (8.6)
Caucasian, *n* (%)	90 (73)	106 (81)	249 (75)	161 (54)	168 (57)
Baseline disease characteristics					
Mean HIV infection duration, years (S.D.)	12.9 (4.68)	12.0 (4.43)	13 (4.2)	9.1 (5.5)	9.1 (5.8)
Mean HIV-1 RNA, $\log_{10}$ copies/mL (S.D.)	4.49 (0.78)	4.61 (0.69)	4.58 (0.8)	4.33 (0.79)	4.28 (0.81)
Median CD4 cell count, cells/mm^3 (range)	163 (3–1274)	153 (3–776)	120 (0–831)	235 (3–831)	230 (2–1096)
CDC[d] category C, *n* (%)	53 (43)	47 (36)	185 (55)	101 (34)	94 (32)
Previous treatment experience					
Median duration previous NRTIs, months (range)	98 (6–219)	92 (5–238)	100 (2–219)	61 (3–226)	62 (1–250)
Median duration previous NNRTIs, months (range)	17 (0–67)	21 (2–164)	23 (1–133)	29 (0–222)	27 (0–115)
Median duration previous PIs, months (range)	73 (5–107)	63 (5–150)	75 (1–151)	41 (0–119)	41 (0–202)
Baseline genotype and phenotype, median (range)					
Median number of primary PI mutations	3.0 (0–8)	3.0 (0–7)	4.0 (0-8)	0 (0–6)	0 (0–6)
Median DRV FC[e] (range)	3.3 (0.2–362.9)	4.3 (0.2–503.2)	N.D.[f]	0.6 (0.1–37.4)	0.6 (0.1–43.8)
Median LPV FC (range)	82.7 (0.4–130.5)	83.9 (0.8–125.4)	N.D.	0.7 (0.4–74.4)	0.8 (0.3–74.5)

Source: [33,34,36,38], copyright © 2006, with permission from Wolters Kluwer Health and Elsevier.
[a]CPI(s) baseline data derived from POWER 1 and 2.
[b]S.D., standard deviation.
[c]Median age, years (range) in POWER 3.
[d]CDC, Centers for Disease Control and Prevention.
[e]FC, fold change in EC_{50}.
[f]N.D., not determined.

POWER 1 (TMC114-C213) and 2 (TMC114-C202) (performance of TMC114/r when evaluated in treatment-experienced patients with PI resistance) were international multicenter randomized controlled open-label 144-week phase IIb trials. The efficacy and safety of DRV/r (400/100 mg q.d., 800/100 mg q.d., 400/100 mg b.i.d., and 600/100 mg b.i.d.) were compared with investigator-selected control PIs (CPI). All patients received an optimized background regimen (OBR) [33,34].

In both trials, a dose–response relationship was observed for the primary endpoint (viral load reduction $\geq$ 1.0 $\log_{10}$ HIV-1 RNA copies/mL) at week 24. All values (range: 45 to 77%) were significantly higher than in the CPI arm (25% and 14%, POWER 1 and 2, respectively). A similar trend was noted for HIV-1 RNA < 50 copies/mL. The mean increase in CD4 cell count was also dose-related. DRV/r 600/100 mg b.i.d provided the greatest virologic suppression and immunologic improvement. Thus, from week 24 all patients on DRV/r received 600/100 mg b.i.d. [35]. Pooled data analyses included only patients on 600/100 mg b.i.d. from baseline (de novo patients, $n = 131$).

Baseline characteristics were well balanced between the CPI and de novo groups (Table 2). At week 24, 53% (vs. 18%; $p < 0.001$) and 39% (vs. 7%; $p < 0.001$) of patients in POWER 1 and 2, respectively, reached HIV-1 RNA < 50 copies/mL, (DRV/r vs. CPI, respectively) [33,34]. Week 24 pooled analyses showed that the virological response was 45% (DRV/r) and 12% (CPIs; $p < 0.0001$). At week 48, the responses were 45% and 10%, respectively ($p < 0.0001$) (Fig. 2a) [35]. The incidence of AEs was comparable between the DRV/r and CPI arms [33–35]. The most common AEs were very similar in nature to those reported for the TITAN (TMC114/r in treatment-experienced patients naive to lopinavir) trial, which is described later in the chapter.

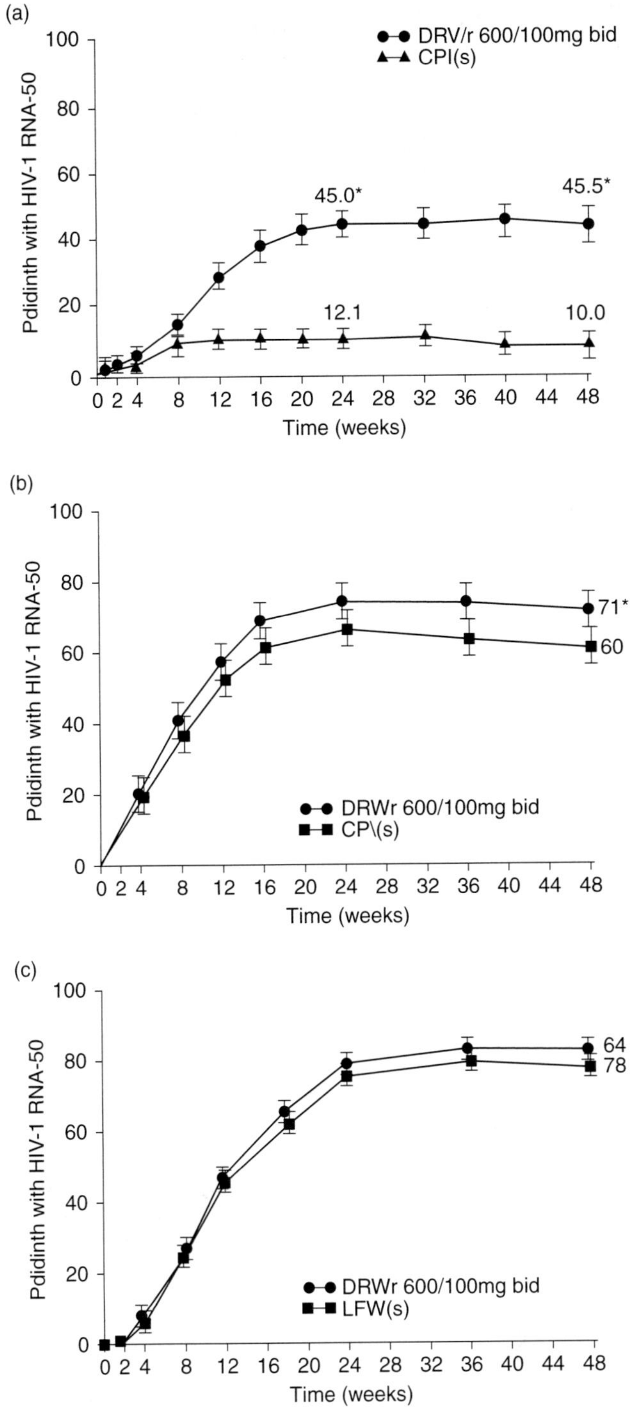

FIGURE 2 Virological response (< 50 copies/mL) to DRV/r from baseline to week 48 in (a) POWER 1 and 2 (pooled data) (from [35], copyright © 2007, with permission from Elsevier), (b) TITAN (from [36], copyright © 2007, with permission from Elsevier), and (c) ARTEMIS (from [37], copyright © 2008, with permission from Wolters Kluwer Health).

Phase IIb Program Revisions Antiviral activity of 600/100 mg b.i.d. DRV/r vs. CPIs and with other ARVs showed a large and robust effect at weeks 16 and 24 in both POWER trials. Discussions with U.S. (Food and Drug Administration) and EU (European Medicines Agency) regulators led to revision of the development program, enabling an application for early conditional approval of DRV/r based on phase IIb data. Further safety data were required to meet the International Conference on Harmonization of Technical Requirements for Registration of Pharmaceuticals for Human Use.

Expansion of Patient Population (POWER 3) Failing control patients from POWER 1 and 2 continued in a rollover trial (TMC114-C215), and this trial also recruited new patients. A second open-label nonrandomized phase IIb rollover trial (TMC114-C208) was also conducted. The combined analysis of these trials, POWER 3 (TMC114-C215 and TMC114-C208), provided additional safety and efficacy data on DRV/r 600/100 mg b.i.d. to support accelerated regulatory approval.

Over 200 patients were rapidly recruited (within one month) into TMC114-C215. Baseline characteristics for the three POWER trials were similar (Table 2). Comparable efficacy endpoints were also achieved with DRV/r 600/100 mg b.i.d. in POWER 3: at week 24, 65% had a reduction ≥ 1.0 $\log_{10}$ HIV-1 RNA copies/mL and 40% achieved < 50 HIV-1 RNA copies/mL. CD4 cell counts increased by a mean of 80 cells/mm^3 [38]. The AE profile of DRV/r 600/100 mg b.i.d. was similar across the POWER trials at week 24. Longer-term follow-up at weeks 96 [39] and 144 [40,41] have since confirmed the durability of efficacy and the tolerability findings from the earlier time points.

Accelerated Approval of DRV DRV/r was first licensed in the United States in June 2006 following priority review, and in the EU in February 2007 for the treatment of HIV-1 in ARV-experienced adult patients. This license was based on the impressive phase IIb 24-week results of POWER 1 and 2, supported by safety data from POWER 3. This data set has resulted in over 80 regulatory approvals to date, including Japan and China, Brazil, Mexico, and Argentina. The approval of a drug based on phase IIb data is rare and demonstrates that DRV answered an urgent unmet medical need.

Confirmation of POWER Data Results from the DUET trials confirmed the POWER efficacy data. These randomized placebo-controlled phase III trials evaluated the efficacy and safety of ETR vs. placebo in highly treatment-experienced patients, a population similar to that employed in the POWER trials. Both arms received a background regimen (BR) including DRV/r (600/100 mg b.i.d.). In the pooled DUET 24-week analysis, 41% of patients in the placebo/BR arm achieved a viral load < 50 HIV-1 RNA copies/mL [42]. Further details on DUET are included in Chapter 6 [43].

Resistance Profile of DRV The DRV resistance profile was determined initially from the pooled 24-week POWER 1 and 2 data. Eleven DRV RAMs were identified: V11I, V32I, L33F, I47V, I50V, I54L/M, G73S, L76V, I84V, and L89V [44]. These DRV RAMs were more likely to occur when a high number of PI RAMs [generally, ≥ [10]: International AIDS Society–USA (IAS-USA)] were present at baseline. Five DRV RAMs were associated with virological failure (VF; V32I, L33F, I47V, I54L, and L89V). However, ≥ 3 DRV RAMs, together with a high number of background mutations, are required for DRV resistance [44]. Updated analysis of the POWER data pooled with the placebo group of the DUET data confirmed the list of DRV RAMs, with one exception: G73S was replaced by T74P. The prevalence of DRV RAMs in routine clinical practice is low (e.g. in > 98,000 isolates with reduced PI susceptibility, 74% had no DRV RAMs) [45].

Redefining Treatment Goals Excellent results with DRV/r in highly treatment-experienced, HIV-1-infected patients, RESIST (randomized evaluation of strategic intervention in multidrug resistant patients with tipranavir) results with TPV/r [46], and new active ARVs developed in this population (ETR, RAL, MRV) played a pivotal role in major international treatment guidelines revisions [47]. Although the original therapeutic goal for treatment-experienced patients was viral load reduction, potent ARVs such as DRV/r showed that HIV-1 RNA < 50 copies/mL is now a realistic treatment goal [48,49].

Phase III Trials

The favorable efficacy and safety profiles of DRV/r described above led to DRV/r evaluation in the wider population of less treatment-experienced and treatment-naive HIV-infected patients. These two phase III trials were under way during the accelerated approval process for DRV/r.

Treatment-Experienced Patients

TITAN Study Design Treatment-experienced patients in TITAN were representative of patients commonly encountered in the clinical setting. TITAN is an international multicenter randomized controlled open-label 96-week phase III trial, which enrolled treatment-experienced but LPV-naive patients [36]. The dosing regimens (DRV/r 600/100 mg b.i.d. vs. LPV/r 400/100 mg b.i.d.) were selected to obtain long-term data for DRV/r vs. a standard-of-care comparator (LPV/r). The primary objective was to demonstrate noninferiority of DRV/r for < 400 HIV-1 RNA copies/mL at week 48. Secondary efficacy objectives included a superiority test in the event of noninferiority and the proportion of patients with plasma < 50 HIV-1 RNA copies/mL.

Efficacy in TITAN The baseline characteristics were well balanced and showed that the population in TITAN was clearly less treatment experienced and PI resistant than in the POWER studies (Table 2). At week 48, significantly more patients treated with DRV/r than those on LPV/r achieved < 400 HIV-1 RNA copies/mL [77% vs. [68]%; difference [9]%, 95% confidence interval (CI) [2 to 16], establishing noninferiority of DRV/r. The superiority of DRV/r over LPV/r (77% vs. 67%; difference 10%, 95% CI 2 to 17; $p = 0.008$) was confirmed. For HIV-1 RNA < 50 copies/mL, significantly more DRV/r patients achieved this endpoint than LPV/r patients (71% vs. 60%; difference 11%, 95% CI 3 to 19; $p = 0.005$; Fig. 2b) [36]. The superiority of DRV/r over LPV/r persisted at week 96 for viral load < 400 HIV-1 RNA copies/mL (66.8% vs. 58.9%, difference 7.9%, 95% CI 0.1 to 5.6; noninferiority $p < 0.001$; superiority $p = 0.034$). Week 48 response rates (HIV-1 RNA < 50 copies/mL) were consistently higher for DRV/r than for LPV/r, irrespective of baseline subgroup [36]. The virologic efficacy of DRV/r was also supported by the increase in median CD4 cell count from baseline to week 48 (88 cells/mm^3 vs. 81 cells/mm^3; DRV/r vs. LPV/r, respectively) [36]. Similar immunological benefits at week 96 were also seen (DRV/r 81; LPV/r 93 cells/mm^3, increase from baseline) [50].

Resistance Profile of DRV/r in TITAN In the 48-week analysis, fewer patients had VF (HIV-1 RNA ≥ 400 copies/mL) on DRV/r (10%) than on LPV/r (22%; $p < 0.001$) [36]. Fewer VF patients developed primary PI mutations and NRTI mutations on DRV/r than on LPV/r [51].

Susceptibility analysis (Antivirogram data) showed that more DRV/r patients with VF retained susceptibility to other PIs than LPV/r patients after failure compared to baseline [51]. TITAN also showed that DRV/r protects the background regimen (BR) better than does LPV/r. After failure, 32% (LPV/r) and 14% (DRV/r) of VF patients harbored virus that was susceptible to fewer NRTIs than at baseline [51]. TITAN 96-week findings are consistent with the 48-week analyses [52].

Safety Analysis in TITAN Safety data were generally similar between groups in TITAN at week 48 (Table 3); the majority of AEs were grade 1 or 2 [36]. The incidence of treatment-related diarrhea ≥ grade 2 was lower with DRV/r than with LPV/r (8% vs. 15%, $p = 0.007$). Discontinuations due to GI-related events (DRV/r, $n = 2$; LPV/r, $n = 5$) and lipid-related events (DRV/r, $n = 0$; LPV/r, $n = 6$) were less frequent for DRV/r than for LPV/r at week 48 [36]. Median changes in triglycerides and total cholesterol from baseline to week 48 were less pronounced in DRV/r than in LPV/r patients (Fig. 3a). By week 96, the AE profile for both drug regimens was similar to that noted at week 48 [50].

TABLE 3 TITAN: Summary of Safety Results in the Week 48 Analysis

	DRV/r ($n = 343$)	LPV/r ($n = 346$)
Mean treatment exposure (weeks)	53.5	51.5
AEs, *n* (%)		
≥1 AE	277 (93)	273 (92)
≥1 serious AE	28 (9)	31 (10)
≥1 grade 3 or 4 AE	80 (27)	89 (30)
≥1 AE leading to permanent discontinuation	20 (7)	21 (7)
Grade 2–4 AEs at least possibly related to study treatment (incidence ≥ 2%)	110 (37)	121 (41)
Diarrhea	23 (8)	43 (15)
Nausea	12 (4)	11 (3)
Rash	12 (4)	10 (3)
Grade 2–4 laboratory abnormalities (incidence ≥ 2%)		
ALT increased	26 (9)	26 (9)
AST increased	20 (7)	26 (9)
Triglycerides increased	57 (19)	75 (25)
Total cholesterol increased	94 (32)	86 (29)
LDL increased	56 (19)	50 (17)
Hyperglycemia	26 (9)	28 (9)
Pancreatic amylase increased	33 (11)	26 (9)
Pancreatic lipase increased	14 (5)	11 (4)
Platelet count decreased	4 (1)	7 (2)
Neutrophil count decreased	9 (3)	17 (6)

Source: [36], copyright © 2007, with permission from Elsevier.

Treatment-Naive Patients

Once-Daily Dosing in Treatment-Naive Patients The feasibility of once-daily DRV/r (800/100 mg) dosing was demonstrated in the 24-week dose–response phase of POWER 1 and 2 [33,34]. Consequently, ARTEMIS (antiretroviral therapy with TMC114 examined in naive subjects) was conducted to evaluate efficacy and safety of once-daily DRV/r vs. LPV/r in treatment-naive patents.

ARTEMIS Study Design ARTEMIS is an ongoing international randomized controlled open-label 192-week phase III trial. The primary objective was to demonstrate the noninferiority of DRV/r (800/100 mg q.d.) to LPV/r (800/200 mg total daily dose) in the primary endpoint of viral load < 50 HIV-1 RNA copies/mL at week 48 [37]. Secondary objectives included testing for superiority in the event that noninferiority was shown, durability of response, immunological response, resistance characteristics, adherence, quality of life, safety, and tolerability. A significant proportion of women and non-Caucasians were enrolled in this trial.

Efficacy in ARTEMIS Baseline demographics and disease characteristics were well balanced [37]. In the primary efficacy analysis, DRV/r was noninferior to LPV/r, as 84 and 78% of patients, respectively, achieved confirmed HIV-1 RNA < 50 copies/mL at 48 weeks (Fig. 2c; estimated difference 5.6%, 95% CI –0.1 to 11). The estimated difference in response for superiority of DRV/r over LPV/r was 5.5% (95% CI –0.3 to 11; $p = 0.062$) [37]. At week 96, DRV/r also demonstrated noninferiority ($p < 0.001$) and superiority ($p = 0.012$) to LPV/r with 79% (DRV/r) vs. 71% (LPV/r) patients achieving undetectable viral load [53]. In the non-VF censored population (censoring patients who discontinued for reasons other than VF), the efficacy of DRV/r (82%) was also superior to that of LPV/r (74%) ($p = 0.016$), indicating that the difference in response at week 96 was not driven by discontinuations due to AEs [54].

In addition to a strong virologic response to DRV/r, the median CD4 cell count was increased from baseline to week 48 in both treatment arms (DRV/r: 137 cells/mm^3; LPV/r 141 cells/mm^3) [37]. At week 96, the immunological response was also comparable for both treatment groups [53].

Resistance Profile of DRV/r in ARTEMIS VF (HIV-1 RNA ≥ 50 copies/mL) occurred in 10% of ARV-naive patients receiving DRV/r and 14% on LPV/r in the 48-week analysis [37]. In the 10 DRV/r patients with VF (for whom genotypic data were available), no new IAS-USA PI RAMs had developed. The VF rate was lower in DRV/r patients (12%) vs. LPV/r (17.1%) patients in the 96-week analysis [55]. Furthermore, at this time point, 31 of 40 DRV/r patients with VF had genotypic information available, and none developed primary PI mutations at failure [55].

Safety Analysis in ARTEMIS The overall tolerability profile of once-daily DRV/r (800/100 mg) in treatment-naive patients was generally similar to that reported in POWER and TITAN in treatment-experienced patients (600/100 mg b.i.d.), with the exception of lipid abnormalities that were less commonly observed with the once-daily dose [37], [53]. A more favorable safety profile was associated with DRV/r than with LPV/r. Most AEs were grade 1 or 2 [37].

Key PI-associated AEs are liver-, gastrointestinal (GI)-, and lipid-related [56]. In ARTEMIS, liver abnormalities were comparable between the two groups, with similar incidences of grades 2 to 4 of ALT and AST elevations at weeks 48 and 96. For GI- and lipid-related AEs, both types occurred less frequently in DRV/r patients than in LPV/r patients at 48 weeks [37] and 96 weeks [53]. The incidence of treatment-related, grades 2 to 4 diarrhea in DRV/r patients was less than half that for LPV/r at both week 48 (4% vs. 10%, respectively; $p < 0.01$ [37]) and week 96 (4% vs. 11%, respectively; $p < 0.001$ [53]).

DRV/r treatment resulted in significantly fewer ≥ grade 2 triglyceride (3% vs. 11%; $p < 0.0001$) and total cholesterol (13% vs. 23%; $p < 0.01$) elevations reported as AEs at week 48. Similar findings were recorded at week 96 (4% vs. 13%, $p < 0.0001$; 18% vs. 28%, $p = 0.0016$, respectively) [53]. Median lipid levels at baseline and week 48 are shown in

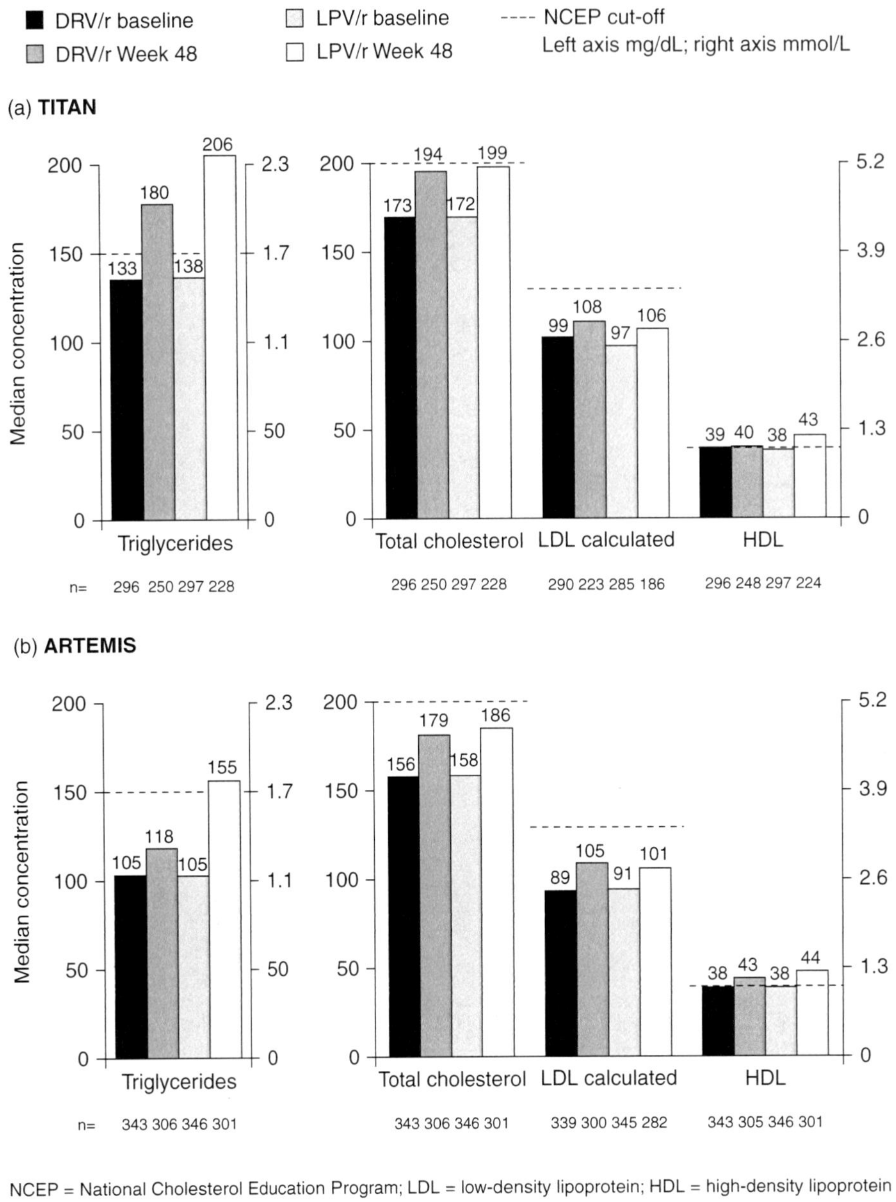

FIGURE 3 Median lipid levels in (a) treatment-experienced and (b) treatment-naive HIV-1-infected patients at baseline and week 48.

Figure 3b. The small increases with time in low- and high-density lipoprotein were similar for both treatment groups. In contrast, the increases in triglycerides and total cholesterol were more pronounced with LPV/r than with DRV/r (Fig. 3b). Indeed, with DRV/r triglycerides, total cholesterol and LDL all remained below the NCEP abnormality cutoffs throughout 48 weeks (Fig. 3b). DRV/r (800/100 mg q.d.) also appears to have a similar lipid profile to ATV/r (300/100 mg q.d.) in healthy volunteers [57].

PK/PD Findings for DRV/r in TITAN and ARTEMIS Trials The in vitro protein binding–corrected EC_{50} value for antiviral activity is 55 and 550 ng/mL for the wild-type and PI-resistant virus, respectively. PK analyses of clinical samples up to week 48 showed that the trough plasma concentrations of DRV remained well above these levels following both 600/100 mg b.i.d. (treatment-experienced patients: TITAN [58] and 800/100 mg q.d. (treatment-naive patients: ARTEMIS [59]) dosing regimens. Thus, these dosing regimens achieve the required drug exposure.

No apparent relationships were observed between DRV/r exposure and efficacy or safety in either TITAN [58] or ARTEMIS [59]. For both trials, there were no clinically relevant differences in exposure to DRV by race, gender, or body weight [60,61]. Furthermore, as the interpatient variation in exposure is low (approximately 30%), predictable

DRV exposure is achieved following administration of both b.i.d. and q.d. dosing regimens. Collectively, these findings indicate that DRV/r in 600/100 mg b.i.d. or 800/100 mg q.d. regimens provide predictable and adequate DRV exposure in those patients likely to benefit from its antiviral activity.

Approval of DRV/r in Less Treatment-Experienced and Treatment-Naive Patients The positive 48-week results from both TITAN and ARTEMIS led to the approval of DRV/r in less treatment-experienced and treatment-naive patients in the United States [11] and Europe (2009). Furthermore, DRV/r has been listed as a preferred PI regimen for treatment-naive patients in the recently revised U.S. Department of Health and Human Services treatment guidelines for HIV infection in adults [48].

Evaluation of DRV/r in Children and Adolescents (DELPHI)

DELPHI (darunavir evaluation in pediatric HIV-1-infected treatment-experienced patients; TMC114-212) is an international multicenter open-label two-part 48-week phase II study in children and adolescents 6 to 18 years of age. In part I (dose selection), randomized patients received either the adult-equivalent dose of DRV/r 600/100 mg b.i.d. (n = 22) or a 20 to 33% higher dose of DRV (n = 22) and an OBR of at least two ARVs [62].

After 2 weeks, DRV/r doses were selected by weight (three bands) based on PK, safety, and change in viral load. In part II (n = 80), all part I patients switched to the selected dose and additional patients were enrolled. Pediatric patients in DELPHI had a treatment experience similar to that of adults in the POWER trials. At week 2, target adult DRV exposure was achieved across the age groups and weight bands, confirming appropriate dose selection in children: $\geq$ 20 to < 30 kg, 375/50 mg b.i.d.; $\geq$ 30 to < 40 kg, 450/60 mg b.i.d.; $\geq$ 40 to < 50 kg, 600/100 mg b.i.d. [62].

At week 24, 64 and 50% of patients achieved a HIV-1 RNA viral load of < 400 and < 50 copies/mL, respectively [63]. Fifty-nine and 48% of patients had HIV-1 RNA < 400 and < 50 copies/mL, respectively, at week 48 [62]. At weeks 24 and 48, the mean absolute CD4 cell count increases from baseline were 117 and 147 cells/mm^3, respectively. Overall, DRV/r was generally well tolerated, and the frequency, type, and severity of the AEs were comparable to those observed in adults [62,63]. Based on these findings, DRV/r was licensed for pediatric use in the United States in December 2008 [11].

FUTURE DIRECTIONS

Studies in Other Populations

The extensive DRV clinical development continues to focus on addressing unmet needs for treating HIV infection. Certain HIV-1-infected patient populations can be underrepresented in registrational clinical trials, especially trials in treatment-experienced patients (e.g., women and non-Caucasians). These populations were well represented in ARTEMIS [37]. The phase IIIb trial, GRACE (gender, race, and clinical experience; NCT00381303) was designed to assess gender and racial differences in the efficacy and safety for DRV/r in treatment-experienced patients. Indeed, 67% of patients were women, 87% of whom were people of color. At week 24 the virologic response rate (HIV-1 RNA < 50 copies/mL) was 51% (intent-to-treat/time-to-loss of virologic response) [64].

Further investigations are under way to evaluate a DRV oral suspension in children from 3 years of age (TMC114-C228; ARIEL, darunavir in treatment-experienced pediatric population), and once daily dosing in treatment-naive adolescents (TMC114-C230; DIONE, darunavir once-daily in treatment-naive adolescents) to help simplify drug administration in this vulnerable population.

HIV is a worldwide disease with significant issues still to be overcome. Trials with DRV/r are being planned in many countries, including those with poorer resource settings (e.g., Africa). Furthermore, collaborations with academia and HIV support groups are important in leading the way to further improvement in HIV treatments.

Once-Daily Dosing

Once-daily dosing has several potential benefits: lower pill count, improved convenience, and a lower daily dose of RTV. ODIN (TMC114-C229; once-daily DRV in treatment-experienced patients), an ongoing phase IIIb trial, is evaluating DRV/r 800/100 mg q.d. vs. 600/100 mg b.i.d. in treatment-experienced patients with no DRV RAMs. The POWER 1 and 2 trials dose–response phase indicated similar results with these dosing regimens in treatment-experienced patients [33,34], particularly in those with no baseline DRV RAMs [65]. Furthermore, the majority of general PI-experienced population in clinical practice have no DRV RAMs [45]. The 48-week results are expected in early 2010.

Refining Treatment Strategies

Significant progress in keeping HIV infection at bay has been made by developing new drugs and by refining treatment strategies. Thus, several ongoing trials are exploring DRV/r in novel treatment paradigms. For example, simplification of treatment (to potentially reduce toxicity and therapy complexity) with DRV/r monotherapy is being explored in maintenance monotherapy trials. MONET (TMC114HIV3006; NCT00458302; maintenance monotherapy in treatment-experienced patients with virological suppression) is currently exploring the effects of DRV/r 800/100 mg q.d. monotherapy vs. a DRV/r-based triple combination therapy in patients with undetectable HIV-1 RNA in their current treatments. Similarly, in MONOI (NCT00421551) patients are switched from stable therapy to either DRV/r monotherapy or a regimen of two NRTIs with DRV/r 600/100 mg b.i.d. Encouraging and comparable results from these two ongoing studies support the further evaluation of DRV/r monotherapy in patients with controlled virologic suppression (HIV-1 RNA < 50 copies/mL) [66,67].

Combining DRV/r with novel therapies, including integrase inhibitors, is also being explored with very encouraging results. As mentioned, DRV/r was being investigated in combination with ETR in the DUET trials [68,69]. Additionally, DRV/r and ETR combined with raltegravir are under investigation in the TRIO (NCT00460382) trial; 86% of patients had HIV-1 RNA levels < 50 copies/mL at week 48 [70].

CONCLUSIONS

DRV/r has demonstrated excellent efficacy and safety in HIV-1 infection across the treatment spectrum, from ARV-naive to highly treatment-experienced adults and in treatment-experienced HIV-1-infected pediatric patients. DRV/r compared favorably in treatment-naive and in less advanced treatment-experienced patients to what was referred to as the "gold-standard," LPV/r, which led to its approval for these populations of HIV-infected patients. DRV/r provided consistently high and durable rates of virologic suppression in highly pretreated patients evaluated in the POWER, DUET, and DELPHI trials. Overall, the phase III trial program has shown and confirmed DRV/r to have a favorable safety profile, being associated with lower rates of diarrhea and lipid changes (triglycerides and cholesterol) than LPV/r. The DDI profiles with DRV/r have been well characterized and demonstrated to be manageable.

Clinical trials to date have shown DRV/r to have a very low propensity for resistance development and could therefore help preserve future options. The lower rate of primary PI mutation development in treatment failures than for LPV/r in ARV-experienced patients (TITAN) has led to a better understanding of emerging resistance. Furthermore, DRV/r protects susceptibility to other PIs and the NRTI backbone more effectively than does LPV/r.

An ongoing development program with DRV/r is exploring the effects of this boosted-PI across different HIV-infected populations and in novel treatment combinations and strategies.

Acknowledgments

The authors wish to acknowledge the medical writer Jackie Phillipson of Gardiner-Caldwell Communications for her assistance in drafting the chapter and coordinating author contributions. This support was funded by Tibotec Pharmaceuticals, Ltd.

REFERENCES

[1] Pomerantz, R. J.; Horn, D. L. Twenty years of therapy for HIV-1 infection. *Nat. Med.* **2003**, *9*, 867–873.

[2] Deeks, S. G.; Hecht, F. M.; Swanson, S.; et al. HIV RNA and CD4 cell count response to protease inhibitor therapy in an urban AIDS clinic. *AIDS* **1999**, *13*, F35-F43.

[3] Heath, K. V.; Singer, J.; O'Shaughnessy, M. V.; et al. Intentional nonadherence due to adverse symptoms associated with antiretroviral therapy. *J. Acquir. Immune Defic. Syndr.* **2002**, *31*, 211–217.

[4] Bartlett, J. A. Addressing the challenges of adherence. *J. Acquir. Immune Defic. Syndr.* **2002**, *29*, S2–S10.

[5] Greub, G.; Cozzi-Lepri, A.; Ledergerber, B.; et al. Intermittent and sustained low-level HIV viral rebound in patients receiving potent antiretroviral therapy. *AIDS* **2002**, *16*, 1967–1969.

[6] Clavel, F.; Hance, A. J. HIV drug resistance. *N. Engl. J. Med.* **2004**, *350*, 1023–1035.

[7] Gupta, G.; Hill, A.; Pillay, D. Drug resistance after virological failure of first-line HAART in resource-rich and resource-poor settings, a meta-analysis. 15th Conference on Retroviruses and Opportunistic Infections, 2008. Abstract 891.

[8] Hill, A.; Sawyer, W. Effect of backbone NRTI on efficacy of first-line boosted PI based HAART: systematic review of 12 clinical trials in 4,896 patients, 48th Interscience Conference on Antimicrobial Agents and Chemotherapy and the 46th Infectious Disease Society of America Joint Meeting, 2008. Abstract H1254.

[9] Scott, J. D. Simplifying the treatment of HIV infection with ritonavir-boosted protease inhibitors in antiretroviral-experienced patients. *Am. J. Health-Syst. Pharm.* **2005**, *62*, 809–815.

[10] Robertson, S. M.; Penzak, S. R.; Pau, A. K. Drug interactions in the management of HIV infection. *Expert Opin. Pharmacother.* **2005**, *6*, 233–253.

[11] Prezista (darunavir) prescribing information, June 2009. Available at http://www.prezista.com. Accessed Oct. 21, 2009.

[12] Ghosh, A. K.; Kincaid, J. F.; Cho, W.; et al. Potent HIV protease inhibitors incorporating high affinity P2-ligands and (*R*)-hydroxyethylamino(sulphonamide) isoestere. *Bioorg. Med. Chem. Lett.* **1998**, *8*, 687–690.

[13] Yoshimura, K.; Kato, R.; Kavlick, M. F.; et al. A potent human immunodeficiency virus type 1 protease inhibitor, UIC-94003 (TMC-216), and selection of a novel (A28S) mutation in the protease active site. *J. Virol.* **2002**, *76*, 1349–1358.

[14] de Béthune, M.-P.; Hertogs, K. Screening and selecting for optimized antiretroviral drugs: rising to the challenge of drug resistance. *Curr. Med. Res. Opin.* **2006**, *22*, 2603–2612.

[15] Surleraux, D. L. N. G.; Tahri, A.; Verschueren, W. G.; et al. Discovery and selection of TMc114, a next generation HIV-1 protease inhibitor. *J. Med. Chem.* **2005**, *48*, 1813–1822.

[16] De Meyer, S. M.; Azijn, A.; Surleraux, D.; et al. TMC114, a novel human immunodeficiency virus type 1 protease inhibitor active against protease inhibitor-resistant viruses, including a broad range of clinical isolates. *Antimicrob. Agents Chemother.* **2005**, *49*, 2314–2321.

[17] Lefebvre, E.; Schiffer, C. A. Resilience to resistance of HIV-1 protease inhibitors: profile of darunavir. *AIDS Rev.* **2008**, *10*, 131–142.

[18] Ghosh, A. K.; Leshchenko, S.; Noetzel, M. Stereoselective photochemical 1,3-dioxolane addition to 5-alkylmethyl-2(5*H*)-furaone: synthesis of bis-tetrahydrofuranyl ligand for HIV protease inhibitor UIC-94017 (TMC114). *J. Org. Chem.* **2004**, *69*, 7822–7829.

[19] Tie, Y.; Boross, P. I.; Wang, Y.F.; et al. High resolution crystal structures of HIV-1 protease with a potent non-peptide inhibitor (UIC-94017) active against multi-drug-resistant clinical strains. *J. Mol. Biol.* **2004**, *338*, 341–352.

[20] Dierynck, I.; De Wit, M.; Gustin, E.; et al. Binding kinetics of darunavir to human immunodeficiency virus type 1 protease explain the potent antiviral activity and high genetic barrier. *J. Virol.* **2007**, *81*, 13845–13851.

[21] Koh, Y.; Nakata, H.; Maeda, K.; et al. Novel bis-tetrahydrofuranylurethane-containing nonpeptidic protease inhibitor UIC-94017 (TMC114) with potent activity against multi-PI-resistant HIV in vitro. *Antimicrob. Agents Chemother.* **2003**, *47*, 3123–3129.

[22] Kovalevsky, A. Y.; Tie, Y.; Liu, F.; et al. Effectiveness of nonpeptide clinical inhibitor TMC-114 on HIV-1 protease with highly drug resistant mutations D30N, I50V, and L90M. *J. Med. Chem.* **2006**, *49*, 1379–1387.

[23] King, N.; Prabu-Jeyabalan, M.; Nalivaika, E.; Wigerinck, P.; de Béthune, M.P.; Schiffer, C. Structural and thermodynamic basis for the binding of TMC114, a next-generation HIV-1 protease inhibitor. *J. Virol.* **2004**, *78*, 12012–12021.

[24] Koh, Y.; Matsumi, S.; Das, D.; et al. Potent inhibition of HIV-1 replication by novel non-peptidyl small molecule inhibitors of protease dimerization. *J. Biol. Chem.* **2007**, *282*, 28709–28720.

[25] Dierynck, I.; De Meyer, S.; Lathouwers, E.; et al. Comparable in vitro susceptibility and virological outcome to darunavir in patients infected with subtype B and non-subtype B HIV isolates participating in the ARTEMIS phase III trial, 17th International AIDS Conference, 2008. Abstract TUPE0049.

[26] Tibotec, Inc. Data on file.

[27] De Meyer, S.; Azijn, H.; Fransen, E.; et al. The pathway leading to TMC114 resistance is different for TMC114 compared with other protease inhibitors. *Antivir. Ther.* **2006**, *11*, S24. Abstract 19.

[28] Back, D.; Sekar, V.; Hoetelmans, R. M. W. Darunavir: pharmacokinetics and drug interactions. *Antiviral Ther.* **2008**, *13*, 1–13.

[29] Sekar, V.; Spinosa-Guzman, S.; Lefebvre, E.; Hoetelmans, R. Clinical pharmacology of TMC114: a new HIV protease inhibitor. 16th International AIDS Conference, 2006. Abstract TUPE0083.

[30] Sekar, V.; Spinosa-Guzman, S.; Stevens, T.; De Paepe, E.; Lefebvre, E.; Hoetelmans, R. Absolute bioavailability of TMC114, administered in the absence and presence of low-dose ritonavir. 7th International Workshop on Clinical Pharmacology of HIV Therapy, 2006. Abstract P86.

[31] Sekar, V.; Kestens, D.; Spinosa-Guzman, S.; et al. The effect of different meal types on the pharmacokinetics of darunavir (TMC114)/ritonavir in HIV-negative healthy volunteers. *J. Clin. Pharmacol.* **2007**, *47*, 479–484.

[32] Aratésh, K.; Clumeck, N.; Pozniak, A.; et al. TMC114/ritonavir substitution for protease inhibitor(s) in a non-suppressive antiretroviral regimen: a 14-day proof-of-principle trial. *AIDS* **2005**, *19*, 943–947.

[33] Katlama, C.; Esposito, R.; Gatell, J. M.; et al. Efficacy and safety of TMC114/ritonavir in treatment-experienced HIV patients: 24-week results of POWER 1. *AIDS* **2007**, *21*, 395–402.

[34] Haubrich, R.; Berger, D.; Chiliade, P.; et al. Week 24 efficacy and safety of TMC114/ritonavir in treatment-experienced HIV patients. *AIDS* **2007**, *21*, F11–F18.

[35] Clotet, B.; Bellos, N.; Molina, J.-M.; et al. Efficacy and safety of darunavir–ritonavir at week 48 in treatment-experienced patients with HIV-1 infection in POWER 1 and 2: a pooled subgroup analysis of data from two randomised trials. *Lancet* **2007**, *369*, 1169–1178.

[36] Madruga, J. V.; Berger, D.; McMurchie, M.; et al. Efficacy and safety of darunavir–ritonavir compared with that of lopinavir–ritonavir at 48 weeks in treatment-experienced, HIV-infected patients in TITAN: a randomised controlled phase III trial. *Lancet* **2007**, *370*, 49–58.

[37] Ortiz, R.; DeJesus, E.; Khanlou, H.; et al. Efficacy and safety of once-daily darunavir/ritonavir versus lopinavir/ritonavir in treatment-naive HIV-1-infected patients at week 48. *AIDS* **2008**, *22*, 1389–1397.

[38] Molina, J. M.; Cohen, C.; Katlama, C.; et al. Safety and efficacy of darunavir (TMC114) with low-dose ritonavir in treatment-experienced patients: 24-week results of POWER 3. *J. Acquir. Immune Defic. Syndr.* **2007**, *46*, 24–31.

[39] Arastéh, K.; Yeni, P.; Pozniak, A.; et al. Efficacy and safety of darunavir/ritonavir in treatment-experienced HIV type-1 patients in the POWER 1, 2 and 3 trials at week 96. *Antiviral Ther.* **2009**, *14*, 859–864.

[40] Katlama, C.; Bellos, N.; Grinsztejn, B.; et al. POWER 1 and 2: combined final 144-week efficacy and safety results of darunavir/ritonavir 600/100 mg bid in treatment-experienced HIV patients. 9th International Congress on Drug Therapy in HIV Infection, 2008. Abstract P21.

[41] Pozniak, A.; Arastéh, K.; Molina, J. M.; et al. Power 3 analysis: 144-week efficacy and safety results for darunavir/ritonavir 600/100 mg bid in treatment-experienced patients. 9th International Congress on Drug Therapy in HIV Infection, 2008. Abstract P24.

[42] Cahn, P.; Haubrich, R.; Leider, J.; et al. Pooled 24-week results of DUET-1 and DUET-2: TMC125 (etravirine; ETR) versus placebo in treatment-experienced HIV-1-infected patients. 47th Interscience Conference on Antimicrobial Agents and Chemotherapy, 2007. Abstract H-717.

[43] Andries, K.; Debunne, A.; Kakuda, T. N.; et al. Etravirine: from TMC125 to INTELENCE: a shift in treatment paradigm for HIV patients. Chapter 6, this volume.

[44] De Meyer, S.; Vangeneugden, T.; van Baelen, B.; et al. Resistance profile of darunavir: combined 24-week results from the POWER trials. *AIDS Res. Hum. Retroviruses* **2008**, *24*, 379–388.

[45] Lathouwers, E.; De Meyer, S.; Dierynck, I.; et al. Update on the prevalence of the 2007 darunavir resistance-associated mutations in samples received for routine clinical resistance testing. 6th European HIV Drug Resistance Workshop, 2008. Abstract 68.

[46] Hicks, C. B.; Cahn, P.; Cooper, D. A.; et al. Durable efficacy of tipranavir–ritonavir in combination with optimised background regimen of antiretroviral drugs for treatment experienced HIV-1-infected patients at 48 weeks in the RESIST studies: an analysis of combined data from two randomised open-label trials. *Lancet* **2006**, *368*, 466–475.

[47] DHHS 2007 Panel on Antiretroviral Guidelines for Adult and Adolescents. Guidelines for the use of antiretroviral agents in HIV-infected adults and adolescents. Department of Health and Human Services, Dec. 1, 2007. Available at http://aidsinfo.nih.gov/contentfiles/AdultandAdolescentGL000721.pdf. Accessed Mar. 31, 2009.

[48] DHHS 2008 Panel on Antiretroviral Guidelines for Adult and Adolescents. Guidelines for the use of antiretroviral agents in HIV-infected adults and adolescents. Department of Health and Human Services, Nov. 3, 2008. Available at http://aidsinfo.nih.gov/contentfiles/AdultandAdolescentGL.pdf. Accessed Jan. 13, 2009.

[49] Committee for Medicinal Products for Human Use, European Medicines Agency. Guideline on the clinical development of medicinal products for the treatment of HIV infection, Nov. 2008. Available at http://www.emea.europa.eu/htms/human/humanguidelines/efficacy.htm. Accessed Feb. 19, 2009.

[50] Bánhegyi, D.; Katlama, C.; Da Cunha, C.; et al. Phase III TITAN week 96 final analysis: efficacy/safety of darunavir/r (DRV/r) vs. lopinavir/r (LPV/r) in LPV/r-naive, treatment-experienced patients. 9th International Congress on Drug Therapy in HIV Infection, 2008. Abstract P022.

[51] De Meyer, S.; Lathouwers, E.; Dierynck, I.; et al. Characterization of virologic failure patients on darunavir/ritonavir in treatment-experienced patients. *AIDS* **2009**, *23*, 1829–1840.

[52] De Meyer, S.; Lathouwers, E.; Dierynck, I.; et al. Resistance development in virological failures with DRV/r or LPV/r: 96-week analysis of the phase III TITAN trial in treatment-experienced patients. 9th International Congress on Drug Therapy in HIV Infection, 2008. Abstract 0424.

[53] Mills, A.; Nelson, M.; Jayaweera, D.; et al. Once-daily darunavir/ritonavir vs. lopinavir/ritonavir in treatment-naive, HIV-1-infected patients: 96-week analysis. *AIDS* **2009**, *23*, 1679–1688.

[54] Nelson, M.; Yeni, P.; Sension, M.; et al. Factors affecting virologic response to darunavir/ritonavir and lopinavir/ritonavir in treatment-naive HIV-1-infected patients in ARTEMIS at 96 weeks. 16th Conference on Retroviruses and Opportunistic Infections, 2009. Abstract 575.

[55] Dierynck, I.; De Meyer, S.; Lathouwers, E.; et al. Characterization of virologic failures in the randomized, controlled, phase III ARTEMIS trial in treatment-naive patients (week 96 analysis). 16th Conference on Retroviruses and Opportunistic Infections, 2009. Abstract 655.

[56] Walmsley, S. Protease-inhibitor based regimens for HIV therapy: safety and efficacy. *J. Acquir. Immune Defic. Syndr.* **2007**, *45*, S5–S13.

[57] Tomaka, F.; Lefebvre, E.; Sekar, V.; et al. Effects of ritonavir-boosted darunavir versus ritonavir-boosted atazanavir on lipid and glucose parameters in HIV-negative, healthy volunteers. *Future HIV Med.* **2009**, *10*, 318–327.

[58] Sekar, V.; De Paepe, E.; Van Baelen, B.; et al. Pharmacokinetic/pharmacodynamic (PK/PD) analysis of darunavir in the TITAN study. 11th European AIDS Conference, 2007. Abstract P4.1/10.

[59] Sekar, V.; Vanden Abeele, C.; Van Baelen, B.; et al. Pharmacokinetic–pharmacodynamic analyses of once-daily darunavir in the ARTEMIS study. 15th Conference on Retroviruses and Opportunistic Infections, 2008. Abstract L-103.

[60] Sekar, V.; De Paepe, E.; Van Baelen, B.; et al. Effect of extrinisic and intrinsic factors on the pharmacokinetics of darunavir/ritonavir (DRV/r) in HIV-1 patients: results of a randomised, controlled, phase III study (TITAN). 11th European AIDS Conference, 2007. Abstract PS4/5.

[61] Sekar, V.; Vanden Abeele, C.; Van Baelen, B.; et al. The effect of extrinsic and intrinsic factors on the pharmacokinetics of darunavir/ritonavir in HIV-1 infected patients: results of a randomized, controlled, phase III study (ARTEMIS). 9th International Workshop on Clinical Pharmacology of HIV Therapy, 2008. Abstract P41.

[62] Blanche, S.; Bologna, R.; Cahn, P.; et al. Pharmacokinetics, safety and efficacy of darunavir/ritonavir in treatment-experienced children and adolescents. *AIDS* **2009**, *23*, 2005–2013.

[63] Bologna, R.; Rugina, S.; Cahn, P.; et al. Safety and efficacy of darunavir coadministered with low-dose ritonavir (DRV/r) in treatment-experienced children and adolescents at week 24. 15th Conference on Retroviruses and Opportunistic Infections, 2008. Abstract 78LB.

[64] Currier, J.; Squires, K.; Averrit Bridge, D.; et al. Safety, tolerability and efficacy of darunavir/ritonavir in treatment-experienced women with HIV infection: 24-week interim analysis of GRACE (gender, age, and clinical experience). 17th International AIDS conference, 2008. Abstract TH-PDB202.

[65] De Meyer, S. M.; Spinosa-Guzman, S.; Vangeneugden, T.; et al. Efficacy of once-daily darunavir/ritonavir 800/100 mg in HIV-infected, treatment-experienced patients with no baseline resistance-associated mutations to darunavir. *J. Acquir. Immune Defic. Syndr.* **2008**, *49*, 179–182.

[66] Arribas, J., Horban, A., Gerstoff, J.; et al. The MONET trial: darunavir/ritonavir with or without nucleoside analogues, for patients with HIV RNA below 50 copies/mL on prior antiretroviral treatment. *AIDS*. **2010**, *24*, 223–230.

[67] Katlama, C., Valentin, M. A., Algarte-Genin, M.; et al. Efficacy of darunavir/ritonavir as single-drug maintenance therapy in patients with HIV-1 viral suppression: a randomized open-label non-inferiority trial, MONOI-ANRS 136. 5th IAS Conference on HIV Pathogenesis, Treatment and Prevention, 2009. Abstract WELBB102.

[68] Lazzarin, A.; Campbell, T.; Clotet, B.; et al. Efficacy and safety of TMC125 (etravirine) in treatment-experienced HIV-1-infected patients in DUET-2: 24-week results from a randomised, double-blind, placebo-controlled trial. *Lancet* **2007**, *370*, 39–48.

[69] Madruga, J.; Cahn, P.; Grinsztejn, B.; et al. Efficacy and safety of TMC125 (etravirine) in treatment-experienced HIV-1-infected patients in DUET-1: 24-week results from a randomised, double-blind, placebo-controlled trial. *Lancet* **2007**, *370*, 29–38.

[70] Yazdanpanah, Y.; Fagard, C.; Descamps, D.; et al. High rate of virologic suppression with raltegravir plus etravirine and darunavir/ritonavir among treatment-experienced patients infected with multidrug-resistant HIV: results of the ANRS 139 TRIO trial. *Clin. Infect. Dis.* **2009**, *49*, 1441–1449.

4

DISCOVERY AND DEVELOPMENT OF TIPRANAVIR

KAREN R. ROMINES
Pathfinder Pharmaceuticals, Inc., Durham, North Carolina

INTRODUCTION

The HIV protease inhibitor tipranavir is one of several approved HIV protease inhibitors, but it has a unique origin. It is the only drug in the class derived from a low-molecular-weight screening hit rather than from peptidic inhibitors. That difference provides a rare opportunity to consider and contrast two very different strategies for starting a drug discovery program, screening a collection of low-molecular-weight compounds, or designing compounds based on peptidic inhibitors.

The project that produced tipranavir began in the early 1990s at the Upjohn Company. At that point, the HIV mortality rate in the United States was climbing steadily, seemingly unhindered by the first antiretroviral agent approved, the nucleoside HIV reverse transcriptase inhibitor zidovudine, which was approved in 1987. At the time, HIV protease inhibitor research was a very active field, and several drug companies had sizable research programs. There were two major reasons for this widespread interest. First, HIV protease is necessary for the production of infectious virus. Without the protease, only harmless, immature viral particles are produced by the infected cells [1]. Second, HIV protease is an aspartyl protease [2,3], quite similar to the human enzyme renin, which plays a role in blood pressure regulation. Peptidomimetic renin inhibitors in the literature and pharmaceutical companies' collections provided useful starting points for HIV protease researchers, and the availability of HIV crystal structures facilitated the design of additional inhibitors [4].

The first HIV protease inhibitors were approved in late 1995 (saquinavir) and early 1996 (ritonavir and indinavir). In 1995, something quite amazing happened: The U.S. mortality rate for HIV began to drop [5]. A positive HIV test shifted dramatically from a terminal diagnosis to a chronic infection that could be controlled for many years if the patient had access to state-of-the-art care and antiretroviral therapy. By the time that tipranavir was approved in 2005, HIV treatment was a very different, and far more promising, endeavor than in the early 1990s, but the protease inhibitors that had been a key part of this change still had significant drawbacks. Two issues were class specific. First, the HIV protease inhibitors had very poor oral bioavailability, and they required high doses to achieve efficacy. For example, the recommended dose of indinavir was 2400 mg/day (800 mg t.i.d.). This issue was well known from the beginning of the HIV protease research programs. Second, these drugs were associated with side effects, including gastrointestinal effects, liver enzyme and cholesterol elevation, and lipodystrophy. This issue was not apparent until the first protease inhibitors were used in large clinical studies, so these data were not available at the beginning of the tipranavir project. The third issue was not confined to the protease inhibitors, but it was, and still is, a significant issue for all HIV inhibitors: development of resistance. HIV replication mechanisms emphasize quantity rather than quality, and the resulting diverse population of viral strains facilitates efficient selection of drug-resistant strains. Any antiretroviral drug is subject to development of viral resistance, and protease resistance was already a significant concern as tipranavir began clinical development. In this chapter we trace the discovery and development of tipranavir and discuss its performance on all three of these clinical issues.

Antiviral Drugs: From Basic Discovery Through Clinical Trials, First Edition. Edited by Wieslaw M. Kazmierski.

DISCOVERY

Many HIV protease research programs started from peptide-derived renin inhibitors. The advantage of this approach was that it readily produced potent HIV protease inhibitors. The disadvantage was found in the pharmacokinetics, and the primary motivation for screening was the poor pharmacokinetic profile of the peptide-derived inhibitors. The hypothesis was that screening could identify a small molecule with better oral bioavailability. The screening hits would probably have much lower potency than the peptide-derived compounds, but x-ray crystal structures of inhibitors bound to HIV protease could be used to guide the optimization of the new molecules and improve the potency. This is exactly what scientists at Upjohn did.

Screening and Identification of Lead Structures

The tipranavir program started with a fluorescence-based assay, and the team screened a set of 5000 dissimilar compounds [6]. At this writing, almost 20 years later, a set of 5000 compounds seems absurdly small for a screen. For many research programs in the current era of high-throughput and ultrahigh-throughput screening, this set is smaller than a validation set. But the Upjohn scientists found a valid hit in that 5000-compound set, which suggests that the set was well designed, and raises the question of how much screening is enough. In this case, a screen of 5000 compounds led to an approved drug, although not without quite a bit of effort. If the Upjohn scientists later screened larger sets of compounds to search for additional hits, they did not report the results, so in this case there is no direct comparison of screening a larger set.

The screening hit was warfarin (**1**, Fig. 1), a potent anticoagulant that inhibited HIV protease with an IC_{50} value of about 30 μM. Based on this result, the Upjohn scientists did a similarity search of the company's compound collection, and tested a number of 4-hydroxycoumarins. That worked led to the identification of another anticoagulant, phenprocoumon (**2**, Fig. 2), which was approximately 30-fold more potent in the HIV protease assay (K_i = 1 μM) and even demonstrated weak antiviral activity in a cell culture assay [ED_{50} = 100 to 300 μM in HIV-1-infected PBMCs (peripheral blood

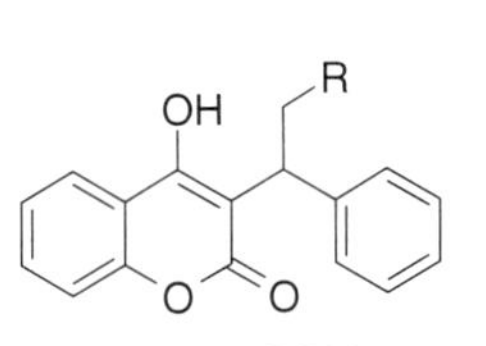

1 Warfarin, R=COMe
2 Phenprocoumon, R=Me

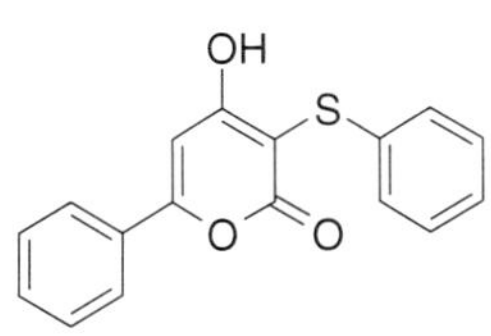

3

FIGURE 1 Screening hits from HIV-1 protease inhibitor assays.

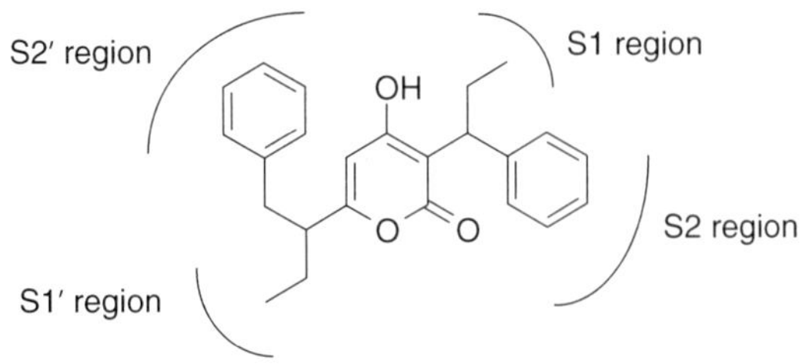

4 PNU-96988

FIGURE 2 Interactions of clinical candidate PNU-96988 with HIV-1 protease.

mononuclear cells)]. Phenprocoumon is a competitive inhibitor, and the Upjohn team was able to get an x-ray crystal structure of **2** bound to HIV-1 protease. The pharmacokinetics of these hits were very encouraging, and sharply contrasted with the peptide-derived inhibitors. Both warfarin and phenprocoumon have been used clinically as oral anticoagulants [6]. Thus, the first step in the screening approach was successful. The team identified a low-molecular-weight inhibitor with oral bioavailability. The next step was to recover at least a portion of the potency lost with this approach, and the x-ray crystal structures proved to be an excellent tool for this optimization work.

It is interesting to note that the Upjohn team was not the only group to pursue a screening strategy in the early 1990s. Scientists at Parke-Davis identified a similar low-molecular-weight inhibitor, the 4-hydroxypyranone **3** (Fig. 1) [7]. Using x-ray crystal structures of the pyranones bound to HIV-1 protease, the Parke-Davis scientists optimized the series to produce very potent inhibitors [8], but no drug candidates from the series have been approved or are in clinical development at this time.

First-Generation Clinical Candidate: PNU-96988

The x-ray crystal structure of the phenprocoumon-HIV-1 protease complex provided valuable information for the optimization of the screening hits. First, the crystal structure demonstrated the importance of the 4-hydroxypyranone ring, which binds with the active site of the enzyme. The lactone oxygen atoms form direct hydrogen bonds with the isoleucine residues on the flap of the HIV protease, thus removing the need for the water molecule found in complexes of HIV protease with peptide-derived inhibitors. This pharmacophore was retained throughout the project and is found at the center of tipranavir. Second, the crystal structure showed that the C3α substituents ethyl and phenyl reached into the S1 and S2 pockets of the enzyme. The benzene ring of the coumarin, however, did not interact well with the S1′ and S2′ regions, and benzene ring substituents were also unable to interact well with those regions of the enzyme. Upjohn chemists removed the benzene ring and replaced it with a C6 substituent containing two groups at the C6α position. Optimization led to PNU-96988 (**4**, Fig. 2), a pseudosymmetric compound able to interact with the S2′ through S2 regions of the HIV protease [6].

PNU-96988 was a far more potent inhibitor of HIV protease than phenprocoumon. The K_i value of PNU-96988 in the enzyme assay was 38 nM, and the compound was selective relative to human aspartyl proteases. PNU-96988 had antiviral activity in cell culture assays with ED_{50} values of 3 to 4 μM, and oral bioavailability levels in rats and dogs were 76 and 45%, respectively. The compound does have two asymmetric centers, and thus it is a mixture of four stereoisomers. These components were separated using chiral high-performance liquid chromatography (HPLC), and all four isomers were active in the enzyme assay, with K_i values ranging from 14 to 109 nM [6]. PNU-96988 was advanced into phase I clinical trials as a stereoisomer mixture, and the compound reportedly was well tolerated and gave the expected blood levels. The company did not pursue further clinical development, however, because more potent candidates were identified [9].

Second-Generation Clinical Candidate: PNU-103017

Discovery of the second generation of HIV protease inhibitors derived from the 4-hydroxycoumarins relied on two structural changes, each of which increased the potency of the inhibitors. First, the benzene ring of the coumarin was saturated. Simple saturation had little impact on the enzyme inhibition (**5b**, Fig. 3), but changing the ring size led to a dramatic increase in potency. The eight-membered ring proved to be the optimal size (**5d,** Fig. 3), and a later x-ray crystal structure showed that this ring folded in a low-energy conformation right into the S1′ pocket of the protease [10].

The second structural change was substitution of a sulfonamide on the C3α phenyl ring (Fig. 4). This sulfonamide group formed an interaction with the S3 pocket of the HIV-1 protease and increased the potency further. The same interaction and corresponding increase in enzyme inhibition potency was also observed with amide substitution, but the sulfonamide had significantly better antiviral activity in cell culture assays, as measured by inhibition of HIV-1 in H9 cells. The Upjohn team identified several potent compounds

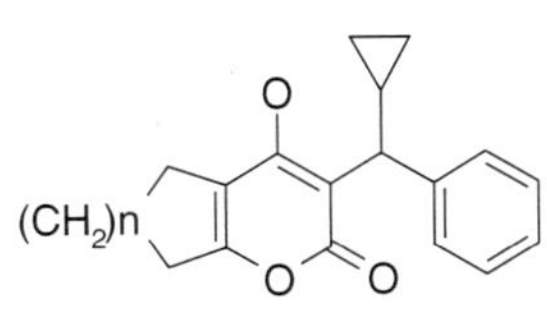

	n=	K_i (μM)
5a	1	>1
5b	2	0.18
5c	3	0.096
5d	4	0.015
5e	5	0.037
5f	6	0.56
5g	7	>1

FIGURE 3 Impact of cycloalkyl ring size on HIV-1 protease inhibition.

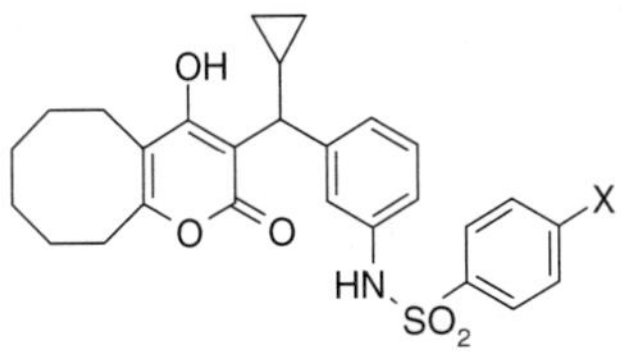

	X	Enzyme Inhibition K_i (nM)	Antiviral Activity ED_{50} (μM)
6a	F	3.1	2.0
6b	CN	0.8	1.3

FIGURE 4 Sulfonamide-substituted cyclooctylpyranones.

in this series, including **6a** and **6b** (Fig. 4). These two compounds demonstrated similar in vitro potency in both enzyme (K_i value) and cell culture (ED_{50} value) assays (Fig. 4), and their pharmacokinetic profiles in rats and dogs were similar. Oral bioavailability in rats was 42 to 50%, and it was even better in dogs (77 to 100%). The choice of clinical candidate was, in the end, based on a single-dose toxicity study in rats, in which **6a** showed severe toxicity at a lower dose than **6b** (360 mg/kg vs. 720 mg/kg). These cyclooctylpyranones have one asymmetric center, and the racemate **6b** was separated into its component enantiomers using chiral HPLC. The *S* enantiomer was more potent than the *R* enantiomer, but the difference was modest, and the racemate **6b** was selected for development [11]. PNU-103017 completed phase I single- and multidose studies in healthy volunteers, but did not advance further. The compound was highly protein bound, and there were some concerns that this would limit its efficacy. More important, some liver enzyme elevations were seen in healthy volunteers during the multidose study [9].

Discovery of Tipranavir

The third-generation clinical candidate, tipranavir, resulted from one more change in the pyranone-based template. This series of compounds retained the substitution at the 3-position, including the sulfonamide that extends into the S3 pocket of the protease, and the team focused on replacing the cyclooctyl ring. The cyclooctyl ring had a very effective interaction with the S1′ region of the enzyme, but it was unable to interact with the S2′ region, and substitution to gain that interaction was not practical. The solution was to remove the cyclooctyl ring, saturate the 5,6-bond of the resulting 4-hydroxypyrone, and then disubstitute at the C6 position. Compounds with phenyl or benzyl substitution at the C6 position were not particularly good inhibitors, but analogs with phenethyl substitution at C6 were quite potent [12]. Optimization of the new lead series led to the discovery of several potent inhibitors, including tipranavir (**7**, Fig. 5) [13].

Compounds with symmetric substitution at the C6 position were less potent than those with asymmetric substitution [12], and consequently, the most promising compounds in the dihydropyrone series had two asymmetric centers. The analogs were all prepared without control of either asymmetric center, resulting in a mixture of four stereoisomers. The component stereoisomers of several potent inhibitors

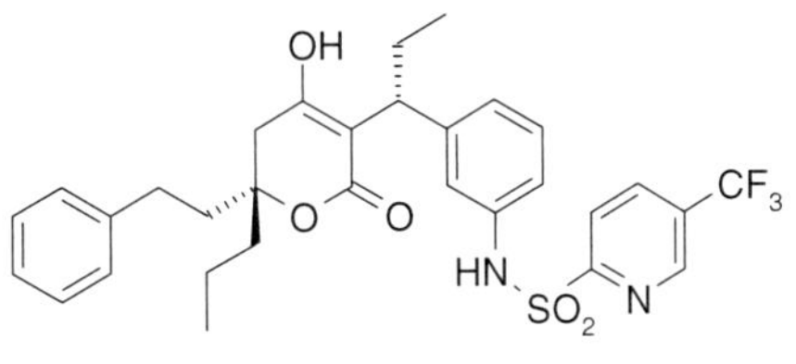

7 tipranavir

FIGURE 5 Structure of tipranavir.

TABLE 1 Stereoisomers of Tipranavir (*R*,*R* Configuration)

C3α,C6 Configuration	Enzyme Inhibition K_i (nM)	Antiviral Activity ED_{50} (μM)
R,*S*	0.018	0.14
R,*R*	0.008	0.03
S,*S*	0.22	1.70
S,*R*	0.032	0.41

were evaluated by separating the CBZ derivatives of a late-stage intermediate amine using chiral HPLC, and results for tipranavir stereoisomers are shown in Table 1. The configuration of the C3α position was important, and the *R* configuration was significantly more potent. The C6 configuration had less impact, but again, the *R* configuration was more potent [13].

The initial preclinical profiling of tipranavir included testing against HIV-2 protease (K_i < 1 nM) and testing against other human aspartyl proteases (K_i > 2 μM). Initial pharmacokinetics in rats showed an oral bioavailability of 30%. This was lower than in earlier-generation candidates, but the studies indicated that plasma levels were over 1 μM, the protein-adjusted IC_{90} estimate, for 8 to 12 h [13].

SYNTHESIS

The chiral HPLC separation technique facilitated the analog studies and allowed the initial DMPK screening, but any further development of tipranavir required a more practical synthesis. Tipranavir is a challenging molecule to synthesize. It contains two remote asymmetric centers, the dihydropyrone core has low chemical stability, and compounds with the tertiary alkoxy C6 center have poor crystallinity.

The first asymmetric synthesis of tipranavir, shown in Scheme 1, was developed in the medicinal chemistry group. The team started by setting the C3α asymmetric center via 1,4-addition of an organocuprate to an unsaturated chiral acylimide (**9**). The chiral auxiliary (*R*)-4-phenyl-2,5,-oxazolidinone (**8**) worked very well, giving a single diastereomer in the 1,4-addition step. The aniline protecting groups were switched from trimethylsilyl to benzyl to give the crystalline intermediate **10**.

The second phase of the synthesis began building in the atoms which eventually formed the dihydropyone ring. First, an acetyl group was installed via addition of a dioxolane derivative to the titanium enolate of **10**. As above, the addition produced a single diastereomer. Cleavage of the dioxolane then gave the acetyl intermediate **11**.

The next challenge was to install the C6 asymmetric center. Since the chiral auxiliary was still present, along with two additional asymmetric centers, the team experimented with adding a ketone containing the two C6 substitutents to the titanium enolate of intermediate **11**. Use of 1-phenylhexan-3-one gave a 3 : 2 mixture of diastereomers, which was an encouraging result, but it was not practical for preparation of tipranavir on a multigram scale. To optimize the reaction, the team switched to an acetylenic ketone (**14**) to help differentiate between the propyl and phenethyl substituents at C6, and they changed from Ti(*i*-Pr)Cl_3 to Ti(O-*n*-Bu)Cl_3. This produced a 25 : 1 mixture of diastereomers, with the major component as the desired isomer **12**. The desired diastereomer was purified using silica gel chromatography, then cyclized to the dihydropyrone **13**. The cyclization step also removed the chiral auxiliary. The synthesis of tipranavir was then completed in two steps: a hydrogenation to saturate the acetylene at C6 and cleave the benzyl protecting groups on the aniline, followed by formation of the sulfonamide. This synthesis was used to make the first 100-g lot of tipranavir for preclinical studies, and it allowed drug development to continue while the synthetic route for process chemistry was being developed. Often, the medicinal chemistry route is used to provide compound for the initial preclinical studies, but since that was not a practical option in this case, the development of this first asymmetric synthesis was critical [14].

The synthesis in Scheme 1 was far more practical for preparation of a chiral drug candidate than the HPLC separation used in the initial preparation of tipranavir, but it was not well suited for process work. Fors et al. developed a convergent approach, in which each of the remote asymmetric centers was prepared separately. The team then constructed the dihydropyrone ring by first forming the C3–C4 bond, then closing the ring at the C2–O1 bond. This convergent strategy avoids preparation of diastereomers in the intermediates, but the team had to overcome the difficulty of constructing the dihydropyrone ring from two pieces with limited reactivity [15].

The strategy for the C6 asymmetric center was a classical resolution, as shown in Scheme 2. The team added 1-phenyl-3-hexanone to the lithium enolate of ethyl acetate to construct the C4–C6 section of the molecule. Cleavage of the resulting ester gave the acid **16**, which was resolved by crystallization with chiral norephedrine. The desired enantiomer **17** was then protected with [(*p*-phenylphenyl)oxy]methyl (POM) ether to give intermediate **18**. The POM protecting group was developed and selected because of its crystallinity. The ester was then converted to an aldehyde in two steps

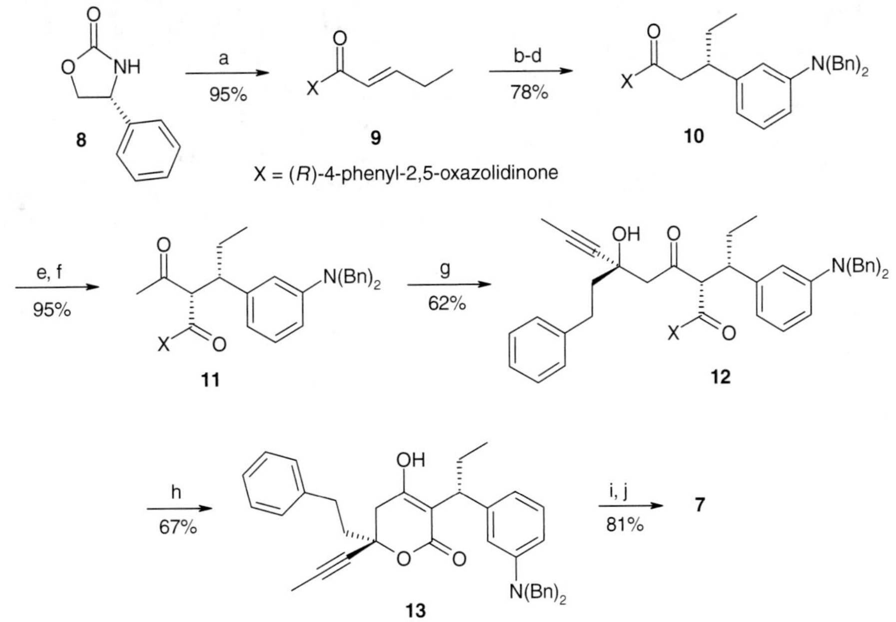

SCHEME 1 Asymmetric synthesis of tipranavir: (a) *n*-BuLi, THF, −78°C, then ClC(O)CH=CHCH$_2$CH$_3$; (b) CuBr, DMS, THF, 0°C, 1 h, then 3-[N(TMS)$_2$]PhMgBr; (c) silica gel, CH$_2$Cl$_2$; (d) Na$_2$CO$_3$, PhCH$_2$Br, H$_2$O, CH$_2$Cl$_2$; (e) TiCl$_4$, CH$_2$Cl$_2$, −78°C, then Hunig's base, then 2-methyl-2-methoxy-1,3-dioxolane; (f) aqueous HClO$_4$; (g) Ti(O-*n*-Bu)Cl$_3$, CH$_2$Cl$_2$, −78°C, then Hunig's base, then PhCH$_2$CH$_2$COCCCH$_3$ (**14**); (h) K-O*t*-Bu, THF, 0°C; (i) H$_2$, Pd/C, MeOH, EtOAc; (j) ArSO$_2$Cl, pyridine, CH$_2$Cl$_2$.

to give the key intermediate **19**. The oxidation-state adjustment was necessary to enhance the reactivity of this intermediate and allow later construction of the dihydropyrone ring.

The first decision in the synthesis of the C3 component, shown in Scheme 3, was to use an aryl nitro derivative rather than a protected aniline derivative for the N atom that will eventually become tipranavir's sulfonamide. The nitro intermediates were selected for their crystallinity. The C3 asymmetric center was obtained by resolution of 1-(3-nitrophenyl)propane (**20**). The team used lipase to acylate the undesired enantiomer selectively, then isolated the desired enantiomer **22** by chromatography. Intermediate **22** was then converted to its mesylate, and the mesylate group was displaced with sodium enolate of diethyl malonate to give **23**. Acid-promoted cleavage of the esters was followed by decarboxylation, and subsequent formation of the methyl ester gave the second key intermediate, **24**.

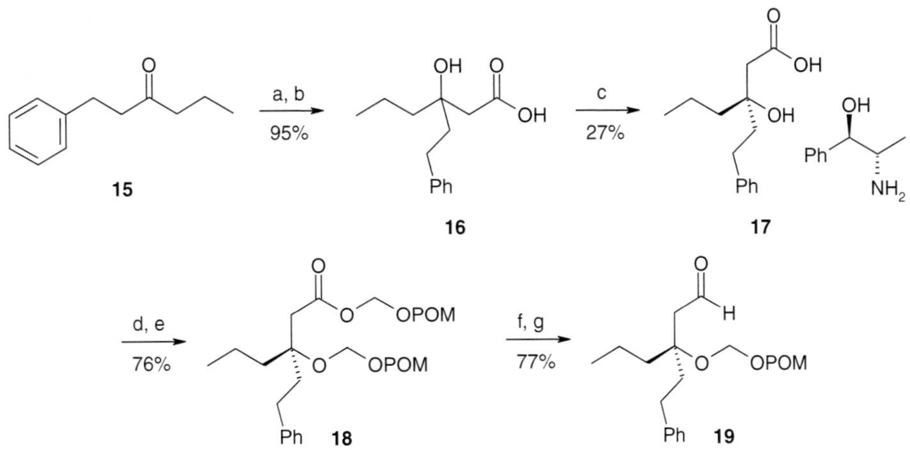

SCHEME 2 Synthesis of the C4–C6 component of tipranavir: (a) H$_2$C=C(OLi)OEt, THF, −30°C; (b) NaOH, MeOH; (c) (1*R*,2*S*)-norephedrine, MeCN, 0°C; (d) HCl, MTBE, H$_2$O; (e) POMOCH$_2$Cl, *i*-Pr$_2$NEt, toluene, 110°C; (f) DIBALH, toluene, −20°C; (g) NaOCl, TEMPO, CH$_2$Cl$_2$, 1 to 5°C.

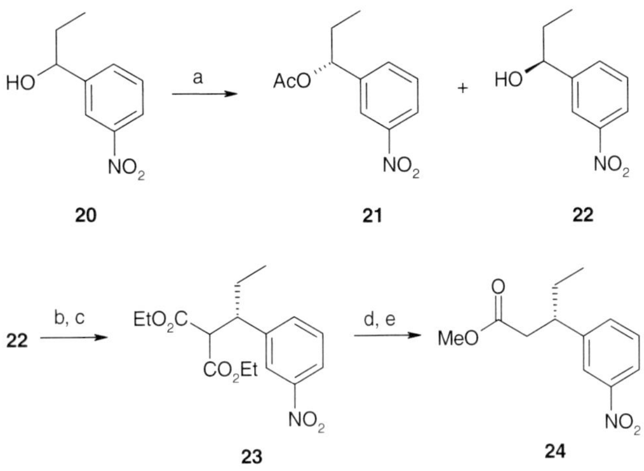

SCHEME 3 Synthesis of the C2–C3 component of tipranavir: (a) isopropenyl acetate, Amano P30 lipase, MTBE, room temperature, 2 days; (b) *i*-Pr_2NEt, CH_2Cl_2; then MsCl, −20 to 0°C; (c) $(EtO_2C)_2CHNa$; (d) 6 N HCl; (e) HCl, MeOH.

Once the two key intermediates were prepared, tipranavir was assembled as shown in Scheme 4. First, the C4–C6 component **19** was added to the sodium anion of the C2–C3 component **24** to form the C3–C4 bond, as a mixture of diastereomers **25**. Since the C4–C6 component was converted to an aldehyde to get the necessary reactivity for the addition of the C3–C4 anion, the oxidation state had to be reset to the ketone **26**. The remainder of the synthesis was straightforward. The POM protecting group was cleaved, and the dihydropyrone ring **27** was formed. The nitro group was then reduced to the aniline, and the sulfonamide was formed to give tipranavir (**7**).

PRECLINICAL DEVELOPMENT

Virology

Tipranavir was the first small-molecule inhibitor of HIV protease to reach the potency range of its contemporary peptide-derived protease inhibitors. Against lab strains, tipranavir had an average IC_{90} value of 0.16 μM and a selectivity index of over 500. Similar results were seen with a panel of clinical isolates, including strains resistant to the NRTI AZT or the NNRTI delavirdine. In vitro combination studies in cell culture assays showed an additive-synergistic effect of using tipranavir with other classes of HIV replication inhibitors, which indicated that tipranavir was probably appropriate for combination therapy. One concern, due to the high protein binding of pyranone and dihydropyrone-based inhibitors, was the potential attenuation of tipranavir's potency in the presence of human proteins. In vitro studies using human plasma, human plasma albumin, or α_1-acid glycoprotein in cell culture to assess the effect of protein binding on antiviral activity showed that the IC_{50} value increased 1.7- to 6.2-fold, and these estimates of the protein binding effect were used to interpret preclinical pharmacokinetic data [16].

Several groups assessed the tipranavir sensitivity of both laboratory strains and clinical isolates that were resistant to other protease inhibitors. These results showed consistently that tipranavir was able to inhibit replication effectively. For example, laboratory strains resistant to indinavir, ritonavir, and nelfinavir had an average IC_{90} of 0.18 μM, and studies with multidrug-resistant clinical isolates gave IC_{90} values of 0.31 to 0.86 μM [17].

During the development of tipranavir, the practice of boosting protease inhibitors with ritonavir was beginning to show promise for reducing the drug burden of peptide-derived protease inhibitors. As part of the effort to assess the feasibility of boosting tipranavir, Upjohn virologists examined the impact of tipranavir on ritonavir-resistant strains of HIV. The study used a pair of isolates from a patient, obtained before and after the patient failed a drug regimen that included ritonavir. The ritonavir-resistant strain was 50-fold less sensitive to ritonavir than the pretreatment strain, but both strains were sensitive to tipranavir [18].

Upjohn virologists attempted to generate a tipranavir-resistant HIV strain by exposing two HIV strains to increasing concentrations of drug. In the initial studies, less than threefold resistance was observed after 30 passages, leading to the conclusion that generation of a tipranavir-resistant strain in vitro was difficult, particularly compared to generating strains resistant to reverse transcriptase inhibitors [16]. Later work did produce a strain with > 10-fold resistance to tipranavir, and it had six mutations in the protease, at

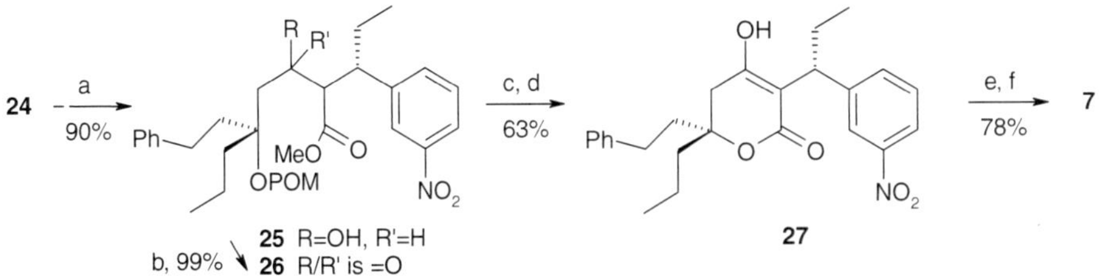

SCHEME 4 Convergent synthesis of tipranavir: (a) NaHMDS, THF, −80°C, then **19**; (b) PCC, NaOAc, Florisil, CH_2Cl_2, −80°C to room temperature; (c) H_2SO_4, MeOH, THF; (d) NaOH, MeOH; (e) H_2, Pd/C, THF; (f) $ArSO_2Cl$, DMSO, pyridine, CH_2Cl_2.

positions 13, 32, 33, 45, 82, and 84 [19]. These results suggested that tipranavir's genetic barrier for development of resistance was relatively high.

Pharmacokinetics

The data reported on preclinical studies of tipranavir are limited. Turner et al. reported that the oral bioavailability in rats was 30% and the half-life was 5.4 h, and they noted that plasma concentrations were over 1 μM for 8 to 12 h after a 10-mg/kg oral dose [13]. Other reports noted that the oral bioavailability in rats, dogs, mice, and rabbits ranged from 6.5 to 28% after a single dose, but exposure increased upon repeat dosing [19].

Some of the preclinical studies examined the effects of ritonavir boosting on tipranavir pharmacokinetics. Exposures increased significantly because the ritonavir boost both increased the absorption of tipranavir and decreased its metabolism [19]. For example, a study of ^{14}C-labeled tipranavir in rats showed absorption over 50% when a 10-mg/kg oral dose was given with a 10-mg/kg dose of RTV. The drug was mainly excreted in the feces (over 75%), and the major component in both plasma and feces was the parent compound, which reflected the decreased metabolism of the tipranavir when coadministered with ritonavir [20].

Toxicology

Preclinical toxicology studies were done in mice, rats, dogs, and cynomologus monkeys. Long-term studies were done in rats and dogs, and some studies were done with the coadministration of ritonavir. The results of all these studies were fairly consistent. The target organs were the gastrointestinal tract and the liver. The thyroid gland was also affected in rodent studies, but that was attributed to rodent-specific metabolites [19].

CLINICAL DEVELOPMENT

The first clinical study of tipranavir dosed the candidate as a single agent. A phase I single-dose study in healthy volunteers reported early in development included the result that doses of 500 mg and above gave plasma drug concentrations over 1 μM for over 8 h [13]. Development of tipranavir alone, however, was soon replaced by coadministration with ritonavir. Three phase I and phase II studies clearly demonstrated the advantages of using ritonavir boosting.

Phase I–IIa

The formulation selected for development was a self-emulsifying drug delivery system (SEDDS) capsule. In a key phase I study, the pharmacokinetics of twice-daily (b.i.d.) tipranavir doses were compared with and without coadministration of ritonavir. Healthy volunteers took tipranavir alone for 11 days and then added ritonavir to the regimen for another 21 days. Coadministration of ritonavir gave over an 20-fold increase in the steady-state trough tipranavir concentrations. This study also provided evidence that tipranavir induces the cytochrome P450 3A4, but addition of the ritonavir inhibited that cytochrome's activity [21].

TABLE 2 Comparison of Tipranavir (TPV) Efficacy with and Without Ritonavir (r) Coadministration in Treatment-Naive HIV-1 Patients

TPV/r Dose (mg, b.i.d.)	Viral Load Drop ($\log_{10}$)	Tipranavir Exposure
1250/0	0.77	1×
300/200	1.43	24×
1200/200	1.64	70×

A subsequent phase I study in healthy volunteers examined the fate of radiolabeled tipranavir when coadministered with ritonavir. The results were consistent with the preclinical study of ^{14}C-labeled tipranavir in rats described above. Most of the tipranavir remained in its parent form in both the plasma and the feces, and the feces was the primary extraction route [22].

Finally, a phase IIa study demonstrated that the increased exposure of boosted tipranavir correlated with increased efficacy. In this study, treatment-naive HIV-1 patients were treated with either boosted or unboosted tipranavir monotherapy for 14 days. The viral load results were very clear: The boosted doses were more efficacious, and the efficacy correlated with the tipranavir exposure levels (Table 2) [23].

A number of phase II studies indicated efficacy in various populations, including PI-experienced patients. These studies also indicated that it was feasible to use tipranavir in combination with other antiretroviral drugs as part of combination therapy [19]. The data from numerous phase I and phase II studies suggested that tipranavir was ready for registration studies.

Phase IIb–III

During the phase II studies, tipranavir changed hands. Pharmacia and Upjohn, which had done all of the discovery and early development work, licensed tipranavir to Boehringer Ingelheim (BI) in 2000. The BI team faced some significant challenges as they developed the design of their registration studies. Tipranavir had been studied in several trials, and there were many encouraging results. The formulation and advantages of boosting were well established, but at least two important issues were unresolved. First, the optimal dose was not known. Second, the clinical practices for HIV therapy were changing rapidly. At this time, in the early 2000s, the number of protease inhibitors on the market was increasing, and ritonavir boosting was becoming routine. The BI team needed to discern how tipranavir could meet medical needs in this evolving market, and they needed to design a clinical program that would clearly demonstrate tipranavir's value. The answer to the first part of the problem was fairly obvious: Tipranavir was well suited to treat HIV strains resistant to other protease inhibitors. It was a promising second- or third-line drug. The question of how best to design the clinical trials to demonstrate tipranavir's ability to treat resistant virus was more challenging.

The first step in getting approval for tipranavir was to determine the best dose to use in phase III studies, and the BI team designed a short, efficient phase IIb study to answer this question. This study was designed to resemble the planned phase III in terms of patient population and background therapy, but the dose-finding study was only 2 weeks long. The study compared, in double-blind fashion, the performance of three different b.i.d. doses of tipranavir/ritonavir (TPV/r): 500/100, 500/200, and 750/200 mg. Patients changed the protease component of their therapy to one of the boosted tipranavir doses but maintained the other components of their regimen. The BI team selected the TPV/r 500/200-mg dose, based on safety, pharmacokinetics, and antiviral activity. The study also noted that patients with virus containing three or more mutations in the HIV protease at positions 33, 82, 84, or 90 were not likely to respond to tipranavir or other protease inhibitors, and these criteria were incorporated into the phase III study design [19].

The BI team chose to use open-label studies for their phase III development program, which is unusual for registration studies. Rather than selecting a single standard comparator protease inhibitor, patients randomized to the comparator groups of the studies used the optimal protease inhibitor, based on the genotype of the patient's virus, dosed in its most convenient fashion, which was not compatible with double-blinding the studies. The BI team expected this design to lead to faster enrollment and a broader comparison of protease inhibitors. In this design it was not necessary to use placebo to supplement lower-dose protease regimens and make them appear to match the highest-dose protease regimens. The investigators simply selected the best protease inhibitor for the patient, and the patients used the drugs in their approved doses [19]. It is interesting to note that this trial design also allows any advantages associated with more convenient dosing regimens to contribute to the efficacy of the drugs. Adherence can play a significant role in the efficacy of a regimen, so this factor could be relevant to the clinical experience of patients, particularly outside the structure of clinical trials.

The problem with open-label studies is that it is very difficult to eliminate bias. The BI team took several steps to address this issue. They preselected an objective endpoint that would be difficult to bias: viral load drop of at least 1 $\log_{10}$. They required care providers and patients to select their optimal background and comparator protease inhibitor before randomization to a tipranavir or comparator groups. This also facilitated the randomization, allowing similar proportions of enfuvirtide users to be assigned to the tipranavir and comparator groups. Finally, the BI team offered patients in the comparator arm an opportunity to leave the study after week 8 and receive tipranavir if the patient had a confirmed virologic failure. The option was not offered to patients who left the trial for safety reasons [19].

For the initial submission to the U.S. Food and Drug Administration (FDA), the BI team used 24-week data from two similar phase III studies. Both of these were large, randomized studies in patients with a history of at least two protease inhibitor regimens, and these studies demonstrated the expected efficacy of tipranavir against protease-resistant HIV-1. The RESIST 1 study ($n = 620$) was done in North America and Australia [24], and the RESIST 2 study was done in Europe and Latin America [25]. As shown in Table 3, both studies showed a clear advantage of tipranavir over comparator protease inhibitors. The FDA was concerned about bias in the open-label trial using patients with quite limited treatment options who had an opportunity (at week 8) to switch to tipranavir treatment. To address this potential bias, the FDA analysis used all subjects who met the virologic failure criteria at week 8 as virologic failures at week 24, regardless of whether they took the option to switch treatments. The results of this analysis also indicated an efficacy advantage for tipranavir (Table 3) [26], and based on the 24-week data, tipranavir received accelerated approval from the FDA on June 22, 2005. Based on the 48-week data, also

TABLE 3 Treatment Response, as Defined by $\geq 1 \log_{10}$ Drop in Viral Load, in the Phase III Clinical Trials of Tipranavir[a]

Trial	Time Point (weeks)	TPV/r (%)	CPI/r (%)	Source
RESIST 1	24	41.5	22.3	Published analysis [24]
	24	36	16	FDA analysis [26]
RESIST 2	24	41	14.9	Published analysis [25]
	24	32	13	FDA analysis [26]
RESIST 1 and 2	48	33.6	15.3	Published analysis [27]

[a]TPV/r, tipranavir/ritonavir; CPI/r, comparator protease inhibitor/ritonavir. Both groups also received optimized background therapy.

shown in Table 3 [27], the drug received traditional approval on October 4, 2007.

Although it has a high genetic barrier to resistance, tipranavir is not immune to the development of clinical resistance. Neuger's analysis of the RESIST 1 and 2 24-week data indicated that patients with five or more baseline mutations in the protease were less likely to have a sustained virologic response unless they were also taking enfuvirtide. Tipranavir-treated patients who stopped responding most often had mutations at 101, 13, 33, 36, 82, and 84 [28]. This list of mutation sites is similar to that associated with the resistant strain generated in vitro, and it is similar to the list of predominant mutation sites emerging during tipranavir treatment (33, 82, and 84) identified by the BI development team [19].

Safety

Part of the reason that ritonavir is so effective at boosting the exposure of other protease inhibitors is its ability to inhibit cytochrome P450 3A (CYP3A). This does not, however, just slow the metabolism of the protease inhibitor. It affects the exposure levels of any drug whose metabolism is mediated by CYP3A. Thus, boosted protease inhibitors typically have a number of drug interactions, and tipranavir is no exception. Tipranavir is a potent inducer of CYP3A, but the inhibitory effects of the co-dosed ritonavir overcome this effect, and many of the drug interactions and contraindications are a result of this inhibition. At steady state, boosted tipranavir also inhibits CYP2D6, but it induces two other cytochromes, CYP1A2 and CYP2C19. A number of drug interaction studies have been done, and a listing of drugs that are affected or may be affected by boosted tipranavir is included in the current tipranavir drug label [29].

The adverse events profile of tipranavir is, for the most part, typical of the boosted protease inhibitor class, although the risk of experiencing these events appears to be consistently more frequent for tipranavir than the comparator protease inhibitors used in the phase III studies. The most common events were gastrointestinal side effects, such as diarrhea, nausea, and vomiting, and these usually resolved without discontinuing treatment. Other events that were more common in the tipranavir-treatment groups were grade 3–4 elevations in ALT/AST and hepatic adverse events, which generally did not limit treatment. The tipranavir group also had more grade 3–4 elevations in cholesterol and triglycerides, and more cases of lipdystrophy were observed. These were not associated with an increased risk of pancreatitis, but the long-term risks of these events are unknown [19].

Two risks associated with tipranavir, both of which are potentially fatal, have been included in a box warning on the tipranavir label [29]. The first, a warning of hepatitis and hepatic decompensation, was included on the initial label in 2005, and increased monitoring of patients with hepatitis B or hepatitis C coinfection is advised. The second, a warning of intracranial hemorrhage (ICH), was added to the label in August 2006. Although the mechanism of ICH is not known, a recent publication reports reduced platelet aggregation in humans receiving tipranavir [30]. In all the cases of liver-associated deaths and ICH, the patients had additional risk factors, but additional cases of both these adverse events have been reported for tipranavir patients since the drug was approved [31].

Other Clinical Studies

An oral solution formulation (100 mg/mL) of tipranavir was approved in 2008 for use in pediatric populations. Two other ongoing trials, one in a diverse male and female population of treatment-experienced patients and one in patients coinfected with hepatitis B or C, were recently terminated, due to low enrollment [32]. There is no indication of any development studies targeting additional indications for tipranavir. The drug does not appear to be in development for treatment-naive HIV patients.

CONCLUSIONS

Tipranavir obviously started in a very different place from other approved protease inhibitors, but the interesting question is: Where did it end up? The drug shows a clear advantage in treating protease-resistant viruses. It has a high genetic barrier for resistance, and it is able to inhibit many viral strains resistant to other protease inhibitors. The side-effect profile is similar to other boosted protease inhibitors, but tipranavir appears to have some additional risks, at least relative to the comparator protease inhibitors used in the phase III studies. All of this is consistent with its approved indication for use in highly treatment-experienced patients.

What about the pharmacokinetics of tipranavir? Finding protease inhibitors with good oral exposure was the primary motivation behind the screening effort at Upjohn. The team had potent peptide-derived compounds, but these compounds had very poor oral bioavailability. The initial results of the screen were very promising. The first hit, warfarin, is still widely used as an oral drug, and an x-ray crystal structure of the second hit, phenprocoumon, identified the pharmacophore and facilitated the optimization. Unfortunately, much of the pharmacokinetic advantage was lost as the optimization progressed. As shown in Table 4, the addition of substituents increased interaction with the pockets of the HIV protease adjacent to the active site and led to much better potency, but it also correlated with increased the molecular weight and *c* log *p* values and with lower oral bioavailability. Tipranavir was the first compound derived from a non-peptidic lead structure to achieve the impressive potency of peptide-derived compounds, but the origin of the structure did not remove the need for ritonavir boosting to achieve efficacious exposure levels.

TABLE 4 Comparison of HIV Protease Inhibitors Derived from Screening Hits

	Enzyme Interactions	Enzyme Inhibition, K_i (nM)	Molecular Weight (Da)	$c \log p$	Oral Bioavailability, Rats (%)
5d	S1′–S1–S2	15	324	4.71	99
6b	S1′–S1–S2–S3	0.8	505	5.06	42
7	S2′–S1′–S1–S2–S3	0.008	603	7.14	30

Despite its imperfections, tipranavir is a valuable addition to the antiretroviral tool set. Its well-documented ability to inhibit the drug-resistant virus strains commonly found in highly treatment-experience patients makes it a reasonable option for second- or third-line protease inhibitor therapy, and for many patients, it has been a lifesaver. The strategy of using antiretroviral drugs to control a virus that readily develops resistance is ultimately a stopgap measure. This strategy requires the continual introduction of new antiretroviral drugs. In this respect, the news has been very good in the recent past. Since the approval of tipranavir, another potent protease inhibitor, darunavir, and the first drugs in two new classes—integrase inhibitors (raltegravir) and entry inhibitors (maraviroc)—have also been approved, providing a number of good options for treatment-experienced patients. The true breakthrough in HIV treatment, however, will not come until scientists find the keys, probably in the virus–host interactions, that lead to treatments that help the host immune system either to clear the HIV infection or to neutralize its pathogenic effects. Since neither of these challenges is likely to be met quickly, drugs such as tipranavir will continue to play an important role for patients who need help now. In that most important respect, the tipranavir experiment of starting from a small-molecule screen is a success.

REFERENCES

[1] Peng, C., et al. Role of human immunodeficiency virus type 1-specific protease in core protein maturation and viral infectivity. *J. Virol.* **1989**, *63*, 2550–2556.

[2] Navia, M. A., et al. Three-dimensional structure of aspartyl protease from human immunodeficiency virus HIV-1. *Nature* **1989**, *337*, 615–620.

[3] Richards, A. D., et al. Effective blocking of HIV-1 proteinase activity by characteristic inhibitors of aspartic proteinases. *FEBS Lett.*, **1989**, *247*, 113–117.

[4] Blundell, T. L., et al. The 3-D structure of HIV-1 proteinase and the design of antiviral agents for the treatment of AIDS. *Trends Biochem. Sci.* **1990**, *15*, 425–430.

[5] Centers for Disease Control. http://www.cdc.gov/hiv/topics/surveillance/resources/slides/mortality/slides/mortality.pdf.

[6] Thaisrivongs, S., et al. Structure-based design of HIV protease inhibitors: 4-hydroxycoumarins and 4-hydroxy-2-pyrones as non-peptidic inhibitors. *J. Med. Chem.* **1994**, *37*, 3200–3204.

[7] Vara Prasad, J. V. N., et al. Novel series of achiral, low molecular weight, and potent HIV-1 protease inhibitors. *J. Am. Chem. Soc.* **1994**, *116*, 6989–6990.

[8] Hagen, S. E., et al. 4-Hydroxy-5,6-dihydropyrones as inhibitors of HIV protease: the effect of heterocyclic substituents at C-6 on antiviral potency and pharmacokinetic parameters. *J. Med. Chem.* **2001**, *44*, 2319–2332.

[9] Chrusciel, R. A.; Strohbach, J. W. Non-peptidic HIV protease inhibitors. *Curr. Top. Med. Chem.* **2004**, *4*, 1097–1114.

[10] Romines, K. R., et al. Use of medium-sized cycloalkyl rings to enhance secondary binding: discovery of a new class of human immunodeficiency virus (HIV) protease inhibitors. *J. Med. Chem.* **1995**, *38*, 1884–1891.

[11] Skulnick, H. I., et al. Structure-based design of nonpeptidic HIV protease inhibitors: the sulfonamide-substituted cyclooctylpyranones. *J. Med. Chem.* **1997**, *40*, 1149–1164.

[12] Thaisrivongs, S., et al. Structure-based design of HIV protease inhibitors: 5,6-dihydro-4-hydroxy-2-pyrones as effective, nonpeptidic inhibitors. *J. Med. Chem.* **1996**, *39*, 4630–4642.

[13] Turner, S. R., et al. Tipranavir (PNU-140690): a potent, orally bioavailable nonpeptidic HIV protease inhibitor of the 5,6-dihydro-4-hydroxy-2-pyrone sulfonamide class. *J. Med. Chem.* **1998**, *41*, 3467–3476.

[14] Judge, T. M., et al. Asymmetric syntheses and absolute stereochemistry of 5,6-dihydro-α-pyrones, a new class of potent HIV protease inhibitors. *J. Am. Chem. Soc.* **1997**, *119*, 3627–3628.

[15] Fors, K. S., et al. Convergent, scalable synthesis of HIV protease inhibitor PNU-140690. *J. Org. Chem.* **1998**, *63*, 7348–7356.

[16] Poppe, S. M., et al. Antiviral activity of the dihydropyrone PNU-140690, a new nonpeptidic human immunodeficiency virus protease inhibitor. *Antimicrob. Agents Chemother.* **1997**, *41*, 1058–1063.

[17] Rusconi, S., et al. Susceptibility to PNU-140690 (tipranavir) of human immunodeficiency virus type 1 isolates derived from patients with multidrug resistance to other protease inhibitors. *Antimicrob. Agents Chemother.* **2000**, *44*, 1328–1332.

[18] Chong, K.-T.; Pagano, P. J. In vitro combination of PNU-140690, a human immunodeficiency virus type 1 protease inhibitor, with ritonavir against ritonavir-sensitive and -resistant clinical isolates. *Antimicrob. Agents Chemother.* **1997**, *41*, 2367–2373.

[19] Boehringer Ingelheim Pharmaceuticals, Inc. Tipranavir. Antiviral Drugs Advisory Committee Briefing Document NDA

21-814, Apr. 19, 2005. Available at: http://www.fda.gov/ohrms/dockets/ac/05/briefing/2005-4139b1-02-boehringer.pdf.

[20] Macha, S., et al. Biotransformation and mass balance of tipranavir, a nonpeptidic protease inhibitor, when co-administered with ritonavir in Sprague–Dawley rats. *J. Pharm. Pharmacol*. **2007**, *59*, 1223–1233.

[21] MacGregor, T. R., et al. Pharmacokinetic characterization of different dose combinations of coadministered tipranavir and ritonavir in healthy volunteers. *HIV Clin. Trials*, **2004**, *5*, 371–382.

[22] Chen, L., et al. Steady-state disposition of the nonpeptidic protease inhibitor tipranavir when coadministered with ritonavir. *Antimicrob. Agents Chemother*. **2007**, *51*, 2436–2444.

[23] McCallister, S., et al. A 14-day dose–response study of the efficacy, safety, and pharmacokinetics of the nonpeptidic protease inhibitor tipranavir in treatment-naive HIV-1-infected patients. *J. Acquir. Immune Defic. Syndr*. **2004**, *35*, 376–382.

[24] Gathe, J., et al. Efficacy of the protease inhibitors tipranavir plus ritonavir in treatment-experienced patients: 24-week analysis from the RESIST-1 Trial. *Clin. Infect. Dis*. **2006**, *43*, 1337–1346.

[25] Cahn, P., et al. Ritonavir-boosted tipranavir demonstrates superior efficacy to ritonavir-boosted protease inhibitors in treatment-experienced HIV-infected patients: 24-week results of the RESIST-2 trial. *Clin. Infect. Dis*. **2006**, *43*, 1347–1356.

[26] FDA briefing memo. Aptivus (tipranavir) 250 mg capsules, Apr. 22, 2005. Available at http://www.fda.gov/ohrms/dockets/ac/05/briefing/2005-4139b1-01-fda.pdf.

[27] Hicks, C. B., et al. Durable efficacy of tipranavir–ritonavir in combination with an optimized background regimen of antiretroviral drugs for treatment-experienced HIV-1-infected patients at 48 weeks in the randomized evalution of strategic intervention in multi-drug resistant patients with tipranavir (RESIST) studies: an analysis of combined data from two randomized open-label trials. *Lancet* **2006**, *368*, 466–475.

[28] Naeger, L. K.; Struble, K. A. Food and Drug Administration analysis of tipranavir clinical resistance in HIV-1-infected treatment-experienced patients. *AIDS* **2007**, *21*, 179–185.

[29] Labeling information for tipranavir (Aptivus). Available at http://www.fda.gov/cder/foi/label/2008/021814s005, 022292lbl.pdf.

[30] Graff, J., et al. Significant effects of tipranavir on platelet aggregation and thromboxane B_2 formation in vitro and in vivo. *J. Antimicrob. Chemother*. **2008**, *61*, 394–399.

[31] Chan-Tack, K. M., et al. Intracranial hemorrhage and liver-associated deaths associated with tipranavir/ritonavir: review of cases from the FDA's adverse event reporting system. *AIDS Patient Care STDS* **2008**, *22*, 843–850.

[32] Tipranavir trials close unexpectedly. *AIDS Patient Care STDS*, **2008**, *22*, 833.

5

TMC278 (RILPIVIRINE): A NEXT-GENERATION NNRTI IN PHASE III CLINICAL DEVELOPMENT FOR TREATMENT-NAIVE PATIENTS

JÉRÔME GUILLEMONT
Johnson & Johnson Pharmaceutical Research and Development, Val de Reuil, France

KATIA BOVEN
Tibotec, Inc., Titusville, New Jersey

HERTA CRAUWELS AND MARIE-PIERRE DE BÉTHUNE
Tibotec BVBA, Beerse, Belgium

INTRODUCTION

The last two decades have seen remarkable progress in the management of human immunodeficiency virus type 1 (HIV-1) infections, with the discovery and clinical development of more than 20 anti-HIV-1 agents in six different classes: nucleoside and nucleotide reverse transcriptase inhibitors [N(t)RTIs], non-nucleoside reverse transcriptase inhibitors (NNRTIs), protease inhibitors (PIs), integrase inhibitors, CCR5 antagonists, and fusion inhibitors. Combination therapy for treatment-naive patients usually comprises three drugs, consisting of two NRTIs with either an NNRTI or a PI [1,2], and provides long-term viral suppression. However, the development of these highly active antiretroviral therapy (HAART) regimens with durable efficacy has highlighted existing needs in the treatment-naive patient population, related primarily to tolerability, safety, transmitted and treatment-emergent resistance, and safety in women of childbearing potential.

Side effects and complex dosing schedules are major obstacles to long-term compliance and treatment adherence. The NNRTIs efavirenz (EFV) and nevirapine (NVP) are among the frequently prescribed antiretrovirals (ARVs) for treatment-naive patients because of their effectiveness and their availability as fixed-dose combinations. The first-generation NNRTIs are, however, associated with issues related to tolerability, safety, and resistance. The use of EFV has been associated with central nervous system events and teratogenicity [3,4], and NVP may cause severe and potentially fatal hepatotoxicity and skin reactions [4]. Higher baseline CD4 cell counts (> 250 cells/mm^3 in females and > 400 cells/mm^3 in males) increase the risk of hepatotoxicity and rash, so NVP is not recommended for use in these patient populations. First-generation NNRTIs have a low genetic barrier to resistance, and cross-resistance between these NNRTIs can be brought on by a single mutation in the HIV reverse transcriptase (RT) enzyme [5–7]. EFV and NVP may not be clinically useful in treatment-naive individuals with primary resistance to NNRTIs [8,9].

The investigational next-generation NNRTI, TMC278 (rilpivirine), is a good candidate for treatment-naive patients because its pharmacokinetic (PK) profile enables once-daily (q.d.) dosing, and this together with the low-dose and compatibility with other agents make this agent highly suitable for possible formulation in fixed-dose combinations with other ARVs. In this chapter we summarize the history, preclinical

Antiviral Drugs: From Basic Discovery Through Clinical Trials, First Edition. Edited by Wieslaw M. Kazmierski.

TABLE 1 Antiviral Activity of Analogs of R131459 Against Wild-Type and Mutant HIV-1 Viruses

$EC_{50}{}^{a}$ (nM)

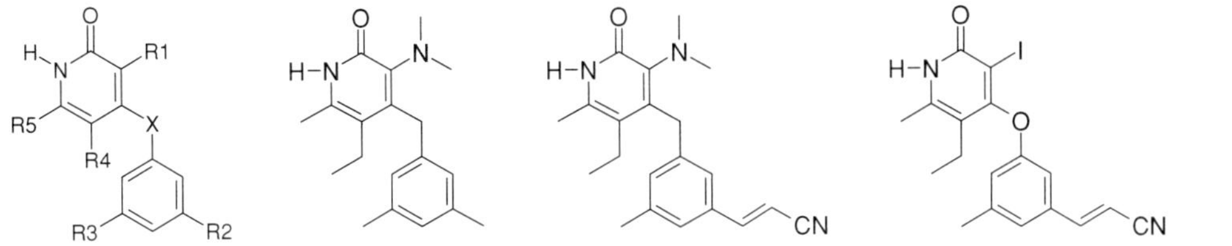

Wild-type	10	0.4	0.8
K103N	32	1.6	0.63
Y181C	125	20	1.3
Y188L	251	125	5.0
F227C/V106F	2512	2512	20

Source: [16].
[a] EC_{50} = 50% effective concentration.

and pharmacologic profile, and clinical development to date of this next-generation NNRTI.

DISCOVERY

Over 30 families of NNRTIs have been developed in the last two decades [10,11]. The marked structural diversity that is displayed by these classes of compounds would suggest that there are still ample opportunities to discover new highly potent NNRTIs. Johnson & Johnson pharmaceutical research and development, in partnership with Institut-Curie (France), contributed to the discovery of the arylpyridone class, with 4-benzyl-3-dimethylamino-2-pyridone (R131459) as the first representative compound [12]. This compound, a hybrid of the Merck pyridone L-697,661 and HEPT derivative, is active at submicromolar concentrations against wild-type HIV-1 and maintains a good level of activity against NVP-resistant HIV-1 strains. To build a structure–activity relationship, a research program was established by medicinal chemists to synthesize and evaluate a wide range of analogs [13] from R131459. The introduction of a *meta*-acrylonitrile moiety on the phenyl ring and replacement of the dimethylamino group in the C3 position by an iodine atom dramatically improved antiviral activity against wild-type and mutant viruses (Table 1) [14,15]. Whereas modifications of the C3, C5, and C6 centers of the pyridinone core formed a solid basis for continued exploration of the iodopyridinone class (IOPY), the poor solubility and bioavailability of the best derivatives led the team to stop its optimization.

A second option was to combine the medicinal chemistry expertise that had been built between the IOPY class [13–16] and the diarylpyrimidine (DAPY) series [17,18] (see Chapter 6). R152929 was selected as a starting point to build a straightforward strategy [19,20]. As suggested by molecular modeling [21], the first approach was based on the modulation of the *para*-substituent on the R152929 tri-substituted phenyl ring. It was decided to evaluate the effect on the activity of the introduction of a G-spacer group between the tri-substituted phenyl ring and the cyano group [19] to significantly increase the interaction with the W229 region of the RT enzyme (Scheme 1). Due to the butterfly-like conformation, DAPY compounds with a cyano group at position 4 on the left wing are very well oriented in the direction of the indole ring of W229. The introduction of a G-spacer group between the cyano group and the tri-substituted phenyl ring optimized hydrophobic interactions among the aromatic rings of Y181, Y188, and W229. The consequence of the extension of this interaction with W229 (CN —CH=CH—CN) was the improvement in the activity against the wild-type and mutant HIV-1 strains. In molecular studies, interaction energies have been calculated and support this explanation. As for the IOPY class, the introduction of the G-spacer groups into the R152929 derivative led to very potent compounds demonstrating high activity against the

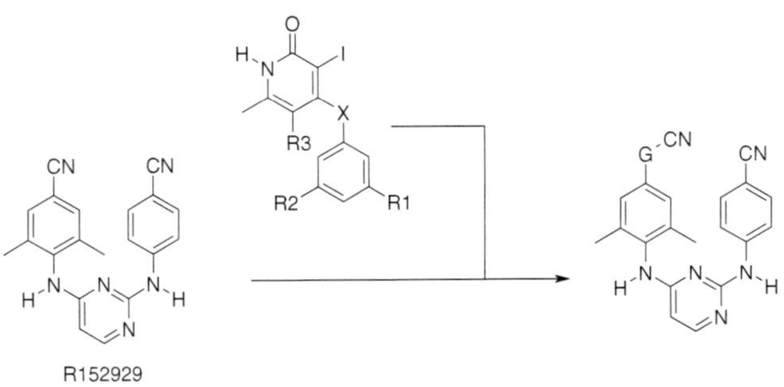

SCHEME 1 Chemical strategy. (From [19].)

TABLE 2 Cytotoxicity and Inhibition of HIV-1: EC_{50} (nM)

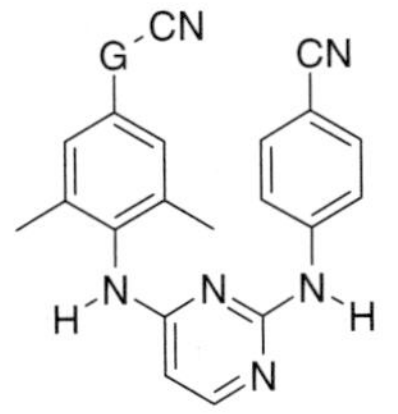

Compound	G-CN	*E/Z*	Type IIIB	CC_{50}	SI[a]	103N	181C	188L	100I	227C	103N + 181C	100I + 103N	227L + 106A
R152929	—CN	—	0.4	5,000	12,500	2	6.3	7.9	31	100	31	1000	12.6
TMC278	—CH=CH—CN	100/0	0.5	30,000	60,000	0.3	1.3	2	0.4	2	1	7.95	1
1	—CH=CH—CN	0/100	0.6	30,000	50,000	1.6	5	31	6.3	4	39.8	794	4
2	—CH=C(Me)—CN	100/0	0.8	20,000	25,000	0.6	1.6	3.1	0.6	2.5	2	31.6	4
3	—CH=C(Me)—CN	0/100	0.8	3,000	3,750	1	4	31.6	3.2	5	20	>10, 000	5
4	—C(Me)=CH—CN	100/0	1	30,000	30,000	1	2.51	4	0.8	5	2.51	25.1	5
5	—CH=CH—CH_2—CN	100/0	1	10,000	10,000	2.5	31.6	20	40	40	N.D.[b]	251	50

Source: [19].
[a]SI, 50% in vitro cytotoxicity concentration (CC_{50})/EC_{50}.
[b]N.D., not determined.

wild-type IIIB virus and the panel of mutant strains (Table 2) with a high selectivity index (SI).

The replacement of the cyano substituent (R152929) by an acrylonitrile group (TMC278: G = vinyl, pure *E*-isomer) [19] led to a very potent compound with EC_{50} values equal to or lower than 1 nM against wild-type IIIB virus and single- and double-mutant NNRTI-resistant strains. Differences of potency between the *E* form (TMC278) and the *Z* form (compound **1**) were in agreement with the docking studies, which showed stronger interactions of the cyano group in the *E*-orientation than in the *Z*-orientation with the W229 region in the binding site of the RT enzyme. Except for compound **3**, substituents in the alpha or beta position on the cyanovinyl group [10,12,13] did not modify the potency against the wild-type single- and double-mutant strains. The introduction of a methylene group between the vinyl and the cyano group was detrimental to the activity.

This study clearly demonstrated the importance of the G-spacer group in DAPY derivatives. With this major modification on the DAPY scaffold, significant progress has been made, especially at the level of the antiviral profile, compared with EFV and its DAPY predecessors. In parallel to the in vitro virologic profiling, preliminary simple experiments in rats and dogs were conducted to select compounds with the best oral bioavailability.

SYNTHESIS

As outlined in Scheme 2, the synthetic method for the preparation of TMC278 involves the two following key building blocks: (**1**) chloropyrimidine and (**2**) 3-(4-amino-3,5-dimethylphenyl) acrylonitrile [19]. TMC278 was prepared by heating the two components in *N*-methylpyrrolidone as solvent in the presence of hydrobromic acid solution in acetic acid. The chloropyrimidine intermediate (**1**) was synthesized in three steps from commercially available 2-thiouracil (**3**) (Scheme 3). The methylsulfanyl intermediate (**4**) was obtained by heating thiouracil (**3**) with sodium hydroxide and methyl iodide at 60°C for 3 h. A 4-aminobenzonitrile (**5**) moiety was added to the pyrimidinone core heterocycle by heating at 150°C for 2 h. A standard chlorination with $POCl_3$ was finally performed to achieve the synthesis of intermediate **1**. The synthesis of the cyanovinyl aniline (**2**) derivative was based on a Heck coupling between a halogenated aniline and acrylonitrile using low loading of Pd/C (0.5 mol%) as a catalyst [22] (Scheme 4).

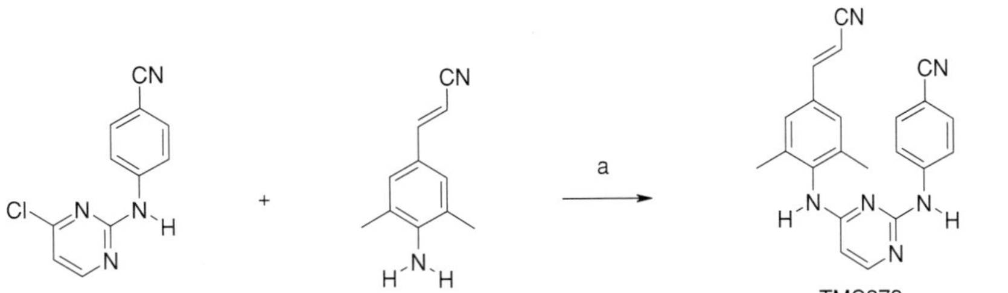

1 2 TMC278

SCHEME 2 Reagents and conditions: (a) NMP, HBr/AcOH, reflux, yield = 80%. (From [19].)

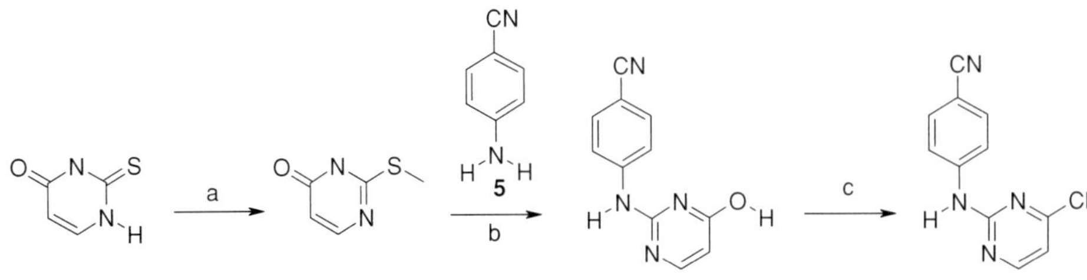

SCHEME 3 Reagents and conditions: (a) NaOH and MeI, 60°C, 3 h, yield = 90%; (b) diglyme, 150°C, 2 h, yield = 80%; (c) $POCl_3$, CH_3CN, reflux, 1 h, yield = 90%. (From [19].)

Therefore, TMC278, as a free base, was synthesized in six high-yield reaction steps. The *E*-isomer of 4-[[4-[[4-(2-cyanoethenyl)-2,6-dimethylphenyl]amino]-2-pyrimidinyl]amino]benzonitrile was obtained and crystallized as a slightly yellow crystalline powder. TMC278 hydrochloride was prepared from aqueous hydrochloric acid in aqueous acetic acid as solvent and recrystallized from an aqueous acetic acid solution.

PRECLINICAL DEVELOPMENT

In Vitro Characterization of TMC278

TMC278 was selected for clinical development based on its potent in-vitro anti-HIV-1 activity against wild-type and NNRTI-resistant strains [23]. The key to the activity of TMC278 lies in the unique structural flexibility of the DAPY class and the plasticity of the TMC278 interaction with the highly flexible NNRTI binding site of RT. This was confirmed by crystal structure analysis of the binding site from the TMC278/HIV-1 RT complex and analyses of the freedom of motion of TMC278 at its binding site. These analyses have revealed the positioning of the compound's cyanovinyl group in a hydrophobic tunnel connecting the NNRTI-binding pocket to the nucleic acid–binding cleft [24,25]. TMC278 has conformational or torsional internal flexibility ("wiggling"), and is able to reposition itself within the flexible NNRTI-binding site ("jiggling"). Adaptation to changes in the RT-binding site has been demonstrated in crystal structures of TMC278 in complexes with the HIV-1 double mutants K103N/Y181C and L100I/K103N [24].

TMC278 was active against wild-type HIV-1 in MT4 human T-lymphoblastoid cells with an EC_{50} value of 0.5 nM [23], which was 2- and 170-fold lower than EC_{50} values obtained for EFV and NVP, respectively (Table 3). In the presence of 50% human serum, the fold change in EC_{50} value (FC) of TMC278 was 9, a shift comparable to that observed for EFV [23]. TMC278 showed a median CC_{50} value of 8.1 μM, resulting in a selectivity index (CC_{50}/EC_{50}) of 16,000. This indicates that TMC278 is a potent and specific inhibitor of HIV-1.

This activity of TMC278, EFV, and NVP was tested against a panel of 22 HIV-1 strains harboring the most prevalent NNRTI resistance-associated mutations (RAMs) constructed using site-directed mutagenesis and homologous recombination techniques [23]. TMC278 retained activity against viral strains that were highly resistant to the first-generation NNRTIs (Table 3). The EC_{50} values for TMC278 against single and double mutants were consistently lower than those for NVP and EFV. Even in the HIV-1 mutant strain with the lowest sensitivity to TMC278, the double mutant L100I + K103N, the EC_{50} for TMC278 was 2.7 nM compared with > 10,000 nM for EFV and NVP.

The antiviral activity of TMC278 was examined using a panel of more than 3500 HIV-1 recombinant clinical

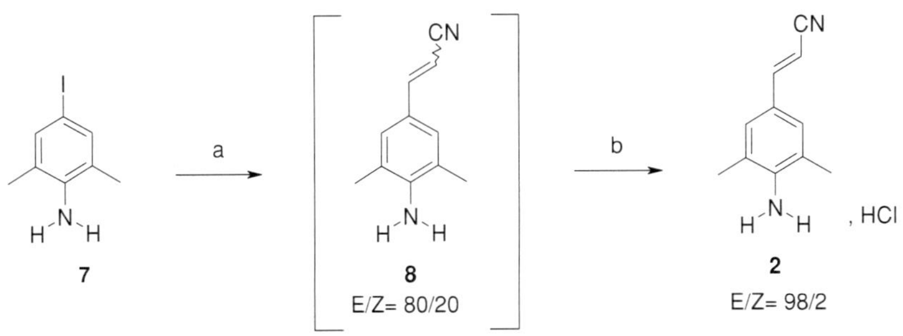

SCHEME 4 Reagents and conditions: (a) Pd/C (0.5 mol%), NaOAc (1.2 equiv), acrylonitrile (1.5 equiv), DMA, 140°C, yield = 80%; (b) EtOH, 6-N HCl in-*i* PrOH, 60°C, yield = 70%. (From [19].)

TABLE 3 In Vitro Activity of TMC278, EFV, and NVP Against Wild-Type and NNRTI-Resistant Site-Directed Mutant HIV-1 Strains

			TMC278	
NNRTI RAMs[b]	NVP[a] Median EC_{50} (nM)	EFV[a] Median EC_{50} (nM)	Median EC_{50} (nM)	FC[c]
Wild-type	85	1.0	0.51	1.0
L100I	638	38	0.37	0.7
K101E	2,467	5.6	1.30	2.5
K103N	5,351	39	0.35	0.7
V106A	2,410	36	0.29	0.6
Y181C	5,351	2.0	1.20	2.4
Y188L	6,722	138	1.60	2.7
G190A	3,465	11	0.30	0.6
G190S	>10,000	344	0.10	0.2
L100I + K103N	>10,000	>10,000	2.70	5.4
K101E + K103N	>10,000	183	0.92	1.8
K103N + Y181C	>10,000	43	1.70	3.2

Source: [23].
[a]Results for NVP and EFV were generated previously.
[b]RAM, resistance-associated mutation.
[c]FC is the ratio median EC_{50} value of the mutant/median EC_{50} of wild type.

isolates, including more than 1500 that were resistant to the first-generation NNRTIs [i.e., having an FC greater than the biologic cutoff for NVP (FC > 8) or EFV (FC > 6)] [23]. Percentages of HIV-1 recombinant clinical isolates with sensitivity to TMC278, EFV, and NVP were determined (Fig. 1). Overall, 89% of these HIV-1 recombinant clinical isolates that were resistant to one or more first-generation NNRTIs had an EC_{50} < 10 nM for TMC278 compared with 33% for EFV and 0% for NVP.

Selection experiments starting from wild-type HIV-1 demonstrated that TMC278 had a higher genetic barrier to resistance development than the first-generation NNRTIs in-vitro [23]. No virus breakthrough was observed at TMC278 concentrations ≥ 40 nM within 30 days after an infection at high multiplicity of infection, whereas breakthrough occurred at 7 or 14 days in the presence of 1 μM NVP or EFV, respectively. Virus breakthrough was observed in some, but not all experiments after 10 days in the presence of 10 nM TMC278. Viruses selected at 10 nM TMC278 contained up to eight mutations, including L100L/I, V106V/I, Y181Y/C, and M230M/I, and showed seven and four FC for EFV and TMC278, respectively. A more comprehensive virology characterization will be published later (manuscript submitted for publication).

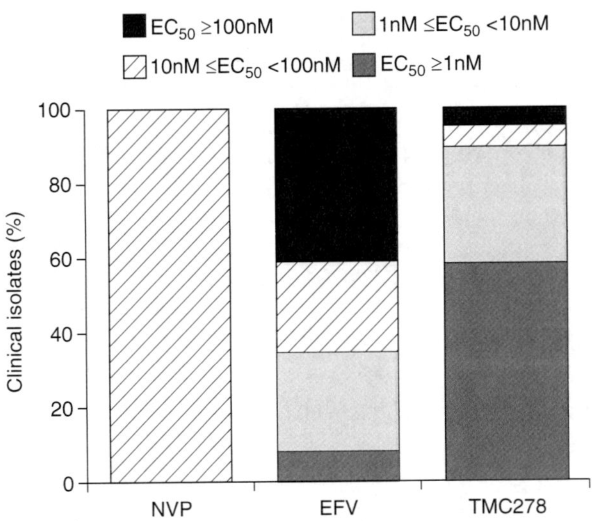

FIGURE 1 Activity of TMC278, EFV, or NVP vs. more than 1500 HIV-1 recombinant clinical isolates resistant to at least one first-generation NNRTI. (From [23].)

Nonclinical Pharmacokinetic Properties

On the basis of in vitro metabolism studies in hepatocytes and in vivo studies of oral TMC278 in dogs (oral bioavailability of 80% with addition of citric acid; elimination half-life of 39 h), slow metabolic clearance of TMC278 was anticipated in humans, with good exposure, long half-life, and potential for once-daily dosing [21]. In vitro studies showed that TMC278 is extensively (> 99%) bound to animal and human plasma proteins, primarily albumin [21].

CLINICAL DEVELOPMENT

Clinical Pharmacology Studies

The pharmacokinetics of TMC278 have been investigated in a number of healthy volunteer studies as well as in patients in proof-of-concept studies, the phase IIb dose-finding study, and will be investigated further in the ongoing phase III studies. TMC278 is well absorbed after oral administration as a tablet formulation. The time to reach maximum plasma concentrations (C_{max}) was consistently around 4 h across studies. The specific PK characteristics of TMC278 in healthy volunteers and patients, with a terminal elimination half-life ($t_{1/2}$) of 45 h on average, have confirmed that it is a good candidate for a once-daily dosing regimen [23]. Steady-state conditions are achieved in 11 days. The major route for elimination of TMC278 is via the feces, with only a very minor role for renal clearance [26]. The phase I metabolism of TMC278 is mediated primarily by CYP3A.

The oral bioavailability of TMC278 formulated as the phase III tablet is approximately 45% lower when administered under fasted conditions than when administered with food [27]. Therefore, TMC278 should always be administered with a meal. Administration of TMC278 after a high-fat breakfast or after a standard breakfast resulted in similar exposures [27]. TMC278 exhibited linear pharmacokinetics after single- and multiple-dose administration up to a dose of 150 mg q.d. in healthy volunteers [28]. The steady-state exposure to TMC278 is somewhat lower in HIV-1-infected patients compared with healthy volunteers, and the exposure to TMC278 in HIV-1-infected patients increased less than proportionally to the dose. The average exposure [area under the plasma concentration–time curve from time of administration to 24 h after dosing (AUC_{24h})] to TMC278 after repeated administration (96 weeks) of 25, 75, and 150 mg q.d. in HIV-1-infected patients, was 2767, 5906, and 10,281 ng·h/mL, respectively [26].

Drug–Drug Interactions (DDIs) Several DDI studies with TMC278 have been performed in healthy volunteers. Additional studies are ongoing, including a DDI study with methadone. TMC278 has no clinically relevant effects on the exposure of ethinylestradiol/norethindrone-based oral contraceptives [26], atorvastatin [29], chlorzoxazone [30], ritonavir (RTV)-boosted darunavir (DRV) [31], ketoconazole [32], RTV-boosted lopinavir (LPV) [33], omeprazole [34], paracetamol [30], rifabutin [35], rifampin [32], or sildenafil [36], specifically at the dose of 25 mg q.d., currently being evaluated in phase III trials. All except two of the DDI studies (sildenafil DDI study [36] and oral contraceptives DDI study [26]) have been performed with TMC278 at a dose of 150 mg q.d., which was the highest dose evaluated in the phase IIb dose-ranging trial, to assess the maximal effect of TMC278 on other drugs within the dose range studied. With the TMC278 dose studied in phase III (25 mg q.d.), any effect on the pharmacokinetics of other agents observed would be either similar or lower because of the lower exposure to TMC278 when dosed at 25 mg q.d. The studies demonstrate that in vivo, TMC278 does not affect CYP2E1 activity [30] or CYP3A activity at lower doses [36,37]. A weak induction of CYP2C19 activity observed after repeated administration of TMC278 150 mg q.d. [34] is unlikely to cause clinically relevant changes in the pharmacokinetics of coadministered drugs that are metabolized by this enzyme.

TMC278 is a CYP3A substrate, and its pharmacokinetics can therefore be affected by inhibitors and inducers of CYP3A. Several studies confirmed the key role of CYP3A in the metabolism of TMC278. The CYP3A inducers rifabutin [35] and rifampin [32] reduced the steady-state exposure (AUC_{24h}) to TMC278 by 46 and 80%, respectively, and should not be coadministered with TMC278 25 mg q.d. The CYP3A inhibitors ketoconazole [32], RTV-boosted LPV [33], and RTV-boosted DRV [31] enhanced the steady-state exposure (AUC_{24h}) to TMC278, by 49, 52, and 130%, respectively.

TMC278 has a low solubility, especially at higher pH. The solubility and hence the absorption of TMC278 may thus be influenced by drugs that increase the gastric pH. The steady-state exposure (AUC_{24h}) to TMC278 150 mg q.d. decreased when coadministered with the proton pump inhibitor omeprazole (40%) [34] or the H_2-antagonist famotidine when administered 2 h before TMC278 (76%), but not 12 h before or 4 h after TMC278 [38]. Thus, separated intake of TMC278 and H_2-antagonists (i.e., 12 h before or 4 h after TMC278) or antacids such as aluminum hydroxide and magnesium hydroxide (i.e., 2 h before or 4 h after TMC278) is a suitable option for patients on TMC278 who require gastric acid–reducing therapy. Atorvastatin [29], chlorzoxazone [30], paracetamol [30], sildenafil [36], or ethinylestradiol/norethindrone-based oral contraceptives [26] had no clinically significant effects on the exposure to TMC278.

In the absence of saturation of metabolic pathways, as suggested by the linear pharmacokinetics of TMC278 at dosages up to 150 mg q.d. in healthy volunteers, it is anticipated that the results of DDI trials performed with TMC278 150 mg q.d. can be extrapolated to a dose of 25 mg q.d.

TMC278 and NRTIs Based on the metabolic profiles and elimination routes, interaction of TMC278 with NRTIs is unlikely. Tenofovir (TDF), emtricitabine (FTC), and lamivudine (3TC) are eliminated mainly via the kidney. In an interaction study, TMC278 150 mg q.d. modestly increased TDF exposure (AUC_{24h}) by 23%, which is not considered clinically relevant. TDF did not affect the exposure to TMC278 [39]. The results of a PK substudy of the phase IIb dose-finding trial demonstrated that the TMC278 dose level had no influence on the pharmacokinetics and metabolism of zidovudine (AZT) [26]. For abacavir (ABC), the primary route for elimination is metabolism via alcohol dehydrogenase, which is not inhibited by TMC278 in vitro at concentrations well above those observed with a dose of 25 mg q.d. [26].

Phase IIa Proof-of-Concept Study in Treatment-Naive Patients

TMC278-C201 was a randomized double-blind placebo-controlled dose-escalating trial designed to evaluate the short-term (7-day) antiviral and immunologic efficacy, safety and tolerability, pharmacokinetics, and viral phenotypic/genotypic patterns of monotherapy with TMC278 25, 50, 100, or 150 mg q.d. in 47 treatment-naive HIV-1-infected patients [40]. All dosages of TMC278 gave statistically significant reductions in plasma viral load from baseline to day 8 (primary endpoint). The median change ranged from –1.1 to –1.3 $\log_{10}$ HIV-1 RNA copies/mL. There was no apparent dose relationship for antiviral activity. Compared with placebo (median change from baseline at day 8 was +0.002 $\log_{10}$ HIV-1 RNA copies/mL), all dosages were statistically significantly different ($p < 0.01$; Wilcoxon rank-sum test for pairwise comparisons). Changes in CD4 and CD8 cell counts were highly variable and not clinically relevant overall. No NNRTI-associated resistance was observed, and TMC278 was well tolerated with no relevant differences in tolerability profiles between active treatment and placebo.

Phase IIb Development

TMC278-C204 Study Design The phase IIb TMC278-C204 trial (ClinicalTrials.gov identifier NCT00110305) is an ongoing multinational (54 centers in 14 countries) randomized active-controlled dose-ranging study that has now been extended to 5 years. A total of 368 treatment-naive HIV-1-infected patients were randomized 1 : 1 : 1 : 1 to receive three-blinded, once-daily doses of TMC278 [25] mg (n = 93), 75 mg (n = 95), 150 mg (n = 91)] or an open-label control EFV 600 mg q.d. (n = 89), all in combination with two backbone NRTIs [41,42]. Investigators selected one of two NRTI regimens (AZT/3TC or TDF/FTC) administered as fixed-dose combinations where available. The primary objective of the study was to evaluate the dose–response relationships for efficacy and safety for TMC278 over 96 weeks (primary analysis at week 48). Secondary objectives included immunological and PK analyses and a resistance analysis.

TMC278-C204 Efficacy Results At week 48, high response rates (proportion of patients with viral load < 50 copies/mL at week 48 according to the time to loss of virological response algorithm, primary objective) of 80, 80, 77, and 81% were seen in the TMC278 25-, 75-, and 150-mg, and EFV groups, respectively [41]. Mean changes from baseline to week 48 in $\log_{10}$ viral load were similar between groups (–2.63, –2.65, –2.63, and –2.64 copies/mL).

The virological response rates were well maintained across groups from week 48 to week 96 (Fig. 2). Proportions of patients with plasma viral loads < 50 HIV-1 RNA copies/mL were 76, 72, 71, and 71% at week 96 [43,44]. Of note, mean CD4 cell counts increased further from baseline over the period from week 48 (122, 145, 143, and 127 cells/mm^3) to week 96 (146, 172, 159, and 160 cells/mm^3).

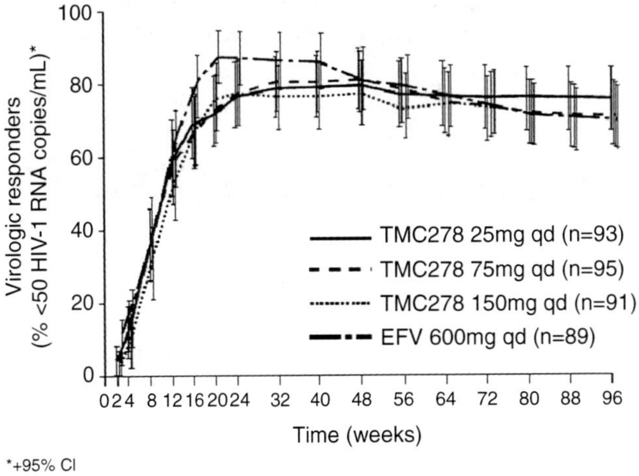

FIGURE 2 Virological response rates (% plasma viral load < 50 HIV-1 copies/mL) over time in study TMC278-C204. (From [44,45].)

Overall, there were no statistically significant differences in efficacy, either among the TMC278 groups or in comparison with EFV, at either week 48 or 96. Rates of virologic failure (defined as patients with loss of virologic response, patients who never achieved confirmed plasma viral load < 50 HIV-1 RNA copies/mL or patients who discontinued before reaching week 96 due to lack of virologic efficacy) were low and were not statistically significantly different between groups at either week 48 (10, 5, 7, and 6%) or week 96 (9, 10, 7, and 8%). Among the failing patients, the proportions developing NNRTI RAMs were similar for TMC278 and EFV [53% (n = 9) vs. 50% (n = 3), respectively] [43,44]. Eight NNRTI RAMs (L100I, K101E, K103N, V108I, E138K, E138R, Y181C, and M230L) were noted in nine patients receiving TMC278, while in the three patients receiving EFV, the NNRTI RAMs K103N and V106M were observed. The most frequent NNRTI RAMs observed in patients receiving TMC278 and EFV were E138K and K103N, respectively.

TMC278-C204 Safety Results TMC278 was generally well tolerated [43,44]. There were few AEs for which there was a difference among the TMC278 doses, although discontinuations due to AEs and rash appeared more frequent in the two higher dose groups than in the 25-mg q.d. group. Most discontinuations on TMC278 were related to laboratory tests. There were no relevant changes in types of AE or noteworthy increases in the incidence of AEs between weeks 48 and 96.

Most EFV withdrawals were due to skin and subcutaneous tissue disorders, psychiatric disorders, and pregnancy.

Incidences of the most commonly reported ($\geq$ 2% of patients in either the combined TMC278 or EFV groups) grade 2 to 4 AEs that were at least possibly related to study medication, including nausea, dizziness, abnormal dreams/nightmare, dyspepsia, asthenia, rash, somnolence, and vertigo, were low in general and were lower with all TMC278 doses than with EFV. Overall, the incidence of any grade 2 to 4 AE that was at least possibly related to TMC278 was 20% in both the TMC278 combined group and the TMC278 25-mg group, which was significantly ($p <$ 0.05, Fisher's exact test) lower than the rate of 37% with EFV.

The overall rate of serious AEs was similar with all TMC278 doses and EFV. The incidence of serious AEs was 12% in the TMC278 combined group, 13% in the TMC278 25-mg group, and 15% in the EFV group. Six patients reported serious AEs at least possibly related to study medication during the first 48 weeks, of which one was reported with EFV (arthralgia) and five with TMC278 (hepatic enzyme increases or cytolytic hepatitis, blood amylase increase, abdominal pain/constipation in the TMC278 25-mg q.d. group, suicide attempt and anemia in the TMC278 150-mg q.d. group). Two deaths, reported in the TMC278 75-mg q.d. group (pneumonia followed by septic shock and cardiopulmonary arrest, and a motor vehicle accident) were deemed not related to study medication.

Incidences of grade 3 to 4 events that were at least possibly related to study medication were not statistically significantly different among TMC278 groups and compared with EFV, occurring in 5% of patients in the TMC278 combined group, in 8% of patients in the TMC278 25-mg q.d. group, and in 8% of EFV-treated patients. Most grade 3 to 4 events were laboratory abnormalities, with overall similar incidences in the TMC278 and EFV groups.

Both neurological and psychiatric AEs were generally less frequent in the TMC278 groups than in the EFV group, with no indication of relationship to dosage. Grade 2 to 4 neurologic events of interest irrespective of relationship to treatment were noted in 7% of patients in the TMC278 combined group, 6% of patients in the TMC278 25-mg q.d. group, and in 15% of patients in the EFV group, with corresponding rates of 8, 10, and 11% for psychiatric events. There were no grade 3 or 4 neurological AEs in patients receiving TMC278 vs. an incidence of 1% grade 3 AEs in patients receiving EFV. The incidence of grade 3 or 4 psychiatric events was low in the TMC278 combined group (2%), TMC278 25-mg q.d. group (1%), and EFV group (1%).

All rashes were of grade 1 or 2 severity, except for one case of grade 3 rash in the TMC278 75-mg q.d. group at approximately 24 weeks on treatment associated with dapsone treatment. This was the only patient in the TMC278 groups who discontinued because of rash. Two patients in the EFV group withdrew because of skin disorders. All other rashes resolved with continuing treatment. No severe (grade 4) rashes were reported. Rashes appeared more common in the TMC278 150- and 75-mg q.d. groups than in the 25-mg q.d. group. The incidence of rash of severity grade 2 or above regardless of relationship to study medication was significantly lower in the TMC278 combined group (3%) or TMC278 25-mg q.d. group (2%) than in the EFV group (11%, $p < 0.05$, TMC278 vs. EFV). There was no association between rash and gender or CD4 cell count for TMC278.

Mean changes from baseline at week 96 in levels of total cholesterol, low–density lipoprotein–cholesterol, high-density lipoprotein–cholesterol, and triglycerides were lower in the TMC278 groups than in the EFV group. There were no TMC278 dose relationships for mean changes in lipid parameters. The TMC278 25-mg q.d. dose was selected for further clinical development in treatment-naive HIV-1-infected patients because it offered the best benefit–risk balance.

Phase III Development

The efficacy and tolerability profile of TMC278 in phase II trials has led to further investigation of this next-generation NNRTI in two fully enrolled ongoing phase III clinical studies in 1374 treatment-naive patients, TMC278-TiDP6-C209 (efficacy comparison in treatment-naive HIV-infected subjects of TMC278 and EFV; ECHO; ClinicalTrials.gov identifier NCT00540449) and TMC278-TiDP6-C215 (TMC278 against HIV, in a once-daily regimen vs. efavirenz; THRIVE; ClinicalTrials.gov identifier NCT00543725). Each of these is a 96-week double-blind double-dummy randomized trial designed to compare TMC278 25 mg q.d. (n = 347 in ECHO; n = 340 in THRIVE) with EFV 600 mg q.d. (n = 347 in ECHO; n = 340 in THRIVE). In ECHO, the background regimen (BR) is fixed to FTC/TDF. In THRIVE, the BR is an investigator choice of ABC/3TC, TDF/FTC, or AZT/3TC. The primary analysis in both trials is at week 48, and the primary objective is to demonstrate noninferiority of TMC278 relative to EFV with regard to the proportion of patients achieving a confirmed plasma viral load < 50 HIV-1 RNA copies/mL at that time point.

FUTURE DIRECTIONS

Pediatrics

The pharmacokinetics, efficacy, and safety of TMC278 25 mg q.d. (phase III tablet formulation) will be investigated in treatment-naive adolescents (aged from 12 to < 18 years) in the 48-week phase II trial TMC278-TiDP38-C213 (pediatric study in adolescents investigating a new NNRTI TMC278; PAINT; ClinicalTrials.gov identifier NCT00799864). In parallel, a pediatric formulation of TMC278 is being developed which will be investigated in children aged less than 12 years of age.

TMC278 Long-Acting Formulation

In addition to the oral tablet and pediatric formulations, TMC278 is being investigated as an innovative, slow-release injectable formulation. The pharmacokinetics and injection-site tolerability of this novel formulation were evaluated after single doses in rats (up to 20 mg/kg) and dogs (up to 400 mg per dog) and after a single subcutaneous or intramuscular injection in healthy human volunteers (doses of 200 to 600 mg) [45]. TMC278 was slowly released from the injection site, resulting in sustained plasma levels for up to 8 weeks in rats and up to 24 weeks in dogs and humans. While injection-site reactions were slightly more common with TMC278 than with placebo, there were no serious AEs, grade 3 or 4 AEs, or rashes.

Potential for Fixed-Dose Combinations with Other ARV Agents

TMC278 is currently still in clinical development but has shown potential for future advantages in terms of dosing requirements in HAART regimens and patient acceptability. Selection of an ARV regimen depends not only on susceptibility of HIV-1 infection to the drugs chosen, but also on other factors, including pill burden and frequency of dosing and tolerability [1]. Despite well-established and well-documented mortality reduction with long-term management of HIV, clinical challenges remain in the real-world clinical setting [46,47]. Regimens are often complex and contain multiple tablets with the need for frequent administration. Maintenance of adherence under these circumstances can be difficult, and failure to adhere to therapy over the long term can adversely influence clinical outcomes [48,49].

Once-daily dosing and the use of fixed-dose combination therapy simplify treatment for treatment-naive patients starting therapy. Evidence is emerging to suggest that simplification of treatment can influence outcomes and enable patients to maintain virologic suppression at least as effectively upon switching to less complex treatment schedules [50]. TMC278 is a small tablet that is given once daily, and as well as the fixed-dose combination with TDF/FTC in development, it could be used in the future in fixed-dose combinations with a range of other ARVs for once-daily dosing.

CONCLUSIONS

NNRTIs as part of a triple regimen are a key component of HAART for treatment-naive patients, provide long-term viral suppression, and are recommended by clinical treatment guidelines [1,2]. The needs for this patient population are safety, tolerability, and convenience, all of which have a bearing on long-term compliance and treatment adherence.

The investigational next-generation NNRTI TMC278 has favorable pharmacological and PK characteristics, including good oral bioavailability and a long half-life. This allows the drug to be administered orally as a convenient, once-daily single pill and in fixed-dose combinations with other ARVs. In the phase II TMC278-C204 trial, TMC278 demonstrated durable and robust antiviral efficacy in treatment-naive patients over 96 weeks, similar to that seen with EFV-based treatment. TMC278 appeared to be generally better tolerated than EFV, with lower incidences of neuropsychiatric AEs, rash, and fewer lipid disturbances. Confirmation of the encouraging observations from the phase II TMC278-C204 trial is being sought in two ongoing phase III double-blind comparisons of TMC278 25 mg q.d. with EFV 600 mg q.d. in treatment-naive patients. TMC278 is also being investigated in children and adolescents, and as a long-acting parenteral formulation.

Acknowledgments

The authors wish to acknowledge the medical writers Ian Woolveridge and Christopher J. Dunn of Gardiner-Caldwell Communications for their assistance in drafting the chapter and in coordinating author contributions. This support was funded by Tibotec. The authors would also like to express gratitude to Andrew Clark, Yaswant Dayaram, Ralph DeMasi, Stephan Marks, Hans Vanavermaete, Kati Vandermeulen, Simon Vanveggel, Dirk Wante, Peter Williams, and Brian Woodfall for their input.

REFERENCES

[1] Hammer, S. M.; Eron, J. J., Jr.; Reiss, P.; et al. Antiretroviral treatment of adult HIV infection: 2008 recommendations of the International AIDS Society–USA panel. *JAMA* **2008**, *300*, 555–570.

[2] European AIDS Clinical Society. Guidelines for the clinical management and treatment of HIV infected adults in Europe, Version 4, Oct. 2008. Available at http://www.eacs.eu/guide/index.htm. Accessed Feb. 6, 2009.

[3] Pérez-Molina, J. A. Safety and tolerance of efavirenz in different antiretroviral regimens: results from a national multicenter prospective study in 1,033 HIV-infected patients. *HIV Clin. Trials* **2002**, *3*, 279–286.

[4] DHHS Panel on Antiretroviral Guidelines for Adult and Adolescents. Guidelines for the use of antiretroviral agents in HIV-infected adults and adolescents. Department of Health and Human Services, Jan. 29, 2008; pp. 1–133. Available at http://www.aidsinfo.nih.gov/ContentFiles/AdultandAdolescentGL.pdf. Accessed Feb. [5], 2009.

[5] Vingerhoets, J.; Azijn, H.; Fransen, E.; et al. TMC125 displays a high genetic barrier to the development of resistance:

evidence from in vitro selection experiments. *J. Virol.* **2005**, *79*, 12773–12782.

[6] Bacheler, L.; Jeffrey, S.; Hanna, G.; et al. Genotypic correlates of phenotypic resistance to efavirenz in virus isolates from patients failing nonnucleoside reverse transcriptase inhibitor therapy. *J. Virol.* **2001**, *75*, 4999–5008.

[7] Antinori, A.; Zaccarelli, M.; Cingolani, A.; et al. Cross-resistance among nonnucleoside reverse transcriptase inhibitors limits recycling efavirenz after nevirapine failure. *AIDS Res. Hum. Retroviruses* **2002**, *18*, 835–838.

[8] Geretti, A. M. Epidemiology of antiretroviral drug resistance in drug-naive persons. *Curr. Opin. Infect. Dis.* **2007**, *20*, 22–32.

[9] Leigh Brown, A. J.; Frost, S. D.; Mathews, W. C.; et al. Transmission fitness of drug-resistant human immunodeficiency virus and the prevalence of resistance in the antiretroviral-treated population. *J. Infect. Dis.* **2003**, *187*, 683–686.

[10] De Clercq, E. Perspectives of nonnucleoside reverse transcriptase inhibitors (NNRTIs) in the therapy of HIV-1 infection. *Farmaco* **1999**, *54*, 26–45.

[11] De Clercq, E. New developments in anti-HIV chemotherapy. *Biochim. Biophys. Acta* **2002**, *1587*, 258–275.

[12] Benjahad, A.; Courte, K.; Guillemont, J.; et al. 4-Benzyl- and 4-benzoyl-3-dimethylaminopyridin-2(1*H*)-ones, a new family of potent anti-HIV agents: optimization and in vitro evaluation against clinically important HIV mutant strains. *J. Med. Chem.* **2004**, *47*, 5501–5514.

[13] Benjahad, A.; Croisy, M.; Monneret, C.; et al. 4-Benzyl and 4-benzoyl-3-dimethylaminopyridin-2(1*H*)-ones: in vitro evaluation of new C-3-amino-substituted and C-5,6-alkyl-substituted analogues against clinically important HIV mutant strains. *J. Med. Chem.* **2005**, *48*, 1948–1964.

[14] Benjahad, A.; Guillemont, J.; Andries, K.; Nguyen, C. H.; Grierson, D. S. 3-Iodo-4-phenoxypyridinones (IOPY's), a new family of highly potent non-nucleoside inhibitors of HIV-1 reverse transcriptase. *Bioorg. Med. Chem. Lett.* **2003**, *13*, 4309–4312.

[15] Benjahad, A.; Oumouch, S.; Guillemont, J.; et al. Structure–activity relationship in the 3-iodo-4-phenoxypyridinone (IOPY) series: the nature of the C-3 substituent on anti-HIV activity. *Bioorg. Med. Chem. Lett.* **2007**, *17*, 712–716.

[16] Himmel, D. M.; Das, K.; Clark, A. D., Jr.; et al. Crystal structures for HIV-1 reverse transcriptase in complexes with three pyridinone derivatives: a new class of non-nucleoside inhibitors effective against a broad range of drug-resistant strains. *J. Med. Chem.* **2005**, *48*, 7582–7591.

[17] Guillemont, J. Discovery of TMC278: a next generation NNRTI drug, highly active against human immunodeficiency virus type-1. XXth International Symposium on Medicinal Chemistry, Vienna, Austria. 2008. Abstract LO9.

[18] Heeres, J., Lewi, P. J. The medicinal chemistry of the data and DAPY series of HIV-1 non-nucleoside reverse transcriptase inhibitors (NNRTIS). *Adv. Antiviral Drug. Des.* **2007**, *5*, 213–242.

[19] Guillemont, J.; Pasquier, E.; Palandjian, P.; et al. Synthesis of novel diarylpyrimidine analogues and their antiviral activity against human immunodeficiency virus type 1. *J. Med. Chem.* **2005**, *48*, 2072–2079.

[20] Mordant, C.; Schmitt, B.; Pasquier, E.; et al. Synthesis of novel diarylpyrimidine analogues of TMC278 and their antiviral activity against HIV-1 wild-type and mutant strains. *Eur. J. Med. Chem.* **2007**, *42*, 567–579.

[21] Janssen, P. A. J.; Lewi, P. J.; Arnold, E.; et al. In search of a novel anti-HIV drug: multidisciplinary coordination in the discovery of 4-[[4-[[4-[(1*E*)-cyanoethenyl]-2,6-dimethylphenyl]amino]-2-pyrimidinyl]amino]benzonitrile (R278474, rilpivirine). *J. Med. Chem.* **2005**, *48*, 1901–1909.

[22] Schils, D.; Stappers, F.; Solberghe, G.; et al. Ligandless heck coupling between a halogenated aniline and acrylonitrile catalyzed by Pd/C: development and optimization of an industrial-scale Heck process for the production of a pharmaceutical intermediate. *Org. Process Res. Dev.* **2008**, *12*, 530–536.

[23] de Béthune, M.-P.; Andries, K.; Azijn, H.; et al. TMC278, a new potent NNRTI, with an increased barrier to resistance and favourable pharmacokinetic profile. 12th Conference on Retroviruses and Opportunistic Infections, Boston, 2005. Abstract 556.

[24] Das, K.; Bauman, J. B.; Clark, A. D., Jr.; et al. High-resolution structures of HIV 1 reverse transcriptase/TMC278 complexes: strategic flexibility explains potency against resistance mutations. *Proc. Natl. Acad. Sci. USA* **2008**, *105*, 1466–1471.

[25] Fang, C.; Bauman, J. D.; Das, K.; Remorino, A.; Arnold, E.; Hochstrasser, R. M. Two-dimensional infrared spectra reveal relaxation of the nonnucleoside inhibitor TMC278 complexed with HIV-1 reverse transcriptase. *Proc. Natl. Acad. Sci. USA* **2008**, *105*, 1472–1477.

[26] Tibotec, Inc. Data on file.

[27] Crauwels, H. M.; van Heeswijk, R. P. G.; Bollen, A.; et al. The effect of different types of food on the bioavailability of TMC278, an investigational non-nucleoside reverse transcriptase inhibitor (NNRTI). 9th International Workshop on Clinical Pharmacology of HIV Therapy, New Orleans, LA, 2008. Poster P32.

[28] Hoetelmans, R.; Van Heeswijk, R.; Kestens, D.; et al. Effect of food and multiple-dose pharmacokinetics of TMC278 as an oral tablet formulation. 3rd IAS Conference on HIV Pathogenesis and Treatment, Rio de Janeiro, Brazil, 2005. Poster TuPe3.1B10.

[29] van Heeswijk, R. P. G.; Hoetelmans, R. M. W.; Aharchi, F.; et al. The pharmacokinetic (PK) interaction between atorvastatin (AVS) and TMC278, a next-generation non-nucleoside reverse transcriptase inhibitor (NNRTI), in HIV-negative volunteers. 11th European AIDS Conference, Madrid, Spain, 2007. Poster P4.3/04.

[30] van Heeswijk, R. P. G.; Hoetelmans, R. M. W.; Kestens, D.; et al. The effects of TMC278, a next-generation NNRTI, on the pharmacokinetics of acetaminophen and CYP2E1 activity in HIV-negative volunteers. 8th International Workshop on Clinical Pharmacology of HIV Therapy, Budapest, Hungary, 2007. Poster P67.

[31] van Heeswijk, R. P. G.; Hoetelmans, R. M. W.; Kestens, D.; et al. The pharmacokinetic (PK) interaction between TMC278, a next-generation NNRTI, and once-daily (qd) darunavir/ritonavir (DRV/r) in HIV-negative volunteers. 47th Interscience Conference on Antimicrobial Agents and Chemotherapy, Chicago, 2007. Poster H-1042.

[32] van Heeswijk, R. P. G.; Hoetelmans, R. M. W.; Kestens, D.; et al. The effects of CYP3A4 modulation on the pharmacokinetics of TMC278, an investigational non-nucleoside reverse transcriptase inhibitor (NNRTI). 7th International Workshop of Clinical Pharmacology, Lisbon, Portugal, 2006. Poster P74.

[33] Hoetelmans, R. M. W.; van Heeswijk, R. P. G.; Kestens, D.; et al. Pharmacokinetic interaction between TMC278, an investigational non-nucleoside reverse transcriptase inhibitor (NNRTI) and lopinavir/ritonavir (LPV/r) in healthy volunteers. 10th European AIDS Conference, Dublin, Ireland, 2005. Poster PE4.3/1.

[34] Crauwels, H. M.; van Heeswijk, R. P. G.; Kestens, D.; et al. The pharmacokinetic (PK) interaction between omeprazole and TMC278, an investigational non-nucleoside reverse transcriptase inhibitor (NNRTI). 9th International Congress on Drug Therapy in HIV Infection, Glasgow, UK, 2005. Poster P239.

[35] Crauwels, H. M.; van Heeswijk, R. P. G.; Kestens, D.; et al. The pharmacokinetic interaction between rifabutin and TMC278, an investigational NNRTI. XVIIth International Aids Conference, Mexico City, Mexico, 2005. Poster TUPE0080.

[36] Crauwels, H. M.; van Heeswijk, R. P. G.; Bollen, A.; et al. TMC278, a next-generation non-nucleoside reverse transcriptase inhibitor (NNRTI), does not alter the pharmacokinetics of sildenafil. 10th International Workshop on Clinical Pharmacology of HIV Therapy, Amsterdam, The Netherlands, 2005. Poster P22.

[37] Crauwels, H. M.; van Heeswijk, R. P. G.; Stevens, T.; et al. The effect of TMC278, a next-generation non-nucleoside reverse transcriptase inhibitor (NNRTI), on CYP3A activity in vivo. 10th International Workshop on Clinical Pharmacology of HIV Therapy, Amsterdam, The Netherlands, 2005. Poster P28.

[38] van Heeswijk, R. P. G.; Hoetelmans, R. M. W.; Kestens, D.; et al. The pharmacokinetic interaction between famotidine and TMC278, a next-generation NNRTI, in HIV-negative volunteers. 24th IAS Conference on HIV Pathogenesis, Treatment and Prevention, Sydney, Australia, 2005. Poster TUPDB01.

[39] Hoetelmans, R.; Kestens, D.; Stevens, M.; et al. Pharmacokinetic interaction between the novel non-nucleoside reverse transcriptase inhibitor (NNRTI) TMC278 and tenofovir disoproxil fumarate (TDF) in healthy volunteers. 6th International Workshop on Clinical Pharmacology of HIV Therapy, Québec City, Canada, 2005. Poster P2.11.

[40] Goebel, F.; Yakovlev, A.; Pozniak, A. L.; et al. Short-term antiviral activity of TMC278—a novel NNRTI—in treatment-naive HIV-1-infected subjects. *AIDS* **2006**, *20*, 1721–1726.

[41] Pozniak, A.; Morales-Ramirez, J.; Mohapi, L.; et al. 48-week primary analysis of trial TMC278-C204: TMC278 demonstrates potent and sustained efficacy in ARV-naïve patients. 14th Conference on Retroviruses and Opportunistic Infections, Los Angeles, 2005. Abstract: 144LB.

[42] Yeni, P.; Goebel, F.; Thompson, M.; et al. TMC278, a next-generation NNRTI, demonstrates potent and sustained efficacy in antiretroviral (ARV)-naive patients: Week 48 primary analysis of study TMC278-C204. 11th European AIDS Conference, Madrid, Spain, 2005. Poster P7.2/08.

[43] Santoscoy, M.; Cahn, P.; Gonzales, C.; et al. TMC278, an investigational next-generation NNRTI, demonstrates long-term efficacy and tolerability in ARV-naïve patients: 96-week results of study C204. XVIIth International AIDS Conference, Mexico City, Mexico, 2008. Abstract TUAB0103.

[44] Molina, J.-M.; Cordes, C.; Ive, P.; et al. Efficacy and safety of TMC278 in treatment-naive, HIV-infected patients: Week 96 data from TMC278-C204. 9th International Congress on Drug Therapy in HIV Infection, Glasgow, UK, 2005. Poster P002.

[45] van't Klooster, G.; Verloes, R.; Baert, L.; et al. Long acting TMC278, a parenteral depot formulation delivering therapeutic NNRTI concentrations in preclinical and clinical settings. 15th Conference on Retroviruses and Opportunistic Infections, Boston, 2008. Abstract 134.

[46] Palella, F. J. Jr.; Delaney, K. M.; Moorman, A. C.; et al. Declining morbidity and mortality among patients with advanced human immunodeficiency virus infection. HIV Outpatient Study Investigators. *N. Engl. J. Med.* **1998**, *338*, 853–860.

[47] Mocroft, A.; Ledergerber, B.; Katlama, C.; et al. Decline in the AIDS and death rates in the EuroSIDA study: an observational study. *Lancet* **2003**, *362*, 22–29.

[48] Paterson, D. L.; Swindells, S.; Mohr, J.; et al. Adherence to protease inhibitor therapy and outcomes in patients with HIV infection. *Ann. Intern. Med.* **2000**, *133*, 21–30.

[49] Nieuwkerk, P. T., Oort, F. J. Self-reported adherence to antiretroviral therapy for HIV-1 infection and virologic treatment response: a meta-analysis. *J. Acquir. Immune Defic. Syndr.* **2005**, *38*, 445–448.

[50] Ruane, P.; Lang, J.; DeJesus, E.; et al. Pilot study of once-daily simplification therapy with abacavir/lamivudine/zidovudine and efavirenz for treatment of HIV-1 infection. *HIV Clin. Trials* **2006**, *7*, 229–236.

6

ETRAVIRINE: FROM TMC125 TO INTELENCE: A TREATMENT PARADIGM SHIFT FOR HIV-INFECTED PATIENTS

Koen Andries and Ann Debunne
Johnson & Johnson Pharmaceutical Research and Development, Beerse, Belgium

Thomas N. Kakuda
Tibotec, Inc., Titusville, New Jersey

Michael Kukla
Johnson & Johnson Pharmaceutical Research and Development, Spring House, Pennsylvania

Ruud Leemans
Johnson & Johnson Pharmaceutical Research and Development, Beerse, Belgium

Johan Vingerhoets, Brian Woodfall, and Marie-Pierre de Béthune
Tibotec BVBA, Beerse, Belgium

INTRODUCTION

Recommended treatment of human immunodeficiency virus (HIV) employs a combination of agents designed to suppress viral replication and slow disease progression [1]. Cells infected with HIV copy the viral single-stranded RNA genome into a double-stranded viral DNA via the HIV reverse transcriptase (RT) enzyme. RT inhibitors prevent completion of the synthesis of the double-stranded viral DNA, which prevents viral replication. There are currently two types of RT inhibitors: nucleoside/nucleotide RT inhibitors [N(t)RTIs] and nonnucleoside RT inhibitors (NNRTIs). N(t)RTIs and NNRTIs target the same enzyme but have different mechanisms of action. N(t)RTIs are competitive inhibitors of reverse transcription, which are incorporated into the growing DNA chain, causing viral DNA synthesis to terminate prematurely. NNRTIs are noncompetitive, allosteric inhibitors of RT; they bind directly to the RT, inducing a conformational change that generates the NNRTI pocket and disrupts the active site [2].

The NNRTIs efavirenz (EFV) and nevirapine (NVP) are generally recommended for initial therapy as a result of their efficacy, generally favorable safety and tolerability profiles, and simplicity of dosing [3,4]. Although first-generation NNRTIs do not require pharmacokinetic (PK) boosting with ritonavir (RTV; r), they are associated with some drawbacks, including a low genetic barrier to the development of resistance and cross-resistance due to single amino acid substitutions in the RT. This restricts sequential use of these agents in treatment-experienced patients [5–8]. In addition, specific toxicity issues, such as central nervous system side effects, teratogenicity, hepatotoxicity, and hypersensitivity reactions, including severe and potentially fatal rash, have been reported [9,10]. There is, therefore, a major clinical

Antiviral Drugs: From Basic Discovery Through Clinical Trials, First Edition. Edited by Wieslaw M. Kazmierski.

need for antiretrovirals (ARVs) with higher genetic barriers to the development of resistance, improved safety and tolerability profiles, and activity against NNRTI-resistant virus.

The NNRTI etravirine (ETR; Intelence, formerly TMC125) has been approved for use in combination with other ARV agents for the treatment of HIV-1 in treatment-experienced adult patients [11]. In this chapter we discuss the history of its discovery and development progress in clinical trials to date.

DISCOVERY

Researchers from Janssen Pharmaceutica and the University of Louvain discovered the first HIV-1 NNRTI compound, the tetraimidazobenzodiazepinone (TIBO), in 1987 [12]. A sustained effort to improve on these compounds eventually led to the discovery of ETR. In the early 1990s, a second class of NNRTIs, chemically unrelated to the TIBO derivatives, was discovered, culminating in the synthesis of loviride [13].

During the optimization phase of loviride, a synthetic intermediate was used to synthesize other simple analogs, portrayed by the generic structure **1** (Table 1). Highlighting a few variations of E and Y illustrates how a subtle observation evolved into a significant discovery. The lead structure discovered in the loviride series (**2**; Fig. 1), had an *ortho*-nitro group, and structure–activity relationship (SAR)

TABLE 1 Activity (EC_{50}, nM) vs. HIV-1[a]

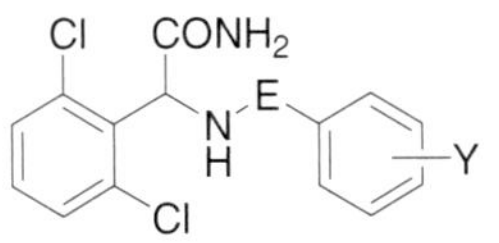

1

Compound	E	Y	EC_{50} (nM)
2	—	*o*-NO_2	100
3	—	*o*-Cl	400
4	—	*p*-Cl	>160,000
5	CSNH	*o*-Cl	>60,000
6	CSNH	*m*-Cl	5,200
7	CSNH	*p*-Cl	160

Source: [14].

[a]All compounds were tested for potency (EC_{50}, nM) to achieve 50% protection of MT-4 cells from HIV-1 cytopathicity as determined by the MTT method [15]. Unless noted otherwise, the IIIB strain of HIV-1 was the infecting virus. Other infecting mutant (in the RT) strains of virus are characterized by the mutated amino acid position and the one-letter codes. For example, Y181C refers to replacement of tyrosine at position 181 with cysteine. Although the data are not reported, in the same experiment mock-infected cells were tested with compound to determine the dose to reduce cells to 50% viability (CC_{50}). Thus, a selectivity index (CC_{50}/IC_{50}) could be determined. All determinations are the result of multiple tests. EC_{50}, 50% effective concentration; IC_{50}, 50% inhibitory concentration.

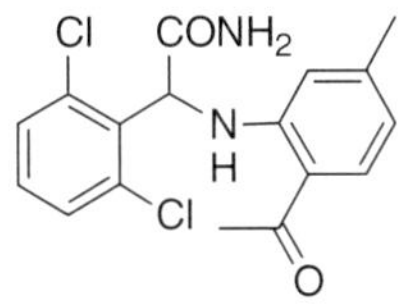

Loviride

FIGURE 1

studies established that compounds in this series were most potent when an *ortho*-substituted phenyl group was present. For example, *ortho*-chlorine substituent **3** was more than 400 times as active as the corresponding *para* substitution **4** (Table 1).

However, when varying E, insertion of a thioamide in combination with Y as a *meta*- or *para*-chlorine (**6** and **7**) resulted in compounds that were much more active than the *ortho* analog (**5**). The level of antiviral activity was modest, but this result was in contrast to previous observations that *ortho* substitution was preferred over *para* substitution. Even though structures **4** and **7** were seemingly very similar, this anomaly in the expected SAR led to the belief that these structures might bind differently in the NNRTI pocket. Consequently, the possibility of a unique SAR for **7** from the loviride series was rationalized and a limited program of structural optimization was undertaken.

To increase the likelihood of identifying new compounds active against NNRTI-resistant strains and which have interesting druglike properties, the SAR, traditionally limited to activity against the wild-type virus, was expanded to include concurrent evaluation of several NNRTI-resistant strains. To facilitate an understanding of the effect of new chemical substituents on the binding of the compounds to wild-type and resistant RT, a panel of mutants was constructed harboring various NNRTI resistance-associated mutations (RAMs) within exactly the same genetic background.

One of the interesting structural attributes of this "new" lead was its flexible nature relative to other NNRTIs. Normally, the best and most potent inhibitor is a rigid structure that fits into the intended site. However, it was reasoned that a flexible structure had a greater likelihood to change slightly, through bond rotations or conformational change, to "refit" into the NNRTI binding pocket that was altered as a result of viral mutation. Consequently, an optimized structure might avoid the loss of activity that other NNRTIs experienced from those mutations.

No substantial improvement in anti-HIV-1 activity was seen until the phenyl acetamide portion of **7** was replaced with benzylimidoyl to give an imidoylthiourea (ITU) structure (**8**, Fig. 2; X = Cl, EC_{50} = 13 nM) [14]. The 10-fold improvement in potency (compared to **7** in Table 1) suggested that the structure could be optimized, giving activity levels similar to those of previous NNRTIs. In fact, when

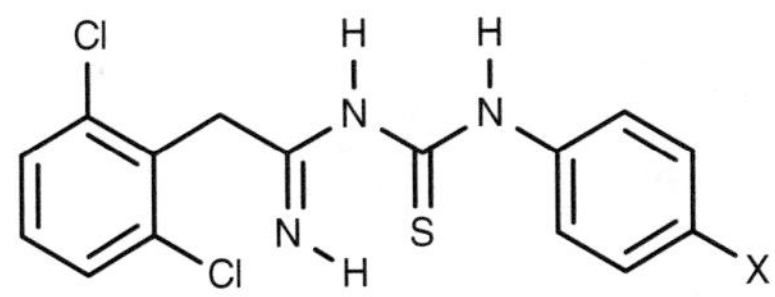

ITU

8

FIGURE 2

X = CN (**9**, Fig. 3), the level of activity (see "ITU" in Table 2) was comparable to the then-marketed products NVP and delavirdine (DLV).

With the ITU compound (**9**), a high level of activity had been attained against the IIIB strain of HIV-1 (EC_{50} = 2.5 nM), but more importantl, when tested against the panel of single amino acid mutant strains of HIV-1, activity was superior to that of NVP and DLV in every instance (Table 2), possibly substantiating the hypothesis that flexible structures might overcome resistance imparted by mutations of the NNRTI binding pocket.

However, it was quickly established that this structure was prone to both hydrolytic and oxidative instability. The latter was shown by the facile conversion to the thiadiazole **10**, a compound completely devoid of RT inhibitory activity. Therefore, an assessment of metabolic stability was included early in the discovery process, thereby establishing a structure–metabolism relationship. The combination of SAR (against wild-type virus and mutants) and structure–metabolism relationship allowed for the concurrent optimization of structures for broad-spectrum anti-HIV activity and metabolic stability.

Preparation of cyanoguanidine analog **11** (Fig. 4), a well-known thiourea bioisostere, was attempted to try to circumvent the instability of the ITU structure. A reaction to form **11** resulted in cyclic DATA **12** and not the desired ITU derivative, which had presumably formed but cyclized spontaneously under the reaction conditions.

Considering the inactivity of the thiadiazole (**10**), it was surprising that **12** was a very potent inhibitor of HIV-1_{IIIB} (EC_{50} = 6.3 nM). Indeed, it was nearly as active as ITU and it was also highly active against a battery of HIV-1 mutant strains (Table 2). The combination of potent biological activity and greatly enhanced structural stability led to a thorough SAR investigation around generic structure **13** (Fig. 5), in which variations of X, Y, and Ar_1 were investigated [16].

Many substituents were acceptable for Ar_1, but derivatives with 2,4,6-trisubstitution were generally the most potent against HIV-1_{IIIB} and were significantly more active

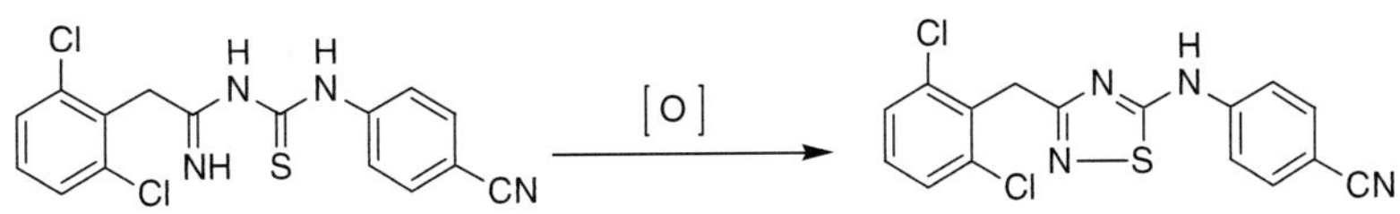

9 **10**

FIGURE 3

TABLE 2 Inhibition of HIV-1 (EC_{50}, nM) by NNRTIs[a]

Compound	IIIB[b]	L100I	K103N	Y181C	Y188L	L100I + K103N	K103N + Y181C
NVP	32	316	6,310	10,000	>100,000	N.D.	>100,000
DLV	63	2,512	2,512	1,995	1,259	N.D.	19,953
EFV	1	40	40	2	158	>10,000	40
Loviride	50	50	63	15,800	1,260	N.D.	N.D.
ITU (X = CN)	2.5	513	589	511	318	N.D.	N.D.
Initial DATA	6.3	398	40	200	316	N.D.	N.D.
Final DATA	0.3	13	3	8	40	1,260	50
ETR	1.4	3.3	1.2	7	4.6	19	4.3

[a]All compounds were tested for potency (EC_{50}, nM) to achieve 50% protection of MT-4 cells from HIV-1 cytopathicity as determined by the MTT method [15]. Unless noted otherwise, the IIIB strain of HIV-1 was the infecting virus. Other infecting mutant (in the RT) strains of virus are characterized by the mutated amino acid position and the one-letter codes. For example, Y181C refers to replacement of tyrosine at position 181 with cysteine. Although the data are not reported, in the same experiment mock-infected cells were tested with compound to determine the dose to reduce cells to 50% viability (CC_{50}). Thus, a selectivity index (CC_{50}/IC_{50}) could be determined. All determinations are the result of multiple tests. N.D., not determined; DATA, diaryltriazine; ITU, imidoylthiourea.

[b]Wild type.

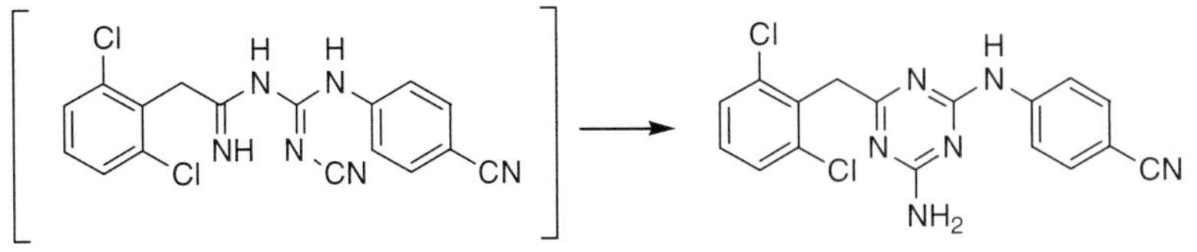

11

12

Initial DATA

FIGURE 4

against all of the HIV-1 mutant strains. The nature of X was not critical, with compounds containing CH_2, NH, O, and S all equally active. Variations of Y were all inactive except NH_2 and NHOH. However, in preclinical studies, the NHOH compound was rapidly dehydroxylated to the original amine. Furthermore, both $Y = NH_2$ and NHOH were readily glucuronidated at the hydroxylamine/amine functionality and excreted.

Many of the analogs with variation of X and substituents at the *para* position of Ar_1 were first synthesized to circumvent metabolic instability. For example, an analog with X = NH and Ar_1 = 2,4,6-trimethylphenyl possessed an excellent potency profile and increased metabolic stability. However, the metabolic vulnerability of $Y = NH_2$ was still a cause for concern.

Contrary to the SAR studies, molecular modeling studies suggested that replacing the 4-NH_2 on the triazine ring with hydrogen should not decrease activity. Indeed, this variation, exemplified as the Final DATA **14** (Fig. 6), was among the most potent of all the DATA compounds against HIV-1_{IIIB} and had a very good profile against all of the HIV-1 mutants tested up to that time (Table 2), as well as good metabolic stability.

New clinically relevant HIV-1 mutations were being identified continuously, including double mutations in the RT. Literature reports indicated that EFV is much more effective than NVP and DLV in most regards (Table 2), but it was ineffective against the double mutant L100I/K103N. In contrast, the most potent DATA analog seemed to show some (albeit weak) activity against the new L100I/K103N double mutant. Simultaneously, replacements for the triazine with other six-membered ring heterocycles, such as pyrimidine, were investigated. Unlike the symmetrical triazine ring, the potential dissymmetry of the pyrimidine ring leads to three possible isomeric structures that were synthesized and are represented by **15a–c** (Table 3). The testing results of **15a–c** compared to the corresponding triazine analog are extremely interesting. Pyrimidines **15a** and **b** were as effective as the triazine **14** in inhibiting HIV-1_{IIIB}, but only **15a** was effective in inhibiting several clinically relevant mutant strains to an even greater degree than the corresponding DATA structure (Table 3).

This led to yet another round of structure–activity variations [17] based on this active pyrimidine. Overall, changes made at the R_1, Y, and R_3 sites on the generic structure **16** (Fig. 7) gave analogs with activity levels very similar to those of the corresponding DATA compounds, including the same weak potency against the L100I/K103N double mutant.

In contrast to a triazine, a pyrimidine has a fourth ring carbon available for substitution, position C5 in this case, indicated here by R_2. The antiviral activities of several variations of R_2 were investigated, and many were found to be ineffective. However, when R_2 was Br, Cl, or acetylene, the activities were comparable to those of the most potent DATA compound. In addition, these analogs had significant activity against the L100I/K103N double mutant.

Many potential clinical candidates resulted from these final SAR studies. ETR (Fig. 8) was chosen based on potency against all the available strains of HIV-1 (Table 2) and its metabolic stability. Early preclinical studies indicated that the solubility and bioavailability of ETR were poor. However, these challenges have since been overcome.

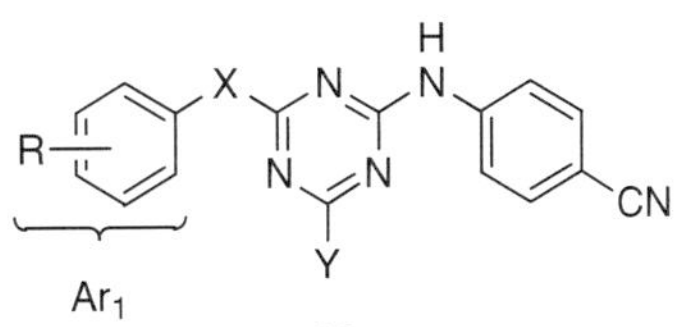

13

FIGURE 5

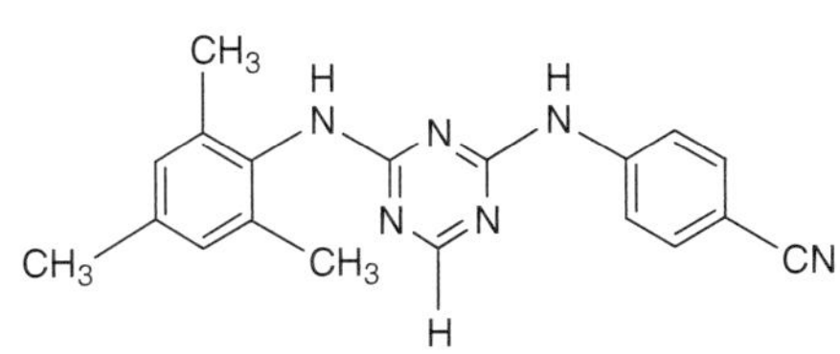

14

FIGURE 6

TABLE 3 Inhibition of HIV-1 (EC_{50}, nM)[a]

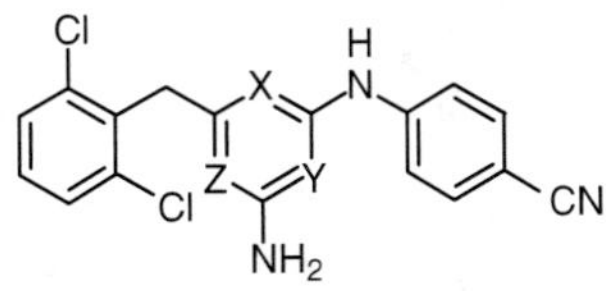

15

Compound	X	Y	Z	IIIB	L100I	K103N	Y181C	Y188L
DATA	N	N	N	6	398	40	200	316
15a	N	N	CH	1	299	12	175	71
15b	CH	N	N	10	96,600	33,300	>100,000	>100,000
15c	N	CH	N	452	>100,000	>100,000	>100,000	>100,000

[a]All compounds were tested for potency (EC_{50}, nM) to achieve 50% protection of MT-4 cells from HIV-1 cytopathicity as determined by the MTT method [15]. Unless noted otherwise, the IIIB strain of HIV-1 was the infecting virus. Other infecting mutant (in the RT) strains of virus are characterized by the mutated amino acid position and the one-letter codes. For examples, Y181C refers to replacement of tyrosine at position 181 with cysteine. Although the data are not reported, in the same experiment mock–infected cells were tested with compound to determine the dose to reduce cells to 50% viability (CC_{50}). Thus, a selectivity index (CC_{50}/IC_{50}) could be determined. All determinations are the result of multiple tests. DATA, diaryltriazine.

FORMULATION

ETR is classified as a Biopharmaceutics Classification System IV compound, characterized by low solubility and low-to-moderate permeability ($\log P > 5$) with a low dissociation constant ($pK_a < 3$). Such compounds typically have low bioavailability when formulated as a conventional oral solid dosage form. In preclinical studies with dogs, low bioavailability was observed when using formulations containing crystalline ETR [18]. Physical modification of crystalline drug to the amorphous state by means of solid dispersion technology was therefore undertaken to improve bioavailability [18]. As ETR degrades chemically during melting, only solvent evaporation methods were evaluated. ETR was initially formulated as a 50-mg capsule with the excipient poly(ethylene glycol) (PEG)-400 for use during early phase I and phase IIa clinical trials. With this formulation, up to 36 capsules/day were administered, representing an unacceptably high pill burden. This formulation was also relatively unstable, thereby limiting the shelf life of the product. Formulation development subsequently focused on increasing bioavailability and/or unit drug load to reduce pill burden while maintaining a robust stability profile. For phase IIb studies, a solid dispersion was prepared via granulo-layering. This approach reduced the pill burden to eight tablets/day [800 mg ETR twice daily (b.i.d.)], acceptable for this stage of development but still unacceptable for late-stage clinical development and commercialization.

For phase III clinical development and commercialization, increased bioavailability and reduced pill number and size were key considerations. Novel methods for manufacturing tablets containing solid dispersions prepared by bead coating or spray drying were therefore pursued. The new formulations were compared with the tablets used in phase IIb studies. Based on the results of the comparative bioavailability studies, spray drying was selected as the manufacturing technique to obtain stable ETR solid dispersions with increased bioavailability. The composition of the spray-dried powder was further optimized, resulting in a fourfold increase in oral bioavailability compared to phase IIb tablets and reducing daily intake to four tablets a day (2 × 100-mg ETR tablets b.i.d.) [19]. This formulation was selected for phase III clinical trials and commercialization.

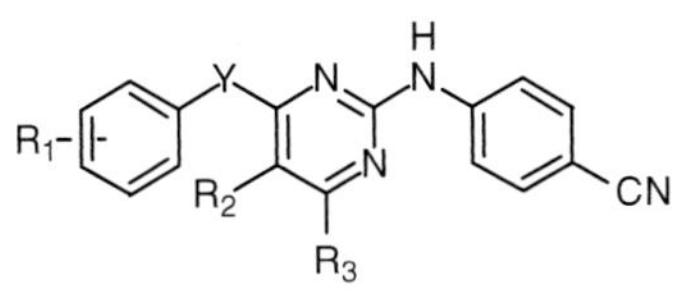

16

FIGURE 7

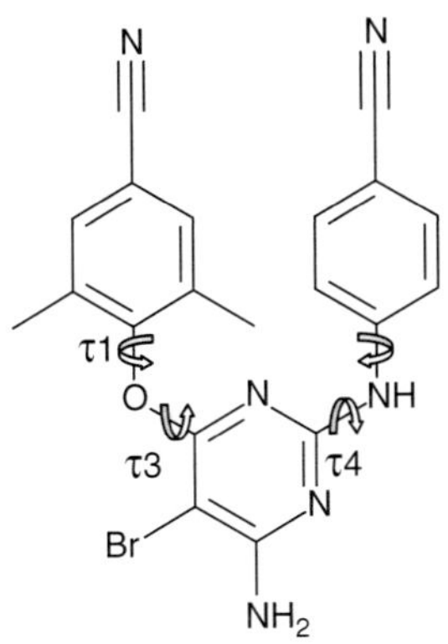

FIGURE 8 Chemical and three-dimensional structure of ETR, showing a highly flexible molecule with four torsion angles ($\tau 1$, $\tau 2$, $\tau 3$ and $\tau 4$), which can accommodate four different mutations in the NNRTI binding pocket.

PRECLINICAL DEVELOPMENT

Resistance to NNRTIs arises because of mutations resulting in altered amino acid positions lining their binding site, with high-level resistance to first-generation NNRTIs often associated with single-point mutations, especially within codon groups 100 to 108 and 181 to 190 [8]. ETR differs from the first-generation NNRTIs in its high degree of molecular flexibility (Fig. 8), which allows the drug to fit the binding site of the RT enzyme when mutations interfering with first-generation NNRTIs are present [20,21]. ETR therefore has an increased genetic barrier to the development of resistance compared with EFV or NVP [5].

ETR displayed excellent activity against panels of NNRTI-resistant viruses, including 82 mutant strains constructed by site-directed mutagenesis and carrying single, double, and triple NNRTI RAMs [22]. The antiviral activity of ETR against NNRTI-resistant HIV-1 was assessed using a panel of 6171 HIV-1 NNRTI-resistant recombinant clinical isolates (Fig. 2a and b). ETR exhibited higher antiviral activity on a larger proportion of viruses from this panel than did the first-generation NNRTIs, having EC_{50} values $\leq$ 10 nM for 83.2% of the viruses and EC_{50} values > 100 nM for only 2% of the viruses (Fig. 9a) [11].

In vitro selection experiments in wild-type and NNRTI-resistant HIV-1 virus strains showed that development of resistance to ETR requires multiple mutations that frequently result in cross-resistance to EFV and NVP [5]. ETR 1 μM completely inhibited the breakthrough of resistant virus from wild-type and NNRTI-resistant HIV-1, in contrast to EFV and NVP. Mutations selected in vitro by ETR included the known NNRTI-associated mutations L100I, Y181C, G190E, M230L, and Y318F and the novel mutations V179I and V179F [5]. These results demonstrated the distinctive profile of antiviral activity of ETR in vitro and its high genetic barrier to the development of resistance.

No concerns relating to carcinogenicity, mutagenesis, or impairment of fertility have been reported with ETR in preclinical animal experiments. Developmental toxicity studies in rats at oral dosages up to 1000 mg/kg daily and in rabbits receiving up to 375 mg/kg daily have shown no treatment-related embryo–fetal effects [23]. ETR had no effect on offspring development or maturation during lactation or post–weaning phases [23]. Hemorrhagic cardiomyopathy has been observed in male mice treated with ETR, however, this is not thought to be directly related to ETR [24]. These preclinical findings have been superseded by the clinical trial results, where no clinically significant cardiac or hematologic effects were observed with ETR.

ETR is extensively protein-bound (99.6% to human albumin and up to 97.7% to α_1-acid glycoprotein [11]). Metabolism takes place predominantly in the liver by methylhydroxylation via cytochrome P450 (CYP) isoenzymes 3A4, 2C9, and 2C19, with subsequent glucuronidation of the metabolites. ETR is a weak inducer of CYP3A and a weak inhibitor of P-glycoprotein, CYP2C9, and CYP2C19. It is not a substrate for P-glycoprotein [11,25].

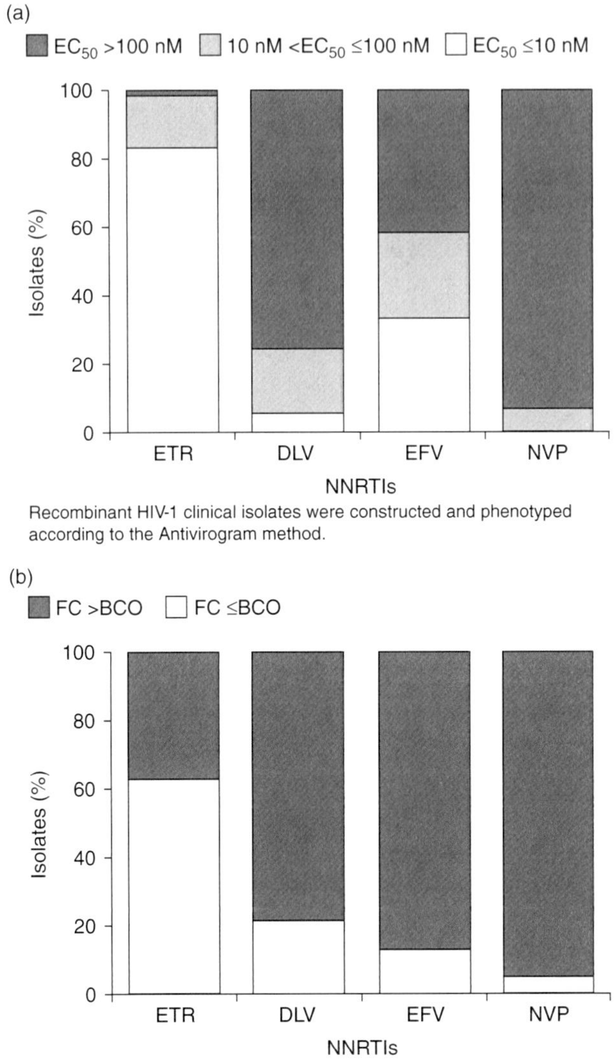

Recombinant HIV-1 clinical isolates were constructed and phenotyped according to the Antivirogram method. Resistance was defined as a FC value greater than the biological cutoff (BCO) as defined by the Antivirogram (version 2.4.00), 3.4 for EFV, 5.5 for NVP, and 10.5 for DLV. In the absence of a BCO value for ETR, the lowest BCO available (3.4) was used.

FIGURE 9 (a) Percentage of the 6171 HIV-1 NNRTI-resistant recombinant clinical isolates clustered by EC_{50} values; (b) percentages of the 6171 HIV-1 NNRTI-resistant recombinant clinical isolates distributed by fold change in EC_{50} (FC).

CLINICAL DEVELOPMENT

Clinical Pharmacology Studies

The pharmacokinetics of ETR have been studied in HIV-negative, healthy adult volunteers, in HIV-1-infected adult patients, and more recently in HIV-1-infected children and adolescents. Currently, the recommended dosage of ETR for adults is 200 mg (2 × 100-mg tablets) b.i.d. following a meal, in combination with other ARV drugs [11]. In a single-dose mass-balance study of radiolabeled ETR in six volunteers, the median time to peak plasma drug concentration (T_{max}) was 3.5 h and median half-life ($t_{1/2}$) was 41 h [26]. Elimination takes place primarily in the feces (94%), with minimal excretion in urine (1.2%). ETR is mostly excreted unchanged (up to 86%) within 24 to 48 h, and 95% of the dose is recovered within 168 h of administration [26]. The phase III/commercial formulation has a distribution $t_{1/2}$ value of 3.9 to 5.4 h after multiple doses, and a terminal elimination $t_{1/2}$ value of 30 to 40 h [25].

ETR does not prolong the QTc interval or cause clinically relevant changes in an electrocardiogram [27]. Neither mild nor moderate hepatic impairment affects the pharmacokinetics of ETR [28]. ETR exposure is increased in the presence of food; overall mean exposure was 51% lower in the fasted state than when dosing after a standard breakfast [29]. Therefore, ETR should be taken following a meal to maximize bioavailability. ETR is readily dispersible in water without compromising its bioavailability [30], offering an alternative dosing option for patients who prefer not to take tablets.

The pharmacokinetics and pharmacodynamics of ETR in HIV-infected patients were investigated in the phase III DUET trials [31]. A population PK model for the phase III formulation of ETR was developed from sparse plasma sampling in the main study and from rich sampling in a substudy. The mean (standard deviation, S.D.) population estimated ETR area under the plasma concentration–time curve over 12 hours (AUC_{12h}) was 5506 (4710) ng·h/mL, and the predose plasma drug concentration (C_{0h}) was 393 (391) ng/mL. The apparent oral clearance was 43.7 L/h, and the interpatient variability of that parameter was 60%. Intrapatient variability for fraction absorbed was 40%. Covariate analysis showed no relevant effect of gender, age, weight, race, renal function, viral hepatitis status, or use of enfuvirtide (ENF) on ETR pharmacokinetics. ETR AUC_{12h} and C_{0h} were not associated with virologic response, and there were no apparent relationships between pharmacokinetics and adverse events (AEs) or laboratory changes. The incidence of rash was not linked to ETR exposure [31].

The pharmacokinetics of ETR in children and adolescents have recently been investigated [32]. ETR doses of 4 and 5.2 mg/kg b.i.d. resulted in comparable exposure in children to that in adults receiving ETR 200 mg b.i.d. [19,31]. There were no tolerability concerns and no apparent association between ETR exposure and two cases of mild-to-moderate rash. Due to the lack of any safety signal in this trial, and to alleviate the general concern related to underdosing in children, a dose of 5.2 mg/kg b.i.d. was chosen for further investigation in an ongoing 48-week phase II trial.

Two phase I studies in healthy HIV-negative volunteers have shown similar exposure to ETR whether the drug is given once daily (q.d.) or b.i.d. [33]. Furthermore, the addition of once-daily DRV/r to once-daily ETR had no effect on ETR pharmacokinetics [34].

Comprehensive drug–drug interaction (DDI) data have been collected for ETR. Briefly, ETR may be coadministered without dose adjustment with a wide range of agents, including N(t)RTIs, most boosted protease inhibitors (PIs), raltegravir, elvitegravir, ENF, pH modifiers, narcotic analgesics, oral contraceptives, and selective-serotonin reuptake inhibitors. Dose adjustment of the coadministered drug may be required when administering ETR with atazanavir/r, fosamprenavir/r, maraviroc, rifabutin, atorvastatin, and sildenafil, and local prescribing information should be consulted. ETR should not be coadministered with EFV, NVP, DLV, tipranavir/r, or unboosted PIs [11,25,35–37].

Phase IIa Proof-of-Concept Studies

The clinical efficacy of ETR has been evaluated in a comprehensive program that started with two proof-of-concept phase II studies, TMC125-C208 in treatment-naive patients [38] and TMC125-C207 in patients with NNRTI-resistant virus [39]. In study TMC125-C208, patients receiving ETR reported a mean decrease from baseline in plasma VL of 1.99 $\log_{10}$ HIV-1 RNA copies/mL, compared with 0.06 $\log_{10}$ HIV-1 RNA copies/mL in patients receiving placebo ($p < 0.001$) [38]. Results from study TMC125-C207 showed a statistically significant reduction in rate of plasma viral load (VL) decay/day (the primary endpoint) of 0.13 $\log_{10}$ HIV-1 RNA copies/mL/day with ETR ($p < 0.001$) [39]. This was the first study to show the successful use of ETR in patients with NNRTI-resistant virus.

Phase IIb Development

Further investigation was undertaken in the phase IIb studies TMC125-C203 [40], TMC125-C223 [41], and TMC125-C227 [42] (Table 4).

TMC125-C203 The primary objective of this trial was to evaluate ETR safety and tolerability with long-term dosing. In general, there was no evidence of a relationship between ETR dose and specific AEs. Most AEs were grade 1 or 2 in severity, and the incidence of grade 3 or 4 AEs was comparable between the treatment groups (27.0% and 27.3% in the combined ETR and placebo groups, respectively).

The incidence of rash was higher in the combined ETR groups compared with the placebo group, with no substantial differences between the three ETR dose groups. Most rashes were mild to moderate in severity; six ETR-treated patients discontinued treatment due to rash. The 24-week results of this study assisted with the design of study TMC125-C223

TABLE 4 Phase IIb Studies of ETR in Treatment-Experienced HIV-1-Infected Patients

Trial	Study Design[a]	Study Treatment	Major Results
TMC125-C203 [40]	r, pc, db	Stage 1: ETR 400 or 800 mg b.i.d. or placebo; Stage 2: ETR 800 or 1200 mg b.i.d. or placebo; 48 weeks	Grade 3–4 AEs: 27% ETR vs. 27.3% placebo; neuropsychiatric AEs: 47% vs. 46%; hepatic AEs: 3% vs. 6%; rash 19% vs. 12% Stage 1: no statistically significant difference between ETR groups and placebo for the change in $\log_{10}$ plasma viral load between baseline and weeks 24 and 48 Stage 2: statistical superiority for the change in $\log_{10}$ plasma viral load between baseline and week 24 was observed for 800 and 1200 mg b.i.d. of ETR vs. placebo ($p = 0.009$ and $p = 0.049$, respectively)
TMC125-C223 [41]	r, ac, pb	ETR 400 or 800 mg b.i.d. or ac; 48 weeks	Mean $\log_{10}$ viral load reductions –0.88 ($p = 0.018$ vs. ac), –1.01 ($p = 0.002$ vs. ac) and –0.14 for 400 mg, 800 mg, and control at week 48; ETR retained activity in the presence of multiple NNRTI mutations
TMC125-C227 [42]	r, ac, ol	ETR 800 mg b.i.d. or ac	Mean $\log_{10}$ VL reductions from baseline at week 12: –1.39 (ETR) vs. –2.16 (ac)

[a]r, randomized; pc, placebo-controlled; db, double-blind; ac, active control; pb, partially blinded; ol, open-label.

and led to the abandonment of the 1200-mg twice-daily dosage [40].

TMC125-C223 The primary objective of this trial was to evaluate the dose–response relationship of antiviral activity within the ETR dose regimens. More patients discontinued in the control group (97.5%) than in the ETR groups (38.4%). Most discontinuations were as a result of virologic failure (VF). The primary efficacy parameter was $\log_{10}$ reduction in plasma VL over time, and this was significantly greater at week 48 with either dose of ETR than with the control regimen (Table 4). Significantly more patients achieved plasma VL <50 HIV-1 RNA copies/mL with ETR 400 mg (22.5%) and 800 mg (21.5%) b.i.d. than with active control (0%) ($p < 0.001$). Moreover, 88.2 and 87.5% of patients in the respective ETR groups with undetectable plasma VLs at 24 weeks maintained this level of response to week 48 [41]. This was the first time that sustained antiviral activity of an NNRTI had been demonstrated in a substantial number of patients with NNRTI-resistant HIV-1.

After 48 weeks of treatment, the tolerability profile of ETR was generally favorable, with no differences in AE profiles related to dosage. Median treatment duration was 48 weeks in both ETR groups vs. 18 weeks in the control group. Discontinuation due to AEs was reported in 15.0 and 19.0% of patients in the ETR 400- and 800-mg groups, respectively. Incidences of rash were 22.5 and 17.7%, compared with 7.5% in the active control group. Most rashes were mild to moderate in severity; six patients (3.8%) in the ETR group discontinued treatment as a result of rash.

As a result of the additional virologic benefit of the 800-mg bid dose in some patient subgroups and an acceptable tolerability profile, this dose equivalent was chosen for further development.

TMC125-C227 ETR was also evaluated in the exploratory TMC125-C227 trial, comparing the efficacy of ETR with investigator-selected PI therapy in NNRTI-resistant, PI-naive patients with HIV-1 infection [42]. Patients in the TMC125-C227 trial were randomized to treatment with either ETR 800 mg b.i.d. or control PI, both in combination with two investigator-selected N(t)RTIs.

Analysis of changes in plasma VL showed a rapid and sustained reduction when patients in the control group who were PI-naive started PI-based treatment. An interim analysis also showed that there was an initial robust decline in plasma VL in the ETR group (–1.3 $\log_{10}$ copies/mL at week 8), but this was not sustained relative to the control regimen beyond 8 weeks. This suboptimal response halted recruitment to TMC125-C227, and ETR was discontinued after a median 14 weeks.

Overall, the results showed that the combination of ETR and N(t)RTIs alone may not be optimal in patients having previously virologically failed an N(t)RTI + NNRTI–containing regimen.

Phase III Development: The DUET Trials

The DUET (TMC125 to demonstrate undetectable viral load in patients experienced with ARV therapy) trials (TMC125-C206 and TMC125-C216) were identically designed double-blind placebo-controlled phase III clinical trials to investigate the efficacy, tolerability, and safety of the phase III formulation of ETR in a large population of treatment-experienced patients with HIV-1 infection.

Study Design Patients aged $\geq$ 18 years and receiving a stable ARV regimen for $\geq$ 8 weeks before screening, with plasma VL > 5000 HIV-1 RNA copies/mL, $\geq$ 3 primary PI mutations, and at least one NNRTI RAM were randomized to ETR 200 mg or placebo b.i.d. plus a background regimen (BR) of DRV/r 600/100 mg, investigator-selected N(t)RTIs, and optional ENF. Patients were stratified according to ENF use, previous DRV/r use, and plasma VL at screening (below or above 30,000 HIV-1 RNA copies/mL) [43].

The primary endpoint was the proportion of patients attaining a confirmed plasma VL < 50 HIV-1 RNA copies/mL at 24 weeks, the first studies to examine "undetectable" plasma VL as the primary endpoint in this patient population. The two trials differed only in geographic location, and a pooled analysis was prespecified. Secondary endpoints in DUET included proportions of patients attaining plasma VL < 400 HIV-1 RNA copies/mL, plasma VL reductions at least 1 $\log_{10}$ copies/mL from baseline, change in plasma VL and CD4 cell count from baseline, proportions of patients with a clinical endpoint (death and/or reporting a new AIDS-defining illness as adjudicated by an independent panel), safety and tolerability, and changes in health-related quality of life [43].

In total, 599 and 604 patients were randomized to the ETR and placebo groups, respectively, in the pooled DUET trials. Baseline characteristics were similar between treatment groups (Table 5).

Efficacy A significantly higher proportion of patients reached confirmed plasma VL < 50 HIV-1 RNA copies/mL at week 48 with ETR compared with placebo (61% vs. 40%, respectively, $p < 0.0001$) (Fig. 10a). In addition, 92% of patients who were undetectable at week 24 sustained that response to week 48 [43]. ETR therapy was also associated with significantly increased CD4 cell counts, again with response being maintained to week 48 (Fig. 10b). The mean plasma VL reduction from baseline was also significantly greater with ETR than with placebo at both weeks 24 and 48 [43].

Subgroup analyses at week 48 showed no significant effect of gender, race, and previous NNRTI use. Higher baseline plasma VL and lower baseline CD4 cell count were associated with lower response in both treatment groups; however, ETR provided superior virologic response than did placebo in each subgroup. Hepatitis coinfection status had no effect on response to ETR [44]. The proportion of patients achieving undetectable VL was higher in the ETR group than in the placebo group, irrespective of number of active background agents, baseline DRV fold change in 50% effective concentration (FC), and ETR FC [43].

TABLE 5 Baseline Characteristics of the Pooled DUET Cohort

	ETR + BR ($n = 599$)	Placebo + BR ($n = 604$)
Male (%)	90	89
Plasma VL ($\log_{10}$ HIV-1 RNA copies/mL), median (range)	4.8 (2.7–6.8)	4.8 (2.2–6.5)
CD4 cell count (cells/mm^3), median (range)	99 (1–789)	109 (0–912)
Prior ARV use		
NNRTIs at screening (%)	12	12
10–15 ARV %	66	65
DRV/r use (%)	4	5
Detectable RAMs		
$\geq$ 3 ETR RAMs (%)	14	13
$\geq$ 2 NNRTI RAMs %	69	69
$\leq$ 3 primary PI RAMs (%)	38	37
BR		
Used ENF (total) (%)	46	47
Used ENF for the first time (de novo use) (%)	26	26
Active background agents = 0 (%)	17	16
Active background agents = 1 (%)	37	39

Source: [43].

Importantly, statistically significant reductions in adjudicated clinical endpoints were also observed with ETR vs. placebo at week 48 (5.8% vs. 9.8% respectively; $p = 0.0408$) [43]. In addition, time to an AIDS-defining event or death was also significantly shorter with placebo than with ETR ($p = 0.0108$) [43].

Resistance Analyses Clinical cutoffs (CCOs) are used to interpret phenotypic susceptibility in HIV-infected, treatment-experienced patients by giving an indication, based on FC values, of how response is affected by viral resistance. A preliminary upper CCO of 13 was identified for ETR, based on a 1 $\log_{10}$ greater response at week 24 than the response with placebo. A lower CCO of 3, below which patients exhibited the highest response rate, was also identified [45]. At baseline in the DUET studies, 67, 18, and 15% of patients had FC values for ETR of $\leq$ 3, 3 to 13, and > 13, respectively. At week 24, the highest response rate (71%) was seen in patients with baseline ETR FC $\leq$ 3, while 50 and 37% response rates were reported in patients with baseline FCs of 3 to 13 and > 13, respectively [54]. The 24-week response rate among patients receiving placebo was 36%. Of note, this was the first time that CCOs could be determined for an NNRTI.

Impact of Baseline Genotype The most recent analysis of the impact of baseline genotype on virologic response to ETR in DUET focused on patients not using de novo

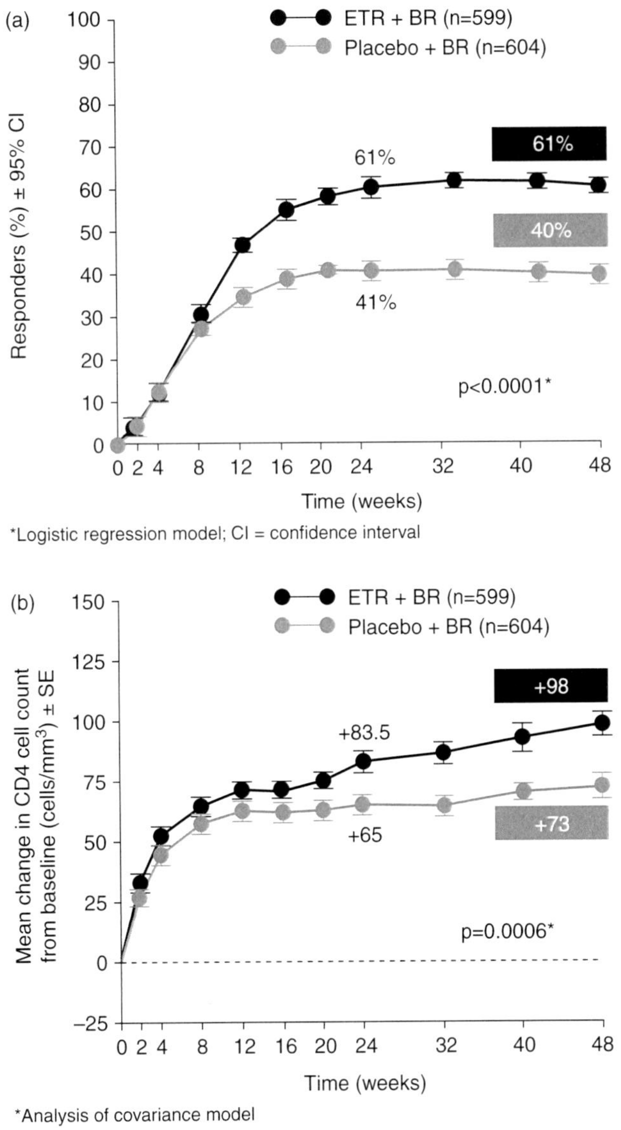

FIGURE 10 (a) Virological response (HIV-1 RNA < 50 copies/mL) at 48 weeks; (b) mean [standard error (S.E.)] change in CD4 cell count from baseline.

ENF and excluded those who discontinued for reasons other than VF [46]. This analysis identified 17 RAMs associated with diminished response to ETR ($\geq$ 25% reduction compared with patients with no detectable NNRTI RAMs at baseline): V90I, A98G, L100I, K101E/H/P, V106I, E138A, V179D/F/T, Y181C/I/V, G190A/S, and M230L. The mutations with the greatest univariate effect on response, V179F/T, Y181V, and G190S, were present in fewer than 5% of patients in the pooled DUET trials at baseline. Of note, K103N, the most prevalent NNRTI RAM in DUET, is not an ETR RAM.

A weighted scoring system reflecting the influence of each mutation was developed to improve correlation with ETR phenotypic susceptibility interpretations [46]. Of the 17 ETR RAMs, Y181I and Y181V were found to have the highest relative weights, followed by L100I, K101P, Y181C, and M230L. The mutations with the highest weights typically had low prevalence. The relative weights of each baseline mutation are added together to give a weighted genotypic score.

This scoring system showed that the virologic response to ETR is a function of weighted genotypic score at baseline. Three score ranges have been described (0 to 2, 2.5 to 3.5, and $\geq$ 4), which relate to highest (74%), intermediate (52%), and lowest (38%) average response rates (i.e., < 50 HIV-1 RNA copies/mL at week 24) [46].

Safety and Tolerability Treatment with first-generation NNRTIs is associated in some patients with specific AEs, including skin reactions, nervous system and psychiatric disorders, and hepatic toxicity. Skin reactions are usually mild to moderate and resolve with continued treatment, but more severe reactions, such as Stevens–Johnson syndrome (SJS) and toxic epidermal necrolysis (TEN), have been observed in some patients receiving NVP [47] and more rarely with EFV [48]; no such reactions were seen with ETR in the DUET trials.

ETR demonstrated a safety–tolerability profile similar to that of placebo, with the exception of rash, at week 48 (Table 6) [43]. Although there was a higher incidence of

TABLE 6 Summary of AEs at Week 48 in the Pooled DUET Trials

	ETR + BR (n = 599)	Placebo + BR (n = 604)
Median Treatment Duration (weeks; range)	52.3 (2–85)	51.0 (3–80)
Any AE (any cause, %)		
Total AEs	96.0	96.0
Grade 3 or 4 AE	33.0	34.9
Discontinuation due to AE	7.2	5.6
Serious AE	19.7	23.3
Death (any cause)	2.0	3.3
Most common AEs ($\geq$ 10% incidence in the ETR + BR group)		
Rash (any type)	19.2	10.9
Diarrhea	18.0	23.5
Nausea	14.9	12.7
Headache	10.9	12.7
Nasopharyngitis	11.0	10.4
AEs of interest (by class)		
Nervous system[a]	17.2	19.7
Psychiatric	16.7	19.5
Hepatic	6.5	6.1
Cardiac	7.0	7.3

Source: [43].
[a]Based on MedDRA system classes "nervous system disorders" and "psychiatric disorders."

rash with ETR, it was generally mild to moderate in severity, occurred early (median time to onset 14 days) and was of limited duration (median duration 15 days), infrequently lead to discontinuation, and was self-limiting with continued treatment. There were no grade 4 skin reactions (SJS, erythema multiforme, or TEN) reported with ETR in the DUET trials [43]. SJS was rarely reported in the ETR early access program (< 0.1%); with broader use of ETR following marketing authorization, severe cutaneous and hypersensitivity reactions, including SJS and TEN, have been reported rarely. Since these reactions can be life-threatening, clinical guidance requires immediate discontinuation of the drug when such severe reactions are suspected. Previous history of NNRTI-related rash did not predict rash with ETR, and there was no link between incidence of rash and baseline CD4 cell count or systemic drug exposure. The incidence of rash was higher in women than in men in the ETR group (30% vs. 18%); however, there were no clear differences in median time to rash onset or median duration of rash, and discontinuation due to rash was low in both males and females (2% vs. 5%) [43]. Pooled results at week 48 showed evidence of lipid neutrality and lack of any clinically relevant hepatic effects [43]. Rates of grade 3 or 4 increased triglycerides and total cholesterol, and low-density lipoprotein cholesterol levels ranged from 5 to 9%, with no significant differences between ETR and placebo.

The incidence of neuropsychiatric events at 48 weeks was similar between the treatment groups and decreased over time [43]. There were no grade 4 neuropsychiatric events with ETR, and rates of discontinuation due to nervous system and psychiatric events ranged from 0 to 0.5% across groups. In addition, the incidence of hepatic and cardiac events was similar between the treatment groups after 48 weeks of treatment [43].

Pooled DUET Week 96 Results Efficacy and safety results from the pooled 96-week DUET data set have been presented [49]. These long-term results confirm the durable efficacy and safety of ETR; 57% of patients achieved VL < 50 HIV-1 RNA copies/mL through 96 weeks of treatment with ETR + BR compared with 36% of placebo + BR patients. In addition, no new safety concerns were reported with ETR through 96 weeks of treatment.

Clinical Development: Conclusions

Treatment choices for ARV-experienced patients are expanding continually, offering new options where none existed previously. In addition to DUET, data have been reported from several trials investigating new ARV combinations, including RESIST [50], TORO [51], POWER [52], MOTIVATE [53], BENCHMRK [54], DUO [55], and TRIO [56]. ETR has been shown to be an effective and well-tolerated option for treatment-experienced patients with NNRTI-resistant HIV-1 infection. The findings of the DUET studies show that clinical benefit is not restricted by patient baseline characteristics or by the choice of BR. In addition, ETR has a favorable pharmacologic, safety, and tolerability profile that makes it suitable for use in combination with many other ARVs.

FUTURE DIRECTIONS

Once-daily dosing was not considered realistic with the phase II formulation of ETR, due to concerns over pill burden, and a switch to once-daily dosing with the phase III formulation prior to the start of the DUET trials was not possible. However, the phase III formulation, with its improved bioavailability and reduced pill burden, is under investigation for its suitability in a once-daily dosing regimen.

Further pilot studies to assess the feasibility of once-daily dosing are under way in ARV-naive HIV-1-infected patients. In addition, the development of a 200-mg tablet is under investigation to simplify dosing and to reduce pill burden, and further exploration of ETR in younger patients is under way.

CONCLUSIONS

ETR is believed to be among the first ARV compounds to have been developed by a systematic process involving structure–activity and structure–metabolism relationships and the use of drug-resistant clinical isolates. In the course of its development, ETR has overcome major hurdles. First, the physicochemical properties of the molecule made formulation very difficult. Application of the spray-dry technology, used in the food industry, addressed this problem and resulted in an acceptable pill size and burden. Second, there was a high level of skepticism in the clinical community about the feasibility of an NNRTI active in patients with NNRTI-resistant HIV-1. This resulted in a development program that was more complicated and longer than that with other ARVs. Clinical results, particularly the phase III DUET studies, show ETR to be an effective and well-tolerated treatment option. ETR has a high genetic barrier to the development of resistance and demonstrates sustained efficacy in treatment-experienced patients, regardless of baseline characteristics or BR. ETR also demonstrates a significant reduction in clinical endpoints vs. placebo. With the exception of rash, which is generally mild to moderate and occurs early, the tolerability profile of ETR is generally similar to that of placebo, without the neuropsychiatric and hepatic concerns that have been associated with the use of first-generation NNRTIs. Representing the first compound to highlight the translational research paradigm, and following the culmination of an extensive preclinical development program, ETR is the first NNRTI to demonstrate clinically relevant and sustained efficacy against NNRTI-resistant HIV-1.

Acknowledgments

The authors wish to acknowledge the medical writers Christopher J. Dunn and Karen Runcie of Gardiner-Caldwell Communications for their assistance in drafting the chapter and coordinating author contributions. This support was funded by Tibotec Pharmaceuticals.

REFERENCES

[1] Cohen, M. S.; Hellman, N.; Levy, J. A.; DeCock, K.; Lange, J. The spread, treatment, and prevention of HIV-1: evolution of a global pandemic. J. Clin. Invest. **2008**, *118*, 1244–1254.

[2] Sluis-Cremer, N.; Temiz, N. A.; Bahar, I. Conformational changes in HIV-1 reverse transcriptase induced by nonnucleoside reverse transcriptase inhibitor binding. *Curr. HIV Res.* **2004**, *2*, 323–332.

[3] Hammer, S. M.; Eron, J. J., Jr.; Reiss, P.; et al. Antiretroviral treatment of adult HIV infection: 2008 recommendations of the International AIDS Society–USA panel. *JAMA* **2008**, *300*, 555–570.

[4] Gazzard, B. G. BHIVA Treatment Guidelines Writing Group. British HIV association guidelines for the treatment of HIV-1-infected adults with antiretroviral therapy 2008. *HIV Med.* **2008**, *9*, 563–608.

[5] Vingerhoets, J.; Azjin, H.; Fransen, E.; et al. TMC125 displays a high genetic barrier to the development of resistance: evidence from in vitro selection experiments. *J. Virol.* **2005**, *79*, 12773–12782.

[6] Bacheler, L.; Jeffrey, S.; Hanna, G.; et al. Genotypic correlates of phenotypic resistance to efavirenz in virus isolates from patients failing nonnucleoside reverse transcriptase inhibitor therapy. *J. Virol.* **2001**, *75*, 4999–5008.

[7] Antinori, A.; Zaccarelli, M.; Cingolani, A.; et al. Cross-resistance among nonnucleoside reverse transcriptase inhibitors limits recycling efavirenz after nevirapine failure. *AIDS Res. Hum. Retroviruses* **2002**, *18*, 835–838.

[8] Delaugerre, C.; Rohban, R.; Simon, A.; et al. Resistance profile and cross-resistance of HIV-1 among patients failing a non-nucleoside reverse transcriptase inhibitor-containing regimen. *J. Med. Virol.* **2001**, *65*, 445–448.

[9] Pérez-Molina, J. A. Safety and tolerance of efavirenz in different antiretroviral regimens: results from a national multicenter prospective study in 1,033 HIV-infected patients. *HIV Clin. Trials* **2002**, *3*, 279–286.

[10] DHHS Panel on Antiretroviral Guidelines for Adult and Adolescents. Guidelines for the use of antiretroviral agents in HIV-infected adults and adolescents. Department of Health and Human Services, Nov. 3, 2008; pp. 1–133. Available at http://www.aidsinfo.nih.gov/ContentFiles/AdultandAdolescentGL.pdf. Accessed Apr. 9, 2009.

[11] Intelence™ (etravirine) tablets: full prescribing information. Tibotec, Inc., Raritan, NJ, Jan. 2008. Available at http://www.intelence-info.com/intelence/full-prescribing-info.html. Accessed Apr. 9, 2009.

[12] Pauwels, R.; Andries, K.; Desmyter, J.; et al. Potent and selective inhibition of HIV-1 replication in vitro by a novel series of TIBO derivatives. *Nature* **1990**, *343*, 470–474.

[13] Pauwels, R.; Andries, K.; Debyser, Z.; et al. Potent and highly selective human immunodeficiency virus type 1 (HIV-1) inhibition by a series of alpha-anilinophenylacetamide derivatives targeted at HIV-1 reverse transcriptase. *Proc. Natl. Acad. Sci. USA* **1993**, *90*, 1711–1715.

[14] Ludovici, D. W.; Kukla, M. J.; Grous, P. G.; et al. Evolution of anti-HIV drug candidates: 1. From α-anilinophenylacetamide (α-APA) to imidoyl thiourea (ITU). *Bioorg. Med. Chem. Lett.* **2001**, *11*, 2225–2228.

[15] Pauwels, R.; Balzarini, J.; Baba, M.; et al. Rapid and automated tetrazolium-based colorimetric assay for the detection of anti-HIV compounds. *J. Virol. Methods* **1988**, *20*, 309–321.

[16] Ludovici, D. W.; Kavash, R. W.; Kukla, M. J.; et al. Evolution of anti-HIV drug candidates: 2. Diaryltriazine (DATA) analogues. *Bioorg. Med. Chem. Lett.* **2001**, *11*, 2229–2234.

[17] Ludovici, D. W.; De Corte, B. L.; Kukla, M. J.; et al. Evolution of anti-HIV drug candidates: 3. Diarylpyrimidine (DAPY) analogues. *Bioorg. Med. Chem. Lett.* **2001**, *11*, 2235–2239.

[18] European Medicines Agency. CHMP Assessment Report for Intelence. Available at http://www.emea.europa.eu/humandocs/PDFs/EPAR/intelence/H-900-en6.pdf. Accessed Apr. 9, 2009

[19] Kakuda, T. N.; Schöller-Gyüre, M.; Workman, C.; et al. Single- and multiple-dose pharmacokinetics of etravirine administered as two different formulations in HIV-1-infected patients. *Antiviral. Thera.* **2008**, *13*, 655–661.

[20] Andries, K.; Azijn, H.; Thielemans, T.; et al. TMC125, a novel next-generation nonnucleoside reversetranscriptase inhibitor active against nonnucleoside reverse transcriptase inhibitor-resistant human immunodeficiency virus type 1. *Antimicrob. Agents Chemother.* **2004**, *48*, 4680–4686.

[21] Das, K.; Clark, A. D., Jr.; Lewi, P. J.; et al. Roles of conformational and positional adaptability in structure-based design of TMC125-R165335 (etravirine) and related non-nucleoside reverse transcriptase inhibitors that are highly potent and effective against wild-type and drug-resistant HIV-1 variants. *J. Med. Chem.* **2004**, *47*, 2550–2560.

[22] Vingerhoets, J.; De Baere, I.; Azijn, H.; et al. Antiviral activity of TMC125 against a panel of site-directed mutants encompassing mutations observed in vitro and in vivo. 16th Conference on Retroviruses and Opportunistic Infections, San Francisco, Feb. 8–11, **2004**. Abstract 621.

[23] Raoof, A.; Lachau-Durand, S.; Verbeeck, J.; Bailey, G.; Mark Martens, M. Etravirine has no effect on fetal development in rats and rabbits. XVIIth International AIDS Conference, Mexico City, Mexico, Aug. 3–8, **2008**. Poster TUPE0013.

[24] De Jonghe, S.; Verbeeck, J.; Vinken, P.; et al. Hemorrhagic cardiomyopathy in male mice treated with an NNRTI: the role of vitamin K. *Toxicol. Pathol.* **2008**, *36*, 321–329.

[25] Kakuda, T. N.; Schöller-Gyüre, M.; Woodfall, B.; et al. TMC125 in combination with other medications: summary of drug–drug interaction studies. 8th International Congress on Drug Therapy in HIV Infection; Glasgow, UK, Nov. 12–16, **2006**. Abstract PL5.2.

[26] Schöller-Gyüre, M.; Raoof, A.; Mannens, G.; et al. Mass-balance of ^{14}C-labelled TMC125 in healthy volunteers. 8th International Workshop on Clinical Pharmacology of HIV Therapy, Budapest, Hungary, Apr. 16–18, **2007**. Abstract 78.

[27] Peeters, M.; Janssen, K.; Kakuda, T. N.; et al. Etravirine (TMC125) has no effect on QT and corrected QT interval in HIV-negative volunteers. *Ann. Pharmacother.* **2008**, *42*, 757–765.

[28] Schöller-Gyüre, M.; Kakuda, T. N.; De Smedt, G.; et al. Pharmacokinetics of TMC125 in HIV-negative volunteers with mild or moderate hepatic impairment. 47th Interscience Conference on Antimicrobial Agents and Chemotherapy, Chicago, Sept. 17–20, **2007**. Abstract A-1428.

[29] Schöller-Gyüre, M.; Boffito, M.; Pozniak, A.; et al. Effect of meals of different composition on the pharmacokinetics of etravirine. *Pharmacotherapy* **2008**, *28*, 1215–1222.

[30] Schöller-Gyüre, M.; Kakuda, T. N.; Van Solingen-Ristea, R. M.; et al. Bioavailability of the 100mg etravirine tablet dispersed in water and of the 25mg pediatric tablet formulation. XVIIth International AIDS Conference, Mexico City, Mexico, Aug. 3–8, **2008**. Abstract MOPE0184.

[31] Kakuda, T. N.; Peeters, M.; Corbett, C.; et al. Pharmacokinetics (PK) and pharmacodynamics (PD) of etravirine (ETR; TMC125) in treatment-experienced HIV-1 infected patients: pooled 48-week results of DUET-1 and DUET-2. 48th Interscience Conference on Antimicrobial Agents and Chemotherapy, and the 46th Meeting of the Infectious Diseases Society of America, Washington, DC, Oct. 25–28, **2008**. Poster H-4056.

[32] Königs, C.; Feiterna-Sperling, C.; Esposito, S.; et al. Pharmacokinetics and dose selection of etravirine in HIV-infected children between 6 and 17 years, inclusive. 16th Conference on Retroviruses and Opportunistic Infections, Montréal, Quebec Canada, Feb. 8–11, **2009**. Abstract S-167.

[33] Schöller-Gyüre, M.; Kakuda, T. N.; De Smedt, G.; et al. Pharmacokinetics of TMC125 in once- and twice-daily regimens in HIV-1-negative volunteers. 47th Interscience Conference on Antimicrobial Agents and Chemotherapy, Chicago, Sept. 17–20, **2007**. Abstract A-1427.

[34] Lalezari, J.; DeJesus, E.; Osiyemi, O.; et al. Pharmacokinetics of once-daily etravirine (ETR) without and with once-daily darunavir/ritonavir (DRV/r) in antiretroviral-naive HIV-1 infected adults. Ninth International Congress on Drug Therapy in HIV Infection (HIV9), Glasgow, UK, Nov. 9–13, **2008**. Poster 0413.

[35] Anderson, M. S.; Kakuda, T. N.; Hanley, W.; et al. Minimal pharmacokinetic interaction between the human immunodeficiency virus nonnucleoside reverse transcriptase inhibitor etravirine and the integrase inhibitor raltegravir in healthy subjects. *Antimicrob. Agents Chemother.* **2008**, *52*, 4228–4232.

[36] Davis, J.; Schöller-Gyüre, M.; Kakuda, T. N.; et al. An open, randomized, two-period, crossover study in two cohorts to investigate the effect of steady-state TMC125 (etravirine) and the combination of TMC125/darunavir/ritonavir on the steady-state pharmacokinetics of oral maraviroc in healthy subjects. 11th European AIDS Conference, Madrid, Spain, Oct. 24–27, **2007**. Poster P4.3/02.

[37] Ramanathan, S.; Kakuda, T. N.; Mack, R.; West, S.; Kearney, B. P. Pharmacokinetics of elvitegravir following coadministration of ritonavir-boosted elvitegravir and etravirine. *Antiviral Ther.* **2008**, *13*, 1011–1017.

[38] Gruzdev, B.; Rakhmanova, A.; Doubovskaya, E.; et al. A randomized, double-blind, placebo-controlled trial of TMC125 monotherapy in antiretroviral naive, HIV-1 infected subjects. *AIDS* **2003**, *17*, 2487–2494.

[39] Gazzard, B. G.; Pozniak, A. L.; Rosenbaum, W.; et al. An open-label assessment of TMC125: a new, next-generation NNRTI, for 7 days in HIV-1 infected individuals with NNRTI resistance. *AIDS* **2003**, *17*, 49–54.

[40] Montaner, J.; Yeni, P.; Clumeck, N. N.; et al. Safety, tolerability, and preliminary efficacy of 48 weeks of etravirine therapy in a phase IIb dose-ranging study involving treatment-experienced patients with HIV-1 infection. *Clin. Infect. Dis.* **2008**, *47*, 969–978.

[41] Cohen, C.; Berger, D. S.; Blick, G.; et al. Efficacy and safety of etravirine (TMC125) in treatment-experienced HIV-1-infected patients: 48-week results of a phase IIb trial. *AIDS* **2009**, *23*, 423–426.

[42] Ruxrungtham, K.; Pedro, R. J.; Latiff, G. H.; et al. Impact of reverse transcriptase resistance on the efficacy of TMC125 (etravirine; ETR) with two NRTIs in PI-naive, NNRTI-experienced patients: Study TMC125-C227. *HIV Med.* **2008**, *9*, 883–896.

[43] Katlama, C.; Haubrich, R.; Lalezari, J.; et al. Efficacy and safety of etravirine in treatment-experienced, HIV-1 patients: pooled 48 week analysis of two randomized, controlled trials. *AIDS*. **2009**, *13*, 2289–22300.

[44] Cahn, P.; Molina, J. M.; Towner, W.; et al. 48-week pooled analysis of DUET-1 and DUET-2: the impact of baseline characteristics on virologic response to etravirine. XVIIth International AIDS Conference, Mexico City, Mexico, Aug. 3–8, **2008**. Abstract and poster TUPE0047.

[45] Peeters, M.; Nijs, S.; Vingerhoets, J.; et al. Determination of phenotypic clinical cut-offs for etravirine (ETR): pooled week 24 results of the DUET-1 and DUET-2 trials. XVIIth International Drug Resistance Workshop, Sitges, Spain, June 10–14, **2008**. Abstract 121.

[46] Vingerhoets, J.; Peeters, M.; Azijn, H.; et al. An update of the list of NNRTI mutations associated with decreased virologic response to etravirine: multivariate analyses on the pooled DUET-1 and DUET-2 clinical trial data. XVIIth International Drug Resistance Workshop, Sitges, Spain, June 10–14, **2008**. Abstract 24.

[47] Viramune® (nevirapine) tablets 200mg. Viramune® (nevirapine) oral suspension 50 mg/5 mL. Available at http://bidocs.boehringer-ingelheim.com/BIWebAccess/ViewServlet.ser?docBase=renetnt&folderPath=/Prescribing+Information/PIs/Viramune/Viramune.pdf. Accessed Feb. 23, 2008.

[48] Sustiva® (efavirenz) capsules and tablets. Available at http://packageinserts.bms.com/pi/pi_sustiva.pdf. Accessed Feb. 23, 2008.

[49] Trottier, B.; Mills, A.; Cahn, C.; et al. Durable efficacy and safety of etravirine (ETR; TMC125) in treatment-experienced, HIV-1-infected patients: pooled week 96 results from the phase III DUET-1 and DUET-2 trials. 18th Annual Canadian Conference on HIV/AIDS Research, Vancouver, British Columbia, Canada, April 23–26 **2009**. Abstract P148.

[50] Hicks, C. B.; Cahn, P.; Cooper, D. A.; et al. Durable efficacy of tipranavir-ritonavir in combination with an optimised background regimen of antiretroviral drugs for treatment-experienced HIV-1-infected patients at 48 weeks in the randomized evaluation of strategic intervention in multi-drug resistant patients with Tipranavir (RESIST) studies: an analysis of combined data from two randomised open-label trials. *Lancet* **2006**, *368*, 466–475.

[51] Reynes, J.; Arastéh, K.; Clotet, B.; et al. TORO: ninety-six-week virologic and immunologic response and safety evaluation of enfuvirtide with an optimized background of antiretrovirals. *AIDS Patient Care STDS* **2007**, *21*, 533–543.

[52] Clotet, B.; Bellos, N.; Molina, J. M. ; et al. Efficacy and safety of darunavir-ritonavir at week 48 in treatment-experienced patients with HIV-1 infection in POWER 1 and 2: a pooled subgroup analysis of data from two randomised trials. *Lancet* **2007**, *369*, 1169–1178.

[53] Gulick, R. M.; Lalezari, J.; Goodrich, J.; et al. Maraviroc for previously treated patients with R5 HIV-1 infection. *N. Engl. J. Med.* **2008**, *359*, 1429–1441.

[54] Steigbigel, R. T.; Cooper, D. A.; Kumar, P. N.; et al. Raltegravir with optimized background therapy for resistant HIV-1 infection. *N. Engl. J. Med.* **2008**, *359*, 339–354.

[55] Canestri, A.; Blanc, C.; Wirden, M.; et al. Efficacy and safety of an antiretroviral regimen containing etravirine plus raltegravir in HIV-1 treatment-experienced patients failing darunavir. *J. Int. AIDS Soc.* **2008**, *11*(Suppl. 1), P38.

[56] Yazdanpanah, Y.; Fagard, C.; Descamps, D.; et al. ANRS 139 TRIO Trial Group. High rate of virologic suppression with raltegravir plus etravirine and darunavir/ritonavir among treatment-experienced patients infected with multidrug-resistant HIV: results of the ANRS 139 TRIO trial. *Clin. Infect. Dis.* **2009**, *49*, 1441–1449.

7

DISCOVERY AND DEVELOPMENT OF TENOFOVIR DISOPROXIL FUMARATE

Erik De Clercq
Rega Institute for Medical Research, Leuven, Belgium

INTRODUCTION

The discovery and clinical development of tenofovir should be viewed in context of the discovery and the development of the acyclic nucleoside phosphonates, a new era in the antiviral drug field which started in 1986, now more than 20 years ago, with the description of the broad-spectrum anti-DNA viral activity of (*S*)-9-(3-hydroxy-2-phosphonylmethoxypropyl)adenine [(*S*)-HPMPA] [1] and the antiretroviral activity of its sister compound 9-(2-phosphonylmethoxyethyl) adenine (PMEA) [1]. In fact, (*S*)-HPMPA could be envisaged as a kind of adduct [2,3] between phosphonoacetic acid, predecessor of the antiviral agent phosphonoformic acid (foscarnet, Foscavir), and the acyclic nucleoside analog (*S*)-9-(2,3-dihydroxypropyl)adenine [(*S*)-DHPA], which was described 30 years ago, in 1978, as the first acyclic nucleoside analog with broad-spectrum antiviral activity [4].

Starting with (*S*)-HPMPA and PMEA, as the result of a close collaboration that I began with Anthonin Holý [Institute of Organic Chemistry and Biochemistry of the Czechoslovak (now Czech) Academy of Sciences in Prague] in 1976, several other acyclic nucleoside phosphonates were described as a key class of antiviral drugs [5], which yielded a wealth of acyclic nucleoside (mostly adenosine) phosphonate analogs, the full potential as antiviral agents in both medical and veterinarian virology, as well as plant virology, still to be fully explored. These compounds are depicted in Figure 1.

After we had shown PMEA (now known as adefovir) to be markedly effective against retroviruses [i.e., HIV and murine (Moloney) sarcoma virus] in vitro [6] and in vivo [7], we showed this to be the case for the (*R*,*S*)-9-(3-fluoro-2-phosphonylmethoxypropyl)adenine (FPMPA) as well [8]. However, FPMPA was not developed further, as shortly after its description, (*R*)-PMPA (later named tenofovir) was discovered [9], and although the 2,6-diamino counterpart (*R*)-PMPDAP proved to be more effective than (*R*)-PMPA against HIV in both in vitro and in vivo antiretrovirus systems [9,10], it was the adenine analog (*R*)-PMPA that was selected for further development.

ANTIVIRAL ACTIVITY SPECTRUM

Tenofovir has an activity spectrum that is slightly different from that of adefovir but fundamentally different from that of cidofovir [11]. Cidofovir [(*S*)-HPMPC], the first acyclic nucleoside phosphonate developed and licensed for clinical use, was first described by De Clercq et al. in 1987 [12] and has, akin to its predecessor (*S*)-HPMPA, a broad antiviral activity spectrum against virtually all DNA viruses, including papova (polyoma and papilloma)-, adeno-, herpes-, and poxviridae (Table 1). Adefovir retains some activity against the herpesviridae but gains significant activity against the hepadnaviridae [e.g. hepatitis B virus (HBV)] and retroviridae [e.g. human immunodeficiency virus (HIV)], whereas tenofovir is principally active only against hepadnaviruses (HBV) and retroviruses (HIV) (Table 1). As an important spin-off, adefovir and tenofovir have been found to be highly efficient in eradicating the episomal form of banana streak virus (BSV) [13], a member of the badnaviruses, which are

Antiviral Drugs: From Basic Discovery Through Clinical Trials, First Edition. Edited by Wieslaw M. Kazmierski.

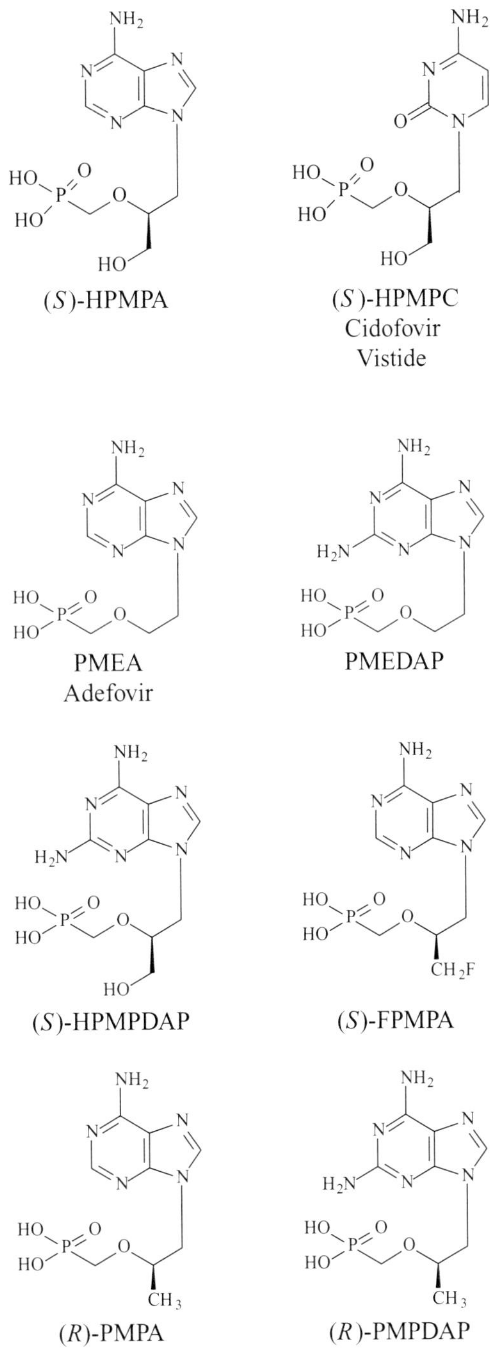

FIGURE 1 Structural formulas of acyclic nucleoside phosphonates.

believed to follow a replication machinery process similar to that of the hepadnaviruses. Treatment with adefovir and tenofovir rendered up to 90% of the plants regenerated from the BSV-infected meristems completely virus-free, an observation that may have far-reaching agricultural implications for the production of healthy banana plants [5]. This economically attractive application of both adefovir and tenofovir has so far remained untapped. An equally interesting observation, shown only for adefovir, is that in its diphosphate form, it specifically blocks the adenylylcyclase activity associated with the edema factor (EF) secreted by *Bacillus anthracis* [14]. Adefovir may therefore have potential in the treatment of anthrax and other bacterial infections caused by bacteria that secrete adenylylcyclase toxins such as *Bordetella pertussis* (whooping cough), *Pseudomonas aeruginosa* (nosocomial infections), and *Yersinia pestis* (plague) [14]. Whether these potential applications extend to tenofovir has not yet been ascertained.

TABLE 1 Antiviral Activity Spectrum of the Acyclic Nucleoside Phosphonates[a]

	Cidofovir [(*S*)-HPMPC]	Adefovir (PMEA)	Tenofovir [(*R*)-PMPA]
Papovaviridae			
Polyoma	×		
Papilloma	×		
Adenoviridae			
Adeno	×		
Herpesviridae			
HSV-1	×	×	
HSV-2	×	×	
VZV	×	×	
CMV	×	×	
EBV	×	×	
HHV-6	×	×	
HHV-7	×	×	
HHV-8	×	×	
Poxviridae			
Variola	×		
Cowpox	×		
Monkeypox	×		
Camelpox	×		
Vaccinia	×		
MCV	×		
Orf	×		
Hepadnaviridae			
HBV		×	×
Retroviridae			
HIV-1		×	×
HIV-2		×	×
SIV		×	×
FIV		×	×

Source: [11], with modifications.
[a]CMV, cytomegalovirus; EBV, Epstein–Barr virus; FIV, feline immunodeficiency virus; HHV, human herpes virus; HSV, herpes simplex virus; MCV, molluscum contagiosum virus; SIV, simian immunodeficiency virus; VZV, varicella-zoster virus.

MECHANISM OF ANTI-HIV ACTIVITY AND RESISTANCE DEVELOPMENT

In contrast to the acyclic guanosine analogs (acyclovir, ganciclovir, and penciclovir) and 2′,3′-dideoxynucleoside analogs

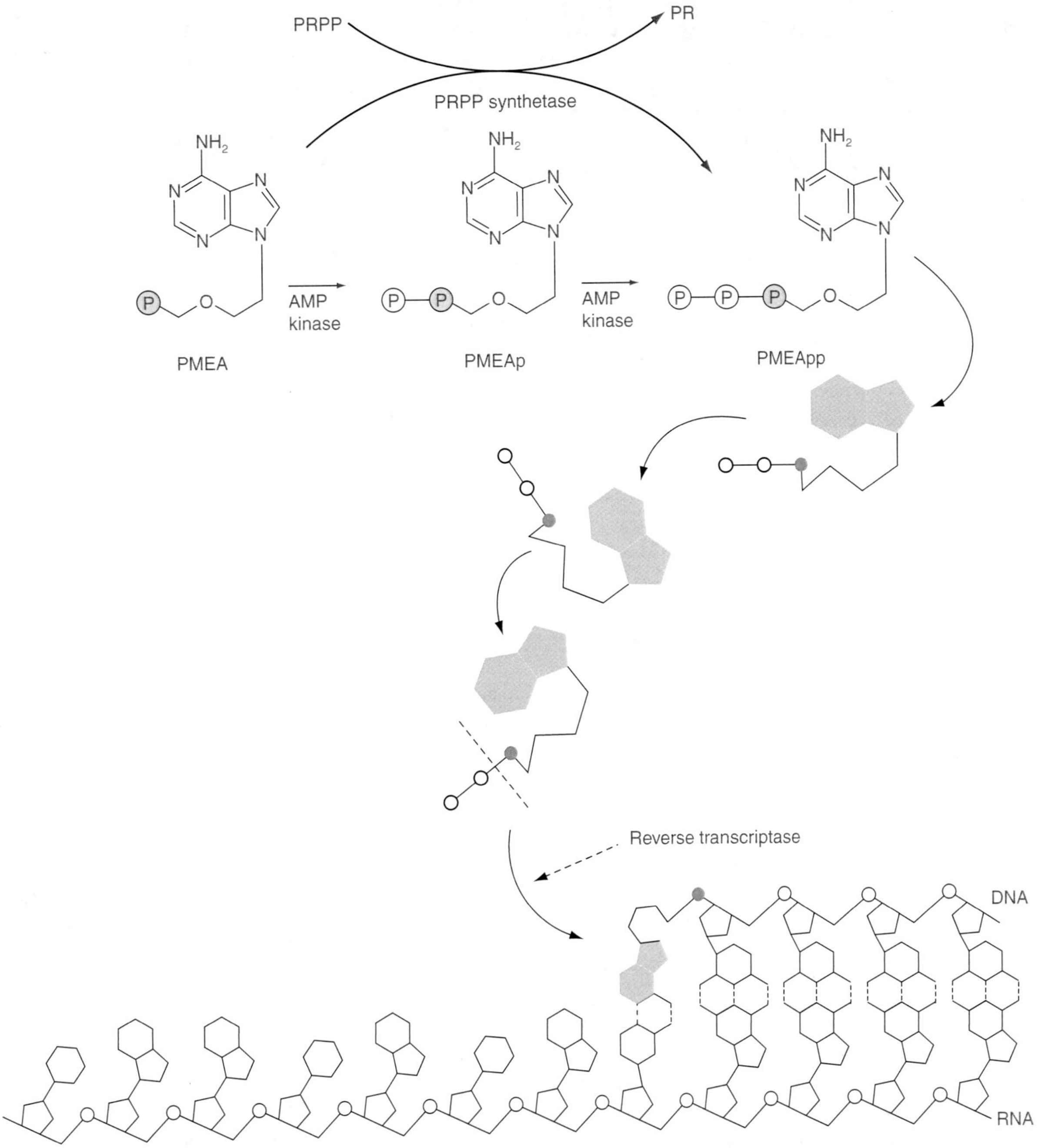

FIGURE 2 Mechanism of antiviral action of tenofovir (PMPA). (From [11], with modifications.)

[azidothymidine (AZT), zalcitabine, didanosine, stavudine, lamivudine, abacavir, and emtricitabine], which require three phosphorylation steps to be converted to their active (i.e., triphosphate) forms, adefovir (PMEA) and tenofovir (PMPA) need only two phosphorylations to be converted to their active (i.e., diphosphate) forms, termed PMEApp and PMPApp, respectively. Both phosphorylations could be carried out in two consecutive steps by AMP kinase or in one step by PRPP synthase (Fig. 2). Unlike AZT, the NtRTIs (PMEA, PMPA) do not alter the endogenous nucleotide pool levels [15]. PMPApp akin to PMEApp would act as competitive inhibitors/alternate substrates with respect to the natural substrate dATP, and when incorporated (following removal of the diphosphate group) into the DNA chain, PMPA akin to PMEA would shut off further DNA synthesis, thereby acting obligatorily as a chain terminator (Fig. 2).

PMPApp acts as a selective inhibitor of the HIV-1 reverse transcriptase (RT): It is 800-fold less inhibitory toward DNA polymerase-β than is HIV-1 RT [16]. Also, PMPApp and its 2,6-diaminopurine counterpart, PMPDAPpp, are much less (or virtually not at all) inhibitory to the mitochondrial DNA polymerase-γ [17]. In fact, very low incorporation efficiencies with human DNA polymerases α, β, and γ were found for PMPApp (0.06 to 1.4%) and PMPDAPpp (0.075 to 2.2%) [18]. Exposure of various human cell types to tenofovir at concentrations that greatly exceeded those required for in vitro anti-HIV-1 activity in peripheral blood mononuclear cells (EC_{50} = 0.2 μM) and to achieve therapeutically relevant plasma levels (0.8 to 1.3 μM) was not associated with mitochondrial toxicity [19]. Additionally, when mitochondrial DNA (mtDNA) content was monitored in tissues from rats, monkeys, or woodchucks treated with tenofovir disoproxil fumarate (TDF), no changes in mtDNA content or mitochondrial enzyme activity were observed [20].

The signature resistance mutations for tenofovir disoproxil fumarate (TDF) is the RT mutation K65R [21]. This mutation causes a variable, yet not complete, loss in susceptibility to TDF, and also to the NRTIs didanosine and abacavir. Typically, the K65R mutation leads to only a three- to four-fold reduction in tenofovir susceptibility, and has been detected in up to 3% of the patients receiving TDF [22].

The RT K65R mutation engendering resistance to TDF and the M184V mutation engendering resistance to lamivudine (3TC) and emtricitabine [(−)FTC] are mutually antagonistic, which means that the K65R mutation could increase the susceptibility of the virus to 3TC or (−)FTC, and, vice versa, the M184V mutation may increase the virus's susceptibility toward tenofovir [23–26]. These observations justify the use of the combination of TDF with (−)FTC, as in Truvada and Atripla.

Resistance development to NRTIs such as AZT depends primarily on the ATP-dependent phosphorolytic excision of the nucleotide analog (i.e., AZT 5′-monophosphate). Excision can occur only when the RT complex exists in its pretranslocational state. Binding of the next complementary nucleotide causes the formation of a stable dead-end complex in the posttranslocational state, which blocks the excision reaction. This would explain why tenofovir would lead less readily to resistance development than would, say, azidothymidine [27].

Although the K65R mutation (in the HIV RT) is unquestionably linked to the emergence of resistance to tenofovir and some NRTIs (other than AZT, i.e., didanosine and abacavir) [28], it is still unclear why the K65R mutation is doing so and whether this resistance is due to an increased excision rate of PMPA from the DNA product. From an epidemiological viewpoint, the incidence of the K65R mutation has decreased in the last couple of years despite increased use of TDF in anti-HIV drug combination regimens [29]. In clinical isolates, K65R is frequently accompanied by the A62V and S68G RT mutations; these mutations serve as (partially) compensatory mutations to improve the viral replication capacity associated with the K65R mutation [30].

In addition to the K65R mutation, the K70E mutation has been reported in a small number of patients failing on antiretroviral drug regimens, including TDF [31]. Apparently, the K70E mutation antagonizes the K65R mutation, and a molecular basis for this antagonism has been provided [32]. Both the K70E and K65R mutations antagonize the thymidine analog mutations (TAMs) M41L, L210W, and T215Y associated with ATP-mediated excision of nucleotide analogs such as AZT 5′-monophosphate [33].

Sequential emergence of viral mutants with K70E and K65R during prolonged tenofovir monotherapy has been noted in rhesus macaques with chronic SHIV infection [34]. Given the antagonism between the K70E and K65R mutations, even in the presence of K65R virus, continuation of tenofovir treatment as part of highly active antiretroviral therapy (HAART) may be justified [34].

ORAL PRODRUG APPROACH: TENOFOVIR DISOPROXIL FUMARATE

Acyclic nucleoside phosphonates have poor, if any, oral bioavailability. This explains why for cidofovir the oral alkoxyalkyl prodrug derivatives HDP (hexadecyloxypropyl)-cidofovir and ODE (octadecyloxyethyl)-cidofovir have been conceived (as reviewed by De Clercq [35,36]). These cidofovir prodrugs could be most useful in the treatment and/or prophylaxis of pox- and herpesvirus infections by the oral route, but have not yet been licensed for this purpose.

For adefovir (PMEA), the oral prodrug bis(pivaloyloxymethyl)-9-(2-phosphonylmethoxyethyl)adenine [bis(POM) PMEA] was successfully developed [37,38] and finally approved in 2002 for clinical use as Hepsera (adefovir dipivoxil) for the treatment of chronic hepatitis B (Fig. 3).

The same oral prodrug approach could have been applied to PMPA. However, pivaloyl-containing compounds may generate pivaloyl acid when releasing the parent drug, and this could cause increased urinary carnitine loss [39]. To avoid this potential problem, a novel series of alkyl methyl carbonate esters of PMPA were synthesized [40], and bis(isopropyloxycarbonyloxymethyl)-[(*R*)-9-(2-phosphonylpropyl)adenine] (Fig. 3) was selected for further development [39]. The favorable pharmacokinetic profile, marked antiviral efficacy, and low toxicity made bis(POC)-PMPA an attractive oral prodrug of PMPA, cited by Naesens et al. [41] as being worth pursuing further in clinical studies in patients infected with HIV or HBV. Actually, bis(POC)PMPA or tenofovir disoproxil fumarate was formally approved for the treatment of HIV infections in 2001, and for the treatment of HBV infections in 2008, thus fulfilling our prophecy in 1998 [41].

CLINICAL EFFICACY OF TDF

Initial studies with TDF had pointed to its durable antiviral activity, potent efficacy against virus strains with RT mutations conferring resistance to NRTIs, infrequent emergence of resistance, a convenient dosing schedule, and placebo-like tolerability for a period of both 24 weeks [42] and 48 weeks [43]. When the combination of TDF with emtricitabine ((−)FTC) and efavirenz (EFV) was compared with that of zidovudine, 3TC, lamivudine, and EFV, the TDF arm was clearly superior in terms of both virologic response (Fig. 4) and safety (lipid profile, risk for lipodystrophy) [44]. This difference was already noted after 48 weeks (Fig. 4) but was sustained for 144 weeks. In particular, the percentage of patients with HIV RNA levels below 400 copies/mL after 48 weeks of treatment was 84% in the TDF + emtricitabine + efavirenz group, compared with 73% in the zidovudine + lamivudine + efavirenz group [44].

Earlier studies had indicated that TDF + lamivudine (3TC) + efavirenz, although comparable in antiviral efficacy with stavudine + lamivudine (3TC) + efavirenz, had a better safety profile based on the occurrence of dyslipidemia [45].

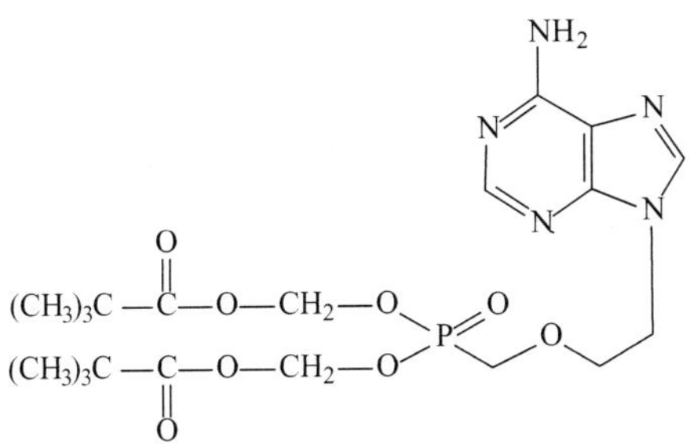

Bis(POM)PMEA
Adefovir dipivoxil
Hepsera

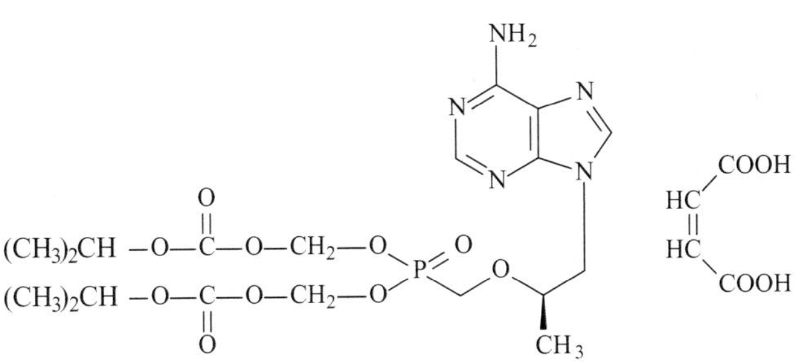

Bis(POC)PMPA
Tenofovir disoproxil fumarate
Viread

FIGURE 3 Prodrugs of adefovir and tenofovir.

In fact, several studies have indicated that switching from, for example, AZT + 3TC or abacavir + 3TC to TDF + (−)FTC resulted in an improvement in dyslipidemia (or a decrease in triglyceride and LDL-cholesterol levels) [46–48].

Safety data from the compassionate use/expanded access programs of TDF over a 4-year period indicated that the drug is well tolerated in HIV patients with a serious renal adverse event incidence rate of 0.57% among 10,695 patients in the expanded access program (cited by De Clercq [49]). Through seven years of therapy in antiretroviral-naive patients, TDF + 3TC + efavirenz demonstrated (1) sustained durable antiretroviral efficacy, (2) continued CD4 cell count increases, (3) no discontinuations due to renal adverse events, (4) no evidence of clinically relevant bone effects, and (5) significant increases in limb fat through year 7 [50].

In the mean time, TDF has been used more frequently in combination with emtricitabine, and this dual-drug combination has recently been extended to a triple-drug combination with the addition of efavirenz (see the next section). Yet TDF may be coadministered with several other anti-HIV drugs such as darunavir (boosted by ritonavir) [51] and raltegravir [52] without the risk of drug–drug interactions requiring dose adjustments.

Similarly, there are no clinically relevant drug–drug interactions between TDF–emtricitabine when combined with elvitegravir (GS-9137) (boosted by ritonavir) [53], and once-daily atazanavir–ritonavir, in combination with TDF–emtricitabine, demonstrated similar antiviral efficacy to that of lopinavir–ritonavir administered twice daily in combination with TDF–emtricitabine, albeit with less gastrointestinal toxicity, in the management of antiretroviral-naive HIV-1-infected patients [54].

FROM VIREAD VIA TRUVADA TO ATRIPLA

Viread (tenofovir disoproxil fumarate) (Fig. 5) was licensed in 2001. As the combination of TDF and emtricitabine [which corresponds to (−)FTC, the 5-fluoro-substituted derivative of 3TC] proved mutually beneficial (in terms of antiviral action and resistance development), both compounds were combined at a fixed dose [TDF at 300 mg and (−)FTC at 200 mg] in a single once-daily tablet (Truvada) (Fig. 5) which was approved by the U.S. Food and Drug Administration (FDA) in 2004. In 2006, the triple-drug combination or "three-in-one" tablet Atripla, became available. Atripla (Fig. 5) contains three active ingredients, representing three different classes of HIV RT inhibitors: an NRTI (nucleoside RT inhibitor: emtricitabine), an NtRTI (nucleotide RT inhibitor: tenofovir), and an NNRTI (nonnucleoside RT inhibitor: efavirenz) [49]. Of pivotal importance for the development and eventual licensing of Atripla for the first-line treatment of HIV infections were the clinical studies of Gallant et al. [44] and Pozniak et al. [55] (see also [56,57]).

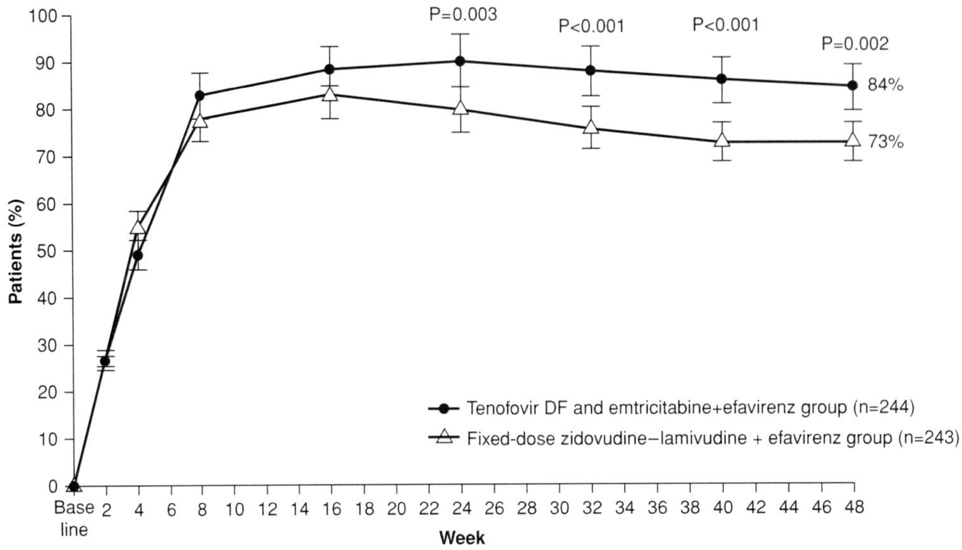

No. of Patients with <400 HIV RNA copies/mL

Tenofovir DF–emtricitabine group	64	119	202	215	219	214	209	206
Zidovudine–lamivudine gruop	66	134	189	202	194	184	177	177

FIGURE 4 Percentage of patients with HIV RNA levels below 400 copies/mL: comparison of Viread [tenofovir disoproxil fumarate (TDF)] + emtricitabine + efavirenz group *vs.* Combivir (zidovudine + lamivudine) + efavirenz group. (Data from [44].)

The coformulation of TDF/(−)FTC/efavirenz, as in Atripla, is bioequivalent to administration of its individual compounds [58]. Cumulative results from three years of follow-up indicated that when compared with the zidovudine (AZT)/lamivudine (3TC)/efavirenz combination, the TDF/(−)FTC/efavirenz combination demonstrated superior durability of viral load suppression and improved safety (fewer adverse events) [59].

The efficacy (virologic suppression) and safety [renal function, limb fat, and triglyceride and cholesterol levels of the triple-drug combination TDF/(−)FTC/efavirenz] has been attested to further in patients receiving HAART after switching their therapy to a single-tablet once-daily regimen of Atripla [TDF/(−)FTC/efavirenz] [60,61].

TDF combined with emtricitabine and efavirenz is apparently an ideal coformulation, achieving optimal virus suppression. Other combinations—TDF plus didanosine [62], TDF plus didanosine and efavirenz [63], and TDF plus abacavir and lamivudine [64]—yielded a high rate of early virologic failure. The triple-drug combination TDF with abacavir and lamivudine was also accompanied by an increased incidence of the K65R and M184V/I mutations [65], which may have contributed to the poor virological performance of this drug combination strategy. Apparently, no evidence was found for metabolic drug interactions among TDF, abacavir, and lamivudine [66].

High rates of early virological failure have been reported with drug regimens consisting of TDF, lamivudine (or emtricitabine), and nevirapine [67,68]. As a consequence of increased recognition of the toxicity of thymidine analogs (i.e., zidovudine or stavudine) regimens comprising TDF, either lamivudine or emtricitabine, and nevirapine are presently used more commonly in treatment programs in resource-constrained settings. These regimens have an excellent long-term toxicity profile and would result in viral suppression rates of $\geq 75\%$ at 12 months or later [69]. Hence, these authors concluded that the available evidence did not support changing the current use of TDF plus emtricitabine (or lamivudine) and nevirapine to treat antiretroviral-naive patients [69].

THE MAJOR PITFALL IN THE CLINICAL USE OF TDF: KIDNEY TOXICITY

The clinical use of NRTIs stavudine, didanosine and zidovudine has been associated with lipoatrophy (loss of fat mass, e.g., of the face, limbs, and buttocks) and an increase in serum lactic acid and triglyceride levels. These effects may be initiated by the mitochondrial toxicity (i.e., inhibition of mitochondrial DNA polymerase γ) caused by these NRTIs [70]. Tenofovir does not cause these effects. On the contrary, switching from stavudine to tenofovir results in a normalization of the triglyceride levels and reversal of the lipoatrophy [71,72].

TDF has been formally approved for use in HIV-infected adults but not in HIV-infected children, one of the potential pitfalls being the possible adverse effects of TDF on bone mineral acquisition during childhood. A decreased bone mineral density (BMD) has been observed in a

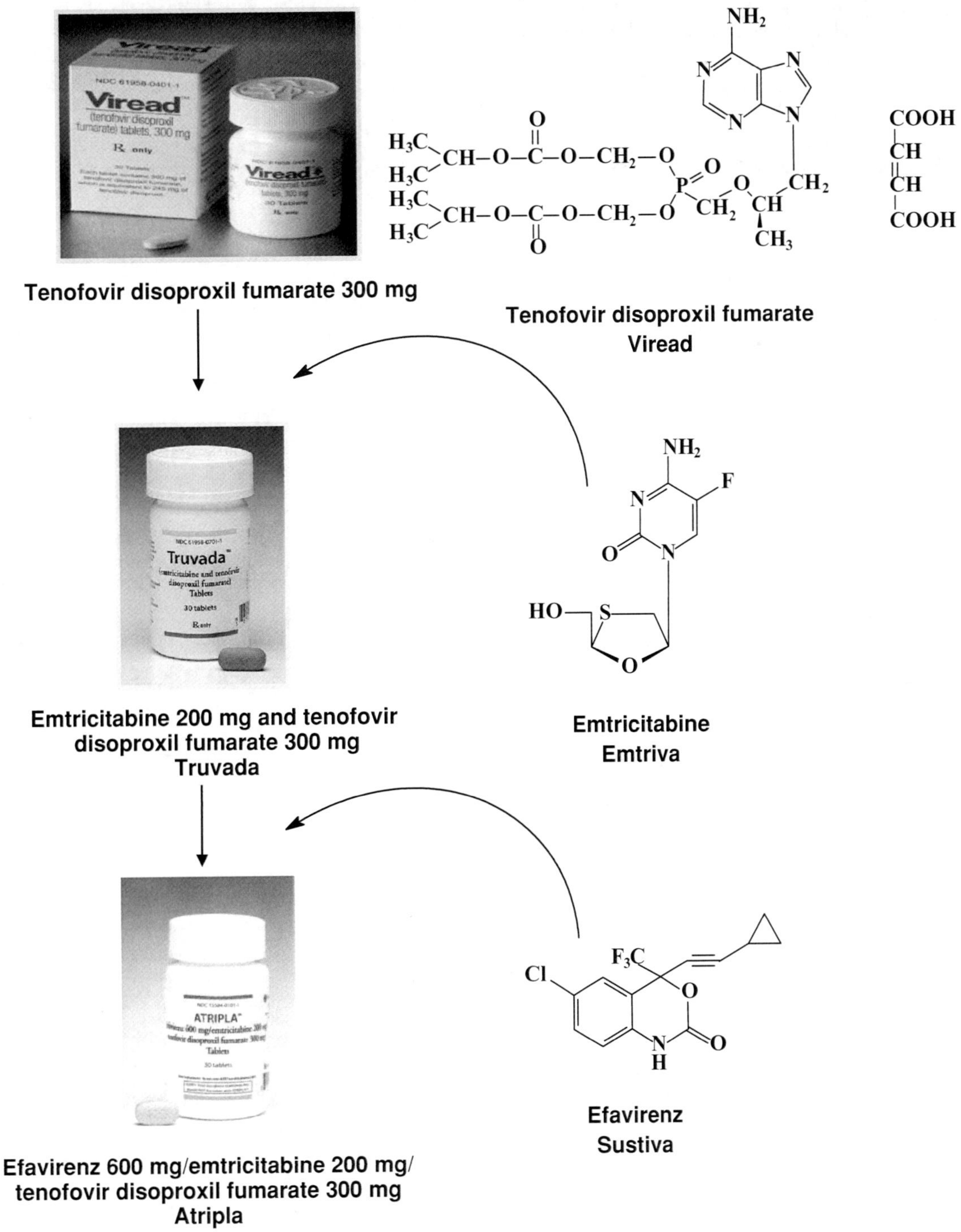

FIGURE 5 Development of Atripla from Viread via Truvada. (*See insert for color representation of the figure.*)

recent study [73], although a previous study did not reveal an effect of TDF on BMD [74]. Clearly, BMD monitoring of HIV-infected children requiring TDF treatment seems to be warranted.

The presence of the phosphonate moiety in tenofovir can be envisaged as the "hallmark" for many of its unique features, including its prolonged antiviral action, allowing infrequent dosing and low resistance profile, but also makes it prone to possible toxicity, especially nephrotoxicity. Yet no TDF-related toxic side effects were noted with the TDF/emtricitabine/efavirenz drug combination regimens [44,45,55].

In two randomized, controlled trials, no clinically relevant renal disease or adverse events were demonstrated in antiretroviral-naive patients treated with TDF over a three-year period (144 weeks) [75]. The renal safety of tenofovir has also been demonstrated in a prospective 96-week longitudinal study in HIV-infected children [76].

Yet there have been several case reports on renal tubular dysfunction [77,78], Fanconi syndrome [79,80], and acute renal failure [81–84] in AIDS patients treated with TDF. In two double-blind placebo-controlled studies, the incidence of renal events was similar among the TDF groups and the placebo groups [85]. In earlier studies, severe complications such as Fanconi syndrome [86], pancreatitis [87,88], and lactic acidosis [89] were observed only after combination of TDF with didanosine—a clear example of a drug combination that should be avoided.

Acute renal failure in HIV patients has remained an important issue [90]. Nephrotoxicity in patients receiving tenofovir seems to be associated with the presence of co-morbidities and with advanced HIV infection [91]. Although the safety of TDF for the treatment of HIV infection in adults has been proven over a period of four years [92], risk factors for the development of nephrotoxicity should be monitored carefully, and baseline renal insufficiency should, of course, argue against the use of TDF [93].

There might be a greater (risk for) decline of renal function if tenofovir is associated with a protease inhibitor–based rather than an NNRTI-based therapy [94]. Recently, a peroxisome proliferator–activated receptor-γ (PPAR-γ) agonist, rosiglitazone, has been identified that may reverse tenofovir-induced nephrotoxicity at the tubular level [95].

TDF FOR THE TREATMENT OF HEPATITIS B

As could be predicted from their antiretroviral activity, PMEA (adefovir) and PMEDAP also proved active against HBV replication [96,97], and, shortly after their anti-HIV activity had been described, (*R*)-PMPA (tenofovir) and (*R*)-PMPDAP were also reported as potent inhibitors of HBV replication [98]. In fact, adefovir and tenofovir were about equipotent in inhibiting in vitro replication [99], including replication of the lamivudine-resistant variant of HBV [containing the M550V (now referred to as the rt M204V) mutation] [100]. The in vitro susceptibility of lamivudine-resistant HBV to adefovir and tenofovir was later confirmed by Lada et al. [101].

After adefovir dipivoxil had initially been pursued for the treatment of HIV infections but was found to be nephrotoxic at the doses (125 or 62.5 mg/day) required to inhibit HIV infections, it was further pursued for the treatment of HBV infections. Here a daily dose of 10 mg sufficed for adefovir dipivoxil to achieve significant histological, virologic and biochemical improvement without the emergence of adefovir-resistant HBV DNA polymerase mutations following 48 weeks of treatment in both HBV e antigen-negative chronic hepatitis B patients [102] and HBV e antigen-positive HBV patients [103]. In patients with antigen-negative chronic hepatitis B, the virus stayed suppressed if treatment was continued for another 96 weeks (following the initial 48 weeks), although the signature adefovir-resistant rt N236T and rt A181V mutations were identified in 5.9% of the patients [104]. The rt N236T mutation also conferred a three- to four-fold reduced susceptibility to tenofovir in cell culture, but the clinical significance of this susceptibility change remains unknown [105].

In the past few years, TDF has been recommended for the treatment of chronic HBV infections in HBV HIV-coinfected patients [106–110]. As compared to patients treated with adefovir dipivoxil, patients treated with TDF reached the threshold of HBV undetectability at a faster rate and in larger proportions than did those taking adefovir dipivoxil [110]. In HIV/HBV-coinfected patients with cirrhosis, TDF might lead to sustained HBV suppression and result in cirrhosis reversal [111,112].

For the past five years or so, TDF has also been considered an attractive treatment option for patients with lamivudine (3TC)-resistant HBV infection [113,114]. TDF has been licensed since 2008 for the treatment of chronic hepatitis B in the European Union, the United States, and several other countries. Not surprisingly, when TDF was given (orally) at a daily dose of 300 mg, it proved (far) superior to adefovir dipivoxil in achieving HBV DNA suppression when given (orally) at a daily dose of 10 mg for a period of 48 weeks in both HBe Ag-negative and HBe Ag-positive chronic hepatitis B patients (Fig. 6) [115].

Of the HBe Ag-negative patients, 99% had HBV DNA $<$ 400 copies/mL after 96 weeks of TDF therapy without evidence of resistance to TDF monotherapy [116]. Of the HBe Ag-positive patients, 88% had HBV DNA $<$ 400 copies/mL (6% achieving HBe Ag loss) after 96 weeks of TDF therapy, again without evidence of resistance to TDF monotherapy [117]. That no resistance to tenofovir was detected following 96 weeks of TDF monotherapy was further substantiated by Snow-Lampart et al. [118] and will be followed up for eight years (384 weeks).

Tenofovir was equally active in vitro against wild-type HBV clinical isolates representing viral genotypes A-H [119]. Studies carried out in Asian patients with HBe Ag-negative or HBe Ag-positive hepatitis B yielded results similar to those reported by Marcellin et al. [115,120]. Deniz and Everhard [121] concluded that TDF is predicted to provide a better health outcome at a lower cost than with entecavir, lamivudine, or adefovir dipivoxil, and should therefore be used as first-line treatment for chronic hepatitis B.

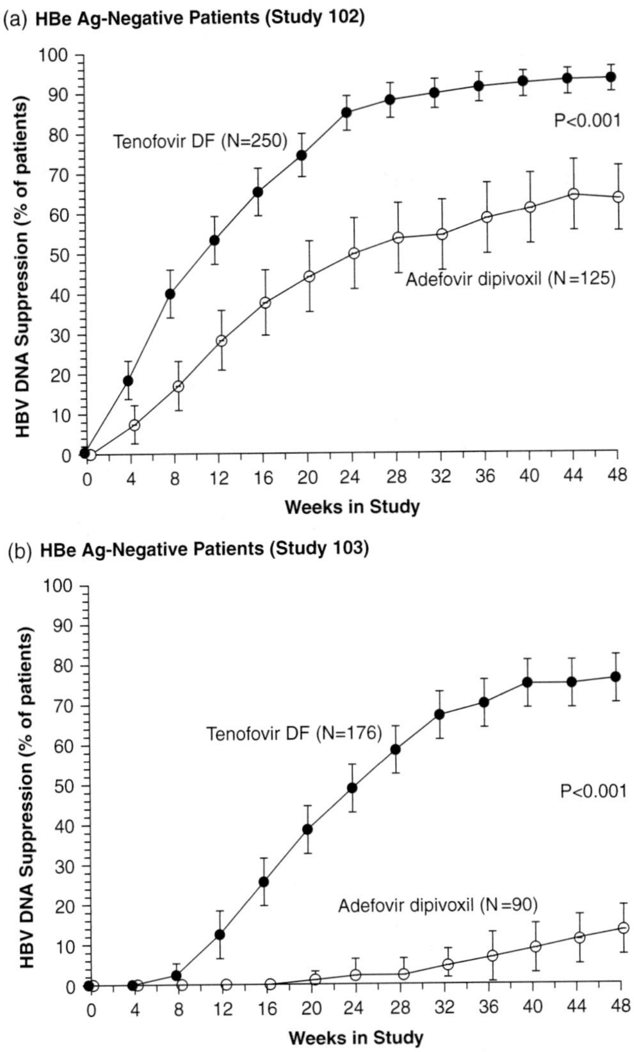

FIGURE 6 Suppression of HBV DNA levels by tenofovir disoproxil fumarate (daily dose: 300 mg through week 48) and adefovir dipivoxil (daily dose: 10 mg through week 48) in (a) HBe Ag-negative and (b) HBe Ag-positive patients. Viral suppression was defined as an HBV DNA level of less than 400 copies/mL. (Data from [115].)

Given the convincing results obtained with TDF in the treatment of chronic HBV infections, the only question remaining is whether TDF should be used as monotherapy or combination therapy [122]. TDF combination therapy should be considered in patients with resistance to adefovir (dipivoxil) [123], but, in their comment to Marcellin et al.'s paper [115], Lai and Yuen [124] stated their belief that if the long-term resistance to TDF turns out to be very low, similar to the 1.2% resistance rate after five years of entecavir treatment, long-term monotherapy with TDF would be a feasible option, comparable to the combination of a nucleotide analog such as adefovir dipivoxil or TDF with a nucleoside analog such as lamivudine or telbivudine [124].

PROPHYLACTIC USE OF TDF IN THE PREVENTION OF HIV INFECTIONS

While the prospects for an effective vaccine to prevent HIV infection have remained daunting, one should seriously consider the potential of TDF (Viread), whether or not combined with emtricitabine (Truvada), and emtricitabine and efavirenz (Atripla), in the pre- and/or postexposure prophylaxis of HIV infections. There are three routes by which HIV could be transmitted: parenterally (e.g., needle stick accidents), sexually (intravaginal, anal, or oral intercourse), and perinatally (from mother to child, during pregnancy, at birth, or through breast feeding). There is compelling experimental evidence that tenofovir can completely prevent retrovirus infections by either the parenteral, sexual, or perinatal route. First, Tsai and colleagues [125] demonstrated that tenofovir, administered subcutaneously starting 48 h before, or 4 or 24 h after, intravenous simian immunodeficiency virus (SIV) inoculation, could completely prevent SIV infection in macaques. Second, Otten and colleagues [126] reported that tenofovir, administered subcutaneously 12 or 36 h after intravaginal HIV-2 inoculation in macaques, could completely prevent HIV infection. Third, Van Rompay and colleagues [127] demonstrated that tenofovir, when administered subcutaneously at two doses of 4 mg/kg either 4 h before or 20 h after, 1 and 24 h after, or as a single dose of 30 mg/kg at 1 h after SIV inoculation, could completely prevent SIV infection in newborn macaques inoculated orally with the virus by 3 days of age.

It is obvious that tenofovir could also be used as a vaginal gel to prevent HIV infection in sexually active women [128], and tenofovir gel has proven effective in the prevention of SIV rectal transmission in macaques after local preexposure application [129], but it should be admitted that topical use would not be as convenient or widely protective as the daily use of a single pill (Viread, Truvada, or Atripla), which should prevent HIV transmission by any route. Defined clinical studies in humans on the use of either Viread, Truvada, or Atripla in the prevention (preexposure prophylaxis) of HIV infection are eagerly awaited.

Preexposure prophylaxis with TDF/(−)FTC prevents vaginal HIV-1 transmission in humanized bone marrow–liver–thymus (BLT) mice [130] as well as rectal SHIV transmission in macaques [131]. Although preexposure prophylaxis will not be able to rid the world of HIV [132], it deserves full support for continued pursuit [133]. Daily oral use of TDF in HIV-infected women was not associated with increased adverse clinical or laboratory adverse events, but its effectiveness could not be evaluated conclusively because of the (too) small number of HIV infections observed during this study [134].

The use of TDF in pregnancy is under surveillance: Findings from the antiretroviral pregnancy registry have indicated that the birth-defect prevalence with exposure during the first trimester to the NtRTIs (28%) was similar to that of other antiretrovirals (2.9%) or the general population-based surveillance data (2.72%) [135].

In a preliminary study, the use of tenofovir in HIV-infected pregnant women may have prevented mother-to-child transmission of HIV [136], although longer prospective studies of tenofovir in pregnant women are warranted to substantiate these observations.

Remarkably, in rhesus macaques, the safety and sustained benefits of prolonged tenofovir-containing regimens have been noted from infancy to adulthood, including during pregnancy [137].

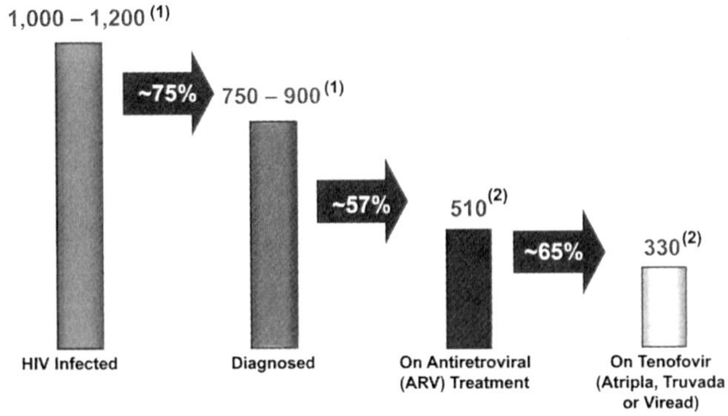

FIGURE 7 U.S. HIV market dynamics (thousands of patients). Less than half of HIV-infected persons are currently on ARV therapy. (*See insert for color representation of the figure.*)

CONCLUSIONS

Twenty-five anti-HIV medicines have been formally licensed for the treatment of AIDS [138]: seven nucleoside RT inhibitors (NRTIs: zidovudine, didanosine, zalcitabine, stavudine, lamivudine, abacavir, emtricitabine), one nucleotide RT inhibitor [NtRTI: tenofovir in its oral prodrug form, tenofovir disoproxil fumarate (TDF), Viread], four nonnucleoside RT inhibitors (NNRTIs: nevirapine, delavirdine, efavirenz, etravirine), 10 protease inhibitors (PIs: saquinavir, ritonavir, indinavir, nelfinavir, amprenavir, lopinavir, atazanavir, fosamprenavir, tipranavir, darunavir), one fusion inhibitor (FI: enfuvirtide), one coreceptor inhibitor (CRI: maraviroc) and one integrase inhibitor (INI: raltegravir). Fixed-dose drug combinations, consisting of zidovudine with lamivudine, or abacavir with zidovudine and lamivudine, or abacavir with lamivudine, or TDF with emtricitabine (Truvada), or TDF with emtricitabine and efavirenz (Atripla), are also available for the treatment of HIV infections.

Of the HIV-infected individuals, about 75% have been diagnosed as such, and about 57% of those are on antiretroviral (ARV) treatment, but the majority (about two-thirds) of those that are on treatment do receive tenofovir in one of its three prescription forms: Viread, Truvada, or Atripla (Fig. 7).

Recommendations about when to initiate antiretroviral therapy (depending on the CD4 cell counts) and what to use for treatment-naive HIV-infected persons are constantly evolving [139]. Once begun, treatment probably should be continued indefinitely. Several regimens are acceptable as initial therapy, with TDF/(−)FTC/efavirenz (Atripla) favored because of potency and ease of administration [139].

The durability of contemporary once-daily fixed-dose antiretroviral regimens [e.g., TDF/(−)FTC/efavirenz (Atripla)] has significantly eclipsed the duration of earlier antiretroviral drug options [140]. This is due to both more convenient dosing and improved tolerability of the modern antiretroviral drug regimens. In fact, the single-tablet Atripla regimen represents a significant simplification in the management of HIV infections, yielding high rates of virologic suppression and low rates of treatment discontinuations [141,142].

Over 1 million years of patient experience has established tenofovir as a key component of HIV treatment [143]. Tenofovir has demonstrated potent antiviral efficacy with a low risk of developing resistance when used as part of an effective combination regimen. It is generally well tolerated, with a low (if any) risk of lipoatrophy or lipid abnormalities such as those seen with nucleoside analogs such as stavudine or zidovudine [143]. On the contrary, switching from the thymidine analogs (such as stavudine) to a tenofovir-containing regimen can benefit patients with lipid abnormalities or lipoatrophy.

From a cost-effectiveness viewpoint, TDF combined with (−)FTC is predicted to provide better health outcomes at lower costs as opposed to lamivudine (3TC) combinations with either abacavir or zidovudine in treatment-naive adults with HIV infection [144,145].

What remains to be taken into account, however, is the cost-effectiveness of switching from stavudine to tenofovir in first-line antiretroviral regimens in developing countries such as South Africa [146]. Rosen et al. [146] estimated that the price of TDF would have to fall from the current $ 17.00 per month to $ 6.17 per month to make it cost neutral (for South Africa), but it would be highly cost-effective at a price of $ 12.94 per month, slightly less than is currently available [146].

Acknowledgment

I am most grateful to Christiane Callebaut for her proficient editorial assistance.

REFERENCES

[1] De Clercq, E.; Holý, A.; Rosenberg, I.; Sakuma, T.; Balzarini, J.; Maudgal, P. C. A novel selective broad-spectrum anti-DNA virus agent. *Nature* **1986**, *323*, 464–467.

[2] De Clercq, E. The acyclic nucleoside phosphonates from inception to clinical use: historical perspective. *Antiviral Res.* **2007**, *75*, 1–13.

[3] De Clercq, E. Acyclic nucleoside phosphonates: past, present and future. Bridging chemistry to HIV, HBV, HCV, HPV, adeno-, herpes-, and poxvirus infections: the phosphonate bridge. *Biochem. Pharmacol.* **2007**, *73*, 911–922.

[4] De Clercq, E.; Descamps, J.; De Somer, P.; Holý, A. (*S*)-9-(2,3-Dihydroxypropyl)adenine: an aliphatic nucleoside analog with broad-spectrum antiviral activity. *Science* **1978**, *200*, 563–565.

[5] De Clercq, E.; Holý, A. Acyclic nucleoside phosphonates: a key class of antiviral drugs. *Nat. Rev. Drug Discov.* **2005**, *4*, 928–940.

[6] Pauwels, R.; Balzarini, J.; Schols, D.; Baba, M.; Desmyter, J.; Rosenberg, I.; Holý, A.; De Clercq, E. Phosphonylmethoxyethyl purine derivatives, a new class of anti-human immunodeficiency virus agents. *Antimicrob. Agents Chemother.* **1988**, *32*, 1025–1030.

[7] Balzarini, J.; Naesens, L.; Herdewijn, P.; Rosenberg, I.; Holý, A.; Pauwels, R.; Baba, M.; Johns, D. G.; De Clercq, E. Marked in vivo antiretrovirus activity of 9-(2-phosphonylmethoxyethyl)adenine, a selective anti-human immunodeficiency virus agent. *Proc. Natl. Acad. Sci. USA* **1989**, *86*, 332–336.

[8] Balzarini, J.; Holý, A.; Jindrich, J.; Dvorakova, H.; Hao, Z.; Snoeck, R.; Herdewijn, P.; Johns, D. G.; De Clercq, E. 9-[(2*R*,*S*)-3-fluoro-2-phosphonylmethoxypropyl] derivatives of purines: a class of highly selective antiretroviral agents in vitro and in vivo. *Proc. Natl. Acad. Sci. USA* **1991**, *88*, 4961–4965.

[9] Balzarini, J.; Holý, A.; Jindrich, J.; Naesens, L.; Snoeck, R.; Schols, D.; De Clercq, E. Differential antiherpesvirus and antiretrovirus effects of the (*S*) and (*R*) enantiomers of acyclic nucleoside phosphonates: potent and selective in vitro and in vivo antiretrovirus activities of (*R*)-9-(2-phosphonomethoxypropyl)-2,6-diaminopurine. *Antimicrob. Agents Chemother.* **1993**, *37*, 332–338.

[10] Balzarini, J.; Aquaro, S.; Perno, C. -F.; Witvrouw, M.; Holý, A.; De Clercq, E. Activity of the (*R*)-enantiomers of 9-(2-phosphonylmethoxypropyl)adenine and 9-(2-phosphonylmethoxypropyl)-2,6-diaminopurine against human immunodeficiency virus in different human cell systems. *Biochem. Biophys. Res. Commun.* **1996**, *219*, 337–341.

[11] De Clercq, E. Potential of acyclic nucleoside phosphonates in the treatment of DNA virus and retrovirus infections. *Expert Rev. Anti-Infect. Ther.* **2003**, *1*, 21–43.

[12] De Clercq, E.; Sakuma, T.; Baba, M.; Pauwels, R.; Balzarini, J.; Rosenberg, I.; Holý, A. Antiviral activity of phosphonylmethoxyalkyl derivatives of purine and pyrimidines. *Antiviral Res.* **1987**, *8*, 261–272.

[13] Helliot, B.; Panis, B.; Frison, E.; De Clercq, E.; Swennen, R.; Lepoivre, P.; Neyts, J. The acyclic nucleoside phosphonate analogues, adefovir, tenofovir and PMEDAP, efficiently eliminate banana streak virus from banana (*Musa* spp.). *Antiviral Res.* **2003**, *59*, 121–126.

[14] Shen, Y.; Zhukovskaya, N. L.; Zimmer, M. I.; Soelaiman, S.; Bergson, P.; Wang, C. R.; Gibbs, C. S.; Tang, W. J. Selective inhibition of anthrax edema factor by adefovir, a drug for chronic hepatitis B virus infection. *Proc. Natl. Acad. Sci. USA* **2004**, *101*, 3242–3247.

[15] Vela, J. E.; Miller, M. D.; Rhodes, G. R.; Ray, A. S. Effect of nucleoside and nucleotide reverse transcriptase inhibitors of HIV on endogenous nucleotide pools. *Antiviral Ther.* **2008**, *13*, 789–797.

[16] Suo, Z.; Johnson, K. A. Selective inhibition of HIV-1 reverse transcriptase by an antiviral inhibitor,(*R*)-9-(2-phosphonylmethoxypropyl)adenine. *J. Biol. Chem.* **1998**, *273*, 27250–27258.

[17] Cherrington, J. M.; Allen, S. J. W.; Bischofberger, N.; Chen, M. S. Kinetic interaction of the diphosphates of 9-(2-phosphonylmethoxyethyl)adenine and other anti-HIV active purine congeners with HIV reverse transcriptase and human DNA polymerases α, β and γ. *Antiviral Chem. Chemother.* **1995**, *6*, 217–221.

[18] Cihlar, T.; Chen, M. S. Incorporation of selected nucleoside phosphonates and anti-human immunodeficiency virus nucleotide analogues into DNA by human DNA polymerases α, β and γ. *Antiviral Chem. Chemother.* **1997**, *8*, 187–195.

[19] Birkus, G.; Hitchcock, M. J.; Cihlar, T. Assessment of mitochondrial toxicity in human cells treated with tenofovir: comparison with other nucleoside reverse transcriptase inhibitors. *Antimicrob. Agents Chemother.* **2002**, *46*, 716–723.

[20] Biesecker, G.; Karimi, S.; Desjardins, J.; Meyer, D.; Abbott, B.; Bendele, R.; Richardson, F. Evaluation of mitochondrial DNA content and enzyme levels in tenofovir DF-treated rats, rhesus monkeys and woodchucks. *Antiviral Res.* **2003**, *58*, 217–225.

[21] Gallant, J. E.; Deresinski, S. Tenofovir disoproxil fumarate. *Clin. Infect. Dis.* **2003**, *37*, 944–950.

[22] Margot, N. A.; Isaacson, E.; McGowan, I.; Cheng, A. K.; Schooley, R. T.; Miller, M. D. Genotypic and phenotypic analyses of HIV-1 in antiretroviral-experienced patients treated with tenofovir DF. *AIDS* **2002**, *16*, 1227–1235.

[23] Murry, J. P.; Higgins, J.; Matthews, T. B.; Huang, V. Y.; Van Rompay, K. K.; Pedersen, N. C.; North, T. W. Reversion of the M184V mutation in simian immunodeficiency virus reverse transcriptase is selected by tenofovir, even in the presence of lamivudine. *J. Virol.* **2003**, *77*, 1120–1130.

[24] Wolf, K.; Walter, H.; Beerenwinkel, N.; Keulen, W.; Kaiser, R.; Hoffmann, D.; Lengauer, T.; Selbig, J.; Vandamme, A. M.; Korn, K.; Schmidt, B. Tenofovir resistance and resensitization. *Antimicrob. Agents Chemother.* **2003**, *47*, 3478–3484.

[25] Deval, J.; White, K. L.; Miller, M. D.; Parkin, N. T.; Courcambeck, J.; Halfon, P.; Selmi, B.; Boretto, J.; Canard, B. Mechanistic basis for reduced viral and enzymatic fitness of HIV-1 reverse transcriptase containing both K65R and M184V mutations. *J. Biol. Chem.* **2004**, *279*, 509–516.

[26] Miller, M. D.; Margot, N.; Lu, B.; Zhong, L.; Chen, S. S.; Cheng, A.; Wulfsohn, M. Genotypic and phenotypic

predictors of the magnitude of response to tenofovir disoproxil fumarate treatment in antiretroviral-experienced patients. *J. Infect. Dis.* **2004**, *189*, 837–846.

[27] Marchand, B.; White, K. L.; Ly, J. K.; Margot, N. A.; Wang, R.; McDermott, M.; Miller, M. D.; Götte, M. Effects of the translocation status of human immunodeficiency virus type 1 reverse transcriptase on the efficacy of excision of tenofovir. *Antimicrob. Agents Chemother.* **2007**, *51*, 2911–2919.

[28] von Wyl, V.; Yerly, S.; Böni, J.; Bürgisser, P.; Klimkait, T.; Battegay, M.; Bernasconi, E.; Cavassini, M.; Furrer, H.; Hirschel, B.; et al. Factors associated with the emergence of K65R in patients with HIV-1 infection treated with combination antiretroviral therapy containing tenofovir. *Clin. Infect. Dis.* **2008**, *46*, 1299–1309.

[29] de Mendoza, C.; Jiménez-Nacher, I.; Garrido, C.; Barreiro, P.; Poveda, E.; Corral, A.; Zahonero, N.; González-Lahoz, J.; Soriano, V. Changing patterns in HIV reverse transcriptase resistance mutations after availability of tenofovir. *Clin. Infect. Dis.* **2008**, *46*, 1782–1785.

[30] Svarovskaia, E. S.; Feng, J. Y.; Margot, N. A.; Myrick, F.; Goodman, D.; Ly, J. K.; White, K. L.; Kutty, N.; Wang, R.; Borroto-Esoda, K.; Miller, M. D. The A62V and S68G mutations in HIV-1 reverse transcriptase partially restore the replication defect associated with the K65R mutation. *J. Acquir. Immune Defic. Syndr.* **2008**, *48*, 428–436.

[31] Delaugerre, C.; Roudiere, L.; Peytavin, G.; Rouzioux, C.; Viard, J. P.; Chaix, M. L. Selection of a rare resistance profile in an HIV-1-infected patient exhibiting a failure to an antiretroviral regimen including tenofovir DF. *J. Clin. Virol.* **2005**, *32*, 241–244.

[32] Kagan, R. M.; Lee, T. S.; Ross, L.; Lloyd, R. M., Jr.; Lewinski, M. A.; Potts, S. J. Molecular basis of antagonism between K70E and K65R tenofovir-associated mutations in HIV-1 reverse transcriptase. *Antiviral Res.* **2007**, *75*, 210–218.

[33] Sluis-Cremer, N.; Sheen, C. W.; Zelina, S.; Torres, P. S.; Parikh, U. M.; Mellors, J. W. Molecular mechanism by which the K70E mutation in human immunodeficiency virus type 1 reverse transcriptase confers resistance to nucleoside reverse transcriptase inhibitors. *Antimicrob. Agents Chemother.* **2007**, *51*, 48–53.

[34] Van Rompay, K. K.; Johnson, J. A.; Blackwood, E. J., Singh, R. P.; Lipscomb, J.; Matthews, T. B.; Marthas, M. L.; Pedersen, N. C.; Bischofberger, N.; Heneine, W.; North, T. W. Sequential emergence and clinical implications of viral mutants with K70E and K65R mutation in reverse transcriptase during prolonged tenofovir monotherapy in rhesus macaques with chronic RT-SHIV infection. *Retrovirology* **2007**, *4*, 25.

[35] De Clercq, E. Antivirals: current state of the art. *Future Virol.* **2008**, *3*, 393–405.

[36] De Clercq, E. Emerging antiviral drugs. *Expert Opin. Emerging Drugs* **2008**, *13*, 393–416.

[37] Naesens, L.; Balzarini, J.; Bischofberger, N.; De Clercq, E. Antiretroviral activity and pharmacokinetcs in mice of oral bis(pivaloyloxymethyl)-9-(2-phosphonylmethoxyethyl) adenine, the bis(pivaloyloxymethyl) ester prodrug of 9-(2-phosphonylmethoxyethyl)adenine. *Antimicrob. Agents Chemother.* **1996**, *40*, 22–28.

[38] Naesens, L.; Snoeck, R.; Andrei, G.; Balzarini, J.; Neyts, J.; De Clercq, E. HPMPC (cidofovir), PMEA (adefovir) and related acyclic nucleoside phosphonate analogues: a review of their pharmacology and clinical potential in the treatment of viral infections. *Antiviral Chem. Chemother.* **1997**, *8*, 1–23.

[39] Robbins, B. L.; Srinivas, R. V.; Kim, C.; Bischofberger, N.; Fridland, A. Anti-human immunodeficiency virus activity and cellular metabolism of a potential prodrug of the acyclic nucleoside phosphonate 9-*R*-(2-phosphonomethoxypropyl) adenine (PMPA), bis(isopropyloxymethylcarbonyl)-PMPA. *Antimicrob. Agents Chemother.* **1998**, *42*, 612–617.

[40] Arimilli, M. N.; Kim, C. U.; Dougherty, J.; Mulato, A.; Oliyai, R.; Shaw, J. P.; Cundy, K. C.; Bischofberger, N. Synthesis, in vitro biological evaluation and oral bioavailability of 9-[2-(phosphonomethoxy)propyl]adenine (PMPA) prodrugs. *Antiviral Chem. Chemother.* **1997**, *8*, 557–564.

[41] Naesens, L.; Bischofberger, N.; Augustijns, P.; Annaert, P.; Van den Mooter, G.; Arimilli, M. N.; Kim, C. U.; De Clercq, E. Antiretroviral efficacy and pharmacokinetics of oral bis(isopropyloxycarbonyloxymethyl)-9-(2-phosphonylmethoxypropyl)adenine in mice. *Antimicrob. Agents Chemother.* **1998**, *42*, 1568–1573.

[42] Schooley, R. T.; Ruane, P.; Myers, R. A.; Beall, G.; Lampiris, H.; Berger, D.; Chen, S. S.; Miller, M. D.; Isaacson, E.; Cheng, A. K. Tenofovir DF in antiretroviral-experienced patients: results from a 48-week, randomized, double-blind study. *AIDS* **2002**, *16*, 1257–1263.

[43] Squires, K.; Pozniak, A. L.; Pierone, G. Jr.; Steinhart, C. R.; Berger, D.; Bellos, N. C.; Becker, S. L.; Wulfsohn, M.; Miller, M. D.; Toole, J. J.; et al. Tenofovir disoproxil fumarate in nucleoside-resistant HIV-1 infection: a randomized trial. *Ann. Intern. Med.* **2003**, *139*, 313–320.

[44] Gallant, J. E.; DeJesus, E.; Arribas, J. R.; Pozniak, A. L.; Gazzard, B.; Campo, R. E.; Lu, B.; McColl, D.; Chuck, S.; Enejosa, J.; et al. Tenofovir DF, emtricitabine, and efavirenz vs zidovudine, lamivudine, and efavirenz for HIV. *N. Engl. J. Med.* **2006**, *354*, 251–260.

[45] Gallant, J. E.; Staszewski, S.; Pozniak, A. L.; DeJesus, E.; Suleiman, J. M.; Miller, M. D.; Coakley, D. F.; Lu, B.; Toole, J. J.; Cheng, A. K. Efficacy and safety of tenofovir DF vs. stavudine in combination therapy in antiretroviral-naive patients: a 3-year randomized trial. *JAMA* **2004**, *292*, 191–201.

[46] Valantin, M.-A.; De Truchis, P.; Bittar, R.; Bollens, D.; Slama, L.; Lebouché, B.; Pétour, P.; Aubron-Olivier, C.; Costagliola, D.; Katlama, C. Early improvement of triglycerides and LDL-cholesterol levels in dyslipidemic HIV-infected patients after switching NRTI backbone to tenofovir plus emtricitabine: the TOTEM randomised trial. 10th International Workshop on Adverse Drug Reactions and Lipodystrophy in HIV, London, Nov. 6–8, 2008. Poster P30.

[47] Gathe, Jr. J. C. Switching HIV-infected, suppressed patients from ABC/3TC to FTC/TDF improves lipids: the SETTLE study. 10th International Workshop on Adverse Drug Reactions and Lipodystrophy in HIV, London, Nov. 6–8, 2008. Poster P37.

[48] Ribera, E.; Clotet, B.; Martinez, E.; Estrada, V.; Sanz, J.; Berenguer, J.; Rubio, R.; Pulido, F.; Larrouse, M.;

Curran, A.; et al. 48 Week outcomes following switch from AZT/3TC to FTC/TDF (TVD) vs continuing on AZT/3TC: 48 week interim analysis of the RECOMB trial. 9th International Congress on Drug Therapy in HIV Infection, Glasgow, U.K, Nov. 9–13, 2008. Poster P054.

[49] De Clercq, E. From adefovir to Atripla™ via tenofovir, Viread™ and Truvada™. *Future Virol.* **2006**, *1*, 709–715.

[50] Madruga, J. V. R.; Cassetti, I.; Etzel, A.; Suleiman, J.; Zhou, Y.; Cheng, A. K.; Enejosa, J. The safety and efficacy of tenofovir DF (TDF) in combination with lamivudine (3TC) and efavirenz (EFV) in antiretroviral-naïve patients through seven years. 9th International Congress on Drug Therapy in HIV Infection, Glasgow, U.K, Nov. 9–13, 2008. Poster P004.

[51] Hoetelmans, R. M.; Mariën, K.; De Pauw, M.; Hill, A.; Peeters, M.; Sekar, V.; De Doncker, P.; Woodfall, B.; Lefebvre, E. Pharmacokinetic interaction between TMC114/ritonavir and tenofovir disoproxil fumarate in healthy volunteers. *Br. J. Clin. Pharmacol.* **2007**, *64*, 655–661.

[52] Wenning, L. A.; Friedman, E. J.; Kost, J. T.; Breidinger, S. A.; Stek, J. E.; Lasseter, K. C.; Gottesdiener, K. M.; Chen, J.; Teppler, H.; Wagner, J. A.; et al. Lack of a significant drug interaction between raltegravir and tenofovir. *Antimicrob. Agents Chemother.* **2008**, *52*, 3253–3258.

[53] Ramanathan, S.; Shen, G.; Cheng, A.; Kearney, B. P. Pharmacokinetics of emtricitabine, tenofovir, and GS-9137 following coadministration of emtricitabine/tenofovir disoproxil fumarate and ritonavir-boosted GS-9137. *J. Acquir. Immune Defic. Syndr.* **2007**, *45*, 274–279.

[54] Molina, J. N.; Andrade-Villanueva, J.; Echevarria, J.; Chetchotisakd, P.; Corral, J.; David, N.; Moyle, G.; Mancini, M.; Percival, L.; Yang, R.; et al. Once-daily atazanavir/ritonavir versus twice-daily lopinavir/ritonavir, each in combination with tenofovir and emtricitabine, for management of antiretroviral-naive HIV-1-infected patients: 48 week efficacy and safety results of the CASTLE study. *Lancet* **2008**, *372*, 646–655.

[55] Pozniak, A. L.; Gallant, J. E.; DeJesus, E.; Arribas, J. R.; Gazzard, B.; Campo, R. E.; Chen, S. S.; McColl, D.; Enejosa, J.; Toole, J. J.; Cheng, A. K. Tenofovir disoproxil fumarate, emtricitabine, and efavirenz versus fixed-dose zidovudine/lamivudine and efavirenz in antiretroviral-naive patients: virologic, immunologic, and morphologic changes: a 96-week analysis. *J. Acquir. Immune Defic. Syndr.* **2006**, *43*, 535–540.

[56] De Clercq, E. AIDS in the Third World: How to stop the HIV infection? *Verh. K. Acad. Geneesk. Belg.* **2007**, *64*, 65–80.

[57] De Clercq, E. Anti-HIV drugs. *Verh. K. Acad. Geneesk. Belg.* **2007**, *64*, 81–104.

[58] Matthias, A. A.; Hinkle, J.; Menning, M.; Hui, J.; Kaul, S.; Kearney, B. P. Bioequivalence of efavirenz/emtricitabine/tenofovir disoproxil fumarate single-tablet regimen. *J. Acquir. Immune Defic. Syndr.* **2007**, *46*, 167–173.

[59] Arribas, J. R.; Pozniak, A. L.; Gallant, J. E.; DeJesus, E.; Gazzard, B.; Campo, R. E.; Chen, S. S.; McColl, D.; Holmes, C. B.; Enejosa, J.; et al. Tenofovir disoproxil fumarate, emtricabine, and efavirenz compared with zidovudine/lamivudine and efavirenz in treatment-naive patients: 144-week analysis. *J. Acquir. Immune Defic. Syndr.* **2008**, *47*, 74–78.

[60] DeJesus, E.; Young, B.; Flaherty, J.; Ebrahimi, R.; Maa, J.-F.; McColl, D.; Seekins, D.; Farajallah, A. Simplification of antiretroviral therapy with efavirenz/emtricitabine/tenofovir DF single tablet regimen vs. continued unmodified antiretroviral therapy in virologically-suppressed, HIV-1-infected patients. 48th Annual ICAAC/IDSA and 46th Annual Meeting, Washington, DC, Oct. 25–28, 2008. Poster H-1234.

[61] DeJesus, E.; Pozniak, A.; Gallant, J.; Arribas, J.; Zhou, Y.; Cheng, A.; Enejosa, J. The 48-week efficacy and safety of switching to fixed-dose efavirenz/emtricitabine/tenofovir DF in HIV-1-infected patients receiving HAART. 48th Annual ICAAC/IDSA and 46th Annual Meeting, Washington, DC, Oct. 25–28, 2008. Poster H-1235.

[62] Léon, A.; Mallolas, J.; Martinez, E.; De Lazzari, E.; Pumarola, T.; Larrousse, M.; Milincovic, A.; Lonca, M.; Blanco, J. L.; Laguno, M.; et al. High rate of virological failure in maintenance antiretroviral therapy with didanosine and tenofovir. *AIDS* **2005**, *19*, 1695–1697.

[63] Maitland, D.; Moyle, G.; Hand, J.; Mandalia, S.; Boffito, M.; Nelson, M.; Gazzard, B. Early virologic failure in HIV-1-infected subjects on didanosine/tenofovir/efavirenz: 12-week results from a randomized trial. *AIDS* **2005**, *19*, 1183–1188.

[64] Gallant, J. E.; Rodriguez, A. E.; Weinberg, W. G.; Young, B.; Berger, D. S.; Lim, M. L.; Liao, Q.; Ross, L.; Johnson, J.; Shaefer, M. S. Early virologic nonresponse to tenofovir, abacavir, and lamivudine in HIV-infected antiretroviral-naive subjects. *J. Infect. Dis.* **2005**, *192*, 1921–1930.

[65] Delaunay, C.; Brun-Vézinet, F.; Landman, R.; Collin, G.; Peytavin, G.; Trylesinski, A.; Flandre, P.; Miller, M.; Descamps, D. Comparative selection of the K65R and M184V/I mutations in human immunodeficiency virus type 1-infected patients enrolled in a trial of first-line triple-nucleoside analog therapy. *J. Virol.* **2005**, *79*, 9572–9578.

[66] Ray, A. S.; Myrick, F.; Vela, J. E.; Olson, L. Y.; Eisenberg, E. J.; Borroto-Esodo, K.; Miller, M. D.; Fridland, A. Lack of a metabolic and antiviral drug interaction between tenofovir, abacavir and lamivudine. *Antiviral Ther.* **2005**, *10*, 451–457.

[67] Rey, D.; Hoen, B.; Chavanet, P.; Schmitt, M. P.; Hoizey, G.; Meyer, P.; Peytavin, G.; Spire, B.; Allavena, C.; Diemer, M.; et al. High rate of early virological failure with the once-daily tenofovir/lamivudine/nevirapine combination in naive HIV-1-infected patients. *J. Antimicrob. Chemother.* **2009**, *63*, 380–388.

[68] Lapadula, G.; Costarelli, S.; Quiros-Roldan, E.; Calabresi, A.; Izzo, I.; Carosi, G.; Torti, C. Risk of early virological failure of once-daily tenofovir–emtricitabine plus twice-daily nevirapine in antiretroviral therapy-naive HIV-infected patients. *Clin. Infect. Dis.* **2008**, *46*, 1127–1129.

[69] Redfield, R. R.; Morrow, J. S. Combination antiretroviral therapy with tenofovir, emtricitabine or lamivudine, and nevirapine. *Clin. Infect. Dis.* **2008**, *47*, 984–985.

[70] Sattler, F. R. Pathogenesis and treatment of lipodystrophy: what clinicians need to know. *Top. HIV Med.* **2008**, *16*, 127–133.

[71] Milinkovic, A.; Martinez, E.; López, S.; de Lazzari, E.; Miró, O; Vidal, S.; Blanco, J. L.; Garrabou, G.; Laguno, M.; Arnaiz, J. A.; et al. The impact of reducing stavudine dose versus switching to tenofovir on plasma lipids, body composition and mitochondrial function in HIV-infected patients. *Antiviral Ther.* **2007**, *12*, 407–415.

[72] van Griensven, J.; Zachariah, R.; Rasschaert, F.; Atté, E. F.; Reid, T. Weight evolution in HIV-1-infected women in Rwanda after stavudine substitution due to lipoatrophy: comparison of zidovudine with tenofovir/abacavir. *Trans. R. Soc. Trop. Med. Hyg.* **2009**, *103*, 613–619.

[73] Purdy, J. B.; Gafni, R. I.; Reynolds, J. C.; Zeichner, S.; Hazra, R. Decreased bone mineral density with off-label use of tenofovir in children and adolescents infected with human immunodeficiency virus. *J. Pediatr.* **2008**, *152*, 582–584.

[74] Giacomet, V.; Mora, S.; Martelli, L.; Merlo, M.; Sciannamblo, M.; Viganò, A. A 12-month treatment with tenofovir does not impair bone mineral accrual in HIV-infected children. *J. Acquir. Immune Defic. Syndr.* **2005**, *40*, 448–450.

[75] Gallant, J. E.; Winston, J. A.; DeJesus, E.; Pozniak, A. L.; Chen, S. S.; Cheng, A. K.; Enejosa, J. V. The 3-year renal safety of a tenofovir disoproxil fumarate vs. a thymidine analogue-containing regimen in antiretroviral-naive patients. *AIDS* **2008**; *22*, 2155–2163.

[76] Viganò, A.; Zuccotti, G. V.; Martelli, L.; Giacomet, V.; Cafarelli, L.; Borgonovo, S.; Beretta, S.; Rombolà, G.; Mora, S. Renal safety of tenofovir in HIV-infected children: a prospective, 96-week longitudinal study. *Clin. Drug Invest.* **2007**, *27*, 573–581.

[77] Peyrière, H.; Reynes, J.; Rouanet, I.; Daniel, N.; de Boever, C. M.; Mauboussin, J. M.; Leray, H.; Moachon, L.; Vincent, D.; Salmon-Céron, D. Renal tubular dysfunction associated with tenofovir therapy: report of 7 cases. *J. Acquir. Immune Defic. Syndr.* **2004**, *35*, 269–273.

[78] Barrios, A.; García-Benayas, T.; González-Lahoz, J.; Soriano, V. Tenofovir-related nephrotoxicity in HIV-infected patients. *AIDS* **2004**, *18*, 960–963.

[79] Karras, A.; Lafaurie, M.; Furco, A.; Bourgarit, A.; Droz, D.; Sereni, D.; Legendre, C.; Martinez, F.; Molina, J. M. Tenofovir-related nephrotoxicity in human immunodeficiency virus-infected patients: three cases of renal failure, Fanconi syndrome, and nephrogenic diabetes insipidus. *Clin. Infect. Dis.* **2003**, *36*, 1070–1073.

[80] Rifkin, B. S.; Perazella, M. A. Tenofovir-associated nephrotoxicity: Fanconi syndrome and renal failure. *Am. J. Med.* **2004**, *117*, 282–284.

[81] Gaspar, G.; Monereo, A.; García-Reyne, A.; de Guzmán, M. Fanconi syndrome and acute renal failure in a patient treated with tenofovir: a call for caution. *AIDS* **2004**, *18*, 351–352.

[82] Hynes, P.; Urbina, A.; McMeeking, A.; Barisoni, L.; Rabenou, R. Acute renal failure after initiation of tenofovir disoproxil fumarate. *Ren. Fail.* **2007**, *29*, 1063–1066.

[83] Kapitsinou, P. P.; Ansari, N. Acute renal failure in an AIDS patient on tenofovir: a case report. *J. Med. Case Rep.* **2008**, *2*, 94.

[84] Patel, S. M.; Zembower, T. R.; Palella, F.; Kanwar, Y. S.; Ahya, S. N. Early onset of tenofovir-induced renal failure: case report and review of the literature. *Sci. World J.* **2007**, *7*, 1140–1148.

[85] Izzedine, H.; Isnard-Bagnis, C.; Hulot, J. S.; Vittecoq, D.; Cheng, A.; Jais, C. K.; Launay-Vacher, V.; Deray, G. Renal safety of tenofovir in HIV treatment-experienced patients. *AIDS* **2004**, *18*, 1074–1076.

[86] Rollot, F.; Nazal, E. M.; Chauvelot-Moachon, L.; Kélaïdi, C.; Daniel, N.; Saba, M.; Abad, S.; Blanche, P. Tenofovir-related Fanconi syndrome with nephrogenic diabetes insipidus in a patient with acquired immunodeficiency syndrome: the role of lopinavir–ritonavir–didanosine. *Clin. Infect. Dis.* **2003**, *37*, e174–e176.

[87] Martinez, E.; Milinkovic, A.; de Lazzari, E.; Ravasi, G.; Blanco, J. L.; Larrousse, M.; Mallolas, J.; García, F; Miró, J. M.; Gatell, J. M. Pancreatic toxic effects associated with co-administration of didanosine and tenofovir in HIV-infected adults. *Lancet* **2004**, *364*, 65–67.

[88] Callens, S.; De Schacht, C.; Huyst, V.; Colebunders, R. Pancreatitis in an HIV-infected person on tenofovir, didanosine and stavudine containing highly active antiretroviral treatment. *J. Infect.* **2003**, *47*, 188–189.

[89] Murphy, M. D.; O'Hearn, M.; Chou, S. Fatal lactic acidosis and acute renal failure after addition of tenofovir to an antiretroviral regimen containing didanosine. *Clin. Infect. Dis.* **2003**, *36*, 1082–1085.

[90] Izzedine, H.; Baumelou, A.; Deray, G. Acute renal failure in HIV patients. *Nephrol. Dial. Transplant.* **2007**, *22*, 2757–2762.

[91] Madeddu, G.; Bonfanti, P.; De Socio, G. V.; Carradori, S.; Grosso, C.; Marconi, P.; Penco, G.; Rosella, E.; Miccolis, S.; Melzi, S.; et al. Tenofovir renal safety in HIV-infected patients: results from the SCOLTA Project. *Biomed. Pharmacother.* **2008**, *62*, 6–11.

[92] Nelson, M. R.; Katlama, C.; Montaner, J. S.; Cooper, D. A.; Gazzard, B.; Clotet, B.; Lazzarin, A.; Schewe, K.; Lange, J.; Wyatt, C.; et al. The safety of tenofovir disoproxil fumarate for the treatment of HIV infection in adults: the first 4 years. *AIDS* **2007**, *21*, 1273–1281.

[93] Mulenga, L. B.; Kruse, G.; Lakhi, S.; Cantrell, R. A.; Reid, S. E.; Zulu, I.; Stringer, E. M.; Krishnasami, Z.; Mwinga, A.; Saag, M. S.; et al. Baseline renal insufficiency and risk of death among HIV-infected adults on antiretroviral therapy in Lusaka, Zambia. *AIDS* **2008**, *22*, 1821–1827.

[94] Goicoechea, M.; Liu, S.; Best, B.; Sun, S.; Jain, S.; Kemper, C.; Witt, M.; Diamond, C.; Haubrich, R.; Louie, S. Greater tenofovir-associated renal function decline with protease inhibitor–based versus nonnucleoside reverse-transcriptase inhibitor–based therapy. *J. Infect. Dis.* **2008**, *197*, 102–108.

[95] Libório, A. B.; Andrade, L.; Pereira, L. V.; Saches, T. R.; Shimizu, M. H.; Seguro, A. C. Rosiglitazone reverses tenofovir-induced nephrotoxicity. *Kidney Int.* **2008**, *74*, 910–918.

[96] Yokota, T.; Mochizuki, S.; Konno, K.; Mori, S.; Shigeta, S.; De Clercq, E. Inhibitory effects of selected antiviral

compounds on human hepatitis B virus DNA synthesis. *Antimicrob. Agents Chemother.* **1991**, *35*, 394–397.

[97] Heijtink, R. A.; de Wilde, G. A.; Kruining, J.; Berk, L.; Balzarini, J.; De Clercq, E.; Holý, A.; Schalm, S. W. Inhibitory effect of 9-(2-phosphonylmethoxyethyl)adenine (PMEA) on human and duck hepatitis B virus infection. *Antiviral Res.* **1993**, *21*, 141–153.

[98] Heijtink, R. A.; Kruining, J.; de Wilde, G. A.; Balzarini, J.; De Clercq, E.; Schalm, S. W. Inhibitory effects of acyclic nucleoside phosphonates on human hepatitis B virus and duck hepatitis B virus infections in tissue culture. *Antimicrob. Agents Chemother.* **1994**, *38*, 2180–2182.

[99] Ying, C.; De Clercq, E.; Neyts, J. Lamivudine, adefovir and tenofovir exhibit long-lasting anti-hepatitis B virus activity in cell culture. *J. Viral Hepatitis* **2000**, *7*, 79–83.

[100] Ying, C.; De Clercq, E.; Nicholson, W.; Furman, P.; Neyts, J. Inhibition of the replication of the DNA polymerase M550V mutation variant of human hepatitis B virus by adefovir, tenofovir, L-FMAU, DAPD, penciclovir and lobucavir. *J. Viral Hepatitis* **2000**, *7*, 161–165.

[101] Lada, O.; Benhamou, Y.; Cahour, A.; Katlama, C.; Poynard, T.; Thibault, V. In vitro susceptibility of lamivudine-resistant hepatitis B virus to adefovir and tenofovir. *Antiviral Ther.* **2004**, *9*, 353–363.

[102] Hadziyannis, S. J.; Tassopoulos, N. C.; Heathcote, E. J.; Chang, T. T.; Kitis, G.; Rizzetto, M.; Marcellin, P.; Lim, S. G.; Goodman, Z.; Wulfsohn, M. S.; et al. Adefovir dipivoxil for the treatment of hepatitis B e antigen-negative chronic hepatitis B. *N. Engl. J. Med.* **2003**, *348*, 800–807.

[103] Marcellin, P.; Chang, T. T.; Lim, S. G.; Tong, M. J.; Sievert, W.; Shiffman, M. L.; Jeffers, L.; Goodman, Z.; Wulfsohn, M. S.; Xiong, S.; et al. Adefovir dipivoxil for the treatment of hepatitis B e antigen-positive chronic hepatitis B. *N. Engl. J. Med.* **2003**, *348*, 808–816.

[104] Hadziyannis, S. J.; Tassopoulos, N. C.; Heathcote, E. J.; Chang, T. T.; Kitis, G.; Rizzetto, M.; Marcellin, P.; Lim, S. G.; Goodman, Z.; Ma, J.; et al. Long-term therapy with adefovir dipivoxil for HBeAg-negative chronic hepatitis B. *N. Engl. J. Med.* **2005**, *352*, 2673–2681.

[105] Delaney, W. E. IV; Ray, A. S.; Yang, H.; Qi, X.; Xiong, S.; Zhu, Y.; Miller, M. D. Intracellular metabolism and in vitro activity of tenofovir against hepatitis B virus. *Antimicrob. Agents Chemother.* **2006**, *50*, 2471–2477.

[106] Ristig, M. B.; Crippin, J.; Aberg, J. A.; Powderly, W. G.; Lisker-Melman, M.; Kessels, L.; Tebas, P. Tenofovir disoproxil fumarate therapy for chronic hepatitis B in human immunodeficiency virus/hepatitis B virus-coinfected individuals for whom interferon-alpha and lamivudine therapy have failed. *J. Infect. Dis.* **2002**, *186*, 1844–1847.

[107] Dore, G. J.; Cooper, D. A.; Pozniak, A. L.; DeJesus, E.; Zhong, L.; Miller, M. D.; Lu, B.; Cheng, A. K. Efficacy of tenofovir disoproxil fumarate in antiretroviral therapy-naive and -experienced patients coinfected with HIV-1 and hepatitis B virus. *J. Infect. Dis.* **2004**, *189*, 1185–1192.

[108] Peters, M. G.; Andersen, J.; Lynch, P.; Liu, T.; Alston-Smith, B.; Brosgart, C. L.; Jacobson, J. M.; Johnson, V. A.; Pollard, R. B.; Rooney, J. F.; et al. Randomized controlled study of tenofovir and adefovir in chronic hepatitis B virus and HIV infection: ACTG A5127. *Hepatology* **2006**, *44*, 1110–1116.

[109] Matthews, G. V.; Avihingsanon, A.; Lewin, S. R.; Amin, J.; Rerknimitr, R.; Petcharapirat, P.; Marks, P.; Sasadeusz, J.; Cooper, D. A.; Bowden, S.; et al. A randomized trial of combination hepatitis B therapy in HIV/HBV coinfected antiretroviral naive individuals in Thailand. *Hepatology* **2008**, *48*, 1062–1069.

[110] Lacombe, K.; Gozlan, J.; Boyd, A.; Boelle, P. Y.; Bonnard, P.; Molina, J. M.; Miailhes, P., Lascoux-Combe, C.; Serfaty, L.; Zoulim, F.; Girard, P. M. Comparison of the antiviral activity of adefovir and tenofovir on hepatitis B virus in HIV-HBV-coinfected patients. *Antiviral Ther.* **2008**, *13*, 705–713.

[111] Matthews, G. V.; Cooper, D. A.; Dore, G. J. Improvements in parameters of end-stage liver disease in patients with HIV/HBV-related cirrhosis treated with tenofovir. *Antiviral Ther.* **2007**, *12*, 119–122.

[112] Mallet, V. O.; Dhalluin-Venier, V.; Verkarre, V.; Correas, J. M.; Chaix, M. L.; Viard, J. P.; Pol, S. Reversibility of cirrhosis in HIV/HBV coinfection. *Antiviral Ther.* **2007**, *12*, 279–283.

[113] van Bömmel, F. ; Wünsche; T.; Mauss, S.; Reinke, P.; Bergk, A.; Schürmann, D.; Wiedenmann, B.; Berg, T. Comparison of adefovir and tenofovir in the treatment of lamivudine-resistant hepatitis B virus infection. *Hepatology* **2004**, *40*, 1421–1425.

[114] Kuo, A.; Dienstag, J. L.; Chung, R. T. Tenofovir disoproxil fumarate for the treatment of lamivudine-resistant hepatitis B. *Clin. Gastroenterol. Hepatol.* **2004**, *2*, 266–272.

[115] Marcellin, P.; Heathcote, E. J.; Buti, M.; Gane, E.; de Man, R. A.; Krastev, Z.; Germanidis, G.; Lee, S. S.; Flisiak, R.; Kaita, K.; et al. Tenofovir disoproxil fumarate versus adefovir dipivoxil for chronic hepatitis B. *N. Engl. J. Med.* **2008**, *359*, 2442–2455.

[116] Marcellin, P.; Buti, M.; Krastev, Z.; Gurel, S.; Balabanska, R.; Dusheiko, G.; Myers, R.; Heathcote, E. J.; Sorbel, J.; Anderson, J.; et al. Two year tenofovir disoproxil fumarate (TDF) treatment and adefovir dipivoxil (ADV) switch data in HBeAg-negative patients with chronic hepatitis B (Study 102). 59th Annual Meeting of the American Association for the Study of the Liver Diseases (AASLD), San Francisco, Oct. 31–Nov. 4, 2008. Oral Presentation 146.

[117] Heathcote, E. J.; Gane, E.; deMan, R.; Chan, S.; Sievert, W.; Mauss, S.; Marcellin, P.; Sorbel, J.; Anderson, J.; Mondou, E.; et al. Two year tenofovir disoproxil fumarate (TDF) treatment and adefovir dipivoxil (ADV) switch data in HBeAg-positive patients with chronic hepatitis B (Study 103). 59th Annual Meeting of the American Association for the Study of the Liver Diseases (AASLD), San Francisco, Oct. 31–Nov. 4, 2008. Oral Presentation 158.

[118] Snow-Lampart, A.; Chappell, B.; Curtis, M.; Zhu, Y.; Heathcote, J.; Marcellin, P.; Borroto-Esoda, K. Week 96 resistance surveillance for HBeAg positive and negative subjects with chronic HBV infection randomized to receive tenofovir DF 300 mg QD. 59th Annual Meeting of the American Association for the Study of the Liver Diseases (AASLD), San Francisco, Oct. 31–Nov. 4, 2008. Poster 977.

[119] Curtis, M.; Hinkle, J.; Harris, J.; Borroto-Esoda, K.; Zhu, Y. Tenofovir is equally active in vitro against wild-type HBV clinical isolates of genotypes A–H. 59th Annual Meeting of the American Association for the Study of the Liver Diseases (AASLD), San Francisco, Oct. 31–Nov 4, 2008. Poster 955.

[120] Lee, S.; Heathcote, E. J.; Sievert, W.; Rinh, H.; Kaita, K.; Younossi, Z.; George, M.; Shiffman, M.; Marcellin, P.; Sorbel, J.; et al. Tenofovir disoproxil fumarate (TDF) versus adefovir dipivoxil (ADV) in Asians with HBeAg-positive and HBeAg-negative chronic hepatitis B participating in Studies 102 and 103. 59th Annual Meeting of the American Association for the Study of the Liver Diseases (AASLD), San Francisco, Oct. 31–Nov. 4, 2008. Poster 980.

[121] Deniz, B.; Everhard, F. Cost effectiveness simultation analysis of tenofovir disoproxil fumarate (TDF), lamivudine (LAM), adefovir dipivoxil (ADV) and entecavir (ETV) in HBeAg negative patients with chronic hepatitis B (CHB) in the USA. 59th Annual Meeting of the American Association for the Study of the Liver Diseases (AASLD), San Francisco, Oct. 31–Nov. 4, 2008. Poster 976.

[122] Reijnders, J. G.; Janssen, H. L. Potency of tenofovir in chronic hepatitis B: mono or combination therapy. *J. Hepatol.* **2008**, *48*, 383–386.

[123] Tan, J.; Degertekin, B.; Wong, S. N.; Husain, M.; Oberhelman, K.; Lok, A. S. Tenofovir monotherapy is effective in hepatitis B patients with antiviral treatment failure to adefovir in the absence of adefovir-resistant mutations. *J. Hepatol.* **2008**, *48*, 391–398.

[124] Lai, C. L.; Yuen, M. F. Chronic hepatitis B: new goals, new treatment. *N. Engl. J. Med.* **2008**, *359*, 2488–2491.

[125] Tsai, C.-C.; Follis, K. E.; Sabo, A.; Beck, T. W.; Grant, R. F.; Bischofberger, N.; Benveniste, R. E.; Black, R. Prevention of SIV infection in macaques by (*R*)-9-(2-phosphonylmethoxypropyl)adenine. *Science* **1995**, *270*, 1197–1198.

[126] Otten, R. A.; Smith, D. K.; Adams, D. R.; Pullium, J. K.; Jackson, E.; Kim, C. N.; Jaffe, H.; Janssen, R.; Butera, S.; Folks, T. M. Efficacy of postexposure prophylaxis after intravaginal exposure of pig-tailed macaques to a human-derived retrovirus (human immunodeficiency virus type 2). *J. Virol.* **2000**, *74*, 9771–9775.

[127] Van Rompay, K. K.; McChesney, M. B.; Aguirre, N. L.; Schmidt, K. A.; Bischofberger, N.; Marthas, M. L. Two low doses of tenofovir protect newborn macaques against oral simian immunodeficiency virus infection. *J. Infect. Dis.* **2001**, *184*, 429–438.

[128] Mayer, K. H.; Masiankowski, L. A.; Gai, F.; El-Sadr, W. M.; Justman, J.; Kwiecien, A.; Masse, B.; Eshleman, S. H.; Hendrix, C.; Morrow, K.; et al. Safety and tolerability of tenofovir vaginal gel in abstinent and sexually active HIV-infected and uninfected women. *AIDS* **2006**, *20*, 543–551.

[129] Cranage, M.; Sharpe, S.; Herrera, C.; Cope, A.; Dennis, M.; Berry, N.; Ham, C.; Heeney, J.; Rezk, N.; Kashuba, A.; et al. Prevention of SIV rectgal transmission and priming of T cell responses in macaques after local pre-exposure application of tenofovir gel. *PLoS Med.* **2008**, *5*, e157.

[130] Denton, P. W.; Estes, J. D.; Sun, Z.; Othieno, F. A.; Wei, B. L.; Wege, A. K.; Powell, D. A.; Payne, D.; Haase, A. T.; Garcia, J. V. Antiretroviral pre-exposure prophylaxis prevents vaginal transmission of HIV-1 in humanized BLT mice. *PLoS Med.* **2008**, *5*, e16.

[131] Garcia-Lerma, J. G.; Otten, R. A.; Qari, S. H.; Jackson, E.; Cong, M. E.; Masciotra, S.; Luo, W.; Kim, C.; Adams, D. R.; Monsour, M.; et al. Prevention of rectal SHIV transmission in macaques by daily or intermittent prophylaxis with emtricitabine and tenofovir. *PLoS Med.* **2008**, *5*, e28.

[132] Paxton, L. A.; Hope, T.; Jaffe, H. W. Pre-exposure prophylaxis for HIV infection: What if it works ? Lancet **2007**, *370*, 89–93.

[133] Kersh, E. N.; Luo, W.; Adams, D. R.; Mitchell, J.; Garcia-Lerma, J. G.; Heneine, W.; Folks, T. M.; Butera, S.; Otten, R. A. Short communication: no evidence of occult SHIV infection as demonstrated by $CD8^+$ cell depletion after chemoprophylaxis-induced protection from mucosal infection in rhesus macaques. *AIDS Res. Hum. Retrovir.* **2008**, *24*, 543–546.

[134] Peterson, L.; Taylor, D.; Roddy, R.; Belai, G.; Phillips, P.; Nanda, K.; Grant, R.; Clarke, E. E.; Doh, A. S.; Ridzon, R.; et al. Tenofovir disoproxil fumarate for prevention of HIV infection in women: a phase 2, double-blind, randomized, placebo-controlled trial. *PLoS Clin. Trials* **2007**, *2*, e27.

[135] Olmscheid, B.; Zhang, S. Use of tenofovir disoproxil fumarate (TDF) in pregnancy: findings from the Antiretroviral Pregnancy Registry (APR). 48th Annual ICAAC/IDSA and 46th Annual Meeting, Washington, DC, Oct. 25–28, 2008. Posters H-456 and 976.

[136] Nurutdinova, D.; Onen, N. F.; Hayes, E.; Mondy, K.; Overton, E. T. Adverse effects of tenofovir use in HIV-infected pregnant women and their infants. *Ann. Pharmacother.* **2008**, *42*, 1581–1585.

[137] Van Rompay, K. K.; Durand-Gasselin, L.; Brignolo, L. L.; Ray, A. S.; Abel, K.; Cihlar, T.; Spinner, A.; Jerome, C.; Moore, J.; Kearney, B. P.; et al. Chronic administration of tenofovir to rhesus macaques from infancy through adulthood and pregnancy: summary of pharmacokinetics and biological and virological effects. *Antimicrob. Agents Chemother.* **2008**, *52*, 3144–3160.

[138] De Clercq, E. Anti-HIV drugs: 25 compounds approved witin 25 years after the discovery of HIV. *Int. J. Antimicrob. Agents* **2009**, *33*, 307–320.

[139] Hirsch, M. S. Initiating therapy: when to start, what to use. *J. Infect. Dis.* **2008**, *197* (Suppl. 3), S252–S260.

[140] Willig, J. H.; Abroms, S.; Westfall, A. O.; Routman, J.; Adusumilli, S.; Varshney, M.; Allison, J.; Chatham, A.; Raper, J. L.; Kaslow, R. A.; et al. Increased regimen durability in the era of once-daily fixed-dose combination antiretroviral therapy. *AIDS* **2008**, *22*, 1951–1960.

[141] Young, B.; DeJesus, E.; Morales-Ramirez, J.; Flaherty, J.; Ebrahimi, R.; Maa, J.-F.; McColl, D.; Seekins, D.; Farajallah, A. Simplification of antiretroviral therapy with efavirenz/emtricitabine/tenofovir DF single tablet regimen vs. continued antiretroviral therapy in suppressed HIV-1-infected patients. 9th International Congress on Drug

Therapy in HIV Infection, Glasgow, UK, Nov. 9–13, 2008. Poster P061.

[142] Hodder, S.; Mounzer, K.; DeJesus, E.; Maa, J.-F.; Ebrahimi, R.; Grimm, K.; Flaherty, J.; Farajallah, A. Patient reported outcomes after simplification to a single tablet regimen of efavirenz (EFV)/emtricitabine (FTC)/tenofovir DF (TDF). 9th International Congress on Drug Therapy in HIV Infection, Glasgow, UK, Nov. 9–13, 2008. Poster P063.

[143] Pozniak, A. Tenofovir: What have over 1 million years of patient experience taught us? *Int. J. Clin. Pract.* **2008**, *62*, 1285–1293.

[144] Brogan, A. J.; Everhard, F.; Talbird, S. E.; Hutt, E.; Zimovetz, E. NRTI Backbone pairs for treatment-naive adults with HIV infection: a UK economic evaluation. 9th International Congress on Drug Therapy in HIV Infection, Glasgow, UK, Nov. 9–13, 2008. Poster P306.

[145] Brogan, A. J.; Everhard, F.; Talbird, S. E.; Hutt, E. Cost-effectiveness of tenofovir/emtricitabine compared with other NRTI pairs in treatment-naïve adults with HIV infection in the United States. 9th International Congress on Drug Therapy in HIV Infection, Glasgow, UK, Nov. 9–13, 2008. Poster P309.

[146] Rosen, S.; Long, L.; Fox, M.; Sanne, I. Cost and cost-effectiveness of switching from stavudine to tenofovir in first-line antiretroviral regimens in South Africa. *J. Acquir. Immune Defic. Syndr.* **2008**, *48*, 224–344.

8

DISCOVERY AND DEVELOPMENT OF APRICITABINE

Susan Cox, John Deadman, Justine Southby, and Jonathan Coates
Avexa Ltd., Richmond, Victoria, Australia

INTRODUCTION

Highly active antiretroviral therapy (HAART) has been shown to suppress HIV-1 replication and improve immune function, and its use has led to a significant decrease in the morbidity and mortality associated with HIV disease [1,2]. The essence of HAART is the use of a combination of medications from different classes of anti-HIV drugs to maximally suppress viral replication and prevent the emergence of drug-resistant strains of virus. Current guidelines recommend the use of two nucleoside reverse transcriptase inhibitors (NRTIs) with a ritonavir-boosted protease inhibitor or two NRTIs with a nonNRTI (NNRTI) for the initial treatment of HIV infection in adults [3,4]. At the time that clinical development of apricitabine (ATC) began, seven NRTIs were approved: zidovudine (AZT), didanosine (ddI), zalcitabine (ddC), stavudine (d4T), lamivudine (3TC), abacavir (ABC), and emtricitabine (FTC), and one nucleotide reverse transcriptase inhibitor (NtRTI), tenofovir (TDF). Although these approved NRTIs are active in regimens for treatment-naive HIV-1-infected patients, they may be less effective in treatment-experienced patients, depending on which NRTI resistance mutations have arisen in the patient's virus during previous treatment. For example, one of the most common drug-resistant mutations found in treatment-experienced patients is the M184V mutation, which confers high-level resistance to 3TC and the related oxathiolane FTC and low-level resistance to ddI and ABC [5–9].

Around the time that clinical development of ATC began, there were five NRTIs in development with varying degrees of activity against HIV with known NRTI resistance mutations (alovudine, amdoxovir, dexelvucitabine, elvucitabine, racemic emtricitabine). None of these has entered phase III development, due primarily to concerns over safety and efficacy. Thus, there is still a need for the development of NRTIs that are active in the presence of NRTI resistance mutations. In addition, given the extended nature of treatment for HIV infection, the long-term safety and tolerability of the treatment regimen are of great importance, and some existing NRTIs are associated with poor long-term tolerability. The development of new NRTIs, with different resistance profiles and improved long-term safety, is therefore warranted to allow the construction of a new treatment regimen when the previous one has failed.

ATC (formerly known as BCH-10618, SPD754, and AVX754) is the (–)-enantiomer of 2*R*-hydroxymethyl-4*R*-(cytosin-1′-yl)-1,3-oxathiolane and has the molecular formula $C_8H_{11}N_3O_3S$ and a molecular weight of 229.26 Da. ATC is a deoxycytidine analog NRTI that is structurally similar to 3TC but has important differences in the spatial organization of the oxathiolane ring (Fig. 1). The absolute stereochemistry of ATC is 2*R*,4*R* and of 3TC is 2*R*,5*S*.

In common with other NRTIs, ATC undergoes a series of intracellular phosphorylation reactions to produce the active triphosphate form [10], which competes with the corresponding endogenous deoxynucleoside triphosphate for binding to the HIV reverse transcriptase. Since ATC lacks the 3′ hydroxyl group necessary for further DNA elongation, its incorporation into the nascent DNA chain instead of deoxycytidine triphosphate leads to the inhibition of reverse transcription, thereby inhibiting HIV replication. The triphosphate form of ATC (ATC-TP) is a potent and highly selective inhibitor of HIV-1 reverse transcriptase in vitro. It has been found to inhibit wild-type HIV-1 reverse transcriptase in vitro with a

Antiviral Drugs: From Basic Discovery Through Clinical Trials, First Edition. Edited by Wieslaw M. Kazmierski.

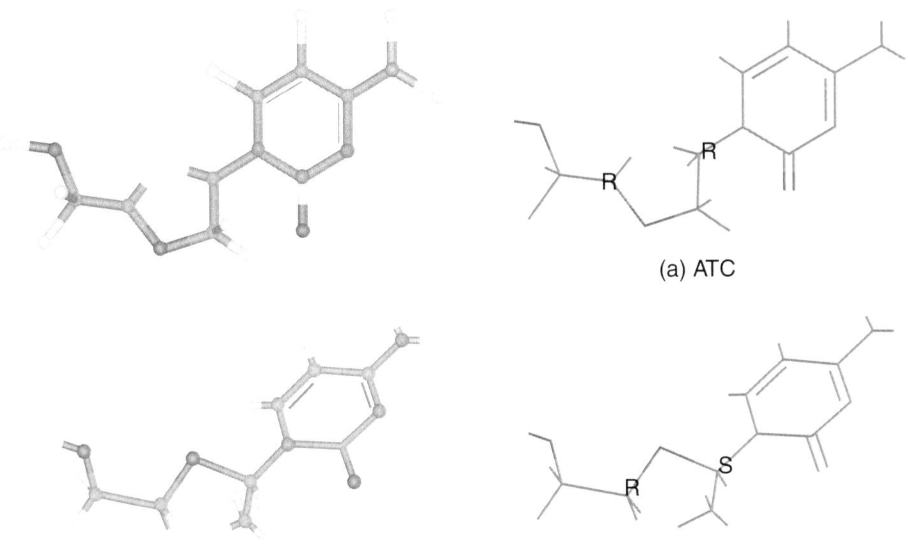

FIGURE 1 Three-dimensional representation of ATC in comparison to 3TC. (*See insert for color representation of the figure.*)

K_i value of 0.08 μM, which is half that of 3TC-TP under the same conditions (0.16 μM) and 150- to 3750-fold lower than for human DNA polymerases, including the mitochondrial DNA polymerase γ [10].

Despite the structural similarity of ATC to 3TC and FTC, ATC retains antiretroviral activity against clinical isolates and laboratory strains of HIV-1 containing the M184V mutation, unlike 3TC and FTC. In vitro studies have shown M184V-containing virus to have only an approximately twofold reduction in susceptibility to ATC compared to the wild-type virus [10–13]. ATC also retains a high level of activity against viruses containing thymidine analog mutations (TAMs) in the reverse transcriptase, which are associated with resistance to the thymidine analogs AZT and d4T [12,14]. These results suggest that ATC may have a place in the treatment of HIV-1-infected patients with NRTI resistance, including as a replacement deoxycytidine analog for 3TC or FTC in patients with the M184V mutation who have failed a regimen containing one of these two NRTIs.

DISCOVERY

The first anti-HIV nucleoside analog demonstrated to have clinical activity was AZT. Later nucleoside analogs (e.g., ddC, d4T, and ddI) acted in a manner similar to AZT, but these agents were found to have some degree of activity against the host cell polymerases (particularly the mitochondrial polymerase γ) and are therefore prone to adverse side effects in some patients. The goal in anti-HIV nucleoside analog discovery thereafter was to discover nucleosides with more selective activity at the reverse transcriptase active site than at that of the host polymerases. The discovery of the activity of the oxathiolane nucleosides against HIV was the first step toward the discovery and development of 3TC and FTC, which have both proven to be highly selective inhibitors of HIV and, as a consequence, are used widely in HIV therapy.

As part of the exploration of the oxathiolane ring as a substitute for the nucleoside analog sugar, which resulted in the identification of 3TC as a potent and noncytotoxic anti-HIV agent, a number of close analogs were also made. These analogs explored the effects on antiviral activity of varying the structure of the oxathiolane ring. A number of different approaches were taken, such as synthesizing the dioxalane analogs and varying the position on the oxathiolane where the base was attached. A single carbon "hop" migrating the cytidine base to the carbon at position 4 results in the oxathiolane sulfur being the only heteroatom between the base-linked carbon and the 5′-hydroxyl–linked carbon and produced a novel oxathiolane-containing nucleoside analogue subsequently named BCH-10618 [ATC]. BCH-10618 was shown to be slightly less active in vitro against HIV compared to 3TC, and for that reason 3TC was the more appropriate clinical development candidate and was developed by Glaxo to market. However, since the widespread uptake and clinical use of 3TC and its related analog FTC has resulted in the selection of the M184V mutation, which renders 3TC and FTC ineffective, a novel, safe, and active compound to treat patients with the M184V mutation has been an unmet medical need. ATC has been demonstrated both in vitro and in the clinic to have potent activity against HIV containing the M184V mutation and also against HIV containing TAMs.

SYNTHESIS

Synthesis of ATC, 2*R*-hydroxymethyl-4*R*-(cytosin-1′-yl)-1,3-oxathiolane

ATC as the free base exists as a single polymorph, which when administered orally in a simple dosage form achieves bioavailability of > 80% with no food effect.

Achiral Synthesis of Oxathiolane Analogs

The original med-chem route to *cis*(±)2-hydroxymethyl-(4-cytosin-1′-yl)-1,3-oxathiolane by Belleau and Nguyen-Ba (WO 92/08717, US5,587,480) gave an approximately equal percentage of the two *cis* and two *trans* forms after separation by flash chromatography. The synthesis used a Pummerer rearrangement of the sulfoxide, but with tetrabutyl ammonium acetate and Ac_2O in this case to give the 4*R* and 4*S* OAc intermediate. Optimization of the Pummerer reaction by Belleau et al. [15] involved maintaining a high concentration of acetate ions in the acetic anhydride, whereby tetra-*n*-butylammonium was found to be superior as a counterion to sodium. In the subsequent Vorbruggen step the coupling gave 60% yield of the *cis* and *trans* isomers (see Scheme 1).

Adaptation of Routes Applicable to 3TC

Whilst 3TC and ATC are clearly isomers, formation of an O—CH—N bond compared to an S—CH—N bond is extremely different, so the mechanism of synthesis differs. For example, 3TC synthesis can be achieved via racemic mixture of *cis*- and *trans*-5-*O*-acetyl with a final separation by fractional crystallization to give the *trans*-(2*S*,5*R*) compound as described by Mansour et al. [16]. However, to use this route for ATC requires five additional steps to move the leaving group to the 4 position [17], and by then the 4 position is enantiomerized to 4*R* and 4*S* in overall 42% yield.

Mansour used the strategy of stereospecific formation of the 2-center by utilizing a menthol chiral auxiliary (WO 92/20669, EP 1153924). This was then converted by an SN2 coupling to a mixture of *cis* and *trans* isomers in a 1 : 1.5 ratio. Subsequently, however, we have shown that when the 2-methyloxathiolane derivative was made directly, the chiral auxiliary on C7 makes the oxathiolane ring unstable during the Pummerer–Vorbruggen coupling step leading to decomposition, and no product was observed. Due to the same mechanism, it was impossible to introduce the OAc leaving group at C4 directly by a Pummerer reaction on this derivative.

Lewis Acids and Stereoinduction of the Vorbruggen Coupling

At this time the combined groups of Mansour at BiochemPharma and Beels at Glaxo [18] disclosed the enhancement of enantiomeric excess in the Vorbruggen coupling step of silyl nucleoside to dioxolane rings, by use of Lewis acids. In the case of oxathiolanes, the excellent *cis*-to-*trans* selectivity of $SnCl_4$ in the Vorbruggen coupling [19] (U.S. Patent 5204466) was attributed to coordination of the metal to the softer sulfur. Thereby, upon reaction with bis-silylated cytosine, in accordance with Hilbert–Johnson-type coupling conditions (see [20] for a review), use of the Lewis acid $SnCl_4$ gave selectivity for the *cis* (β-anomer)-to-*trans* isomer of > 300 : 1 where R = TBDPS, but only 1.3 : 1 *cis* to *trans* where R = BzO.

Subsequently, Yu of Shire-Biochem disclosed (2003/0135048) that catalysts could be derived from metals of group 1B or 11B. Yu tested a number of different copper salts in the combined Pummerer–Vorbruggen step with 2-chiral 2(*R*)-benzyloxymethyl-1,3-oxathiolane without any noticeable change in the *cis*-to-*trans* ratio. Only where the copper catalyst is reduced from 20 mol% to 2 mol% did the *cis*-to-*trans* ratio drop from 3.9 : 1 to 2.4 : 1 (Scheme 2). The result for the same experiment without the addition of copper catalyst is 2.0 : 1.

Additional evidence for such a mechanism was observed for the pentacyclic oxathiolane system whereby 4′,5′-dehydro-1,3-oxathiolane has been observed to form as a by-product at about 10% of all couplings and as the major product if the cytosine base is not added (S. Marcuccio, AMT, unpublished results). Such eliminations also explain the decomposition observed in the 2-carboxy-1,3-oxathiolane system in routes attempted using chiral esters.

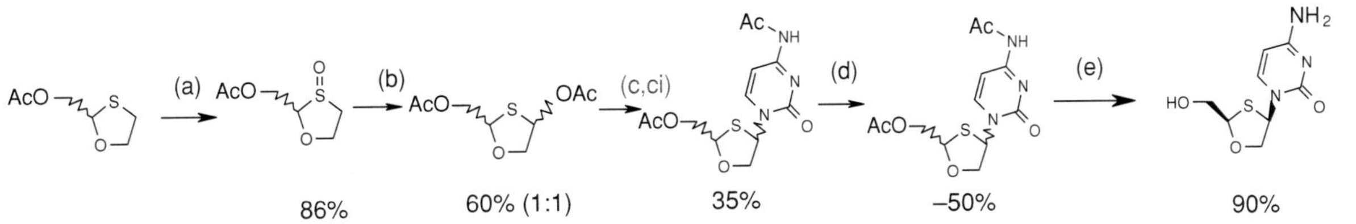

SCHEME 1 Chiral synthesis of ATC, (–)2-hydroxymethyl-(4-cytosin-1′-yl)-1,3-oxathiolane: (a) monoperoxyphtalic acid, $(Bu)_4NHBr$, DCM, water, 30 min; (b) $(Bu)_4NHOAc$, Ac_2O, 110 to 120°C, Ar(g), 14 h; (c) NH_4SO_4, HMDS, reflux, Ar(g); (ci) SnCl4, DCM, 0°C to room temperature, O/N, reflux 3 h; (d) flash column; (e) NH_3/MeOH, room temperature, 16 h.

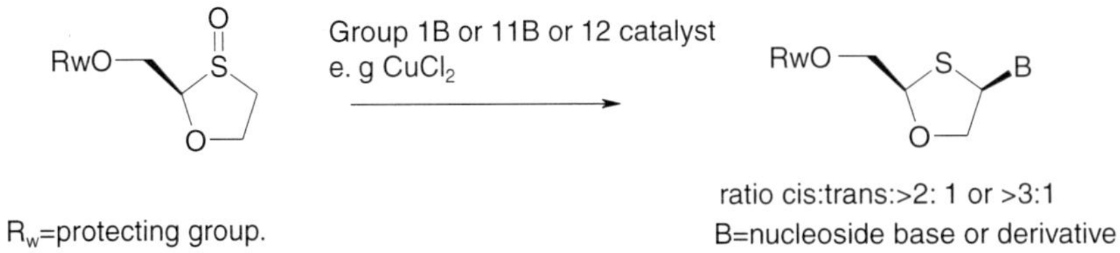

SCHEME 2 Synthesis of ATC.

Trimethylsilyl Iodide as Activating Agent for the Cytosine Base in Stage 2

Trimethylsilyl iodide (TMSI) is required in 3 equivalents and is corrosive, difficult to sample for assay, and expensive. A range of Lewis acids have been evaluated, but to date, TMSI is the most suitable.

Mechanism of the Pummerer Reaction

Preparation of 2-benzoyloxymethyl-4-(*N*-acetylcytosin-1-yl)-1,3-oxathiolane [17] was investigated to optimize the synthesis. The preparative method required two further rounds of process development to get to the 100-kg scale (Raylo and Rhodia, unpublished results for S. Tenjarla and A. Cimpoia, Shire). The method is a plant-scale procedure and uses the quantities of reagents shown in Table 1. 2% H_3PO_4 was used in the workup instead of 2% HCl. A final extra water wash was also carried out. 1,3-Oxathiolane–*S*-oxide was prepared as in the plant and *N*-acetylcytosine [20] was prepared by reaction of cytosine [23] with acetic anhydride in the presence of DMAP in DMF at 50°C (Scheme 3).

Plant-Scale Chiral Synthesis of ATC

The plant-scale route gives the desired compound contaminated typically with up to 30% of the (–)-*trans* isomer formed during the coupling step and with a small percentage of the (+)-*cis* isomer, carried through from any (+)-BOMO in the starting material and the corresponding (+)-*trans* formed from the (+)-BOMO also. These could be separated by chromatography. A program led by A. Cimpoia (Shire) showed that the deprotected ATC [(±)2-hydroxymethyl-(±)4-(cytosin-1′-yl)-1,3-oxathiolane] could be resolved by formation of diastereomeric salts with chiral acids (WO/2006/096954).

In particular, as part of this program it was observed surprisingly that formation of the salt with the achiral tosic acid gave a conglomerate form (U.S. Patent 7,501,514), allowing the isomers to be separated by preferential crystallization (for reviews of conglomerate behavior, see [21] and [22]). This is a highly fruitful observation since less than 10% of all racemate salts exhibit conglomerate behavior [23]. Typical of the conglomerate behavior, where the compound crystallizes as a single enantiomer in the crystal lattice, is the fact that the melting point of the racemic conglomerate tosylate salt (186.8°C) is lower than that of the crystals of either single enantiomer [213.2°C for the (–)*cis* and 214.2°C for (+)*cis*]. At scale this process also has the advantage that toluenesulfonic acid is inexpensive compared to chiral salts. The acid counterion itself can then simply be removed by mixing the salt with an ion-exchange resin such as Dowex 550A-OH (140% w/w). To summarize, the industrial-scale process is then carried out in four steps from (–)BOMO, giving ATC in greater than 99% chiral purity (Scheme 4).

TABLE 1 Reagent Consumption in Plant-Scale Synthesis of ATC

Reagent		
Dichloromethane	530 L	of sulfoxide solution
Triethylamine	485 mol	2.2 equiv
TMSI	486 mol	2.2 equiv
2-Benzoyloxymethyl-1,3-oxathiolane-*S*-oxide [19]	220 mol	1 equiv
TMSI	199 mol	0.9 equiv
$CuCl_2$	44.6 mol	0.2 equiv
N-Acetylcytosine [20]	221 mol	1 equiv
Water	320 L	
Dichloromethane	100 L	
2% HCl	320 L	
Aqueous NH_3	320 L × 2	

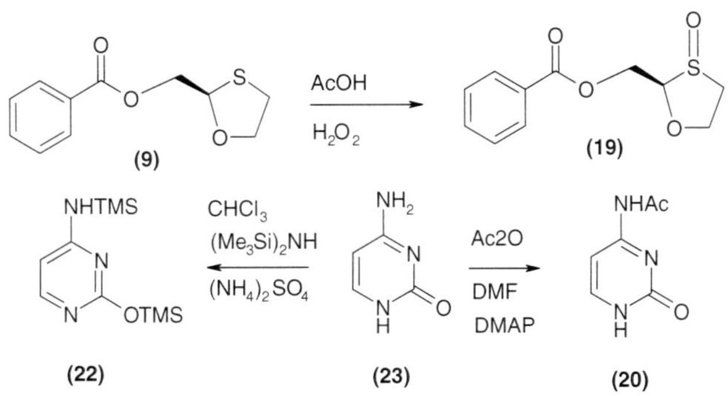

SCHEME 3 Step 1 of ATC synthesis.

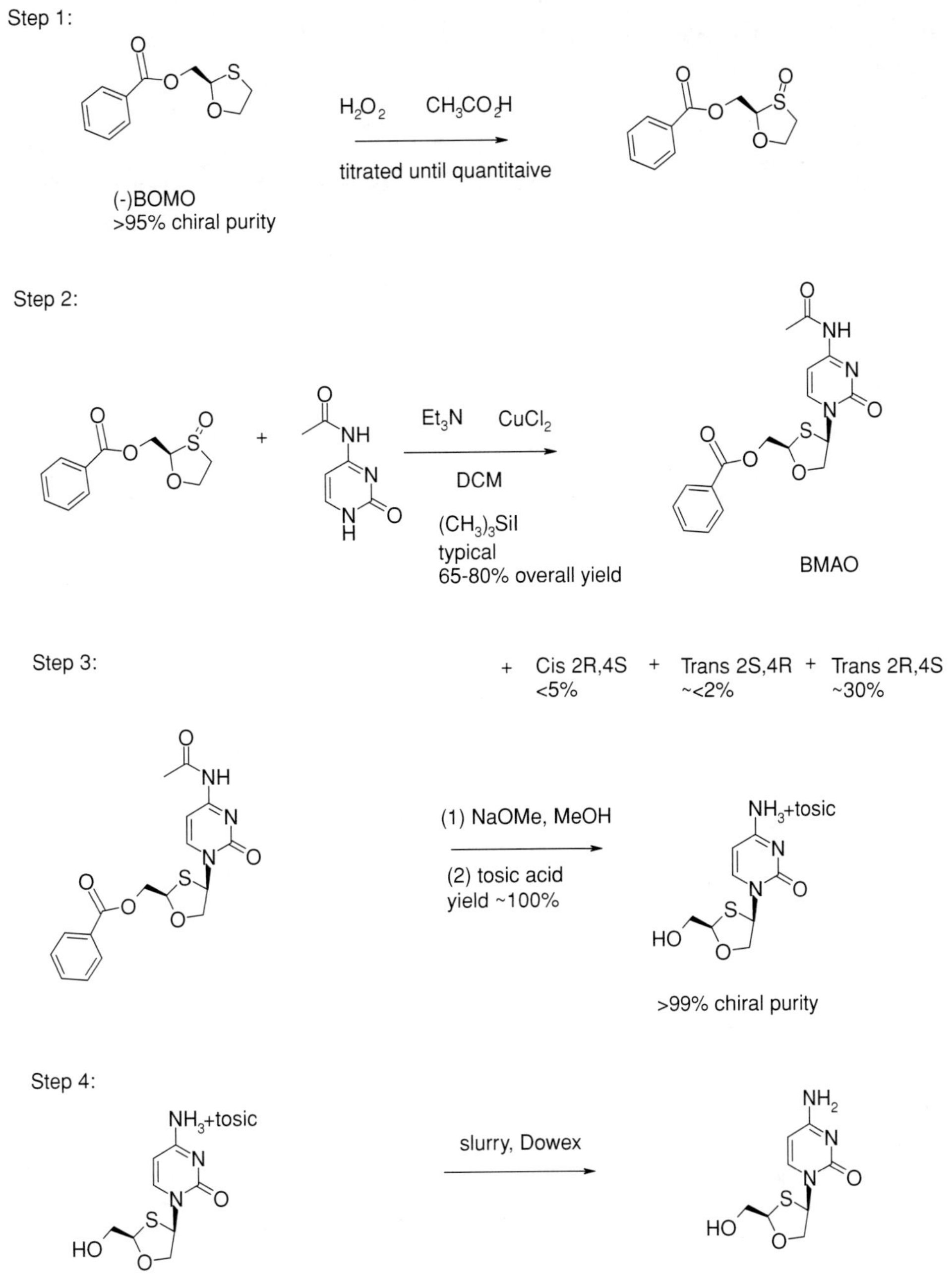

SCHEME 4 Plant-scale synthesis of ATC.

Plant-Scale Method

Reaction Step 1 Hydrogen peroxide is added slowly to a mixture of 2-(*R*)-benzoyloxymethyl-1,3-oxathiolane and acetic acid at about 55°C until the reaction is complete, by high-performance liquid chromatographic (HPLC) analysis for (–)BOMO consumption. The reaction mixture is cooled to room temperature and then charged with methylene chloride. The mixture is quenched successively by addition of a dilute solution of sodium metabisulfite, dilute sodium carbonate solution, and dilute sodium chloride solution. The water content of the layer is reduced by azeotropic distillation at constant volume and analyzed by HPLC for *R*-BOMO oxide.

Reaction Step 2 *R*-BOMO-*S*-oxide stock solution, methylene chloride, and triethylamine are charged to a reactor and cooled to within the range –20 to –10°C. TMSI is added while maintaining the temperature below –10°C and agitated at −10°C until the reaction is complete by HPLC analysis for *R*-BOMO-*S*-oxide consumption. Copper(II) chloride, *N*-acetyl cytosine, and triethylamine are added while maintaining the mixture at about −10°C. The mixture is agitated at about −5°C until the reaction is complete. The reaction mixture is added to water and agitated for about 1 h. Copper salts are partially eliminated by filtration. The layers are separated and the organic phase is washed successively with diluted aqueous ammonia, water, diluted phosphoric acid, and diluted aqueous ammonia. The solution is dried by azeotropic distillation at constant volume and analyzed by HPLC for 2-benzoyloxymethyl-4-(*N*-acetylcytosin-1-yl)-1,3-oxathiolane in methylene chloride.

Reaction Step 3 2-Benzoyloxymethyl-4-(*N*-acetylcytosin-1-yl)-1,3-oxathiolane in methylene chloride is concentrated at atmospheric pressure. Methanol is charged and the mixture is concentrated at atmospheric pressure. A solution of 30% sodium methoxide in methanol is charged to the concentrated solution while maintaining the contents at about 40 to 45°C. The reaction mixture is cooled to about 20 to 25°C and agitated until the reaction is complete by the absence of starting material. The reaction mixture is filtered, *p*-toluenesulfonic acid monohydrate is added, and the mixture is agitated at about 20 to 25°C. The resulting slurry is cooled, agitated, and rinsed forward with methanol, cake dried, then warmed to 65°C to recrystallize from methanol/isopropanol. The 2*R*-hydroxymethyl-4*R*-cytosinyl-1-yl-1,3-oxathiolane *p*-toluenesulfonic acid salt is analyzed by HPLC.

Reaction Step 4 Dowex OH resin (prewashed with methanol), methanol, and 2*R*-hydroxymethyl-4*R*-cytosinyl-1-yl-1,3-oxathiolane *p*-toluenesulfonic acid salt are charged into the reactor and the mixture is heated at about 40 to 45°C and agitated until reaction is deemed complete by HPLC for consumption of starting material. The methanolic solution is filtered and concentrated to reduced volume, isopropanol added, the slurry cooled, and the resulting cake dried.

Conclusions

ATC can be prepared in four steps from (–)BOMO at the 200-kg batch scale without the requirement for chiral auxiliaries.

Recent Developments

Avexa has continued to pursue process development work in the scale manufacture of ATC and has developed a novel patented process that prepares ATC in three steps from (–)BOMO in greater than 99% chiral purity. This does not require any new reagents and, in particular, any other chiral auxiliaries, and from the regulatory perspective will therefore be equivalent.

PRECLINICAL PHARMACOKINETICS AND TOXICITY

Investigation of the pharmacokinetics of ATC showed ATC to be rapidly absorbed, with T_{max} achieved within 2 h following single or multiple dosing in rats and monkeys. There was no accumulation of ATC following multiple dosing in either rats or monkeys. When administered orally to rats, ATC was found to have a bioavailability of approximately 77%, with levels in the cerebrospinal fluid approximately 16.5% of that found in the serum.

There is little evidence of metabolism of ATC in rats or monkeys. Excretion studies with [^{14}C]ATC showed the radioactivity to be excreted rapidly by both species, with the vast majority being recovered in the first 24 h, and the major component observed in both urine and feces was the unchanged drug. Studies using the isolated rat perfused kidney suggest that the renal elimination of ATC occurs by a mixture of glomerular filtration and active tubular secretion [24]. In monkeys, a metabolite identified as the product of deamination of ATC and representing 8 to 15% of the dose administered was observed in the urine and feces. This metabolite was also observed in the rat, although in smaller amounts (2.8% in urine, 1.1% in feces), and has shown neither antiviral nor pharmacological activity.

In vitro tests using human liver microsomes found that neither ATC nor its metabolite showed any significant inhibition of major cytochrome P450 isozymes (CYP1A2, CYP2A6, CYP2C9, CYP2D6, CYP2E1, and CYP3A4) [25]. In addition, ATC showed no induction of CYP1A2 or CYP3A4 in cultured human hepatocytes. ATC is only a weak inhibitor of P-glycoprotein and has no effect on the activity of the glucuronidating enzyme UGT1A1 in vitro (Avexa, unpublished results). These results indicate that significant interactions between ATC and drugs that undergo hepatic metabolism are unlikely.

The initial phosphorylation of ATC to produce the monophosphate form is catalyzed by deoxycytidine kinase [10,26]. This enzyme is also responsible for the initial intracellular phosphorylation of 3TC and FTC, raising the possibility of competition for phosphorylation between ATC and other deoxycytidine analogs. In vitro experiments to investigate this possibility showed that coadministration of ATC and 3TC resulted in concentration-dependent decreases in ATC phosphorylation in peripheral blood mononuclear cells (PBMCs), whereas ATC had no effect on the phosphorylation of 3TC or FTC [26]. The activity of ATC against M184V-containing HIV-1 was reduced when ATC was administered with 3TC, suggesting that coadministration of ATC and 3TC would result in reduced effectiveness of the ATC. The potential for this intracellular interaction between ATC and 3TC to occur clinically is discussed in the following section.

The NRTI class of drugs has been associated with mitochondrial toxicity [27]. NRTIs act by inhibiting the HIV-1 reverse transcriptase; however, they may similarly inhibit human DNA polymerases, including DNA polymerase γ, the enzyme responsible for replication of mitochondrial DNA. Inhibition of this polymerase results in mitochondrial DNA depletion and mitochondrial dysfunction, which may be manifested as lipoatrophy, hepatic steatosis, lactic acidosis, mitochondrial myopathy, and peripheral neuropathy. In vitro studies have shown that ATC has a low propensity for mitochondrial toxicity, with no effect observed at concentrations of up to 200 μM on the mitochondrial content of HepG2 and Molt-4 cells after continuous exposure for 7 to 28 days [13]. In a subsequent study, ATC had no effect on the mitochondrial content of HepG2 cells cultured for up to 16 days with concentrations of 0.3 to 300 μM, in contrast to ddC, ddI, and d4T, which markedly reduced mitochondrial DNA content, while 3TC, FTC, AZT, and ABC produced slight increases in mitochondrial DNA content, possibly due to an adaptive cellular response to partial mitochondrial dysfunction [28]. The favorable mitochondrial toxicity profile of ATC is consistent with its high level of selectivity for HIV-1 reverse transcriptase relative to human DNA polymerase γ [10] and has been reflected in clinical trials to date, with no reports of peripheral neuropathy, lipoatrophy, lactic acidosis, hepatotoxicity, or hyperlipasemia leading to pancreatitis attributed to ATC, including in a 48-week phase II study of ATC [29,30]. ATC has a low propensity for cellular toxicity in vitro [10,13], including a low potential for myelotoxicity against human bone marrow cells in vitro [13]. In addition, neither ATC nor its metabolite has shown any effect on hERG potassium channel activity in vitro.

ATC (50 to 1000 mg/kg per day) was also found to have a favorable toxicity profile during a 52-week study in monkeys [31]. The main effects were mild and reversible hyperpigmentation, gastrointestinal effects, and marginal changes in red blood cell parameters in males only. In line with the in vitro findings, there was no evidence of mitochondrial toxicity in the liver, heart, or skeletal muscle and no bone marrow toxicity.

In vitro experiments have shown that as well as being a potent and highly selective inhibitor of the wild-type HIV-1 reverse transcriptase, ATC has substantial activity against HIV-1 strains with a variety of reverse transcriptase mutations associated with NRTI resistance, including M184V and TAMs (Table 2). In one study, the activity of ATC against 50 HIV-1 clinical isolates consisting of five wild-type isolates and 45 NRTI-resistant isolates was tested using the Antivirogram recombinant virus assay [13]. The susceptibility to ATC compared to the wild-type isolates was reduced only 1.2- to 2.2-fold against HIV-1 isolates resistant to AZT [M41L and T215Y or T215F and a median of three additional nucleoside-associated mutations (NAMs)], 3TC (M184V), or both AZT and 3TC (M184V plus at least two TAMs) and 1.3- to 2.8-fold against isolates resistant to ABC (L74V, Y115F, M184V plus a median of one other NAM) or d4T (V75T or V75M, M41L, T215F, or T215Y and a median of four other NAMs). In contrast, insertions at position 69 of the reverse transcriptase resulted in a more substantial 5.6-fold reduction in susceptibility to ATC and multidrug-resistant isolates with the Q151 mutation showed a 14- to 16-fold reduction in susceptibility. In another study, the PhenoSense assay was used to test the activity of ATC against a panel of 215 HIV-1 isolates with different patterns of TAMs [12]. The presence of five TAMs in the 41–215 pathway (codons 41, 67, 210, 215, and 219 of the reverse transcriptase) was found to confer a median 1.8-fold reduction in susceptibility to ATC, and the presence of five TAMs in the 67–70–219 pathway (codons 41, 67, 70, 215, and 219) resulted in a median 1.3-fold reduction in ATC susceptibility. The M184V mutation reduced susceptibility to ATC by approximately 1.8-fold in this study, in both the absence and presence of TAMs.

The K65R mutation, which is selected by ABC, ddI, d4T, and TDF and is associated with decreased susceptibility to these drugs [32–35], has been found to result in reductions in ATC susceptibility in vitro ranging from 2.6- to 4.6-fold [36,37]. This reduced susceptibility appears to be due to a reduction in binding or incorporation of ATC rather than to increased excision of incorporated ATC monophosphate [38]. The L74V mutation, associated with decreased susceptibility to ABC and ddI [9,39], does not appear to affect susceptibility to ATC [37] or the efficiency of chain termination by ATC-TP [38].

Resistance to ATC is slow to emerge in vitro, as shown by repeated passaging of MT-2 cells (with the HIV-1_{LAI} virus), MT-4 cells (wild-type HXB2-D), and C8166 cells (HIV-1_{RF}) in the presence of ATC [36]. Following 18 to 20 serial drug passages of ATC, three reverse transcriptase mutations—M184V, V75I, or K65R—were selected individually in separate experiments. The resulting mutants generally had a low level of resistance to ATC, with a 1.1-, 1.6-, and 3.6-fold change in susceptibility to ATC for the M184V, V75I, and K65R mutants, respectively. Continuous passaging of HIV-1 already containing the M184V or K65R mutation in the presence of ATC for 38 weeks did not result in any additional mutations, nor did continuous passaging of HIV-1 containing the M41L, M184V, and T215Y mutations in the presence of ATC for 28 weeks [40]. The original mutations were maintained under ATC drug pressure but generally lost in the absence of ATC. Thus, ATC appears to maintain mutations in the HIV-1 reverse transcriptase associated with reduced replicative fitness, such as M184V, while not selecting additional resistance mutations.

PHASE I–III SAFETY AND EFFICACY

Phase I Studies

Phase I studies have been conducted to assess the pharmacokinetics and safety of ATC, for ATC given alone and in combination with other drugs likely to be administered to HIV-1-infected patients. ATC showed largely linear

TABLE 2 Summary of In Vitro Antiviral Activity of ATC Against Drug-Resistant Strains and Clinical Isolates of HIV-1

Virus Profile[a]	Mean/Median Fold-Change Susceptibility to ATC vs. Wild Type	Ref.
3TC-resistant		
3TC-resistant	1.5	[14]
3TC-resistant	1.8	[15]
M184V	1.6	[16]
3TC-resistant	0.84	[17]
AZT-resistant		
5 TAMs (41–215 pathway)	1.8	[16]
5 TAMs (67–70–219 pathway)	1.3	[16]
AZT-resistant	1.2	[17]
3TC- and AZT-resistant		
3TC- and AZT-resistant	1.7	[14]
41,215 + M184V	2.1	[16]
67,70,219 + M184V	1.8	[16]
3TC- and AZT-resistant	2.2	[17]
ABC-resistant		
ABC-resistant	1.3	[17]
d4T-resistant		
d4T-resistant	2.8	[17]
K65R		
K65R	2.6	[52]
K65R + M184V	3.6	[52]
L74V		
L74V	1.1	[52]
L74V + M184V	1.9	[52]
L74V + 3 TAMs	1.8	[52]
L74V + 5 TAMs	2.4	[52]
Multidrug resistant		
Q151M	14	[17]
Q151M + M184V	16	[17]
T69 insertions	5.2	[17]

[a]3TC, lamivudine; AZT, zidovudine; ABC, abacavir; d4T, stavudine.

pharmacokinetics following oral administration of single doses (400, 800, and 1600 mg) during a phase I dose escalation study in 26 healthy adult volunteers [41]. Plasma concentrations of ATC reached a peak at approximately 1.5 to 2 h after dosing and then declined in a log-linear manner over 12 h with a half-life of approximately 3 h. The majority of the dose (65 to 80%) was excreted in the urine as unchanged drug within 24 h. After adjustment for body weight, the pharmacokinetic properties of ATC were similar in the male and female participants of the study. The pharmacokinetic profile for multiple doses of ATC was found to be similar to that of single-dose ATC in healthy adult subjects [42]. In addition, a phase I study in 20 healthy male volunteers showed that the pharmacokinetics of ATC are not significantly affected by food, indicating that no dosing restrictions are necessary with respect to food intake [43]. The pharmacokinetic profile of ATC in HIV-1-infected patients is similar to that observed in healthy subjects [44,45].

ATC must be phosphorylated intracellularly to its triphosphate form to exert its antiviral activity. In a phase I study with 21 healthy male volunteers, maximum intracellular concentrations of ATC-TP in PBMCs were reached around 3.5 h after dosing, with an intracellular half-life of approximately 6 to 7 h [46]. Similar intracellular pharmacokinetics for ATC were observed in a phase II trial in HIV-1-infected patients [45]. The intracellular half-life of ATC-TP of 6 to 7 hour and plasma elimination half-life of approximately 3 h support twice-daily dosing of ATC.

A phase I study was conducted in 18 healthy male volunteers to assess the effect of the coadministration of ATC and the HIV protease inhibitor tipranavir [47]. Administration of ATC in the presence of steady-state levels of tipranavir (ritonavir-boosted) resulted in a modest increase in the ATC area under the curve (AUC; $\sim$ 40%) and C_{max} ($\sim$ 25%). The magnitude of this interaction was considered unlikely to be clinically significant, and therefore no dose adjustment for

ATC is required when administered with ritonavir-boosted tipranavir. A phase I study with 16 healthy adult volunteers found that coadministration of ATC with trimethoprim-sulfamethoxazole (widely used in HIV-1-infected patients for the prophylaxis of *Pneumocystis jiroveci* pneumonia) increased the ATC AUC (65.8%) and C_{max} (32.5%). It was also concluded that this increase in ATC exposure was not likely to be clinically significant and that no adjustment of ATC dose is considered necessary when ATC is given in combination with trimethoprim–sulfamethoxazole [42].

Coadministration of ATC with 3TC was found to have no effect on the plasma pharmacokinetics of either drug in a phase I study of 21 healthy male volunteers [46]. However, the intracellular level of ATC-TP in PBMCs was reduced to approximately 15% of that observed with ATC alone, while the intracellular concentration of 3TC-TP was unaffected by the coadministration. These results are consistent with the in vitro findings that coadministration of ATC and 3TC inhibited the intracellular phosphorylation of ATC [26] and suggest that such coadministration would reduce the efficacy of ATC. As a consequence, ATC should not be coadministered with 3TC or any other deoxycytidine analog that is phosphorylated by deoxycytidine kinase.

In a phase I clinical study to investigate the cardiovascular safety of ATC in 37 healthy subjects, there were no significant changes to the QT/QTc intervals following doses of ATC of 800 or 1600 mg when compared to placebo at the time of individual T_{max} for ATC, at the time of individual T_{max} for the primary metabolite of ATC, or when averaged over 1 to 4 h after dosing [48]. Thus, ATC does not induce any clinically significant effect upon electrocardiogram parameters at therapeutic or supratherapeutic doses consistent with maximum exposure expected to occur in clinical practice. ATC was well tolerated during these phase I studies, both alone and in combination with tipranavir, trimethoprim–sulfamethoxazole, or 3TC [41–43,46–48].

Phase II Studies

Phase II studies of ATC have been conducted in both treatment-naive [49] and treatment-experienced [30,50,51] HIV-1-infected patients. The safety and efficacy of ATC were assessed in a double-blind randomized placebo-controlled study of 63 antiretroviral-naive HIV-1-infected patients (mean plasma viral load level 4.3 $\log_{10}$ HIV-1 RNA copies/mL; mean $CD4^+$ T-cell count 505.7 cells/mm^3) in which ATC was administered as monotherapy for 10 days [49]. Four doses of ATC, given as six dosing regimens, were evaluated: 200 mg twice daily (b.i.d.) (400 mg/day), 400 mg b.i.d. (800 mg/day), 800 mg once daily (q.v.) (800 mg/day), 600 mg b.i.d. (1200 mg/day), 1200 mg q.v. (1200 mg/day), or 800 mg b.i.d. (1600 mg/day). There were approximately equal numbers of patients randomized to each total dose; patients randomized to the 800- and 1200-mg/day groups were then randomly assigned to either a once- or twice-daily schedule. After 7 days of treatment, there were statistically significant reductions in plasma viral load levels from baseline relative to placebo in all dosage groups ($p \leq 0.0001$). After 10 days of treatment, the mean reductions in viral load in the 1200- and 1600-mg per day dosage groups (-1.65 and -1.58 $\log_{10}$ HIV-1 RNA copies/mL, respectively) were significantly greater than the reduction observed in the 400-mg/day group (-1.18 $\log_{10}$ copies/mL, $p < 0.05$) and were suggestive of a plateau in the dose–response curve being reached at the upper doses (Fig. 2). The proportion of patients with at least a 1.0 $\log_{10}$ reduction in viral load after 10 days of ATC monotherapy was 64, 75, 86, and 92% at doses of 400, 800, 1200, and 1600 mg, respectively. Within the 800- and 1200-mg/day groups, ATC appeared to be similarly effective when administered as a single daily or twice-daily dose. All doses of ATC in this study were well tolerated, and the safety profile of ATC was similar to that of the placebo [49]. There were no severe or serious treatment-emergent adverse events and no adverse events that led to discontinuation. In addition, ATC did not select any particular mutation during the 10 days of monotherapy.

In a second double-blind randomized phase II study, the efficacy and safety of ATC were compared to that of 3TC in 51 treatment-experienced HIV-1-infected patients failing treatment with 3TC and harboring the reverse transcriptase mutation M184V. Patients stopped their existing 3TC treatment and were randomized to receive twice-daily 600 mg ATC, 800 mg ATC, or 150 mg 3TC. Randomization was stratified according to the number of TAMs at screening (<3 TAMs, ≥ 3 TAMs). At day 21, the background antiretroviral therapy (ART) could be optimized according to genotype at screening and patients continued to receive ATC or 3TC until week 24. At week 24, all patients switched to receiving open-label ATC 800 mg twice daily, to week 48.

At day 21 (the primary endpoint of the study), after 3 weeks of functional monotherapy with ATC, the mean reductions in viral load in the 600- and 800-mg ATC groups (0.90 and 0.71 $\log_{10}$ HIV-1 RNA copies/mL, respectively) were significantly greater than in the 150-mg 3TC group (0.03 $\log_{10}$ HIV-1 RNA copies/mL) [50]. From day 21 to week 24, with optimization of the background ART at day 21, there were greater reductions in viral load in the 600- and 800-mg ATC groups compared to the 3TC group, although by week 24 the differences among the three groups were small, as might be expected since the study was powered for the primary endpoint at day 21 [51] (Fig. 3). The mean reduction in viral load at week 24 was 2.14, 2.13, and 1.88 $\log_{10}$ copies/mL for the 600-mg ATC, 800-mg ATC, and 150-mg 3TC groups, respectively (Table 3). In the two ATC groups, approximately 70% of patients had achieved a viral load of <50 copies/mL at week 24 and there were clinically meaningful mean increases in $CD4^+$ cells of 145 and 211 cells/μL in the 600- and 800-mg ATC groups, respectively.

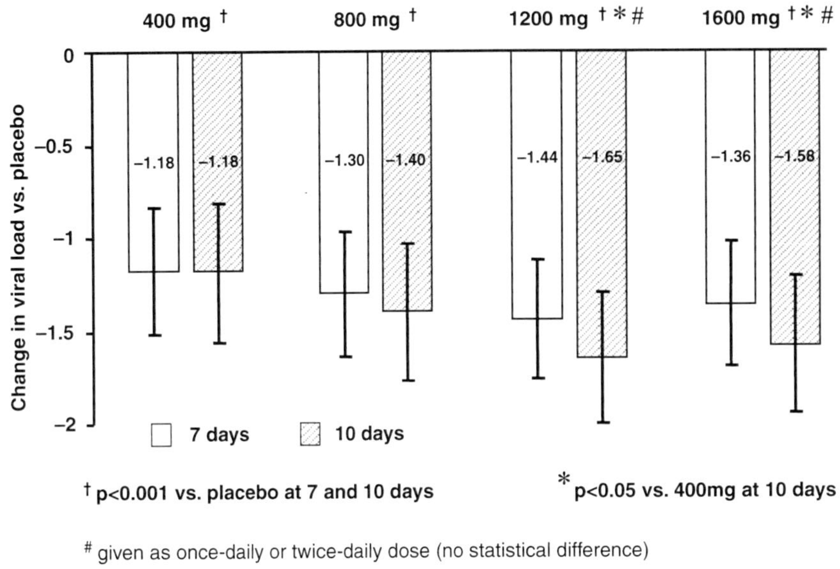

FIGURE 2 Mean change from baseline in plasma HIV-1 viral load vs. placebo after treatment with varying doses of ATC monotherapy for 7 or 10 days in antiretroviral-naive HIV-1-infected patients (intent-to-treat population).

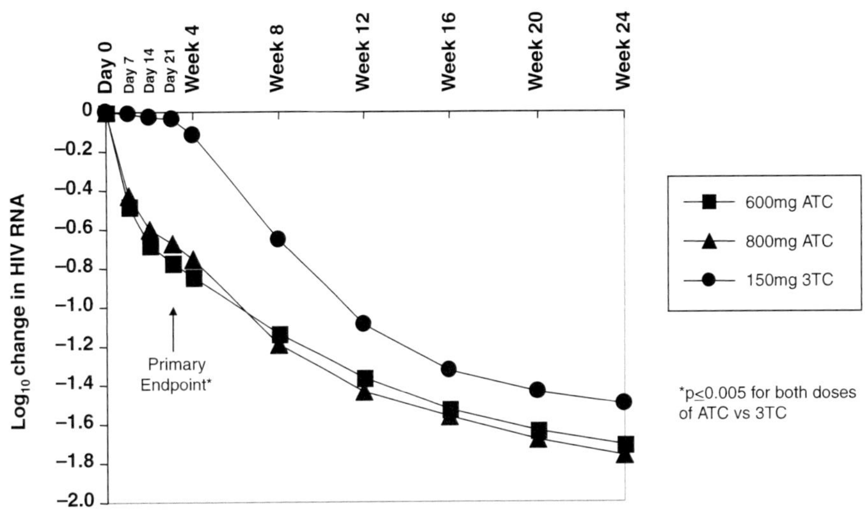

FIGURE 3 Time-weighted average $\log_{10}$ change in HIV RNA from day 0 to week 24 for week 24 per protocol population during treatment with twice-daily 600 mg ATC, 800 mg ATC, or 150 mg 3TC in treatment-experienced HIV-1-infected patients with the M184V mutation.

TABLE 3 Efficacy of ATC at Weeks 24 and 48 in Treatment-Experienced Patients with the M184V Mutation

	600 mg ATC	800 mg ATC	150 mg 3TC
Week 24 per protocol population	$n = 14$	$n = 15$	$n = 12$
% of patients with < 50 copies/mL	71.4	73.3	58.3
% of patients with < 400 copies/mL	85.7	80.0	66.7
$\Delta CD4^+$ cells (cells/μL)	145	211	113
Decrease in viral load ($\log_{10}$ HIV-1 RNA copies/mL)	2.14	2.13	1.88
Week 48 per protocol population	$n = 13$	$n = 14$	$n = 11$
% of patients with < 50 copies/mL	69.2	85.7	90.9
$\Delta CD4^+$ cells (cells/μL)	261	277	200
ITT population	$n = 17$	$n = 17$	$n = 16$
No. of patients undergoing ART reoptimization	2 (11.8%)	2 (11.8%)	7 (43.8%)

For the 150-mg 3TC group, approximately 58% of patients had achieved a viral load of < 50 copies/mL at week 24 and there was a mean increase in $CD4^+$ cells of 113 cells/μL. The 800-mg ATC dose appeared to be more effective than the 600-mg dose for patients with ≥ 3 TAMs at the start of the study.

The improvements in viral load observed at week 24 were maintained or enhanced at week 48, after all three groups had received 24 weeks of twice-daily open-label 800 mg ATC [30] (Table 3). The group of patients who switched from 150 mg 3TC to 800 mg ATC at week 24 showed improvements in both their viral load and $CD4^+$ cell count at week 48, with 90.9% of patients having a viral load of < 50 copies/mL at week 48 and there being a mean increase in $CD4^+$ cells (from day 0) of 200 cells/μL. This would suggest that patients who do not achieve undetectable viral loads while on 3TC may be able to switch to ATC and achieve improvements in viral load without necessarily having to change their background regimen. More patients in the 150-mg 3TC group (7 of 16 patients) had their ART reoptimized between day 21 and week 48 than in the 600-mg ATC (2 of 17) and 800-mg ATC (2 of 17) groups.

Both the 600- and 800-mg twice-daily doses of ATC were well tolerated, and ATC had a similar safety profile than 3TC over the first 24 weeks of the study [29,50]. ATC continued to be well tolerated over the second 24 weeks of the study, when all patients received 800 mg ATC twice daily [30]. There were no serious adverse events related to ATC, no discontinuations from the study due to an ATC-related adverse event, and no deaths in this study. The adverse events related to ATC were generally gastrointestinal in nature (e.g., diarrhea, nausea, dyspepsia, gastric disorder) and mild or moderate in severity (Table 4). There were no changes in serum lipids or creatinine associated with ATC and no cases of rash, hypersensitivity, hyperlactemia, lactic acidosis, pancreatitis, or increases in liver function tests. The most common treatment-emergent adverse events were diarrhea ($n = 17$), nausea ($n = 10$), nasopharyngitis ($n = 9$), hypertriglyceridemia ($n = 9$), and upper respiratory tract infection ($n = 8$), which occurred equally in the ATC and 3TC arms. The long-term safety and efficacy of ATC in this study population will be assessed in the follow-up extension study.

TABLE 4 Treatment-Related Adverse Events Occurring Between Day 0 and Week 48[a]

Adverse Event	600 mg ATC ($n = 17$)	800 mg ATC ($n = 18$)	150 mg 3TC ($n = 16$)
Diarrhea	1 (5.9%)	1 (5.6%)	
Dyspepsia	—	1 (5.6%)	—
Gastric disorder	—	1 (5.6%)	—
Nausea	1 (5.9%)	—	—
Vomiting	—	—	1 (6.3%)
Increased lipase levels	—	1 (5.6%)	—
Weight loss	—	1 (5.6%)	—
Anorexia	—	1 (5.6%)	—
Dizziness	1 (5.9%)		
Peripheral neuropathy	—	—	1 (6.3%)
Facial wasting	—	—	1 (6.3%)
Lipoatrophy	—	—	1 (6.3%)

[a]All patients received ATC 800 mg twice daily from week 24 to week 48. The treatment-related adverse events in the 150 3TC group all occurred during the first 24 weeks of the study (i.e., during 3TC treatment).

There was no evidence of development of resistance to ATC over the course of the 48-week study, including during 21 days of functional monotherapy with ATC [30,50,52]. No patients were found to have developed K65R, L74V, or other NAMs at day 21, week 24, or week 48. The M184V mutation appeared to be maintained during ATC treatment in this study, as has been observed in vitro [40,53]. At day 21, the M184V mutation was present in all 24 patients receiving ATC whose virus could be genotyped, and at week 12 it was present in the majority of patients receiving ATC (in combination with optimized background ART) in whom a genotype could be obtained (7/11 patients plus two patients had the partial reversion M184V/M) [50,52]. It has been suggested that it may be of benefit to maintain the M184V mutation, given that it is associated with reduced replicative fitness and that it appears to protect against further NRTI resistance mutations and restore sensitivity to AZT and TDF [54–56].

Phase III Studies

A phase III study to assess the efficacy and safety of ATC plus optimized background regimen (OBR) compared to 3TC plus OBR in treatment-experienced HIV-1-infected patients with the M184V mutation is currently in progress.

FUTURE DIRECTIONS

The HIV-1 reverse transcriptase is an essential enzyme for viral replication and a proven target in the treatment of HIV infection, with two classes of drugs, NRTIs and NNRTIs, exerting their antiviral activity by inhibiting the action of this enzyme. The value of NRTIs in the treatment of HIV infection is underscored by their widespread use in HAART regimens. However, the rapid replication rate of HIV-1 combined with the lack of an efficient proofreading system mean that mutations occur readily in the HIV-1 reverse transcriptase that can cause the virus to become resistant to the NRTI plus any cross-resistant NRTI, which may ultimately result in treatment failure. There is therefore a need for new NRTIs that are active against NRTI-resistant HIV-1.

The good antiviral activity of ATC in treatment-experienced HIV-1-infected patients with the M184V mutation (and up to five TAMs) indicates that ATC may have a role as a replacement deoxycytidine analog in patients who have developed resistance to the deoxycytidine analogs 3TC or FTC via the M184V mutation. As with all antiviral drugs, there is the potential that the virus could also develop resistance to ATC, through addition of further mutations beyond M184V, which could open up possibilities for follow-on compounds after ATC. However, to date no resistance to ATC and no ATC resistance mutations have been identified in the clinic up to 96 weeks of treatment. Resistance development to ATC therefore appears to be slow, and it is tempting to speculate that adding further mutations beyond M184V that would enable resistance to ATC is difficult to achieve without significantly impairing the ability of the enzyme to function. The lack of significant development of resistance to ATC, together with its excellent safety, tolerability, and pharmacokinetic properties, means that an obvious need for a follow-on series beyond ATC has not been identified. Rather, given the lack of interaction observed between ATC and other drugs (apart from 3TC/FTC), a more appropriate area for future progress would be the development of a single coformulated tablet containing ATC together with other appropriate drugs.

REFERENCES

[1] Palella, F. J., et al. Declining morbidity and mortality among patients with advanced human immunodeficiency virus infection. *N. Engl. J. Med.* **1998**, *338*, 853–860.

[2] Murphy, E. L., et al. Highly active antiretroviral therapy decreases mortality and morbidity in patients with advanced HIV disease. *Ann. Intern. Med.* **2001**, *135*, 17–26.

[3] Hammer, S. M., et al. Antiretroviral treatment of adult HIV infection. 2008 recommendations of the International AIDS Society–USA Panel. *JAMA* **2008**, *300*, 555–570.

[4] Panel on Antiretroviral Guidelines for Adults and Adolescents. Guidelines for the use of antiretroviral agents in HIV-1-infected adults and adolescents. Department of Health and Human Services, Nov. 3, 2008, pp 1–139. Available at http://www.aidsinfo.nih.gov/ContentFiles/AdultandAdolescentGL.pdf. Accessed Feb. 12, 2009.

[5] Boucher, C. A. B., et al. High-level resistance to (–)enantiomeric 2′-deoxy-3′-thiacytidine in vitro is due to one amino acid substitution in the catalytic site of human immunodeficiency virus type I reverse transcriptase. *Antimicrob. Agents Chemother.* **1993**, *37*, 2231–2234.

[6] Schuurman, R., et al. Rapid changes in human immunodeficiency virus type 1 RNA load and appearance of drug-resistant virus populations in persons treated with lamivudine (3TC). *J. Infect. Dis.* **1995**, *171*, 1411–1419.

[7] Schinzai, R. F., et al. Characterization of human immunodeficiency viruses resistant to oxathiolane–cytosine nucleosides. *Antimicrob. Agents Chemother.* **1993**, *37*, 875–881.

[8] Gu, Z., et al. Novel mutation in the human immunodeficiency virus type 1 reverse transcriptase gene that encodes cross-resistance to 2′,3′-dideoxyinosine and 2′,3′-dideoxycytidine. *J. Virol.* **1992**, *66*, 7128–7135.

[9] Tisdale, M.; Alnadaf, T.; Cousens, D. Combination of mutations in human immunodeficiency virus type 1 reverse transcriptase required for resistance to the carbocyclic nucleoside 1592U89. *Antimicrob. Agents Chemother.* **1997**, *41*, 1094–1098.

[10] de Muys, J.-M., et al. Anti-human immunodeficiency virus type 1 activity, intracellular metabolism, and pharmacokinetic evaluation of 2′-deoxy-3′-oxa-4′-thiocytidine. *Antimicrob. Agents Chemother.* **1999**, *43*, 1835–1844.

[11] Taylor, D. L., et al. Drug resistance and drug combination features of the human immunodeficiency virus inhibitor, BCH-10652 [(±)-2′-deoxy-3′-oxa-4′-thiocytidine, dOTC. *Antivir. Chem. Chemother.* **2000**, *11*, 291–301.

[12] Bethell, R. C.; Lie, Y. S.; Parkin, N. T. In vitro activity of SPD754, a new deoxycytidine nucleoside reverse transcriptase inhibitor (NRTI), against 215 HIV-1 isolates resistant to other NRTIs. *Antivir. Chem. Chemother.* **2005**, *16*, 295–302.

[13] Gu, Z., et al. In vitro antiretroviral activity and in vitro toxicity profile of SPD754, a new deoxycytidine nucleoside reverse transcriptase inhibitor for treatment of human immunodeficiency virus infection. *Antimicrob. Agents Chemother.* **2006**, *50*, 625–631.

[14] Gallant, J. E., et al. Nucleoside and nucleotide analogue reverse transcriptase inhibitors: a clinical review of antiretroviral resistance. *Antivir. Ther.* **2003**, *8*, 489–506.

[15] Belleau, B., et al. A novel class of 1,3-oxathiolane nucleoside analogues having potent anti-HIV activity. *Bioorg. Med. Chem. Lett.* **1993**, *3*, 1723–1728.

[16] Mansour, T. S., et al. Anti-human immunodeficiency virus and anti-hepatitis-B virus activities and toxicities of the enantiomers of 2′-deoxy-3′-oxa-4′-thiocytidine and their 5-fluoro analogues in vitro. *J. Med. Chem.* **1995**, *38*, 1–4.

[17] Wang, W.; Jin, H.; Mansour, T. S. Synthesis of optically active 2′,3′-dideoxy-3′-oxa-4′-thio-ribonucleoside analogues by transposition of a leaving group on chiral oxathiolanes via a reductive–oxidative process. *Tetrahedron Lett.* **1994**, *35*, 4739–4742.

[18] Humber, D. C., et al. Expeditious preparation of (−)-2′-deoxy-3′-thiacytidine (3TC). *Tetrahedron Lett.* **1992**, *33*, 4625–4628.

[19] Choi, W. B., et al. In situ complexation directs the stereochemistry of N-glycosylation in the synthesis of thialanyl and dioxolanyl nucleoside analogs. *J. Am. Chem. Soc.* **1991**, *113*, 9377–9379.

[20] Vörbruggen, H.; Ruh-Pohlenz, C.; Eds. *Handbook of Nucleoside Synthesis*, Wiley, New York, 2001.

[21] Wang, Y.; Chen, A. M. Enantioenrichment by crystallization. *Org. Process Res. Dev.* **2008**, *12*, 282–290.

[22] Lorenz, H., et al. Crystallization based separation of enantiomers (review). *J. Univ. Chem. Technol. Metall.* **2007**, *42*, 5–16.

[23] Jacques, J.; Collet, A.; Wilen, S. H.; Eds. *Enantiomers, Racemates and Resolutions*, 3rd ed., Krieger Publishing, Malabar, FL, 1994.

[24] Nakatani-Freshwater, T., et al. Effects of trimethoprim on the clearance of apricitabine, a deoxycytidine analog reverse transcriptase inhibitor, and lamivudine in the isolated rat perfused kidney. *J. Pharmacol. Exp. Ther.* **2006**, *319*, 941–947.

[25] Sawyer, J.; Cox, S. In vitro pharmacology of apricitabine, a new NRTI for HIV. 16th International AIDS Conference, 2006. Abstract CDB0046.

[26] Bethell, R., et al. In vitro interactions between apricitabine and other deoxycytidine analogues. *Antimicrob. Agents Chemother.* **2007**, *51*, 2948–2953.

[27] Brinkman, K., et al. Adverse effects of reverse transcriptase inhibitors: mitochondrial toxicity as common pathway. *AIDS* **1998**, *12*, 1735–1744.

[28] de Baar, M. P., et al. Effects of apricitabine and other nucleoside reverse transcriptase inhibitors on replication of mitochondrial DNA in HepG2 cells. *Antiviral Res.* **2007**, *76*, 68–74.

[29] Cox, S., et al. Safety profile of apricitabine, a novel NRTI, during 24-week dosing in experienced HIV-1 infected patients. 17th International AIDS Conference, 2008. Abstract TUAB0106.

[30] Cahn, P., et al. 48-Week data from study AVX-201: a randomised phase 2b study of apricitabine in treatment-experienced patients with M184V and NRTI resistance. 9th International Congress on Drug Therapy in HIV Infection, 2008. Abstract 0414.

[31] Locas, C.; Ching, S.; Damment, S. Safety profile of SPD754 in cynomolgus monkeys treated for 52 weeks. 11th Conference on Retroviruses and Opportunistic Infections, 2004. Abstract 527.

[32] García-Lerma, J. G., et al. A novel genetic pathway of human immunodeficiency virus type 1 resistance to stavudine mediated by the K65R mutation. *J. Virol.* **2003**, *77*, 5685–5693.

[33] Harrigan, P. R., et al. Resistance profile of the human immunodeficiency virus type 1 reverse transcriptase inhibitor abacavir (1592U89) after monotherapy and combination therapy. CNA2001 Investigative Group. *J. Infect. Dis.* **2000**, *181*, 912–920.

[34] Wainberg, M. A., et al. In vitro selection and characterization of HIV-1 with reduced susceptibility to PMPA. *Antiviral. Ther.* **1999**, *4*, 87–94.

[35] Winters, M. A., et al. Human immunodeficiency virus type 1 reverse transcriptase genotype and drug susceptibility changes in infected individuals receiving dideoxyinosine monotherapy for 1 to 2 years. *Antimicrob. Agents Chemother.* **1997**, *41*, 757–762.

[36] Gu, Z., et al. BCH-10618, a new heterosubstituted nucleoside analogue against HIV-1 infection. *Antiviral. Ther.* **2001**, *6*(Suppl. 1), 8.

[37] Cox, S., et al. Antiviral activity of ATC in vitro against HIV isolates with combinations of NRTI resistance mutations. 11th European AIDS Conference, 2007. Abstract P7.1/02.

[38] Frankel, F. A., et al. Kinetics of inhibition of HIV type 1 reverse transcriptase-bearing NRTI-associated mutations by apricitabine triphosphate. *Antiviral. Chem. Chemother.* **2007**, *18*, 93–101.

[39] St Clair, M. H., et al. Resistance to ddI and sensitivity to AZT induced by a mutation in HIV-1 reverse transcriptase. *Science* **1991**, *253*, 1557–1559.

[40] Oliveira, M., et al. Apricitabine does not select additional drug resistance mutations in tissue culture in HIV-1 variants containing K65R, M184V or M184V plus thymidine analogue mutations. *Antimicrob. Agents Chemother.* **2009**, *53*, 1683–1685.

[41] Holdich, T.; Shiveley, L.; Sawyer, J. Pharmacokinetics of single oral doses of apricitabine, a novel deoxycytidine analogue reverse transcriptase inhibitor, in healthy volunteers. *Clin. Drug Invest.* **2006**, *26*, 279–286.

[42] Shiveley, L., et al. Pharmacokinetics of apricitabine, a novel nucleoside reverse transcriptase inhibitor, in healthy volunteers treated with trimethoprim–sulphamethoxazole. *J. Clin. Pharm. Ther.* **2008**, *33*, 45–54.

[43] Holdich, T.; Sawyer, J. Influence of food on the pharmacokinetics of apricitabine, a novel deoxycytidine analogue reverse transcriptase inhibitor. *Expert Opin. Pharmacother.* **2008**, *9*, 1–5.

[44] Sawyer, J.; Struthers-Semple, C. Pharmacokinetics of apricitabine in healthy volunteers and HIV-infected individuals. 16th International AIDS Conference, 2006. Abstract TUPE0077.

[45] Cahn, P., et al. Multiple-dose pharmacokinetics of apricitabine, a novel nucleoside reverse transcriptase inhibitor, in patients with HIV-1 infection. *Clin. Drug Invest.* **2008**, *28*, 129–138.

[46] Holdich, T.; Shiveley, L. A.; Sawyer, J. Effect of lamivudine on the plasma and intracellular pharmacokinetics of apricitabine, a novel nucleoside reverse transcriptase inhibitor, in healthy volunteers. *Antimicrob. Agents Chemother.* **2007**, *51*, 2943–2947.

[47] Moore, S. M., et al. Comparison of the pharmacokinetics of apricitabine in presence and absence of ritonavir boosted tipranavir. 8th International Workshop on Clinical Pharmacology of HIV Therapy, 2007. Abstract 68.

[48] Moore, S. M., et al. A thorough QT/QTc study in healthy volunteers of two doses of apricitabine compared to placebo and a moxifloxacin positive control. 8th International Workshop on Clinical Pharmacology of HIV Therapy, 2007. Abstract 29.

[49] Cahn, P., et al. Efficacy and tolerability of 10-day monotherapy with apricitabine in antiretroviral-naive, HIV-infected patients. *AIDS* **2006**, *20*, 1261–1268.

[50] Cahn, P., et al. Superior activity of apricitabine compared to 3TC over 21 days in treatment experienced HIV-1 infected patients failing therapy with M184V and NRTI resistance. 4th IAS Conference on HIV Pathogenesis, Treatment and Prevention, 2007. Abstract WESS203.

[51] Cahn, P., et al. 24 week data from study AVX-201: a prospective, randomised, double-blind, dose-ranging phase 2b study of apricitabine in treatment-experienced patients with M184V and NRTI resistance. 15th Conference on Retroviruses and Opportunistic Infections, 2008. Abstract 793.

[52] Cox, S.; Southby, J.; Moore, S. Genotypic analysis of patients enrolled in study AVX-201 and treated with apricitabine for 24 weeks. *Antiviral Ther.* **2008**, *13*(Suppl. 3), A22.

[53] Petrella, M., et al. Differential maintenance of the M184V substitution in the reverse transcriptase of human immunodeficiency virus type 1 by various nucleoside antiretroviral agents in tissue culture. *Antimicrob. Agents Chemother.* **2004**, *48*, 4189–4194.

[54] Back, N.; et al. Reduced replication of 3TC-resistant HIV-1 variants in primary cells due to a processivity defect of the reverse transcriptase enzyme. *EMBO J.* **1996**, *15*, 4040–4049.

[55] Petrella, M.; Wainberg, M. A. Might the M184V substitution in HIV-1 RT confer clinical benefit? *AIDS Rev.* **2002**, *4*, 224–232.

[56] Miller, M. D., et al. Antiviral activity of tenofovir (PMPA) against nucleoside-resistant clinical HIV samples. *Nucleosides Nucleotides Nucleic Acids* **2001**, *20*, 1025–1028.

9

DISCOVERY AND DEVELOPMENT OF MARAVIROC AND PF-232798: CCR5 ANTAGONISTS FOR THE TREATMENT OF HIV-1 INFECTION

Patrick Dorr

Abbott Laboratories, Berkshire, UK

Paul Stupple

Pfizer Global R&D, Kent, UK

INTRODUCTION

Acquired immunodeficiency syndrome (AIDS) was recognized as a disease in 1981 [1] with the discovery of the causative viral pathogen, later to be known as the human immunodeficiency virus 1 (HIV-1), shortly afterward [2,3]. HIV-1 infection and AIDS soon became a worldwide pandemic and the biggest infectious disease killer globally. Current estimates of the pandemic indicate 33 million infected, 2.1 million deaths from AIDS last year, and 2.7 million newly infected patients [4].

At the time the first treatments [nucleoside reverse transcriptase inhibitors, (NRTIs)] became available, AIDS was a more acute disease which was usually rapidly progressive and almost invariably lethal. The first generation of NRTIs, requiring complex dosing schedules, were soon followed by the non-nucleoside reverse transcriptase inhibitors (NNRTIs), and in the mid-1990s, the advent of the first HIV-1 protease inhibitors and the highly active antiretroviral therapy (HAART) combination dosing regimens. This brought a sea change to the treatment of the infection, with HAART for the first time achieving impressive sustained drops in viral load (VL), to levels that were undetectable even to the most sensitive technologies. Under HAART, patients' immune functions are largely (albeit not completely) restored, provided that they adhere to what can be complex, and at times, unpleasant treatments. Such patients, unfortunately, can remain infectious, capable of transmitting the virus by the usual modes (unprotected sex, and intravenous drug use with blood-contaminated needles), but are able to return to a much improved day-to-day lifestyle. Pharmacological treatment by HAART regimens has, in general, transformed AIDS from an acute, rapidly fatal condition to a chronic disease.

Despite the effectiveness of HAART regimens and the continuous improvements made to the dosing frequency and side-effect profiles of their components [5,6], emergence of resistance to one or more classes of antiretroviral remains a problem, and can be enhanced by issues surrounding compliance to a dosing regimen (for a recent review, see [7]). In one large study of HIV-1-positive adults who received treatment yet were viremic with > 500 HIV-1 RNA copies/mL within 3 years, it was estimated that approximately 76% had resistance to one or more HIV-1 drugs [8]. In addition, HIV-1 resistant to one or more classes of drugs is transmitted increasingly to treatment-naive patients, dramatically limiting their treatment options from the outset [9,10]. It was against this background in 1996 that CCR5 was identified as the predominant and essential coreceptor for HIV-1 cell entry, thereby triggering a widespread search for new ligands to find new therapeutic agents against HIV-1 that targeted a host rather than a viral factor in order to offer new treatments. The rationale for cell entry as a target per se was, however, pharmacologically validated by HIV-gp41 binding peptides prior to the development of CCR5 antagonists. Elucidation of

Antiviral Drugs: From Basic Discovery Through Clinical Trials, First Edition. Edited by Wieslaw M. Kazmierski.

the mechanism of viral entry led to the development of fusion inhibitors [11,12]. The HIV-1 entry process into host immune cells, associated antiviral targets, and their respective leading inhibitors has been summarized previously [13].

The first licensed drug in this class, enfuvirtide (Fuzeon, Trimeris/Roche; formerly known as T-20) acts at the point of virus entry into cells by binding to the viral envelope protein gp41 and preventing a postattachment step of the viral entry [14]. The drug has excellent efficacy in treatment-experienced patients, but the mode of administration and cost of goods associated with a complex peptide drug have restricted its use [15]. However, this represented groundbreaking research demonstrating HIV-1 entry to be a valid therapeutic target. Efforts since have predominantly focused on small-molecule HIV-1 entry disrupters to enable oral delivery. Some milestones in this effort have included the discovery of gp120-CD4-binding inhibitors, such as BMS-378806 [16], and blockade of CXCR4 via the antagonists AMD3100 and AMD070 [17]. These approaches have met with various challenges in efficacy and potential for significant side effects, respectively. However, the greatest tangible success in targeting HIV-1 entry as a new mechanism for new antiretroviral agents, has been the discovery, clinical development, and very recently, the approval of the CCR5 antagonist maraviroc (MVC) for the treatment of HIV-1 infection.

Chemokine receptors are a large family of G-protein-coupled receptors (GPCRs) that regulate leukocyte activation and migration to sites of inflammation via interaction with a family of secreted chemoattractant cytokines or "chemokines" [18]. Aminergic GPCRs recognize small-molecule ligands, and are attractive drug targets as reflected by the success pharmaceutical companies have had in modulating them with small molecules for the successful treatment of many diseases [19]. However, chemokine receptors belong to the family of peptidergic GPCRs, which have proven far more challenging to develop drugs against, and are bound by large peptides. The chemokine receptors most commonly utilized by HIV-1 in vivo are CCR5 and/or CXCR4, with CCR5 being almost exclusively the essential and sole coreceptor for infection of a person previously uninfected [20–23].

The rationale behind the development of CCR5 inhibitors was provided by the discovery of a natural 32-bp deletion (CCR5-Δ32, or Δ32) within the coding sequence of the gene, which results in the complete absence of CCR5 expression on the cell surface. Subjects (approximately 1% of northern European Caucasians, and of lower frequencies in other races) who are homozygotes for this deletion are protected genetically from HIV-1 infection [24–27] while heterozygotes have delayed disease progression. The absence of an overt phenotype associated with CCR5-Δ32 homozygosity provided considerable support to the confidence in safety of a CCR5 antagonist. Observations that CCR5 promoter polymorphisms also provided considerable resistance to HIV-1 progression following infection also attracted interest [28]. Cognate agonist ligands for CCR5 that caused receptor internalization, thereby making it unavailable for CCR5-tropic (R5) HIV strains, also helped elucidate this receptor as a valid antiviral target [29–31]. Finally, R5 HIV-1 strains are overwhelmingly the most commonly transmitted [32–34]; they usually predominate throughout asymptomatic infection. Approximately 50% of patients who develop AIDS carry only R5 strains [35,36], and appear to be the predominant phenotype in HIV-positive children [37] . The translation between genetic absence of CCR5 vs. "blocked" CCR5 as an antiviral mechanism was borne out more recently with the observation from clinical trials that numerous CCR5 antagonists safely reduced viral load in humans [38–41].

CCR5 is a 352-amino acid protein with a basic structure that is typical of a seven-transmembrane GPCR. It consists of three extracellular loops (ECL1, ECL2, and ECL3) and the N terminus, which are involved in chemokine binding and interactions with the viral protein gp120 (following an initial complex formation with CD4 to enable HIV-1 entry as described above), and three intracellular loops and the C terminus, which participate in G protein–mediated signal transduction.

Chemokine interaction with CCR5 initiates several events. The receptor associates with G proteins, leading to activation of signaling processes: changes in receptor conformation, G-protein interaction and GTP binding, intracellular Ca^{2+} redistribution, activation of MAP kinase and Jun-N-terminal kinase, and receptor internalization. A number of cognate/endogenous CC chemokines (see Table 1) bind to CCR5 with different affinities and abilities to activate the receptor [42–46]. The observation that CCR5 ligands can inhibit HIV-1 entry [29] influenced the identification of CCR5 as a coreceptor for the virus.

The physiological function of CCR5 in a fully developed organism remains to be fully elucidated. For target research and development with a drug as the intended outcome, it was reassuring that Δ32 homozygotes have no major apparent deficiencies, and prolonged therapy with maraviroc suggests continued and sudden CCR5 functional blockade, and viral suppression has highlighted a high correlation with the Δ32 phenotype in terms of efficacy and safety. A better understanding of the physiological role of CCR5 may

TABLE 1 Cognate Ligands for CCR5

Systematic Ligand Name	Original Ligand Name
CCL3	MIP-1α (macrophage inflammatory protein 1α)
CCL4	MIP-1β (macrophage inflammatory protein 1α)
CCL5	RANTES (regulated on activation, normally T-cell expressed and secreted)
CCL7	
CCL8	MCP-2 (monocyte chemoattractant protein 1)
CCL14	HCC-1 (hemofiltrate CC chemokine 1)
CCL3L1	LD78β

also provide alternative development indications for CCR5 inhibitors, possibly against one or more of the pathologies that have been negatively associated with CCR5 knockout or inhibition (see the section "Future Directions"). In 1996, when CCR5 was shown to be an essential and dominant coreceptor for HIV-1 cell entry, however, none of this was known. The identification of CCR5 as a putative anti-HIV-1 target prompted widespread discovery activities across academia and industry, which have resulted in many clinical candidates [47,48]. Antiviral analogs and peptide-based mimics of cognate ligands have been reported [49,50], and antibodies against CCR5 were reported and continue to progress through clinical trials (e.g., HGS004 [51], PRO-140 [52]). However, the limitations posed by antibodies and peptides (e.g., lack of oral delivery), the lack of other known ligands, and breakthroughs in GPCR assays have, led to high-throughput screening approaches to initiate medicinal chemistry for small-molecule antagonists (agonists were not so highly sought, due to perceived risk of an inflammatory trigger and coreceptor switch [49]). A range of antagonists were subsequently discovered, and some progressed into clinical trials. Many have met with attrition for various reasons (idiosyncratic liver toxicity, QT prolongation, lack of oral bioavailability, and inherent polypharmacology (for a review, see [53]). Maraviroc is the first and to date only CCR5 antagonist to meet with formal approval for therapeutic antiretroviral use, having avoided all these attritional factors. The targeted second-generation follow-up clinical candidate to maraviroc, PF-232798, is progressing well in phase II. A recent review describing the leading CCR5 antagonists across the pharmaceutical and biotechnology industries has been published [53] . The background, use, and future of maraviroc and PF-232798 from the Pfizer laboratories at Sandwich are described specifically here.

DISCOVERY OF MARAVIROC AND PF-232798

In the absence of convenient, high-throughput assays mimicking the many events in HIV-1 cell entry at the time of CCR5 discovery as coreceptor, radioligand-binding assays using iodinated chemokines adapted from reported techniques [54] were used successfully to identify initial chemical leads [55–61]. These hits, in turn, progressed through bespoke screening cascades of virology, primary and selectivity pharmacology assays, and pharmacokinetic (PK) studies, prior to toxicological and clinical evaluation.

HTS AND BIOLOGICAL SCREENING TO GUIDE MEDICINAL CHEMISTRY

The Pfizer CCR5 antagonist program began with a high-throughput screen of the corporate screening file (about 500,000 compounds at the time) based on inhibition of the binding of [^{125}I]MIP-1β to human CCR5 as stably integrated and expressed on HEK-293 cells. Several hits emerged from the screen, most prominently UK-107543 (Scheme 1), which had reasonable inhibitory activity against [^{125}I]MIP-1β binding (IC_{50} = 0.6 μM). However, this was devoid of antiviral activity, and proved to be a CCR5 agonist, as assessed using calcium signaling (FLIPR) assays [58]. It was also found to be a potent (IC_{50} = 40 nM) inhibitor of the polymorphic human CYP2D6 enzyme, putatively via coordination of the pyridine N atom to the heme group. Two strategies were adopted to circumvent CYP2D6 inhibition: first, simple replacement of the pyridine N atom with C-retained potent CCR5 receptor binding but with much reduced CYP inhibition, and second, steric crowding of the piperidine N atom by incorporation into a tropane ring, which gave further improvements in potency in both the CCR5 binding and signaling assays, gp120-CD4-CCR5 complex formation screen, and HIV fusion assay [58]. This also effectively ablated CYP inhibition [62].

These screens eventually guided chemistry to the further replacement of one phenyl group from the benzhydryl moiety with an amide function that drove a significant reduction in lead lipophilicity, and in combination with the tropane ring design, instilled significant and, importantly R5-HIV-specific antiviral activity (no cytotoxicity) within the series (UK-372673; see Scheme 1). It was proposed that reducing the conformational flexibility of the propylamino linking group through *syn*-pentane interactions contributed to the enhanced performance of the tropane group. Structure–activity relationship (SAR) studies showed activity in the series to reside within the *S*-phenyl configuration, while both the endo- and exo-benzimidazole diastereoisomers showed largely equivalent receptor binding and antiviral potencies. The Pfizer program then turned to focus on overcoming high and unacceptable affinity for the hERG potassium channel, which was not entirely unexpected in light of the series being basic with a positive log P.

A number of strategies directed toward all locations of the lead structure were deployed, predominantly guided by compound-competition screening against labeled dofetilide binding to hERG-subunit-containing cell membranes [63]. The most successful of these sought to introduce polarity in peripheral aromatic regions and optimize substitution patterns for CCR5 binding affinity. The polarity introduced, as exemplified by UK-395859 (Scheme 1), achieved impressive antiviral activity [$IC_{90} \sim 1$ nM HIV-1 (BaL) in peripheral blood lymphocytes (PBL)] and reduced the affinity for hERG ($IC_{50} > 10$ μM), but showed extremely low penetration of Caco-2 cell layers (< 1 cm/s) and no evidence of absorption in rat PK studies (oral dosing and hepatic portal vein and systemic exposure determination). This was presumed to be a consequence of water coating due to hydrogen binding. The morpholino analog UK-396794 (Scheme 1) retained the impressive antiviral/hERG profile and was fully absorbed in rat. However, this compound was very

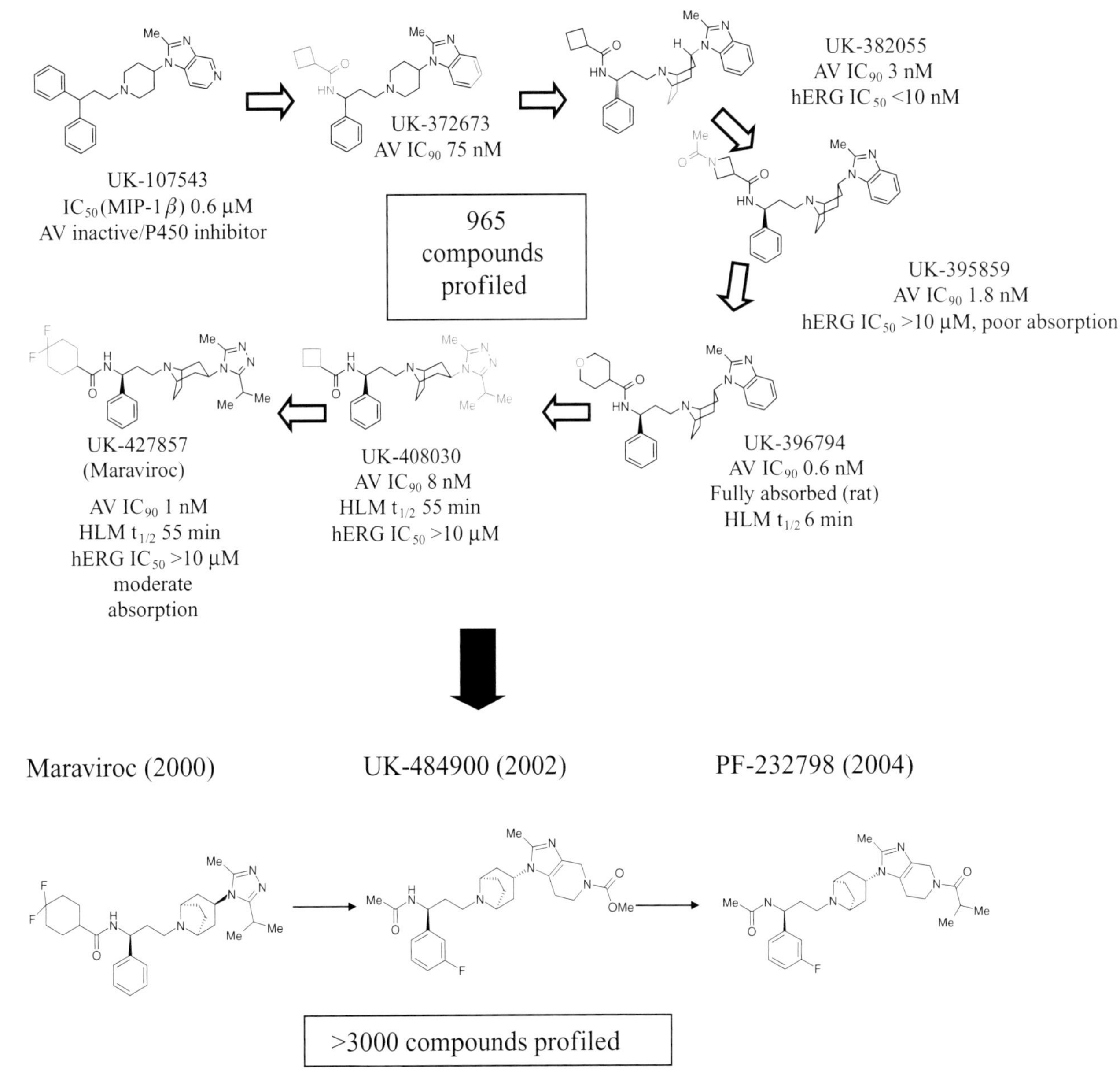

SCHEME 1 Key stages and overarching SAR enabling guidance of the maraviroc medicinal chemistry program, and subsequent generation of PF-232798 (nomination year for clinical evaluation highlighted).

susceptible to p450 degradation in isolated human liver microsomes (HLMs), suggesting the likelihood of a poor PK profile (potential for a high peak/trough ratio and unacceptable drug–drug interactions). Synthetic effort led to the triazole UK-408030 (Scheme 1), a series within which antiviral activity of the exo- and endo-tropanes began to very much favor the exo diastereoisomer and balanced somewhat the profile for favorable absorption, stability, hERG, and CCR5-mediated antiviral activity. Evolution of the cyclobutyl group, powered by parallel chemistry techniques, then provided the difluorocyclohexyl group in UK-427857 (later known as maraviroc; Fig. 1), which showed excellent antiviral potency (R5 HIV-1 cross-clade primary isolate in PBL culture geometric mean $IC_{90} = 1$ nM [58,64]), with low activity against hERG ($IC_{50} > 10$ μM). Profiling in vitro highlighted broad anti R5 HIV-1 spectrum in a range of assays and either additive or synergistic properties in combination with other antiretroviral drugs [58].

In preclinical absorption, distribution, metabolism, and excretion (ADME) studies (for full details, see [65]), maraviroc had high clearance in rat and moderate clearance in dog, which appeared to be mediated by a combination of renal, metabolic, and biliary processes. Maraviroc exhibited moderate tissue distribution, in keeping with its basic

TABLE 2 Predicted and Measured Human Pharmacokinetic Profile for Maraviroc

Parameter	Maraviroc Predicted from Rat and Dog	Maraviroc Measured (30 mg i.v. single dose or 100 mg b.i.d. oral)
Clearance (mL/min/kg)	11	10.5 ± 1.3
Vd (L/kg)	2	2.8 ± 0.9
$t_{1/2}$ (h)	3	13.2 ± 2.8
Absorption (%)	30	55
Bioavailability (%)	20	23 (19.2 – 27.8)
C_{min} (nM unbound) at 100 mg b.i.d.	1	5.4 ± 1.4

and moderately lipophilic nature. The ratio of CSF to free plasma concentration is 0.1, indicating a low level, but potentially some distribution to the central nervous system (CNS). Maraviroc was slowly metabolized by human liver microsomes (HLMs). Using expressed human cytochrome P450 enzymes only, CYP2D6 and CYP3A4 metabolized the compound with five-fold higher turnover by CYP3A4. Maraviroc showed only weak inhibition of CYP2D6 ($IC_{50} = 87$ μM) using recombinant CYPs and fluorescent probe substrates. No inhibition of CYP1A2, CYP2C9, CYP2C19, or CYP3A4 by maraviroc (up to 100 μM) was observed. Maraviroc also showed inherently low membrane permeability in Caco-2 flux studies that predict incomplete absorption in general, with transcellular flux enhanced in the presence of P-glycoprotein inhibitors [65]. It was 20 to 30% absorbed in rats, but well absorbed in dogs and shows nonlinear pharmacokinetics (PK) in oral dose escalation studies in humans (see below). Predicting human PK from animal studies and in vitro models is challenging. At the time of nomination to clinical evaluation, it was estimated that a convenient dosing regime of about 100 mg twice daily (b.i.d.) should be well tolerated and maintain unbound compound levels above the geometric mean, cross-clade antiviral IC_{90} in native cell assays [58]. Retrospectively, the actual absorption and subsequent PK in humans was superior to that of the profile predicted (see Table 2). The discovery of the slow physical and functional dissociation of maraviroc and, indeed, all antagonists reported to date from the CCR5 receptor [64,66,67] suggested that receptor occupancy might be retained following clearance of free drug, although the turnover of CCR5 and its expressing cells might limit the effectiveness of prolonged receptor occupancy in driving viral load reduction [58].

Maraviroc was characterized extensively in pharmacology-based assays prior to a regulatory-based preclinical toxicology package to enable evaluation in human phase 1 clinical trials. These studies highlighted the potent and selective CCR5 inhibitory potency of maraviroc, specific anti R5-HIV-1 cross-clade activity, and inactivity (see Table 3) against a range of Th1 and Th2 immune functions [58]. Maraviroc was profiled extensively in

TABLE 3 In Vitro Immune Selectivity Profile of Maraviroc

Immune Function Assay	Maraviroc Potency
MCP-3-induced intracellular Ca^{2+} release (CCR2)	$IC_{50} > 10$ μM
IL-2-stimulated T-cell proliferation	$IC_{50} > 10$ μM
LPS-stimulated TNF-α release by differentiated THP-1 cell	$IC_{50} > 4$ μM
Antigen-stimulated lymphocyte proliferation	$IC_{50} > 10$ μM
MIP-1α-induced chemotaxis of THP-1 cells (CCR1)	$IC_{50} > 25$ μM
MCP-1-induced chemotaxis of THP-1 cells (CCR2)	$IC_{50} > 25$ μM
ITAC-induced chemotaxis by H9 cells (CCR3)	$IC_{50} > 25$ μM
SLC-induced chemotaxis by H9 cells (CCR7)	$IC_{50} > 25$ μM
IL-8-induced chemotaxis of neutrophils (CXCR1/CXCR2)	$IC_{50} > 25$ μM
Gro-α-induced chemotaxis of neutrophils (CXCR2)	$IC_{50} > 25$ μM
MIP-1α binding to CCR1	$IC_{50} > 10$ μM
Eotaxin binding to CCR3	$IC_{50} > 10$ μM
TARC binding to CCR4	$IC_{50} > 10$ μM
rhMIP-3β binding to CCR7	$IC_{50} > 10$ μM
I309 binding to CCR8	$IC_{50} > 10$ μM
Superoxide production in neutrophils	$IC_{50} > 10$ μM
IL-4-stimulated IgE synthesis in lymphocytes	$IC_{50} \geq 10$ μM (two donors); $IC_{50} = 1$ to 10 μM (one donor)

Source: [58].

hERG-associated assays in vitro and in vivo (dog hemodynamics), highlighting a low risk of QT prolongation [58,65]. The overall outcome of this preclinical study was to conclude that maraviroc showed a profile that was deemed potent enough to enable viral load reduction under a convenient dosing regime, without obvious or apparent off-target pharmacology. However, and in common with many discovery projects, a strategy to mitigate against unforeseen and idiosynchratic toxicity included the discovery of follow-up clinical candidates. This led to the discovery and clinical evaluation of PF-232798.

DISCOVERY AND CHARACTERIZATION OF PF-232798, A SECOND-GENERATION CCR5 ANTAGONIST

PF-232798 evolved from a medicinal chemistry campaign guided by a bespoke biological screening cascade, essentially as described previously [58,64], aimed at increasing the absorption, and improving the PK vs. maraviroc, while retaining the favorable pharmacological and antiviral properties, in a significantly differentiated chemotype. This was also deemed appropriate to mitigate against potential compound-specific toxicity or potential adverse events for maraviroc. It was also felt that such differentiation might drive differential occupancy of the CCR5 antagonist binding pocket and enable activity against any R5-HIV isolates that mutated to acquire resistance to maraviroc in the longer term (remaining R5-tropic), and thereby offer the potential for additional lines of therapy (see the section "Resistance to Maraviroc"). The PF-232798 structure arose from an alternative means of circumventing the CYP2D6 and hERG activity associated with the original high-throughput screening hit UK-107543 by simple reduction of the pyridine ring to give an imidazopiperidine. Incorporation of SAR learning from the maraviroc medicinal chemistry program, and optimization of the amide and imidazopiperidine substituents, in within the endo tropane diastereoisomer series, as distinct from the maraviroc series, was undertaken. By maintaining a small amount of amide substitution, this allowed the identification of UK-484900, the original clinical candidate follow-up compound to maraviroc, and then PF-232798 (Scheme 1). This culminated in over 3000 compounds being synthesized and screened in a bespoke cascade for the eventual nomination and clinical profiling of PF-232798. Both compounds showed a primary and selectivity pharmacological profile similar to that of maraviroc [64,93]. Comparative antiviral profiling showed UK-484900 to be at least as potent in the recombinant pseudotyped antiviral PhenoSense assay [69] as maraviroc, and with the same spectrum.

In PBL assays it proved to be two- to seven-fold more active, with the same cross-clade spectrum. This encouraging profile, coupled with preclinical pharmacokinetic properties, showed improvements over maraviroc (three-fold higher flux in Caco-2 penetration studies, complete absorption in rat and dog, with longer $t_{1/2}$) and potential for improved pharmacokinetics and subsequent dosing regime in humans. This prompted plans to advance UK-484900 to toxicology studies and clinical evaluation. UK-484900 was inherently more active than maraviroc against the hERG ion channel ($IC_{50} = 2.1$ μM vs. > 10 μM, dofetlide-binding inhibition), although its potential for a reduced peak/trough ratio for systemic exposure (unbound or "free" compound) in humans, led to postulation that the QT window would be at least as favorable as it is with maraviroc. Clinical studies confirmed the validity of this hypothesis, and retrospective comparison with the clinical exposure PK data (steady state) for maraviroc highlighted essential equivalent free compound exposure above antiviral IC_{90} values at 30 mg q.d. for UK-484900 vs. 300 mg b.i.d. for maraviroc. To mitigate against unexpected attrition, PF-232798 was also nominated for clinical evaluation shortly afterward, as it showed a similar preclinical PK profile and pharmacology to UK-484900. This proved to be a sensible strategy, as UK-484900 showed an effect in preclinical regulatory embryo–fetal toxicity studies, whereas maraviroc and PF-232798 both showed clean profiles. For this reason, PF-232798 was selected as the second-generation CCR5 antagonist to follow maraviroc, ahead of UK-484900. UK-484900 remains a useful tool for investigating CCR5's role in non-HIV indications and the inflammatory associations of HIV infections in light of its potent pharmacological profile and ability to occupy CCR5 in preclinical in vivo models of disease in mice (see the section "Future Directions"). PF-232798 showed a significantly improved PK profile in clinical studies compared to maraviroc, highlighting the potential for a lower dose and a less frequent dosing regime in clinical practice (see Fig. 1).

PF-232798 is estimated to be at 2.5-fold (95% CI 2.3 to 2.7-fold) less antiviral than maraviroc, based on comparative highly powered high-throughput recombinant in vitro antiviral assays (PhenoSense), which show PF-232798 to have the same antiviral spectrum [64]. This is deemed to be a conservative estimate of PF-232798 antiviral activity, as it was equally potent in low-throughput native-cell-based assays [64]. PF-232798, like maraviroc, showed inherently low affinity for the hERG ion channel (IC_{50} > 10 μM, dofetilide binding) and in all QT-associated preclinical studies in vitro and in vivo. In addition to superior PK relative to maraviroc, potential to provide additional lines of therapy to address emergent maraviroc-resistant HIV-1 strains (MVC^{RES} HIV-1) in the clinic is another driver for the development of PF-232798. Intuitively, CCR5 offers an attractive target for antiviral drug discovery, in that targeting a host protein creates an additional hurdle for HIV-1 to gain resistance, as the virus cannot simply mutate rapidly to moderate drug binding to one of its own proteins, as seen for all other

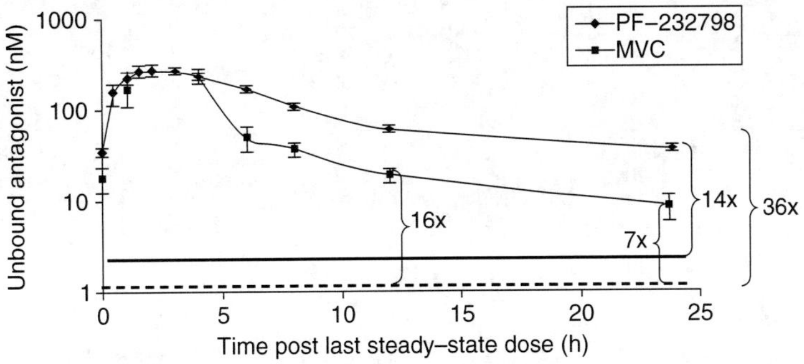

FIGURE 1 Data represent the mean unbound antagonist concentration in plasma ± S.E.M. PF-232798 dosed at 250 mg q.d., 7 days dosing ($n = 6$ volunteers); MVC dosed at 300 mg b.i.d., 10 days ($n = 8$ volunteers). Total plasma levels were measured by HPLC-MS and corrected for in vitro plasma protein binding (75 and 94% for MVC and PF-232798, respectively). The fold antiviral IC_{90} values estimated for maraviroc and PF-232798 are described. The dashed line represents both the unbound antiviral geometric IC_{90} for MVC against 43 primary isolates [1], and the IC_{90} for PF-232798 vs. HIV BaL in PBL culture. The solid bold line represents the estimated IC_{90} potency for PF-232798 vs. primary isolate HIV in PBL based on the 2.5-fold lower activity vs. MVC observed against a panel of primary isolates in the PhenoSense assay.

anti-HIV targets. Indeed, preclinical in vitro studies have shown that gaining resistance to CCR5 antagonists is relatively difficult [70]. HIV-1 does not mutate to enable entry via the CXCR4 coreceptor switch as observed in animal models, in vitro systems, or indeed, in clinically derived isolates [70–72]. As opposed to selection of X4 virus, resistance to CCR5 antagonists has been demonstrated in the clinic (see the section "Resistance to Maraviroc in Clinical Trials") and in preclinical studies, and is achieved following mutation to enable gaining entry via antagonist-occupied receptor rather than by mutation to enable entry via an alternative coreceptor [70,72–75].

Although some of those mutations can confer resistance to chemically related CCR5 antagonists [73,74,76], class resistance is not inevitable [77], and there is considerable weight of evidence that the resistant strains cannot utilize CCR5 that is occupied by an antagonist that has not been used as the selecting agent for generating the resistant isolate [66,75,78–81]. Indeed, PF-232798 retained full activity against an expanded clone of the B-clade MVC^{RES} HIV-1 isolate CC185 in PBL culture (Fig. 2). Partial retention (> 50%) of activity was observed against an expanded clone of the G-clade MVC^{RES} HIV-1 isolate RU570, although a lowered plateau effect was observed. This was deemed significant in light of full retention being observed with saquinavir and alternative CCR5 antagonist templates aplaviroc and vicriviroc [64]. It remains to be seen if this encouraging trend is seen with clinically derived MVC^{RES} HIV-1. This is a promising observation for this new class, suggesting that class resistance may not be achieved as readily as for traditional antiretroviral targets. To understand the observations and SAR associated with CCR5 antagonist resistance in relationship with

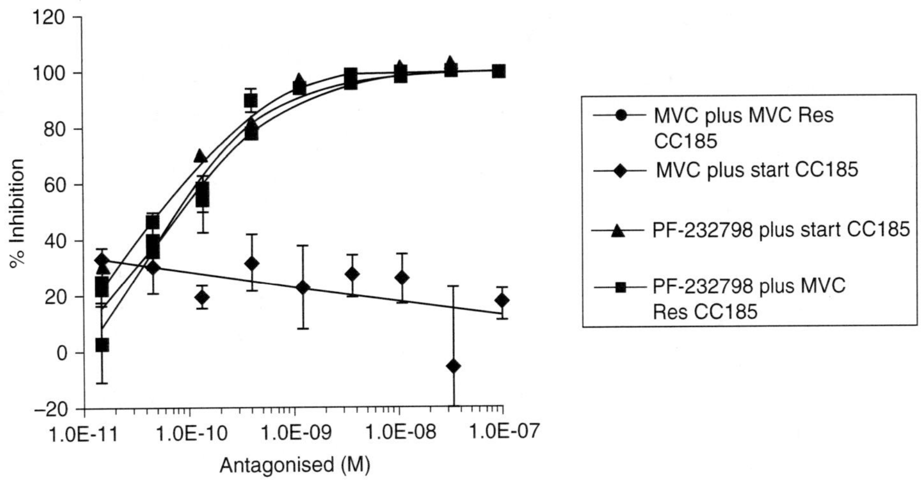

FIGURE 2 All assays performed in parallel PBL cultures comparing maraviroc-passaged (resistant-strain CC185) and vehicle-passaged controlled cultures. Data points represent mean values ± S.E.M. (From [64].)

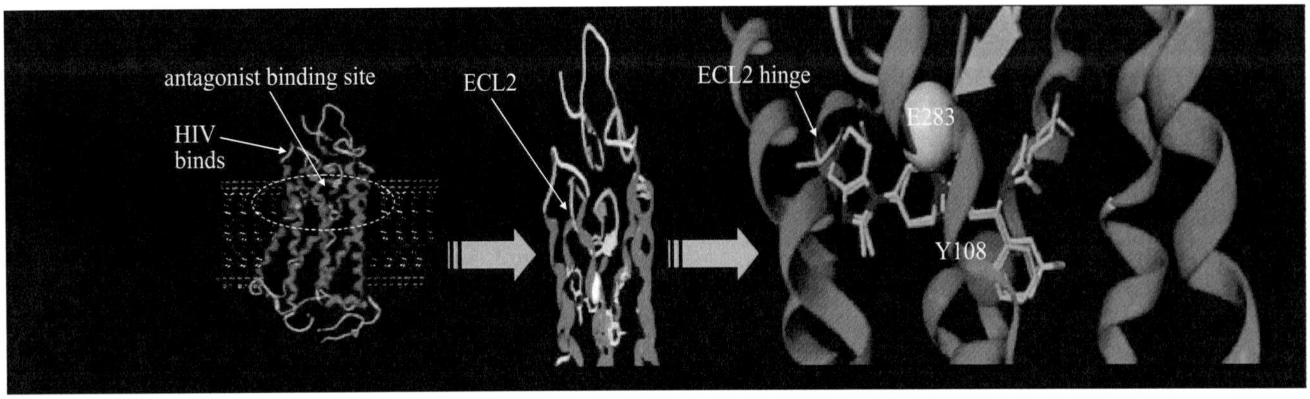

FIGURE 3 Diagrammatic representation of CCR5 in the cytoplasmic membrane of an immune cell. Overlaps of PF-232798 (pale blue) and MVC (green) are highlighted. Interaction of the ionic interaction between the basic nitrogen of the antagonists and hydrophobic interaction of their phenyl moieties with the E283 and Y108 residues, respectively, in the transmembrane pocket are highlighted. All images generated using the computer modeling Pfizer software package FLOPS (flexes ligands optimizing property similarity) and Pfizer crystal structure database, as guided by assay data from site-directed alanine mutagenesis, where loss of functional binding was observed for E238A and Y108A mutants for maraviroc and PF-232798. (*See insert for color representation of the figure.*)

maraviroc and PF-232798 as a second-generation candidate, a study designed to investigate the binding mode of these compounds was undertaken.

CCR5 antagonists are commonly referred to as *allosteric antagonists* in that they bind to the site equivalent to the retinol-binding site of the structurally characterized GPCR rhodopsin (for a review of CCR5 antagonist binding, see [82]). This binding mode is allosteric with respect to the gp120-CD4 complex binding site to CCR5, which binds the extracellular N-terminal and extracellular loop (ECL) regions (especially the second loop; see [83–85]). However, the antagonist binding site might be considered as orthosteric with respect to chemokines, part of which bind at sites within the transmembrane "retinol equivalent" site [86]. The basic mechanism of CCR5 antagonist antiviral activity is to binding the receptor to drive rearrangement of the extracellular loops into a conformation that is no longer recognized by the gp120-CD4 complex. Offset of the antagonist, and in particular the functional recovery of the receptor to enable either chemokine or HIV-1, binding, appears to be extremely slow thereafter, as judged by the small reduction in potency in wash and chase experiments [64,66].

CCR5 antagonist resistance seen in vitro and observed in clinical practice is underpinned by the mutation of viral envelope to a form that can recognize the extracellular pattern of the antagonist-occupied receptor N-terminus and loops. Different CCR5 antagonists appear to stablize significantly different conformations of the CCR5 ECLs. The SAR for this has been in part characterized through compound screening against MVC^{RES} HIV-1 CC185, coupled with computer-assisted antagonist-receptor docking models based on data from site-directed mutagenesis mapping of antagonists, as reported previously for the maraviroc program [53,66,68]. These identified the essential hydrophobic interaction between the phenyl moieties of maraviroc and PF-232798 with Y108, and the ionic interactions between the basic tropane nitrogen and the acidic residues E283 (also observed independently; see [82]). Modeling studies highlight the fact that additional occupancy of the imidazopiperidine group of PF-232798 relative to the triazole moiety of maraviroc around the ECL2 hinge region appears to enable sufficient change in conformation that laboratory-generated MVC^{RES} HIV-1 cannot bind, highlighting a nonoverlapping resistant profile (see Fig. 3).

SYNTHESIS

The chemistry for large-scale preparation of maraviroc as the active ingredient in the Censentri/Zelsentry has four steps. In step 1, ethyl (*S*)-3-[(4,4-difluorocyclohexyl) carboximido]-3-phenylpropanoate (UK-453464) is reduced with sodium borohydride and methanol in tetrahydrofuran to give alcohol UK-453465, which is isolated from either tetrahydrofuran and cyclohexane or from acetone and water. In step 2, UK-453465 is oxidized with aqueous sodium hypochlorite catalyzed by 2,2,6,6-tetramethyl-1-piperidinyloxy free radical in dichloromethane to give aldehyde (UK-453,453), which is isolated from toluene and/or heptane. In step 3, exo-8-benzyl-3-(3-isopropyl-5-methyl-4*H*-1,2,4-triazol-4-yl)-8-azabicyclo[3.2.1]octane (UK-408,026) is hydrogenolyzed over a palladium-on-carbon catalyst in the presence of *p*-toluenesulfonic acid and carbon in methanol or aqueous propan-2-ol to give amine (UK-408,027-15), which is isolated from propan-2-ol. In step 4, the aldehyde (UK-453,453) is reductively coupled with the amine (UK-408,027-15) in the presence of sodium triacetoxy-borohydride in tetrahydrofuran and/or ethyl acetate to give

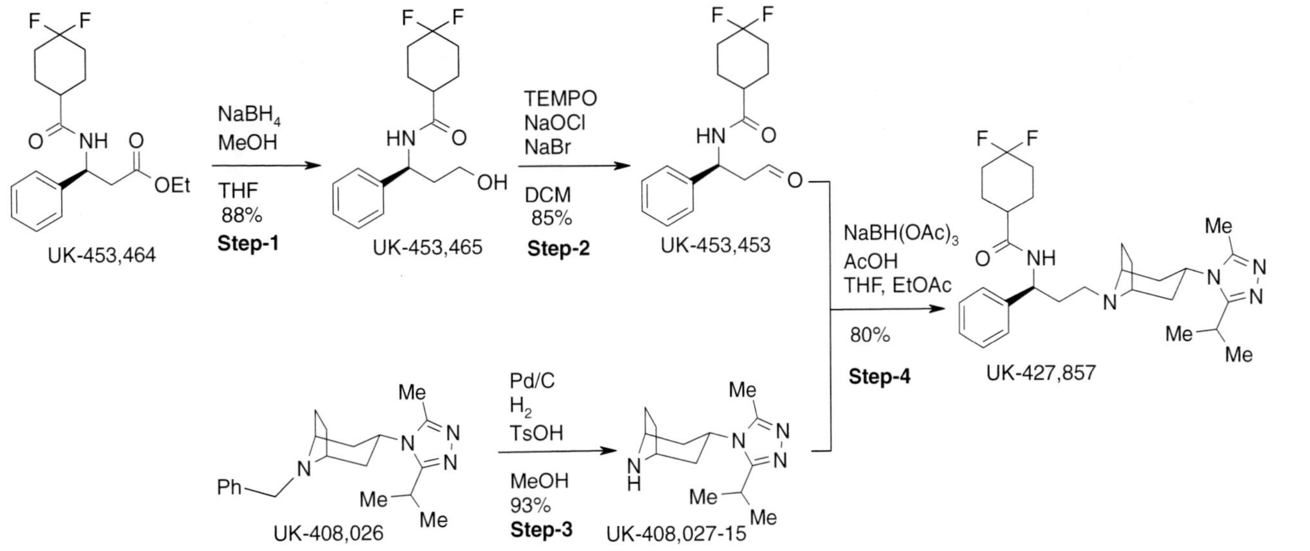

SCHEME 2 Process chemistry synthesis of maraviroc.

maraviroc, which is isolated from ethyl acetate. This is shown in Scheme 2 with associated conditions and yields.

The left-hand side of PF-232798 was constructed starting from a known enantiomerically pure amine (**7**) (Scheme 3). Acetylation, followed by reduction of the ester **8** and subsequent oxidation, furnished the required aldehyde (**10**). Reaction of a known aminotropane (**11**) with 4-chloro-3-nitropyridine, formed a 4-aminopyridine (**12**). Reduction of the nitro functionality followed by imidazopyridine formation resulted in a switch of the tropane protecting group from Boc (*tert*-butoxycarbonyl) to acetyl. Carbamate (**15**) was prepared in three steps: (1) quaternization of the pyridyl group followed by sodium borohydride reduction, (2) hydrogenation of the alkene, and (3) acid-mediated removal of the acetyl protecting group. Reductive amination of the aldehyde **10** with tropane **15** gave carbamate **16**, which after deprotection and reaction with isobutyryl chloride furnished PF-232798 (**18**).

NONCLINICAL SAFETY AND TOXICITY STUDIES

The studies to investigate the toxicity of maraviroc were particularly extensive and rigorous in light of the intention to treat an immune-compromised population through inhibition of a receptor that mediates immune cell signaling, with a first-in-mechanism and structurally completely novel compound. The toxicological profile of maraviroc is detailed here rather than that of PF-232798 for the sake of brevity, the high degree of similarity between the two compounds, and the greater characterization of maraviroc in light of its more advanced status and pioneering nature. A regulatory-based toxicity–safety phamacology package involving numerous regulatory toxicity species showed maraviroc to have an extremely well-tolerated profile, with no significant adverse findings at systemic free drug exposure levels at multiples of the intended therapeutic exposure levels. Maraviroc had little interaction with physiologically important receptors, binding sites, enzymes, or ion channels apart from a weak affinity for the human μ-opioid receptor ($K_i = 0.6$ μM) and human α2A adrenergic receptor ($K_i = 10$ μM), which exceeded by > 30-fold the $C_{\max}$ free drug levels achieved at therapeutic dosing in humans.

The basic nature and positive log *D* of CCR5 antagonists, and more specifically the attrition for the Sch-C (the first compound reported in HIV monotherapy trials) due to QT prolongation, have ensured extensive scrutiny of CCR5 antagonists at the hERG channel. Results from in vitro hERG channel studies showed maraviroc to have very weak effects ($IC_{50} > 10$ μM) on IKr current and only affect cardiac repolarization in vivo at unbound plasma concentrations greater than 3 μM (approximately 10-fold the mean unbound $C_{\max}$ value in HIV-positive patients at the later-established clinical dose of 300 mg b.i.d.) [58,65].

The toxicity of single and repeated doses of maraviroc was studied in mouse, rat, dog, and cynomolgous monkey. In terms of metabolism and general pharmacokinetics, these species can all be considered as useful models for humans, but considering pharmacology at the target receptor level, the macaque is by far closest to humans in sequence and function, especially because maraviroc has a similar affinity for this isoform and human CCR5, whereas it is essentially inactive (binding and signaling) against the isoform from the other species (see Table 4) [67]. In short, it was only possible to achieve functional occupancy of CCR5 in macaques, and dosing regimes to ensure total functional occupancy in this species were tested to fully ascertain mechanistic toxicity.

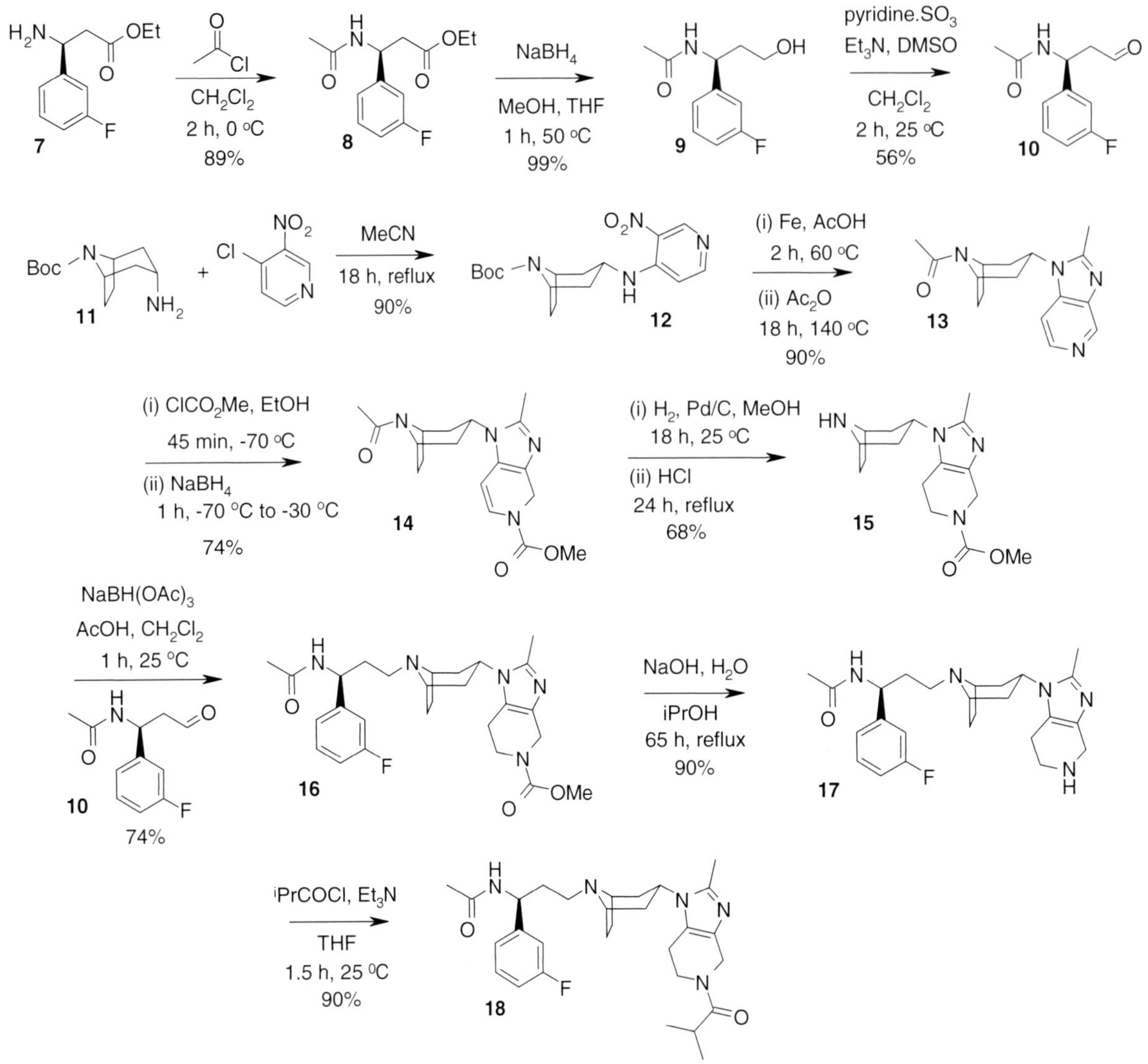

SCHEME 3 Laboratory synthetic route for PF-232798.

TABLE 4 Comparative Pharmacology of Maraviroc Against CCR5 Isoforms from Various Species

Experiment	Human CCR5	Macaque CCR5
K_d	0.9 nM	1.4 nM
[3H]MVC binding	(95% CI 0.7–1.1 nM)	(95% CI 1.1–1.7 nM)
IC_{50}	7.2 nM	17.5 nM
[125I]MIP-1β binding to cell membranes	(95% CI 5.5–9.5 nM)	(95% CI 14.1–21.0 nM)
IC_{50}	14 nM	17.5 nM
MIP-1β-induced intracellular calcium release	(95% CI 10–20 nM)	(95% CI 9.6–32.9 nM)
$t_{1/2}$	16.0 h	1.5 h
[3H]MVC dissociation	(95% CI 9.0–27.0 h)	(95% CI 1.3–1.9 h)

Pivotal toxicity studies after repeated doses included 3-month mouse, 6-month rat, 6-month dog, and a 9-month cynomolgus monkey. Doses shown to yield unbound maraviroc exposure levels at many multiples of expected therapeutic exposure resulted in an encouraging unremarkable profile. Due to the relatively high physiological similarities between cynomolgus monkeys and humans, and the total functional CCR5 blockade achieved in this species (unlike the other species), data from this study were deemed the most relevant. The NOAEL levels (QTc interval increase) were three- to five-fold the clinically relevant equivalent in humans. With respect to clinical observations and significance, reduced systolic and diastolic blood pressure was observed at high exposure. This may be related to the dose-limiting adverse event for humans of postural hypotension, which is a significantly more difficult effect to observe in animals than in humans.

Detailed immunological and hematology analysis in these toxicity studies showed no maraviroc-dependent effects on general hematology or serum globulins; no effects of histology changes in bone marrow, lymph nodes, spleen, thymus; and no increase in the incidence of infections. Specific immunotoxicology studies in monkeys (at 100% CCR5 functional blockade) showed no changes in lymphocyte subset distribution; NK cell activity, phagocytosis activity/oxidative burst, or humoral response (IgM and IgG). In short, blockade of CCR5 and maraviroc exposure per se were deemed to have a clean profile with no measurable adverse effects on immune function.

PHASE I–III CLINICAL PK SAFETY AND EFFICACY EVALUATION OF MARAVIROC

Phase I PK studies on maraviroc demonstrated oral bioavailability and a terminal half-life of 16 to 23 h [87,88]. Single doses of up to 900 mg and multiple doses of up to 300 mg b.i.d. for 28 days were well tolerated and gave unbound exposure levels far in excess of the measured antiviral IC_{90} [89]. Drug–drug interaction studies showed maraviroc effects to be easily managed [94–97]. Proof of pharmacology that maraviroc was blocking CCR5 in humans was also demonstrated (estimated EC_{50} for in vivo CCR5 functional blockade in humans = 0.13 nM [68,90–93]). In phase IIa studies, treatment-naive HIV-1 patients who received maraviroc monotherapy at doses ranging from 25 mg q.d. to 300 mg b.i.d. for 10 days experienced a maximum reduction of up to 1.84 $\log_{10}$ copies/mL [38]. Phase IIb/III development program included long-term studies of maraviroc in combination with other antiretroviral drugs in both R5-treatment-naive and treatment-experienced patients infected with CCR5 tropic HIV-1, as well as patients with non-R5 HIV-1 (X4/dual tropic/nonphenotypable- HIV-1) [98]. Maraviroc [at 300 mg b.i.d. in combination with an optimized background therapeutic (OBT) regimen] received approval from the U.S. Food and Drug Administration (FDA) in August 2007, and subsequently from multiple regulatory authorities around the world, for use in combination with other antiretroviral agents in treating adults with R5-HIV-1 infection [39,41,99]. The MOTIVATE trials concluded all subjects with R5- HIV-1 receiving maraviroc (300 mg b.i.d. + OBT provided significantly superior virologic control and increases in CD4 cell count compared with placebo + OBT without any safety issues) [99–103].

Clinical development studies for maraviroc in antiretroviral-naive subjects infected with CCR5-tropic HIV-1 only [109] met with approval by the FDA in 2009 following extensive studies [107,108]. Treatment-naive patients are arguably the most appropriate patient population to study, since the vast majority (80 to 90%) of patients who are antiretroviral-naive are infected with CCR5-tropic virus only, compared to 50 to 60% in ART drug-experienced patients [104–106].

RESISTANCE TO MARAVIROC IN CLINICAL TRIALS: OBSERVATIONS AND IMPLICATIONS

As outlined above, preclinical in vitro studies have shown that gaining resistance to CCR5 antagonists is relatively difficult [70]. HIV-1 does not mutate to enable entry via the CXCR4 coreceptor switch as observed in animal models, in vitro systems, or indeed, in clinically derived isolates [70,72,110]. In clinical studies, preliminary virologic analyses have identified two phenotypic pathways associated with virologic failure in the phase III studies of maraviroc. Either CXCR4-using virus was detected on maraviroc treatment or virus was selected that was able to infect cells using maraviroc-bound CCR5 [111]. CXCR4-mediated entry is not a consequence of mutation of previously CCR5-using virus but of selection of preexisting (yet undetected at baseline/patient screening) CXCR4-using virus, with return of R5 phenotype upon cessation of maraviroc therapy [112,113]. Shifts in tropism resulting from maraviroc therapy have not been associated with decreasing $CD4^{+}$ cell counts or clinical deterioration therapy [103,113,114]. Resistance to CCR5 antagonists, as opposed to selection of X4 virus, has been demonstrated in the clinic and in preclinical studies, and is achieved following mutation to enable gaining entry via antagonist-occupied receptor rather than by mutation to enable entry via an alternative coreceptor [70,72–75]. It has been reported that some envelope mutations can confer resistance to chemically related CCR5 antagonists [73,74,76]. However, class resistance is not inevitable [77], and there is a considerable weight of evidence that the resistant strains cannot utilize CCR5 that is occupied by an antagonist that has not been used as the selecting agent for generating the resistant isolate [66,75,78–81]. Maraviroc is active against isolates resistant to other drug classes, and laboratory-generated maraviroc-resistant isolates appear not to show reduced susceptibility against other drug classes [58,75].

Laboratory generation of resistant isolates to numerous advanced CCR5 antagonists has been widely reported following selection using a given CCR5 antagonist in relatively long serial passage experiments. In these studies, and consistent with studies using maraviroc, R5-HIV-1 gains the ability to bind antagonist-occupied CCR5 via various mutations in gp120 which enable recognition of the antagonist-occupied and free receptor and are therefore deemed "fit" [73,78,114,115]. The efficiency of the resistant viruses to use the different CCR5 configurations underlies how resistance is diagnosed in the PhenoSense assay (susceptibility dose–response testing uses $E_{\max}$ plateaus rather than shifts in EC_{50} values to define resistance [75]).

FUTURE DIRECTIONS

Treatment options for HIV-1 are much improved in recent years, and options for establishing highly efficacious first-line therapeutic combinations with those that are exceptionally well tolerated are being sought. This, together with ongoing studies in naive patient populations with maraviroc, may highlight its (and PF-232798) utility in first-line therapy, especially in progress toward personalized medicine.

With gene therapy at an early stage for HIV-1 therapy, and the disappointing outcome to date in HIV vaccine research, much debate on the use of anti-HIV drugs as prophylactic agents has been apparent. This follows the phenomenal success in preexposure prophylaxis to prevent vertical mother-to-child transmission, and prophylactic strategies have been widely discussed (for a review, see [116]). A significant initiative has been the establishment in 2002 of the International Partnership for Microbicides (IPM), aimed at accelerating the development and accessibility of microbicides to prevent HIV-1 transmission in women [117]. The favorable pharmacology of CCR5 antagonists strongly supports the use of these compounds by this approach, and many companies have agreed to a free license to evaluate their respective CCR5 antagonists with respect to prophylactic activity in clinical trials. Maraviroc is among those scheduled for topical evaluation. Potential for oral prophylaxis, although currently not being evaluated in a clinical setting, is also an exciting prospect, and follows encouraging PK studies highlighting high concentrations of maraviroc in the female genital tract following oral dosing [118], and some encouraging data on CCR5 antagonists [119,120] and peptide analogs of cognate ligands in small-primate studies [121]. Similar studies have been undertaken with other mechanistic classes [122]. CCR5 antagonists are also compelling for either oral or topical prophylactic therapy, due to their mechanism of early-stage entry inhibition, barriers to resistance, the lack of infectivity of CXCR4 utilizing virus, and the slow physical and functional offset of CCR5 antagonists, yielding a favorable pharmacodynamic effect.

HIV-1 infection under the management of HAART is broadly considered a chronic (indeed, lifelong) rather than an acute disease, and it is the complications of age-related problems that are providing significant new burdens on patients and health care systems. This is double-edged, as it reflects the overall success or HAART in enabling life expectancy to be near-normal, but the morbidity of liver, kidney, cardiac, and dementia-associated diseases, for example are becoming more prevalent in this population [7,123,124]. Antiretroviral therapy inhibits HIV-1 replication, allowing recovery of $CD4^+$ T-cell numbers and the restoration of immune function. However, it has been observed that some people responding to HAART experience clinical deterioration, with symptoms and signs of an inflammatory illness known as *immune reconstitution inflammatory syndrome* (IRIS [125]). This results from pathological immune responses occurring during immune reconstitution. Clinicians working in the field of HIV-1 medicine can expect to encounter persons with IRIS [126–128]. This is a relatively new area of HIV-1 medicine and one for which CCR5 antagonists generally could provide utility in treatment (i.e., reduction of IRIS) in light of the mechanism of action involving antagonism of an immune signaling receptor. This remains fairly speculative, but monitoring of inflammatory or, indeed, cited IRIS biomarkers (see [129]) for retrospective and prospective maraviroc-associated studies has merit. Non-HIV indications arguably offer a more compelling and widespread new utility for maraviroc [93]. Discovering drugs for indications other than those for which they were originally designed has a very fruitful track record and is associated with low-cost R&D success [130]. This is inherently compelling, due to maraviroc being an approved and safe medicine, but also because a host of correlations and supportive data from pharmacogenomic, ex vivo, and preclinical studies have directly highlighted, or at least implicated, the use of CCR5 antagonists for many indications [131,132]. Specifically, these include inflammation [133,134], multiple sclerosis [135–138], rheumatoid arthritis [139–141], graft rejection [142–144], IBD [145], endometriosis [146], diabetes [133,147], renal diseases [148–150], liver fibrosis [151,152], pancreatitis [145,153], respiratory disease [154–157], heart disease [158–160], psoriasis and dermatitis [161,162], stroke [163], obesity [164], Alzheimer's disease [165] atherosclerosis [166–170], cancer [145,171], and pain [134,172]. Evaluation of clinical candidates for efficacy or proof of concept is fraught with high financial risk, so data to evidence utility of maraviroc in IRIS or non-HIV indications from retrospective and prospective HIV-1 trials by appropriate endpoint and biomarker studies is compelling. Preclinical studies on animal disease using CCR5 antagonists are challenging and also pose translational risks, especially as maraviroc and other selective CCR5 antagonists to date do not bind rodent CCR5. However, human CCR5 "knock-in" mice (where the human receptor ORF supplants the endogenous murine CCR5 sequence) have been constructed and a dosing regime to ensure complete CCR5 blockade with UK-484900, due to its favorable PK in mice (relative to maraviroc) [68,93]. By examining the effect of UK-484900-induced CCR5 blockade in disease models using these mice, a useful steppingstone to clinical trials to examine the potential utility of maraviroc and PF-232798 in IRIS and non-HIV might be enabled.

Acknowledgments

The authors wish to thank all the CCR5- and HIV-associated team members at Pfizer, together with collaborators, clinical trials volunteers, and patients, for their contributions to the maraviroc and PF-232798 projects that have provided the substrate for this chapter. Particular thanks are due to Hernan Valdez for his constructive review of the chapter and his enthusiastic support for CCR5-based initiatives. We also thank Sebastien Galan, Gary O'Connor, and Olivier Dirat for their detailed review and contributions to the synthesis sections.

REFERENCES

[1] Masur, H.; Michelis, M. A.; Greene, J. B.; Onorato, I.; Stouwe, R. A.; Holzman, R. S.; Wormser, G.; Brettman, L.; Lange, M.; Murray, H. W.; Cunningham-Rundles, S. An outbreak of community-acquired *Pneumocystis carinii* pneumonia: initial manifestation of cellular immune dysfunction. *N. Engl. J. Med.* **1981**, *305*, 1431–1438.

[2] Barre-Sinoussi, F.; Chermann, J. C.; Rey, F.; Nugeyre, M. T.; Chamaret, S.; Gruest, J.; Dauguet, C.; Axler-Blin, C.; Vezinet-Brun, F.; Rouzioux, C.; et al. Isolation of a T-lymphotropic retrovirus from a patient at risk for acquired immune deficiency syndrome (AIDS). *Science* **1983**, *220*, 868–871.

[3] Gallo, R. C.; Sarin, P. S.; Gelmann, E. P.; Robert-Guroff, M.; Richardson, E.; Kalyanaraman, V. S.; Mann, D.; Sidhu, G D.; Stahl, R. E.; Zolla-Pazner, S.; et al. Isolation of human T-cell leukemia virus in acquired immune deficiency syndrome (AIDS). *Science* **1983**, *220*, 865–867.

[4] 2007 AIDS pandemic update. 2008. http://www.unaids.org/en/KnowledgeCentre/HIVData/EpiUpdate/EpiUpdArchive/2007/default.asp.

[5] Vercauteren, J.; Deforche, K.; Theys, K.; Debruyne, M.; Duque, L. M.; Peres, S.; Carvalho, A. P.; Mansinho, K.; Vandamme, A. M.; Camacho, R. The incidence of multidrug and full class resistance in HIV-1 infected patients is decreasing over time (2001–2006) in Portugal. *Retrovirology* **2008**, *5*, 12.

[6] Carr, A. Toxicity of antiretroviral therapy and implications for drug development. *Nat. Rev. Drug Discov.* **2003**, *2*, 624–634.

[7] Lunzen, J. Treatment of heavily antiretroviral-experienced HIV-infected patients. *AIDS Rev.* **2007**, *9*, 246–253.

[8] Richman, D. D.; Morton, S. C.; Wrin, T.; Hellmann, N.; Berry, S.; Shapiro, M. F.; Bozzette, S. A. The prevalence of antiretroviral drug resistance in the United States. *AIDS* **2004**, *18*, 1393–1401.

[9] Little, S. J.; Holte, S.; Routy, J. P.; Daar, E. S.; Markowitz, M.; Collier, A. C.; Koup, R. A.; Mellors, J. W.; Connick, E.; Conway, B.; et al. Antiretroviral-drug resistance among patients recently infected with HIV. *N. Engl. J. Med.* **2002**, *347*, 385–394.

[10] Shet, A.; Berry, L.; Mohri, H.; Mehandru, S.; Chung, C.; Kim, A.; Jean-Pierre, P.; Hogan, C.; Simon, V.; Boden, D.; Markowitz, M. Tracking the prevalence of transmitted antiretroviral drug-resistant HIV-1: a decade of experience. *J. Acquir. Immune Defic. Syndr.* **2006**, *41*, 439–446.

[11] Derdeyn, C. A.; Decker, J. M.; Sfakianos, J. N.; Zhang, Z.; O'Brien, W. A.; Ratner, L.; Shaw, G. M.; Hunter, E. Sensitivity of human immunodeficiency virus type 1 to fusion inhibitors targeted to the gp41 first heptad repeat involves distinct regions of gp41 and is consistently modulated by gp120 interactions with the coreceptor. *J. Virol.* **2001**, *75*, 8605–8614.

[12] Pierson, T. C.; Doms, R. W.; Pohlmann, S. Prospects of HIV-1 entry inhibitors as novel therapeutics. *Rev. Med. Virol.* **2004**, *14*, 255–270.

[13] Moore, J. P.; Doms, R. W. The entry of entry inhibitors: a fusion of science and medicine. *Proc. Natl. Acad. Sci. USA* **2003**, *100*, 10598–10602. Epub 12003 Sep 10595.

[14] Chen, R. Y.; Kilby, J. M.; Saag, M. S. Enfuvirtide. *Expert Opin. Invest. Drugs* **2002**, *11*, 1837–1843.

[15] Greenberg, M. L.; Cammack, N. Resistance to enfuvirtide, the first HIV fusion inhibitor. *J. Antimicrob. Chemother.* **2004**, *54*, 333–340.

[16] Lin, P. F.; Blair, W.; Wang, T.; Spicer, T.; Guo, Q.; Zhou, N.; Gong, Y. F.; Wang, H. G.; Rose, R.; Yamanaka, G.; et al. A small molecule HIV-1 inhibitor that targets the HIV-1 envelope and inhibits CD4 receptor binding. *Proc. Natl. Acad. Sci. USA* **2003**, *100*, 11013–11018.

[17] Hendrix, C. W.; Collier, A. C.; Lederman, M. M.; Schols, D.; Pollard, R. B.; Brown, S.; Jackson, J. B.; Coombs, R. W.; Glesby, M. J.; Flexner, C. W.; et al. Safety, pharmacokinetics, and antiviral activity of AMD3100, a selective CXCR4 receptor inhibitor, in HIV-1 infection. *J. Acquir. Immune Defic. Syndr.* **2004**, *37*, 1253–1262.

[18] Charo, I. F.; Ransohoff, R. M. The many roles of chemokines and chemokine receptors in inflammation. *N. Engl. J. Med.* **2006**, *3540*, 610–621.

[19] Wise, A.; Gearing, K.; Rees, S. Target validation of G-protein coupled receptors. *Drug Discov. Today* **2002**, *7*, 235–246.

[20] Choe, H.; Farzan, M.; Sun, Y; Sullivan, N.; Rollins, B.; Ponath, P. D.; Wu, L.; Mackay, C. R.; LaRosa, G.; Newman, W.; et al. The beta-chemokine receptors CCR3 and CCR5 facilitate infection by primary HIV-1 isolates. *Cell* **1996**, *85*, 1135–1148.

[21] Deng, H.; Liu, R.; Ellmeier, W.; Choe, S.; Unutmaz, D.; Burkhart, M.; Di Marzio, P.; Marmon, S.; Sutton, R. E.; Hill, C. M.; et al. Identification of a major co-receptor for primary isolates of HIV-1. *Nature* **1996**, *381*, 661–666.

[22] Dragic, T.; Litwin, V.; Allaway, G. P.; Martin, S. R.; Huang, Y.; Nagashima, K. A.; Cayanan, C.; Maddon, P. J.; Koup, R. A.; Moore, J. P.; Paxton, W. A. HIV-1 entry into $CD4^+$ cells is mediated by the chemokine receptor CC-CKR-5. *Nature* **1996**, *38*, 667–673.

[23] Feng, Y.; Broder, C. C.; Kennedy, P. E.; Berger, E. A. HIV-1 entry cofactor: functional CDNA cloning of a seven-transmembrane, G protein-coupled receptor. *Science* **1996**, *272*, 872–877.

[24] Dean, M.; Carrington, M.; Winkler, C.; Huttley, G. A.; Smith, M. W.; Allikmets, R.; Goedert, J. J.; Buchbinder, S. P.; Vittinghoff, E.; Gomperts, E.; et al. Genetic restriction of HIV-1 infection and progression to aids by a deletion allele of the CKR5 structural gene: hemophilia growth and development study, multicenter aids cohort study, multicenter hemophilia cohort study, San Francisco city cohort, alive study. *Science* **1996**, *273*, 1856–1862.

[25] Huang, Y.; Paxton, W. A.; Wolinsky, S. M.; Neumann, A. U.; Zhang, L.; He, T.; Kang, S.; Ceradini, D.; Jin, Z.; Yazdanbakhsh, K.; et al. The role of a mutant CCR5 allele in HIV-1 transmission and disease progression. *Nat. Med.* **1996**, *2*, 1240–1243.

[26] Liu, R.; Paxton, W. A.; Choe, S.; Ceradini, D.; Martin, S. R.; Horuk, R.; MacDonald, M. E.; Stuhlmann, H.; Koup, R. A.; Landau, N. R. Homozygous defect in HIV-1 coreceptor accounts for resistance of some multiply-exposed individuals to HIV-1 infection. *Cell* **1996**, *86*, 367–377.

[27] Samson, M.; Libert, F.; Doranz, B. J.; Rucker, J.; Liesnard, C.; Farber, C. M.; Saragosti, S.; Lapoumeroulie, C.; Cognaux, J.; Forceille, C.; et al. Resistance to HIV-1 infection in Caucasian individuals bearing mutant alleles of the CCR-5 chemokine receptor gene. *Nature* **1996**, *382*, 722–725.

[28] Ometto, L.; Bertorelle, R.; Mainardi, M.; Zanchetta, M.; Tognazzo, S.; Rampon, O.; Ruga, E.; Chieco-Bianchi, L.; De Rossi, A. Polymorphisms in the CCR5 promoter region influence disease progression in perinatally human immunodeficiency virus type 1-infected children. *J. Infect. Dis.* **2001**, *183*, 814–818.

[29] Cocchi, F.; DeVico, A. L.; Garzino-Demo, A.; Arya, S. K.; Gallo, R. C.; Lusso, P. Identification of rantes, mip-1 alpha, and mip-1 beta as the major HIV-suppressive factors produced by $CD8^+$ T cells. *Science* **1995**, *270*, 1811–1815.

[30] Cocchi, F.; DeVico, A. L.; Garzino-Demo, A.; Cara, A.; Gallo, R. C.; Lusso, P. The V3 domain of the HIV-1 gp120 envelope glycoprotein is critical for chemokine-mediated blockade of infection. *Nat. Med.* **1996**, *2*, 1244–1247.

[31] Raport, C. J.; Gosling, J.; Schweickart, V. L.; Gray, P. W.; Charo, I. F. Molecular cloning and functional characterization of a novel human CC chemokine receptor (CCR5) for rantes, mip-1beta, and mip-1alpha. *J. Biol. Chem.* **1996**, *271*, 17161–17166.

[32] Schuitemaker, H.; Kootstra, N. A.; de Goede, R. E.; de Wolf, F.; Miedema, F.; Tersmette, M. Monocytotropic human immunodeficiency virus type 1 (HIV-1) variants detectable in all stages of HIV-1 infection lack T-cell line tropism and syncytium-inducing ability in primary T-cell culture. *J. Virol.* **1991**, *65*, 356–363.

[33] Shankarappa, R.; Margolick, J. B.; Gange, S. J.; Rodrigo, A. G.; Upchurch, D.; Farzadegan, H.; Gupta, P.; Rinaldo, C. R.; Learn, G. H.; He, X.; et al. Consistent viral evolutionary changes associated with the progression of human immunodeficiency virus type 1 infection. *J. Virol.* **1999**, *73*, 10489–10502.

[34] Zhu, T.; Mo, H.; Wang, N.; Nam, D. S.; Cao, Y.; Koup, R. A.; Ho, D. D. Genotypic and phenotypic characterization of HIV-1 patients with primary infection. *Science* **1993**, *261*, 1179–1181.

[35] Karlsson, I.; Antonsson, L.; Shi, Y.; Karlsson, A.; Albert, J.; Leitner, T.; Olde, B.; Owman, C.; Fenyo, E. M. HIV biological variability unveiled: frequent isolations and chimeric receptors reveal unprecedented variation of coreceptor use. *AIDS* **2003**, *17*, 2561–2569.

[36] Koning, F. A.; Kwa, D.; Boeser-Nunnink, B.; Dekker, J.; Vingerhoed, J.; Hiemstra, H.; Schuitemaker, H. Decreasing sensitivity to rantes (regulated on activation, normally T cell-expressed and -secreted) neutralization of CC chemokine receptor 5–using, non-syncytium-inducing virus variants in the course of human immunodeficiency virus type 1 infection. *J. Infect. Dis.* **2003**, *188*, 864–872.

[37] Sullivan, W. M.; Dorr, P.; Perros, M.; Hudson, R.; Leif, J.; Luzuriaga, K.; Clapham, P. R. Lack of alternative coreceptor use by pediatric HIV-1 R5 isolates for infection of primary cord or adult peripheral blood mononuclear cells. *Arch. Virol.* **2008**, *153*, 363–366. Epub 2007 Dec 2013.

[38] Fatkenheuer, G.; Pozniak, A. L.; Johnson, M. A.; Plettenberg, A.; Staszewski, S.; Hoepelman, A. I.; Saag, M. S.; Goebel, F. D.; Rockstroh, J. K.; Dezube, B. J.; et al. Efficacy of short-term monotherapy with maraviroc, a new CCR5 antagonist, in patients infected with HIV-1. *Nat. Med.* **2005**, *11*, 1170–1172.

[39] Lalezari, J.; Goodrich, J.; DeJesus, E.; Lampiris, H.; Gulick, R.; Saag, M.; Ridgway, C.; McHale, M.; Van der Ryst, E.; Mayer, H. Efficacy and safety of maraviroc plus optimized background therapy in viremic art-experienced patients infected with CCR5-tropic HIV-1: 24-week results of a phase 2b/3 study in the US and Canada. 14th Conference on Retroviruses and Opportunistic Infections, 2007. Abstract 104bLB.

[40] Lalezari, J.; Thompson, M.; Kumar, P.; Piliero, P.; Davey, R.; Patterson, K.; Shachoy-Clark, A.; Adkison, K.; Demarest, J.; Lou, Y.; et al. Antiviral activity and safety of 873140, a novel CCR5 antagonist, during short-term monotherapy in HIV-infected adults. *AIDS* **2005**, *19*, 1443–1448.

[41] Nelson, M.; Fätkenheuer, G.; Konourina, I.; Lazzarin, A.; Clumeck, N.; Horban, A.; Tawadrous, M.; Sullivan, J.; Mayer, H.; Van der Ryst, E. Efficacy and safety of maraviroc plus optimized background therapy in viremic, art-experienced patients infected with CCR5-tropic HIV-1 in

Europe, Australia, and North America: 24-week results. 14th Conference on Retroviruses and Opportunistic Infections, 2007. Abstract 104aLB.

[42] Mueller, A.; Mahmoud, N. G.; Goedecke, M. C.; McKeating, J. A.; Strange, P. G. Pharmacological characterization of the chemokine receptor, CCR5. *Br. J. Pharmacol.* **2002**, *135*, 1033–1043.

[43] Mueller, A.; Mahmoud, N. G.; Strange, P. G. Diverse signaling by different chemokines through the chemokine receptor CCR5. *Biochem. Pharmacol.* **2006**, *72*, 739–748. Epub 2006 Jul 2017.

[44] Mueller, A.; Strange, P. G. The chemokine receptor, CCR5. *Int. J. Biochem. Cell Biol.* **2004**, *36*, 35–38.

[45] Mueller, A.; Strange, P. G. CCL3, acting via the chemokine receptor CCR5, leads to independent activation of janus kinase 2 (jak2) and gi proteins. *FEBS Lett.* **2004**, *570*, 126–132.

[46] Thelen, M. Dancing to the tune of chemokines. *Nat. Immunol.* **2001**, *2*, 129–134.

[47] Westby, M.; Van der Ryst, E. CCR5 antagonists: host-targeted antivirals for the treatment of HIV infection. *Antiviral Chem. Chemother.* **2005**, *16*, 339–354.

[48] Emmelkamp, J. M.; Rockstroh, J. K. CCR5 antagonists: comparison of efficacy, side effects, pharmacokinetics and interactions: review of the literature. *Eur. J. Med. Res.* **2007**, *12*, 409–417.

[49] Mosier, D. E.; Picchio, G. R.; Gulizia, R. J.; Sabbe, R.; Poignard, P.; Picard, L.; Offord, R. E.; Thompson, D. A.; Wilken, J. Highly potent rantes analogues either prevent CCR5-using human immunodeficiency virus type 1 infection in vivo or rapidly select for CXCR4-using variants. *J. Virol.* **1999**, *73*, 3544–3550.

[50] Gaertner, H.; Lebeau, O.; Borlat, I.; Cerini, F.; Dufour, B.; Kuenzi, G.; Melotti, A.; Fish, R. J.; Offord, R.; Springael, J. Y.; et al. Highly potent HIV inhibition: engineering a key anti-HIV structure from psc-rantes into mip-1 beta/ccl4. *Protein Eng. Des. Sel.* **2008**, *21*, 65–72.

[51] Lalezari, J.; Yadavalli, G. K.; Para, M.; Richmond, G.; DeJesus, E.; Brown, S. J.; Cai, W.; Chen, C.; Zhong, J.; Novello, L. A.; et al. Safety, pharmacokinetics, and antiviral activity of hgs004, a novel fully human igg4 monoclonal antibody against CCR5, in HIV-1-infected patients. *J. Infect. Dis.* **2008**, *197*, 721–727.

[52] Poli, G. Pro-140 (progenics). *IDrugs* **2001**, *4*, 1068–1071.

[53] Dorr, P.; Perros, M. CCR5 inhibitors in HIV therapy. *Expert Opin. Drug Discov.* **2008**, *3*, 1345–1361.

[54] Combadiere, C.; Ahuja, S. K.; Tiffany, H. L.; Murphy, P. M. Cloning and functional expression of CC CKR5, a human monocyte CC chemokine receptor selective for mip-1(alpha), mip-1(beta), and rantes. *J. Leukoc. Biol.* **1996**, *60*, 147–152.

[55] Armour, D. R.; de Groot, M. J.; Price, D. A.; Stammen, B. L.; Wood, A.; Perros, M.; Burt, C. The discovery of tropane-derived CCR5 receptor antagonists. *Chem. Biol. Drug Des.* **2006**, *67*, 305–308.

[56] Baba, M.; Nishimura, O.; Kanzaki. N.; Okamoto, M.; Sawada, H.; Iizawa, Y.; Shiraishi, M.; Aramaki, Y.; Okonogi, K.; Ogawa, Y.; et al. A small-molecule, nonpeptide CCR5 antagonist with highly potent and selective anti-HIV-1 activity. *Proc. Natl. Acad. Sci. USA* **1999**, *96*, 5698–5703.

[57] Castonguay, L. A.; Weng, Y.; Adolfsen, W.; Di Salvo, J.; Kilburn, R.; Caldwell, C. G.; Daugherty, B. L.; Finke, P. E.; Hale, J. J.; Lynch, C. L.; et al. Binding of 2-aryl-4-(piperidin-1-yl)butanamines and 1,3,4-trisubstituted pyrrolidines to human CCR5: a molecular modeling-guided mutagenesis study of the binding pocket. *Biochemistry* **2003**, *42*, 1544–1550.

[58] Dorr, P.; Westby, M.; Dobbs, S.; Griffin, P.; Irvine, B.; Macartney, M.; Mori, J.; Rickett, G.; Smith-Burchnell, C.; Napier, C.; et al. Maraviroc (UK-427,857), a potent, orally bioavailable, and selective small-molecule inhibitor of chemokine receptor CCR5 with broad-spectrum anti-human immunodeficiency virus type 1 activity. *Antimicrob. Agents Chemother.* **2005**, *49*, 4721–4732.

[59] Maeda, K.; Yoshimura, K.; Shibayama, S.; Habashita, H.; Tada, H.; Sagawa, K.; Miyakawa, T.; Aoki, M.; Fukushima, D.; Mitsuya, H. Novel low molecular weight spirodiketopiperazine derivatives potently inhibit R5 HIV-1 infection through their antagonistic effects on CCR5. *J. Biol. Chem.* **2001**, *276*, 35194–35200.

[60] Shiraishi, M.; Aramaki, Y.; Seto, M.; Imoto, H.; Nishikawa, Y.; Kanzaki, N.; Okamoto, M.; Sawada, H.; Nishimura, O.; Baba, M.; Fujino, M. Discovery of novel, potent, and selective small-molecule CCR5 antagonists as anti-HIV-1 agents: synthesis and biological evaluation of anilide derivatives with a quaternary ammonium moiety. *J. Med. Chem.* **2000**, *43*, 2049–2063.

[61] Strizki, J. M.; Xu, S.; Wagner, N. E.; Wojcik, L.; Liu, J.; Hou, Y.; Endres, M.; Palani, A.; Shapiro, S.; Clader, J. W.; et al. Sch-c (sch 351125), an orally bioavailable, small molecule antagonist of the chemokine receptor CCR5, is a potent inhibitor of HIV-1 infection in vitro and in vivo. *Proc. Natl. Acad. Sci. USA* **2001**, *98*, 12718–12723.

[62] Armour, D. R.; de Groot, M. J.; Price, D. A.; Stammen, B. L.; Wood, A.; Perros, M.; Burt, C. The discovery of tropane-derived CCR5 receptor antagonists. *Chem. Biol. Drug Discov.* **2006**, *67*, 305–308.

[63] Price, D. A.; Armour, D.; de Groot, M.; Leishman, D.; Napier, C.; Perros, M.; Stammen, B. L.; Wood, A. Overcoming herg affinity in the discovery of the CCR5 antagonist maraviroc. *Bioorg. Med. Chem. Lett.* **2006**, *16*, 4633–4637. Epub 2006 Jun 4616.

[64] Dorr, P.; Westby, M.; McFadyen, L.; Mori, J.; Davis, J.; Perruccio, F.; Jones, R.; Stupple, P.; Middleton, D.; Perros, M. PF-232798, a second generation oral CCR5 antagonist. 15th Conference on Retroviruses and Opportunistic Infections, 2008. Abstract 737.

[65] Napier, C.; Dorr, P.; Gladue, P.; Halliday, R.; Leishman, D.; Machin, I.; Mitchell, R.; Nedderman, A.; Perros, M.; Roffey, S.; et al. The preclinical pharmacokinetics and safety pharmacology of the anti-HIV CCR5 antagonist, UK-427,857. 10th Conference on Retroviruses and Opportunistic Infections, 2003. Abstract H137.

[66] Dorr, P.; Todd, K.; Irvine, B.; Robas, N.; Thomas, A.; Fidock, M.; Sultan, H.; Mills, J.; Perrucio, F.; Burt, C.; et al.

Site-directed mutagenesis studies of CCR5 reveal differences in the interactions between the receptor and various CCR5 antagonists. 45th Interscience Conference on Antimicrobial Agents and Chemotherapy, 2005. Abstract H411.

[67] Napier, C.; Sale, H.; Mosley, M.; Rickett, G.; Dorr, P.; Mansfield, R.; Holbrook, M. Molecular cloning and radioligand binding characterization of the chemokine receptor CCR5 from rhesus macaque and human. *Biochem. Pharmacol.* **2005**, *71*, 163–172.

[68] Mansfield, R.; Able, S.; Griffin, P.; Irvine, R.; James, I.; Macartney, M.; Miller, K.; Napier, C.; Navratilova, I.; Perros, M.; et al. CCR5 pharmacology methodologies and associated applications. *Methods Enzymol.* **2009**, *460*, 17–55.

[69] Whitcomb, J. M.; Huang, W.; Fransen, S.; Limoli, K.; Toma, J.; Wrin, T.; Chappey, C.; Kiss, L. D.; Paxinos, E. E.; Petropoulos, C. J. Development and characterization of a novel single-cycle recombinant-virus assay to determine human immunodeficiency virus type 1 coreceptor tropism. *Antimicrob. Agents Chemother.* **2007**, *51*, 566–575.

[70] Westby, M.; Smith-Burchnell, C.; Mori, J.; Lewis, M.; Whitcomb, J.; Petropoulos, C.; Perros, M. In vitro escape of R5 primary isolates from the CCR5 antagonist, UK-427,857, is difficult to achieve and involves continued use of the CCR5 receptor. XIII International HIV Drug Resistance Workshop, 2004. Abstract S10.

[71] Stoddart, C.; Xu, S.; Wojcik, J.; Riley, J.; Strizki, J. Evaluation of in vivo HIV-1 escape from SCH-c (SCH 351125). 13th Conference on Retroviruses and Opportunistic Infections, 2003. Abstract 614.

[72] Trkola, A.; Kuhmann, S. E.; Strizki, J. M.; Maxwell, E.; Ketas, T.; Morgan, T.; Pugach, P.; Xu, S.; Wojcik, L.; Tagat, J.; et al. HIV-1 escape from a small molecule, CCR5-specific entry inhibitor does not involve CXCR4 use. *Proc. Natl. Acad. Sci. USA* **2002**, *99*, 395–400.

[73] Marozsan, A. J.; Kuhmann, S. E.; Morgan, T.; Herrera, C.; Rivera-Troche, E.; Xu, S.; Baroudy, B. M.; Strizki, J.; Moore, J. P. Generation and properties of a human immunodeficiency virus type 1 isolate resistant to the small molecule CCR5 inhibitor, SCH-417690 (SCH-d). *Virology* **2005**, *338*, 182–199.

[74] Pugach, P.; Marozsan, A. J.; Ketas, T. J.; Landes, E. L.; Moore, J. P.; Kuhmann, S. E. HIV-1 clones resistant to a small molecule CCR5 inhibitor use the inhibitor-bound form of CCR5 for entry. *Virology* **2007**, *361*, 212–228.

[75] Westby, M.; Smith-Burchnell, C.; Mori, J.; Lewis, M.; Mosley, M.; Stockdale, M.; Dorr, P.; Ciaramella, G.; Perros, M. Reduced maximal inhibition in phenotypic susceptibility assays indicates that viral strains resistant to the CCR5 antagonist maraviroc utilize inhibitor-bound receptor for entry. *J. Virol.* **2007**, *81*, 2359–2371.

[76] Tsibris, A. M.; Sagar, M.; Gulick, R. M.; Su, Z.; Hughes, M.; Greaves, W.; Subramanian, M.; Flexner, C.; Giguel, F.; Leopold, K. E.; et al. In vivo emergence of vicriviroc resistance in a human immunodeficiency virus type 1 subtype c-infected subject. *J. Virol.* **2008**, *82*, 8210–8214.

[77] Kuhmann, S. E.; Hartley, O. Targeting chemokine receptors in HIV: a status report. *Annu. Rev. Pharmacol. Toxicol.* **2008**, *48*, 425–461.

[78] Kuhmann, S. E.; Pugach, P.; Kunstman, K. J.; Taylor, J.; Stanfield, R. L.; Snyder, A.; Strizki, J. M.; Riley, J.; Baroudy, B. M.; Wilson, I. A.; et al. Genetic and phenotypic analyses of human immunodeficiency virus type 1 escape from a small-molecule CCR5 inhibitor. *J. Virol.* **2004**, *78*, 2790–2807.

[79] Ogert, R. A.; Wojcik, L.; Buontempo, C.; Ba, L.; Buontempo, P.; Ralston, R.; Strizki, J.; Howe, J. A. Mapping resistance to the CCR5 co-receptor antagonist vicriviroc using heterologous chimeric HIV-1 envelope genes reveals key determinants in the c2-v5 domain of gp120. *Virology* **2008**, *373*, 387–399.

[80] Westby, M.; Mori, J.; Smith-Burchnell, C.; Lewis, M.; Mosley, M.; Perruccio, F.; Mansfield, R.; Dorr, P.; Perros, M. Maraviroc (UK-427,857)-resistant HIV-1 variants are sensitive to CCR5 antagonists and enfuvirtide. XIV International HIV Drug Resistance Workshop, 2005. Abstract 65.

[81] Westby, M.; Smith-Burchnell, C.; Hamilton, D.; Robas, N.; Irvine, B.; Fidock, M.; Mills, J.; Perruccio, F.; Mori, J.; Macartney, M.; et al. UK-427,857-resistant primary isolates are susceptible to structurally-related CCR5 antagonists. 12th Conference on Retroviruses and Opportunistic Infections, 2005. Abstract 96.

[82] Kondru, R.; Zhang, J.; Ji, C.; Mirzadegan, T.; Rotstein, D.; Sankuratri, S.; Dioszegi, M. Molecular interactions of CCR5 with major classes of small-molecule anti-HIV CCR5 antagonists. *Mol. Pharmacol.* **2008**, *73*, 789–800.

[83] Liu, S.; Fan, S.; Sun, Z. Structural and functional characterization of the human CCR5 receptor in complex with HIV gp120 envelope glycoprotein and CD4 receptor by molecular modeling studies. *J. Mol. Model.* **2003**, *9*, 329–336.

[84] Navenot, J. M.; Wang, Z. X.; Trent, J. O.; Murray, J. L.; Hu, Q. X.; DeLeeuw, L.; Moore, P. S.; Chang, Y.; Peiper, S. C. Molecular anatomy of CCR5 engagement by physiologic and viral chemokines and HIV-1 envelope glycoproteins: differences in primary structural requirements for rantes, mip-1 alpha, and vmip-ii binding. *J. Mol. Biol.* **2001**, *313*, 1181–1193.

[85] Zhou, N.; Luo, Z.; Hall, J. W.; Luo, J.; Han X.; Huang, Z. Molecular modeling and site-directed mutagenesis of CCR5 reveal residues critical for chemokine binding and signal transduction. *Eur. J. Immunol.* **2000**, *30*, 164–173.

[86] Blanpain, C.; Doranz, B. J.; Bondue, A.; Govaerts, C.; De Leener, A.; Vassart, G.; Doms, R. W.; Proudfoot, A.; Parmentier, M. The core domain of chemokines binds ccr5 extracellular domains while their amino terminus interacts with the transmembrane helix bundle. *J. Biol. Chem.* **2003**, *278*, 5179–5187.

[87] Abel, S.; Van der Ryst, E.; Muihead, G. J.; Rosario, A.; Edgington, A.; Weissgerber, G. Pharmacokinetics of single and multiple oral doses of UK-427,857-a novel CCR5 antagonist in healthy volunteers. 10th Conference on Retroviruses and Opportunistic Infections, 2003. Abstract 547.

[88] Walker, D.; Abel, S.; Comby, P.; Muirhead, G. J.; Nedderman, A. N.; Smith, D. A. Species differences in the disposition of the CCR5 antagonist, UKk-427,857, a new potential treatment for HIV. *Drug. Metab. Dispos.* **2005**, *33*, 587–595.

[89] Russell, D.; Bakhtyari, A.; Jazrawi, R. P.; Whitlock, L.; Ridgway, C.; McHale, M.; Abel, S. Multiple dose study to investigate the safety of UK-427,857 (100mg or 300mg) bid for 28 days in healthy males and females. 43rd Interscience Conference on Antimicrobial Agents and Chemotherapy, 2003. Abstract H-874.

[90] Dorr, P.; Rickett, G.; Perros, M. Method for identifying CCR5 receptor antagonists by measuring residency time. U.S. Patent Application 20040023845, 2004.

[91] Rosario, M. C.; Jacqmin, P.; Dorr, P.; James, I.; Jenkins, T. M.; Abel, S.; van der Ryst, E. Population pharmacokinetic/pharmacodynamic analysis of CCR5 receptor occupancy by maraviroc in healthy subjects and HIV-positive patients. *Br. J. Clin. Pharmacol.* **2008**, *65*, 86–94.

[92] Rosario, M. C.; Jacqmin, P.; Dorr, P.; van der Ryst, E.; Hitchcock, C. A pharmacokinetic–pharmacodynamic disease model to predict in vivo antiviral activity of maraviroc. *Clin. Pharmacol. Ther.* **2005**, *78*, 508–519.

[93] Dorr, P. Maraviroc outlook in HIV and non-HIV diseases. HIV-Infection and Organ Transplantation Symposium, 2008.

[94] Abel, S.; Jenkins, T. M.; Whitlock, L. A.; Ridgway, C. E.; Muirhead, G. J. Effects of cyp3a4 inducers with and without cyp3a4 inhibitors on the pharmacokinetics of maraviroc in healthy volunteers. *Br. J. Clin. Pharmacol.* **2008**, *65*, 38–46.

[95] Abel, S.; Russell, D.; Whitlock, L. A.; Ridgway, C. E.; Muirhead, G. J. Effect of maraviroc on the pharmacokinetics of midazolam, lamivudine/zidovudine, and ethinyloestradiol/levonorgestrel in healthy volunteers. *Br. J. Clin. Pharmacol.* **2008**, *65*, 19–26.

[96] Abel, S.; Russell, D.; Whitlock, L. A.; Ridgway, C. E.; Muirhead, G. J. The effects of cotrimoxazole or tenofovir co-administration on the pharmacokinetics of maraviroc in healthy volunteers. *Br. J. Clin. Pharmacol.* **2008**, *65*, 47–53.

[97] Abel, S.; Russell, D.; Whitlock, L. A.; Ridgway, C. E.; Nedderman, A. N.; Walker, D. K. Assessment of the absorption, metabolism and absolute bioavailability of maraviroc in healthy male subjects. *Br. J. Clin. Pharmacol.* **2008**, *65*, 60–67.

[98] Fätkenheuer, G.; Nelson, M.; Lazzarin, A.; Konourina, I.; Hoepelman, A. I.; Lampiris, H.; Hirschel, B.; Tebas, P.; Raffi, F.; Trottier, B.; et al. Subgroup analyses of maraviroc in previously treated R5 HIV-1 infection. *N. Engl. J. Med.* **2008**, *359*, 1442–1455.

[99] Ayoub, A.; Van der Ryst, E.; Turner, K.; McHale, M. A review of the markers of immune function during the maraviroc phase I and IIa studies. 14th Conference on Retroviruses and Opportunistic Infections, 2007. Abstract 509.

[100] Hoepelman, I.; Ayoub, A.; Heera, J. The incidence of severe liver enzyme abnormalities and hepatic adverse events in the maraviroc clinical development programme. 11th European AIDS Conference, 2007. Abstract H2/5.

[101] Fätkenheuer, G.; Konourina, I.; Nelson, M. Efficacy and safety of maraviroc (mvc) plus optimized background therapy (obt) in varaemic, antiretroviral treatment-experienced patients infected with CCR5-tropic (R5) HIV-1 in Europe, Australia and North America (Motivate 2): 48-week results. 11th European AIDS Conference, 2007. Abstract PS3/5.

[102] Lalezari, J.; Mayer, H. Efficacy and safety of maraviroc in antiretroviral treatment-experienced patients infected with CCR5-tropic HIV-1: 48-week results of Motivate 1. 47th Annual Interscience Conference on Antimicrobial Agents and Chemotherapy, 2007. Abstract H-718a.

[103] Mayer, H.; van der Ryst, E.; Saag, M.; Clotet, B.; Fätkenheuer, G.; Clumeck, M.; Turner, K.; Goodrich, J. Safety and efficacy of maraviroc (MVC), a novel CCR5 antagonist, when used in combination with optimized background therapy (OBT) for the treatment of antiretroviral-experienced subjects infected with dual/mixed-tropic HIV-1: 24-week results of a phase 2b exploratory trial. 16th International AIDS Conference, 2006. Abstract THLB0215.

[104] Lusso, P. HIV and the chemokine system: 10 years later. *EMBO J.* **2006**, *25*, 447–456.

[105] Demarest, J.; Vavro, C.; Labranche, C.; Kitrinos, K.; McDanal, C.; Sparks, S.; Chavers, S.; Castillo, S.; Elrick, D.; McCarty, L.; et al. HIV-1 co-receptor tropism in treatment naive and experienced subjects. 44th Interscience Conference on Antimicrobial Agents and Chemotherapy, 2004. Abstract H-1136.

[106] Hoffmann, C. The epidemiology of HIV coreceptor tropism. *Eur. J. Med. Res.* **2007**, *12*, 385–390.

[107] Saag, M.; Ive, P.; Heera, J.; Tawadrous, M.; DeJesus, E.; Clumeck, N.; Cooper, D.; Horban, A.; Mohapi, L.; Mingrone, H.; et al. A multicenter, randomized, double-blind, comparative trial of a novel CCR5 antagonist, maraviroc versus efavirenz, both in combination with combivir (zidovudine/lamivudine), for the treatment of antiretroviral-naive subjects infected with R5 HIV-1: week 48 results of the merit study. 4th International AIDS Symposium, 2007. AbstractWESS104.

[108] Bredeek, U. F.; Harbour, M. CCR5 antagonists in the treatment of treatment-naive patients infected with CCR5 tropic HIV-1. *Eur. J. Med. Res.* **2007**, *12*, 427–434.

[109] Trinh, L.; Han, D.; Huang, W.; Wrin, T.; Larson, J.; Kiss, L.; Coakley, E.; Petropoulos, C.; Parkin, N.; Whitcomb, J.; Reeves, J. Technical validation of an enhanced sensitivity trofile HIV co-receptor tropism assay for selecting patients for therapy with entry inhibitors targeting CCR5. XVII International HIV Drug Resistance Workshop, Sitges, Spain, 2008.

[110] Stoddart, S.; Wojcik, J.; Riley, J.; Strizki, J. Evaluation of in vivo HIV-1 escape from SCH-c (SCH 351125). 13th conference on Retroviruses and Opportunistic Infections, 2003. Abstract 614.

[111] Heera, J.; Saag, M.; Ive, P.; Whitcomb, J.; Lewis, M.; McFadyen, L.; Goodrich, J.; Mayer, H.; van der Ryst, E.; Westby, M. Virological correlates associated with treatment failure at week 48 in the phase 3 study of maraviroc in treatment-naive patients. 15th Conference on Retroviruses and Opportunistic Infections, 2008. Abstract 40LB.

[112] Lewis, M.; Simpson, P.; Fransen, S.; Westby, M. CXCR4-using virus detected in patients receiving maraviroc in the phase III studies motivate 1 and 2 originates from a pre-existing minority of cxcr4-using virus. XVI International HIV Drug Resistance Workshop, 2007. Abstract 56.

[113] van der Ryst, E.; Wood, A.; Dorr, P.; Westby, M.; Mansfield, M.; Mayer, H.; Perros, M. Challenges in the design and development of maraviroc, a novel CCR5 antagonist for the treatment of CCR5-tropic HIV-1 infection. Chemokines and Chemokine Receptors Symposium, 2008.

[114] Lewis, M.; Mori, J.; Simpson, P.; Whitcomb, J.; Li, X.; Roberston, D.; Westby, M. Changes in v3 loop sequence associated with failure of maraviroc treatment in patients enrolled in the motivate 1 and 2 trials. 15th Conference on Retroviruses and Opportunistic Infections. 2008. Abstract 871.

[115] Ogert, R.; Buontempo, O.; Wojcik, L.; Ba, L.; Buontempo, L.; Ralston, R.; Strizki, J.; Howe, J. A. Mapping of vicriviroc resistance mutations in HIV-1 gp120 generated by in vitro selection of a primary HIV-1 isolate in PM-1 cells. 16th International HIV Drug Resistance Workshop, 2007. Abstract S35.

[116] Buchbinder, S. HIV testing and prevention strategies. *Top. HIV Med.* **2008**, *16*, 9–14.

[117] International Partnership for Microbicides. http://www.ipm-microbicides.org/. **2008**.

[118] Dumond, J.; Patterson, K.; Pecha, A.; Werner, R.; Andrews, E.; Damle, B.; Tressler, R.; Worsley, J.; Boggess, K.; Kashuba, A. Maraviroc (MVC) pharmacokinetics (PK) in blood plasma (BP), genital tract (GT) fluid and tissue in healthy female volunteers. 15th Conference on Retroviruses and Opportunistic Infections, 2008. Abstract 135LB.

[119] Veazey, R. S.; Klasse, P. J.; Schader, S. M.; Hu, Q.; Ketas, T. J.; Lu, M.; Marx, P. A.; Dufour, J.; Colonno, R. J.; Shattock, R. J.; et al. Protection of macaques from vaginal SHIV challenge by vaginally delivered inhibitors of virus-cell fusion. *Nature* **2005**, *438*, 99–102.

[120] Veazey, R. S.; Springer, M. S.; Marx, P. A.; Dufour, J.; Klasse, P. J.; Moore, J. P. Protection of macaques from vaginal SHIV challenge by an orally delivered CCR5 inhibitor. *Nat. Med.* **2005**, *11*, 1293–1294.

[121] Lederman, M. M.; Veazey, R. S.; Offord, R.; Mosier, D. E.; Dufour, J.; Mefford, M.; Piatak, M.; Lifson, J. D.; Salkowitz, J. R.; Rodriguez, B.; et al. Prevention of vaginal SHIV transmission in rhesus macaques through inhibition of CCR5. *Science* **2004**, *306*, 485–487.

[122] Dumond, J. B.; Yeh, R. F.; Patterson, K. B.; Corbett, A. H.; Jung, B. H.; Rezk, N. L.; Bridges, A. S.; Stewart, P. W.; Cohen, M. S.; Kashuba, A. D. Antiretroviral drug exposure in the female genital tract: implications for oral pre- and post-exposure prophylaxis. *AIDS* **2007**, *21*, 1899–1907.

[123] Lunzen J. State of the art 2008. HIV-Infection and Organ Transplantation Symposium, 2008.

[124] Selik, R. M.; Byers, R. H.; Dworkin, M. S. Trends in diseases reported on U.S. death certificates that mentioned HIV infection, 1987–1999. *J. Acquir. Immune Defic. Syndr.* **2002**, *29*, 378–387.

[125] Lederman, M. M.; Este, J. Targeting a host element as a strategy to block HIV replication: Is it nice to fool with Mother Nature? *Curr. Opin. HIV AIDS* **2009**, *4*, 79–81.

[126] Crothers, K.; Huang, L. Pulmonary complications of immune reconstitution inflammatory syndromes in HIV-infected patients. *Respirology* **2009**, *23*, 23.

[127] Crum-Cianflone, N. F. Immune reconstitution inflammatory syndromes: What's new? *AIDS Read.* **2006**, *16*, 199–206, 213, 216–217; discussion 214–197.

[128] Elston, J. W.; Thaker, H. Immune reconstitution inflammatory syndrome. *Int. J. STD AIDS* **2009**, *20*, 221–224.

[129] Bonham, S.; Meya, D. B.; Bohjanen, P. R.; Boulware, D. R. Biomarkers of HIV immune reconstitution inflammatory syndrome. *Biomark. Med.* **2008**, *2*, 349–361.

[130] Chong, C. R.; Sullivan, D. J. New uses for old drugs. *Nature* **2007**, *448*, 645–646.

[131] Ribeiro, S.; Horuk, R. The clinical potential of chemokine receptor antagonists. *Pharmacol. Ther.* **2005**, *107*, 44–58.

[132] Wells, T. N.; Power, C. A.; Shaw, J. P.; Proudfoot, A. E. Chemokine blockers: Therapeutics in the making? *Trends Pharmacol. Sci.* **2006**, *27*, 41–47.

[133] Navratilova, Z. Polymorphisms in ccl2&ccl5 chemokines/chemokine receptors genes and their association with diseases. *Biomed. Pap. Med. Fac. Palacky Univ. Olomouc Czech Repub.* **2006**, *150*, 191–204.

[134] Schroder, C.; Pierson, R. N.; Nguyen, B. N.; Kawka, D. W.; Peterson, L. B.; Wu, G.; Zhang, T.; Springer, M. S.; Siciliano, S. J.; Iliff, S.; et al. CCR5 blockade modulates inflammation and alloimmunity in primates. *J. Immunol.* **2007**, *179*, 2289–2299.

[135] Eikelenboom, M. J.; Killestein, J.; Izeboud, T.; Kalkers, N. F.; van Lier, R. A.; Barkhof, F.; Uitdehaag, B. M.; Polman, C. H. Chemokine receptor expression on T cells is related to new lesion development in multiple sclerosis. *J. Neuroimmunol.* **2002**, *133*, 225–232.

[136] Otaegui, D.; Ruiz-Martinez, J.; Olaskoaga, J.; Emparanza, J. I.; Lopez de Munain, A. Influence of CCR5-delta32 genotype in Spanish population with multiple sclerosis. *Neurogenetics* **2007**, *8*, 201–205.

[137] Sellebjerg, F.; Madsen, H. O.; Jensen, C. V.; Jensen, J.; Garred, P. CCR5 delta32, matrix metalloproteinase-9 and disease activity in multiple sclerosis. *J. Neuroimmunol.* **2000**, *102*, 98–106.

[138] Szczucinski, A.; Losy, J. Chemokines and chemokine receptors in multiple sclerosis: potential targets for new therapies. *Acta Neurol. Scand.* **2007**, *115*, 137–146.

[139] Aggarwal, A.; Agarwal, S.; Misra, R. Chemokine and chemokine receptor analysis reveals elevated interferon-inducible protein-10 (ip)-10/cxcl10 levels and increased number of $CCR5^+$ and $CXCR3^+$ CD4 T cells in synovial fluid of patients with enthesitis-related arthritis (ERA). *Clin. Exp. Immunol.* **2007**, *148*, 515–519.

[140] Prahalad, S. Negative association between the chemokine receptor CCR5-delta32 polymorphism and rheumatoid arthritis: a meta-analysis. *Genes Immun.* **2006**, *7*, 264–268.

[141] Wheeler, J.; McHale, M.; Jackson, V.; Penny, M. Assessing theoretical risk and benefit suggested by genetic association studies of CCR5: experience in a drug development programme for maraviroc. *Antiviral Ther.* **2007**, *12*, 233–245.

[142] Bogunia-Kubik, K.; Duda, D.; Suchnicki, K.; Lange, A. CCR5 deletion mutation and its association with the risk of developing acute graft-versus-host disease after allogeneic hematopoietic stem cell transplantation. *Haematologica* **2006**, *91*, 1628–1634.

[143] Fischereder, M.; Luckow, B.; Hocher, B.; Wuthrich, R. P.; Rothenpieler, U.; Schneeberger, H.; Panzer, U.; Stahl, R. A.; Hauser, I. A.; Budde, K.; et al. CC chemokine receptor 5 and renal-transplant survival. *Lancet* **2001**, *357*, 1758–1761.

[144] Panzer, U.; Reinking, R. R.; Steinmetz, O. M.; Zahner, G.; Sudbeck, U.; Fehr, S.; Pfalzer, B.; Schneider, A.; Thaiss, F.; Mack, M.; et al. CXCR3 and CCR5 positive T-cell recruitment in acute human renal allograft rejection. *Transplantation* **2004**, *78*, 1341–1350.

[145] Maggs, J. R.; Chapman, R. W. Sclerosing cholangitis. *Curr Opin. Gastroenterol.* **2007**, *23*, 310–316.

[146] Hornung, D.; Bentzien, F.; Wallwiener, D.; Kiesel, L.; Taylor, R. N. Chemokine bioactivity of rantes in endometriotic and normal endometrial stromal cells and peritoneal fluid. *Mol. Hum. Reprod.* **2001**, *7*, 163–168.

[147] Kalev, I.; Oselin, K.; Parlist, P.; Zilmer, M.; Rajasalu, T.; Podar, T.; Mikelsaar, A. V. CC-chemokine receptor CCR5-del32 mutation as a modifying pathogenetic factor in type 1 diabetes. *J. Diabet. Complicat.* **2003**, *17*, 387–391.

[148] Panzer, U.; Schneider, A.; Steinmetz, O. M.; Wenzel, U.; Barth, P.; Reinking, R.; Becker, J. U.; Harendza, S.; Zahner, G.; Fischereder, M.; et al. The chemokine receptor 5 delta32 mutation is associated with increased renal survival in patients with IGa nephropathy. *Kidney Int.* **2005**, *67*, 75–81.

[149] Stasikowska, O.; Danilewicz, M.; Wagrowska-Danilewicz, M. The significant role of rantes and CCR5 in progressive tubulointerstitial lesions in lupus nephropathy. *Pol. J. Pathol.* **2007**, *58*, 35–40.

[150] Teramoto, K.; Negoro, N.; Kitamoto, K.; Iwai, T.; Iwao, H.; Okamura, M.; Miura, K. Microarray analysis of glomerular gene expression in murine lupus nephritis. *J. Pharmacol. Sci.* **2008**, *106*, 56–67.

[151] Hellier, S.; Frodsham, A. J.; Hennig, B. J.; Klenerman, P.; Knapp, S.; Ramaley, P.; Satsangi, J.; Wright, M.; Zhang, L.; Thomas, H. C.; et al. Association of genetic variants of the chemokine receptor CCR5 and its ligands, rantes and MCP-2, with outcome of HCV infection. *Hepatology* **2003**, *38*, 1468–1476.

[152] Schwabe, R. F.; Bataller, R.; Brenner, D. A. Human hepatic stellate cells express CCR5 and RANTES to induce proliferation and migration. *Am. J. Physiol. Gastrointest. Liver Physiol.* **2003**, *285*, G949–G958.

[153] Goecke, H.; Forssmann, U.; Uguccioni, M.; Friess, H.; Conejo-Garcia, J. R.; Zimmermann, A.; Baggiolini, M.; Buchler, M. W. Macrophages infiltrating the tissue in chronic pancreatitis express the chemokine receptor CCR5. *Surgery* **2000**, *128*, 806–814.

[154] Chvatchko, Y.; Proudfoot, A. E.; Buser, R.; Juillard, P.; Alouani, S.; Kosco-Vilbois, M.; Coyle, A. J.; Nibbs, R. J.; Graham, G.; Offord, R. E.; Wells, T. N. Inhibition of airway inflammation by amino-terminally modified rantes/CC chemokine ligand 5 analogues is not mediated through CCR3. *J. Immunol.* **2003**, *171*, 5498–5506.

[155] Kallinich, T.; Schmidt, S.; Hamelmann, E.; Fischer, A.; Qin, S.; Luttmann, W.; Virchow, J. C.; Kroczek, R. A. Chemokine-receptor expression on T cells in lung compartments of challenged asthmatic patients. *Clin. Exp. Allergy* **2005**, *35*, 26–33.

[156] Lun, S. W.; Wong, C. K.; Ko, F. W.; Ip, W. K.; Hui, D. S.; Lam, C. W. Aberrant expression of CC and CXC chemokines and their receptors in patients with asthma. *J. Clin. Immunol.* **2006**, *26*, 145–152.

[157] Srivastava, P.; Helms, P. J.; Stewart, D.; Main, M.; Russell, G. Association of CCR5delta32 with reduced risk of childhood but not adult asthma. *Thorax* **2003**, *58*, 222–226.

[158] Candore, G.; Balistreri, C. R.; Caruso, M.; Grimaldi, M. P.; Incalcaterra, E.; Listi, F.; Vasto, S.; Caruso, C. Pharmacogenomics: a tool to prevent and cure coronary heart disease. *Curr. Pharm. Des.* **2007**, *13*, 3726–3734.

[159] Damas, J. K.; Eiken, H. G.; Oie, E.; Bjerkeli, V.; Yndestad, A.; Ueland, T.; Tonnessen, T.; Geiran, O. R.; Aass, H.; Simonsen, S.; et al. Myocardial expression of CC- and CXC-chemokines and their receptors in human end-stage heart failure. *Cardiovasc. Res.* **2000**, *47*, 778–787.

[160] Kraaijeveld, A. O.; de Jager, S. C.; de Jager, W. J.; Prakken, B. J.; McColl, S. R.; Haspels, I.; Putter, H.; van Berkel, T. J.; Nagelkerken, L.; Jukema, J. W.; Biessen, E. A. CC chemokine ligand-5 (CCL5/rantes) and CC chemokine ligand-18 (ccl18/parc) are specific markers of refractory unstable angina pectoris and are transiently raised during severe ischemic symptoms. *Circulation* **2007**, *116*, 1931–1941.

[161] Kato, Y.; Pawankar, R.; Kimura, Y.; Kawana, S. Increased expression of RANTES, CCR3 and CCR5 in the lesional skin of patients with atopic eczema. *Int. Arch. Allergy Immunol.* **2006**, *139*, 245–257.

[162] Ottaviani, C.; Nasorri, F.; Bedini, C.; de Pita, O.; Girolomoni, G.; Cavani, A. CD56brightcd16(−) nk cells accumulate in psoriatic skin in response to CXCL10 and CCL5 and exacerbate skin inflammation. *Eur. J. Immunol.* **2006**, *36*, 118–128.

[163] Jiang, L.; Newman, M.; Saporta, S.; Chen, N.; Sanberg, C.; Sanberg, P. R.; Willing, A. E. Mip-1alpha and mcp-1 induce migration of human umbilical cord blood cells in models of stroke. *Curr. Neurovasc. Res.* **2008**, *5*, 118–124.

[164] Huber, J.; Kiefer, F. W.; Zeyda, M.; Ludvik, B.; Silberhumer, G. R.; Prager, G.; Zlabinger, G. J.; Stulnig, T. M. CC chemokine and CXC chemokine receptor profiles in visceral and subcutaneous adipose tissue are altered in human obesity. *J. Clin. Endocrinol. Metab.* **2008**, *93*, 3215–3221.

[165] Reale, M.; Iarlori, C.; Feliciani, C.; Gambi, D. Peripheral chemokine receptors, their ligands, cytokines and Alzheimer's disease. *J. Alzheimer's Dis.* **2008**, *14*, 147–159.

[166] Afzal, A. R.; Kiechl, S.; Daryani, Y. P.; Weerasinghe, A.; Zhang, Y.; Reindl, M.; Mayr, A.; Weger, S.; Xu, Q.; Willeit, J. Common CCR5-del32 frameshift mutation associated with serum levels of inflammatory markers and cardiovascular disease risk in the Bruneck population. *Stroke* **2008**, *39*, 1972–1978.

[167] Braunersreuther, V.; Steffens, S.; Arnaud, C.; Pelli, G.; Burger, F.; Proudfoot, A.; Mach, F. A novel rantes antagonist prevents progression of established atherosclerotic lesions in mice. *Arterioscler. Thromb. Vasc. Biol.* **2008**, *28*, 1090–1096.

[168] Braunersreuther, V.; Zernecke, A.; Arnaud, C.; Liehn, E. A.; Steffens, S.; Shagdarsuren, E.; Bidzhekov, K.; Burger, F.; Pelli, G.; Luckow, B.; et al. CCR5 but not CCR1 deficiency reduces development of diet-induced atherosclerosis in mice. *Arterioscler. Thromb. Vasc. Biol.* **2007**, *27*, 373–379.

[169] van Wanrooij, E. J.; Happe, H.; Hauer, A. D.; de Vos, P.; Imanishi, T.; Fujiwara, H.; van Berkel, T. J.; Kuiper, J. HIV entry inhibitor TAK-779 attenuates atherogenesis in low-density lipoprotein receptor-deficient mice. *Arterioscler. Thromb. Vasc. Biol.* **2005**, *25*, 2642–2647.

[170] Zernecke, A.; Shagdarsuren, E.; Weber, C. Chemokines in atherosclerosis: an update. *Arterioscler. Thromb. Vasc. Biol.* **2008**, *19*, 19.

[171] Wu, Y.; Li, Y. Y.; Matsushima, K.; Baba, T.; Mukaida, N. Ccl3–CCR5 axis regulates intratumoral accumulation of leukocytes and fibroblasts and promotes angiogenesis in murine lung metastasis process. *J. Immunol.* **2008**, *181*, 6384–6393.

[172] Bhangoo, S.; Ren, D.; Miller, R. J.; Henry, K. J.; Lineswala, J.; Hamdouchi, C.; Li, B.; Monahan, P. E.; Chan, D. M.; Ripsch, M. S.; White, F. A. Delayed functional expression of neuronal chemokine receptors following focal nerve demyelination in the rat: a mechanism for the development of chronic sensitization of peripheral nociceptors. *Mol. Pain* **2007**, *3*, 38.

10

DISCOVERY OF THE CCR5 ANTAGONIST VICRIVIROC (SCH 417690/SCH-D) FOR THE TREATMENT OF HIV-1 INFECTION

Jayaram R. Tagat, Julie M. Strizki, and Lisa M. Dunkle
Merck Research Laboratories, Kenilworth, New Jersey

INTRODUCTION

The discovery of chemokine receptor-5 (CCR5) antagonists for the treatment of HIV-1 infection exemplifies the success that can be achieved when possible chemical leads are rationally optimized to enhance their druglike properties toward the goal of modulating a valid biological target. Following the discovery of the chemokine receptors CCR5 and CXCR4 as coreceptors that are essential for HIV-1 entry into cells [1,2], it was recognized that persons homozygous for the Δ32 mutation in CCR5, which renders the gene nonfunctional, are strongly protected from infection [3]. Furthermore, this apparently occurs without immunological defects. The identification of CCR5 as a G-protein-coupled receptor (GPCR) prompted the search for new leads from GPCR-directed libraries that had been previously generated by many pharmaceutical companies [4]. Other advances in drug discovery, such as combinatorial synthesis of analogs [5,6], rapid pharmacokinetic screening [7], and early evaluation of drug safety [8], fueled the lead optimization process, resulting in clinical proof of concept [9]. In this chapter we describe one such effort that led to the discovery of the piperazine-based CCR5 antagonist vicriviroc (**1**, Sch 417690, Sch-D).

HIT-TO-LEAD STUDIES

The discovery program began with the establishment of biochemical and cell-based assays for screening and hit validation. Three assays were used to determine coreceptor binding and inhibition of viral entry and viral replication [10]. The primary assay, also used in initial high-throughput library screening, measured the ability of compounds to inhibit ^{125}I-labeled RANTES (regulated upon activation, normal T-cell expressed and secreted) binding to the CCR5 receptor on cell membranes. Selected compounds were then evaluated in a single-cycle viral entry assay in which a pseudo-type virus bearing a reporter gene for luciferase was used to infect cells expressing CD4$^+$ and CCR5. Finally, antiviral activity was assessed by measuring the ability of compounds to inhibit the growth of primary HIV-1 isolates in human peripheral blood mononuclear cells. Supplementary assays (inhibition of calcium flux, GTPγS, and chemotaxis) to confirm the mechanism of action (functional antagonism) were also performed [10].

The discovery of vicriviroc (VCV, **1**) began with high-throughput screening of a compound collection. Several chemotypes, representing various GPCR antagonist families, were found to inhibit the CCR5-RANTES binding interaction. However, only two series of compounds from the piperidino-piperazine-(**3**) and piperidino-piperidine-based (**4**) muscarinic antagonists (Scheme 1) showed activity in antiviral assays at subcytotoxic levels. Interestingly, the structure–activity relationship (SAR) trend developed in parallel showed that similar structural features were required at the two ends of templates **3** and **4**, whereas the structural requirements in the center of the templates were quite distinct. We focus here on the piperazine-based scaffold **3**, which

Antiviral Drugs: From Basic Discovery Through Clinical Trials, First Edition. Edited by Wieslaw M. Kazmierski.

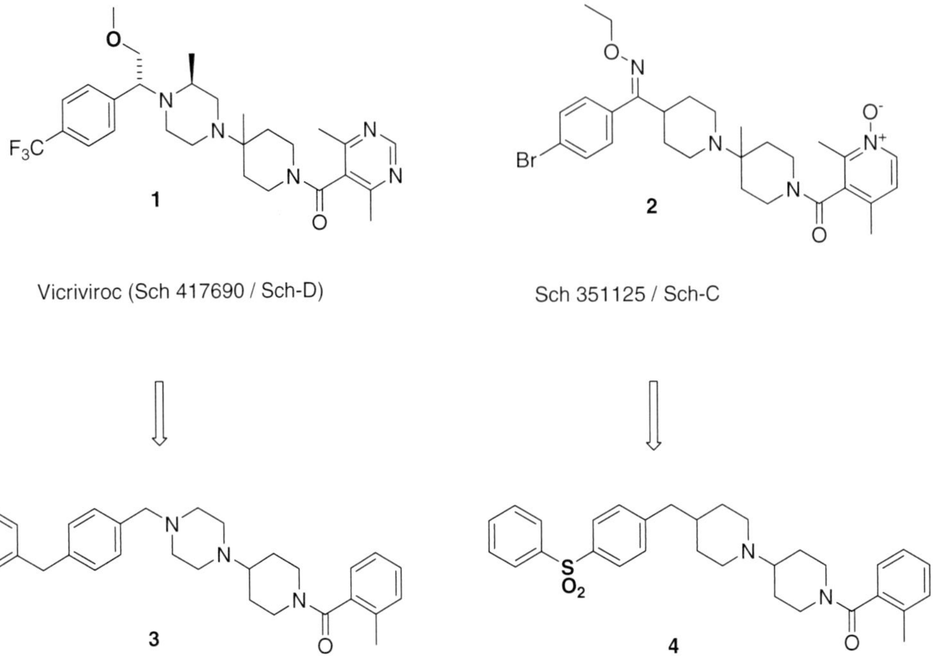

SCHEME 1 Piperazine- and piperidine-based CCR5 antagonists.

led to the discovery of vicriviroc (VCV) (**1**). The discovery of Sch 351125 (**2**, Sch-C) based on the piperidine core is described elsewhere [11].

In the piperidino-piperazine series, initial hits included compounds such as **5** and **6** (Fig. 1), which were potent antagonists of the muscarinic M2 receptor and weak binders of CCR5. The 2(*R*)-methylpiperazine moiety was essential for potent binding in the muscarinic antagonists, whereas the 2(*S*)-methylpiperazine moiety afforded improved affinity for CCR5. Similarly, changing the *ortho*-substituted benzamide group required for potent M2 binding to 2,6-disubstituted benzamide tweaked the selectivity over the M2 receptor further in favor of CCR5 [12].

The early lead compound **7** (Fig. 2), which embodies both key structural features, also showed encouraging activity in the cell-based entry assay ($IC_{50} = 2$ nM). Furthermore, compound **7** inhibited HIV growth in peripheral blood mononuclear cells (PBMCs) with an IC_{50} of 8 nM. It was also shown to be a functional antagonist of the CCR5 receptor. After defining the middle and right side of the template, attention was turned to the left side. The left-side-truncated structure (**8**) (Fig. 3) maintained binding and functional potency similar to that of **7** but showed a twofold improvement in CCR5/M2 selectivity.

LEAD OPTIMIZATION STUDIES

Further probing of minimum requirements for CCR5 affinity (Table 1) showed that the parent piperidino-piperazine (**9**) is only a weak CCR5 inhibitor (K_i = 440 nM). However, introduction of the 2(*S*)-methyl group on the piperazine ring (**11**) improved the potency 15-fold, and this was improved to 30-fold by the new lead (**8**), which also has a benzylic methyl group. Introduction of a quaternary methyl group at the ring junction between the two heterocyclic rings resulted in compound **13** with excellent potency and selectivity. The *R*/*S* diastereomer of compound **13** was eightfold less active,

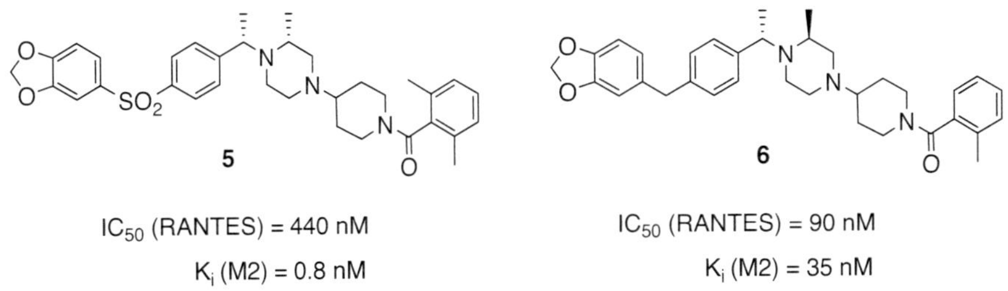

FIGURE 1 Hits from high-throughput screening.

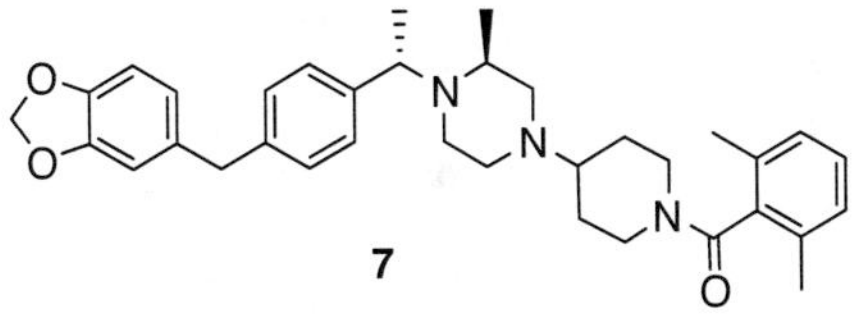

7

Binding (K_i nM)		Entry	PBMC
CCR5	M2	(IC_{50} nM)	IC_{50} (nM)
14	760	2	8

* Functional Antagonist: Ca Flux / GTP-gS assays

FIGURE 2 Pharmacophore identification.

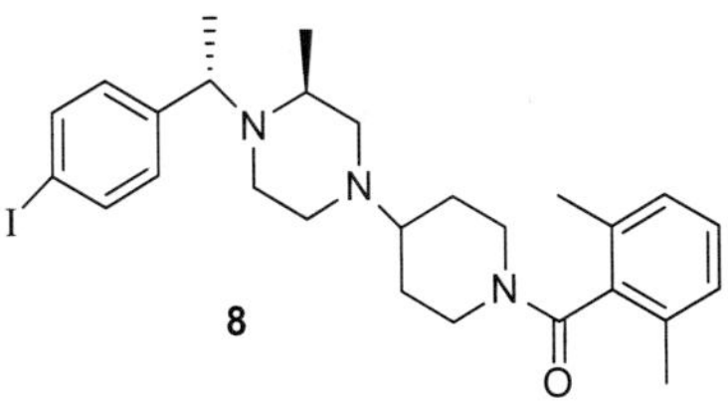

8

CCR5 Binding, K_i = 15 nM
M2 Binding, K_i = 1450 nM
HIV Entry, EC_{50} = 4 nM

FIGURE 3 Lead structure with good CCR5/M2 selectivity.

whereas the *R/R* and the *S/R* diastereomers had little affinity for CCR5 [13].

When the iodo substituent in compound **8** was moved from the *para*-position to the *ortho*- or *meta*-position, the activity was diminished, and it also served as a functional handle to introduce a variety of other substituents. Electron-withdrawing groups such as CF_3 and SO_2CH_3 at the *para*-position were introduced by starting with phenyl rings bearing these substituents. Medium-sized groups were preferred as the *para*-substituent on the left-side phenyl ring (I ~ CF_3 > Br > Cl > CN > Ph > SO_2CH_3 >> H).

The trifluoromethyl group conferred desirable pharmacokinetic properties on the CCR5 pharmacophore, and compound **14** showed a modest blood plasma level [area under the curve (AUC)] in orally dosed rats. The orally administered plasma levels measured in rats were found to improve with the additional polarity conferred by the amide moiety on the right side (Table 2). Thus, by changing the lipophilic benzamide **14** to the anthranilamide **15** or the salicylamide **16**, the AUC values were improved two- to threefold. However, the potency in the entry assay also decreased as polarity increased.

When the phenyl ring of the right-side amide moiety was changed to a pyridine ring, a significant improvement in oral exposure resulted without a concomitant decrease in functional activity (Table 3). The nicotinamide **17** had excellent potency in the CCR5 binding and the viral entry assays, low affinity for the muscarinic receptors, and a fourfold increase in the AUC (rat) over the benzamide derivative **14**. A detailed pharmacokinetic (PK) study in rats showed that the nicotinamide **17** was well absorbed and resulted initially in high plasma concentrations; however, it underwent rapid first-pass metabolism to nicotinamide *N*-oxide (**18**), which is the major circulating metabolite. Synthetically prepared nicotinamide *N*-oxide (**18**) had reduced CCR5 affinity as well as selectivity over the off-target (M2) compared to the nicotinamide **17** but showed excellent oral bioavailability in rat and monkey [13].

The muscarinic M1 receptors are prevalent in the gastrointestinal (GI) tract, while the M2 receptors are widely distributed in the brain and heart tissue. During preliminary safety evaluations, when compound **18** was administered orally to rats, side effects related to heart rate and

TABLE 1 Methylation Patterns Determine CCR5 Affinity

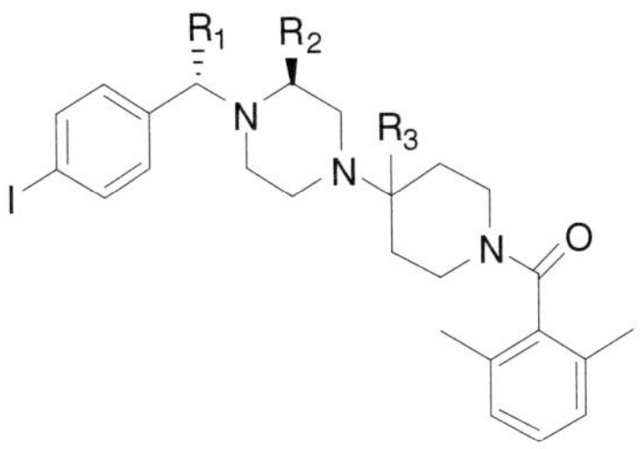

Compound	R_1	R_2	R_3	K_i(nM)	EC_{50}(nM)[a]
9	H	H	H	440	
10	H	H	CH_3	62	
11	H	CH_3	H	30	
8	CH_3	CH_3	H	15	4
12	H	CH_3	CH_3	8	2.7
13	CH_3	CH_3	CH_3	4	1

[a]Entry data are for the JrFl strain of HIV-1.

TABLE 2 Polar Amides Improve Oral Exposure in Rat

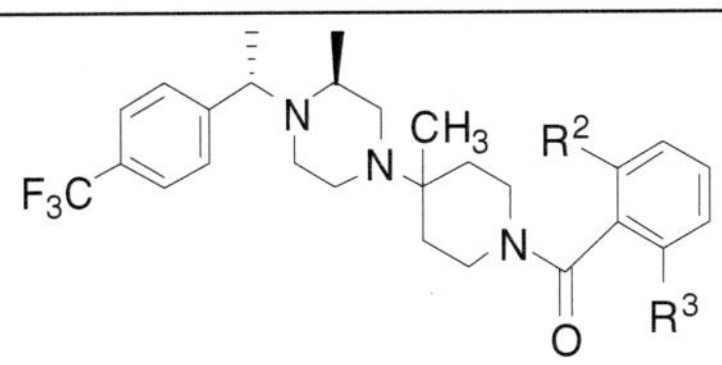

			CCR5 Data		Rapid Rat PK[a]
Compound	R^2	R^3	K_i(nM)	EC_{50} (nM)	AUC (ng·h/mL)
14	CH_3	CH_3	1	0.4	922
15	Cl	NH_2	5	1.2	1872
16	CH_3	OH	5	3.2	2540

[a]Dose = 10 mg/kg, p.o.

TABLE 3 Nicotinamide and Its N-Oxide

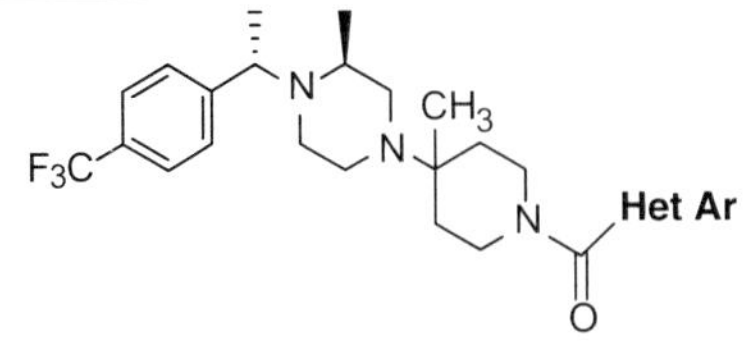

Compound	Het Ar	M2 K_i (nM)	CCR5 Data K_i (nM)	CCR5 Data EC_{50} (nM)	Rapid Rat PK[a] AUC (ng·h/mL)
17	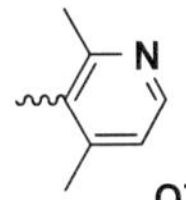	2500	2.3	0.5	3905
18	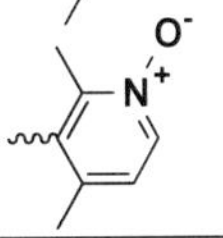	250	7.2	3.2	9243

[a]Dose = 10 mg/kg, p.o.

GI function were observed at doses of 10 mg/kg. The high plasma concentrations of **18** are apparently sufficient to afford exposure to muscarinic receptors, resulting in adverse events. As a consequence, development of compound **18** was discontinued.

The novel nicotinamide **17** and its N-oxide **18**, which has superior pharmacokinetic properties, also posed a unique structural problem. Being unsymmetrical tertiary amides, they exist as four rotational isomers observable by high-performance liquid chromatography (HPLC) (Scheme 2). Two of these rotamers are due to the slow rotation about the N—CO bond that is common in many tertiary amides and is of no consequence. However, the second set of rotamers arises due to hindered rotation about the bond connecting the carbonyl group to the heteroaryl ring and generates a pair of atropisomers. Although mechanistically interesting, this phenomenon poses challenges that need to be overcome during the development of such compounds.

EARLY CLINICAL CCR5 PROGRAM

The oximino-piperidine compound **2** (Sch 351125, Sch-C) was the first CCR5 antagonist to demonstrate clinical proof of concept for the treatment of HIV-1-infected individuals [9]. At oral doses of either 50 or 100 mg b.i.d., Sch 351125 achieved similar reductions in plasma HIV-1 RNA of 1.3 $\log_{10}$ following 10 days of monotherapy. It was safe up to doses of 200 mg b.i.d., but induced QT_c prolongation at the highest tested dose of 400 mg (b.i.d.). The observation of QT_c prolongation in the clinic is thought to be due to the binding of the compound to the human ether a-go-go related gene (hERG) potassium channel. In vitro binding studies showed that Sch 351125 had modest affinity for hERG potassium channels, and at high doses this compound apparently achieves sufficient exposure for in vivo binding. This characteristic was investigated further in the backup program.

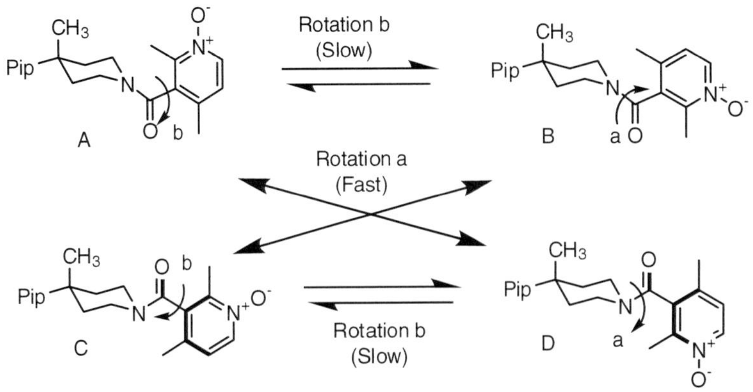

SCHEME 2 Rotational isomers (rotamers) of compounds **2** and **18**.

TABLE 4 Symmetrical Heteroaryl Amides

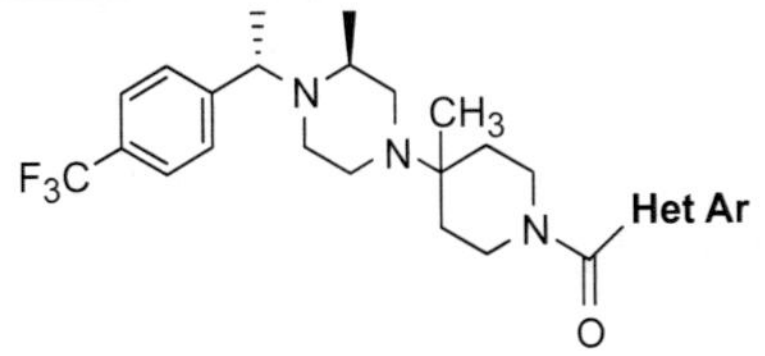

Compound	Het Ar	M2 K_i (nM)	CCR5 Data K_i (nM)	CCR5 Data EC_{50} (nM)	Rapid Rat PK[a] AUC (ng·h/mL)
19	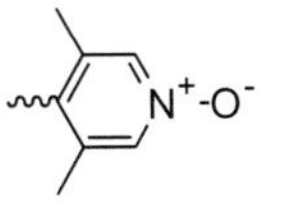	255	18	0.9	6760
20	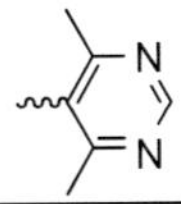	453	3	0.5	6210

[a]Dose = 10 mg/kg, p.o.

BACKUP PROGRAM

The main goals of the backup program were to reduce or eliminate the number of rotamers, minimize the QT_c prolongation issue due to hERG binding, and improve the receptor selectivity (CCR5/M2) while maintaining the functional potency and oral bioavailability associated with the first-generation compounds. For structural diversity, focus was directed to the piperidino-piperazine series. Since the high-energy rotamers (from bond rotation *b* in Scheme 2) stem from the unsymmetrical nature of the nicotinamide moiety, two types of symmetrical heteroaryl amides were developed. While the isonicotinamide **19** was a potent inhibitor of HIV entry and produced sufficient oral exposure in rat, it showed only 10- to 15-fold selectivity over the M2 receptor for CCR5. On the other hand, the pyrimidine carboxamide **20** showed 150-fold selectivity for CCR5 over M2 while maintaining high potency and good oral exposure (Table 4).

The existence of rotational isomers can be observed on chiral HPLC [14]. As shown in Figure 4, the unsymmetrical amide **18** exhibited four peaks, corresponding to the four rotamers depicted in Scheme 2. Experimentally, the high-energy pair of rotamers (from the unsymmetrical nicotinamide *N*-oxide) equilibrated to a steady-state mixture of 2 : 1 in 5 h at 37°C, 18 h at 25°C, and 4 days at 10°C. On the other hand, the symmetrical pyrimidine carboxamide **20** exhibited only two peaks in the chiral HPLC. This is due simply to the hindered rotation about the amide bond, and the rotamers equilibrate in < 2 h at 37°C. In pharmacological evaluation, despite its improved CCR5/M2 ratio, compound **20** still showed some GI side effects at the 30-mg/kg dose in rat, and it became evident that the receptor selectivity needed to be even higher.

Given the structural similarities between templates **2** and **20** and the parallel nature of their structure–activity relationship (SAR), the exceptionally higher receptor selectivity for

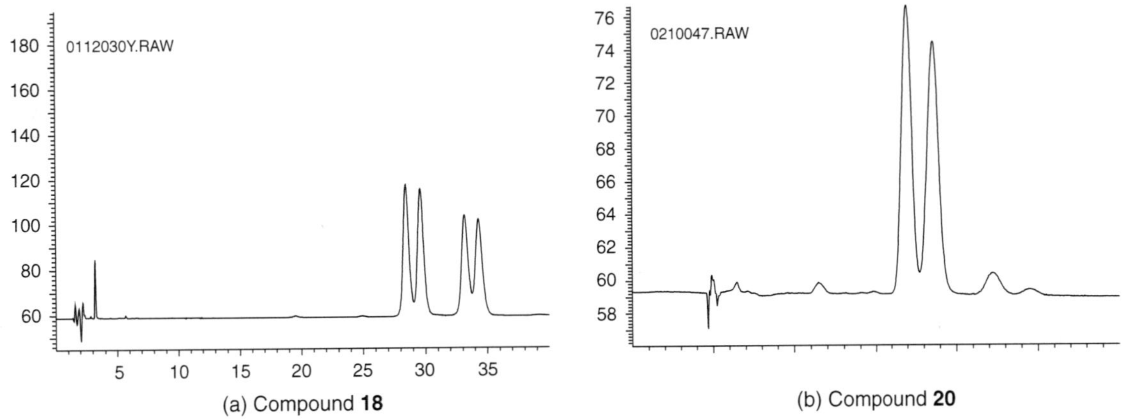

FIGURE 4 Observation of rotamers on chiral HPLC.

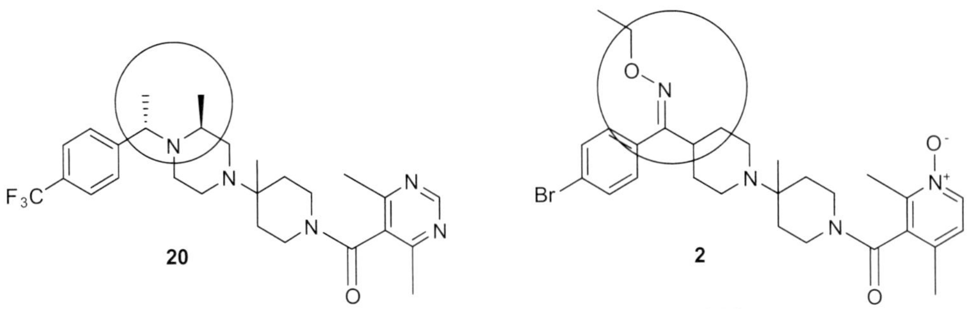

20

K_i (nM)

CCR5	M1	M2
2.8	575	456

2

K_i (nM)

CCR5	M1	M2
2	>1000	>1000

FIGURE 5 Origin of receptor selectivity.

2 pointed toward the central portion of **2** as the origin of receptor selectivity (Fig. 5). Changing the methyl group on the piperazine ring in **20** to an ethyl group resulted in diminished affinity for CCR5, so attention was centered on the benzylic site.

As the size of the benzylic methyl group was increased sequentially to ethyl, propyl, and benzyl groups, the receptor selectivity improved by leaps and bounds [15]. However, the increased lipophilicity of the molecule with the larger benzylic substituent also resulted in a decrease in the level of oral exposure observed in rat PK (Table 5). The propyl derivative **22** had the optimal combinations of excellent potency against a diverse panel of HIV isolates, CCR5/M1-M2 receptor selectivity, and good oral bioavailability in rat and cynomolgus monkey. It did not inhibit or induce cytochrome P450 (CYP) enzymes, but was > 99% protein bound. It also showed 90% inhibition of the hERG channel at 10 μM and formed an acyl glucuronide metabolite via oxidation of the propyl side chain.

To block the oxidation of the propyl side chain, it was replaced by cyclopropyl methyl (**24**), trifluoropropyl (**25**), and methoxy methyl (**1**) groups, respectively (Table 6). The cyclopropyl methyl derivative **24** had excellent potency in the HIV entry and proliferation (PBMC) assays and good oral exposure in rat. However, it showed potent inhibition of hERG (>90% at 10 μM). A similar level of hERG liability and reduced potency in the cell-based HIV entry and PBMC assays knocked trifluoropropyl analog **25** out of contention.

The methoxymethyl analog **1** (vicriviroc, VCV) had the best receptor selectivity (M2/CCR5 > 5000) and excellent oral bioavailability (%F = 100% in rat and 89% in monkey). In a geographically diverse panel of HIV isolates, compound **1** had a mean IC_{90} of 6 nM [16], which is an order of

TABLE 5 Large Benzylic Substituents Improve Receptor Selectivity

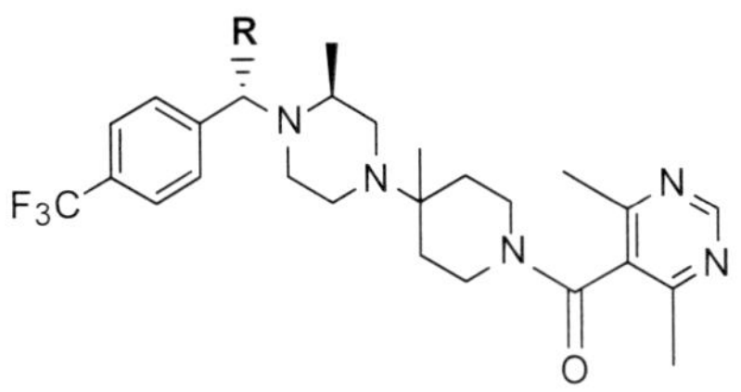

Compound	R	Binding, K_i (nM) CCR5	M1	M2	EC_{50} (nM)[a] Yu-2	Rat PK[b] $AUC_{0\text{-}6h}$
20	Methyl	2.8	575	456	0.39	6210
21	Ethyl	5.2	3900	4750	0.35	7310
22	Propyl	1.1	6075	4760	0.18	4600
23	Benzyl	1.4	>3900	>5700	0.13	2030

[a]HIV entry inhibition.
[b]AUC = ng · h/mL; dose = 10 mg/kg.

TABLE 6 Isosteric Analogs of the Benzylic Propyl Derivative

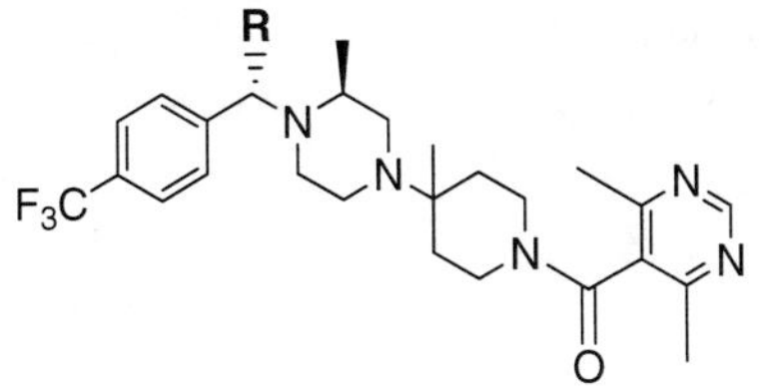

Compound	R	Binding, K_i (nM) CCR5	M1	M2	EC_{50} (nM)[a] Yu-2	IC_{90} (nM)[b] HIV-PBMC	Rat PK $AUC_{0\text{-}6h}$[c]
24	cyc-$PrCH_2$	1.6	1,894	3,512	0.2	0.1–4	5,900
25	$CF_3CH_2CH_2$	N.D.[d]	>3,700	>6,700	1.4	0.5–20	4,600
1	CH_3OCH_2	2.5	>10,000	>10,000	0.45	0.45–10	6,900
26	$CH_3CH_2OCH_2$	N.D.	>5,000	>5,000	0.2	0.2–3.0	3,100
27	$CF_3CH_2OCH_2$	N.D.	>5,000	>5,000	1.1	5–25	4,230
28	Me_2CHOCH_2	N.D.	>5,000	>5,000	0.9	2–12	2,700

[a]HIV entry inhibition.
[b]HIV isolates include JrCSF, ASM57, bal, JV1083, and RU 570.
[c]AUC = ng · h/mL; dose = 10 mg/kg, p.o.
[d]N.D., not determined.

magnitude higher than the first-generation compound **2**. In vitro binding studies showed that the dissociation constant (K_d) for VCV-CCR5 binding is 0.4 nM with a binding half-life of 12 h. In addition, VCV inhibited activation of CCR5 by its natural ligands, RANTES, MIP-1α and MIP-1β, in calcium flux, GTPγS binding, and chemotaxis assays. VCV did not induce expression of CCR5 mRNA in cells and was not cytotoxic in cell culture up to a concentration of 50 μM.

The ethoxy methyl analog **26** was slightly more potent but had only one-half the oral exposure as the methoxy methyl analog **1** in rats. The trifluoroethoxy methyl analog **27,** designed to block the cleavage of the ethyl group, did improve the oral plasma level in rats but suffered in terms of its potency. The branched isopropoxy ether analog **28** was slightly less potent than **1** but had only one-third oral exposure levels in rat. All ether analogs had excellent selectivity for CCR5, with little or no binding to the muscarinic receptors. The methoxy methyl ether (**1**), which had the best combination of potency, receptor selectivity, and oral exposure, was selected for further profiling.

Introduction of the polar ether substituent in **1** modulated the protein binding compared to an isosteric alkyl substituent (84% for **1** compared to 99% for **22**). Significantly, it had reduced affinity for the hERG channel (IC_{50} = 5.8 μM) compared to the oximino piperidine **2** (hERG IC_{50} = 1.1 μM). Accordingly, QT_c prolongation was not observed up to plasma concentrations of 3.5 μM in monkeys and 6 μM in dogs [16]. A chronic dosing study in rats showed that there was neither inhibition nor induction of liver enzymes. VCV is not a Pgp substrate and is unlikely to cause drug interactions when coadministered with Pgp inhibitors [17]. In addition, it showed good central nervous system (CNS) penetration (brain/plasma = 0.86) in animals. The major route of metabolism (rat) for VCV is through the liver, where O-demethylation of the side chain followed by glucuronidation is observed.

In antiviral assays, VCV (**1**) was active against a broad range of HIV isolates from different genetic subtypes and geographic regions. Also, since inhibition of the CCR5 receptor represents a novel mechanism of viral inhibition, VCV was active against HIV mutants that were resistant to fusion, reverse transcriptase, and protease inhibitors as well as multidrug-resistant strains, with EC_{50} values ranging from 8.7 to 32.9 nM, and less than a twofold change from the EC_{50} values for the wild-type virus [16]. However, non-R5 tropic virus strains (X4 and dual) were not inhibited by the action of VCV. In drug combination studies, VCV showed additive to synergistic effects in combination with other classes of anti-HIV agents, including a monoclonal antibody against the CCR5 receptor [16,18].

Since VCV represented a new class of HIV inhibitor with a novel mechanism of action, in vitro studies were initiated to isolate and characterize escape viruses resistant to VCV. Prolonged serial passage of virus (> 16 weeks) in the presence of increasing concentrations of VCV was required to generate resistant mutants [19,20]. In some cases, up to 52 passages in the presence of VCV were required to generate highly resistant isolates. In all but one case, VCV-resistant viruses generated in vitro remained CCR5-tropic and could not infect cells expressing only the CXCR4 receptor. Further characterization showed that these resistant viruses were cross-resistant to other small molecule CCR5 antagonists but were susceptible to other classes of anti-HIV agents. Sequence analysis and site-directed mutagenesis studies showed that multiple mutations in the viral envelope gene, particularly in the V3 loop region, were associated with VCV resistance. However, the specific pattern of amino acid mutations observed are different for each resistant viral isolate; therefore, genotypic testing for VCV resistance is currently not feasible, and phenotypic testing is required to assess VCV susceptibility.

CLINICAL STUDIES

In phase I clinical studies (36 uninfected and 47 HIV-infected subjects) of multiple doses of VCV (10, 25, or 50 mg b.i.d.), exposure to the compound increased in a dose-dependent manner for all subjects. The pharmacokinetic parameters (mean $t_{1/2} \geq 24$ h) supported q.d. dosing. VCV was well tolerated in all patients with no dose-related adverse events. In related studies it was determined that when VCV is coadministered with a potent CYP3A4 inhibitor such as ritonavir, exposure increased significantly over that achieved when VCV was administered as a single agent at the same dose. This is consistent with the observation that VCV is metabolized primarily by CYP3A4. When taken with food, the rate of absorption of VCV decreased slightly, but there was no significant change in overall exposure. Cardiac safety data from several phase I studies, including a thorough QT study, has demonstrated that VCV does not cause QT_c prolongation up to doses of 50 mg b.i.d. or as high as 150 mg q.d. in a ritonavir-containing regimen.

The antiviral activity of VCV (Fig. 6) administered as monotherapy in CCR5-tropic HIV-infected, treatment-naive

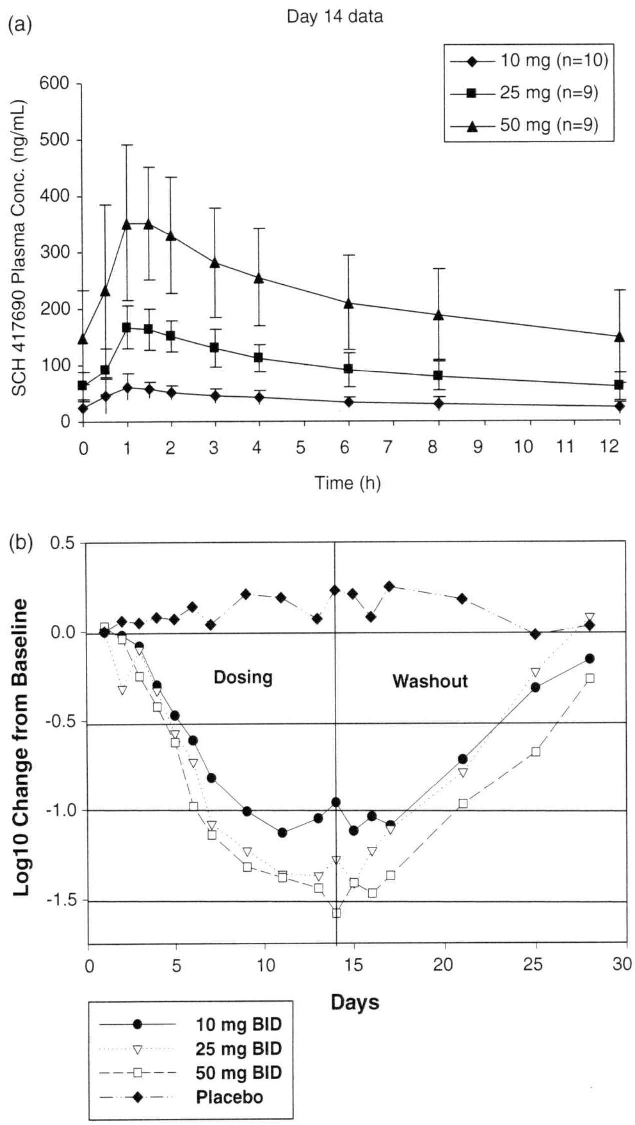

FIGURE 6 (a) Pharmacokinetics and (b) antiviral activity of vicriviroc in HIV-infected subjects.

patients with a $CD4^+$ count greater than 250 cells/mm^3 was demonstrated in a proof-of-concept study [21,22]. HIV-1 RNA levels were monitored closely during 14 days of dosing, washout, and follow-up. The primary clinical endpoint of the study was the mean change from baseline in plasma viral load ($\log_{10}$ HIV-1 RNA) on the last day (14) of treatment. Viral kinetics, onset, and rebound data were also collected. Subjects were randomized to three groups ($n = 16$ per group) and received VCV 10, 25, or 50 mg b.i.d. ($n =$ [12] per dose group) or placebo ($n =$ [4] per dose group) for 14 days. The steady-state $C_{\max}$ values were 120, 270, and 570 nM for the doses of 10, 25, and 50 mg, respectively. Trough ($C_{\min}$) concentrations remained above IC_{90} for more than 12 h. A potent antiviral effect was observed for all groups receiving VCV. The mean reduction in viral load was -1.08, -1.56, and -1.68 $\log_{10}$ copies/mL for the three VCV doses, respectively, compared with no change for placebo recipients. $CD4^+$ counts also increased by an average of 140 cells/mm^3, while no change was seen in the placebo group. The antiviral effect lasted for nearly 2 days after the dosing was stopped, a postantiviral effect that has been observed with other CCR5 antagonists, maraviroc and aplaviroc [23,24].

A subsequent phase II trial (P03802) in 92 CCR5-tropic treatment-naive persons explored once-daily (q.d.) dosing of VCV 25, 50, and 75 mg or placebo. VCV monotherapy was administered for 14 days prior to initiation of zidovudine or lamivudine in all subjects, and switching of placebo recipients to efavirenz [25]. Potent antiviral activity was observed in all three VCV dosage groups at day 14. Virologic breakthrough was observed, however, in the two lower-dose VCV groups after 16 to 24 weeks of treatment. All of the 22 breakthrough subjects had developed resistance mutations characteristic of lamivudine resistance (M184V), suggesting that the regimens had not provided adequate suppression of viral replication. Only four of these subjects demonstrated resistance to VCV. When the study was stopped, efficacy in the VCV 75-mg arm was not statistically different from that in the efavirenz control arm. Subsequent pharmacokinetic analyses suggested that the doses used in the study may have provided suboptimal exposure to VCV. As the promising VCV safety profile did not preclude study of higher exposures, future clinical trials have explored higher VCV exposures.

Two phase II clinical studies in treatment-experienced CCR5-tropic HIV patients with VCV have been completed [26]. In the first study (A5211), patients failing an antiretroviral regimen containing a ritonavir-boosted protease inhibitor were randomized to receive VCV 5, 10, or 15 mg q.d., or placebo. After 14 days, the primary endpoint of change from baseline plasma HIV-1 RNA was determined and subjects then received optimized background therapy (OBT), prescribed based on the susceptibility profile of their virus at the time of screening. At 14 days (prior to optimization of background therapy), potent antiviral activity was observed in all VCV arms. However, after all subjects had reached 16 to 24 weeks of therapy, the 5-mg q.d. VCV dose was discontinued, due to suboptimal antiviral activity. All subjects on that arm were dose-escalated to 10 or 15 mg q.d. Similarly, after 16 weeks of treatment, any subject who experienced virologic failure (largely the placebo group) was allowed to switch to active VCV at a dose of 15 mg. The 10- and 15-mg arms were continued, without the placebo control, until the end of the 48-week study. Overall, the safety profile of VCV was quite promising, with no apparent dose-related adverse events. When the trial had been ongoing for approximately 18 months, five malignancies were diagnosed over the course of approximately 6 months. However, following careful expert and regulatory review, these malignancies were judged not to be clearly related to VCV, and the study was continued to its completion.

Subjects who completed the study were allowed to roll into another trial (P04100) in which they received open-label VCV: 15 mg q.d. at first and subsequently, 30 mg q.d. Seventy-nine subjects entered the rollover study, and over half of those subjects remain on VCV after three to four years of follow-up [27].

In the second trial in treatment-experienced patients (P03672), random patients received VCV at 20 or 30 mg q.d., or placebo, in combination with an OBT regimen containing a ritonavir-boosted protease inhibitor. This trial also demonstrated a very promising safety profile for VCV and potent, sustained antiviral efficacy, which at 48 weeks suggested that the 30-mg q.d. dose provided somewhat better antiviral activity and a reduced likelihood of emergence of VCV resistance [28].

The subjects of both phase II trials were given the opportunity to continue receiving VCV 30 mg q.d. in open-label extensions of the original trials. To date, 205 subjects have been treated. Mean duration of treatment was 116 weeks (range 1 to 250 weeks); total exposure to vicriviroc was 457 patient-years. For the subjects who remain on treatment in these open-label extensions, vicriviroc has demonstrated excellent long-term tolerability; few subjects experienced AIDS-defining complications, malignancies were consistent in type and frequency with expectations in this population, and there was no clearly vicriviroc-related toxicity. These combined data represent the longest treatment experience to date with a CCR5 antagonist [29].

A large global phase III program is ongoing in treatment-experienced patients, all of whom have now been treated for at least 48 weeks. A second phase II study is also ongoing in treatment-naive subjects; it is designed to explore the role of VCV 30 mg in combination with ritonavir-boosted atazanavir as a novel class-sparing regimen for first-line use. The VCV regimen is being compared to one of the standard of care, tenofovir + emtricitabine in combination with atazanavir/ritonavir.

CONCLUSIONS

As noted, recognition of the chemokine coreceptor CCR5 as an essential component of the HIV entry process that can be deactivated without untoward immunotoxicity was the cornerstone of this case history. That it belonged to the class of GPCRs, which has given rise to many therapeutic targets, provided further impetus in support of the program. We were fortunate to take the right path forward when we came to a fork on the road toward the discovery of vicriviroc (**1**). From a handful of hits in the binding screen, assays to evaluate the inhibition of HIV entry and proliferation in PBMCs and eliminate cytotoxic compounds helped in correctly selecting the piperidino-piperazine family as the template for our hit-to-lead work. Pruning the molecule that was fully optimized for a different GPCR target (M2 receptor) generated a lead (**8**) with modest potency, selectivity for the desired target (CCR5), and low molecular weight to start our lead optimization efforts. Designing in structural complexity from this low-molecular-weight fragment, we were able to improve receptor selectivity and pharmacokinetic properties without making the final compound overly bulky. Rapid evaluation of pharmacokinetics and pharmacology profiles led to the selection of candidates for preclinical drug safety evaluation. Feedback from the clinical studies with our first-generation proof-of-concept compound (**2**) defined the criteria and direction of the backup program.

This perspective is dedicated to the entire CCR5 team at Schering-Plough for all their hard work and perseverance in the face of setbacks that led us to the development of vicriviroc.

Acknowledgments

We thank Stuart McCombie, Ashit Ganguly, John Piwinski, William Greenlee, and Bahige Baroudy for many discussions and support. Wieslaw Kazmierski is thanked for the invitation to write this chapter.

REFERENCES

[1] Strizki, J. M. Targeting HIV attachment and entry for therapy. *Adv. Pharmacol.* **2008**, *56*, 93–120.

[2] Kazmierski, W. M.; Gudmundsson, K. S.; Piscitelli, S. C. Small molecule CCR5 and CXCR4-based viral entry inhibitors for anti-HIV therapy currently in development. *Annu. Rep. Med. Chem.* **2007**, *42*, 301–320.

[3] Liu, R.; Paxton, W. A.; Choe, S.; Ceradini, D.; Martin, S. R.; Horuk, R.; MacDonald, M. E.; Stuhlmann, H.; Koup, R. A.; Landau, N. R. Homozygous defect in HIV-1 coreceptor accounts for resistance of some multiply-exposed individuals to HIV-1 infection. *Cell* **1996**, *86*, 367–377.

[4] Schlyer, S.; Horuk, R. I want a new drug: G-protein-coupled receptors in drug development. *Drug Discov. Today* **2006**, *11*, 481–493.

[5] Kennedy, J. P.; Williams, L.; Bridges, T. M.; Daniels, R. N.; Weaver, D.; Lindsley, C. W. Application of combinatorial chemistry science in modern drug discovery. *J. Comb. Chem.* **2008**, *10*, 345–354.

[6] Duffner, J. L.; Clemons, P. A; Koehler, A. N. A pipeline for ligand discovery using small-molecule microarrays. *Curr. Opin. Chem. Biol.* **2007**, *11*, 74–82.

[7] Cox, K. A.; Dunn-Meynell, K.; Korfmacher, W. A.; Broske, L.; Nomeir, A. A.; Lin, C. C.; Cayen, M. N.; Barr, W. H. *Drug Discov. Today* **1999**, *4* (5), 232.

[8] Roberts, R.; Cain, K.; Coyle, B.; Freathy, C.; Leonard, J. F.; Gautier, J. C. Early drug safety evaluation: biomarkers, signatures, and fingerprints. *Drug. Metab. Rev.* **2003**, *35*, 269–275.

[9] Baroudy, B. M. A small molecule antagonist of CCR5 that effectively inhibits HIV-1. Potential as a novel anti-retroviral agent. 7th Conference on Retrovirus and Opportunistic Infections, San Francisco, 2000. Abstract S17.

[10] Palani, A.; Shapiro, S.; Clader, J. W.; Greenlee, W. J.; Cox, K.; Strizki, J.; Endres, M.; Baroudy, B. M. Discovery of 4-[(*Z*)-(4-bromophenyl)(ethoxyimino)methyl]-1′-[(2, 4-dimethyl-3-pyridinyl)carbonyl]-4′-methyl-1,4′-bipiperidine *N*-oxide (1): an orally bioavailable human CCR5 antagonist for the treatment of HIV infection. *J. Med. Chem.* **2001**, *44*, 3339–3342.

[11] Strizki, J. M.; Xu, S.; Wagner, N. E.; Wojcik, L.; Liu, J.; Hou, Y.; Endres, M.; Palani, A.; Shapiro, S.; Clader, J. W.; et al. SCH-C (SCH 351125), an orally bioavailable, small molecule antagonist of the chemokine receptor CCR5, is a potent inhibitor of HIV-1 infection in vitro and in vivo. *Proc. Natl. Acad. Sci.* USA **2001**, *98* (22), 12718–12723.

[12] Tagat, J. R.; McCombie, S. W.; Steensma, R. W.; Lin, S.-I.; Nazareno, D. V.; Baroudy, B.; Vantuno, N.; Xu, S.; Liu, J. Piperazine-based CCR5 antagonists as HIV-1 inhibitors I: 2(*S*)-methyl piperazine as a key pharmacophore element. *Bioorg. Med. Chem. Lett.* **2001**, *11*, 2143–2146.

[13] Tagat, J. R.; Steensma, R. W.; McCombie, S. W.; Nazareno, D. V.; Lin, S.; Neustadt, B. R.; Cox, K.; Xu, S.; Wojcik, L.; Murray, M. G.; et al. Piperazine-based CCR5 antagonists as HIV-1 inhibitors: II. The discovery of 1-[(2, 4-dimethyl-3-pyridinyl)carbonyl]-4-methyl-4-3(*S*)-methyl-4-1(*S*)-4-trifluoro mehtyl)phenyl] ethyl]-1-piperazinyl] piperidine N^1-oxide (Sch 350634), an orally bioavailable, potent CCR5 antagonist. *J. Med. Chem.* **2001**, *44*, 3343–3346.

[14] McCombie, S. W.; Tagat, J. R.; Vice, S.; Lin, S.-I.; Steensma, R.; Palani, A.; Neustadt, B.; Baroudy, B.; Strizki, J.; et al. Piperazine-based CCR5 antagonists as HIV-1 inhibitors: III. Synthesis, anti-viral and pharmacokinetic profiles of symmetrical, heteroaryl carboxamides. *Bioorg. Med. Chem. Lett.* **2003**, *13*, 567–571.

[15] Tagat, J. R.; McCombie, S. W.; Nazareno, D.; Labroli, M. A.; Xiao, Y.; Steensma, R. W.; Strizki, J. M.; Baroudy, B.

M.; Cox, K.; Lachowicz, J.; et al. Piperazine-based CCR5 antagonists as HIV-1 inhibitors: IV. Discovery of 1-[(4, 6-dimethyl-5-pyrimidinyl)carbonyl]-4-4-{2-methoxy-1(*R*)-4-(trifluoromethyl)-phenyl}ethyl-3(*S*)-methyl-1-piperazinyl]-4-methyl piperidine (Sch-417690/Sch-D), a potent, highly selective and orally bioavailable CCR5 antagonist. *J. Med. Chem.* **2004**, *47*, 2405–2408.

[16] Strizki, J. M.; Tremblay, C.; Xu, S.; Wojcki, L.; Wagner, N.; Gonsiorek, W.; Hipkin, W.; Chou, C-C.; Pugliesie-Sivo, C.; Xiao, Y.; et al. Discovery and Characterization of vicriviroc (Sch-417690), a CCR5 antagonist with potent activity against human immunodeficiency virus type-1. *Antimicrob. Agents Chemother.* **2005**, *49*, 4911–4919.

[17] Revill, P.; Bayes, M.; Bozzo, J.; Serradell, N.; Rosa, E.; Bolos, J. Vicriviroc. Anti-HIV agent, viral entry inhibitor, chemokine CCR5 antagonist. *Drugs Future* **2007**, *32*, 417–427.

[18] Murga, J. D.; Franti, M.; Pevear, D. C.; Maddon, P. J.; Olson, W. C. Potent antiviral synergy between monoclonal antibody and small-molecule CCR5 inhibitors of human immunodeficiency virus type 1. *Antimicrob. Agents Chemother.* **2006**, *50*, 3289–3296.

[19] Maroszan, A. J; Kuhmann, S. E.; Morgan, T.; Herrera, C.; Rivera-Troche, E.; Xu, S.; Baroudy, B. M; Strizki, J.; Moore, J. P. Generation and properties of human immuno-deficiency virus type I isolate resistant to the small molecule CCR5 inhibitor, Sch-417690 (Sch-D). *Virology* **2005**, *338*, 182–199.

[20] Ogert, R. A; Wojcik. L.; Buontempo, C.; Ba, L.; Buontempo, P.; Ralston, R.; Strizki, J.; Howe, J. A. Mapping resistance to the CCR5 co-receptor antagonist vicriviroc using heterologous chimeric HIV-1 envelope genes reveals key determinants in the C2-V5 domain of gp120. *Virology* **2008**, *373* (2), 387–399.

[21] Schuermann, D.; Rouzier, R.; Nougarede, R.; Reynes, J.; Fätkenheuer, G.; Raffi, F.; Michelet, C.; Tarral, A.; Hoffman, C.; Kiunke, J. Sch-D (Sch-417690): Anti-viral activity of a CCR5 receptor antagonist. 11th Conference on Retroviruses and Opportunistic Infections, San Fransisco, Feb. 8–11, 2004. Abstract 140 LB.

[22] Schuermann, D.; Pechardscheck, C.; Rouzier, R. Sch 417690: Antiviral activity of a potent new CCR5 antagonist. 3rd IAS Conference on HIV Pathology and Treatment, Rio de Janeiro, Brazil, 2005. Abstract TuOa0205.

[23] Yeni, P.; LaMarca, A.; Berger, D.; Cimoch, P.; Lazzarin, A.; Salvato, P.; Smaill, F. M.; Teofilo, E.; Madison, S. J.; Nichols, W. G.; et al. Antiviral activity and safety of aplaviroc, a CCR5 antagonist, in combination with lopinavir/ritonavir in HIV-infected, therapy-naive patients: results of the EPIC study (CCR100136). *HIV Med.* **2009**, *10*, 116–124.

[24] Gulick, R. M.; Lalezari, J.; Goodrich, J.; Clumeck, N.; DeJesus, E.; Horban, A.; Nadler, J.; Clotet, B.; Karlsson, A.; Wohlfeiler, M.; et al. Maraviroc for previously treated patients with R5 HIV-1 infection. *N. Engl. J. Med.* **2008**, *359*, 1429–1441.

[25] Greaves, W.; Landovitz, R.; Fatkenheuer, G. Late virologic breakthrough in treatment naive patients on a regimen of Combivir® + vicriviroc. 13th Conference on Retrovirus and Opportunistic Infections (CROI), Denver, CO, 2006. Abstract 161LB.

[26] Safety and effectiveness of the oral HIV entry inhibitor vicriviroc in HIV infected patients. Available at http://www.clinicaltrials.gov/ct2/results?term=NCT00082498.

[27] Gulick, R.; Haas, D.; Collier, A. C.; et al. Two-year follow-up of treatment-experienced patients on vicriviroc (VCV). 47th Annual Interscience Conference on Antimicrobial Agents and Chemotherapy (ICAAC), Chicago, 2007. Abstract 2060.

[28] Zingman, B.; Suleiman, J.; DeJesus, E.; et al. Vicriviroc, a next generation CCR5 antagonist, exhibits potent, sustained suppression of viral replication in treatment-experienced adults: VICTOR-E1 48-week results. 15th Conference on Retroviruses and Opportunistic Infections (CROI), Boston, 2008. Abstract 39LB.

[29] Dunkle, L. M.; Greaves, W. L.; McCarthy, M. C.; et al. The long-term safety of vicriviroc. 12th European AIDS Conference, Cologne, Germany, Nov. 11–14, 2009.

11

DISCOVERY AND DEVELOPMENT OF HIV-1 ENTRY INHIBITORS THAT TARGET gp120

John F. Kadow, John Bender, Alicia Regueiro-Ren, Yasutsugu Ueda, Tao Wang, Kap-Sun Yeung, and Nicholas A. Meanwell

Bristol-Myers Squibb Company Research and Development, Wallingford, Connecticut

INTRODUCTION

The identification and characterization of human immunodeficiency virus-1 (HIV-1) as the cause of acquired immunodeficiency syndrome (AIDS) in 1983 triggered a vigorous effort to identify antiviral drugs capable of interrupting replication of a virus that in the absence of therapy represents a death sentence [1–4]. The initial focus sought to capitalize on knowledge of the antiviral properties of nucleoside analogs, with zidovudine (AZT) the first of eight nucleoside reverse transcriptase inhibitors (NRTIs) eventually approved to treat the disease [5]. The first nonnucleoside reverse transcriptase inhibitors (NNRTIs) were described in 1989 [6] and a screening campaign later surfaced TIBO derivatives [7]. These discoveries ultimately spawned four marketed drugs [5] in an arena that continues to be studied with some vigor [8]. The advent of HIV protease inhibitors, heralded by the approval of saquinavir in 1995, and the development of the effective combinations of drugs known as highly active antiretroviral therapy (HAART) have transformed HIV into a more manageable, chronic disease [9,10]. The development of HIV inhibitors culminated with the introduction in 2006 of a fixed-dose combination of tenofovir, emtricitabine, and efavirenz (two NRTIs and one NNRTI) into a convenient once-daily single oral pill marketed as Atripla [11,12].

However, despite the fact that the more recently approved HIV inhibitors are generally better tolerated than the early drugs, leading to improved compliance, 22 of the 25 approved drugs target just two enzymes: the protease and reverse transcriptase (RT) [5]. HIV exhibits poor fidelity of replication, a function of the poor proofreading capability of HIV-RT, leading to the emergence of resistant viruses, a property of the virus that necessitates combination therapy for effective control. It was against this backdrop that we implemented a screening campaign using a virus replication screen to identify new classes of HIV inhibitors that acted against novel drug targets without bias for a particular mechanism [13]. This was viewed as a potential avenue toward addressing the resistance emerging to the most commonly prescribed marketed therapeutics [14]. This initiative produced a number of compounds that interfered with HIV-1 replication in cell culture without overt cytotoxicity. Most of these were characterized as NNRTIs, a drug class that is structurally diverse and for which over 30 distinct chemotypes have now been reported [15]. However, one compound, the simple indole glyoxamide (1) (Fig. 1), a member of a purely prospective library of amide derivatives, emerged as a molecule with a unique mechanistic profile [16,17]. This compound demonstrated excellent specificity for inhibition of both M- and T-tropic HIV-1 (Table 1), assessed by testing against a panel of viruses that included HIV-2, simian immunodeficiency virus, herpes simplex virus, human cytomegalovirus, respiratory syncytial virus, murine leukemia virus, and influenza [17]. Time-of-addition experiments indicated that **1** inhibited an early event in HIV infection that was subsequently determined to be interference with the binding of HIV-1 gp120 to the host-cell receptor CD4 [17].

Antiviral Drugs: From Basic Discovery Through Clinical Trials, First Edition. Edited by Wieslaw M. Kazmierski.

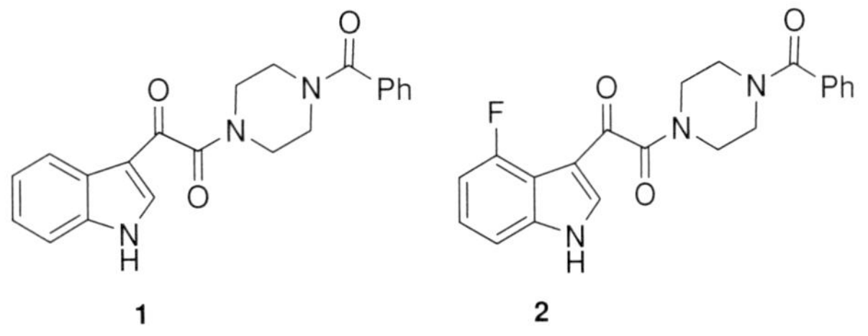

FIGURE 1 Initial indole inhibitors.

INITIAL STRUCTURE–ACTIVITY RELATIONSHIPS

A broad-based approach was adopted to more fully understand the scope of the pharmacophore defined in its most basic form by **1**, with the initial survey focused on an examination of indole and piperazine substitution patterns and structural variation of the phenyl ring of the benzamide moiety. The latter enterprise assessed the effect of substitution of the phenyl ring and its replacement by a range of heterocycles. The structure–activity relationships surrounding the benzamide element were found to be quite sensitive to both structural variation and substitution, with the result that none of the changes examined led to significantly more potent HIV inhibitors [18]. Similarly, an initial survey of known acyclic and cyclic piperazine isosteres failed to identify suitable substitutes, although introduction of a simple methyl substituent was found to offer a potency benefit, although not in a completely predictable fashion [19]. However, the introduction of a fluorine atom at C4 of the indole nucleus enhanced potency in the primary pseudotype assay by almost 60-fold, inspiring a deeper analysis [17,20]. A systematic survey revealed that substitution at C4 with halogens and either methoxy or ethoxy improved potency over the prototype **1**, but larger or more polar moieties were less well tolerated [20]. Substitution at C5 or C6 of the indole ring was generally associated with diminished antiviral activity, either when introduced individually or in combination with substituents at other positions. At C7, alkoxy substituents led to enhanced potency with larger alkyl moieties optimal. Gratifyingly, the combination of C4 and C7 substituents produced a series of compounds with excellent potency and

TABLE 1 Antiviral Activity of Indole Attachment Inhibitors

	Virus (Tropism)			
	SF-2 (T)		JRFL (M)	
Indole Compound	EC_{50} (nM)	CC_{50} (μM)	EC_{50} (nM)	CC_{50} (μM)
1	1,030 ± 29	145 ± 23	153.0 ± 119.0	>200
2	62.4 ± 33.7	146 ± 74	2.39 ± 0.85	52.5 ± 1.2

identified an optimal pattern of substitution that subtended the remainder of the program.

The 4-fluoro derivative **2** was used as a prototype with which to benchmark pharmacokinetic properties and identify potential problems with the chemotype. The oral bioavailability of **2** in dogs and monkeys administered at a dose of 10 mg/kg as a solution in poly(ethylene glycol)-400 (PEG-400) was complete, $F = \sim 100\%$. However, the oral bioavailability of **2** was poor in rats, $F = 9.4\%$ at a dose of 5 mg/kg, where the high clearance observed (48 mL/min/kg) was anticipated based on the low metabolic stability of the compound in rat liver microsomal assays. The maximal plasma concentrations of **2** achieved in all three species exceeded the antiviral EC_{50}, and dose escalation studies in rats and dogs revealed dose-related but not dose-proportional increases in exposure. However, when **2** was administered to rats as a suspension in water containing 0.75% (w/w) Methocel 4AM and 0.5% (w/w) Pluronic F68, drug exposure was not meaningful. A nanoparticulate form of the drug was developed that when administered as a suspension to rats and dogs resulted in only a marginal improvement, with bioavailability of 4 and 36%, respectively [17]. The problems of dissolution-limited exposure were related to the poor physical properties of **2**, which showed a low aqueous solubility of 5 μg/mL, almost 1000-fold lower than the solubility in PEG-400, measured as 4.6 mg/mL [17].

These problems prompted a search for compounds that combined similar or better antiviral activity with improved pharmaceutical properties. A comparative survey was conducted with indole **3** and the four corresponding azaindoles **4** to **7** to assess the potential of the latter to provide inhibitors with better overall profiles than those of the indole series [21]. The indole derivative **3** (Table 2) was a potent, noncytotoxic inhibitor of HIV-1 in cell culture using a pseudovirus (LAI strain) assay and displayed high permeability in a Caco-2 assay (Pc 169 nm/s at pH 6.5). However, this compound exhibited a relatively short half-life when incubated in human-liver microsomes (HLMs, $t_{1/2} = 16.9$ min) and low solubility of 16 μg/mL at pH 6.5 in an aqueous buffer solution. Poor stability in HLM was considered indicative of an increased potential for metabolic instability in humans. Attempts to improve the low solubility and poor stability in HLM of indoles such as **2** and **3** without adversely affecting other properties, particularly membrane permeability, proved challenging.

The profiles of the four possible azaindole derivatives, **4** to **7**, were considerably different than that of indole **3**, as can be seen by the data in Table 2, and encouraged further exploration. Compared to indole **3**, the anti-HIV-1 potency of the 4- and 7-azaindole derivatives, **4** and **7** ($EC_{50} = 1.6$ and 1.65 nM, respectively), was similar but reduced for the 6-azaindole analog, **6** ($EC_{50} = 22$ nM), and markedly more so for the 5-azaindole (5) ($EC_{50} = 576$ nM). However, it was anticipated that the positive effects on potency of the

TABLE 2 Comparison of Indole and Azaindoles

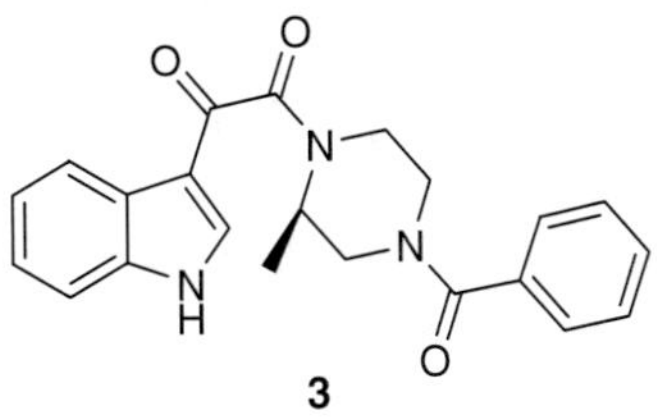

3

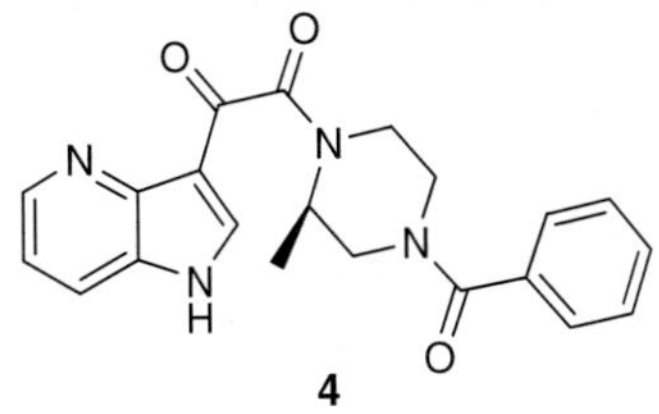

4

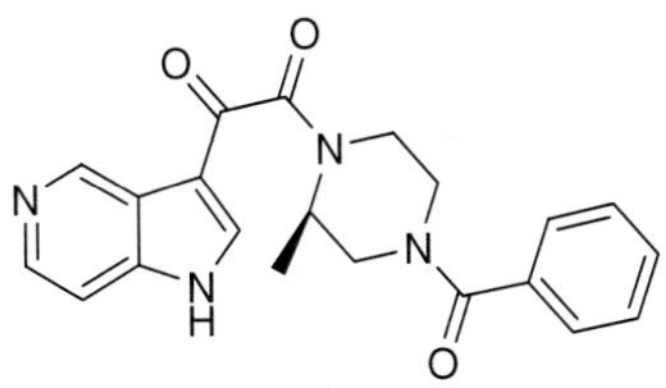

5

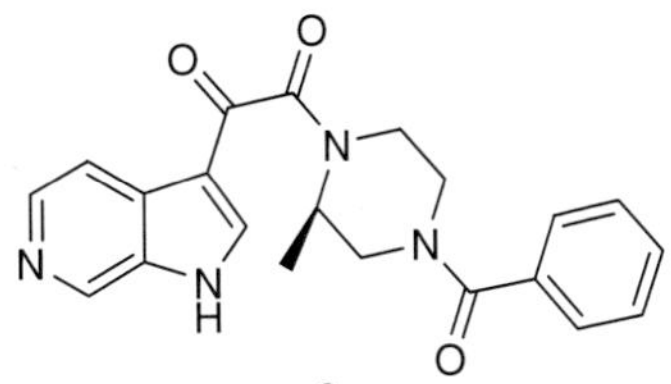

6

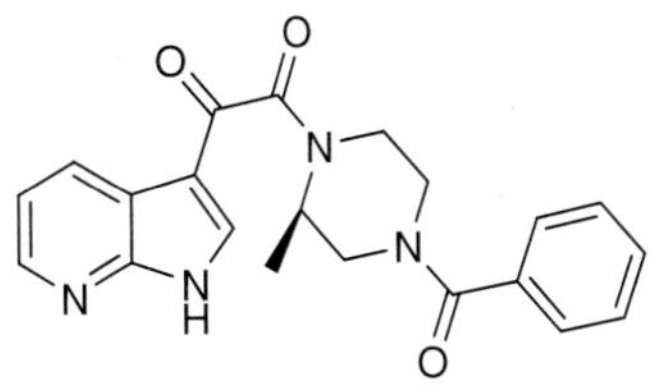

7

	3	4	5	6	7
EC_{50} (nM) (LAI)	4.85 ± 4.06 (n =2)	1.56 ± 0.16 (n = 2)	575.90 ± 87.26	21.55 ± 16.98 (n = 2)	1.65 ± 1.60 (n = 2)
CC_{50} (μM)	195.00 ± 59.47 (n = 2)	>300 (n = 2)	>300 (n = 2)	>300 (n = 2)	280.20 ± 21.92 (n = 11)
HLM, $t_{1/2}$ (min)	16.9	>100	>100	38.5	49.5
Caco-2 Pc at pH 6.5 (nm/s)	169	76	19	<15	168
Crystalline solubility at 25°C and pH 6.5 (mg/mL)	0.016	0.932	0.419	0.487	0.936
pK_a[a]	10.0	9.0, 5.8	6.2, 9.8	6.0, 9.3	2.0, 9.7
Log D at pH 6.5	1.9	0.9	1.2	1.5	1.8

[a] Spectrophotometric analysis.

substitution at positions 4 and 7 described previously might compensate for any differences. The azaindoles uniformly displayed enhanced solubility by more than 25-fold (419 to 936 μg/mL) over that of indole derivative **3**. The azaindoles also displayed enhanced metabolic stability, as measured by half-life in HLM (38.5 to >100 min).

The membrane permeabilities based on Caco-2 studies appeared to correlate approximately with the degree of ionization at pH 6.5, but, again, substitution at the 4- and 7-positions was expected to modulate this property favorably. At the time of these studies, the only core heterocycle readily available commercially was 7-azaindole. The availability of this intermediate helped accelerate efforts in this series while new and reliable syntheses of 4- and 6-azaindoles based on the Bartoli indole synthesis were developed to facilitate SAR work on a laboratory scale [22].

DISCOVERY OF BMS-378806

The incorporation of a methoxy group at the 4-position of 7-azaindole-based HIV-1 attachment inhibitors provided enhanced potency. The (R)-methyl group installed on the piperazine ring does not exert a marked effect on potency in this heterocycle background but contributed to the overall profile of the molecule, which was designated BMS-378806 (Scheme 1, Fig. 2) [17]. This compound proved to be an entry inhibitor that exhibited a virology profile similar to **2** toward HIV-1 but with markedly improved aqueous solubility (170 μg/mL) in crystalline form. The solubility of BMS-378806 improved to 1.3 mg/mL at pH 2.1 and 3.3 mg/mL at pH 11, revealing a U-shaped solubility profile consistent with the measured pK_a values of 2.9 and 9.6 (Table 3). The compound competed with soluble CD4 binding to a monomeric form of gp120 in an ELISA assay with IC_{50} = 100 nM, was not cytotoxic at concentrations > 225 μM, and did not inhibit the HIV-1 enzymes reverse transcriptase, protease, or integrase. BMS-378806 showed no relevant inhibition toward a panel of other viruses, which, along with additional biochemical studies, demonstrated that this azaindole had retained the same mechanism of action as the precursor indoles [17]. The generation of resistant viruses and sequencing identified M426L, M434I/V, and M475I of gp120 as primary resistance mutations in the HIV-1 strains NL4-3 and LAI [17,23,24]. Recombinant viruses containing these individual substitutions display a resistant phenotype [23]. The M426L and M475I mutations map to the pocket on gp120 that interacts with phenylalanine 43 of CD4, a residue that has been shown to be critical to recognition; these data provide additional support for the proposed mode of action [25].

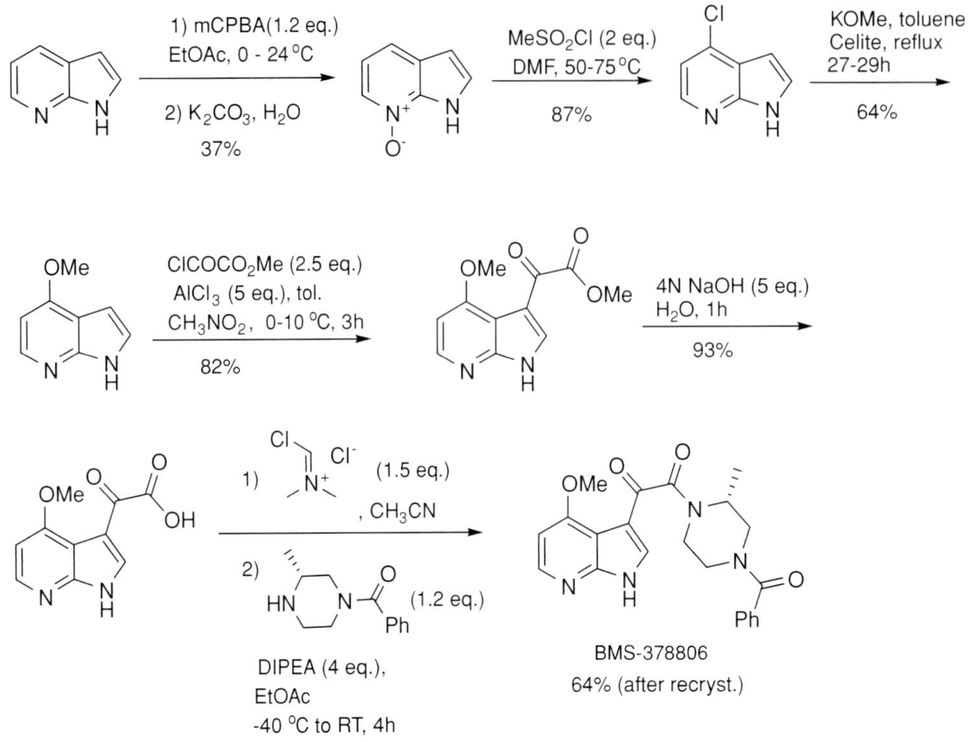

SCHEME 1 Process for the synthesis of BMS-378806.

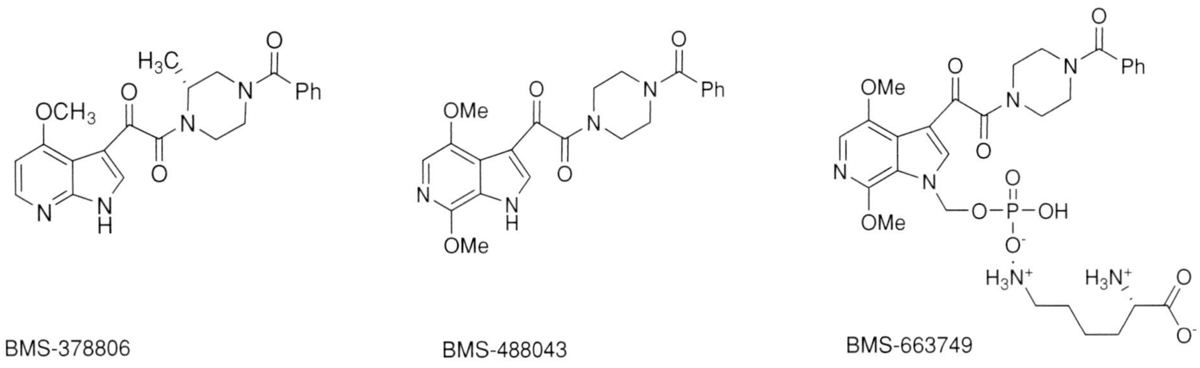

FIGURE 2 HIV attachment inhibitor clinical compounds.

TABLE 3 BMS-488043 vs. BMS-378806: Partial In Vitro Profile

Compound	EC_{50} (nM) (JRFL)	CC_{50} (μM)	HLM $t_{1/2}$ (min)	Caco-2 Pc at pH 6.5 (nm/s)	Crystalline Solubility at 25°C and pH 6.5 (mg/mL)	pK_a	log D at pH 6.5	Protein Binding (Human)
BMS-378806	1.47 ± 0.63	>300 ($n = 6$)	37	51	~0.2 1.3 at pH 2.1 3.3 at pH 11	2.9, 9.6	1.6	73%
BMS-488043	0.88 ± 0.46 ($n = 56$)	>300 ($n = 2$)	>100	178	~0.04 0.9 at pH 1.5 0.25 at pH 10	2.9, 9.3	1.5	95%

A preparative synthesis of BMS-378806 described in a published patent application was initiated with the oxidation of the nitrogen atom of commercially available 7-azaindole using mCPBA (Scheme 1) [26]. Treatment of the resulting *N*-oxide with methanesulfonyl chloride at slightly elevated temperatures yielded 4-chloro-7-azaindole. Conversion of the 4-chloro functionality of the 7-azaindole into a 4-methoxy group was accomplished with potassium methoxide in refluxing toluene. The dicarbonyl functionality was installed at the 3-position of the azaindole using a Lewis acid–mediated Friedel–Crafts acylation with methyl chlorooxoacetate and aluminum chloride as the catalyst. Interestingly, the use of nitromethane as a cosolvent resulted in a notable increase in the yield of this reaction. The resulting methyl ester was hydrolyzed to a carboxylic acid, which, in turn, was converted to an acid chloride using the Vilsmeier reagent. A final coupling of the intermediate acid chloride with (*R*)-(3-methylpiperazin-1-yl) (phenyl)methanone completed the synthesis of BMS-378806.

The plasma protein binding of BMS-378806 was found to be 73, 63, 44 and 54% in human, rat, dog, and monkey plasma, respectively, determined using an ultrafiltration method at a plasma concentration of 1 μg/mL. As predicted by the high free fraction, the presence of 40% human serum increased the EC_{50} value by a modest 1.2-fold in MT-2 cells infected with HIV-1 LAI virus.

The oral bioavailability of BMS-378806 in rats, dogs, and monkeys administered as a solution in PEG-400/EtOH (90 : 10 v/v), was 19, 77, and 24%, respectively, and the pharmacokinetic profiles of the compound in these species are summarized in Table 4. In both rats and monkeys, prolonged absorption increased the P.O. half-life considerably over that observed after intravenous (i.v.) administration, a factor that was taken into consideration for human dose projection calculations. In rats, an aqueous crystalline suspension of free base in 0.75% (w/w) Methocel A4M Premium administered orally at a dose of 25 mg/kg, identical to that used for solution dosing, afforded a relative bioavailability of 61%. Importantly, dose-proportional increases in the AUC and C_{max} were observed between doses of 5 and 25 mg/kg when BMS-378806 was administered either as a solution or suspension. In the rat, brain levels of the drug were found to be very low, but the compound did readily partition beyond plasma based on the volume of distribution, which ranged from 0.4 to 0.6 L/kg [17]. The compound showed moderate permeability in a Caco-2 assay, with a Pc value of 51 nm/s. This value was 3.5-fold lower than the Pc value of 180 nm/s obtained for basolateral to apical transport, shown to be mediated by P-glycoprotein, and these properties could play a role in the low brain levels [27].

The human clearance of BMS-378806 predicted from microsomal stability data was 9.2 mL·min/kg (46% of hepatic blood flow), which indicated intermediate clearance. The rank order of predicted hepatic clearance based on in vitro microsomal stability was monkey > rat > human > dog and a good in vitro-to-in vivo correlation was observed preclinically in all three species [27]. The preclinical studies were used to generate a predicted human oral bioavailability of 20% and human dose projections which suggested that the compound would probably need to be dosed more frequently than once a day, but all of the data suggested that the compound had the potential to be an important first in class compound [27].

Additional preclinical studies revealed that BMS-378806 was not a potent inhibitor of any of the five major human CYP450 enzyme isoforms and was metabolized by CYP450 1A2, 2D6, and 3A4, so the risk of significant drug–drug interactions in a clinical setting was anticipated to be minimal [17,27]. Safety profiling revealed no significant liabilities and supported the advancement of the molecule into clinical studies. The excellent safety, solubility, and protein-binding profiles of BMS-378806 were all positive attributes that supported its development. Unfortunately, exposure in normal healthy volunteers was low and the compound failed to realize targeted plasma concentrations, whereupon development efforts on the compound were halted [28].

FURTHER OPTIMIZATION OF THE CHEMOTYPE: THE DISCOVERY OF BMS-488043

Optimization of the 6-aza series proceeded on an independent course and resulted in the realization of an early target, the 4,7-dimethoxy-6-azaindole BMS-488043 [21]. This compound was a target based on the potency of the 4,7-dimethoxyindole analog [20]. Interestingly, the pK_a values of 2.9 and 9.3 and log D of 1.5 in octanol/water at pH 6.5 found for BMS-488043 were essentially the same as those

TABLE 4 BMS-488043 vs. BMS-378806: Preclinical In Vivo Studies

	Rat		Dog		Monkey	
Parameter	BMS-378806	BMS-488043	BMS-378806	BMS-488043	BMS-378806	BMS-488043
Oral C_{max} (μg/mL)	0.09	1.9	4.5	2.5	0.3	2.5
Oral AUC (μg.h/mL)	0.5	6.3	11	18	1.9	12
IV terminal $t_{1/2}$ (h)	0.3	2.4	1.2	2.6	0.9	4.7
Bioavailability (%)	19	90	77	57	24	60

TABLE 5 BMS-488043 vs. BMS-378806: Antiviral Activity Against HIV-1 B Clade Clinical Isolates

Envelope Subtype	No. Strains Tested	BMS-488043, EC_{50} (nM)	BMS-378806, EC_{50} (nM)
B	40	0.6 to >5000 (med. $EC_{50} = 36.5$)	1.0 to >5000 (med. $EC_{50} = 61.5$)

determined for BMS-378806 (see Table 3). Despite these similarities, BMS-488043 significantly improved on the two preclinical liabilities of BMS-378806 of most concern: HLM stability and Caco-2 permeability. The $t_{1/2}$ value in HLM was > 100 min for BMS-488043 in a system where BMS-378806 had a half-life of 37 min. The Caco-2 Pc for BMS-488043 was 178 nm/s, which compared favorably with 51 nm/s measured for BMS-378806. The lack of a piperazinyl methyl substituent in BMS-488043 contributed to the improved metabolic stability of this compound since the methyl analog was less stable, and studies in related molecules suggested that the methyl group may be a target of oxidative metabolism. To achieve these gains, BMS-488043 sacrificed both the fraction of free unbound drug (human protein binding = 95%) and the crystalline solubility (~0.04 mg/mL at pH 6.5, 0.9 mg/mL at pH 1.5, and 0.25 mg/mL at pH 10) compared to BMS-378806. However, BMS-488043 satisfied the objective of identifying a molecule with the correct balance of permeability, metabolic stability, and potency without fully compromising solubility or the fraction of free protein-unbound drug. As shown in Table 5, both azaindole compounds displayed a range of potency toward HIV-1 B clade clinical isolates, with BMS-488043 possessing a slight overall advantage. Due to the spectrum of activity observed for this class of compound, clinical exposures would need to be sufficient to cover a significant percentage of viruses rather than just the most susceptible ones with the lowest EC_{50} values. Detailed studies of the mechanism of action of BMS-488043 have been published [29–31].

As shown in Scheme 2, a preparative synthesis of BMS-488043 from the patent literature began with the selective bromination of 4-methyl-3-nitropyridin-2-amine and applied Leimgruber–Batcho indole synthesis methodology for construction of the azaindole [32]. The diazonium salt of the 2-aminopyridine intermediate was prepared in situ with *tert*-butylnitrite under acidic conditions, and then displacement with methanol installed the desired 2-methoxy group. Lithium methoxide and *N,N*-dimethylformamide dimethylacetal were employed to provide the desired enamine intermediate. The second methoxy group was installed through a copper(I)-mediated displacement of the bromide under basic conditions at elevated temperature. The 6-azaindole was formed by reduction of the 3-nitro functionality to a primary amine followed by spontaneous cyclization onto the enamine. The desired 4,7-dimethoxy-6-azaindole was isolated as an HCl salt from a solution of TMSCl in isopropanol. As in the synthesis of BMS-378806, the α-ketoester was installed at the 3-position of the azaindole using a Lewis acid–mediated Friedel–Crafts acylation. The final step in the synthesis of BMS-488043 was the direct amide formation from the anion of *N*-benzoylpiperazine and the methyl ester intermediate.

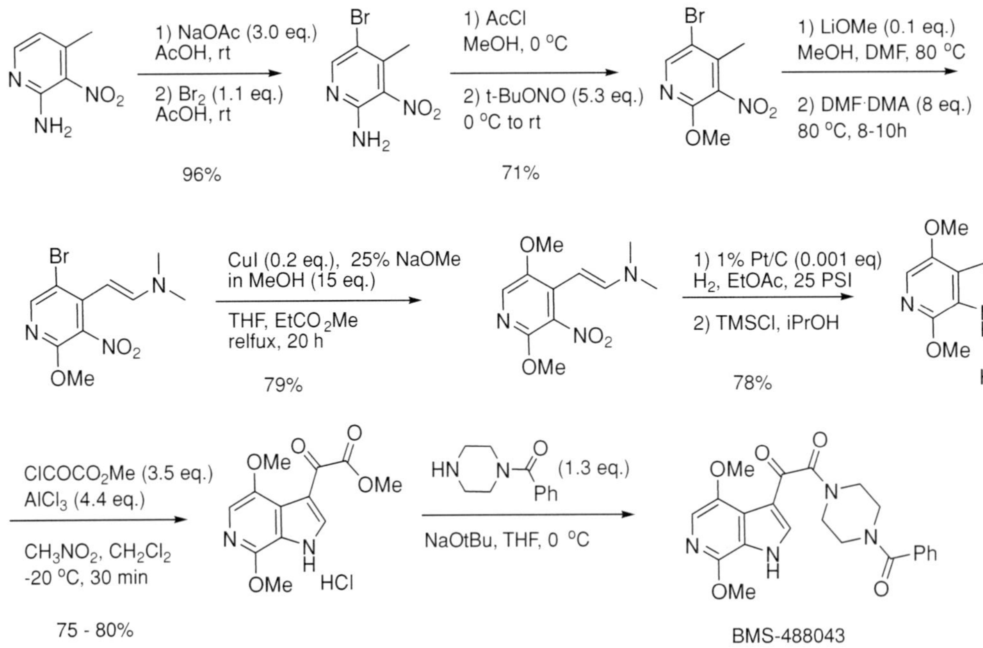

SCHEME 2 Process for the synthesis of BMS-488043.

The in vitro property advantages of BMS-488043 translated into significant improvements in the pharmacokinetic profile [33]. Particularly gratifying was the significant increase in the oral bioavailability and exposure of BMS-488043 observed in rats and monkeys, although exposure (AUC) and i.v. terminal half-lives were higher in all three species than for BMS-378806 (Table 4).

The oral bioavailability of BMS-488043 from solution (90% PEG-400/10% EtOH) was 90, 57, and 60% in rats, dogs, and monkeys, respectively, which compared with 19, 77, and 24% for BMS-378806 (Table 4) [21,33]. A crystalline suspension of BMS-488043 at 5 mg/kg (mean particle size ~7 μm) in rats provided an acceptable bioavailability of 55%. After oral dosing, plasma levels in rat, dog, and monkey measured at 12 h were at least 18-fold higher than the median antiviral EC_{50}. The compound readily distributed out of plasma, but brain levels were very low in rats. The human clearance, based on either human microsomal data or allometric scaling of animal data (where a good in vitro/in vivo correlation was seen), was predicted to be low (1.5 to 3.0 mL/min/kg). The terminal half-life after i.v. administration ranged from 2.4 to 4.7 h in the animal species, with the human half-life predicted to be 3.0 to 4.9 h from allometric scaling of animal data [33].

The pharmacokinetic and metabolic profiles of BMS-488043 predicted that the compound should have better oral exposure in humans than was observed from BMS-378806. In addition, in HLM, the compound was primarily metabolized by CYP3A4, suggesting that its exposure might potentially be enhanced by coadministration of a CYP3A4 inhibitor such as ritonavir. BMS-488043 displayed a pharmaceutical and preclinical toxicology profile that supported further development, and its profile suggested that the compound should not cause significant drug–drug interactions.

In normal healthy volunteers, under fasting conditions, C_{max} and the AUC of BMS-488043 following administration of formulated capsules at single doses of 200, 400, or 800 mg increased in a dose-related but not dose-proportional manner [28]. Exposure did not increase significantly following doses of 1200, 1800, or 2400 mg in capsules, but exposure over a 400 to 1200-mg dose range was increased three- to five-fold when administered concomitantly with a high-fat rather than a low-fat meal. A solution dose of 200 mg increased exposure three-fold over the capsule formulation under fasting conditions and pretreatment with ritonavir at a dose of 400 mg of BMS-488043 increased exposure by 43%. The oral exposure of BMS-488043 in humans was at least 15-fold higher than that of BMS-378806 under similar dosing conditions [33].

The antiviral activity, safety, and tolerability of BMS-488043 were evaluated in a multiple-dose study in HIV-infected adults [28]. Patients received doses of either 800 or 1800 mg of BMS-488043 or placebo every 12 h for 8 days concomitantly with a high-fat meal, which was specified to enhance exposure. Monotherapy was safe and well tolerated, with no serious adverse events observed during the study. Of the drug-treated patients, 67% had a viral load decline of $>0.5 \log_{10}$ copies/mL, while none of the placebo-treated subjects achieved that level of viral load decline. The majority of BMS-488043-treated patients in both groups (7 of 12 in the 800-mg group and 8 of 12 in the 1800-mg group) saw their HIV viral loads decrease by at least $1.0 \log_{10}$. The results of these clinical studies with BMS-488043 demonstrated that an orally bioavailable small-molecule HIV-1 attachment inhibitor can express potent antiviral activity in infected subjects.

BMS-663749: A PHOSPHONOXYMETHYL PRODRUG OF BMS-488043

To achieve targeted plasma exposure levels in humans, a large dose of BMS-488043 administered concomitantly with a high-fat meal was required to overcome problems arising from dissolution- or solubility-limited absorption. The necessity for a high-fat meal and the excessive pill burden required to achieve targeted exposure multiples precluded further development of the initial clinical capsule formulation. Development of a prodrug and improvements to the formulation were considered suitable approaches to enhancing the exposure of BMS-488043 in humans and to eliminating the high-fat-meal requirement. Recently, several successful approaches to improving the oral bioavailability via alternative formulation of BMS-488043 have been described [34,35].

Phosphate prodrugs, either as direct derivatives or with incorporation via linkers, have been used to successfully enhance the solubility and exposure of a range of compounds by both i.v. and oral routes [36,37]. A recent successful application of this type of prodrug approach to the antifungal agent ravuconazole from our own laboratories was a factor in the decision to explore the potential of this as a solution to the issue of dissolution- or solubility-limited absorption [38]. However, the record of success for orally administered phosphate-based prodrugs has been less impressive than for i.v. applications, and several studies have attempted to elucidate the physicochemical properties predictive of success [36,37]. In general, compounds with high permeability and low solubility (BCS class 2) for which the projected dose is not extremely low are compounds for which a phosphate prodrug approach is predicted to offer an opportunity to significantly enhance oral exposure. BMS-488043 fits this profile and was thus deemed an excellent candidate with which to examine this approach to providing an improved formulation. However, prodrug design is still an experimental science since the success of a phosphate prodrug approach is also dependent on empirical properties, including the ability of the parent compound to remain supersaturated in intestinal fluids, the propensity for crystallization in vivo, and the stability

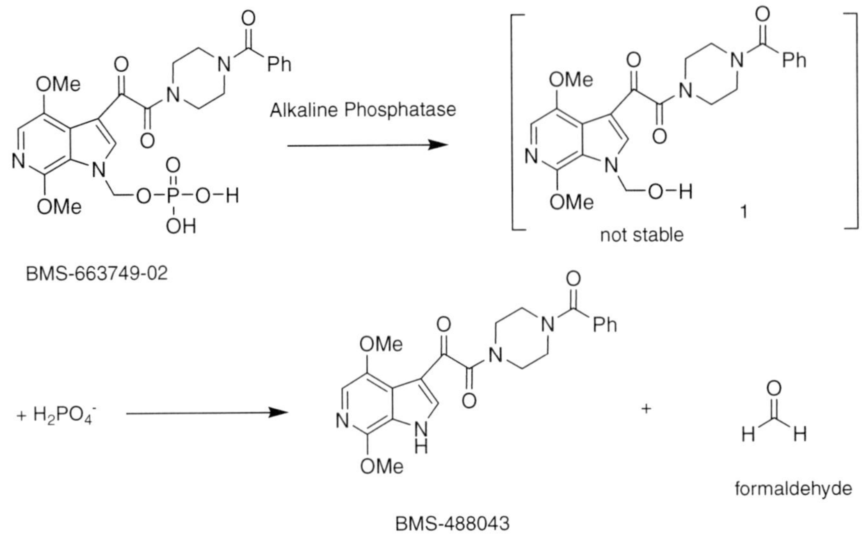

SCHEME 3 Generation of BMS-488043 from BMS-663749.

of both the phosphate prodrug and linker intermediates. The azaindole nitrogen of BMS-488043 provides a convenient functionality to introduce prodrug moieties, but the direct attachment of a phosphate group to the azaindole nitrogen was not promising. Therefore, a methylene phosphate prodrug moiety was attached to the indole nitrogen since this moiety offered considerable potential to provide a functional phosphate prodrug.

BMS-663749 is the methylene phosphate prodrug of BMS-488043 and could be isolated as either the free acid or in salt form [39,40]. The hydroxymethyl indole intermediate arising from enzyme-mediated dephosphorylation of BMS-663749 in vivo was expected to collapse spontaneously to BMS-488043, simultaneously liberating one molecule of formaldehyde per molecule of BMS-488043 (Scheme 3). Literature precedent suggests that hydroxymethylindole derivatives are unstable when the pK_a of the indole N—H is less than 11 [41]. As mentioned earlier, the pK_a measured for the azaindole N—H of BMS-488043 is 9.3. Consistent with this, the intermediate hydroxymethylazaindole has not been isolated or detected. BMS-663749, crystallized as a monolysine salt, was an off-white powder containing a small amount of amorphous material. The aqueous solubility of BMS-663749 at room temperature increases from 0.22 mg/mL at pH 1.4 to >12 mg/mL at pH 5.4 and pH 8.9. Concentrations of >100 mg/mL have been achieved in water. In contrast, the aqueous solubility of BMS-488043 in the pH range 4 to 8, as mentioned earlier, is 40 μg/mL. The prodrug exhibits satisfactory aqueous solution stability under acidic and neutral conditions for at least 24 h at 37°C.

The initial synthetic route to BMS-663749 (Scheme 4) is comprised of four steps, the last two of which can be accomplished without isolation of the penultimate free acid intermediate. To ensure reproducible reactivity, di-*tert*-butylchloromethyl phosphate was freshly prepared from *tert*-butylammonium bis-protected phosphate and chloroiodomethane for each run performed. An early survey of conditions revealed that deprotonation of BMS-488043 could be carried out with 3 equivalents of sodium hydride and that the subsequent iodine-catalyzed alkylation was optimally executed with 5 equivalents of di-*tert*-butylchloromethyl phosphate. Silica gel chromatography provided the diester in sufficient purity to allow subsequent deprotection, salt formation, and crystallization steps to reliably produce pure material. A broad survey of organic and inorganic salts identified the monolysine salt, monohydrate, as the best candidate for advancing to key in vivo studies with a crystalline form that could reproducibly be prepared to meet purity and stability targets. The overall yield from BMS-488043 was about 56% using this discovery chemistry procedure, and a more efficient synthesis will be disclosed elsewhere.

Following oral administration, BMS-663749 is thought to be hydrolyzed by alkaline phosphatase (ALP) present at the brush border membrane of the intestinal lumen to form BMS-488043, which is subsequently rapidly absorbed, due to its high membrane permeability. This hypothesis is supported by the fact that good-to-excellent oral bioavailabilities (62 to 94%) of BMS-488043 were observed after administration of BMS-663749 to rats, dogs, and monkeys, and very little or no BMS-663749 was found to be present in plasma. Phosphate prodrug BMS-663749 was hydrolyzed to form parent in the presence of human placental alkaline phosphatase, a number of cell lines, and hepatocytes, suggesting that it should function similarly in humans.

In a food-effect study (crossover design) comparing a BMS-663749-filled capsule and the BMS-488043 clinical capsule (at 20-mg/kg equivalent doses of BMS-488043), the

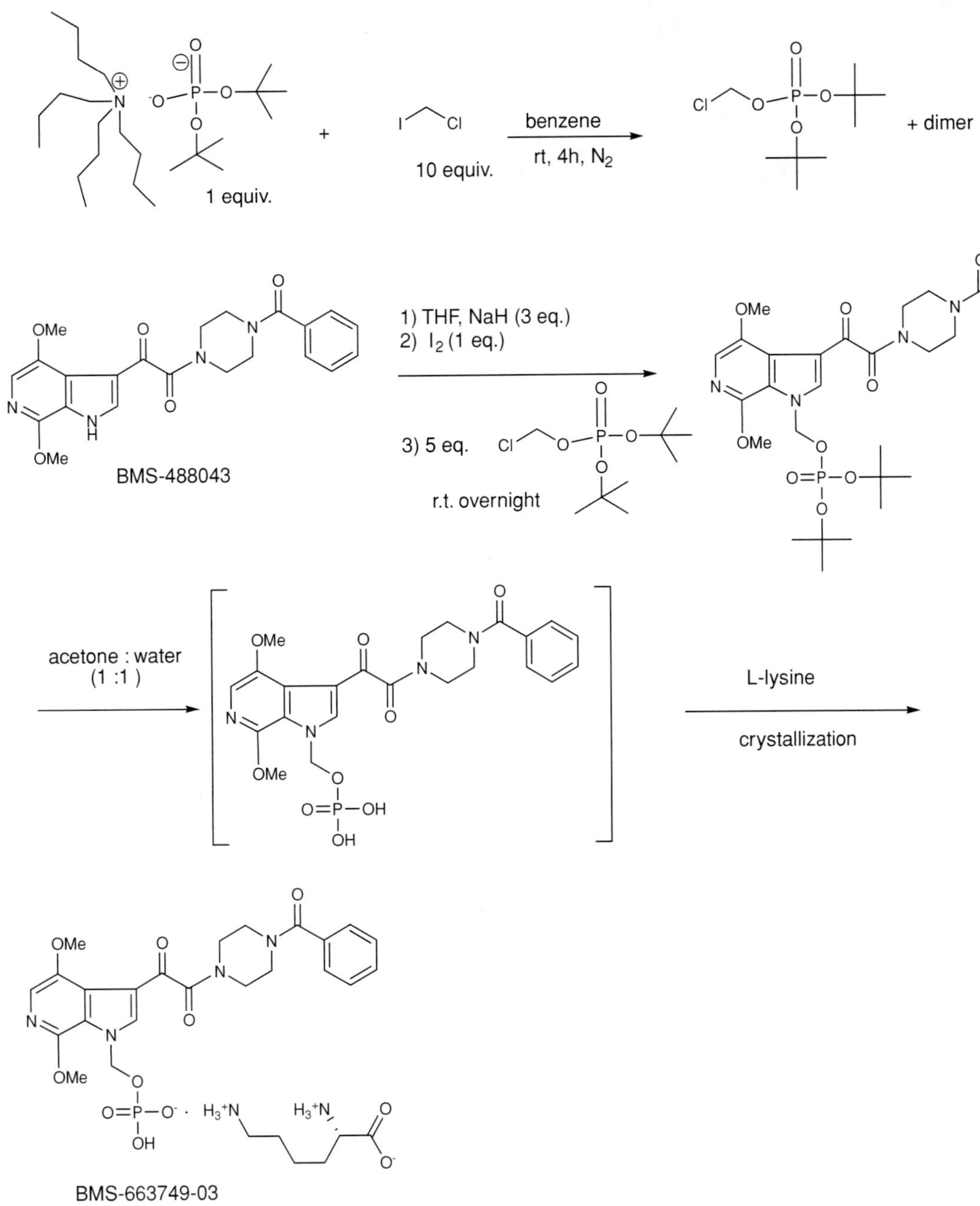

SCHEME 4 Synthesis of BMS-663749.

AUC of BMS-488043 in fasted dogs given BMS-663749 was about 4.3-fold higher than that obtained from a clinical capsule of BMS-488043 in the fed animals and 38-fold higher than that obtained in the fasted dogs [39,42]. The AUC and C_{max} values of BMS-488043 after dosing with BMS-663749 were similar in both fasted and fed dogs (there was a ninefold increase in AUC in fed dogs administered BMS-488043 as the clinical capsule compared to fasted dogs). This demonstrated that after oral administration of the prodrug, a significant increase in the exposure of parent drug was achieved without a food effect. Furthermore, the enhanced in vivo exposure from BMS-663749-filled capsules suggested that a traditional solid oral dosage form of BMS-663749 for systemic delivery of BMS-488043 was feasible. No specific toxicology or safety issues were identified for BMS-663749 during preclinical and pre-IND profiling.

Since preclinical studies with BMS-663749 suggested that it acted as a highly water-soluble source of BMS-488043 with the potential to address the dissolution- or solubility-limited absorption encountered in initial clinical studies, the prodrug was advanced to clinical studies in normal healthy volunteers. In these studies, the prodrug was found to be efficient in delivering parent molecule to plasma after oral dosing and the exposure of parent molecule increased nicely with escalating dose. The pharmacokinetic behavior of a 200-mg equivalent dose of solid prodrug approximated that observed from a 200-mg solution dose of parent molecule. However, although these initial studies demonstrated the viability of the phosphate prodrug approach, both BMS-663749 and parent BMS-488043 were supplanted in development by molecules with superior profiles.

FURTHER SAR: STUDIES OF C7-INDOLE-AMIDES AND HETEROCYCLES

In addition to substitutions at the C7 position of the attachment inhibitor indole or azaindole with simple functional groups, molecules with more elaborated amides and heterocycles at the position were also investigated [43]. As shown in Table 6, the primary carboxamide **8** maintained potency in a single-cycle infection assay using the JRFL-enveloped pseudotype virus, while the methyl amide analog **9** exhibited a modest increase in potency as compared to the C7-unsubstituted parent compound **2**. As exemplified by the pyridin-3-yl carboxamide **10**, substitution with a more bulky or extended amide group often led to a >10-fold decrease in potency. However, certain five-membered heteroaryl amide analogs provided subnanomolar potency, as demonstrated by the thiazol-2-yl analog **11**, which exhibits an EC_{50} of 57 pM in the pseudotype assay. More interestingly, direct incorporation of the indole C7 position with a variety of heterocycles, particularly the five-membered rings, resulted in substantial enhancement in potency to the subnanomolar range (e.g., analogs **12** to **15**). These C7 heteroaryl analogs were at least several fold more potent than their corresponding heteroaryl amide analogs (compare, e.g., **10** and **12**, and **11** and **13**), with **12** showing a dramatic improvement in potency over **10**. Substitution on the heteroaryl appended to position 7 was also well tolerated and usually maintained the subnanomolar potency of the series. Moreover, these C7 heteroaryl inhibitors, including the oxadiazole **14** and the tetrazole analog **15**, also maintained nanomolar activity against M- and T-tropic viruses in cell culture. As mentioned above, a methoxy group also conferred potency to the indole chemotype and was another preferred substituent at C4. In general, the 4-OMe-substituted analogs of the C7 amide and heterocycle series were equipotent to analogs in the 4-F-indole series.

For both the C7 amide and heterocycle series, it was challenging to obtain a balance between human liver microsomal stability and membrane permeability. Analogs that contained less polar amide groups or heterocycles at C7 were permeable, but unstable in human liver microsomes. Analogs with more polar amide groups or heterocycles were metabolically stable, but showed poor Caco-2 membrane permeability. Pharmacokinetic studies of these two classes of inhibitor in rats nevertheless suggested that oral bioavailability correlated with membrane permeability. For example, the C7-1,2,4-oxadiazole analog **14**, which possessed an excellent Caco-2 permeability [Pc (pH 6.5) >300 nm/s], showed an oral bioavailability of 89% and a C_{max} of 2.6 μg/mL when dosed orally as a solution in 90% PEG-400/10% EtOH to rats (i.v. 1 mg/kg, p.o. 5 mg/kg). However, indole **14** was predicted to be a compound of a high clearance class in humans based on its half-life of 17 min in HLM. The stable tetrazole analog **15** ($t_{1/2}$ > 200 min in HLM) had a Caco-2 permeability of 17 nm/s and thus showed negligible oral exposure in rats. Surprisingly, the methyl amide **9** showed good

TABLE 6 Antiviral Activity and Cytotoxicity of 4-F-7-Carboxamide and Heteroaryl-Indole Inhibitors

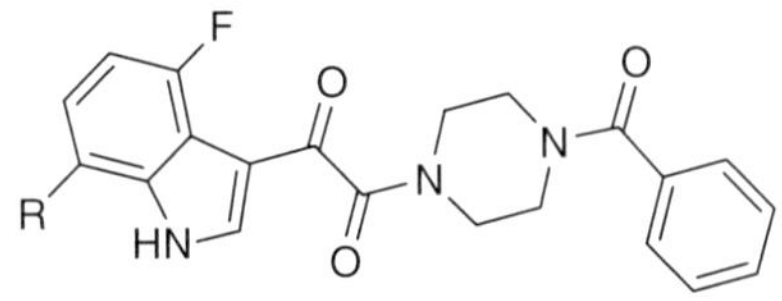

Compound	R =	EC_{50} (nM)	CC_{50} (μM)
8	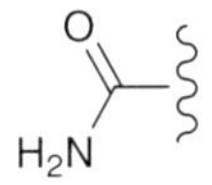	2.03	>300
9	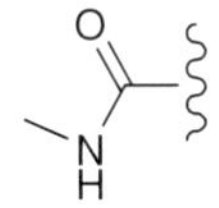	0.52	>300
10	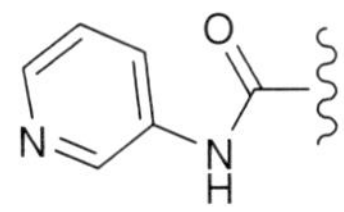	9.09	133
11	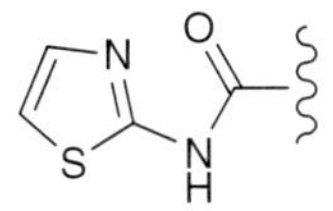	0.057	89
12	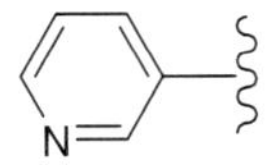	0.06	10
13	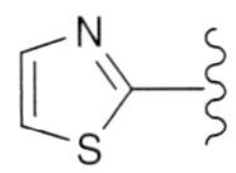	0.0067	23
14	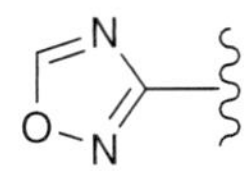	0.05	74
15	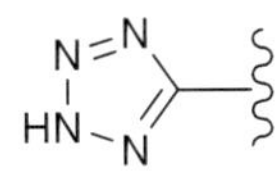	0.08	245

metabolic stability in HLM ($t_{1/2} = 81$ min) and a desirable Caco-2 permeability (112 nm/s), which translated into an oral bioavailability of 65% in rats. Subsequent in vivo evaluations also indicated that inhibitor **9** had high oral exposure in dogs and monkeys. However, the potency of **9** against a range of HIV clinical isolates and laboratory strains in cell culture in the presence of human serum was judged to be insufficient, consistent with high protein binding (98.9%), which precluded development. The profiles of compounds **8** to **15** were insufficient to consider advancing them for further development. However, accounts of additional studies in both the indole and azaindole motif and the discovery of molecules and prodrugs with superior profiles and that supplanted BMS-488043 and BMS-663749 in development will be provided in the future.

OTHER SMALL-MOLECULE HIV INHIBITORS THAT BIND TO gp120

Small-molecule gp120 inhibitors have been reviewed relatively recently [44]. Currently, we are unaware of any additional small molecules that target gp120 from other groups with the potential to advance into clinical studies in the near future. A synthetic bivalent inhibitor composed of two BMS-378806 molecules tethered via the C4 position was reported. The compound was not significantly more potent than BMS-378806, but it was more potent than a monomer core with linker attached (Fig. 3) [45]. Two distinct oxalamide-containing small molecules, NBD-556 and NBD-557 (Fig. 3), that block gp120-CD4 interaction were identified using an HIV syncytium assay [46]. PF-821385 (Fig. 3) an inhibitor of gp120-CD4 interaction was advanced into clinical studies [47,48]. However, development of PF-821385 was abandoned after single-ascending-dose studies in healthy volunteers predicted an efficacious drug dose close to or above the maximum tolerated dose [49,50]. A series of gp120-CD4 inhibitors with a sulfonamide as an isostere for the ketoamide group have also been disclosed [51]. Finally, a patent application claimed molecules that would bind to HIV envelope proteins and cause conformational changes that induced the exposure of cryptic epitopes on the envelope proteins [52].

CONCLUSIONS

In summary, initial optimization of the preclinical in vitro and in vivo profiles of a 6-azaindole series of attachment inhibitors relied upon SAR gleaned in preliminary studies with early indole and 7-azaindole leads and provided a 4,6-dimethoxy-substituted compound BMS-488043. This

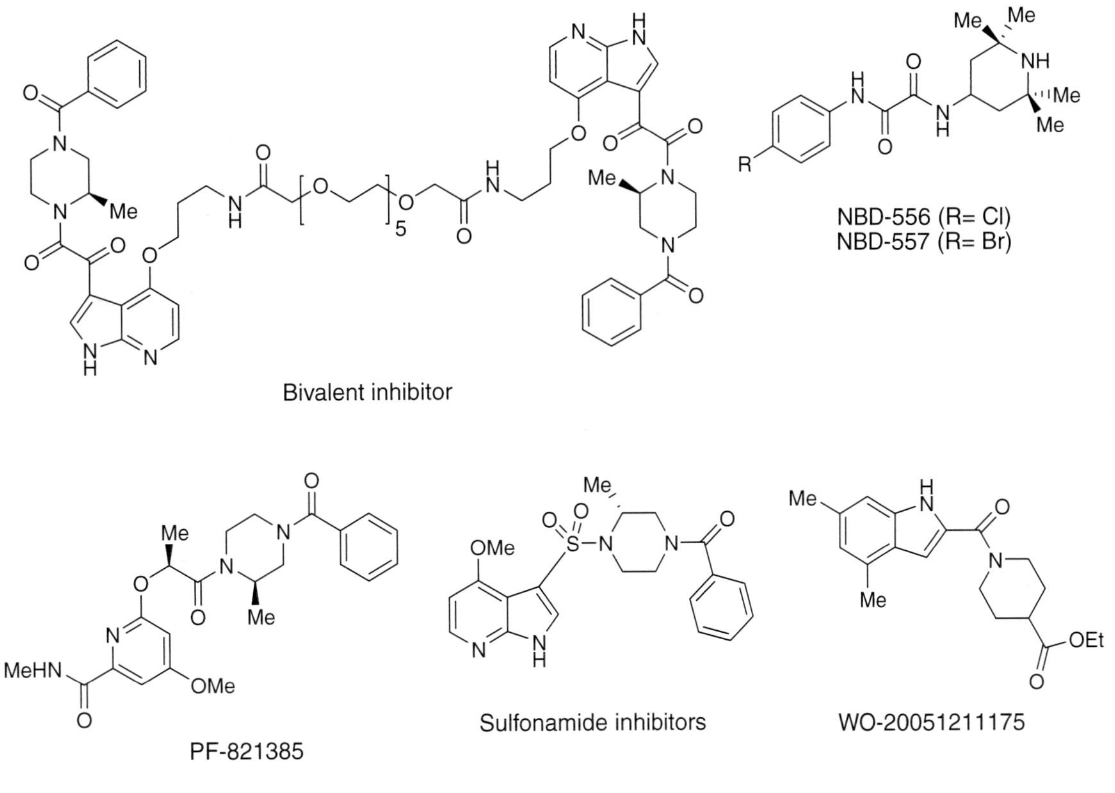

FIGURE 3 HIV gp120 inhibitors.

attachment inhibitor offered improved in vivo pharmacokinetic properties in three species and appeared to address the low permeability and metabolic stability that were considered to be the most serious liabilities associated with BMS-378806, a 7-azaindole compound that had shown insufficient exposure in human clinical studies. BMS-488043 demonstrated proof of concept for this class of HIV inhibitor in HIV-1-infected human subjects. A phosphate prodrug of BMS-488043, BMS-663749, advanced into clinical studies in normal healthy volunteers, and the prodrug methodology was shown to be a workable approach to addressing dissolution- or solubility-limited absorption in this class of compounds.

Acknowledgments

The authors gratefully acknowledge the contributions of all the researchers who contributed to Bristol-Myers Squibb Co.'s HIV attachment program, the majority of whom are cited in the references.

REFERENCES

[1] Gallo, R. C.; Montagnier, L. The discovery of HIV as the cause of AIDS. *N. Engl. J. Med.* **1990**, *349*, 2283–2285.

[2] Pomerantz, R. J.; Horn; D. L. Twenty years of therapy for HIV-1 infection. *Nat. Med.* **2003**, *9*, 867–873.

[3] Barré-Sinoussi, F.. The early years of HIV research: integrating clinical and basic research. *Nat. Med.* **2003**, *9*, 844–846.

[4] Merson, M. H. The HIV-AIDS pandemic at 25: the global response. *N. Engl. J. Med.* **2006**, *354*, 2414–2417.

[5] De Clercq, E. Anti-HIV drugs: 25 compounds approved within 25 years after the discovery of HIV. *Int. J. Antimicrob. Agents* **2009**, *33*, 307–320.

[6] Baba, M.; Tanaka, H.; De Clercq, E.; Pauwels, R.; Balzarini, J.; Schols, D.; Nakashima, H.; Perno, C. F.; Walker, R. T.; Miyasaka, T. Highly specific inhibition of human immunodeficiency virus type 1 by a novel 6-substituted acyclouridine derivative. *Biochem. Biophys. Res. Commun.* **1989**, *165*, 1375–1381.

[7] Pauwels, R.; Andries, K.; Desmyter, J.; Schols, D.; Kukla, M. J.; Breslin, H. J.; Raeymaeckers, A.; Van Gelder, J.; Woestenborghs, R.; Heykants, J.; et al. Potent and selective inhibition of HIV-1 replication in vitro by a novel series of TIBO derivatives. *Nature* **1990**, *343*, 470–474.

[8] Sweeney, Z. K.; Klumpp, K. Improving non-nucleoside reverse transcriptase inhibitors for first-line treatment of HIV infection: the development pipeline and recent clinical data. *Curr. Opin. Drug Discov. Dev.* **2008**, *11*, 458–470.

[9] Hammer, S. M.; Squires, K. E.; Hughes, M. D.; Grimes, J. M.; Demeter, L. M.; Currier, J. S.; Eron, J. J.; Feinberg, J. E.; Balfour, H. H.; Deyton, L. R.; et al. A controlled trial of two nucleoside analogs plus indinavir in persons with human immunodeficiency virus infection and CD4 cell counts of 200 per cubic millimeter or less. *N. Engl. J. Med.* **1997**, *337*, 725–733.

[10] Hammer, S. M.; Eron; J., J., Jr.; Reiss, P.; Schooley, R. T.; Thompson, M. A.; Walmsley, S.; Cahn, P.; Fischl, M. A.; Gatell, J. M.; Hirsch, M. S.; et al. Antiretroviral treatment of adult HIV infection: recommendations of the International AIDS Society–USA panel. *JAMA* **2008**, *300*, 555–570.

[11] Frampton, J. E.; Croom, K. F. Efavirenz/emtricitabine/tenofovir disoproxil fumarate: triple combination tablet. *Drugs* **2006**, *66*, 1501–1512.

[12] Killingley, B.; Pozniak, A. The first once-daily single-tablet regimen for the treatment of HIV-infected patients. *Drugs Today* **2007**, *43*, 427–442.

[13] Blair, W.; Spicer, T. P. World Patent Application WO-2001/96610, **2001**.

[14] Richman, D. D.; Morton, S. C.; Wrin, T.; Hellmann, N.; Berry, S.; Shapiro, M. F.; Bozzette, S. A. The prevalence of antiretroviral drug resistance in the United States. *AIDS* **2004**, *18*, 1393–1401.

[15] De Clercq, E. The role of non-nucleoside reverse transcriptase inhibitors (NNRTIs) in the therapy of HIV-1 infection. *Antiviral Res.* **1998**, *38*, 153–179.

[16] Blair, W. S.; Deshpande, M.; Fang, H.; Lin, P.-F.; Spicer, T. P.; Wallace, O. B.; Wang, H.; Wang, T.; Zhang, Z.; Yeung, K.-S. World Patent Application WO-2000/76521, **2000**.

[17] Wang, T.; Zhang, Z.; Wallace, O. B.; Deshpande, M.; Fang, H.; Yang, Z.; Zadjura, L. M.; Tweedie, D. L.; Huang, S.; Zhao, F.; et al. Discovery of 4-benzoyl-1-[(4-methoxy-1*H*-pyrrolo[2,3-*b*]pyridin-3-yl)oxoacetyl]-2-(*R*)-methylpiperazine (BMS-378806): a novel HIV-1 attachment inhibitor that interferes with CD4-gp120 interactions. *J. Med. Chem.* **2003**, *46*, 4236–4239.

[18] Meanwell, N. A.; Wallace, O. B.; Wang, H.; Deshpande, M.; Pearce, B. C.; Trehan, A.; Yeung, K.-S.; Qiu, Z.; Wright, J. J. K.; Robinson, B. A.; et al. Inhibitors of HIV-1 attachment: 3. A preliminary survey of the effect of structural variation of the benzamide moiety on antiviral activity. *Bioorg. Med. Chem. Lett.* **2009**, *19*, 5136.

[19] Wang, T.; Kadow, J. F.; Zhang, Z.; Yin, Z.; Gao, Q.; Wu, D.; DiGuigno Parker, D.; Yang, Z.; Zadjura, L.; Robinson, B. A.; et al. Inhibitors of HIV-1 attachment: 4. A study of the effect of piperazine substitution patterns on antiviral potency in the context of indole-based derivatives. *Bioorg. Med. Chem. Lett.* **2009**, *19*, 5140.

[20] Meanwell, N. A.; Wallace, O. B.; Fang, H.; Wang, H.; Deshpande, M.; Wang, T.; Yin, Z.; Zhang, Z.; Pearce, B. C.; James, J.; et al. Inhibitors of HIV-1 attachment: 2. An initial survey of indole substitution patterns. *Bioorg. Med. Chem. Lett.* **2009**, *19*, 1977–1981.

[21] Wang, T.; Yin, Z.; Zhang, Z.; Bender, J. A.; Yang, Z.; Johnson, G.; Yang, Z.; Zadjura, L. M.; D'Arienzo, C. J.; Parker, D. D.; et al. Inhibitors of HIV-1 attachment: 5. An evolution from indole to azaindoles leading to the discovery of BMS-488043, a drug candidate that demonstrates antiviral activity in HIV-1-infected subjects. *J. Med. Chem.* **2009**, *52*, 7778–7787.

[22] Zhang, Z.; Yang, Z.; Meanwell, N. A.; Kadow, J. F.; Wang, T. A general method for the preparation of 4- and 6-azaindoles. *J. Org. Chem.* **2002**, *67*, 2345–2347.

[23] Guo, Q.; Ho, H.-T.; Dicker, I.; Fan, L.; Zhou, N.; Friborg, J.; Wang, T.; McAuliffe, B. V.; Wang, H.-G. H.; Rose, R. E.; et al. Biochemical and genetic characterizations of a novel human immunodeficiency virus type 1 inhibitor that blocks gp120-CD4 interactions. *J. Virol.* **2003**, *77*, 10528–10536.

[24] Lin, P.-F.; Blair, W.; Wang, T.; Spicer, T.; Guo, Q.; Zhou, N.; Gong, Y.-F.; Wang, H.-G. H.; Rose, R.; Yamanaka, G.; et al. A small molecule HIV-1 inhibitor that targets the HIV-1 envelope and inhibits CD4 receptor binding. *Proc. Natl. Acad. Sci. USA* **2003**, *100*, 11013–11018.

[25] Kwong, P. D.; Wyatt, R.; Robinson, J.; Sweet, R. W.; Sodroski, J.; Hendrickson, W. A. Structure of an HIV gp120 envelope glycoprotein in complex with the CD4 receptor and a neutralizing human antibody. *Nature* **1998**, *393*, 648–659.

[26] Benoit, S.; Gingras, S.; Soundararajan, N., inventors; Bristol-Myers Squibb Co., assignee. Process for the preparation of antiviral 7-azaindole derivatives. WO 2003082289 A1, Oct. 9, **2003**.

[27] Yang, Z.; Zadjura, L.; D'Arienzo, C.; Marino, A.; Santone, K.; Klunk, L.; Greene, D.; Lin, P.-F.; Colonno, R.; Wang, T.; et al. Preclinical pharmacokinetics of a novel HIV-1 attachment inhibitor BMS-378806 and prediction of its human pharmacokinetics. *Biopharm. Drug Dispos.* **2005**, *26*, 387–402.

[28] Hanna, G.; Lalezari, J.; Hellinger, J.; Wohl, D.; Masterson, T.; Fiske, W.; Kadow, J.; Lin, P.-F.; Giordano, M.; Colonno, R.; Grasela D. Antiviral activity, safety, and tolerability of a novel, oral small-molecule HIV-1 attachment inhibitor, BMS-488043, in HIV-1 infected subjects. 11th Conference Retroviruses and Opportunistic Infection, San Francisco, Feb. 8–11, **2004**. Abstract 141.

[29] Ho, H.-T.; Fan, L.; Nowicka-Sans, B.; McAuliffe, B.; Li, C.-B.; Yamanaka, G.; Zhou, N.; Fang, H.; Dicker, I.; Dalterio, R.; et al. Envelope conformational changes induced by human immunodeficiency virus type 1 attachment inhibitors prevent CD4 binding and downstream entry events. *J. Virol.* **2006**, *80*, 4017–4025.

[30] Lin, P. F.; Ho, H. T.; Gong, Y. F.; Dicker, I.; Zhou, N.; Fan, L.; McAuliffe, B.; Kimmel, B.; Nowicka-Sans, B.; Wang, T.; et al. Characterization of a small molecule HIV-1 attachment inhibitor BMS-488043: virology, resistance, and mechanism of action. 11th Conference on Retroviruses and Opportunistic Infections, San Francisco, Feb. 8–11, **2004**. Abstract 534.

[31] Lin, P. F.; Ho, H. T.; Fan, L.; Li, C. B.; Nowicka-Sans, B.; McAuliffe, B.; Zhou, N.; Dalterio, R.; Gong, Y.; Eggers, B.; et al. Inhibition mechanism of small molecule HIV-1 attachment inhibitors. 12th Conference on Retroviruses and Opportunistic Infections, Boston, Feb. 22–25, **2005**. Abstract 544.

[32] Liu, W.; Patel, S. S.; Cuniere, N.; Lear, Y.; Deshpande, P. P.; Simon, J. N.; Lai, C.; Pullockaran, A. J.; Soundararajan, N.; Bien, J. T., inventors; Bristol-Myers Squibb Co., assignee. Method of preparation of azaindole derivatives. US 2007032503 A1, Feb. 8, **2007**.

[33] Yang, Z.; Zadjura, L. M.; Marino, A. M.; D'Arienzo, C. J.; Malinowski, J.; Gesenberg, C.; Lin, P.-F.; Colonno, R. J.; Wang, T.; Kadow, J. F.; et al. *J. Pharm. Sci.* **2010**, *99*, 2135–2152.

[34] Fakes, M. G.; Vakkalagadda, B. J.; Qian, F.; Desikan, S.; Gandhi, R. B.; Lai, C.; Hsieh, A.; Franchini, M. K.; Toale, H.; Brown, J. Enhancement of oral bioavailability of an HIV-attachment inhibitor by nanosizing and amorphous formulation approaches. *Int. J. Pharm.* **2009**, *370*, 167–174.

[35] Tobyn, M.; Brown, J.; Dennis, A. B.; Fakes, M.; Gao, Q.; Gamble, J.; Khimyak, Y. Z.; McGeorge, G.; Patel, C.; Sinclair, W.; Timmins, P. Amorphous drug–PVP dispersions: application of theoretical, thermal, and spectroscopic analytical techniques to the study of a molecule with intermolecular bonds in both the crystalline and pure amorphous state. *J. Pharm. Sci.* **2009** (online early disclosure).

[36] Heimbach, T.; Oh, D.-M.; Li, L. Y.; Rodriguez-Hornedo, N.; Garcia, G.; Fleisher, D. Enzyme-mediated precipitation of parent drugs from their phosphate prodrugs. *Int. J. Pharm.*, **2003**, *261*, 81–92.

[37] Heimbach, T.; Oh, D.-M.; Li, L. Y.; Forsberg, M.; Savolainen, J.; Leppaenen, J.; Matsunaga, Y.; Flynn, G.; Fleisher, D. Absorption rate limit considerations for oral phosphate prodrugs. *Pharm. Res.* **2003**, *20*, 848–856.

[38] Ueda, Y.; Matiskella, J. D.; Golik, J.; Connolly, T. P.; Hudyma, T. W.; Venkatesh, S.; Dali, M.; Kang, S.-H.; Barbour, N.; Tejwani, R.; et al. Phosphonooxymethyl prodrugs of the broad spectrum antifungal azole, ravuconazole: synthesis and biological properties. *Bioorg. Med. Chem. Lett.* **2003**, *13*, 3669–3672.

[39] Ueda, Y.; Connolly, T. P.; Wang, T.; Chen, C.-P. H.; Yeung, K.-S.; Zheng, M.; Bender, J.; Yang, Z.; Lin, P. F.; Colonno, R. P.; et al. Unpublished results.

[40] Ueda, Y.; Connolly, T. P.; Kadow, J. F.; Meanwell, N. A.; Wang, T.; Chen, C.-P. H.; Yeung, K.-S.; Zhang, Z.; Leahy, D. K.; Pack, S. K.; et al., inventors; Bristol-Myers Squibb Co., assignee. Prodrugs based on bicyclic nitrogen-containing heterocyclic antiviral agents having substituted piperazine or piperidine rings. U.S. Patent Application 2005209246 A1, Sept. 22, **2005**.

[41] Zhu, Z.; Chen, H.-G.; Goel, O. P.; Chan, O. H.; Stilgenbauer, L. A.; Stewart, B. H. Phosphate prodrugs of PD 154075. *Bioorg. Med. Chem. Lett.* **2000**, *10*, 1121–1124.

[42] Zheng, M., et al. Unpublished results.

[43] Yeung, K. S.; Kadow, J. F.; Meanwell, N. A. et. al. Unpublished results.

[44] Kadow, J.; Wang, H.-G. H.; Lin, P.-F. Small-molecule HIV-1 gp120 inhibitors to prevent HIV-1 entry: an emerging opportunity for drug development. *Curr. Opin. Invest. Drugs* **2006**, *7*, 721–726.

[45] Wang, J.; Le, N. Heredia, A.; Song, H.; Redfield, R.; Wang, L.-X. Modification and structure–activity relationship of a small molecule HIV-1 inhibitor targeting the viral envelope glycoprotein gp120. *Org. Biomol. Chem.* **2005**, *3*, 1781–1786.

[46] Zhao, Q.; Ma, L.; Jiang, S.; Liu, S.; He, Y.; Strick, N.; Neamati, N.; Debnath, A. K. Identification of *N*-phenyl-*N'*-(2,2,6,6-tetramethyl-piperidin-4-yl)-oxalamides as a new class of HIV-entry inhibitors that prevent gp120 binding to CD4. *Virology* **2005**, *339*, 213–225.

[47] Middleton, D. S.; Mowbray, C. E.; Stephenson, P. T.; Williams, D. H., inventors; Pfizer, Inc., assignee. Preparation of piperazine derivatives for use in pharmaceutical compositions for the treatment of HIV infection. U.S. Patent Application 2005043300, Feb. 24, **2005**.

[48] Fenwick, D. R.; Gillmore, A. T.; Platts, M. Y., inventors; Pfizer Inc., assignee. Preparation of a crystalline form of 5-[[(1*S*)-2-((2*R*)-4-benzoyl-2-methylpiperazin-1-yl)-1-methyl-2-oxoethyl]oxy]-4-methoxypyridine-2-carboxylic acid methylamide for the treatment of HIV. PCT Patent Application. WO2006085199, Aug. 17, **2006**.

[49] Parkinson, T.; Stephenson, P.; Pickford, C.; Tran, D.; Williams, D.; Fenwick, D.; Fok-Seang, J.; Gardner, I.; Westby, M.; Middleton, D.; Perros, M. Characterization of a novel series of gp120 inhibitors. International Conference on Antiretroviral Research, **2008**. Abstract A-24.

[50] Chan, P. L. S.; Schaick, E.; Langdon, J. D.; Parkinson, T.; McFadyen, L. PK-PD modeling to support go/no go decisions for a novel gp120 inhibitor. Population Approach Group in Europe, **2007**. Abstract 1162.

[51] Lu, R.-J.; Tucker, J. A.; Zinevitch, T.; Kirichenko, O.; Konoplev, V.; Kuznetsova, S.; Sviridov, S.; Pickens, J.; Tandel, S.; Brahmachary, E.; et al. Design and synthesis of human immunodeficiency virus entry inhibitors: sulfonamide as an isostere for the α-ketoamide group. *J. Med. Chem.* **2007**, *50*, 6535–6544.

[52] Srivastava, I. K.; Sharma, V.; Barnett, S. W.; Ulmer, J., inventors; Chiron Corp., assignee. Env polypeptide complexes and methods of use. PCT Patent Application WO2005121175, Dec. 22, **2005**.

12

DISCOVERY OF MK-0536: A POTENTIAL SECOND-GENERATION HIV-1 INTEGRASE STRAND TRANSFER INHIBITOR WITH A HIGH GENETIC BARRIER TO MUTATION

MELISSA S. EGBERTSON, JOHN S. WAI, AND MARK CAMERON
Merck Research Laboratories, West Point, Pennsylvania

R. SCOTT HOERRNER
Merck Process Chemistry, Rahway, New Jersey

INTRODUCTION

Raltegravir (MK-0518, **1**) is a potent first-generation HIV integrase inhibitor (Fig. 1). It inhibits integrase-catalyzed strand transfer with an IC_{50} value of 10 nM and is a potent antiviral agent, inhibiting the spread of HIV infection in cell culture with an IC_{95} of 33 ± 23 nM in the presence of 50% normal human serum. It retains activity vs. diverse clinical isolates, including HIV-2, and exhibits a potent antiviral effect in treatment-naive patients and in patients infected with triple-class resistant virus. The compound has few drug–drug interactions and does not require co-dosing with a P450 inhibitor such as ritonavir for good bioavailability [1–4].

A second-generation HIV integrase inhibitor was sought that maintains the good efficacy, tolerability, and lack of drug–drug interactions of **1** while also having improved pharmacokinetics that would allow once-daily dosing, and activity against mutant virus resistant to first-generation inhibitors. In this chapter we describe work leading to the identification of compound **2** as a second-generation integrase inhibitor candidate [5].

Previous experience in developing integrase inhibitors was useful in designing a new chemical class of compounds to achieve these goals. The original diketo acid integrase inhibitor L-731988 (compound **3**, Fig. 2) displays a template of two carbonyl groups flanking a central enol moiety [6–8]. The terminal carboxyl group appears to act as a Lewis base rather than as a Lewis acid, as has been demonstrated by its replacement by functional groups that have Lewis basic but not Lewis acidic character (e.g., by a pyridine moiety) [9]. This is exemplified by two templates explored in two first-generation HIV-1 integrase inhibitors that use a Lewis base heteroatom as a replacement for the carboxyl group. For the early clinical candidate 1,6-naphthyridine L-870810 (compound **4**) [10,11], the Lewis base heteroatom is the 1-naphthyridine nitrogen. For the pyrimidinone **1** [12,13] it is the 6-oxo group. Exploration of the structure–activity relationship (SAR) leading to these series showed that potency is enhanced if these three key structural elements of the pharmacophore are coplanar with one another [12,14,15]. Both the 1,6-naphthyridine and pyrimidinone incorporate a ring nitrogen ortho to the central amide bond, which allows that amide bond to be coplanar with the rest of the template.

Novel templates that took advantage of these features were developed. For example, in the bicyclic template **5**, the central amide bond is forced to be planar relative to the rest of the template through use of a constraining alkyl ring. Compounds of this type were found to be potent inhibitors [16]. In designing analogs to this bicyclic system, it appeared that tetrahydronaphthyridine template **6** would be a good target,

Antiviral Drugs: From Basic Discovery Through Clinical Trials, First Edition. Edited by Wieslaw M. Kazmierski.

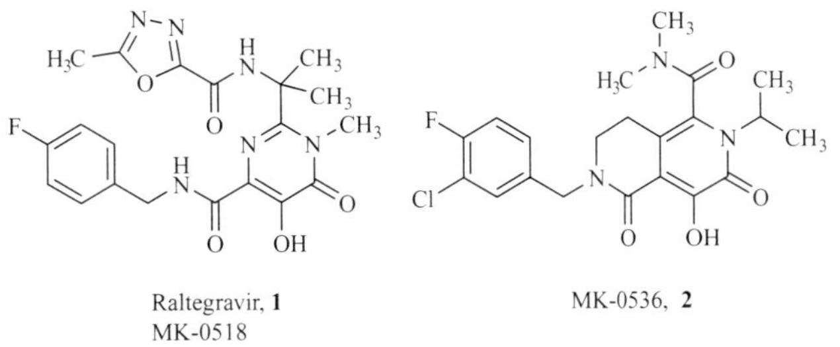

FIGURE 1 First- and second-generation HIV-1 integrase inhibitors.

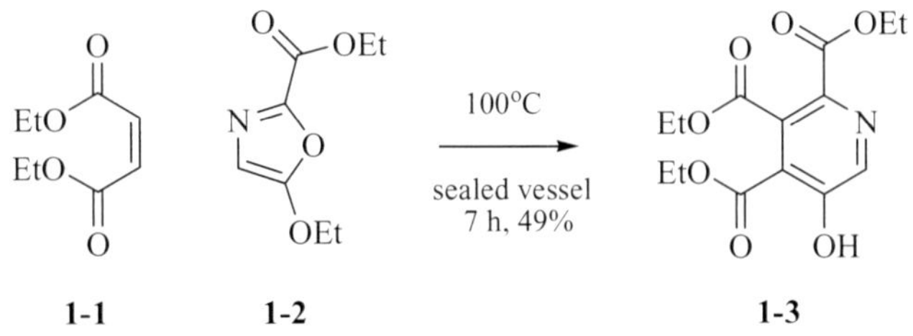

SCHEME 1 Kozikowski–Isobe synthesis of tetra-substituted pyridines.

since it encompasses many of the same structural features as **5**. In addition, the carboxylic amide moiety *para* to the phenolic oxygen was envisioned as an important structural element, since similar substitution in the 1,6-naphthyridine series had resulted in greatly improved metabolic stability [10,11,17].

RESULTS

The synthesis of the carboxamide-substituted tetrahydronaphthyridine template **6** was accomplished using chemistry similar to that first reported by Kozikowski and Isobe for the synthesis of tetra-substituted pyridine **1-3** from the Diels–Alder reaction of diethyl maleate **1-1** and 5-ethoxy-2-(pent-1-en-2-yl)-1,3-oxazole **1-2** (Scheme 1) in 49% isolated yield [18]. When we explored this type of reaction, it was observed that the ethoxy-substituted oxazole **1-2** was a very volatile reagent and that even under sealed reaction conditions it has a tendency to evaporate out of the liquid phase of the reaction and condense at the top of the reaction vessel. This type of Diels–Alder reaction appears underutilized in the literature, perhaps because the high volatility of the ethoxyoxazole precludes efficient conversions. In planning the synthesis of template **6**, it was proposed to decrease the volatility of the diene and thus make it a more compatible reactant with the dienophile **2-3** (Scheme 2). This was accomplished by simply adding molecular weight to the diene in the form of an extended alkyl substituent on the ester to give *n*-butyloxyoxazole **2-6**. Dienophile **2-3** and the oxazole **2-6** were prepared as outlined in Scheme 2.

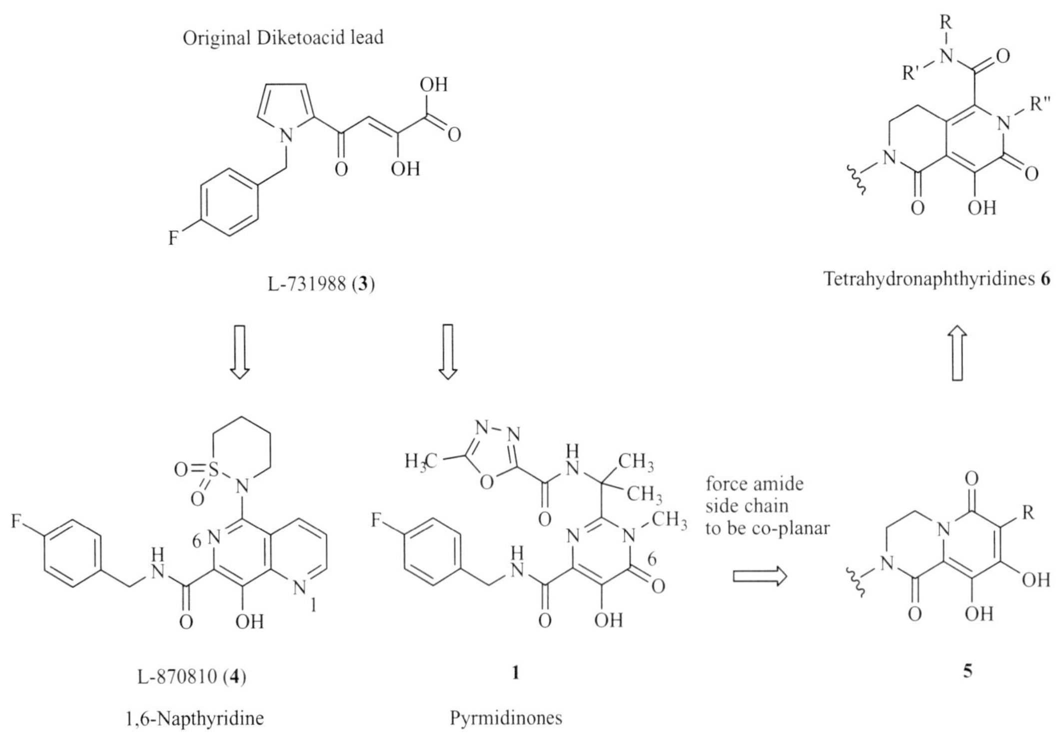

FIGURE 2 Evolution of tetrahydronaphthyridine target **6**.

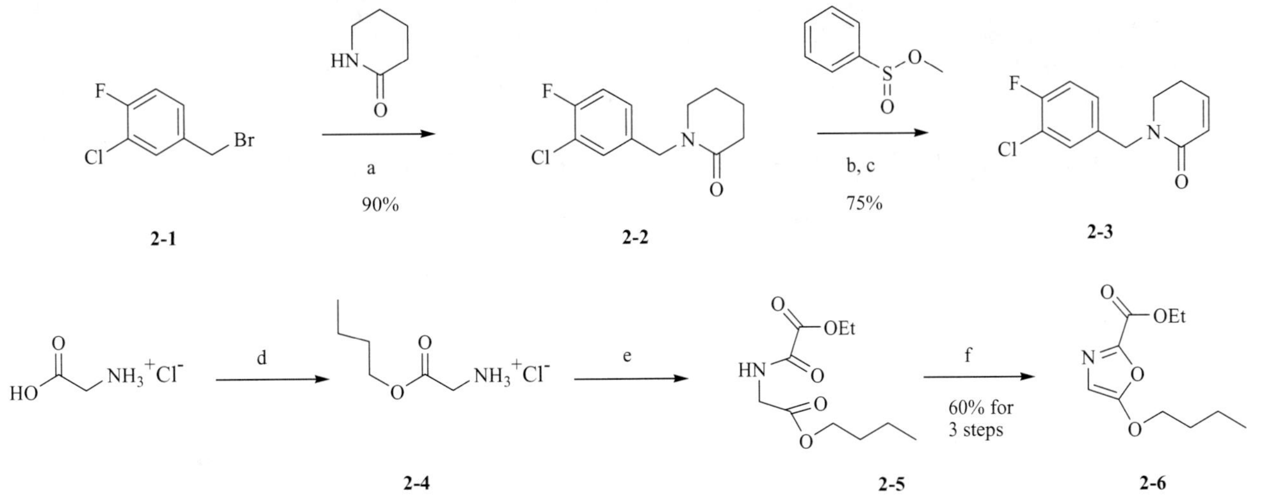

SCHEME 2 Synthesis of the Diels–Alder reaction components **2-3** and **2-6**. (a) NaH, NMP, 0°C; (b) LiHMDS, THF, −20°C; (c) toluene, Na_2CO_3, 100°C; (d) 1-butanol, thionyl chloride, room temperature to 70°C; (e) diethyloxalate, TEA, ethanol, room temperature to 50°C; (f) P_2O_5, CH_3CN, room temperature to 60°C.

The Diels–Alder reaction was performed neat in a sealed vessel at 130°C, with about a 2 : 1 ratio of diene to dienophile, for 48 to 72 h (Scheme 3). Initial experiments indicated a modest yield of the desired Diels–Alder product **3-1**; however, the goal of decreasing the volatility of the diene was achieved, and the desired product that formed precipitated from the reaction and could easily be isolated by filtration after the cooled reaction mixture was diluted with ether. It was noticed that batches of oxazole **2-6** that had been chromatographed more than once gave lower yields than batches that had been chromatographed once, raising the possibility that some acidic impurity carried over from the oxazole formation, could potentially catalyze the Diels–Alder reaction. Further experimentation revealed that the conversion of the reactions and the yields could be greatly improved with the addition of a small amount (0.75 equiv) of neat trifluoroacetic acid (TFA). Higher equivalents of TFA led to lower yields, as more of **2-6** reverted to **2-5**. Subsequently, it was found a milder proton source, such as water (1.5 equiv), also produced product, and in better yield (75%). Up to 4 equiv of water produced product in a similar fashion, but larger amounts of water (~0.5 M reaction solution) inhibited the reaction. Only the desired regioisomer was isolated from filtration of the crude reaction mixture slurry with ether. The remaining mass consisted of multiple by-products.

With a robust route to the tetrahydronaphthyridine now available, we sought a synthetic route that would allow us to vary the amide substituents late in the synthesis so that many analogs could readily be prepared. An example is outlined in Scheme 4. Oxidation of the pyridine to the *N*-oxide **4-1**, followed by acetylation, rearrangement, and hydrolysis of the resulting diacetic ester **4-3** gave **4-4** in good yield. Using conditions developed for the synthesis of Raltegravir [19], excellent selection of N-alkylation product **4-6** over the O-alkylation product was possible, presumably because magnesium's coordination of the diol in **4-5** attenuates the nucleophilicity of the tetrahydronaphthyridine

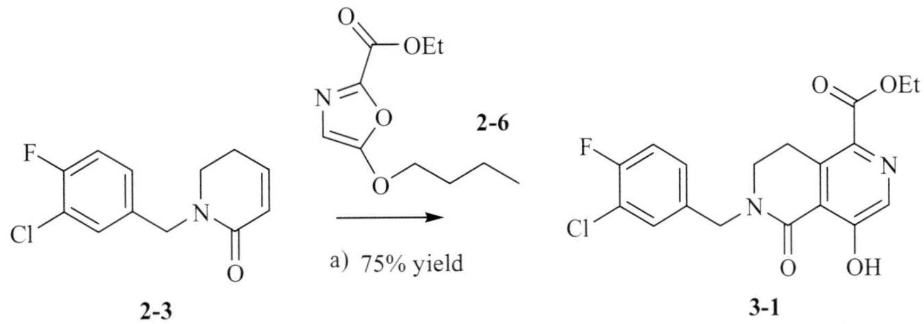

SCHEME 3 Optimized Diels–Alder reaction to form carboxy-substituted tetrahydronaphthyridine template **6**. (a) 1.4 equiv **2-6**, 1.5 equiv H_2O, neat, 130°C, sealed vessel, 48 to 78 h.

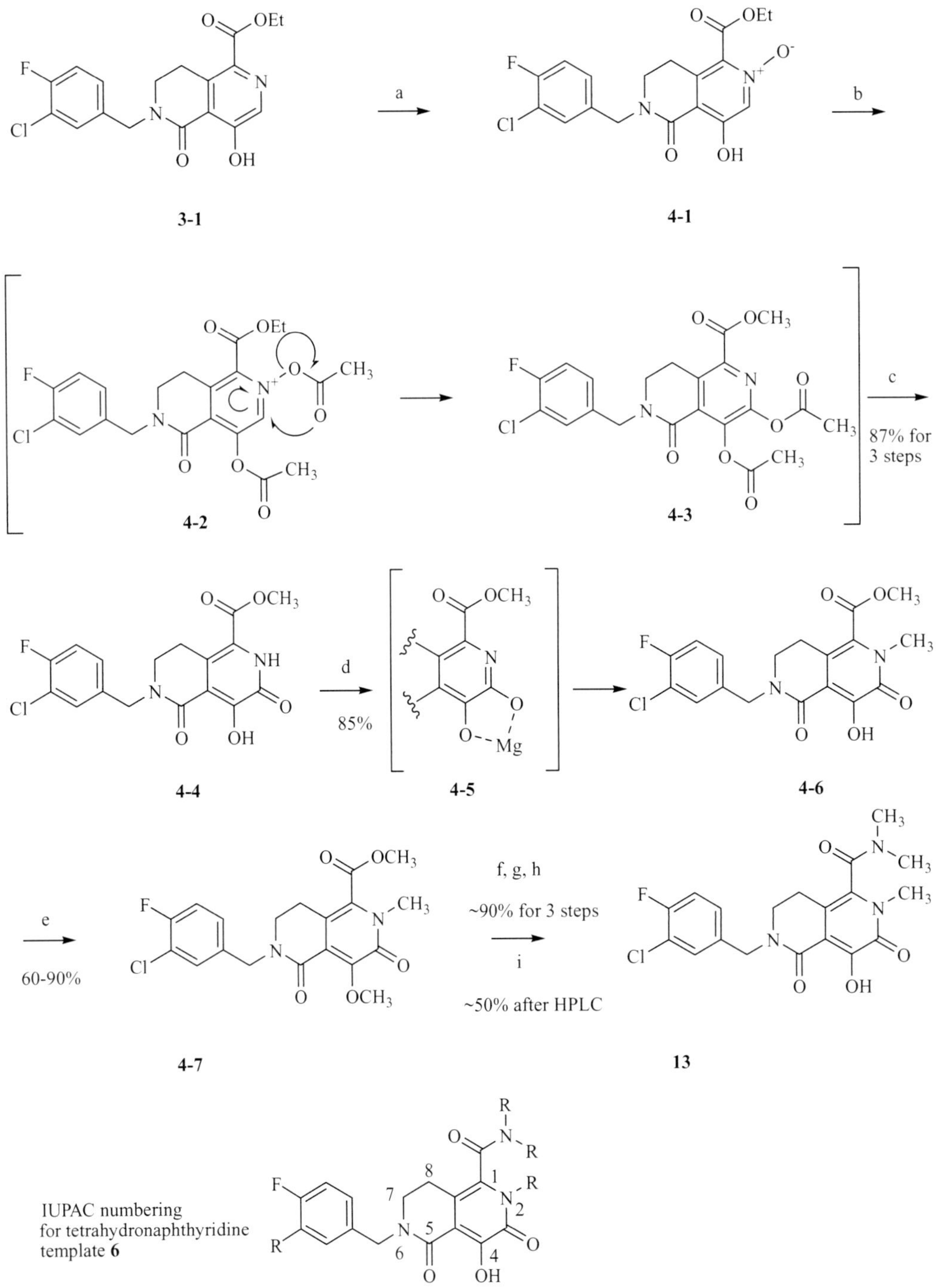

SCHEME 4 Preparation of tetrahydronaphthyridine analogs. Preparation of analog **13**. IUPAC numbering for tetrahydronaphthyridine template **6**. (a) H_2O_2/HOAc 100°C; (b) Ac_2O, 100°C; (c) $NaOCH_3$/THF/CH_3OH 45°C; (d) $Mg(OCH_3)_2$, CH_3I, DMF, 60°C; (e) Cs_2CO_3, CH_3I, DMF; (f) LiOH, THF/CH_3OH/H_2O; (g) oxalyl chloride, DMF (cat.), CH_2Cl_2; (h) $(CH_3)_2NH$; (i) HBr/HOAc.

system. A variety of simple alkyl halides could be used in this reaction [20]. Protection of the phenolic oxygen through methylation gave **4-7**. This step proved somewhat problematic to drive to completion, but the fully protected product proved to be a good candidate for purification midway through the sequence. Hydrolysis of the purified **4-7** followed by formation of the acid chloride and coupling with an appropriate amine gave the amide, which was then deprotected and chromatographed to give final products **7** to **15** (Table 1), such as the compound

TABLE 1 Alkyl Substitution Analogs of Tetrahydronaphthyridine Template 6

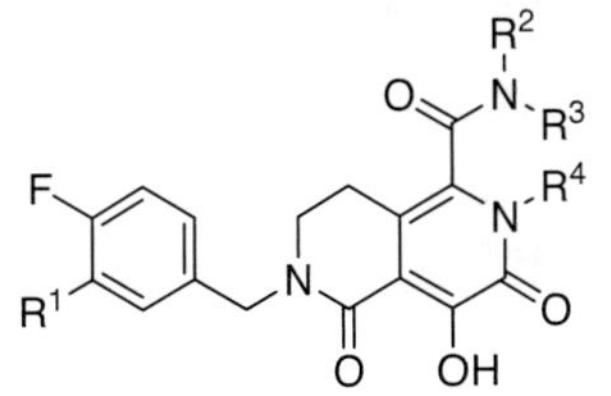

Compound	R^1	R^2	R^3	R^4	Strand Transfer (IC_{50} nM) (0.5 nM Mn)[a]	Antiviral Activity in cell Culture (10% FBS) (IC_{95} nM)[b]	Antiviral Activity in cell culture (50% NHS) (IC_{95} nM)[c]	PB 10% Human[d]	Log P^e
7	H	H	CH_3	H	11	375	645	97.6	0.9
8	H	CH_3	CH_3	H	1	354	539	56	0.56
9	H	CH_3	CH_3	CH_3	11	333	291	51	0.74
10	H	H	CH_3	CH_3	8	> 1000	500[f]	68	0.95
11	Cl	CH_3	CH_3	H	8	10	19	97	1.3
12	Cl	H	CH_3	CH_3	7	250	333	90	1.5
13	Cl	CH_3	CH_3	CH_3	16	73	91	78	1.3
14	Cl	CH_3	CH_3	Et	2	16	33	88	1.7
2	Cl	CH_3	CH_3	iPr	3	16[g]	35[g]	90	2.1
15	Cl	CH_3	CH_3	iBu	7	38	337	97	2.5

[a]Inhibition of strand transfer assay [26], $n \geq 2$.
[b]Antiviral activity in cell culture in the presence of fetal bovine serum (FBS) [27], $n \geq 2$.
[c]Antiviral activity in cell culture in the presence of 50% normal human serum (NHS) [27], $n \geq 2$.
[d]Percent binding to 10% human plasma extrapolated to 100%.
[e]Log of the partition coefficient (octanol/water).
[f]$n = 1$.
[g]$n = 197$.

shown, **13** [6-(3-chloro-4-fluorobenzyl)-4-hydroxy-*N*,*N*-dimethyl-3,5-dioxo-2-(propan-2-yl)-2,3,5,6,7,8-hexahydro-2,6-naphthyridine-1-carboxamide]. In this way a variety of analogs with a different substitution at the amide and N-substitution could be prepared in a convergent fashion.

Different benzyl substituents were either incorporated from the beginning by synthesis of the appropriate N-benzylated dienophile, or *p*-OCH_3-benzyl was used as a protecting group on the dienophile, which could be taken through the Diels–Alder reaction to give intermediate **5-1.** This protecting group was robust enough to survive the subsequent oxidation and amide formation steps, yet could be removed easily at a late stage of the synthesis to give intermediate **5-4**, which could then be selectively N- alkylated with the desired *N*-benzyl groups (Scheme 5).

Examination of the tetrahydronaphthyridine products revealed that they exhibited atropisomerization. The steric bulk of the substituents on the amide nitrogen, the ring nitrogen, and the protons on the methylene of the naphthyridine ring cause steric strain between these substituents. As a result, the amide bond is forced out of the plane of the tetrahydronaphthyridine system (Fig. 3). The steric strain hinders rotation of the amide bond around the carbon–carbon bond, giving rise to long-lived rotational isomers (atropisomers). Similar atropisomer behavior has been reported for 1,2-substituted naphthylene compounds [21]. Experimentally, atropisomerization was revealed by the presence of diastereotopic benzyl-CH_2-proton peaks in the NMR spectra. Also, using chiral HPLC, the enantiomers of analog **13** can be separated under neutral conditions (CH_3OH/HPLC, or CO_2/CH_3OH/SFC conditions) [22].

At pH 5 and lower, racemization of the purified enantiomers was slow; in pH 5 buffer/CH_3OH solution, the $t_{1/2}$ for racemization was about 8.4 h. Long-lived atropisomers can pose a challenge to drug development, since each enantiomer must be characterized separately for safety issues [23,24]. However, it was found that the atropisomers of analog **13** rapidly interconvert in pH 7 buffer with a half-life of only a few minutes, thus diminishing this concern [22]. Deprotonation of the phenolic oxygen will be more pronounced at pH 7 and higher, leading to greater access to the putative transitional intermediate C (Fig. 4), which may help to explain the relative ease of atropisomer interconversion at higher pH.

The greater steric bulk of the isopropyl substituent in compound **2** raised the possibility that it would undergo interconversion of the atropisomers at a significantly slower rate than for compound **13**. MMMF calculations indicated an difference of about 8 kcal between **2** and **13** (26 vs. 18 kcal;

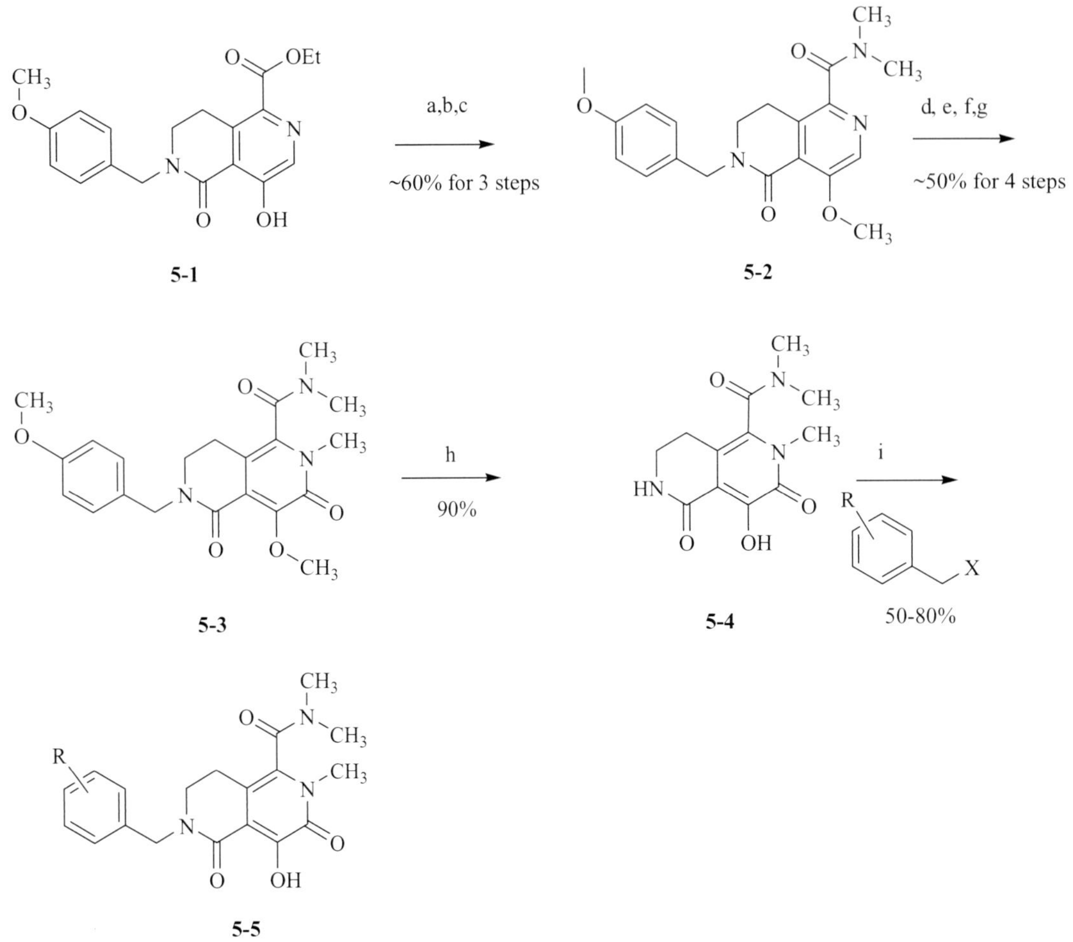

SCHEME 5 Alternative route to analogs with different *N*-benzyl substituents. (a) TMSCHN$_2$, CH$_2$Cl$_2$, CH$_3$OH; (b) LiOH, THF; (c) (CH$_3$)$_2$NH, EDC, HOAT, TEA, THF; (d) mCPBA, CH$_2$Cl$_2$; (e) Ac$_2$O, 110°C, 16 to 24 h; (f) NaOCH$_3$; (g) Mg(OCH$_3$)$_2$, CH$_3$I; (h) 33% HBr/HOAc sealed tube 75°C, 16 h; (i) NaH, DMF, RPhCH$_2$X.

Fig. 5) in the energy barrier for interconversion [25]. The barrier to interconversion was estimated using a torsional drive on the angle indicated in Figure 3.

To extend these investigations into more physiologically relevant conditions, the atropisomers of **2** were incubated in water and in human plasma and the rate of atropisomers interconversion was determined by chiral HPLC. Interconversion of the two atropisomers of **2** in an aqueous environment was strongly influenced by pH. In water, the material became a 15 : 85 mixture of enantiomers in 60 min. Lowering pH slowed the interconversion, and raising the pH gave more rapid interconversion. In human plasma at 9 μM concentration, the $t_{1/2}$ of interconversion is too fast to measure by these methods, with complete interconversion observed in less than 30 min. Similar rates of interconversion were observed in dog, rat, and rhesus plasma. It was concluded that interconversion of the atropisomers *in vivo* was likely to be so rapid as not to pose any developmental hurdle [23].

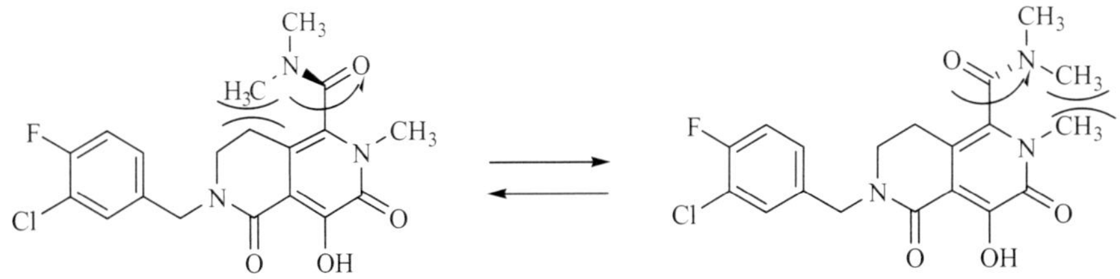

FIGURE 3 Hindered rotation of the external amide bond of tetrahydronaphthyridine analog **13**.

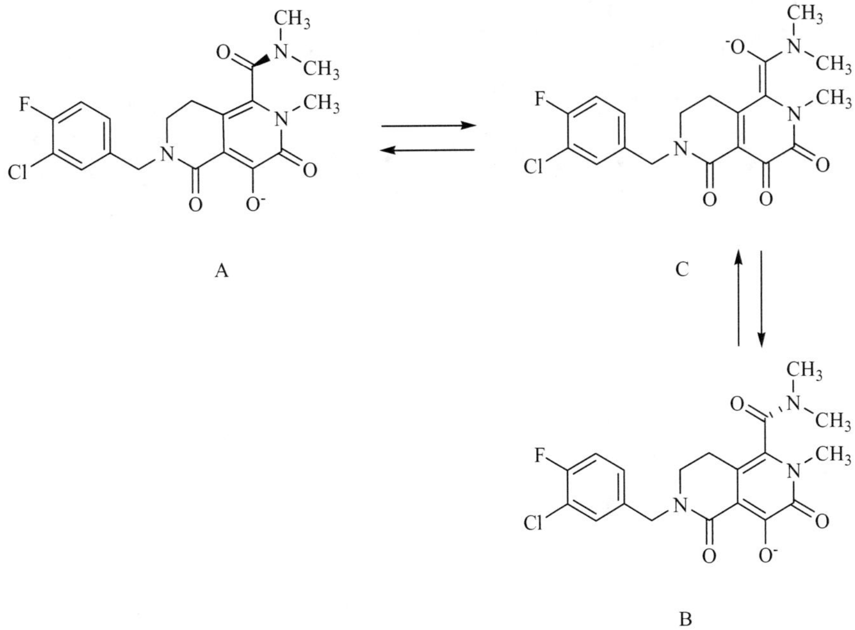

FIGURE 4 Tautomers of deprotonated analog **13**.

The analogs in Table 1 were prepared and evaluated for their strand transfer and antiviral activity in vitro. Strand transfer inhibition and antiviral activity for analogs **7** to **15** are shown in Table 1. The first four analogs (**7** to **10**) possessing a 4-fluorobenzyl group were explored with varying substitution on the amide and pyridine nitrogen. While the compounds were potent inhibitors of strand transfer reaction, they showed > 300 nM antiviral activity in assay conditions with low or high serum concentrations. As a group (compounds **7** to **10**) the compounds possessed a partition coefficient (log *P*) of < 1. Addition of a 3-chloro substituent on the benzyl ring increased the log *P* values into the > 1 to 2.5 range. While the intrinsic strand transfer activity of analogs **7** to **10** was similar to that of the chloro analogs **11** to **13**, the chloro-substituted analogs' antiviral activity was improved two- to 28-fold even in the presence of 50% human serum, perhaps as the result of improved cell permeability.

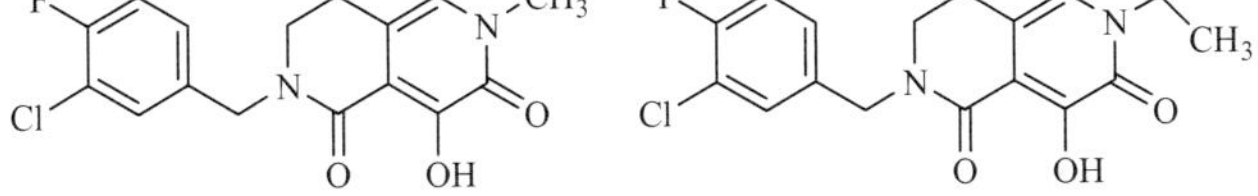

13 18 kcal/mol **2** 26 kcal/mol

FIGURE 5 MMMF calculation of energy barrier for interconversion of atropisomers of compounds **13** and **2**.

Alkylation of the amide NH or the pyrimidinone NH was associated with lowering of protein binding (compare analog **7** to analogs **8** and **10**, and analog **13** to analogs **11** and **12**). Compounds possessing both 4-F,3-Cl-benzyl substitution and per-alkylation of the amide and pyrimidinone showed the best profiles. In particular, compounds **11, 13, 14**, and **2** showed excellent inhibition of integrase activity in the strand transfer inhibition assay and were < 100 nM in the antiviral cell assay in the presence of 50% human serum. Although intrinsically quite potent, the isobutyl analog **15** lost activity in cell culture relative to the other analogs, probably due to its greater affinity for plasma proteins.

The emergence of HIV mutants that exhibit resistance to treatment is a well-documented and worrisome reality of antiviral therapy. To illustrate, the x-ray structure of the catalytic domain of integrase is shown in Fig. 6 [28]. Shown in yellow are the three catalytic residues: aspartic acids 64 and 116 and glutamic acid 152. Aspartic acids 64 and 116 are shown with magnesium bound to them, as it is known that Mg^{2+} is required to catalyze the 3′-processing and strand transfer reactions [29].

Studies were undertaken to better understand the relationship between inhibitor structure and the evolution of mutant viruses. Serial passage experiments with different structural classes of integrase inhibitors have generated drug-resistant viruses, which have been characterized to reveal their amino acid substitution around the catalytic site [30,31]. After serial incubations, the diketo acid **16** [8] (Fig. 7) selects for mutations in the amino acids residues highlighted in green (S153Y, T66I/S153Y, S153Y/N155S). Napthyridine (**4**) selects for those in magenta (F121Y/T125K). Compound **1**

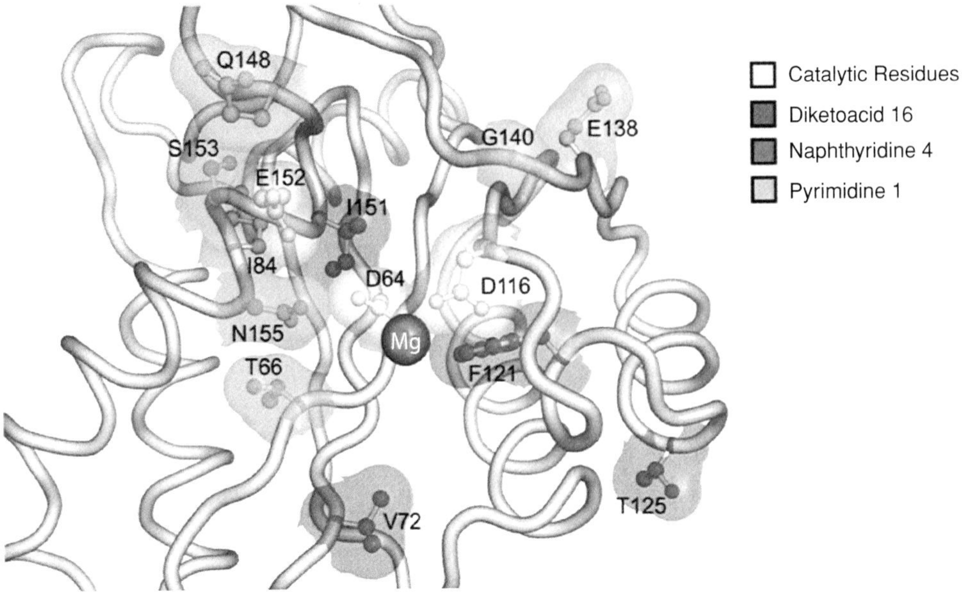

FIGURE 6 Modeling depiction of x-ray data for an HIV integrase active site. Colored residues (magenta, cyan, green) indicate residues found in mutant viruses generated from extended serial passage of cells cultured with integrase inhibitors of different structural classes. Yellow: HIV integrase catalytic residues [28]. Green: amino acids mutated in response to prolonged incubation with a diketo acid inhibitor (compound **16**). Pink: amino acids mutated in response to prolonged incubation with a naphthyridine analog inhibitor (compound **4**). Light blue: amino acids mutated in response to prolonged incubation with a pyrimidine analog inhibitor (compound **1**). (*See insert for color reprensentation of the figure.*)

produces mutations in the amino acids highlighted in light blue (Q148K, E138A/G148K, E138A/G140A/Q148K).

To summarize these findings, these catalytic domain mutations strongly suggest that these inhibitors are binding to the catalytic site. Structurally different inhibitors selected for different sets of mutants, indicating that they appear to be binding in different orientations within the catalytic domain. Mutation residues occur throughout the catalytic site. Interestingly, N155 and Q148 mutations can confer cross-resistance to all structural classes.

As research has progressed, a panel of laboratory mutants was selected to evaluate next-generation inhibitors. Mutant viruses were constructed using site-directed mutagenesis. The ability of integrase inhibitors to inhibit viral reproduction is assessed with a single-cycle infectivity assay [30,31].

Potency against the panel of mutant viruses improves significantly with greater steric bulk of the R1 substituents for **13**, **14**, **2**, and **15** (Table 2). Compound **2** maintains good potency against T66I/S153Y, Q148K, and F121Y, with only a three-fold decrease against these single and double mutants. Compounds **2** and **15** exhibit significant effect against the triple mutant isolated from in vitro passage with **1**. Furthermore, compound **2** demonstrates a significant improvement in mutation profile when compared to the first-generation inhibitors **1** (MK-0518) and Elvitegravir (GS-9137) (Fig. 8) [32].

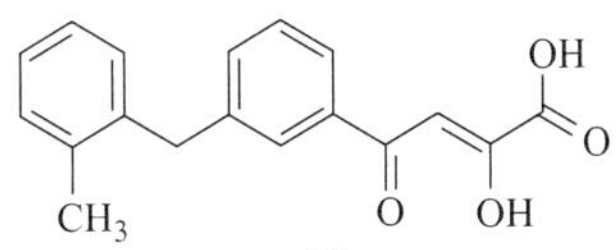

16

FIGURE 7 Structure of diketo acid (**16**) used in serial passage to generate mutant in vitro.

It is generally believed that the key to maintaining suppression of mutant virus is the ability to maintain trough levels of HIV inhibitors that are in excess of the IC_{95} of the inhibitor. Pharmacokinetic (PK) profiles consistent with once- or twice-daily a day dosing that maintain or exceed these trough levels are therefore very important. The PK profile of compound **2** was examined in rats and dogs and was very encouraging (Fig. 9). In rats, the mean trough level at 24 h after an oral dose of 10 mg/kg was 250 nM, 6.25-fold the IC_{95} for the compound (35 nM), and in dogs the mean trough level 24 h after a 2-mg/kg oral dose was 62 nM.

Many HIV-infected patients are treated with HIV protease inhibitors, which either have P450 enzyme inhibitory activity themselves or are co-dosed with ritonavir, a potent P450 inhibitor, to extend their half-life and exposure [33,34]. It has proved relatively straightforward to add compound **1** to the dosing regimens of such patients, as it is eliminated not through the action of P450 enzymes but by the formation of the *O*-glucuronide through UGT enzyme activity [1].

TABLE 2 Mutation Profiles: Inhibition of Mutant Virus by Tetrahydronaphthyridine Integrase Strand Transfer Inhibitors

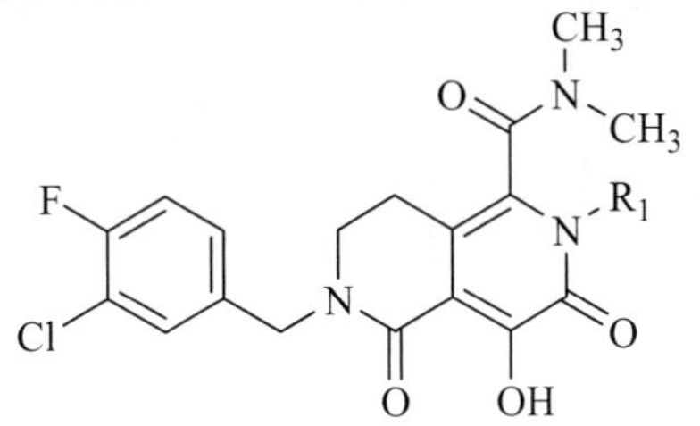

Compound	R_1	Antiviral Activity in Cell Culture (50% NHS) (IC_{95}, nM)	Ratio of IC_{50} in Single-Cycle Infectivity Assay[a] for Mutant Virus vs. Wild-Type Virus				
			T66I/S153Y	N155S	Q148K	E138A/G140A/ Q148K	F121Y
1		52	1	17	48	388	3
4		93	3	18	12	607	8
11	H	19	4	18	N.A.	N.A.	6
13	CH_3	91	6	27	20	462	7
14	Et	34	2	32	4	N.A.	3
2	*i*Pr	35	1	3	1	118	1
15	*i*Bu	337	1	4	1	86	2

[a]See [30,31] for assay details. N.A., not available.

Examination of the metabolism of compound **2** in rats and dogs found that it, too, is eliminated primarily through the UGT pathway and therefore may also be an excellent candidate for addition to the optimized background therapy (OBT) regimen for patients. Incubation of **13** and **2** in dog and human hepatocytes provided a measure of intrinsic stability for these compounds across species (Table 3). Both compounds showed low human hepatocyte clearance, thus producing a low predicted human clearance. For compound **2**, the human clearance predicted is 0.9 ± 0.6 mL·min/kg.

Compounds **13** and **2** were identified as compounds suitable for further exploration in a clinical setting. Their large-scale synthesis therefore became necessary. It was envisaged that a synthetic sequence similar to the medicinal chemistry route could furnish the requisite drug candidate in quantities sufficient to support exploratory clinical trials. The

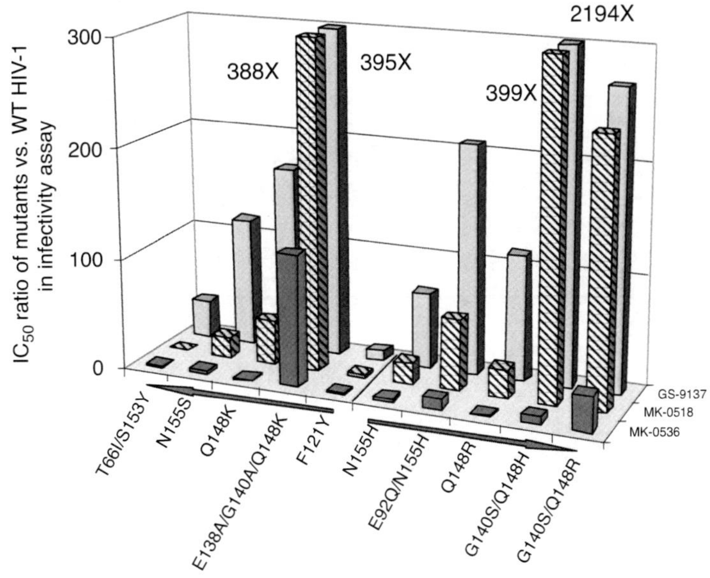

FIGURE 8 Ratios of compound IC_{50s} for laboratory and clinical mutant virus vs. wild-type virus.

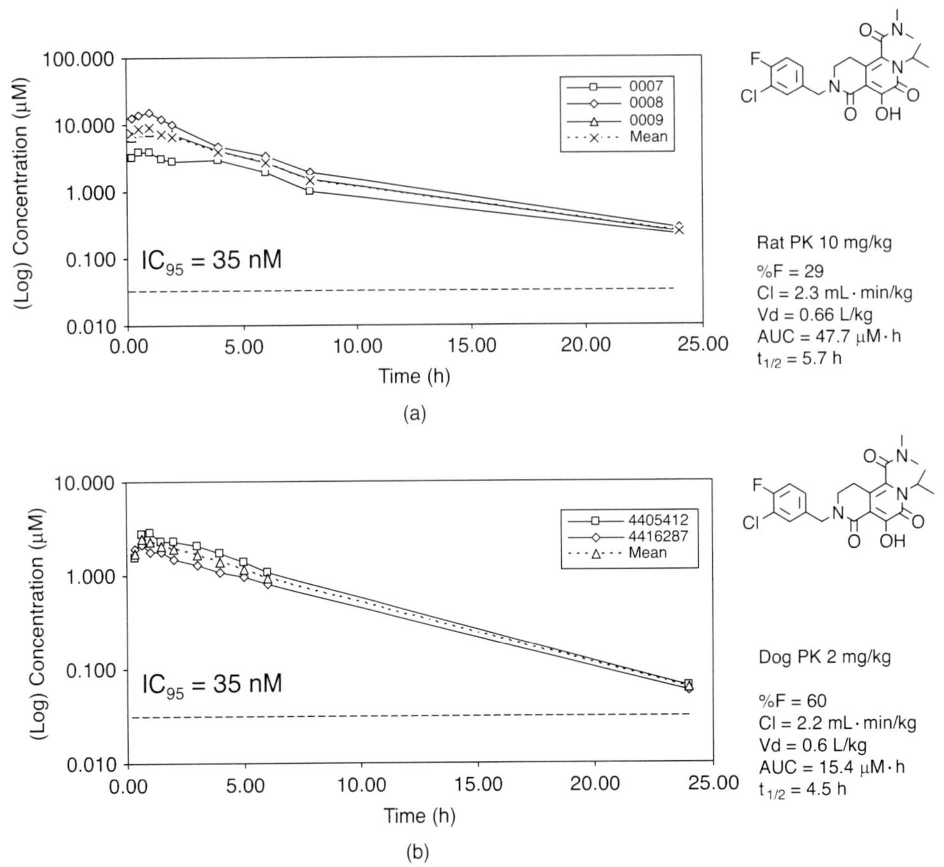

FIGURE 9 (a) Rat and (b) dog PK for compound **2**. Nat salt, P.O., in 0.5% methylcellulose: rat, 10 mg/kg; dog, 2 mg/kg.

TABLE 3 Dog and Human Hepatocyte Stability of Compounds 13 and 2[a]

	Antiviral Assay (IC_{95}, nM) (50% NHS)	Hepatocyte Stability Assay (Cl, mL·min/kg)	
		Dog	Human
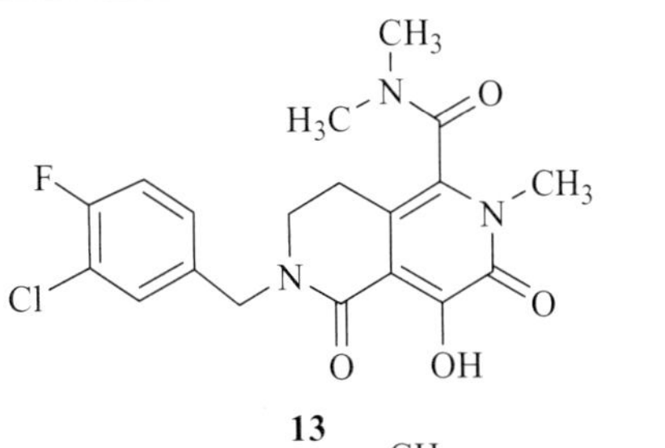 **13**	91	3.6	1.8
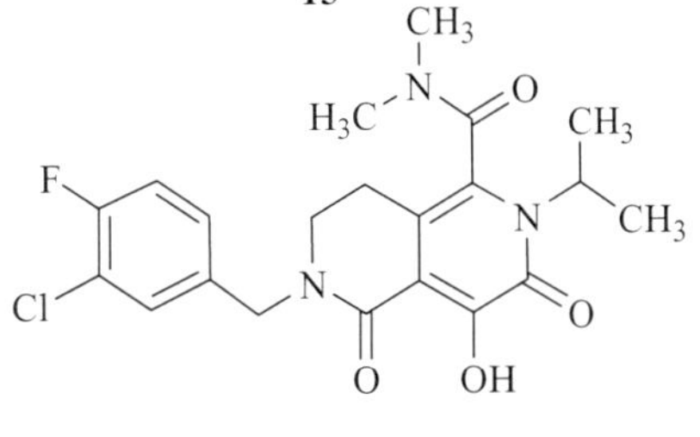 **2**, MK-0536; low predicted human clearance: 0.9 ± 0.6 mL · min/kg	35	10	3

[a]Human clearance predicted, using the well-stirred model [35].

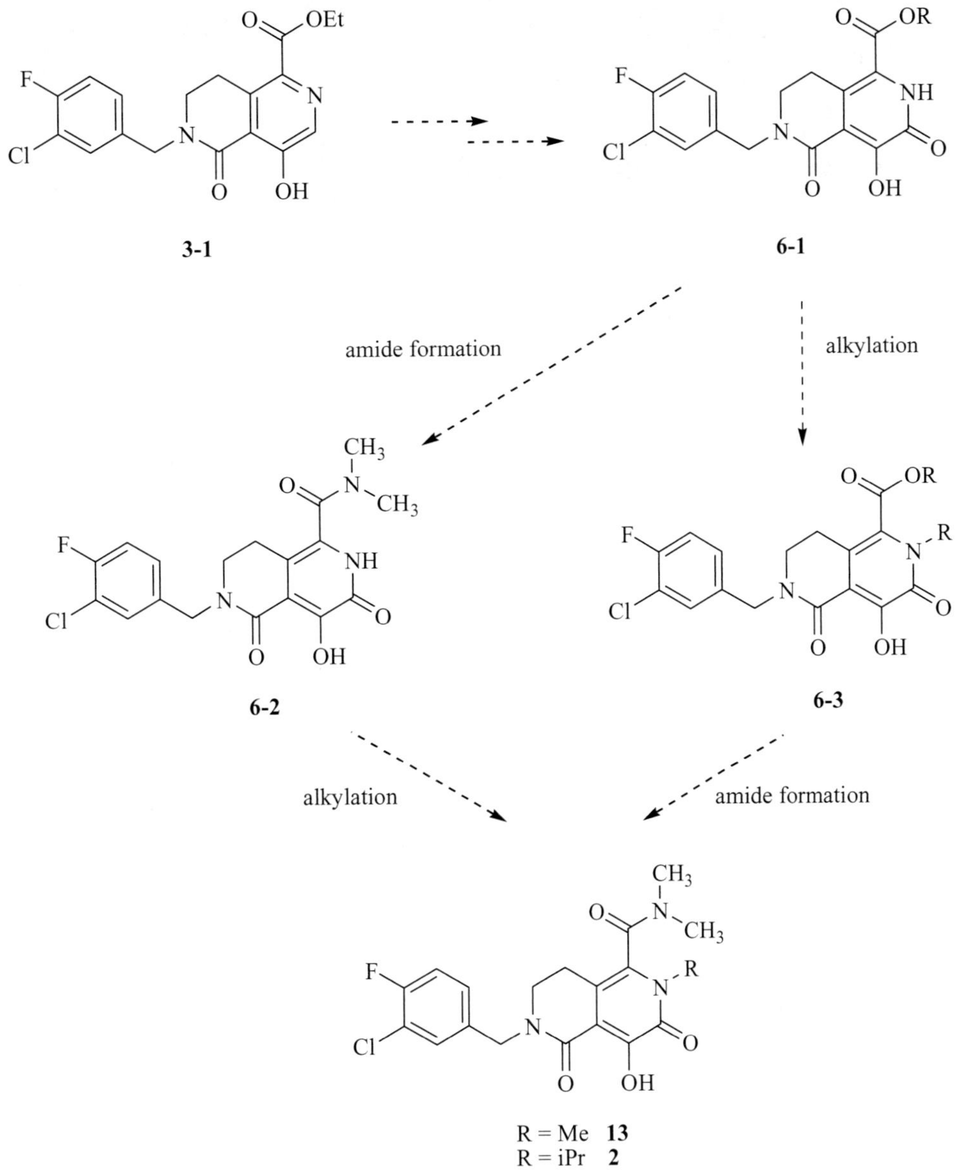

SCHEME 6 Proposed process optimization scheme for synthesis of compounds **13** and **2**.

Diels–Alder product **3-1** was determined to be a key intermediate (Scheme 6). Efficient elaboration to an intermediate like **6-1** would allow flexibility in the final approach, which could explore the medicinal chemistry route of alkylation to give **6-3**, followed by amide formation, or replace it with an alternative scheme of amide formation to give **6-2** followed by alkylation to give the final products.

Before the route could be employed to prepare kilogram quantities of drug, several scalability and reaction safety concerns had to be addressed, including reduction of the number of steps and/or number of isolation steps, elimination of time-consuming chromatographic purifications, and overall yield improvement.

Compound **3-1** is a common intermediate in the syntheses of both **2** and **13** (Scheme 6). Consequently, a robust and efficient synthesis of this compound was paramount to support each delivery of bulk drug. Closer examination of the Diels–Alder reaction of oxazole **2-6** and dienophile **2-3** showed that **3-1** was formed regioselectively in a 9 : 1 ratio over the other possible Diels–Alder product **7-2** (Scheme 7). In developing the large-scale synthesis of **3-1**, several safety and reaction issues had to be overcome. These included: (1) detrimental formation of **7-1** in the reaction between glycine butyl ester **2-4** with diethyl oxalate, which resulted in loss of yield and necessitated chromatographic purification of the oxalate **2-5**; (2) inefficient stirring of the reaction mass due

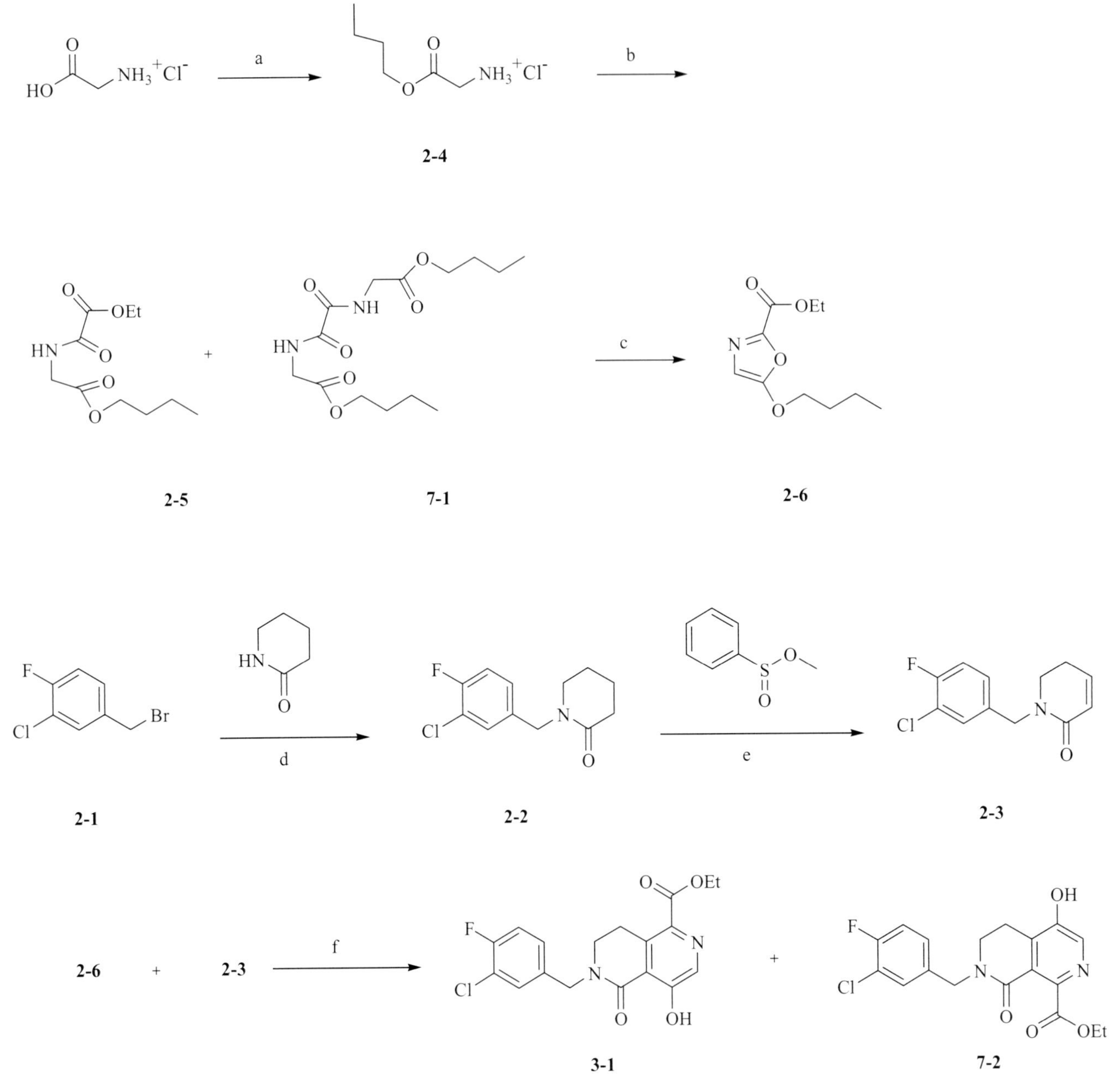

SCHEME 7 Process optimization of intermediate **3-1**: impurities to be avoided and optimized reaction conditions. (a) $SOCl_2$, BuOH, 95% yield; (b) ethyl oxalyl chloride, Et_3N, EtOH, 94% yield; (c) P_2O_5, CH_3CN, 80% yield; (d) 50% NaOH, Bu_4NHSO_4, *tert*-$BuOCH_3$, 93% yield; (e) LiHMDS, $PhS(O)OCH_3$, heat, 90% yield; (f), neat, 1 mol% H_2O, 130°C, 70% yield.

to gel formation in the subsequent cyclization–dehydration step to form **2-6**; (3) evolution of large volumes of hydrogen gas from the use of sodium hydride in the alkylation of valerolactam to give the N-substituted product **2-2**; and (4) difficulty in scaling the cycloaddition step, since this involved a solvent-free reaction in a sealed tube at 130°C and isolation via triturating the solid formed upon cooling, as well as chromatographic purification on a large scale to removed unwanted regioisomer **7-2**.

The first issue was solved when **2-4** was caused to react with commercially available ethyl oxalyl chloride. This resulted in isolation of **2-5** in 94% yield and of sufficient quality to be used in the next step without prior purification, as no bisamide **7-1** was detected. Second, the cyclization–dehydration of **2-5** with P_2O_5 to afford the oxazole **2-6** required precise control of temperature and initial reaction concentration. Mixtures of P_2O_5 aged in acetonitrile with moderate heating (30 to 40°C) are prone to go through a phase-change phenomenon resulting in a gelatinous mass that is difficult to agitate. Adding a portion of the oxalate in acetonitrile (5 to 10% of charge) to the reaction slurry prior to warming overcame gel formation. Alternatively, the addition of an inert filter aid, Solka Floc, prior to heating also alleviated gel formation. Quenching the batch under safe operating conditions was achieved by steady transfer of the reaction mixture to chilled water, resulting in a two-phase mixture. Extraction with ethyl acetate gave a stock solution of **2-6** that was used directly in the next step.

Third, a safer, more efficient formation of **2-2** was achieved under phase transfer conditions (NaOH/Bu_4NHSO_4/MTBE), which provided the added advantage of improved yield and product purity. Finally, formation of **3-1** proved to be an interesting problem to solve at scale. The original small-scale procedure called for the reaction to be run without organic solvent in the presence of 1 mole equivalent of water, and at 130°C in a sealed tube with product solidification upon cooling. Interestingly, the reaction failed in a variety of solvents and was unaffected by the presence of typical Lewis acids employed in Diels–Alder reactions. The confounding issues of product solidifying, variability in yield, and the need to remove the unwanted Diels–Alder regioisomer raised concerns of ease of isolation and reproducibility at scale. Fortunately, we overcame these issues by performing the reaction in a sealed autoclave at 130°C in the presence of 5 to 10% water (the reaction developed 200 psi of pressure at the kilogram reaction scale). Once the reaction was complete, *N*-methylpyrolidine was added to prevent solidification of the reaction upon cooling. After cooling to 20 to 25°C, 1 : 1 water–ethanol was added to the solution and the product was crystallized with complete rejection of undesired regioisomer **7-2**. The desired product **3-1** was isolated in 65 to 70% yield and > 99% purity (Scheme 7).

With a reliable synthesis of **3-1** now in hand, our attention was drawn to the safe and scalable conversion of **3-1** to compound **13** via compound **8-1** (Scheme 8). The original oxidation conditions involved the use of 30 wt% aqueous hydrogen peroxide in glacial acetic acid at 100°C. The *N*-oxide **4-1** formed was then isolated in approximately 95% yield and heated in acetic anhydride at 100°C to give the rearrangement product as the bisacetate **4-3**. Isolation of **4-3** followed by cleavage with sodium ethoxide then gave **8-1** in 86% yield over the two steps. Besides safety concerns connected to performing this reaction at scale, significant amounts (10 to 15%) of unsaturated product **8-2** were formed that could be effectively removed only by chromatography.

For large-scale preparation of intermediate **8-1** a more efficient and safer process was developed (Scheme 8). By carrying out the reaction with commercially available 32% per-acetic acid in acetic acid as the oxidant at 45 to 50°C, **4-1** was formed in > 95% assay yield. To increase efficiency in the oxidation–rearrangement process, **4-1** was not isolated and instead carried through into the next stage as a solution in toluene. Addition of acetic anhydride to the solution, then heating to 100°C, gave the bisacetate **4-3**, and cleavage of the acetate groups with sodium ethoxide afforded the desired product **8-1** in 75 to 80% overall yield from **3-1**. Using these conditions, < 0.5% of **8-2** was observed in the final product.

Scale-up issues also needed to be resolved for the N-methylation step leading to **4-6** (Scheme 8), including the use of copious amounts of methyl iodide, and inconsistent yields due to reaction stalling. Conditions that overcame reaction stalling were developed. By removing excess CH_3OH prior to addition of the alkylating reagent and replacing methyl iodide with methyl tosylate, the reaction consistently gave > 95% conversion, and isolation of crude material, followed by swishing in hot methanol as a purification step, afforded the intermediate **4-6** in 70% yield. The original procedure for conversion of **4-6** to **13** called for four consecutive reactions involving protection of the hydroxyl group, saponification of the ester to the acid, in situ formation of the acid chloride, and then subsequent reaction with dimethylamine. Finally, deprotection of the hydroxyl group and chromatographic purification afforded the desired product **13** in 27% yield from **4-6** (Scheme 8).

To minimize the number of steps involved, an efficient direct conversion of intermediate **4-6** to the desired compound **13** was developed (Scheme 8). No reaction was observed between **4-6** and $(CH_3)_2AlN(CH_3)_2$ or $HN(CH_3)_2/MgCl_2$, and an unclean reaction was observed from the reaction of **4-6** with $LiN(CH_3)_2$. However, efficient direct conversion to **13** was achieved by reacting **4-6** with $(CH_3)_2NMgCl$ (prepared in situ from 2 M dimethylamine in THF and 2 M ^{i}PrMgCl in THF) to afford **13** in 84% yield and 97% purity. The reaction proceeds with concomitant formation of the unsaturated lactam **8-3**, at 1 to 1.5%. Formation of the unsaturated lactam is not understood. NMR evidence clearly suggested that it is not an artifact of previous reactions. Indeed, with a combination of higher reaction temperatures (> 0°C) and longer reaction times, increased levels of the lactam **8-3** (concentrations as high as 10% were observed). Fortunately, the impurity may be removed to acceptable levels (< 0.5%) by treatment of an ethanolic solution of the product with Darco G 60 to give the final product (**13**) in > 99% purity and 71% overall assay yield from **4-6**.

The next goal was to develop a large-scale preparation of compound **2** (Scheme 9). Initial probe reactions exploring the synthesis of compound **2** indicated that an alternative, more efficient route would be required to support multikilogram, bulk drug demands. However, with a change in the order of chemical transformations (i.e., amidation prior to oxidation, then alkylation), judicious application of the final-stage chemistry developed for compound **13** would suffice in delivering initial drug quantities to meet pressing project time lines (Scheme 9). Direct amidation of **3-1** by $(CH_3)_2NMgCl$ gave modest yields, but amidation of the acid chloride, formed in situ from the acid **9-1**, gave pure amide **9-2** in > 95% isolated

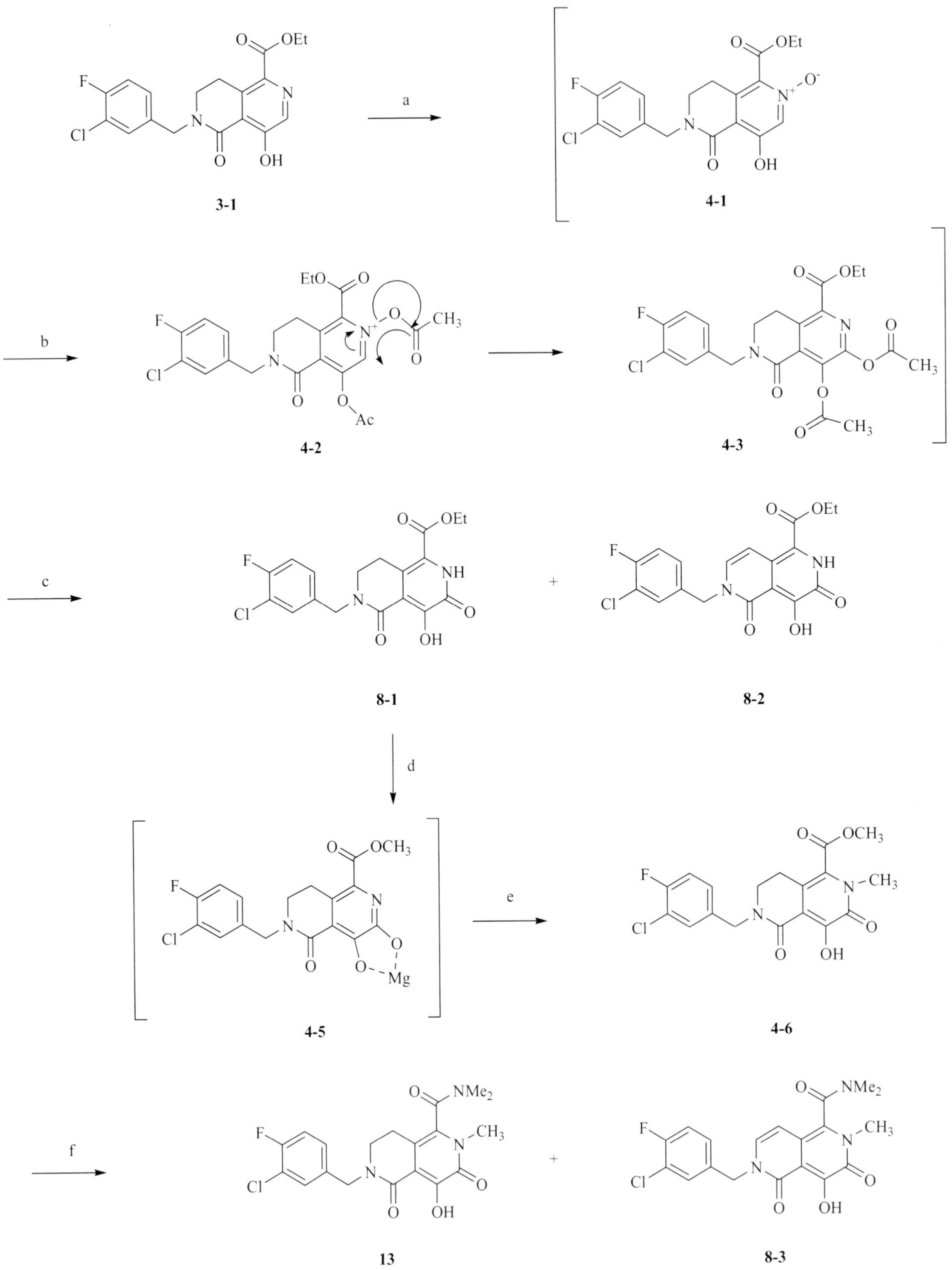

SCHEME 8 Process optimization for the late-stage synthesis of compound **13**. Impurities to be avoided and optimized reaction conditions. (a) CH_3CO_3H, AcOH, NaOAc, 50°C, 99% yield; (b) Ac_2O, C_7H_8, 100°C; (c) NaOEt, 80% yield; (d) $Mg(OCH_3)_2$ in CH_3OH, DMF; (e) CH_3OTs, 45°C; (f) 3 to 4 mol equiv $ClMgN(CH_3)_2$, THF/CH_2Cl_2, −10 to 0°C.

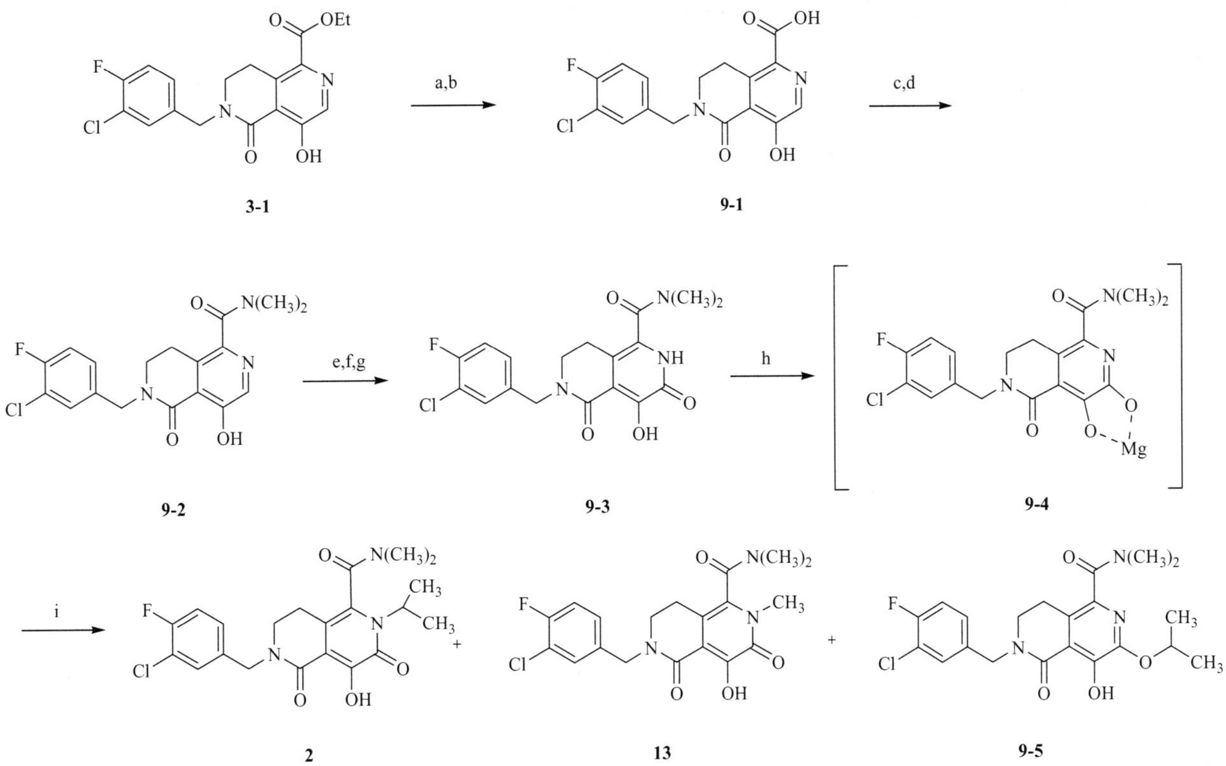

SCHEME 9 Process optimization for the synthetic scheme leading from **3-1** to **2**. Impurities to be avoided and optimized conditions. (a) 10 N NaOH, C_2H_5OH, reflux; (b) 5 N HCl; (c) $(COCl)_2$, cat. DMF, CH_2Cl_2; (d) 2 M $HN(CH_3)_2$ in THF; (e) CH_3CO_3H, NaOAc, AcOH, 50°C; (f) Ac_2O, heat; (g) NaOEt; (h) $Mg(OCH_3)_2$ in CH_3OH; (i) $^{i\text{-}}$PrBr, DMSO, 40°C.

yield. Oxidation and rearrangement under conditions described above afforded **9-3** in 80% yield (Scheme 9).

Scale-up of the final two steps indeed proved to be problematic. In the penultimate step, which utilized transient protection of the hydroxyl groups as the magnesium bis-alkoxide **9-4**, stringent removal of methanol was critical; otherwise, competitive formation of *N*-methyl analog **13** was observed. This presumably resulted from in situ formation of methyl iodide from the reaction between CH_3OH and MgI_2 formed during the reaction. In the final alkylation step, DMSO proved to be the optimal aprotic solvent, and control of reaction temperature was key to obtaining > 95% conversion. With reaction temperatures > 50°C, competitive reaction of isopropyl iodide with DMSO was observed, leading to incomplete reactions and consequently to contamination of final product with **9-3**. Unfortunately, under these conditions unavoidable formation of the *O*-isopropyl product **9-5** was observed. Although significant amounts (~ 45%) of **9-5** were obtained, the desired product (**2**) was isolated from the mixture via selective crystallization from ethyl acetate/cyclohexane, and final re crystallization from acetone/methyl *tert*-butyl ether gave **2** in 42% yield, 99% purity, in sufficient amounts to support early clinical work.

A more efficient and chromatography-free synthesis [36] was later developed to supply bulk drug, whereby N-alkylation is introduced prior to forming the naphthyridone ring (Scheme 10). Conversion of **10-7** to **10-9** was developed as a through process, whereby conjugate addition of diphenylketimine glycine amide **10-4** (prepared in four steps from CBZ-glycine **10-1** in 57% overall yield), followed by reduction amination with acetone, gives isopropyl amine intermediate **10-9**. This is followed by reaction with ethyl oxalyl chloride to furnished the penultimate oxalate intermediate **10-10** in 45% overall yield from **10-7**. Ring closure was caused by treatment of **10-10** with DABCO to afford **2** in 80% isolated yield and > 99% purity.

CONCLUSIONS

In summary, a novel heterocyclic template that combined structural features from earlier classes of integrase compounds can be prepared by an efficient water-catalyzed Diels–Alder reaction. Exploration of the substitution in this series led to the discovery of potent integrase inhibitors with excellent activity against mutant virus raised both in vitro and in the clinic. Compound **2** proved particularly effective. Compound **2** was also found to possess excellent pharmacokinetics, and studies in human hepatocytes led to a low predicted human clearance. Modification of the initial

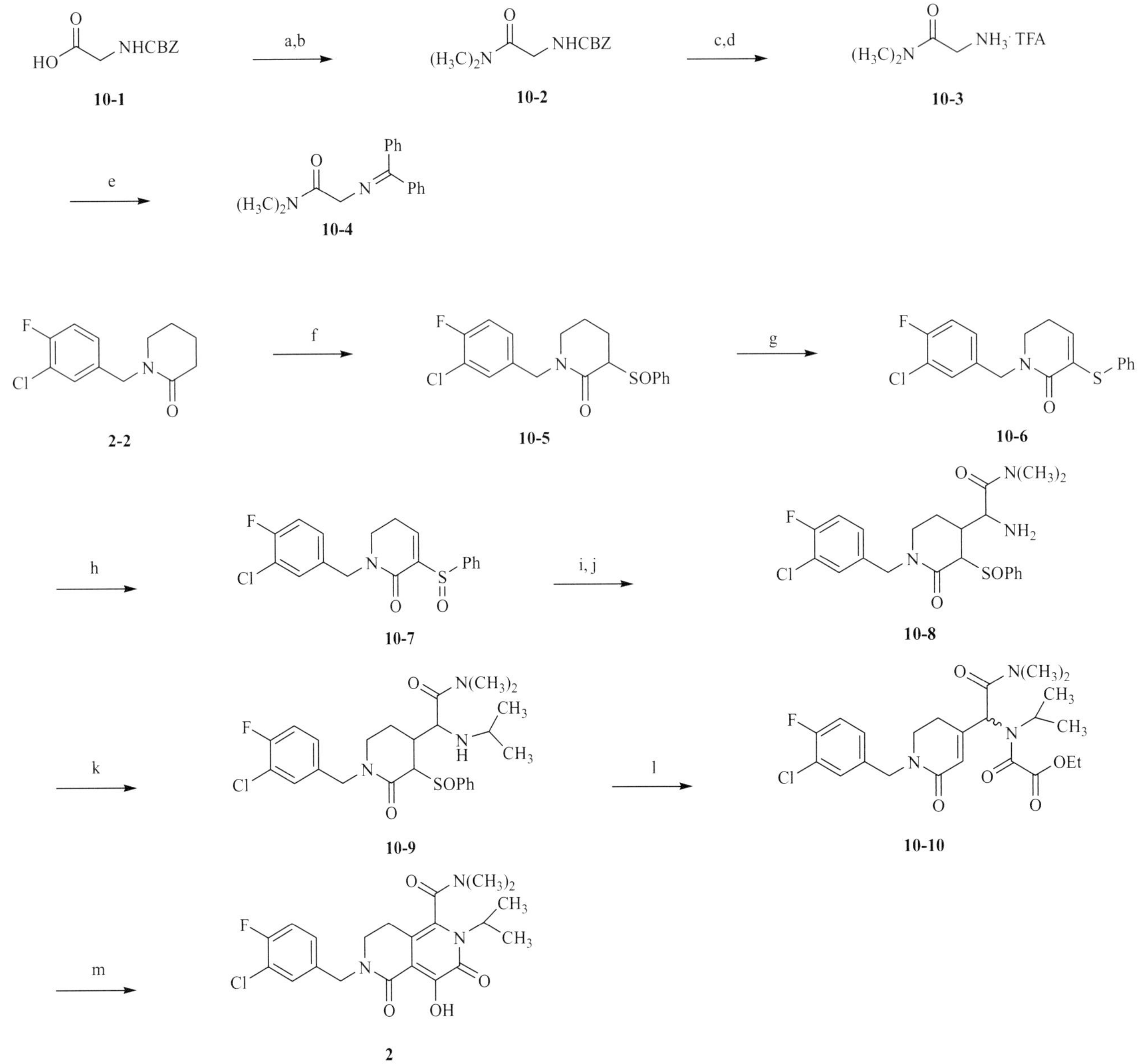

SCHEME 10 Alternative efficient synthetic route to compound **2**. (a) CDI, EtOAc; (b) 2 M $HN(CH_3)_2$ in THF; (c) H_2, Pd/C, CH_3OH; (d) CF_3CO_2H; (e) HN=CPh_2, CH_2Cl_2; (f) $C_6H_5S(O)OCH_3$, LiHMDS, THF; (g) Ac_2O, CH_3SO_3H, CH_3CN; (h) $NaIO_4$, CH_3OH, H_2O; (i) **10-4**; (j) 2 N HCl; (k) $NaHB(OAc)_3$, acetone; (l) EtOCOCOCl, Et_3N, C_7H_8 0 to 90°C; (m) DABCO, LiBr, THF.

synthesis produced an efficient process that allowed large-scale synthesis to support preclinical and clinical studies.

Acknowledgments

We would like to acknowledge the dedicated efforts of the many people who contributed to this work. In particular, we thank those people whose work is featured in this report: Wei Han, who designed the tetrahydronaphthyridine template (**6**); Rowena Ruzek, Cuthbert Martyr, Debbie Perlow, and Lou Anne Neilson, who contributed to the medicinal chemistry routes disclosed; Roger Farr, Bruce Foster, and Ulf Dolling, who contributed to the early process development work; Philip Pye, Remy Angelaud, Danny Mancheno, and Dave Askin, who created the process chemistry scheme outlined in Scheme 10; Kate Holloway, for the modeling and interpretation of the integrase catalytic domain depicted in Fig. 7; Chris Culberson, who provided the MMMF calculations depicted in Fig. 5; Mirlinda Biba and Chris Welch for their work on the separation and characterization of the atropisomers of compound **13**; Carl Homnick and Kristy Hoffman, for their work on separating and characterizing the interconversion of the atropisomers of compound **2**; Rick Woodward, Jim Guare, Joe Pawluczyk, and John Swestock for their synthetic scale-up support for our medicinal chemistry efforts; Marc Witmer, who provided mutation profiling support; and Chris Kochansky and Reza Anari for DMPK support.

REFERENCES

[1] Summa, V.; Petrocchi, A.; Bonelli, F.; Crescenzi, B.; Donghi, M.; Ferrara, M.; Fiore, F.; Gardelli, C.; Paz, O. G.; Hazuda, D. J.; et al. Discovery of Raltegravir, a potent, selective orally bioavailable HIV-integrase inhibitor for the treatment of HIV-AIDS infection. *J. Med. Chem.* **2008**, *51*, 5843–5855.

[2] Grinsztejn, B.; Nguyen, B. Y.; Katlama, C.; Gatell, J. M.; Lazzarin, A.; Vittecoq, D.; Gonzalez, C. J.; Chen, J.; Harvey, C. M.; Isaacs, R. D. Safety and efficacy of the HIV-1 integrase inhibitor raltegravir (MK-0518) in treatment-experienced patients with multidrug-resistant virus: a phase II randomised controlled trial. *Lancet* **2007**, *369*, 1261–1269.

[3] Hazuda, D.; Iwamoto, M.; Wenning, L. Emerging pharmacology: inhibitors of human immunodeficiency virus integration. *Ann. Rev. Pharmacol. Toxicol.* **2009**, *49*, 377–394.

[4] Markowitz, M.; Nguyen, B. Y.; Gotuzzo, E.; Mendo, F.; Ratanasuwan, W.; Kovacs, C.; Prada, G.; Morales-Ramirez, J. O.; Crumpacker, C. S.; Isaacs, R. D.; et al. Rapid and durable antiretroviral effect of the HIV-1 Integrase inhibitor raltegravir as part of combination therapy in treatment-naive patients with HIV-1 infection: results of a 48-week controlled study. *J. Acquir. Immune Defic. Synd.* **2007**, *46*, 125–133.

[5] Han, W.; Egbertson, M.; Wai, J. S.; Zhuang, L.; Ruzek, R. D.; Perlow, D. S.; Isaacs, R. C. A.; Cameron, M.; Foster, B. S.; Dolling, U. H.; et al. Preparation of hydroxynaphthyridinediones as HIV integrase inhibitors. WO 2005087768, Sept. 3, 2005.

[6] Hazuda, D. J.; Felock, P.; Witmer, M.; Wolfe, A.; Stillmock, K.; Grobler, J. A.; Espeseth, A.; Gabryelski, L.; Schleif, W.; Blau, C.; Miller, M. D. Inhibitors of strand transfer that prevent integration and inhibit HIV-1 replication in cells. *Science* **2000**, *287*, 646–650.

[7] Selnick, H. G.; Hazuda, D. J.; Egbertson, M.; Guare, J. P.; Wai, J. S.; Young, S. D.; Clark, D. L.; Medina, J. C. Preparation of nitrogen-containing 4-heteroaryl-2,4-dioxobutyric acids useful as HIV integrase inhibitors. Merck & Co., Inc. 99-US12095[9962513], 287, Dec. 9, 1999; WO, June 1, 1999.

[8] Wai, J. S.; Egbertson, M. S.; Payne, L. S.; Fisher, T. E.; Embrey, M. W.; Tran, L. O.; Melamed, J. Y.; Langford, H. M.; Guare, J. P., Jr.; Zhuang, L.; et al. 4-Aryl-2,4-dioxobutanoic acid inhibitors of HIV-1 integrase and viral replication in cells. *J. Med. Chem.* **2000**, *43*, 4923–4926.

[9] Young, S. D.; Egbertson, M.; Pearson, P. G.; Wai, J. S.; Fisher, T. E.; Guare, J. P.; Embrey, M. W.; Tran, L. O.; Zhuang, L.; Vacca, J.; et al. Preparation of aromatic and heteroaromatic 4-aryl-2,4-dioxobutyric acid derivatives useful as HIV integrase inhibitors. Merck & Co., Inc. 99-US12093[9962520], 319, Dec. 9, 1999; WO, June 1, 1999.

[10] Egbertson, M.; Langford, H. M.; Melamed, J.; Wai, J. S.; Han, W.; Perlow, D. S.; Zhuang, L.; Embrey, M.; Young, S. D. Preparation of *N*-(substituted benzyl)-8-hydroxy-1,6-naphthyridine-7-carboxamides useful as HIV integrase inhibitors for treatment of HIV infection/AIDS. Merck & Co., Inc. 2003-US7671[2003077857], 217, Sept. 25, 2003; WO, Mar. 12, 2003.

[11] Anthony, N. J.; Gomez, R. P.; Young, S. D.; Egbertson, M.; Wai, J. S.; Zhuang, L.; Embrey, M.; Tran, L. O.; Melamed, J.; Langford, H. M.; et al. Preparation of (poly)azanaphthalenyl carboxamides as HIV integrase inhibitors. Merck & Co., Inc. 2001-US31456[2002030930], 434. Apr. 18, 2002. WO, Oct. 9, 2001.

[12] Pace, P.; Di Francesco, M. E.; Gardelli, C.; Harper, S.; Muraglia, E.; Nizi, E.; Orvieto, F.; Petrocchi, A.; Poma, M.; Rowley, M.; et al. Dihydroxypyrimidine-4-carboxamides as novel potent and selective HIV integrase inhibitors. *J. Med. Chem.* **2007**, *50*, 2225–2239.

[13] Pace, P.; Rowley, M. Integrase inhibitors for the treatment of HIV infection. *Curr. Opin. Drug Discov. Dev.* **2008**, *11*, 471–479.

[14] Zhuang, L.; Wai, J. S.; Embrey, M. W.; Fisher, T. E.; Egbertson, M. S.; Payne, L. S.; Guare, J. P., Jr.; Vacca, J. P.; Hazuda, D. J.; Felock, P. J.; et al. Design and synthesis of 8-hydroxy-[1,6]naphthyridines as novel inhibitors of HIV-1 integrase in vitro and in infected cells. *J. Med. Chem.* **2003**, *46*, 453–456.

[15] Zhuang, L.; Wai, J. S.; Payne, L. S.; Young, S. D.; Fisher, T. E.; Embrey, M.; Guare, J. P. Preparation of aza- and polyaza-naphthalenyl ketones useful as HIV integrase inhibitors. Merck & Co., Inc. 2001-US42553[2002036734], 189, May 10, 2002; WO, Oct. 9, 2001.

[16] Wai, J. S.; Kim, B.; Fisher, T. E.; Zhuang, L.; Embrey, M. W.; Williams, P. D.; Staas, D. D.; Culberson, C.; Lyle, T. A.; Vacca, J. P.; et al. Dihydroxypyridopyrazine-1,6-dione HIV-1 integrase inhibitors. *Bioorg. Med. Chem. Lett.* **2007**, *17*, 5595–5599.

[17] Egbertson, M.; Kuo, M. S.; Perlow, D. S.; Langford, H. M.; Melamed, J. Y.; Wai, J. S.; Vacca, J.; Wallace, A.; Leonard, Y.; Hazuda, D.; et al. Potent HIV integrase inhibitor with excellent pharmacokinetics. Abstract of papers, 234th ACS National Meeting, Boston, 2007. Poster 091.

[18] Kozikowski, A. P.; Isobe, K. Oxazoles in organic synthesis: some observations on the use of 5-alkoxyoxazoles in the Diels–Alder process. *Heterocycles* **1978**, *9*, 1271–1275.

[19] Humphrey, G. R.; Miller, R. A.; Maligres, P. E.; Weissman, S. Process for preparing N-substituted hydroxypyrimidinone carboxamides. Merck & Co., Inc. WO 2009088729, 2009.

[20] A similar use of alkali metal carbonates is described in Sugahara, M.; Moritani, Y.; Kuroda, T.; Kondo, K.; Shimadzu, H.; Ukita, T. An efficient synthesis of the anti-asthmatic agent T-440: a selective N-alkylation of 2-pyridone. *Chem. Pharm. Bull.* **2000**, *48*, 589–591.

[21] Ahmed, A.; Bragg, R. A.; Clayden, J.; Lai, L. W.; McCarthy, C.; Pink, J. H.; Westlund, N.; Yasin, S. A. Barriers to rotation about the chiral axis of tertiary aromatic amides. *Tetrahedron* **1998**, *54*, 13277–13294.

[22] Welch, C. J.; Biba, M.; Pye, P.; Angelaud, R.; Egbertson, M. Serendipitous discovery of a pH-dependant atropisomer bond rotation: Toward a write-protectable chiral molecular switch? *J. Chromatogr. B* **2008**, *875*, 118–121.

[23] Zhou, Y. S.; Tay, L. K.; Hughes, D.; Donahue, S. Simulation of the impact of atropisomer interconversion on plasma exposure of atropisomers of an endothelin receptor antagonist. *Clin. Pharmacol.* **2004**, *44*, 680–688.

[24] Ikeura, Y.; Ishichi, Y.; Tanaka, T.; Fujishima, A.; Murabayashi, M.; Kawada, M.; Ishimaru, T.; Kamo, I.; Doi, T.; Natsugari, H. Axially chiral *N*-Benzyl-*N*,7-dimethyl-5-phenyl-1,7-naphthyridine-6-carboxamide derivatives as tachykinin NK1 receptor antagonists: determination of the absolute stereochemical requirements. *J. Med. Chem.* **1998**, *41*, 4232–4239.

[25] Halgren, T. A. Merck molecular force field: I. Basis, form, scope, parameterization, and performance of MMFF94. *J. Comput. Chem.* **1996**, *17*, 490–519.

[26] Hazuda, D. J.; Anthony, N. J.; Gomez, R. P.; Jolly, S. M.; Wai, J. S.; Zhuang, L.; Fisher, T. E.; Embrey, M.; Guare, J. P., Jr.; Egbertson, M. S.; et al. A naphthyridine carboxamide provides evidence for discordant resistance between mechanistically identical inhibitors of HIV-1 integrase. *Proc. Nat. Acad. Sci. USA* **2004**, *101*, 11233–11238.

[27] Vacca, J. P.; Dorsey, B. D.; Schleif, W. A.; Levin, R. B.; McDaniel, S. L.; Darke, P. L.; Zugay, J.; Quintero, J. C.; Blahy, O. M.; Roth, E.; et al. L-735,524: an orally bioavailable human-immunodeficiency-virus type-1 protease inhibitor. *Proc. Nat. Acad. Sci. USA* **1994**, *91*, 4096–4100.

[28] Maignan, S.; Guilloteau, J. P.; Zhou-Liu, Q.; Clement-Mella, C.; Mikol, V. Crystal structures of the catalytic domain of HIV-1 integrase free and complexed with its metal cofactor: high level of similarity of the active site with other viral integrases. *J. Am. Chem. Soc.* **1998**, *282*, 359–368.

[29] Grobler, J. A.; Stillmock, K.; Hu, B.; Witmer, M.; Felock, P.; Espeseth, A. S.; Wolfe, A.; Egbertson, M.; Bourgeois, M.; Melamed, J.; et al. Diketo acid inhibitor mechanism and HIV-1 integrase: implications for metal binding in the active site of phosphotransferase enzymes. *Proc. Nat. Acad. Sci. USA* **2002**, *99*, 6661–6666.

[30] Witmer, M.; Danovich, R. Selection and analysis of HIV-1 integrase strand transfer inhibitor resistant mutant viruses. *Methods* **2009**, *47*, 277–282.

[31] Zahm, J. A.; Bera, S.; Pandey, K. K.; Vora, A.; Stillmock, K.; Hazuda, D.; Grandgenett, D. P. Mechanisms of human immunodeficiency virus type 1 concerted integration related to strand transfer inhibition and drug resistance. *Antimicrob. Agents Chemother.* **2008**, *52*, 3358–3368.

[32] Sato, M.; Motomura, T.; Aramaki, H.; Matsuda, T.; Yamashita, M.; Ito, Y.; Kawakami, H.; Matsuzaki, Y.; Watanabe, W.; Yamataka, K.; et al. Novel HIV-1 integrase inhibitors derived from quinolone antibiotics. *J. Med. Chem.* **2006**, *49*, 1506–1508.

[33] Zeldin, R.; Petruschke, R. A. Pharmacological and therapeutic properties of ritonavir-boosted protease inhibitor therapy in HIV-infected patients. *J. Antimicrob. Chemother.* **2004**, *53*, 4–9.

[34] Merry, C.; Barry, M. G.; Mulcahy, D.; Ryan, M.; Heavey, J.; Tjia, J. F.; Gibbons, S. E.; Breckenridge, A. M.; Back, D. J. Saquinavir pharmacokinetics alone and in combination with ritonavir in HIV-infected patients. *AIDS* **1997**, *11*, F29–F33.

[35] Hepatocyte stability methods. Well-stirred model: Freshly isolated at 1 or 2 million cells/mL and suspended in William's E medium. Substrate concentration was 1 μM and incubations were conducted at 37°C in either a water bath or incubator that contained a 95%/5% O_2/CO_2 atmosphere for 1 or 2 h. The culture was sampled five to six time points over the course of this incubation time. Protein was precipitated from the samples by treatment with a volume of acetonitrile and 0.1% formic acid followed by centrifugation (~ 1800 g). Parent compound was monitored in the supernatant via LC-MS/MS to give percent parent remaining vs. time plots. An elimination rate constant was calculated and then subsequently used to determine in vitro intrinsic clearance values. A similar approach is outlined in Jones, H.M.; Houston, J. B. *Drug Metab. Dispos.* **2004**, *32*(9) 973–982.

[36] Pye, P.; Angelaud, R. Merck process research. Unpublished results, 2005.

13

DISCOVERY AND DEVELOPMENT OF HIV INTEGRASE INHIBITOR RALTEGRAVIR

VINCENZO SUMMA AND PAOLA PACE
Merck Research Laboratories, Rome, Italy

INTRODUCTION

Recent years have been marked by real progress in global responses to the HIV epidemic. Activism created a new norm around the right to access to treatment for people living with HIV worldwide, and 3 million people are now taking antiretroviral medication [1]. UNAIDS and other key actors are redoubling prevention efforts through systematic analysis to determine what works and what can be scaled up. Although there have been some setbacks in research on new prevention technologies, such as vaccines and microbicides, investment and attention continue to grow. At the same time, sobering statistics underscore that neither prevention nor treatment is keeping pace with the epidemic. Every day some 6800 people are newly infected with HIV and over 5700 die from AIDS [2]. For every person newly accessing antiretroviral therapy, more than four people are becoming newly infected. Currently, 25 approved drugs for the treatment of HIV infection exist, and these are categorized into six classes: (1) protease inhibitors, (2) nucleoside reverse transcriptase inhibitors (NRTIs), (3) non-nucleoside reverse transcriptase inhibitors (NNRTIs), (4) integrase inhibitors, (5) chemokine co-receptor (CCR) inhibitors, and (6) fusion inhibitors. The last three classes have recently been approved as treatments for HIV infection, with one marketed drug in each class: maraviroc (Celsentri) for CCR5 [3], the injectable fusion inhibitor peptide enfuvirtide (Fuzeon) [4], and the integrase inhibitor raltegravir (Isentress), the discovery of which is described in this chapter. The most common drug combination given to those beginning treatment consists of two NRTIs combined with either an NNRTI or a "boosted" protease inhibitor. Ritonavir (in small doses) is most commonly used as the booster; it is a strong Cyp450 inhibitor and by this inhibition reduces the oxidative metabolism of the other protease inhibitors, prolonging their plasma half-life. An example of a common antiretroviral combination is the two NRTIs zidovudine and lamivudine, combined with the NNRTI efavirenz. At the beginning of treatment, the combination of drugs that a person is given is called *first-line therapy*. If after awhile HIV becomes resistant to this combination, or if side effects are particularly strong, the combination of the drugs is changed to find a more effective or tolerated therapy, this procedure is continually implemented every time that the therapy becomes ineffective. After several cycles of different combination therapies, there is a shift in the possible therapy, called *second-line therapy*, which will ideally include a minimum of three drugs, and possibly with at least one from a new class, in order to increase the likelihood of treatment success. There is now a considerable patient population with resistance to multiple classes of the traditional drugs, and it is to these patients that the newer drugs were initially targeted. Although over the years a plethora of HIV-1 integrase inhibitors have been discovered [5], raltegravir is the first drug with this mechanism of action approved by the FDA and EMEA. Integrase is required to carry out the insertion of HIV-1 DNA into the genome of the host cell. Integrase assembles on the ends of the viral DNA as one component of the viral preintegration complex (PIC) and catalyzes two sequential catalytic reactions, specifically 3′ endonucleolitic processing of the viral DNA, and strand transfer, which

Antiviral Drugs: From Basic Discovery Through Clinical Trials, First Edition. Edited by Wieslaw M. Kazmierski.

covalently links the viral and cellular DNAs [6]. In vivo proof of concept for the integrase inhibition was first shown in an experimental model of retroviral infection using rhesus macaques infected with SHIV-89.6P with 8-hydroxy [1,6]-naphthyridine carboxamides. The robust antiviral activity in this model supplied evidence of in vivo efficacy for integrase inhibitors in retroviral infections, thereby establishing a solid base for the treatment of HIV-1 infection [7]. Furthermore, proof of concept has also been achieved in humans [8].

DISCOVERY

The medicinal chemistry behind the discovery of raltegravir by Merck Research Laboratories Rome (known as IRBM) relies on an understanding of the similarities of the mechanism of action of HIV integrase and another polynucleotidyl transferase, the NS5b RNA-dependent RNA polymerase of HCV virus. HIV-1 integrase is a 32-kDa enzyme comprised of three structurally and functionally distinct domains, all required for each step of the integration process. Extensive mutagenesis studies mapped the catalytic site to the core domain (residues 50 to 212), which contains the catalytic residues Asp64, Asp116, and Glu152. These residues are highly conserved in the integrase superfamily and polynucleotide transferases, including the RNA-dependent RNA polymerase of HCV. In both enzymes, two metal ions (Mg^{2+}) are present in the active site and hold by the amino acids mentioned above, the cations are required for phosphoryltransferase activities. Early studies using recombinant integrase and high-throughput screening assays have led to the identification of 4-aryl-2,4-diketobutanoic acids (**1**, Fig. 1) as the first class of potent and selective strand transfer HIV integrase inhibitors [6]. Diketo acids (DKAs) compete with host DNA for the binding site on HIV integrase, thus selectively inhibiting the strand transfer process. This inhibition is dependent on the presence of divalent ions, magnesium, or manganese in in vitro assays [9].

It is believed that the diketo acid moiety chelates with two divalent metal ions in the active site of the integrase to form a tertiary ligand–Me^{2+}–integrase complex, thus blocking substrate DNA binding. At IRBM in Rome, we discovered simultaneously that DKAs were also active-site HCV NS5b RNA-dependent RNA polymerase inhibitors [10], with a mechanism of action similarly related to the interaction with metals in the active site. This finding was the basis of an integrated drug discovery program where compounds made as inhibitors of the HCV polymerase were screened also on the HIV integrase, and vice versa. Because the diketoacid group is biologically labile and suffers from other undesirable properties, on both programs we were interested in replacing it with alternative, more stable, metal chelating ligands. Further screening of the sample collection identified a second low-micromolar-specific and reversible inhibitor of NS5b HCV polymerase, competitive with the diketoacid, a meconic acid ester (**2**, Fig. 1) [11]. Whereas the meconic acid lead was unstable and underwent decarboxylation in acidic media, the constraint of the six-membered ring was an attractive template. Therefore, we designed workable replacements for this core structure, maintaining a chelating moiety formed by a carbonyl, an acidic hydroxyl function, and a carboxylic acid.

This work led to the identification of a dihydroxypyrimidine carboxylic acid (**3**, Fig. 1) [12], which was much more stable in acid and basic media and did not have any issue of irreversible covalent binding to protein present in the DKA series, showing great improvement in the druglike properties of this new class of inhibitors. The compound was active against HCV polymerase (30 μM) with good selectivity against other enzymes that have a Mg^{2+} ion in the active site. However, this class of compounds had modest potency in the HCV cell–based assays. This is probably due to the highly polar nature of the pyrimidine carboxylic acid template, which at physiological conditions has the carboxylic acid and the hydroxyl group at the 5 position both deprotonated. Thus, replacement of at least one of these acidic functionalities was sought. Many carboxylic acid isosteres

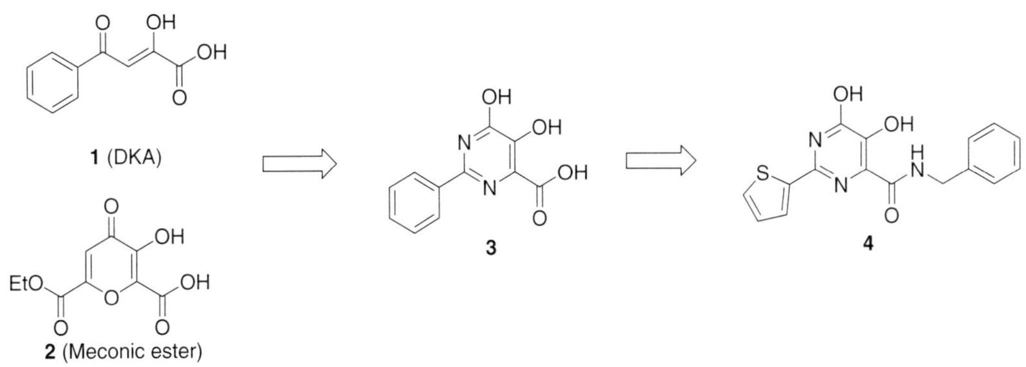

FIGURE 1 From HCV polymerase to HIV integrase: the discovery of the pyrimidine carboxamide lead.

were prepared and tested, including simple amide and esters. Although this work did not give any satisfactory result in the HCV program, it gave a real breakthrough for the HIV integrase. In fact, one of the potential acid replacement, a benzylamide (**4**, Fig. 1), proved to be a potent inhibitor (IC_{50} = 85 nM) of the strand transfer reaction catalyzed by HIV integrase but inactive against HCV NS5b at 50 μM. In pharmacokinetic studies in rat, the compound showed moderate oral bioavailability (15%) and low plasma clearance (5 mL·min/kg). Counterscreening studies to assess selectivity showed that it did not inhibit human DNA polymerase α, β, and γ at 10 μM.

These findings supported the fact that we had discovered a valid lead for the HIV integrase project. However, **4** had a number of issues: It showed modest activity in the cell-based assay, low bioavailability in rat, and was highly plasma protein bound (< 1% unbound in human plasma). In particular, the nonspecific binding of a drug to plasma protein, mostly serum albumin and α-acid glycoprotein, is an important determinant of its biological efficacy since it modulates the availability of the drug to its intended target. Drug–protein complexes in plasma also serves as drug reservoir for free drug concentration, as the drug is removed from the body by various elimination processes and prolong the duration of action. Thus, the physicochemical properties, the effective concentration to be targeted, and the potential side effects influence how much binding to plasma proteins can still be tolerated and precisely how this parameter has to be tuned for a new drug entity. In particular, in the HIV field it is known that compounds with very high protein plasma protein binding show a marginal activity in the cell-based assay in the presence of human serum. To assess the role of serum protein on drug availability at a quantitative level, the inhibitor concentration required to inhibit 95% of the spread of HIV infection in MT4 cell culture was measured in the presence of low-serum (10% fetal bovine serum, 10% FBS) and also in the highest serum feasible conditions (50% normal human serum, 50% NHS) that are considered close to the physiological conditions. Both assays were important for compound selection, since cell-based activity in the low-serum conditions (10% FBS) reflects the ability to cross cell membranes while the high serum conditions (50% NHS) provided efficacy in a physiologically more relevant environment.

We started lead optimization of **4** by exploring the benzylamide moiety, and a focused library of more than 200 amides was synthesized and screened [13]. From this set of compounds, structure–actvity relationship (SAR) trends began to emerge. It was immediately evident that the NH was essential (Table 1, **5**) and an aromatic ring separated by at least one sp^3 atom was essential for the activity since the anilide **6** (IC_{50} = 1 μM) and the cycloalkyl derivative **7** (IC_{50} = 50 μM) lost significant activity. α-Branching on the benzylic amide was also detrimental (**8**, IC_{50} = 0.2 μM). An extensive SAR performed on the benzyl ring (data not shown) showed

TABLE 1 Investigation of the Amide

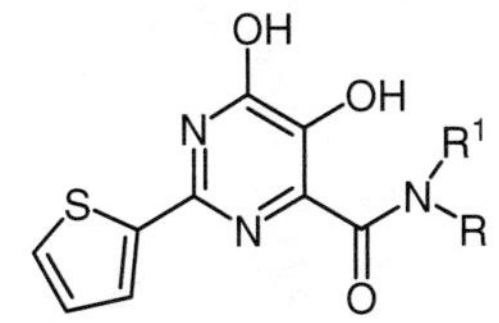

Compound	R	R^1	QI IC_{50} (nM)
4	CH_2Ph	H	85
5	CH_2Ph	Me	530
6	Ph	H	1000
7	CH_2-cyclohexyl	H	>1000
8	$CH(CH_3)Ph$	H	200
9	(4-F)Ph	H	10

that a small electron-withdrawing group in the *para* position was preferred. The 4-fluoro-substituted benzyl amide **9** (IC_{50} = 0.01 μM) was optimal for enzyme inhibition, and by and large this substituent on the amide portion was used throughout the course of the project. However, despite the increased in vitro potency, compound **9** showed weak inhibition of the spread of HIV-1 infection in cell culture. The rat pharmacokinetic profile showed improved oral bioavailability (F = 29%), exposure 1.3 (nAUC μM·h·kg/mg), and plasma clearance (11 mL·min/kg) similar to that of **4**.

The modest cellular activity of **9** can be explained by a combination of factors, such as poor cell permeability, high protein binding, and poor solubility. To improve these parameters, the 2-position of the pyrimidine core became the focus of the subsequent SAR [14]. We found that the thiophene ring of **9** could simply be replaced with an H, generating the minimal template that conserves the intrinsic activity in the enzymatic assay, or substituted by simple small alkyl groups, or benzyl, aryl, or heterocycles, without affecting the activity. We interpreted the small effect that changing the 2-substituent had on in vitro potency as evidence that this part of the molecule does not interact strongly with the enzyme, and therefore this appeared to be the site that would be most likely to tolerate more dramatic changes influencing the physicochemical properties of the inhibitors aiming to develop compounds with activity in the cell-based assays. To address the low activity in the cell-based assays we chose to try to incorporate functional groups with polarity or large dipole moments. We started by including amines, with the thinking that this may also help balance the negative charge on the molecules due to the 5-hydroxyl group, which is deprotonated at physiological pH. Compound **11** (Table 2), in which a dimetylamino group was added to the benzylic methylene, was one of the most interesting compounds in this series: Even if less active on the enzyme than **10**, it showed comparable activity in the cell-based assay under low-serum conditions (QI IC_{50} = 0.20 μM and spread CIC_{95} = 0.31 μM in 10% FBS), indicating that we were moving in a productive direction.

TABLE 2 Effect of the Basic Group

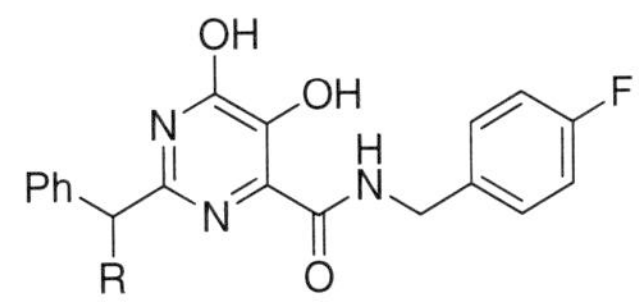

Compound	R	QI IC_{50} (nM)	Spread CIC_{95} 10% FBS (μM)	Spread CIC_{95} 10% FBS (μM)
10	H	50	>10	>10
11	NMe_2	200	0.31	>10

TABLE 3 Simple Acyclic 2-Substituents

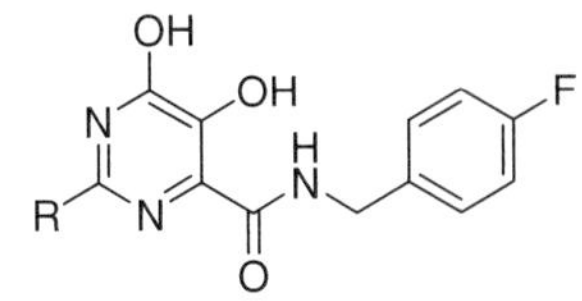

Compound	R	QI IC_{50} (nM)	Spread CIC_{95} (μM) 10% FBS	50% NHS
12	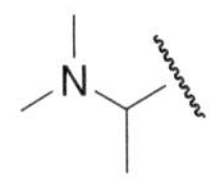	10	0.12	0.50
13	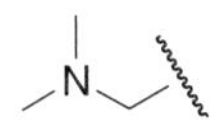	200	1.0	>1.0
14	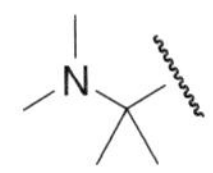	50	0.05	0.078

Compound **11** was characterized further by studying its DMPK properties in vivo and in vitro. In pharmacokinetic studies in rats, **11** showed good oral bioavailability ($F = 59\%$) and low plasma clearance (Clp = 14 mL·min/kg). The profile was even better in dog, with improved oral bioavailability ($F = 93\%$), very low plasma clearance (Clp = 0.5 mL·min/kg), and long terminal plasma half-life ($t_{1/2} = 6.0$ h). Counter-screening studies showed that the compound did not inhibit cytochrome P450s 2C19, 2C9, 2D6, and 3A4. However, the compound was weakly active when tested in spread assay in the presence of the physiologically more relevant 50% normal human serum, and the shift between the low- and high-serum conditions correlated well with a measured human plasma protein binding > 99.9%. To address the high protein binding, we decided to test whether decreasing the molecular weight and lipophilicity of our inhibitors, via removal of the bulky aryl group, would have a favorable impact on cell-based potency in the presence of 50% normal human serum (Fig. 2). It is indeed known that for lipophilic acids plasma protein binding correlates to the water/*n*-octanol distribution coefficient (log *P*). Compounds with low lipophilicity or a basic center usually have lower protein binding. We therefore decided to try to improve the activity of **11** by removing the phenyl group to reduce lipophilicity, while maintaining the presence of the beneficial amino group.

The first approach we tried was to replace the phenyl ring with a simple methyl, such as in compound **12** (Fig. 2 and Table 3); this modification was efficacious in reducing the protein binding (human PPB = 92.5%) and resulted in only a fourfold shift in potency in the spread assay between low- and high-serum conditions. This was the first compound in the series to break the micromolar barrier in the presence of 50% NHS, having an IC_{95} = 0.50 μM. With the added advantage of eliminating the chiral center, we removed the methyl group as in compound **13**, but this modification was detrimental, probably because we had reduced the lipophilicity too far, whereas when we introduced a second methyl substituent, as in **14**, we discovered a very interesting compound. To our great excitement, **14** was equipotent on the enzyme and in the cell-based assay in low-serum conditions with a marginal shift in high-serum concentrations (IC_{50} = 0.05 μM; CIC_{95} = 0.05 μM 10% FBS; 0.08 μM 50% NHS).

The pharmacokinetic profile of **14** was determined in Sprague–Dawley rats, beagle dogs, and rhesus monkeys. In

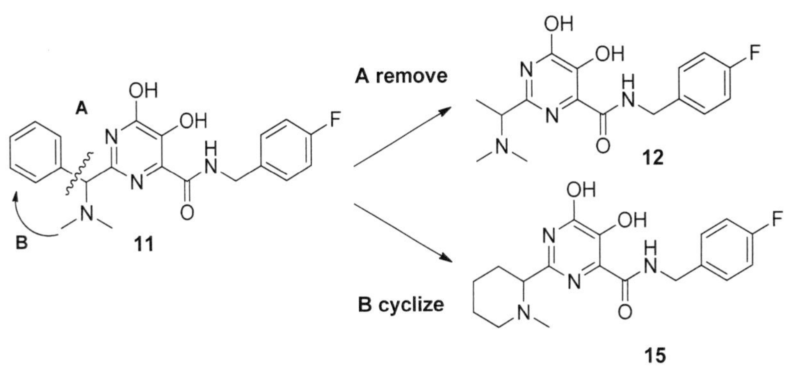

FIGURE 2 Strategies employed to reduce the protein binding.

all three species, the compound had prolonged plasma half-lives, moderate to low clearance and good to excellent oral bioavailability (from 28% in rats to 100% in dogs). The compound is not an inhibitor of major CYP450 isoforms nor an inducer of CYP3A4. It was not metabolized oxidatively (did not show turnover with liver microsomes in the presence of NADPH), and the major metabolites seen in animals and in liver microsomes in the presence of UDPGA and hepatocytes was the 5-*O*-glucuronide. All these findings indicate a low potential for drug–drug interactions, which is very important in HIV therapy, where a combination of drugs is the standard of care. Thus, the compound **14** was selected as a potential preclinical development candidate. Unfortunately, it was quickly found to be toxic to rodents at very high doses, and its development was halted. In the meanwhile we were following an alternative approach and the new strategy was to construct analogs in which the basic group was embedded in an aliphatic cycle. As shown in Table 4, the 2-piperidyl derivative **15** exhibited higher potency in the in vitro enzyme assay than in the 3- (**16**) and 4-piperidyl (**17**) counterparts. However, **15** displayed disappointing cell-based activities, perhaps due to the presence of multiple hydrogen-bond donors. Therefore, the NH was methylated (**18**), giving a very pleasing 10-fold improvement in activity in cell-based assay under both serum conditions ($CIC_{95} = 0.14$ and 0.4 μM 10% FBS and 50% NHS, respectively). The five-membered analog **19** showed a similar profile.

At this point in the project, capitalizing on the experience gained in the HCV polymerase program, where *N*-methylpyrimidones showed improved pharmacokinetic properties with respect to dihydroxypyrimidines and generally lower plasma protein binding, we investigated the effect of methylation of the pyrimidine 2-nitrogen for a small set of HIV integrase compounds. In particular, we prepared **20** (Table 5), the *N*-methylpyrimidone corresponding to **18**. Although the activity was reduced both on the enzyme and in the cell-based assays (QI $IC_{50} = 0.44$ μM, 10% FBS $CIC_{95} =$ 0.8 μM, 50% NHS $CIC_{95} = 1.0$ μM), the plasma protein binding was greatly reduced (hPPB 55% for **20** vs. 95% for **18**) and the rat PK was improved, with higher oral bioavailability and lower clearance ($F = 100\%$, Clp = 31 mL·min/kg for **20** vs. $F = 60\%$, Clp = 60 mL·min/kg for **18**). Encouraged by these preliminary data, we continued the SAR studies on five- and six-membered cyclic amines with the aim to further probe both the cell-based activity and the pharmacological properties of these compounds [15]. Pleasingly, introduction of a heteroatom in the piperidine ring, as in the morpholine derivative **21**, gave a nice increase in cell-based activity. Resolution gave the separate enantiomers, and the (+)**21** was slightly more active than the (−)**21**. The minimal serum-induced shift in the assay was presumably a reflection of low plasma protein binding (81%).

(+)**21** was found to have good pharmacokinetic properties across preclinical species. It showed high oral bioavailability in rat (56%), dog (69%), and rhesus (73%), with low plasma clearance (rat 9, dog 2.2, and rhesus 14 mL/min/kg) and moderate to good plasma half-lives (rat 1.1, dog 7.3, and rhesus 2.0 h). It was stable in rat, dog, and human liver microsomes in the presence of NADPH. The glucuronidation rate in the presence of UDPGA was minimal, and measurement of the rate of formation of glucuronide showed that glucuronidation was faster in rats than in dogs and humans. It was not an inhibitor of the major CYP450 enzymes (3A4, 2D6, 1A2, and 2C19) up to 100 μM and was clean in many other preclinical

TABLE 4 Cyclic 2-Substituents

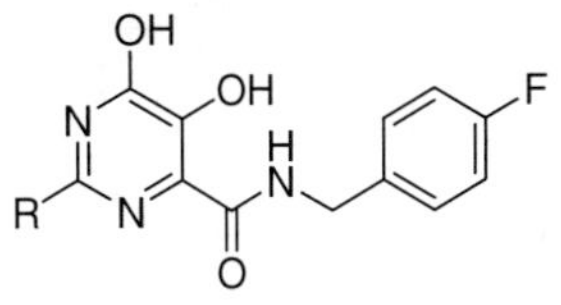

Compound	R	QI IC_{50} (nM)	Spread CIC_{95} (μM)	
			10% FBS	50% NHS
15	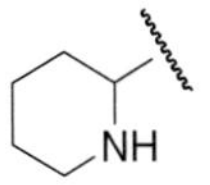	100	1.5	6
16	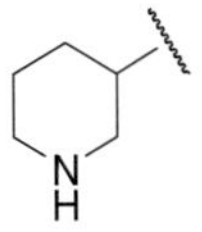	800	>10	>10
17	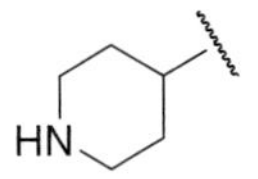	1200	>10	>10
18	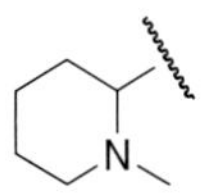	200	0.14	0.40
19	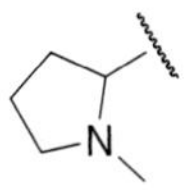	120	0.15	0.62

TABLE 5 *N*-Methylpyrimidones

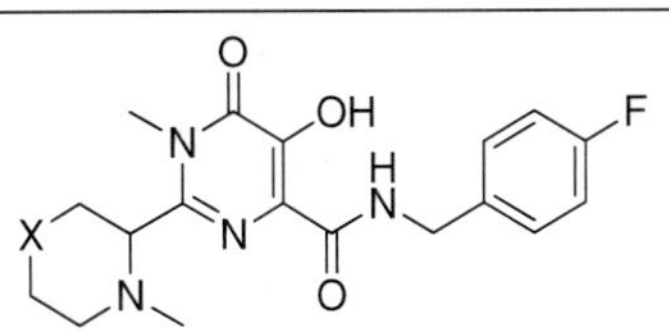

20 (X = CH_2)
21 (X = O)

Compound	QI IC_{50} (nM)	Spread CIC_{95} (μM)		PPB % Bound (Human)
		10% FBS	50% NHS	
20	438	0.8	1.0	55
21	62	0.06	0.10	70
(+)**21**	20	0.04	0.06	81

TABLE 6 Acyclic *N*-Methylpyrimidones

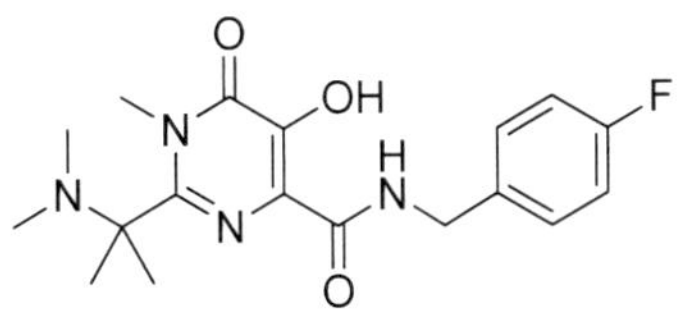

22

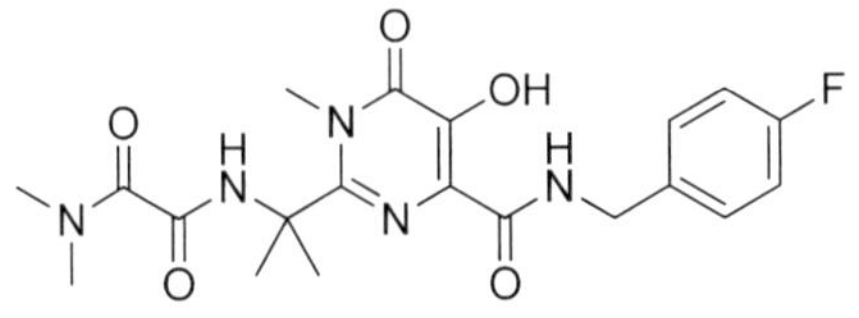

23

Compound	QI IC_{50} (nM)	Spread CIC_{95} (μM) 10% FBS	Spread CIC_{95} (μM) 50% NHS
22	230	>1.0	>1.0
23	10	0.045	0.07

counterscreenings and experiments. Disappointingly, further studies found the compound to be positive in Ames assay, and development of the compound was halted.

Looking for another preclinical candidate, we went on to explore acyclic substituents at the 2-position of the *N*-methylpyrimidone series (Table 6). Given the experience gained in the pyrimidine series, we prepared the *N*-methylpyrimidone corresponding to **14**. However, this modification did not produce a compound with the desired activity, as well as being modestly potent, as are many other compounds bearing simple modifications of the basic amines. Reasoning that perhaps our compounds were getting too polar, we sought to introduce other functional groups not basic which are still known to reduce protein binding [16]. Further rational to attempt this approach was the evidence that the napthyridine inhibitors prepared by our colleagues at Merck West Point, which did not contain basic nitrogen, showed great potency in spread assay under high-serum conditions [17]. In this novel SAR effort we prepared many derivatives, acetamide, sulfonamides, ureas, and sulfonylureas [18]. Among them, the *N*,*N*-dimethyl oxalamide derivative **23** used by our colleagues at West Point [8] proved to be particularly interesting because it showed very good potency in the spread assay, equivalent to that of many HIV drugs on the market.

The oxalamide derivative **23** was dosed in rat, dog, and rhesus, showing good oral bioavailability, moderate plasma clearance, and reasonable terminal half-life (Table 7). In analogy with the previous inhibitors in our hands, the compound is a very weak substrate for CYP450 enzymes and is metabolized primarily by glucuronidation. Higher in vitro metabolism was observed in rhesus and rat microsomes in the presence of UDPGA, which correlated with the moderate in vivo clearance, while the compound showed very low turnover in dog liver microsomes, as mirrored by the low in vivo clearance. The preclinical pharmacokinetic profiles, combined with the in vitro turnover data (rat, dog, rhesus, and human 20, 3, 46, and 8 μL·min/mg, respectively), the plasma protein binding (rat, dog, rhesus, and human 35, 38, 18, and 28% free fraction, respectively), and other parameters were used to extrapolate a low human plasma clearance with a profile similar that for dogs. The agent was then selected as a preclinical candidate and passed safety assessment and genotoxicity studies. These results allowed rapid progression to phase I clinical trials. As the compound was taken forward into humans, we were pleased to see a reasonable correspondence between the predicted and observed pharmacokinetic properties [19].

As the compound was taken into safety assessment, we also profiled it against a panel of resistant HIV mutants (Fig. 3). During several years of research in the HIV integrase field we were able to select a series of mutants by using proprietary and literature-reported HIV integrase inhibitors. We used this panel to evaluate and select the new inhibitors for development. The rapidity with which drug-resistant HIV variants appear in HIV-infected individuals undergoing drug therapy is critical to the usefulness of anti-HIV compounds. Generally, the HIV-integrase inhibitors showed a higher genetic barrier to developing resistances in in vitro systems, so we assumed that a compound with a low shift in potency on this panel of resistant mutants vs. wild-type is likely to be associated with a higher potency against these mutants if they are generated in vivo. In particular, it is relevant that the activity against mutants retaining sufficient activity allows virus propagation while reducing susceptibility to the particular inhibitor under study. The profile of **23** was similar to that of L-870,810, a napthyridine compound developed at West Point and significantly better than S-1360, a

TABLE 7 Pharmacokinetic Profiles for Compound 23[a]

Species	p.o. Dose (mg/kg)	*F* (%)	$t_{1/2}$ (h)	Clp (mL·min/kg)	p.o. AUC (μM·h)
Rat	3	36	6	21	2.2
Dog	10	93	16	8	44
Rhesus	10	24	3	20	5.3

[a]As Na^+ salt for rat and dog dosing, free acid for rhesus.

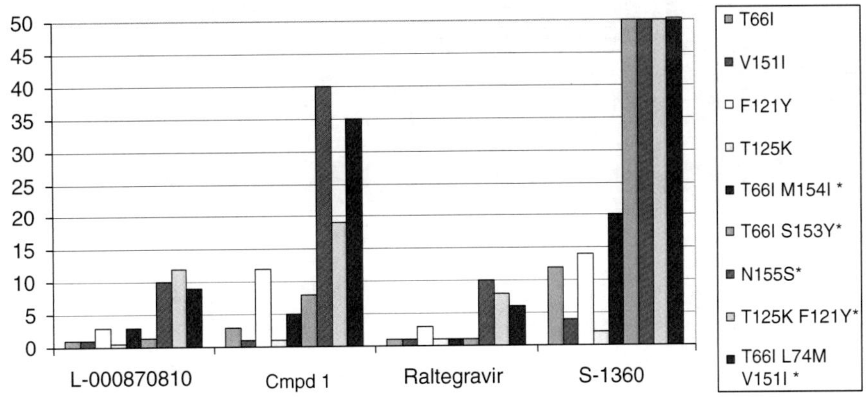

FIGURE 3 Comparative mutation profiles for L-000870810, 23, raltegravir (27), and S1360. Fold shift observed in a single-cycle cell infectivity assay using cell cultures containing HIV-1 possessing site-directed IN mutations compared to cell cultures containing wild-type HIV-1.

compound by Shionogi that underwent clinical development and was subsequently halted. However, the potency of **23** shifted significantly (10- and 40-fold, respectively) against the single-point mutants F121Y and N155S, mutants that were not replication impaired, and for this reason we placed it on hold while a longer-lived variant was sought. In a novel SAR effort, focus was maintained in searching small aromatic heterocycles with a heteroatom pattern similar to that of the oxalamide moiety, as these may maintain the electronic properties while changing the physicochemical properties of the molecule.

In the six-membered heterocycles, the simple 2-pyridine derivative **24** (Table 8) had modest activity in the cell-based assay in the presence of 50% NHS, but the introduction of a second nitrogen, as in the pyrimidine **25**, gave a very potent compound. In the five-membered series, compounds bearing three heteroatoms were more active than those with two. In particular, the oxadiazole **27** had exquisite potency in all assays, while the more polar triazole **28** was much less potent in cells under low-serum conditions, probably due to poor cell penetration. In line with our SAR experience, a more lipophilic heterocycle such as **29** shows a larger shift between low and high serum levels in cells due to high protein binding. When assayed against a panel of integrase mutants, the activity of **27** is much improved over that of previous development candidates, shifting only three- and 10-fold in the presence of F121Y and N155S single mutants (Fig. 3).

Due to its excellent potency, **27** was further profiled in in vitro and in vivo experiments. When tested on an extensive panel of receptor and ion channel binding and enzyme inhibition, assays showed no significant activity. Compound 27 was fully profiled in pharmacokinetic and safety studies on preclinical species, discussed later in the chapter, and advanced into the clinic as MK0518, ultimately to become raltegravir or Isentress [19].

SYNTHESIS

Raltegravir consists of a central hydroxypyrimidinone heterocyclic core that is rapidly assembled by a two-component coupling reaction between the amidoxime **33**, in turn prepared from acetone cyanohydrin **30**, as in Scheme 1, and

TABLE 8 Oxalamide Replacements

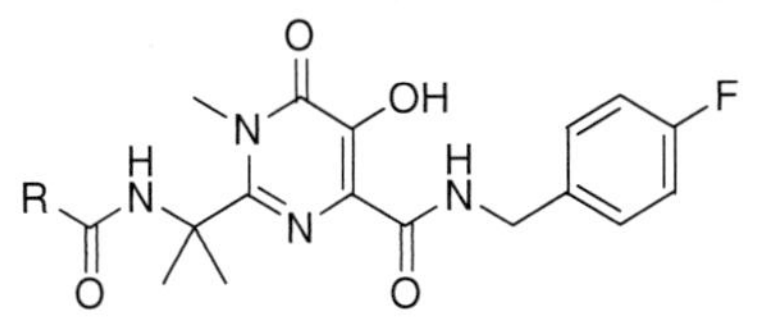

Compound	R	QI IC_{50} (nM)	Spread CIC_{95} (μM) 10% FBS	50% NHS
24	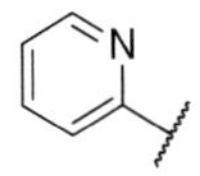	20	0.12	1.0
25	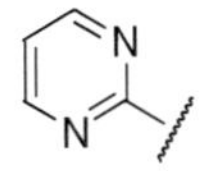	7	0.02	0.05
26	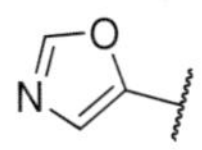	7	0.50	0.50
27	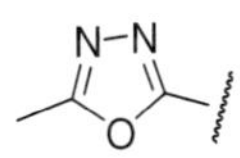	10	0.019	0.031
28	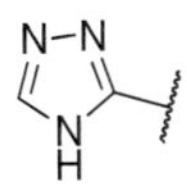	4	0.25	1.0
29	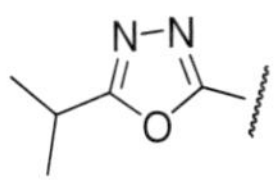	7	0.02	0.16

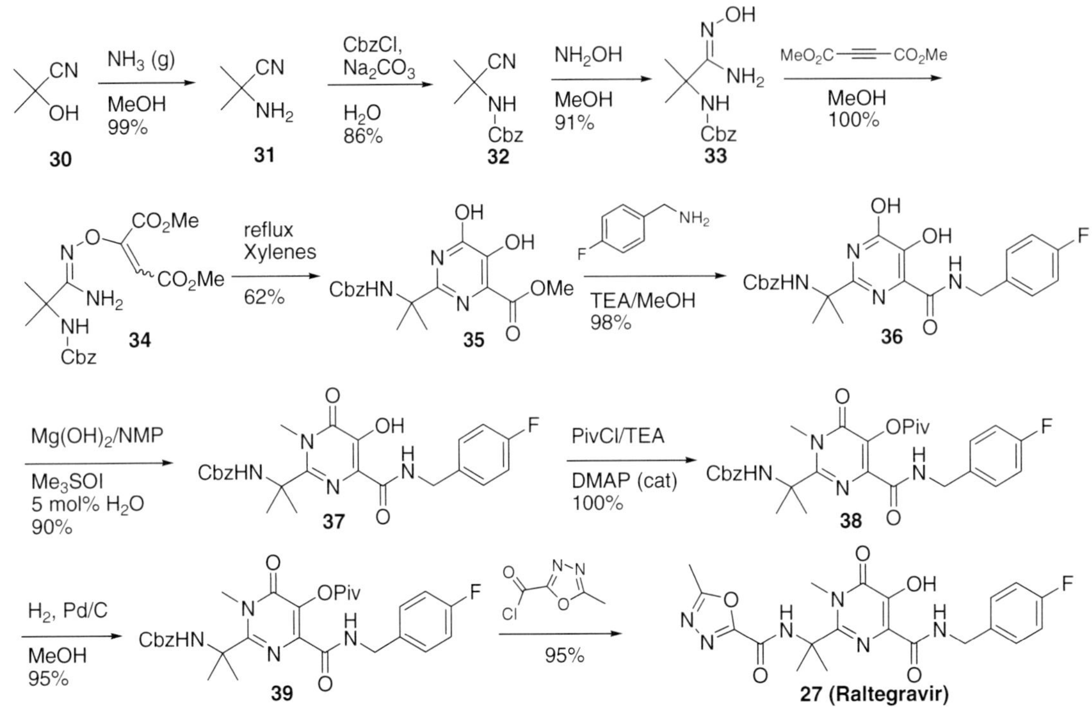

SCHEME 1 Complete synthesis of raltegravir.

dimethylacetylenedicarboxylate (DMAD), to give 34*Z*/34*E*, followed by thermal rearrangement to the pyrimidine moiety **35** [20,21]. The subsequent N-methylation of the dihydroxypyrimidine was carried out on our benches by selective benzoylation of the 5-hydroxyl group, followed by alkylation with methyl sulfate in the presence of LiH in dioxane (Scheme 2). With this procedure we were able to isolate the *N*-methylpyrimidone **41** in 64% yield, together with variable amounts of the O-methylated derivative **42**, which was separated by column chromatography. The methyl ester of the isolated **41** is then converted into the corresponding benzylic amide **37** by reaction with *p*-fluorobenzylamine in methanol. This methodology was significantly improved by our process group, where the *N*-alkylation was carried out on the *p*-fluorobenzylamide without any additional protection step (Scheme 2). $Me_3SO^+I^-$ was used as a methylating agent. This reagent slowly dissociates to MeI and DMSO under the reaction conditions allowing higher conversions to

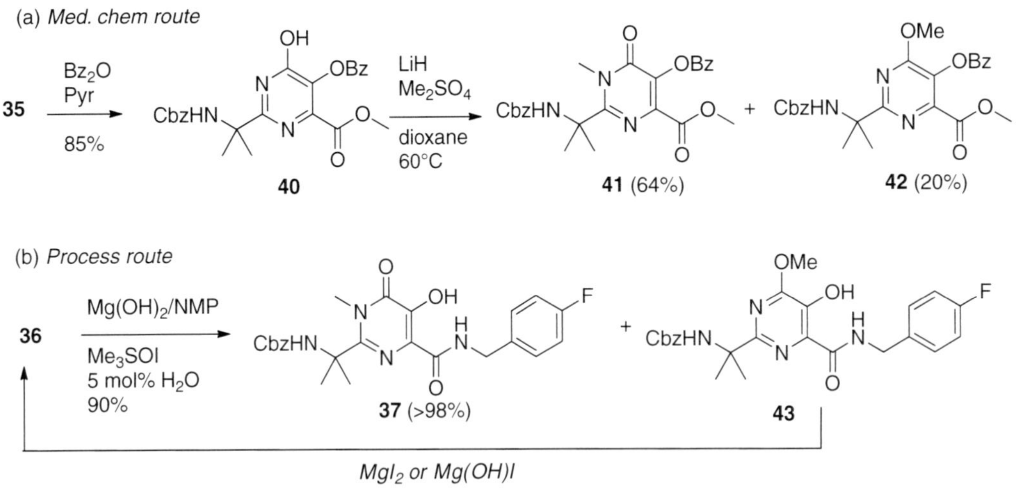

SCHEME 2 Methylation of pyrimidine.

methylated product with fewer equivalents of reagent. Importantly, 2 equiv of $Mg(OH)_2$ are used and the mixture is aged for 5 to 7 h at 100°C in *N*-methylpyrrolidone (NMP). In this way, the ratio of *N*-methyl to *O*-methyl products starts out low (i.e., 60 to 70% of *N*-methyl out of total methylated products), but on continued aging, the *O*-methyl group on **43** is cleaved by magnesium salts to give back the starting material **36**. Since only the *O*-methyl group is cleaved, while the methyl on the *N*-methylpyrimidone **37** is unaffected by reaction conditions, all product is funneled over the N-methylated product **37**. To complete the synthesis, **37** is protected at the 5-hydroxy as pivaloate ester, the Cbz is removed, and the free amine is reacted with oxadiazole acyl chloride with concomitant removal of the pivaloate group. On a process scale, raltegravir is obtained in nine linear steps, with 33% overall yield without chromatography.

PRECLINICAL PHARMACOKINETIC AND TOXICOLOGY

The pharmacokinetic profile of **27** was determined in Sprague–Dawley rat, dog, and rhesus, showing good oral bioavailability, low-to-moderate clearance with multiphasic elimination in all species, and long terminal half-lives. For the i.v. experiments, 20% DMSO/40% PEG-400/40% H_2O was used as a vehicle and the compound was dosed at 3 mg/kg in rat and 1 mg/kg in dog and rhesus. The corresponding plasma clearance (*Clp*) values were 39, 6, and 18 mL·min/kg, and the volume of distribution (*Vd*) values were 2.0, 0.9, and 1.2 L/kg for rat, dog, and rhesus, respectively (Table 9).

The vehicle of choice was 1% methylcellulose for the p.o. dosing. The compound was dosed in rat at 3 mg/kg as Na^+ and K^+ salts and as free acid, with higher exposure achieved with the salts than with the free OH (AUC: $Na^+ = 1.4$, $K^+ = 1.4$, free OH = 1.0 μM·h, respectively). With the K^+ salt, AUC increased linearly in a rat dose proportionality study, increasing the oral dose from 1 to 100 mg/kg (4, 15, and 60 mg/kg were the medium doses, $r^2 = 0.95$, AUC from 0.8 to 35 μM·h). Also, in dog, higher AUC and C_{max} values were observed for the K^+salt than for the free acid with a two-dose regimen of 2 and 10 mg/kg (Table 10).

TABLE 9 Intravenous Pharmacokinetic Parameters for 27

Species	Dose (mg/kg)	Clp^a (mL·min/kg)	$\alpha t_{1/2}{}^b$ (h)	$\beta t_{1/2}{}^c$ (h)	Vd^d (L/kg)
Rat	3	39	N.D.	2	2.0
Dog	1	6	N.D.	11	0.9
Rhesus	1	18	N.D.	4	1.2

[a] Plasma clearance.
[b] Plasma primary phase half-life following i.v. administration (N.D. not determined).
[c] Terminal plasma half-life following i.v. administration.
[d] Volume of distribution.

Looking at the p.o. profile, **27** showed biphasic elimination with a short α-phase and a prolonged β-phase. This behavior was a very important feature in maintaining the plasma concentration well above CIC_{95} at 12 h (for the K^+ salt, C_{12h} in dog is 160 and 350 nM at 2 and 10 mg/kg, respectively). The plasma protein binding was measured for preclinical species and humans, showing modest interspecies variability of the free fraction values (rat 26.6, dog 29.1, rhesus 15.4, and human 17.2%; Table 11) [19]. Consistently with other pyrimidine inhibitors, the rate of metabolism in hepatic microsomes from preclinical species and humans was higher in the presence of the cofactor UDPGA than in the presence of NADPH, showing that oxidative metabolism does not play a significant role. The major route of metabolism proved to be the 5-*O*-glucuronidation of the hydroxypyrimidinone core structure by UDP glucuronosyl transferase (UDP) enzymes. Interestingly, the lower rate of metabolism was observed in human and dog liver microsomes (Table 11). Metabolic turnover was also assessed in intact rat and human hepatocytes, where in agreement with the relative turnover observed in microsomal preparations, the compound was more stable in human than in rat hepatocytes. Taking into account all the in vitro and in vivo data and the antiviral potency of **27**, it was predicted to be suitable for twice-daily dosing, with a pharmacokinetic profile similar to that of dog [20].

The agent did not show any off-target activity in an in-vitro counterscreening panel, or against human polymerases α, β, and γ. It was not an inhibitor of the major CYP450s, did not induce CYP3A4 in human hepatocytes, nor was it an inhibitor of UGT1A1. Thus, it has a low probability to be the perpetrator of drug–drug interactions. It did not react with glutathione after incubation at 37°C for 24 h. [^{3}H]**27** was used to measure the irreversible protein covalent binding in vivo (rat 25 mg/kg p.o.) to liver, kidney, and plasma and in vitro to human and rat liver microsomes. In both assays the covalent binding was <50 pmol equiv/mg protein.

Three GLP-compliant studies were performed to evaluate the effects of raltegravir on the cardiovascular, respiratory, and central nervous systems [22]. A cardiovascular telemetry study performed in dogs after a single 5-,15-, or 45-mg/kg dose resulted in the absence of any change in cardiovascular indices attributable to raltegravir treatment, reaching C_{max} values of 3.6, 10, and 25 μM, respectively, at 1 h after dosing. Raltegravir potential to affect the respiratory or neurobehavioral system was tested following a single oral administration of 30, 90, or 120 mg/kg to Sprague–Dawley rats. Both studies showed that raltegravir does not induce any treatment-related changes. A maximum concentration of approximately 30 μM was reached at the highest dose, as estimated from toxicokinetic data. Ancillary pharmacology was performed to determine the effects of raltegravir in cardiovascular, respiratory, and renal function in dogs, and in

TABLE 10 Per os Pharmacokinetic parameters for 27[a]

Compound	$F\%^b$ Rat/Dog/Rhesus	$C_{max}{}^c$ (μM) Rat/Dog/Rhesus	$t_{1/2}{}^d$ (h) Rat/Dog/Rhesus	AUC[e] (μM·h) Rat/Dog/Rhesus
27 Na^+	N.D./N.D./N.D.	1.0/N.D./N.D.	N.D./N.D./N.D.	$1.4_{(3)}$/N.D./N.D.
27 K^+	45/69–85/N.D.	$1.6/4.6_{(2)}–24_{(10)}$/N.D.	7.5/13/N.D.	$1.3_{(3)}/11_{(2)}–45_{(10)}$/N.D.
27 OH	37/45/8	$1.2_{(3)}/3_{(2)}–8_{(10)}/0.3$	N.D./N.D./7	$1.0_{(3)}/7_{(2)}–21_{(10)}/1.8_{(10)}$

[a]Numbers in parentheses refer to the p.o. dose; N.D., not determined.
[b]Oral bioavailability.
[c]Maximum plasma concentration.
[d]Terminal-phase plasma half-life.
[e]Area under the curve.

central nervous system (CNS) and gastrointestinal motility in mice. The toxicity of raltegravir was studied in mouse, rat, rabbit, and dog models, investigating single- and repeat-dose studies, genotoxicity, carcinogenicity (ongoing), reproductive toxicity studies, and a number of nonpivotal additional toxicity studies. It is not our place in this review to go into the details of all these experiments; suffice it to say that the compound did not produce any negative findings and was therefore advanced into the clinic.

PHASE I–III SAFETY AND EFFICACY

Raltegravir was moved forward in phase I studies to determine the pharmacokinetics after single and multiple doses in healthy HIV-negative subjects as well as for drug–drug interactions studies [23]. In a double-blind single-dose multiple-period study, 24 healthy male volunteers were randomly allocated to one of three groups and received single escalating doses of raltegravir (from 50 to 1600 mg) or placebo. In a multiple-dose study, 40 healthy male volunteers were divided into five groups of eight subjects each. Six subjects in each group received oral raltegravir in escalating doses of 100, 200, 400, 600, and 800 mg b.i.d., and two subjects of each group received placebo twice daily for 10 days [24]. In the multiple-dose studies, AUC and C_{max} were dose proportional over 100 to 1600 mg and there was approximate dose proportionality for C_{12h} over 100 to 800 mg. Plasma concentrations decreased from C_{max} in a biphasic manner, with an initial half-life of 1 h and a terminal half-life of 7 to 12 h. With multiple dosing, steady state was achieved after two days. Different studies investigated the food effect on the pharmacokinetic paramenters. The extent of raltegravir absorption ($AUC_{0-\infty}$) was slightly higher in the fed state, but food slowed the rate and extended the duration of absorption, with a 34% decrease in C_{max}, an 8.5-fold increase in C_{12h}, and a 7.3-h delay in T_{max}. However, considerable interindividual variability was seen, particularly with respect to C_{12h}, and the authors concluded that the effects of food did not appear to be clinically important and that raltegravir could be administered without regard to food. Two studies were also conducted on subjects with renal and hepatic insufficiency, suggesting that no dose adjustment is considered to be necessary in these patients.

The main clinical programme to support the marketing authorization application for Isentress consisted of two identical phase III double-blind randomized placebo-controlled trials investigating the safety, tolerability, and efficacy of raltegravir 400 mg b.i.d. in combination with optimized background therapy (OBT) in treatment-experienced patients who failed antiretroviral therapies with triple-class resistant virus (protocols 018 and 019); one phase II study for dose finding in combination therapy in treatment-experienced patients (protocol 005); and one phase II study for proof-of-concept in monotherapy (part 1) and thereafter, dose finding in combination therapy (part 2), both in treatment-naive patients (protocol 004). Details of these studies are summarized in Table 12.

TABLE 11 In Vitro Metabolism and Plasma Protein Binding

Species	Intrinsic Oxidative Clearance (μL·min/mg)[a]	Intrinsic Glucuronidation Clearance (μL·min/mg)[b]	Unbound Fraction in Plasma
Rat	<1	32 ± 2	0.27
Dog	<1	2.2 ± 3	0.29
Rhesus	<1	33 ± 2	0.15
Rabbit	<1	10 ± 1	0.10
Human	<1	8.3 ± 0.5	0.17

[a]In the presence of NADPH.
[b]In the presence of UDPGA.

TABLE 12 Summary of Main Clinical Studies

Protocol	Design/Duration	Treatment	*n*	Population	Study Objectives	Primary Endpoint
004 (phase IIa), part 1	Multicenter double-blind randomized dose ranging controlled study; 10 days	100 mg b.i.d. 200 mg b.i.d. 400 mg b.i.d. 600 mg b.i.d. Comparator: placebo	7 7 6 8 7	Treatment-naive patients with plasma HIV RNA ≥ 5000 copies/mL and CD4 cell counts ≥ 100 cells/mm^3; at least 18 years of age	Part 1: Dose finding and proof-of-concept (monotherapy)	Change from baseline in plasma HIV RNA on day 10
004 (phase IIa), part 2	Multicenter double-blind randomized dose ranging controlled study; 48 weeks with extension to 144 weeks	100 mg b.i.d. 200 mg b.i.d. 400 mg b.i.d. 600 mg b.i.d. Comparator: EFV	39 40 41 40 38		Part 2: Dose finding (combination therapy: TDF + 3TC)	Proportion of patients with HIV RNA < 400 copies/mL at week 24
005 (phase IIb)	Multicenter double-blind randomized dose ranging placebo-ontrolled study; 48 weeks with extension to 144 weeks	200 mg b.i.d. 400 mg b.i.d. 600 mg b.i.d. Placebo	43 45 45 45	Treatment-experienced patients with plasma HIV RNA > 5000 copies/mL and CD4 cell counts > 50 cells/mm^3 and documented resistant to at least one ART in each of the three classes; at least 18 years of age	Dose finding (combination therapy: OBT)	Change from baseline in HIV RNA at week 24
018 (phase III)	Multicenter double-blind randomized placebo-ontrolled study; 48 weeks with extension to 152 weeks	400 mg b.i.d. Placebo	232 118	Treatment-experienced with plasma HIV RNA ≥ 1000 copies/mL and documented resistance to 3 ART classes; at least 16 years of age	Demonstration of efficacy (combination therapy: OBT)	Proportion of patients with HIV RNA < 400 copies/mL at week 16
019 (phase III)	Multicenter double-blind randomized placebo-ontrolled study; 48 weeks with extension to 152 weeks	400 mg b.i.d. Placebo	230 119	Treatment-experienced with plasma HIV RNA ≥ 1000 copies/mL and documented resistance to 3 ART classes; at least 16 years of age	Demonstration of efficacy (combination therapy: OBT)	Proportion of patients with HIV RNA < 400 copies/mL at week 16

The first part of protocol 004 was conducted in 35 treatment-naive HIV-positive patients and was designed to assess the pharmacokinetics, efficacy, and tolerability of raltegravir monotherapy over 10 days [25]. Eligible subjects were aged > 18 years, were hepatitis B or C negative, had an HIV RNA level > 5000 copies/mL and a CD4$^+$ cell count > 100 cells/mm^3 at screening. Patients were randomly allocated to one of five treatment groups, receiving 100, 200, 400, or 600 mg of raltegravir b.i.d. or placebo. After 10 days, all doses of raltegravir monotherapy were associated with a significant reduction from baseline in HIV RNA compared with placebo. When stratified by baseline HIV RNA > 50,000 copies/mL, those with higher viral loads had a greater decline from baseline, although the slope from day 1 to 10 did not differ. There were no significant differences in reduction in HIV RNA between raltegravir doses. The second part of protocol 004 was a 48-week semirandomized double-blind dose-ranging study in 201 patients receiving raltegravir vs, efavirenz, both administerd in combination with tenofovir and lamivudine [26]. Patients were randomized to receive oral raltegravir 100, 200, 400, or 600 mg b.i.d. or standard-dose efavirenz. Although participants were treatment naive,

35% had AIDS and 54% had HIV RNA levels > 50,000 copies/mL at study entry. At baseline, mean HIV RNA levels ranged from 4.6 to 4.8 $\log_{10}$ copies/mL, and the mean $CD4^+$ cell count ranged from 271 to 338 cells/mm^3. At 24 weeks, 85 to 92% of patients in all groups had achieved an undetectable viral load. A similar proportion of patients in the raltegravir and efavirenz groups achieved an HIV RNA level < 50 copies/mL that was sustained for up to 48 weeks. Patients in the Raltegravir arms achieved an HIV RNA < 50 copies/mL count significantly more rapidly than did those in the efavirenz arm (week 16: 80 vs. 70%, respectively).

From this study, raltegravir-containing regimens appeared to be effective in antiretroviral-naive patients and may be an option for patients who are unable to tolerate standard initial therapies. Another phase II dose-ranging study (protocol 005) that aimed to assess the safety and efficacy of raltegravir in combination with optimized background therapy in treatment-experienced patients infected with multidrug-resistant HIV-1 was conducted in the United States, Europe, Latin America, and Asia [27]. Nonpregnant HIV-1-seropositive patients aged over 18 years with a plasma HIV-1 RNA viral load above 5000 copies/mL and a $CD4^+$ cell count above 50 cells/μL, on stable antiretroviral therapy for more than three months and infected with HIV-1 with documented genotypic or phenotypic resistance to at least one non-nucleoside reverse transcriptase inhibitor (NNRTI), one nucleoside reverse transcriptase inhibitor (NRTI), and one protease inhibitor (PI) were eligible. Before randomization, the investigators selected each patient's optimized background regimen on the basis of the patient's antiretroviral treatment history, with the aim of designing the best possible treatment regimen. Patients were allocated randomly to one of four treatment arms: oral raltegravir 200, 400, or 600 mg b.i.d., or placebo. The primary endpoints were antiretroviral activity as measured by change in viral load from baseline at week 24 and safety. The antiretroviral effects of raltegravir at all doses were better than those with placebo when added to the optimized background regimen. In all raltegravir groups there was a decrease of about 2 $\log_{10}$ copies/mL in HIV-1 RNA from baseline noted as early as two weeks after the initiation of treatment, which was sustained through 24 weeks. The proportion of patients achieving a viral load of fewer than 50 copies/mL was significantly higher in all raltegravir groups than in groups with placebo. The reduction in viral load was accompanied by increases in $CD4^+$ cell counts compared with baseline. Raltegravir at all doses had a safety profile much the same as that of placebo and there were no dose-related toxicities.

Overall, this study has shown that raltegravir has a rapid, potent and sustained antiretroviral effect in patients with advanced HIV-1 infection who had failed previous therapy, with triple-class resistant virus, and with a limited number of active antiretroviral drugs in their background regimen. On the basis of the data from this study, on the data of the previous phase II study (protocol 004), and on the data from drug interaction studies, the dose of 400 mg of raltegravir b.i.d. without dose adjustment when used in combination with other antiretroviral drugs was selected for phase III studies. Two identical phase III studies, BENCHMRK (blocking integrase in treatment-experienced patients with a novel compound against HIV—Merck) 1 and 2, have been conducted to evaluate the safety profile and efficacy of raltegravir (400 mg b.i.d.) in treatment-experienced patients with viral resistance in combination with an optimized background therapy [28,29]. BENCHMRK 1 (protocol 018) was conducted at 65 sites in Europe, the Asia/Pacific, and South America (n = 352). BENCHMRK 2 (protocol 019) was conducted at 53 sites in North and South America (n = 351). Male and female patients at least 16 years of age were enrolled. Patients were to have a screening plasma HIV RNA of > 1000 copies/mL on stable ART for ≥ 2 months and were to be infected with HIV that showed reduced susceptibility to at least one compound in each of NNRTI, NRTI, and PI classes. Based on screening resistance testing results and prior treatment and resistance history, ARTs were revaluated to optimize the background therapy (OBT). Patients were randomized to receive oral raltegravir 400 mg b.i.d. + OBT or placebo + OBT. The primary efficacy objective was to evaluate the antiretroviral activity of raltegravir 400 mg b.i.d. in the study as measured by proportion with < 400 copies/mL at week 16. A secondary analysis at week 48 measured the proportion with HIV RNA < 50 copies/mL, HIV RNA < 400 copies/mL, change from baseline in plasma HIV RNA ($\log_{10}$ copies/mL), and change from baseline in $CD4^+$ cell count (cells/mm^3).

The Treatment effects were similar in the two studies. Inclusion of enfuvirtide or darunavir in the OBT for patients who were naive to these agents improved the responses to raltegravir and placebo groups compared to patients without these agents. It was concluded from these studies that raltegravir 400 mg b.i.d. has potent and superior antiretroviral and immunological efficacy to that of placebo + OBT, which is sustained through week 48; in patients receiving new, active antiretroviral therapies in OBT, up to 89% achieved HIV RNA < 50 copies/mL at week 48; and raltegravir 400 mg b.i.d. + OBT is generally well tolerated compared to placebo in combination with OBT.

A further phase III study called STARTMRK (protocol 021) was conducted by comparing raltegravir- and efavirenz-based combination regimens as initial treatment for adults infected with HIV-1 [30]. STARTMRK is a continuing international double-blind randomized active controlled phase III trial in which 563 patients from 67 study centers on five continents (Australia, Brazil, Canada, Chile, Colombia, France, Germany, India, Italy, Mexico, Peru, Spain, Thailand, and the United States) received either 400 mg of raltegravir administered orally twice daily or 600 mg of efavirenz administered orally once daily, both in combination with tenofovir of emricitabine. The primary endpoint at week 48 was achievement of less than 50 vRNA copies/mL. Secondary endpoints at week 48 were the achievement of less than 400 vRNA copies/mL and the change from baseline in $CD4^+$ cell count. Of the 563 patients, 59 (10%) discontinued treatment mainly because of adverse events. More than half ($n = 297$, 53%) of participants had more than 100,000 vRNA copies/mL. In the main analysis that recorded as failures all patients who did not complete the study, 86·1% ($n = 241$) of the raltegravir group achieved the primary endpoint of fewer than 50 vRNA copies/mL at week 48, compared with 81·9% ($n = 230$) of the efavirenz group, indicating that raltegravir was not inferior to efavirenz. More patients achieved viral suppression to fewer than 50 vRNA copies/mL in the raltegravir group than in the efavirenz group at early time points (weeks 2 to 16). The time to achieve such viral suppression was shorter for patients on raltegravir than for those on efavirenz. The mean change in CD4 cell count from baseline to week 48 was 189 cells/μL [95% confidence interval (CI) 174 to 204] for raltegravir recipients and 163 cells/μL (148 to 178) for efavirenz recipients (difference, 26 cells/μL, 95% CI 4 to 47). The viral load reduction and increase in $CD4^+$ cell count was maintained through 96 weeks; the treatment difference in suppressing vRNA below 50 copies/mL was 2% favoring raltegravir, and patients on the raltegravir arm experienced a statistically similar, yet numerically greater increase in $CD4^+$ cell count (240 cells/mm^3) than those on the efavirenz arm.

Overall, 66 patients (10% on raltegravir and 14% on efavirenz) did not achieve fewer than 50 vRNA copies/mL during the study, defined as virological failure. Of the patients on raltegravir who had virological failure, half had mutations known to confer raltegravir resistance. When resistance to raltegravir was developed, the mutational pattern was consistent with that previously reported in treatment-experienced patients on raltegravir [31]. Raltegravir had a more favorable safety and tolerability profile than than of efavirenz. Of patients taking the regimen containing raltegravir, 47% experienced drug-related clinical-related adverse events and CNS-related adverse events vs. 78% of patients receiving the efavirenz-based regimen. Dyslipidemias are common complications of antiretroviral drugs and are often associated with protease inhibitors and reverse transcriptase inhibitors. Raltegravir had a modest effect on serum lipids between baseline and week 48, including total low-density lipoprotein (LDL) and high-density lipoprotein (HDL) cholesterol levels, as well as triglycerides, but changes were significantly higher for efavirenz recipients. Results from this STARTMRK study supported an expanded indication for raltegravir (Isentress), approved by the U.S. Food and Drug Administration on July 8, 2009, to include the treatment of adult patients starting HIV-1 therapy for the first time.

Drug-interaction studies of raltegravir have been conducted in HIV-negative patients [32]. Raltegravir is not a cytochrome P450 (CYP) substrate, inducer, or inhibitor; therefore, CYP-related interactions are not expected. In addition, raltegravir does not inhibit P-glycoprotein (Pgp)-mediated transport. Raltegravir is a Pgp substrate, although there are no data indicating that it may be affected by Pgp inducers or inhibitors. Some drug interactions have been reported, presumably as a result of induction or inhibition of UGT 1A1 glucuronidation.

Many other clinical studies have been conducted and are still ongoing that highlight raltegravir, the first agent approved in the class of integrase inhibitors, as an important addition to the armamentarium of antiretroviral agents, both in treatment-experienced and treatment-naive patients. Raltegravir has favorable pharmacokinetic properties, a small pill burden, and an acceptable tolerability profile. Raltegravir used in combination with other active antiretrovirals affords the opportunity for achievement of immunologic and virologic recovery in patients.

FUTURE DIRECTIONS

Despite the clear success of raltegravir (Isentress), research for second-generation strand-transfer-specific integrase inhibitors continues to be very active. HIV is a viral pathogen characterized by a high mutational rate, and probably following prolonged clinical use of Isentress the emergence of drug-resistant viral strains can be problematic, causing the loss of drug effectiveness. It is therefore essential to continue to develop new antiretroviral drugs with potency against an ever-wider range of viral isolates to provide novel treatment options. Within this effort to identify second-generation integrase inhibitors with a higher genetic barrier to mutation and limited cross resistance, ongoing studies in Merck's laboratories focused on the design and synthesis of many structurally diverse templates mimicking the diketoacid pharmacophore [33]. In particular, optimization of a series of tricyclic 10-hydroxy-7,8-dihydropyrazinopyrrolopyridazine-1,9-diones [34] led to the discovery of MK-2048 with excellent antiviral activity ($CIC_{95} = 41$ nM in 50% normal human serum) and good pharmacokinetics in preclinical species [35]. This candidate next-generation inhibitor was found to retain excellent activity against four of five types of drug-resistant integrase mutants (N155S, Q148K, F121Y, T66I/S153Y). Experimental data indicated that MK-2048 has a dissociation half-life from the integrase/DNA complex of 32 h on wild-type integrase, more than four times that of raltegravir. This half-life fades almost tenfold, to 4 h, in the face of N155S mutant virus, while for raltegravir it shrinks to 0.7 h, suggesting for MK-2048 a reduced susceptibility to resistance mutations [36]. Apart from Merck, interest in the field of integrase inhibitors continues at a high level, with many companies and academic institutions publishing and patenting in this field.

REFERENCES

[1] WHO/UNAIDS/UNICEF. Towards universal access: scaling up priority HIV(AIDS interventions in the health sector. Progress report, 2008. http://www.who.int/hiv/pub/Towards_Universal_Access _Report_2008.pdf.

[2] UNAIDS. AIDS epidemic update, 2007. Available at http://data.unaids.org/pub/EPISlides/2007/2007_epiupdate_en.pdf.

[3] Wood, A.; Armour, D. The discovery of the CCR5 receptor antagonist UK-427857: a new agent for the treatment of HIV infection and AIDS. *Prog. Med. Chem.* **2005**, *43*, 39–271.

[4] Manfredi, R.; Sabbatani, S. A novel antiretroviral class (fusiion inhibitors) in the management of HIV infection: present features and future perspectives of enfuvirtide (T-20). *Curr. Med. Chem.* **2006**, *13*, 2369–2384.

[5] Pommier, Y.; Johnson, A. A.; Marchand, C. Integrase inhibitors to treat HIV(AIDS. *Nat. Rev. Drug Discov.* **2005**, *4*, 236–248.

[6] Hazuda, D. J.; Felock, P.; Witmer, M.; Wolfe, A.; Stillmock, K.; Grobler, J. A.; Espeseth, A.; Gabryelski, L.; Schleif, W.; Blau, C.; Miller, M. D. Inhibitors of strand transfer that prevent integration and inhibit HIV-1 replication in cells. *Science* **2000**, *287*, 646–650.

[7] Hazuda, D. J.; Young, S. D.; Guare, J. P.; Neville, A. J.; Gomez, R. P.; Wai, J. S.; Vacca, J. P.; Handt, L.; Motzel, S. L.; Klein, H. J.; et al. Integrase inhibitors and cellular immunity suppress retroviral replication in rhesus macaques. *Science* **2004**, *305*, 528–532.

[8] Ramirez, M. 10th European AIDS Conference, Dublin, Ireland, 2006. Abstract LPBS1/6. Beatriz Grinsztejn, B.; Nguyen, B.; Katlama, C.; Gatell, J. M.; Lazzarin, A.; Vittecoq, D; Gonzalez, C. J.; Chen, J.; Harvey, C. M.; Isaacs, R. D. Safety and efficacy of the HIV-1 integrase inhibitor raltegravir (MK-0518) in treatment-experienced patients with multidrug-resistant virus: a phase II randomised controlled trial. *Lancet* **2007**, *369*, 1261–1269.

[9] Grobler, J. A.; Stillmock, K.; Hu, B.; Witmer, M.; Felock, P.; Espeseth, A. S.; Wolfe, A.; Egbertson, M.; Bourgeois, M.; Melamed, J.; et al. Diketo acid inhibitor mechanism and HIV-1 integrase: implications for metal binding in the active site of phosphotransferase enzymes. *Proc. Natl. Acad. Sci. USA* **2002**, *99*, 6661–6666.

[10] Summa, V.; Petrocchi, A.; Pace, P.; Matassa, V. G.; De Francesco, R.; Altamura, S.; Tomei, L.; Koch, U.; Neuner, P. Discovery of α,γ-diketo acids as potent selective and reversible inhibitors of hepatitis C virus NS5b RNA-dependent RNA polymerase. *J. Med. Chem.* **2004**, *47*, 14–17.

[11] Pace, P.; Nizi, E.; Pacini, B.; Pesci, S.; Matassa, V.; De Francesco, R.; Altamura, S.; Summa, V. The monoethyl ester of meconic acid is an active site inhibitor of HCV NS5B RNA-dependent RNA polymerase. *Bioorg. Med. Chem. Lett.* **2004**, *14*, 3257–3261.

[12] Summa, V.; Petrocchi, A.; Matassa, V. G.; Taliani, M.; Laufer, R.; De Francesco, R.; Altamura, S.; Pace, P. HCV NS5b RNA-dependent RNA polymerase inhibitors: from α,γ-diketoacids to 4,5-dihydroxypyrimidine or 3-methyl-5-hydroxypyrimidinonecarboxylic acids—design and synthesis. *J. Med. Chem.* **2004**, *47*, 5336–5339.

[13] Petrocchi, A.; Koch, U.; Matassa, V. G.; Pacini, B.; Stillmock, K. A.; Summa, V. From dihydroxypyrimidine carboxylic acids to carboxamides HIV 1 integrase inhibitors: SAR around the amide mojety. *Bioorg. Med. Chem. Lett.* **2007**, *17*, 350–353.

[14] Pace, P.; Di Francesco, M. E.; Gardelli, C.; Harper, S.; Muraglia, E.; Nizi, E.; Orvieto, F.; Petrocchi, A.; Poma, M.; Rowley, M.; et al. Dihydroxypyrimidines-4-carboxamides as novel potent and selective HIV-integrase inhibitors. *J. Med. Chem.* **2007**, *50*, 2225–2239.

[15] Gardelli, C.; Nizi, E.; Muraglia, E.; Crescenzi, B.; Ferrara, M.; Orvieto, F.; Pace, P.; Pescatore, G.; Poma, M.; Rico Ferreira, R. M.; et al. Discovery and synthesis of HIV integrase inhibitors: development of potent and orally bioavailable *N*-methyl pyrimidones. *J. Med. Chem.* **2007**, *50*, 4953–4975.

[16] Chapman, R. G.; Ostuni, E.; Takayama, S.; Holmlin, R.; Erik, Y. L.; Whitesides, G. M. Surveying for surfaces that resist the adsorption of proteins. *J. Am. Chem. Soc.* **2000**, *122*, 8303–8304.

[17] Guare, J. P.; Wai, J. S.; Gomez, R. P.; Anthony, N. J.; Jolly, S. M.; Cortes, A. R.; Vacca, J. P.; Felock, P. J.; Stillmock, K. A.; Schleif, W. A.; et al. A series of 5-aminosubstituted 4-fluorobenzyl-8-hydroxy[1,6naphthyridine-7-carboxamide HIV-1 integrase inhibitors. *Bioorg. Med. Chem. Lett.* **2006**, *16*, 2900–2904.

[18] Summa, V.; Petrocchi, A.; Bonelli, F.; Crescenzi, B.; Donghi, M.; Ferrara, M.; Fioré, F.; Gardelli, C.; Gonzalez Paz, O.; Hazuda, D. J.; et al. Discovery of raltegravir, a potent, selective orally bioavailable HIV integrase inhibitor for the treatment of HIV-AIDS infection. *J. Med. Chem.* **2008**, *51*, 5843–5855.

[19] Laufer, R.; Gonzalez Paz, O.; Di Marco, A.; Bonelli, F.; Monteagudo, E.; Summa, V.; Rowley, M. Quantitative prediction of human clearance guiding the development of raltegravir (MK-0518, Isentress) and related HIV integrase inhibitors. *Drug Metab. Dispos.* **2009**, *37*, 873–883.

[20] Culbertson, T. P. *J. Heterocycl. Chem.* **1979**, *16*, 1423

[21] Pye, P. J.; Zhong, Y.; Jones, G. O.; Reamer, R. A.; Houk, K. N.; Askin, D. *Angew. Chem. Int. Ed.* **2008**, *47* (22), 4134.

[22] Raltegravir. Scientific discussion. Available at http://www.emea.europa.eu/humandocs/PDFs/EPAR/isentress/H-860-en6.pdf.

[23] Cocohoba, J.; Dong, B. J. Raltegravir: the first HIV integrase inhibitor. *Clin. Ther.* **2008**, *30*, 1747–1765.

[24] Iwamoto, M.; Wenning, L. A.; Petry, A. S.; et al. Safety, Tolerability and pharmacokinetics of raltegravir after single and multiple doses in healthy subjects. *Clin. Pharmacol. Ther.* **2008**, *83*, 293–299.

[25] Markowitz, M.; Morales-Ramirez, J. O.; Nguyen, B. Y.; et al. Antiretroviral activity, pharmacokinetics, and tolerability of MK-0518, a novel inhibitor of HIV-1 integrase, dosed as monotherapy for 10 days in treatmentnaive HIV-1 infected individuals. *J. Acquir. Immune Defic. Syndr.* **2006**, *43*, 509–515.

[26] Markowitz, M.; Nguyen, B. Y.; Gotuzzo, E. Rapid and durable antiretroviral effect of the HIV integrase inhibitor raltegravir

as part of combination therapy in treatment-naive patients with HIV-1 infection: results of a 48-week controlled study. *J. Acquir. Immune Defic. Syndr.* **2007**, *46*, 125–133.

[27] Grinsztejin, B.; Nguyen, B. Y.; Katlama, C.; Gatel, J. M.; Lazzarin, A.; Vittecoq, D.; Gonzalez, C. J.; Chen, J.; Harvey, C. M.; Isaacs, R. D. (Protocol 005 Team). Safety and efficacy of the HIV-1 integrase inhibitor raltegravir (MK-0518) in treatment-experienced patients with multidrug-resistant virus: a phase II randomised controlled trial. *Lancet* **2007**, *369*, 1261–1269.

[28] Cooper, D.; Gatell, J.; Rockstroh, J.; Katlama, C.; Yeni, P.; Lazzarin, A.; Xu, X.; Isaacs, R.; Teppler, H.; Nguyen, B. Y. (BENCHMRK-1 Study Group). 48-Week results from BENCHMRK-1, a phase III study of raltegravir in patients failing ART with triple-class resistant HIV-1. 15th Conference on Retroviruses and Opportunistic Infections, Boston, Feb. 3–6, 2008. Abstract 788.

[29] Steigbigel, R.; Kumar, P.; Eron, J.; Schechter, M.; Markowitz, M.; Loufty, M.; Zhao, J.; Isaacs, R.; Nguyen, B.; Teppler, H. (BENCHMRK-2 Study Group). 48-Week results from BENCHMRK-2, a phase III study of raltegravir in patients failing ART with triple class resistant HIV. 15th Conference on Retroviruses and Opportunistic Infections, Boston, Feb. 3–6, 2008. Abstract 789.

[30] Lennox, J. L.; DeJesus, E.; Lazzarin, A.; Pollard, R. B.; Ramalho Madruga, J. V.; Berger, D. S.; Zhao, J.; Xu, X.; Williams-Diaz, A.; Rodgers, A. J.; et al. (STARTMRK investigators). Safety and efficacy of raltegravir-based versus efavirenz-based combination therapy in treatment-naive patients with HIV-1 infection: a multicentre, double-blind randomised controlled trial. *Lancet* **2009**, *374*, 796–806.

[31] Steitbigel, R. T.; Cooper, D. A.; Kumar, P. N.; et al. Raltegravir with optimized background therapy for resistant HIV-1 infection. *N. Engl. J. Med.* **2008**, *359*, 339–354.

[32] Isentress. Package insert. Available at https://www.merck.com/product/usa/pi_circulars/i/isentress/isentress_pi.pdf.

[33] Egbertson, M. S. HIV Integrase inhibitors: from diketoacids to heterocyclic templates: a history of HIV integrase medicinal chemistry at Merck West Point and Merck Rome (IRBM). *Curr. Top. Med. Chem.* **2007**, *13*, 1251–1272.

[34] Wai, J. S.; Vacca, J. P.; Zhuang, L.; Kim, B.; Lyle, T. A.; Wiscount, C. M.; Egbertson, M. S.; Neilson, L. A.; Embrey, M.; Fisher, T. E.; Staas, D. D. Pyrazinopyrrolopyridazines as HIV integrase inhibitors: their preparation, pharmaceutical compositions, and use to prevent or treat HIV infection. Merck & Co., Inc. WO-2005110415A1, 2005.

[35] Wai, J.; Fisher, T.; Embrey, M.; Egbertson, M.; Vacca, J.; Hazuda, D.; Miller, M.; Witmer, M.; Gabryelski, L.; Lyle, T. Next generation of inhibitors of HIV-1 integrase strand transfer inhibitor: structural diversity and resistance profiles. 14th Conference on Retroviruses and Opportunistic Infections, Los Angeles, 2007. Abstract 87.

[36] Grobler, J. A.; McKenna, P. M.; Ly, S. Functional irreversible inhibition of integration by slowly dissociating strand transfer inhibitors. 10th International Workshop on Clinical Pharmacology of HIV Therapy, Amsterdam, Apr. 15–17, 2009. Abstract O-10.

14

ELVITEGRAVIR: A NOVEL MONOKETO ACID HIV-1 INTEGRASE STRAND TRANSFER INHIBITOR

HISASHI SHINKAI
Central Pharmaceutical Research Institute, JT, Inc., Osaka, Japan
MASANORI SATO
Pharmaceutical Division, JT, Inc., Tokyo, Japan
YUJI MATSUZAKI
Central Pharmaceutical Research Institute, JT, Inc., Osaka, Japan

INTRODUCTION

Three viral enzymes, human immunodeficiency virus type 1 (HIV-1) integrase, HIV-1 reverse transcriptase, and HIV-1 protease, are essential for retroviral replication and comprise important targets for disrupting the viral replication cycle [1]. Reverse transcriptase inhibitors and protease inhibitors have already achieved significant advances in antiretroviral therapy, but at times do not achieve complete suppression and thus risk the production of resistant HIV-1 [2,3]. On the other hand, studies on the integrase inhibitors have advanced only recently. Elvitegravir (EVG), which is also referred to as JTK-303 or GS-9137, represents a structurally novel class of HIV-1 integrase strand transfer inhibitors, and has a monoketo acid motif in a quinolone carboxylic acid core structure. EVG exhibits an IC_{50} value of 7.2 nM in an HIV-1 integrase strand transfer assay using 5 nM of target DNA, and an EC_{50} of 0.9 nM in an acute HIV-1 infection assay. A well-known class of HIV-1 integrase strand transfer inhibitors is the keto-enol acid (often referred to as diketo acid) series, and the keto-enol acid moiety (γ-ketone, α-enol, and carboxylic acid) or its bioisosters is believed to be essential for inhibitory activity [4]. The metal-chelating functions of the keto-enol acid family, in simultaneous coordination with two divalent metal ions, are considered to be relevant to their mechanism of inhibitory action. Nevertheless, the novel quinolone integrase inhibitor EVG described here has only a monoketo acid motif (coplanar β-ketone and carboxylic acid) as an alternative to the keto-enol acid motif. Although the simplified monoketo acid motif has only two coordinating functional groups and cannot fully duplicate the interactions of the reported keto-enol acid series, EVG is nevertheless as potent at inhibiting integrase and displaying antiretroviral activity as are the keto-enol acid integrase inhibitors.

DISCOVERY

Divalent Metal Ions and Integrase Inhibitors

The binding and activity of keto-enol acid HIV-1 integrase inhibitors are divalent metal cation dependent [4–7]. Thus, the interaction of the inhibitors with divalent metal ions in the active site of the enzyme is considered to be a key factor in the inhibition of HIV-1 integrase. Therefore, in the design of integrase inhibitors, it is crucially important to know the number of metals involved in the enzyme activity and in the inhibitory activity, but this has yet to be determined. HIV-1 integrase requires divalent metal ions, such as Mn^{2+} and Mg^{2+}, for catalytic activity [8]. The catalytic core domain of HIV-1 integrase contains two aspartates and one glutamate

Antiviral Drugs: From Basic Discovery Through Clinical Trials, First Edition. Edited by Wieslaw M. Kazmierski.

(the DDE motif consists of aspartic D64, D116, and gultamic E152), which are essential for enzymatic activity [9]. This catalytic triad potentially binds two divalent metals.

HIV-1 integrase belongs to a large family of DNA-processing enzymes (polynucleotidyl transferases) that includes avian sarcoma virus (ASV) integrase and polymerases [10–12]. These enzymes contain the same arrangement of three catalytically essential carboxylates, which are highly conserved in all integrases and polymerases [1,13]. In ASV integrase, an additional metal coordinated by aspartic D64 and glutamic E157 was observed with Zn^{2+} or Cd^{2+} ions [14]. A second such metal has also been observed in DNA polymerase I [15]. Moreover, a dual metal-ion mechanism is proposed as a chemically reasonable mechanism of action for polynucleotidyl transferases [10,16–19]. This information supports the notion that HIV-1 integrase would also contain two divalent metal ions. However, only a single Mg^{2+} ion was observed to be chelated by aspartic D64 and D116 in the crystal structures of the catalytic core domain of HIV-1 integrase [20,21]. HIV-1 integrase consists of three distinct structural domains (the zinc binding N-terminal, the catalytic core, and the DNA binding C-terminal) [9] and performs a two-step reaction: removal of the terminal dinucleotide from each 3′-end of the viral DNA (3′-processing) and subsequent joining of the 3′-end of the viral DNA to host DNA (strand transfer) [9,22]. Both the N- and C-terminal domains are required for the 3′-processing and strand transfer steps [23–29], while the core domain alone can only carry out a disintegration reaction [24,25,30–33]. DNA ending with the sequence CAGT is also required for functional activity in HIV-1 integrase [34]. Therefore, the catalytic core domain by itself is not able to assume the precise structure required for the functional enzyme. Full-length integrase complexed with DNA is essential to achieve the exact conformation of a functional integrase and may allow binding of the second metal ion. Two divalent cations (Mg^{2+} or Mn^{2+}) apparently coordinate the DDE motif of HIV-1 integrase with the phosphodiester backbone of the DNA substrates (the viral donor cDNA and the chromosomal acceptor DNA) during the integration steps [35,36]. However, this cannot be determined until crystal structures for either the complete HIV-1 integrase molecule or the HIV-1 integrase complexed with DNA substrate are made available.

Keto-enol acid inhibitors selectively interrupt the strand transfer step, and in cell-based assays inhibit integration without affecting earlier phases of the HIV-1 replication cycle [4,7,37–39]. In addition, the binding of the keto-enol acid inhibitors was only detected when full-length integrase was assembled onto the viral DNA ends [4]. To explain these observations, it is proposed that the keto-enol acid inhibitors can bind only with the interface of the full-length integrase-DNA-divalent metal complex after 3′-processing [1]. Their ability to bind selectively to the enzyme complexed with the viral DNA and to compete with the host DNA substrate may explain their selectivity for the strand transfer reaction [4,39]. Moreover, the role of a second metal ion in selective strand transfer inhibition is suggested [1]. If the binding of the keto-enol acid inhibitors require a second metal, and this metal is required for forming a strand transfer complex, it is understandable why inhibitors selectively block the strand transfer reaction, and why inhibitor binding is observed only in the context of viral DNA. Although a co-crystal of full-length integrase complexed with DNA substrates and an inhibitor would detail the exact binding mode and allow structure-based approaches for drug design, no useful data have been available [40–43]. Therefore, we undertook modifying the keto-enol acid structure so as to obtain new bioisosters of keto-enol acid, or a new scaffold as an alternative to that of keto-enol acid.

Monoketo and Keto-enol Acids

The keto-enol acid groups are known to have metal-chelating functions, and the ability to coordinate two divalent metal ions simultaneously [44]. In fact, the keto-enol acid reacts with magnesium chloride to give dianionic species under physiological conditions, and complexes form involving two divalent cations and two keto-enol acid ligand molecules [44]. Although it is still unclear whether two metal ions are involved in the inhibitory action of the keto-enol acids, this dual metal-chelating function has been considered relevant to the mechanism of action of the keto-enol acid inhibitors [4]. Thus, the keto-enol acid moiety (γ-ketone, α-enol, and carboxylic acid) is believed to be essential for the inhibitory activity of this series of integrase inhibitors [4], and the structures of keto-enol triazole (S1360) [45], keto-enol tetrazole (5CITEP) [40], 9-carbonyl-1,2-catechol (Catechol) [46], 7-carbamoyl-8-hydroxy-(1,6)-naphthyridine (L-870810) [46,47], and 4-carbamoyl-5-hydroxy-6-pyrimidinone (raltegravir/MK-0518) [48] were synthesized as bioisosters of the keto-enol acid pharmacophore (Fig. 1). The carboxylic acid in the keto-enol acid motif could reasonably be replaced with a triazole or a tetrazole, which are well-known bioisoters of a carboxylic acid group [49]. The triazole derivative S 1360 inhibited the HIV-1 integrase at an IC_{50} of 20 nM and the HIV-1 replication at an EC_{50} of 140 nM, and was the first to be tested in clinical trials [50]. The enolizable α-ketone and carboxylic acid moiety of the keto-enol acid side chain can be replaced with a 1,2-catechol [46]. This result means that an acidic phenolic hydroxyl group can serve as an alternative to the carboxylic acid group in the keto-enol acid motif, and that the enolizable ketone at the α-position can be replaced with a phenol group as an enol mimic. The 1,3-keto-enol acid can enolize at the α-position to a conjugated *Z*-4-oxo-2-hydroxy-2-butenoic structure with a coplanar conformation, and this ability to adopt the coplanar arrangement of the keto-enol acid motif is considered important for the inhibitory activity.

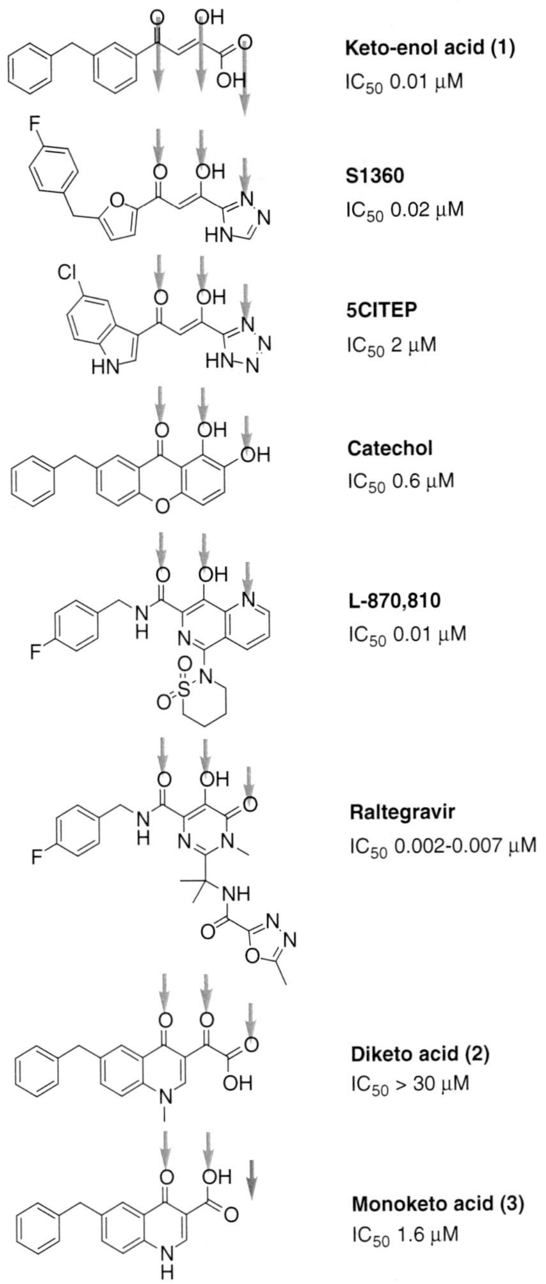

FIGURE 1 Bioisosters of the keto-enol acid, diketo acid, and monoketo acid.

Since the 1,2-catechol is conformationally restricted to a similar arrangement as the planar α-enol form, the planar α-enol form would be a biologically active conformation in the keto-enol acid class of integrase inhibitors. The 2-hydroxyl group in the 1,2-catechol derivative can also be replaced with a heteroaromatic nitrogen [46]. This means that the carboxylic acid in the keto-enol acid motif can be replaced not only by acidic bioisosters but also by a basic heterocycle bearing a lone-pair donor atom such as a pyridine ring [22]. It has been reported that the heteroaromatic nitrogen in the pyridine ring mimics the corresponding carboxyl oxygen in the keto-enol acid motif as a Lewis base equivalent [46]. Moreover, the α-enol and carboxylic acid moiety of the keto-enol acid motif can be replaced with a 5-hydroxy-6-pyrimidinone [51], indicating that the carboxylic acid group can be replaced with a simple carbonyl group. Raltegravir, possessing a 4-carbamoyl-5-hydroxy-6-pyrimidinone core, inhibits strand transfer activity at an IC_{50} value of 2 to 7 nM and has anti-HIV-1 activity at a CIC_{95} of 19 nM in 10% fetal bovine serum and a CIC_{95} of 33 nM in 50% human serum. Recently approved in the United States and in the European Union in 2007, raltegravir is the most advanced compound in the keto-enol acid class of HIV-1 integrase strand transfer inhibitors [48].

All bioisosters of the keto-enol acid motif have the three functional groups that mimic a ketone, enolizable ketone, and carboxyl oxygen, and can assume a coplanar conformation (gray arrows in Fig. 1). Although as yet whether the two metal ions are involved in the enzyme activity and in the inhibitory action remains to be determined, the structural requirements for keto-enol acid integrase inhibitors indicate that the metal-chelating functions of the keto-enol acid motif, which can coordinate two metal ions simultaneously, are relevant to the mechanism of inhibition [4]. Therefore, we designed quinolone-3-glyoxylic acid (diketo acid **2**) as a nonenolizable diketo acid that can assume a planer conformation without forming enol (dashed arrow in Fig. 1). This motif has no central enol group, but still has three functional groups that potentially coordinate with the two metal ions. However, the diketo acid did not exhibit integrase inhibitory activity. This indicates the importance of the central ionizable enol in the keto-enol acid motif. In contrast, we found that 4-quinolone-3-carboxylic acid (monoketo acid **3**) does exhibit integrase inhibitory activity [7]. This novel quinolone integrase inhibitor has only two functional groups, a carboxylic acid and a β-ketone, which are coplanar (Fig. 1). This result shows that the coplanar monoketo acid motif in 4-quinolone-3-carboxylic acid can serve as an alternative to the keto-enol acid motif, even though the down-sized monoketo acid motif is unlikely to fully coordinate with the two divalent metal ions. The carboxylic acid in the monoketo acid motif would be an alternative to the central ionizable enol in the keto-enol acid moiety. A monoketo acid (compound **3**), which has only two functional groups and cannot fully coordinate the two divalent metal ions, is far less potent than are keto-enol acids. Thus, the chelating ability of the monoketo acid motif is weaker than that of the keto-enol acid motif. Although the finding regarding monoketo acid suggests that full functions of the keto-enol acid motif may not be essential for inhibitory activity, the metal-chelating functions are still important for their inhibitory action. The weak metal-chelating ability of the monoketo acid may be preferable from a safety standpoint, since there is a report that reduced cytotoxicity may be related to a weaker affinity for metal ions in the keto-enol acid class of integrase inhibitors [46]. Therefore, we chose the monoketo acid as an initial lead compound and began to modify structures around the core monoketo acid moiety to lead to more potent compounds despite the comparatively low starting potency ($IC_{50} = 1.6\ \mu M$).

The structural optimization process for the monoketo acid integrase inhibitors is shown in Figure 2. The distal aromatic moiety of the keto-enol acid integrase inhibitors can accommodate a wide range of substituents, and structure–activity relationship (SAR) studies have shown the aromatic portion to be crucial for potency [6,52,53]. The distal aromatic moiety is also crucial for potency in the monoketo acid inhibitors. Introduction of 2-fluoro and 3-chloro substituents into the distal benzene ring (compound **4**) led to a significant improvement (approximately a 36-fold increase) of its inhibition of strand transfer ($IC_{50} = 44$ nM) and its antiviral activity ($EC_{50} = 0.81\ \mu M$). Compound **5**, bearing a hydroxyethyl group at the 1-position of the quinolone ring, was 1.8-fold more potent at inhibiting strand transfer ($IC_{50} = 24$ nM) and displayed an approximately 11-fold stronger antiviral activity ($EC_{50} = 76$ nM) than compound **4**. Introduction of a methoxy group at the 7 position of the quinolone ring (compound **6**) led to a significant improvement of inhibition of strand transfer ($IC_{50} = 9.1$ nM) and antiviral activity ($EC_{50} = 17.1$ nM). Compound **7**, bearing an isopropyl group

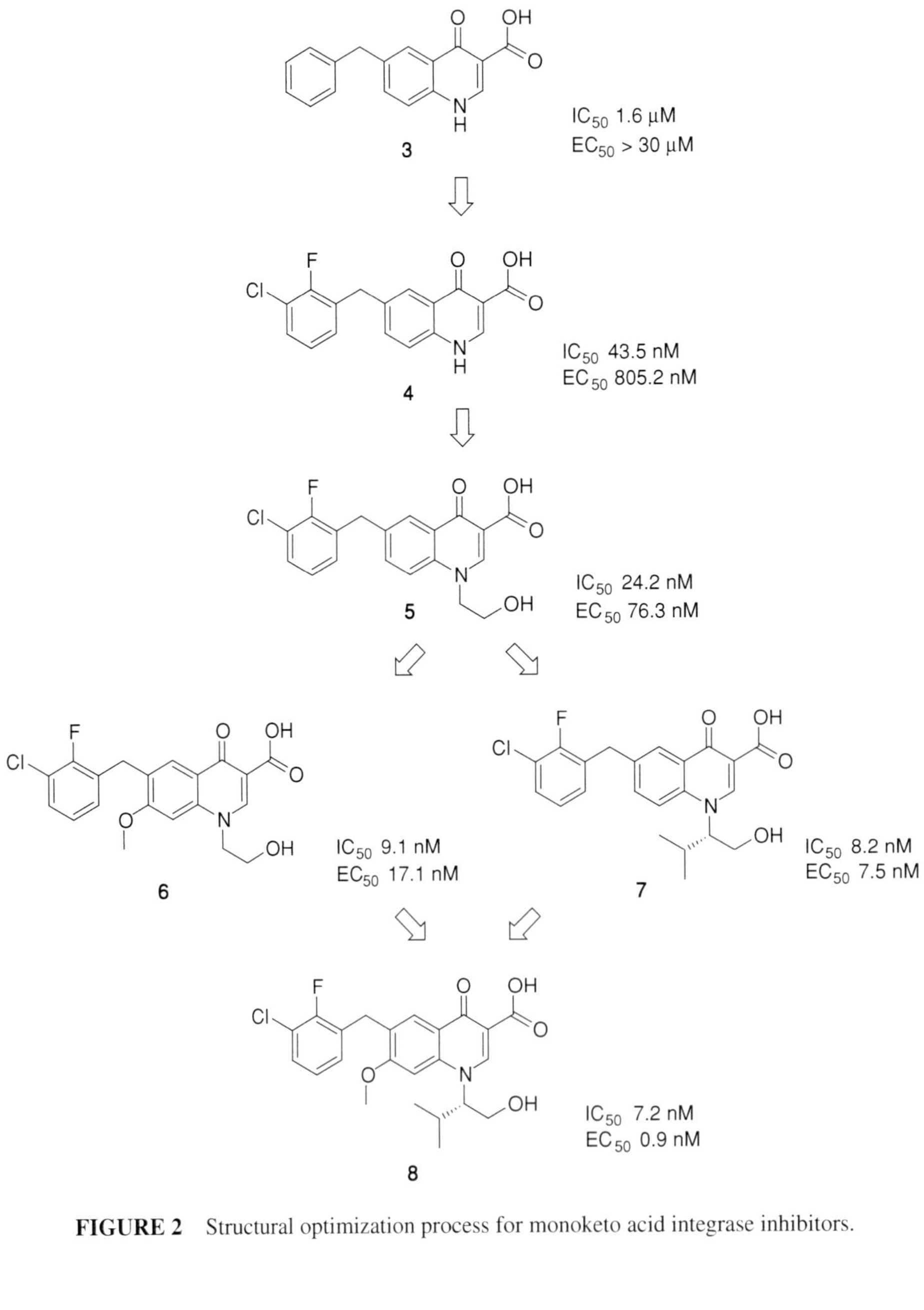

FIGURE 2 Structural optimization process for monoketo acid integrase inhibitors.

at the 1*S* position of the hydroxyethyl moiety, was approximately three-fold more potent at inhibiting strand transfer (IC_{50} = 8.2 nM), and approximately 10-fold stronger at inhibiting HIV replication (EC_{50} = 7.5 nM) than compound **5**, although the introduction of an isopropyl group at the 1*R* position of the hydroxyethyl moiety did not enhance inhibitory activity. The introduction of both a methoxy group at the 7 position of the quinolone ring and an isopropyl group at the 1*S* position of the hydroxyethyl moiety (EVG) led to a synergistic improvement in antiviral activity (EC_{50} = 0.9 nM). Although no additive or synergistic improvement in the inhibition of HIV-1 integrase (IC_{50} = 7.2 nM) was observed, this may be due to the condition of the strand transfer assay using 5 nM of target DNA, which can affect the potency of inhibitors. More detailed SARs have been described in another publication [60].

Keto-enol acid integrase inhibitors are reported to be much more potent, than 3′-processing reactions at inhibiting integrase-catalyzed strand transfer processes [37,54]. Our monoketo acid integrase inhibitor was also confirmed to be a selective strand transfer inhibitor (Fig. 3). A 5′-end-labeled 21-mer double-stranded DNA oligonucleotide, corresponding to the last 21 bases of the U5 viral LTR, is converted via a 19-mer oligonucleotide (3′-processing product) to strand transfer products (> 21-mer oligonucleotides) by HIV-1 integrase. Monoketo acid EVG was more than 100-fold as potent as the 3′-processing reaction at inhibiting integrase-catalyzed strand transfer processes (Fig. 3). The identification of the highly potent HIV-1 integrase strand transfer inhibitor, EVG, which has the monoketo acid motif as an alternative to the keto-enol acid motif, provides novel insights into the structural requirements and the binding mode of this type of inhibitor. The capacity for full coordination with the two divalent metal ions is apparently not always essential for the activity of strand transfer inhibitors. EVG is the most clincally advanced novel quinolone integrase inhibitor.

SYNTHESIS

The preparation of EVG is shown in Scheme 1. After 5-iodonation of 2,4-difluorobenzoic acid, the acid chloride of 2,4-difluoro-5-iodobenzoic acid was coupled with ethyl 3-(dimethylamino)acrylate to produce 2-benzoyl-3-(dimethylamino)acrylate. Substitution with (*S*)-valinol and subsequent cyclization with potassium carbonate and protection of the alcohol with TBS ether gave the 6-iodoquinolone ester. Palladium-catalyzed Negishi coupling of the 3-chloro-2-fluorobenzylzinc bromide derived from the corresponding benzylbromide with 6-iodoquinolone ester led to a 6-benzylquinolone ester. Hydrolysis of the TBS ether and ethyl ester, and subsequent methoxylation with sodium methoxide, produced EVG.

CLINICAL RESULTS

The first human study for EVG was conducted among Japanese healthy male volunteers by Japan Tobacco Inc. [55]. In the study, single oral administration of up to 800 mg of EVG, the highest dose, was safe and well tolerated. The plasma concentration of EVG increased with dose in a proportional manner. Food significantly increased the plasma exposure of EVG by approximately 2.7-fold. After the dose of 400 mg under the fed condition, T_{max} and $t_{1/2}$ were 2.3 and 3.2 h, respectively, and the plasma concentrations of EVG at 12 to 24 h well exceeded the protein binding–adjusted in vitro EC_{90} or EC_{50} concentrations.

Based on these results, Gilead Sciences began a short-term monotherapy study in the United States to evaluate the pharmacokinetics and antiviral activity of EVG [56]. Meanwhile, Kearney et al. [57] reported a significant boosting effect of ritonavir, along with a longer half-life (~ 9 h) of EVG. Therefore, boosting with ritonavir at 50 mg q.d. was

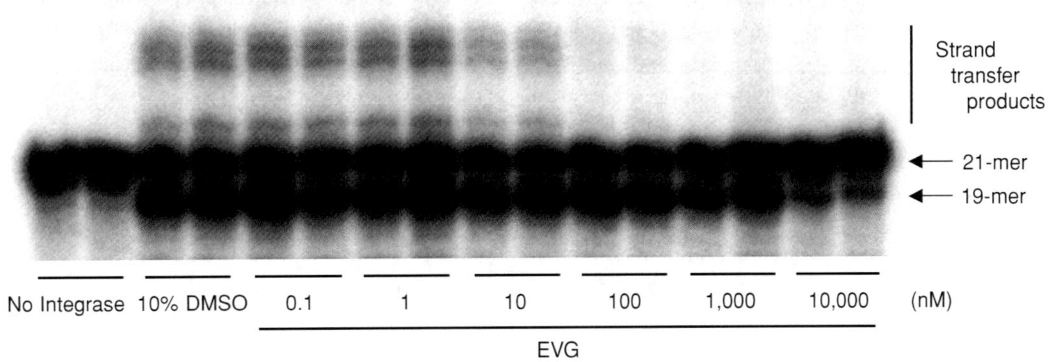

FIGURE 3 Inhibition of 3′-processing and strand transfer by EVG. Gel electrophoresis shows the viral DNA substrate (21-mer oligonucleotide), 3′-processing product (19-mer oligonucleotide), and strand transfer products (> 21-mer oligonucleotides).

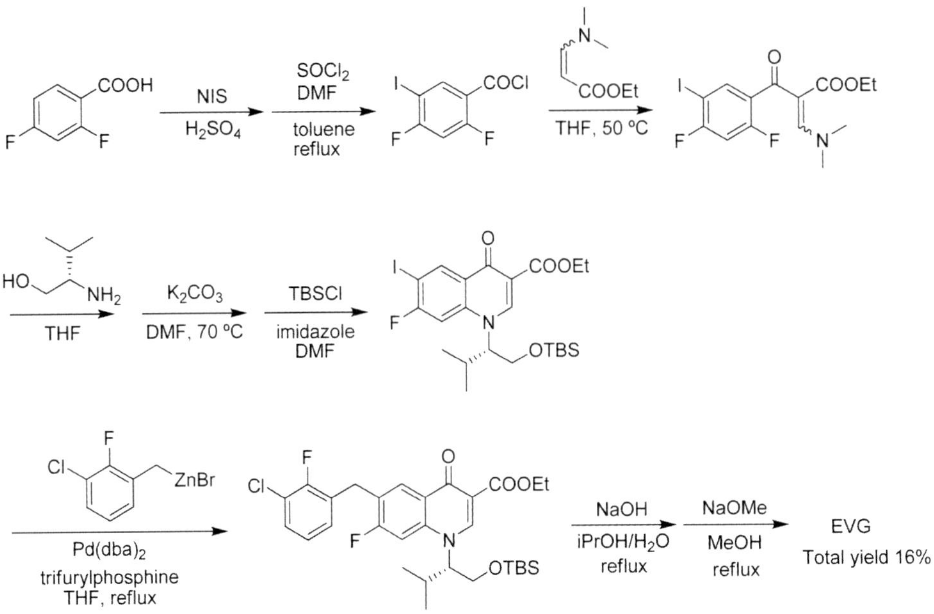

SCHEME 1 Synthesis of elvitegravir.

evaluated, as well as 200, 400 and 800 mg b.i.d. and 800 mg q.d. in the monotherapy study. In the 400 or 800 mg b.i.d. and 50 mg/r q.d. groups, a plasma viral load reduction by approximately 2 $\log_{10}$ copies/mL was observed over 10 days of monotherapy. In pharmacokinetic/pharmacodynamic analysis, Kearney et al. reported that C_{trough} concentration was the most sensitive predictor for antiviral activity. EVG was safe and well tolerated in all the dosing groups.

Following these findings, a 48-week phase IIb dose-ranging study was started at doses of 20, 50, and 125 mg of EVG with 100 mg of ritonavir in combination with more than two nucleos(t)ide reverse transcriptase inhibitors and with or without a fusion inhibitor, enfuvirtide/T-20, in treatment-experienced patients. In the 125-mg/r arm, approximately 2 $\log_{10}$ copies/mL reduction in viral load was observed by 2 weeks after the introduction of the new treatment, which included EVG. However, the durability of viral reduction depended largely on the number of active drugs in the background regimen. The majority of subjects who started without any active drug in the background regimen experienced viral rebound after rapid viral supression. In contrast, subjects who had any active drugs in the background regimen exhibited a longer duration of the viral response [58]. In particular, in subjects who were naive to and started with enfuvirtide, viral suppression was maintained throughout the study period. These findings strongly indicate that EVG has potent and durable antiviral efficacy when used together with other active agents. EVG was also generally safe and tolerable in this study. The emergence of drug-resistant-related mutations was frequent in subjects who experienced virologic failure during EVG-included therapy. Most resistant virus to EVG also showed cross-resistance to raltegravir. Therefore, sequential therapy with raltegravir after viral failure with EVG would not be expected to be an effective option.

Currently, phase III studies by Gilead Sciences are ongoing in the United States, the European Union, Canada, and Australia. These are randomized double-blind double-dummy studies comparing EVG with raltegravir in combination with a ritonavir-boosted protease and another active agent in treatment-experienced HIV-1-infected subjects.

EVG has exhibited both a preferable safety profile and durable antiviral activity to date, and can be administered once daily when coadministered with a pharmacoenhancer such as ritonavir. These profiles could serve as a promising option not only for treatment-experienced patients but also for treatment-naive patients. The risk of treatment-emergent resistance, however, even by a small dose of ritonavir, cannot be eliminated completely. Gilead Sciences is currently developing GS-9350, a pharmacoenhancer without antiviral activity [59]. In the future, a combination with a pure booster, such as GS-9350, could enlarge the clinical use of EVG, including for treatment-naive patients.

CONCLUSIONS

We discovered the coplanar monoketo acid motif in the scaffold, 4-quinolone-3-carboxylic acid, to be an alternative to the keto-enol acid motif in integrase inhibitors. These novel quinolone integrase inhibitors were structurally optimized to provide the highly potent derivative EVG, which was much more potent at inhibiting integrase-catalyzed strand transfer processes than 3′-processing reactions, as reported previously for compounds of the keto-enol acid class [37,54]. The chelating ability of the keto-enol acids, which can coordinate with two divalent metal ions simultaneously, is considered to be important, but structurally modified monoketo acids cannot fully mimic the chelating function of the keto-enol acids. The monoketo acids have potentially weaker affinity for metal ions than the keto-enol acids, and cannot fully coordinate with two metal ions. This would seem to be disadvantageous for achieving activity. In fact, the initial lead compound **3** was less potent than the keto-enol acid compound **1**. However, the highly potent EVG was obtained by structural modification around the monoketo acid moiety. Furthermore, this potentially weaker chelating ability of the monoketo acids might, in fact, be advantageous in terms of selectivity and safety. Indeed, the novel quinolone integrase inhibitor EVG has exhibited a very safe profile in the clinical studies performed to date. EVG has exhibited significant antiviral activities in phase II studies and is currently undergoing phase III trials.

REFERENCES

[1] Pommier, Y.; Johnson, A. A.; Marchand, C. Integrase inhibitors to treat HIV/AIDS. *Nat. Rev. Drug Discov.* **2005**, *4*, 236–248.

[2] Richman, D. D. HIV chemotherapy. *Nature* **2001**, *410*, 995–1001.

[3] Weiss, R. A. HIV and AIDS: looking ahead. *Nat. Med.* **2003**, *9*, 887–891.

[4] Grobler, J. A.; Stillmock, K.; Binghua, H.; Witmer, M.; Felock, P.; Espeseth, A. S.; Wolfe, A.; Egbertson, M.; Bourgeois, M.; Melamed, J.; et al. Diketo acid inhibitor mechanism and HIV-1 integrase: implications for metal binding in the active site of phosphotransferase enzymes. *Proc. Natl. Acad. Sci. USA* **2002**, *99*, 6661–6666.

[5] Neamati, N.; Lin, Z.; Karki, R. G.; Orr, A.; Cowansage, K.; Strumberg, D.; Pais, G. C. G.; Voigt, J. H.; Nicklaus, M. C.; Winslow, H. E.; et al. Metal-dependent inhibition of HIV-1 integrase. *J. Med. Chem.* **2002**, *45*, 5661–5670.

[6] Marchand, C.; Johnson, A. A.; Karki, R. G.; Pais, G. C. G.; Zhang, X.; Cowansage, K.; Patel, T. A.; Nicklaus, M. C.; Burke, T. R., Jr.; Pommier, Y. Metal-dependent inhibition of HIV-1 integrase by β-diketo acids and resistance of the soluble double-mutant (F185K/C280S). *Mol. Pharmacol.* **2003**, *64*, 600–609.

[7] Sato, M.; Motomura, T.; Aramaki, H.; Matsuda, T.; Yamashita, M.; Ito, Y.; Kawakami, H.; Matsuzaki, Y.; Watanabe, W.; Yamataka, K.; et al. Novel HIV-1 integrase inhibitors derived from quinolone antibiotics. *J. Med. Chem.* **2006**, *49*, 1506–1508.

[8] Ellison, V.; Brown, P. O. A Stable complex between integrase and viral DNA ends mediates human immunodeficiency virus integration in vitro. *Proc. Natl. Acad. Sci. USA* **1994**, *91*, 7316–7320.

[9] Esposito, D.; Craigie, R. HIV integrase structure and function. *Adv. Virus Res.* **1999**, *52*, 319–333.

[10] Thomas A.; Steitz, T. A. Structural biology: a mechanism for all polymerases. *Nature* **1998**, *391*, 231–232.

[11] Dyda, F.; Hickman, A. B.; Jenkins, T. M.; Engelman, A.; Craigie, R.; Davies, D. R. Crystal structure of the catalytic domain of HIV-1 integrase: similarity to other polynucleotidyl transferases. *Science* **1994**, *266*, 1981–1986.

[12] Rice, P. A.; Baker, T. A. Comparative architecture of transposase and integrase complexes. *Nat. Struct. Biol.* **2001**, *8*, 302–307.

[13] Yang, W.; Steitz, T. A. Recombining the structures of HIV integrase, RuvC and RNase H. *Structure* **1995**, *3*, 131–134.

[14] Bujacz, G.; Alexandratos, J.; Wlodawer, A.; Merkel, G.; Andrake, M.; Katz, R. A.; Skalka, A. M. Binding of different divalent cations to the active site of avian sarcoma virus integrase and their effects on enzymatic activity. *J. Biol. Chem.* **1997**, *272*, 18161–18168.

[15] Beese, L. S.; Steitz, T. A. Structural basis for the 3′-5′ exonuclease activity of *Escherichia coli* DNA polymerase I: a two metal ion mechanism. *EMBO J.* **1991**, *10*, 25–33.

[16] Wlodawer, A. Crystal structures of catalytic core domains of retroviral integrases and role of divalent cations in enzymatic activity. *Adv. Virus Res.* **1999**, *52*, 335–350.

[17] Thomas, A.; Steitz, T. A. DNA polymerases: structural diversity and common mechanisms. *J. Biol. Chem.* **1999**, *274*, 17395–17398.

[18] Horton, N. C.; Perona, J. J. Making the most of metal ions. *Nat. Struct. Biol.* **2001**, *8*, 290–293.

[19] Feng, M.; Patel, D.; Dervan, J. J.; Ceska, T.; Suck, D.; Haq, I.; Sayers, J. R. Roles of divalent metal ions in flap endonuclease–substrate interactions. *Nat. Struct. Biol.* **2004**, *11*, 450–456.

[20] Goldgur, Y.; Dyda, F.; Hickman, A. B.; Jenkins, T. M.; Craigie, R.; Davies, D. R. Three new structures of the core domain of HIV-1 integrase: an active site that binds magnesium. *Proc. Natl. Acad. Sci. USA* **1998**, *95*, 9150–9154.

[21] Maignan, S.; Guilloteau, J.-P.; Zhou-Liu, A.; Clément-Mella, C.; Mikol, V. Crystal structures of the catalytic domain of HIV-1 integrase free and complexed with its metal cofactor: high level of similarity of the active site with other viral integrases. *J. Mol. Biol.* **1998**, *282*, 359–368.

[22] Hazuda, D. J.; Anthony, N. J.; Gomez, R. P.; Jolly, S. M.; Wai, J. S.; Zhuang, L.; Fisher, T. E.; Embrey, M.; Guare, J. P., Jr.; Egbertson, M. S.; et al. A naphthyridine carboxamide provides evidence for discordant resistance between mechanistically identical inhibitors of HIV-1 integrase. *Proc. Natl. Acad. Sci. USA* **2004**, *101*, 11233–11238.

[23] Drelich, M.; Wilhelm, R.; Mous, J. Identification of amino acid residues critical for endonuclease and integration activities of HIV-1 IN protein in vitro. *Virology* **1992**, *188*, 459–468.

[24] Bushman, F. D.; Engelman, A.; Palmer, I.; Wingfield, P.; Craigie. R. Domains of the integrase protein of human

immunodeficiency virus type 1 responsible for polynucleotidyl transfer and zinc binding. *Proc. Natl. Acad. Sci. USA* **1993**, *90*, 3428–3432.

[25] Yao, Q. Y.; Tierney, R. J.; Croom-Carter, D.; Cooper, G. M.; Ellis, C. J.; Rowe, M.; Rickinson, A. B. Isolation of intertypic recombinants of Epstein–Barr virus from T-cell- immunocompromised individuals. *J. Virol.* **1996**, *70*, 4585–4597.

[26] Vink, C.; Groeneger, A. M. O.; Plasterk, R. H. Identification of the catalytic and DNA-binding region of the human immunodeficiency virus type I integrase protein. *Nucleic Acids Res.* **1993**, *21*, 1419–1425.

[27] Schauer, M.; Billich, A. The N-terminal region of HIV-1 integrase is required for integration activity, but not for DNA-binding. *Biochem. Biophys. Res. Commun.* **1992**, *185*, 874–880.

[28] Kulkosky, J.; Katz, R. A.; Merkel, G.; Skalka, A. M. Activities and substrate specificity of the evolutionarily conserved central domain of retroviral integrase. *Virology* **1995**, *206*, 448–456.

[29] Engelman, A.; Bushman, F. D.; Craigie, R. Identification of discrete functional domains of HIV-1 integrase and their organization within an active multimeric complex. *EMBO J.* **1993**, *12*, 3269–3275.

[30] Engelman, A.; Craigie, R. Identification of conserved amino acid residues critical for human immunodeficiency virus type 1 integrase function in vitro. *J. Virol.* **1992**, *66*, 6361–6369.

[31] Van Gent, D. C.; Vink, C.; Groeneger, A. A.; Plasterk, R. H. Complementation between HIV integrase proteins mutated in different domains. *EMBO J.* **1993**, *12*, 3261–3267.

[32] Mazumder, A.; Engelman, A.; Craigie, R.; Fesen, M.; Pommier, Y. Intermolecular disintegration and intramolecular strand transfer activities of wild-type and mutant HIV-1 integrase. *Nucleic Acids Res.* **1994**, *22*, 1037–1043.

[33] Shibagaki, Y.; Holmes, M. L.; Appa, R. S.; Chow, S. A. Characterization of feline immunodeficiency virus integrase and analysis of functional domains. *Virology* **1997**, *230*, 1–10.

[34] Vink, C.; van Gent, D. C.; Elgersma, Y.; Plasterk, R. H. Human immunodeficiency virus integrase protein requires a subterminal position of its viral DNA recognition sequence for efficient cleavage. *J. Virol.* **1991**, *65*, 4636–4644.

[35] Sechi, M.; Bacchi, A.; Carcelli, M.; Compari, C.; Duce, E.; Fisicaro, E.; Rogolino, D.; Gates, P.; Derudas, M.; Al-Mawsawi, L. Q.; Neamati, N. From ligand to complexes: inhibition of human immunodeficiency virus type 1 integrase by β-diketo acid metal complexes. *J. Med. Chem.* **2006**, *49*, 4248–4260.

[36] Marchand, C.; Johnson, A. A.; Semenova, E.; Pommier, Y. Mechanism and inhibition of HIV integration. *Drug. Discov. Today: Dis. Mech.* **2006**, *3*, 253–260.

[37] Hazuda, D. J.; Felock, P.; Witmer, M.; Wolfe, A.; Stillmock, K.; Grobler, J. A.; Espeseth, A.; Gabryelski, L.; Schleif, W.; Blau, C.; Miller, M. D. Inhibitors of strand transfer that prevent integration and inhibit HIV-1 replication in cells. *Science* **2000**, *287*, 646–650.

[38] Wai, J. S.; Egbertson, M. S.; Payne, L. S.; Fisher, T. E.; Embrey, M. W.; Tran, L. O.; Melamed, J. Y.; Langford, H. M.; Guare, J. P., Jr.; Zhuang, L.; et al. 4-Aryl-2,4-dioxobutanoic acid inhibitors of HIV-1 integrase and viral replication in cells. *J. Med. Chem.* **2000**, *43*, 4923–4926.

[39] Espeseth, A. S.; Felock, P.; Wolfe, A.; Witmer, M.; Grobler, J.; Anthony, N.; Egbertson, M.; Melamed, J. Y.; Young, S.; Hamill, T.; et al. HIV-1 integrase inhibitors that compete with the target DNA substrate define a unique strand transfer conformation for integrase. *Proc. Natl. Acad. Sci. USA* **2000**, *97*, 11244–11249.

[40] Goldgur, Y.; Craigie, R.; Cohen, G. H.; Fujiwara, T.; Yoshinage, T.; Fujishita, T.; Sugimoto, H.; Endo, T.; Murai, H.; Davies, D. R. Structure of the HIV-1 integrase catalytic domain complexed with an inhibitor: a platform for antiviral drug design. *Proc. Natl. Acad. Sci. USA* **1999**, *96*, 13040–13043.

[41] Verschueren, W. G.; Dierynck, I.; Amssoms, K. I. E.; Hu, L.; Boonants, P. M. J. G.; Pille, G. M. E.; Daeyaert, F. F. D.; Hertogs, K.; Surleraux, D. L. N. G.; Wigerinck, P. B. T. P. Design and optimization of tricyclic phtalimide analogues as novel inhibitors of HIV-1 integrase. *J. Med. Chem.* **2005**, *48*, 1930–1940.

[42] Owen, T. C.; Harris, J. N. Unusual deacylations: the 2-acetyl-3-methylbenzothiazolium cation. *J. Am. Chem. Soc.* **2000**, *112*, 6136–6137.

[43] Sotriffer, C. A.; Ni, H. H.; McCammon, J. A. Active site binding modes of HIV-1 integrase inhibitors. *J. Med. Chem.* **2000**, *43*, 4109–4117.

[44] Maurin, C.; Bailly, F.; Buisine, E.; Vezin, H.; Mbemba, G.; Mouscadet, J. F.; Cotelle, P. Spectroscopic studies of diketoacids–metal interactions: a probing tool for the pharmacophoric intermetallic distance in the HIV-1 integrase active site. *J. Med. Chem.* **2004**, *47*, 5583–5586.

[45] Barreca, M. L.; Ferro, S.; Rao, A.; Luca, L. D.; Zappala, M.; Monforte, A. M.; Debyser, Z.; Witvrouw, M.; Chimirri, A. Pharmacophore-based design of HIV-1 integrase strand-transfer inhibitors. *J. Med. Chem.* **2005**, *48*, 7084–7088.

[46] Zhuang, L.; Wai, J. S.; Embrey, M. W.; Fisher, T. E.; Egbertson, M. S.; Payne, L. S.; Guare, J. P., Jr.; Vacca, J. P.; Hazuda, D. J.; Felock, P. J.; et al. Design and synthesis of 8-hydroxy-[1,6]naphthyridines as novel inhibitors of HIV-1 integrase in vitro and in infected cells. *J. Med. Chem.* **2003**, *46*, 453–456.

[47] Hazuda, D. J.; Young, S. D.; Guare, J. P.; Anthony, N. J.; Gomez, R. P.; Wai, J. S.; Vacca, J. P.; Handt, L.; Motzel, S. L.; Klein, H. J.; et al. Integrase inhibitors and cellular immunity suppress retroviral replication in rhesus macaques. *Science* **2004**, *305*, 528–532.

[48] Wang, Y.; Serradell, N.; Bolos, J.; Rosa, E. MK-0518, HIV integrase inhibitor. *Drugs Future* **2007**, *32*, 118–122.

[49] Herr, J. R. 5-Substituted-1H-terazoles as carboxylic acid isosteres: medicinal chemistry and synthetic methods. *Bioorg. Med. Chem.* **2002**, *10*, 3379–3393

[50] De Clercq, E. New approaches toward anti-HIV chemotherapy. *J. Med. Chem.* **2005**, *48*, 1297–1313.

[51] Summa, V.; Petrocchi, A.; Matassa, V. G.; Gardelli, C.; Muraglia, E.; Rowley, M.; Paz, O. G.; Laufer, R.; Monteagudo, E.; Pace, P. 4,5-Dihydroxypyrimidine carboxamides and *N*-alkyl-5-hydroxypyrimidinone carboxamides are

potent, selective HIV integrase inhibitors with good pharmacokinetic profiles in preclinical species. *J. Med. Chem.* **2006**, *49*, 6646–6649.

[52] Pais, G. C. G.; Zhang, X.; Marchand, C.; Neamati, N.; Cowansage, K.; Svarovskaia, E. S.; Pathak, V. K.; Tang, Y.; Nicklaus, M.; Pommier, Y.; Burke, T. R., Jr. Structure activity of 3-aryl-1,3-diketo-containing compounds as HIV-1 integrase inhibitors. *J. Med. Chem.* **2002**, *45*, 3184–3194.

[53] Marchand, C.; Zhang, X.; Pais, G. C. G.; Cowansage, K.; Neamati, N.; Burke, T. R., Jr.; Pommier, Y. Structural determinants for HIV-1 integrase inhibition by β-diketo acids. *J. Biol. Chem.* **2002**, *277*, 12596–12603.

[54] Sechi, M.; Derudas, M.; Dallocchio, R.; Dessi, A.; Bacchi, A.; Sannia, L.; Carta, F.; Palomba, M.; Ragab, O.; Chan, C.; et al. Design and synthesis of novel indole β-diketo acid derivatives as HIV-integrase inhibitors. *J. Med. Chem.* **2004**, *47*, 5298–5310.

[55] Kawaguchi, I.; Ishikawa, T.; Ishibashi, M.; Irie, S.; Kakee, A. Safety and pharmacokinetics of single oral dose of JTK-303/GS-9137, a novel HIV integrase inhibitor, in healthy volunteers. 13th Conference on Retroviruses and Opportunistic Infections 2006. Available at http://www.retroconference.org/2006/pdfs/580.pdf.

[56] DeJesus, E.; Berger, D.; Markowitz, M.; Cohen, C.; Hawkins, T.; Ruane, P.; Elion, R.; Farthing, C.; Zhong, L.; Chen, A. K.; et al. Antiviral activity, pharmacokinetics, and dose response of the HIV-1 integrase inhibitor GS-9137 (JTK-303) in treatment-naive and treatment-experienced patients. *J. Acquir. Immune Defic. Syndr.* **2006**, *43*, 1–5.

[57] Kearney, B.; Mathias, A.; Zhong, L. Pharmacokinetics/pharmacodynamics of GS-9137, an HIV integrase inhibitor in treatment-naive and experienced patients. Proceedings of the 7th International Workshop on Clinical Pharmacology of HIV Therapy, Lisbon, Portugal, 2006. Abstract 73.

[58] Zolopa, A. R.; Lampiris, H.; Blick, G.; Walworth, C.; Zhong, L.; Chuck, S. L.; Enejosa, J.; Kearney, B. P.; Cheng, A. K. The HIV integrase inhibitor elvitegravir (EVG/r) has a potent and durable antiretroviral activity in treatment-experienced patients with active optimized background therapy (OBT). 47th Interscience Conference on Antimicrobial Agents and Chemotherapy, 2007. Abstract H-714.

[59] Mathias, A.; Lee, M.; Callebaut, C.; Xu, L.; Tsai, L.; Murray, B.; Liu, H.; Yale, K.; Warren, D.; Kearney, B. GS-9350: A pharmacoenhancer without anti-HIV activity. 16th Conference on Retroviruses and Opportunistic Infections, **2009**. Abstract 40.

[60] Sato, M.; Kawakami, H.; Motomura, T.; Aramaki, H.; Matsuda, T.; Yamashita, M.; Ito, Y.; Matsuzaki, Y.; Yamataka, K.; Ikeda, S.; Shinkai, H. Quinolone carboxylic acids as a novel monoketo acid class of human immunodeficiency virus type 1 integrase inhibitors. *J. Med. Chem.* **2009**, *52*, 4869–4882.

PART II

HEPATITIS C VIRUS

15

DISCOVERY AND DEVELOPMENT OF TELAPREVIR

ANNE-LAURE GRILLOT, LUC J. FARMER, B. GOVINDA RAO, AND WILLIAM P. TAYLOR
Vertex Pharmaceuticals, Inc., Cambridge, Massachusetts

ILAN S. WEISBERG AND IRA M. JACOBSON
Joan and Sanford I. Weill Medical College of Cornell University, New York, New York

ROBERT B. PERNI
Sirtris, Cambridge, Massachusetts

ANN D. KWONG
Vertex Pharmaceuticals, Inc., Cambridge, Massachusetts

INTRODUCTION

More than 170 million people worldwide are infected with the hepatitis C virus (HCV) [1,2]. Following acute HCV infection, approximately 80% of patients progress to a chronic infected state [3]. HCV infection is the most common risk factor for developing hepatocellular carcinoma and is the main cause of all liver transplants in developed nations [4]. The current standard of care (SoC) for HCV infection is an empirically derived therapy (which does not specifically target HCV), which consists of weekly injections of pegylated interferon (peginterferon) plus daily oral dosing with ribavirin (RBV) [5–8]. These drugs result in a sustained viral response (SVR) in about 42 to 46% of genotype 1–infected patients [9–11].

Multiple steps in the HCV life cycle where HCV replication can be inhibited have been identified [12]. The hepatitis C virus is a single-stranded RNA virus belonging to the Flaviviridae family. After HCV infects the host hepatocyte, the positive-stranded RNA genome is translated directly using the HCV internal ribosomal entry site (IRES) to produce a single 3000-amino acid polyprotein chain that contains all the structural and nonstructural viral proteins required for replication. This viral polyprotein is cleaved by host and viral proteases such as NS3·4A, releasing structural proteins to package progeny virus, and nonstructural proteins to form the multiprotein replicase complex required for viral RNA replication [13–15]. The replicase complex synthesizes negative-stranded replicative HCV RNA intermediates from the genomic positive-stranded RNA template, which in turn are used as a template to synthesize more progeny HCV RNA. Finally, progeny HCV RNA is packaged and matured into infectious virus as it egresses through the endoplasmic reticulum out of the cell.

The HCV nonstructural protein 3 (NS3) is a 631-amino acid bi-functional protein with a catalytic serine protease domain in the N-terminal 181-amino acid portion and a helicase domain in the C-terminal portion. NS3 associates tightly and noncovalently with NS4A, a 54-amino acid cofactor to form the NS3·4A complex [15–22]. Examination of the NS3 catalytic domain in the absence [23] and presence of NS4A [22] indicates that NS4A is buried deeply into the core of NS3 and assists in organizing the active site of the enzyme. The catalytic efficiency of the native NS3·4A complex is an order of magnitude higher than has been reported for the NS3 protease N-terminal domain with a synthetic peptide derived

Antiviral Drugs: From Basic Discovery Through Clinical Trials, First Edition. Edited by Wieslaw M. Kazmierski.

from NS4A [24], which in turn is an order of magnitude higher than the NS3 protease domain alone [25]. The NS3·4A protease is responsible for the cleavage of the viral polyprotein between NS4-NS4A, NS4A-NS4B, NS4B-NS5A, and NS5A-NS5B, to release components of the HCV replicase, and has been shown to be essential for viral replication [26].

Thus, NS3·4A is an attractive target for therapeutic intervention, and drug discovery targeting small-molecule inhibitors of NS3·4A has become a focus of intense interest in the pharmaceutical industry. Vertex Pharmaceuticals entered the HCV drug discovery field in 1997 in collaboration with Eli Lilly, to address the high unmet medical need for this disease using Vertex's core strength in structure-based drug design.

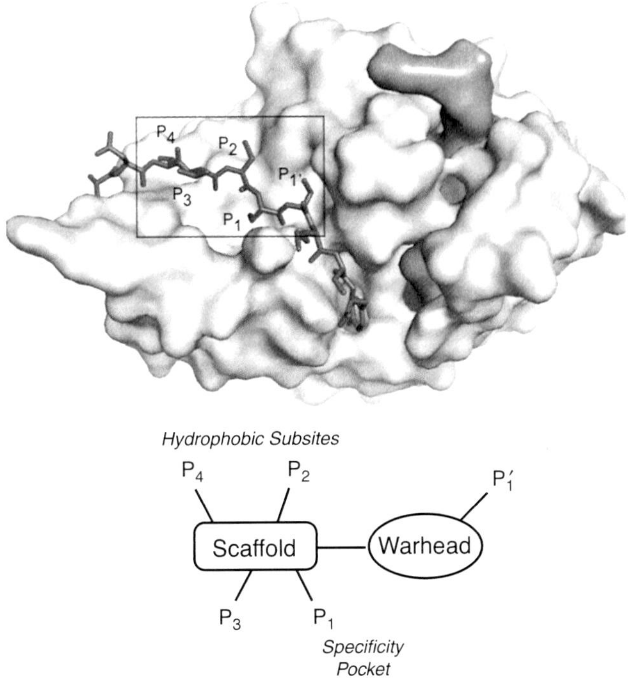

FIGURE 1 Model of substrate (dark sticks) bound to the active site of NS3·NS4A protease. The NS3 protease is shown as a light gray surface and NS4A peptide is shown in a darker gray surface. The schematic shows different hydrophobic subsites that are filled by an inhibitor that spans P'_1 to P_4.

DISCOVERY

During the period of more than a dozen years that has elapsed since the structure of the HCV NS3·4A protease was solved [22], several inhibitors of this enzyme have emerged and entered clinical development for the treatment of HCV-infected patients. The interest surrounding these new therapies is reflected in the publication of a number of reviews on HCV protease inhibitors in development [27–30].

However, back in 1996, medicinal chemists viewed the pursuit of this target for the development of a therapeutic agent as a daunting task, for several reasons [31]. The first hurdle in tackling the target was the lack of assays to drive optimization based on structure–activity relationships (SARs). In particular, there was no robust in vitro cell culture system to assess the ability of HCV NS3·4A protease inhibitors to prevent virus replication. At Vertex, efforts were devoted to the development of a suitable enzyme assay, and later, to implementation of the HCV subgenomic replicon assay [32]. Replicon assay activity and pharmacokinetic profiling were relied upon heavily to evaluate compounds preclinically. Additionally, the target product profile was developed based on our understanding of the HCV life cycle, but there was no readily available small-animal model to validate our approach. Another hurdle in pursuing the target is apparent in a model of the HCV NS3·4A protease complexed with a decamer substrate peptide (Fig. 1). The substrate binding site is a shallow and solvent-exposed cleft that presents no apparent pockets to engineer enzyme affinity. Additionally, the enzyme affinity for peptides based on natural substrates that span the S6 to S4′ subsites of the enzyme dropped significantly when they were truncated to fewer than 10 amino acids in length [25]. Thus, achieving druglike features in inhibitors, such as good affinity with molecular weights below 500 Da, appeared difficult.

Vertex Strategy

Early in Vertex's discovery program, it was decided to pursue compounds that would distribute preferentially to the liver, as this organ is the primary site in the body where HCV replication occurs. Furthermore, targeting a drug to the liver had the advantage of potentially limiting systemic toxicity by lowering systemic exposure. Targeting the liver had implications on compound evaluation and progression. In particular, in addition to evaluating in vitro potency, compound liver levels in rodents were measured routinely, and compounds with high liver exposure were prioritized for advancement. Eventually, a mouse model of protease inhibition was developed at Vertex to help assess the ability of compounds to inhibit HCV protease in the liver after oral administration. Another key aspect of Vertex's strategy was the systematic utilization of co-complex crystal structures of compounds bound in the enzyme active site to guide inhibitor optimization. The use of these principles toward the discovery of telaprevir (VX-950) has been published [33,34].

Inhibitor Design

The natural NS5A-5B substrate 1 was used as a starting point for inhibitor design. Truncation studies on a 10–amino acid-long substrate spanning the S6 to S4′ subsites of the enzyme showed that removal of the P4′ residue resulted in a dramatic loss of activity (~ 100-fold), but that subsequent truncations at P3′ and P2′ had little additional deleterious effects [24], suggesting that these residues were not sites where optimization could lead to significant gains in affinity.

On the nonprime site, removal of the P6 and P5 acidic residues resulted in significant decreases in binding affinities. Additionally, truncation of the hydrophobic residues at P4 and P3 led to further loss in affinity, suggesting that affinity could be gained through hydrophobic contacts at P3 and P4. From these studies it appeared that truncation beyond three or four amino acids on the nonprime substrate binding side would be difficult, as significant hydrophobic contacts would be needed to achieve adequate affinity. Hence, the question that remained was: Was it possible to design a druglike inhibitor with sufficient binding affinity?

A large body of literature exists that pertains to the inhibition of serine proteases such as HCV protease by covalent reversible inhibitors [35]. Attack of the C-terminal electrophilic moiety of these inhibitors by the catalytic serine residue results in the formation of a reversible covalent bond between the enzyme and the inhibitor. The resulting enzyme–inhibitor complex is a transition state–like tetrahedral intermediate that mimics amide bond hydrolysis, and that is stabilized through several ionic interactions. As a result, covalent reversible inhibitors have been shown to be 10 to 1000 times more potent than inhibitors that rely solely on ionic interactions. This strategy appeared feasible for the inhibition of HCV protease, as a way to gain back the affinity lost by necessary truncation of the natural substrate. We therefore decided to pursue covalent reversible inhibitors spanning the S4 to S1′ subsites of the enzyme (Fig. 1). The aldehyde functionality was chosen initially as a warhead surrogate, as shown in hexapeptide aldehyde **2** ($K_i = 0.89$ μM). The P6 and P5 residues were then replaced by a heterocyclic cap, which led to the tetrapeptide aldehyde **3** ($K_i = 12$ μM) as the starting point for further optimization (Scheme 1) [36].

Inhibitor Optimization

Several areas of the tetrapeptide aldehyde were optimized either sequentially or in parallel. To this end, parallel synthesis methods were utilized extensively, to conduct multisite optimization as needed. Early optimization focused on the P2 residue, a site where optimization of hydrophobic contacts could potentially lead to gains in inhibitor affinity. Based on chemistries available from the available 4-hydroxyproline starting material, ethers, esters, and carbamates were investigated (Scheme 2). Crystal structures of example molecules from each class revealed that several orientations of the proline 4-substituent in the P2 pocket were tolerated (Fig. 2). Binding affinity is influenced by interactions with the side chains forming the S2 pocket: Arg181, Asp107, and His83.

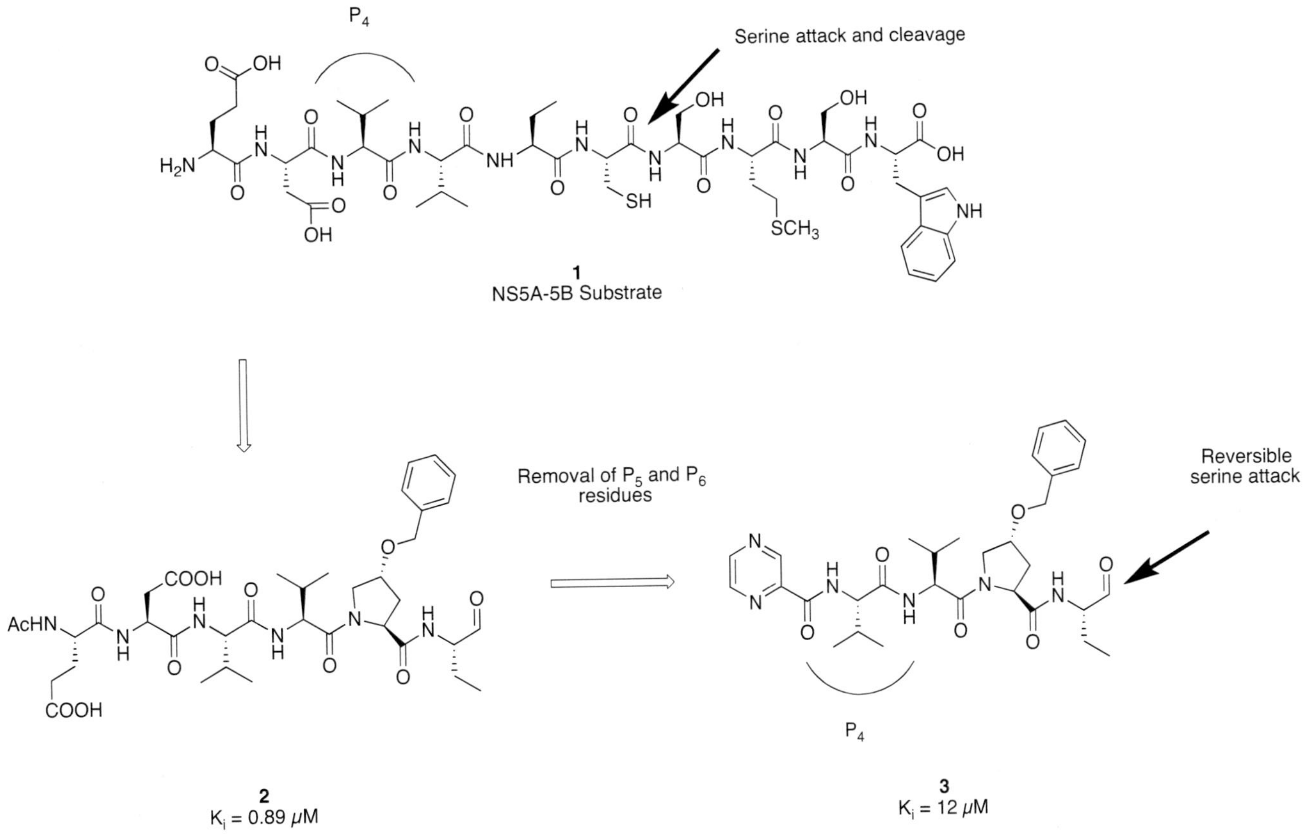

SCHEME 1 Elaboration from a 10-amino acid substrate to a tetrapeptide aldehyde inhibitor.

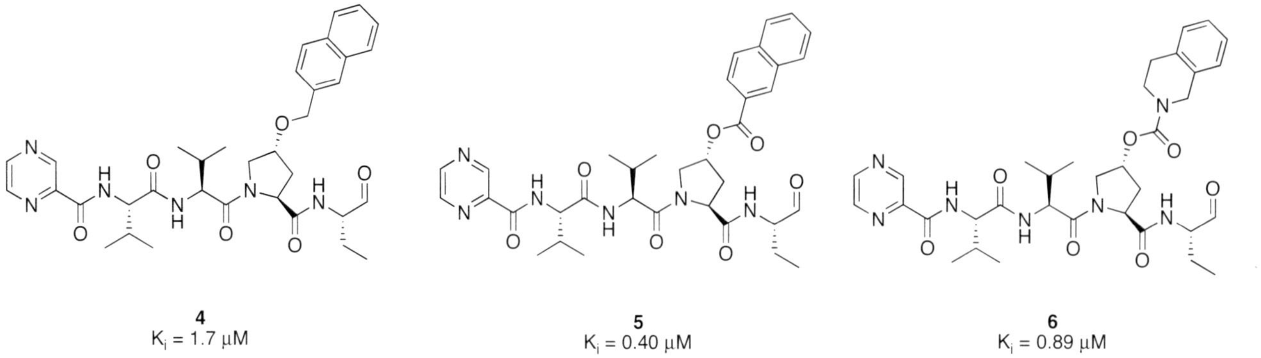

SCHEME 2 Chemical structures of aldehyde inhibitors **4**, **5**, and **6**.

Esters such as **5** (K_i = 0.4 μM) were generally more potent than ethers (e.g., **4**, K_i = 1.7 μM); however, they were too hydrolytically unstable to be of use. Primary carbamates were investigated as an alternative to esters, with varying success. However, replacement of the 2-naphthyl ester with the isosteric tetrahydroisoquinolyl (THIQ) carbamate led to compound **6**, which showed similar affinity for the enzyme (K_i = 0.89 μM) [36].

The S1 specificity pocket, defined by the side chains of Leu135, Phe154, and Ala157, is responsible for selectivity vs. the clotting cascade serine proteases such as thrombin. The consensus sequence for substrates resulting in transcleavage all have a cysteine at P1, a nucleophilic residue incompatible with an electrophilic warhead. Examination of the structure–activity relationship (SAR) at this position showed preference for small hydrophobic side chains, such as ethyl, propyl, and trifluoroethyl. Incorporation of an oxygen atom as well as disubstitution at the geminal position led to loss of affinity. The propyl side chain was chosen as a good compromise between synthetic accessibility and affinity [36].

The initial aldehyde warhead needed to be optimized, as aldehydes perform poorly in drugs and are readily oxidized to carboxylic acids in vivo. A number of warheads (carboxylic acid, trifluoromethyl ketones, chloromethyl ketones, etc.) commonly used in serine protease inhibitors were investigated without success. Successful replacement of the aldehyde was finally accomplished with an α-ketoamide, which resulted in up to 40-fold improvements in binding affinity [37]. X-ray structure analysis of α-ketoamides such as **7** (Scheme 3) showed an unexpected arrangement of the tetrahedral intermediate. Instead of observing the oxyanion hole defined by Ser139 and Gly137 being occupied by the oxygen of the electrophilic carbonyl, we observed occupancy by the oxygen from the nonelectrophilic carbonyl and the negatively charged oxygen pointing out toward solvent [37].

Various ketoamide substitutions were investigated. Additional affinity could be gained by introducing a carboxylic acid in the prime side (**8**, K_i = 26 nM, Scheme 3). However, these compounds generally displayed no potency in the replicon assay, presumably due to their charged character

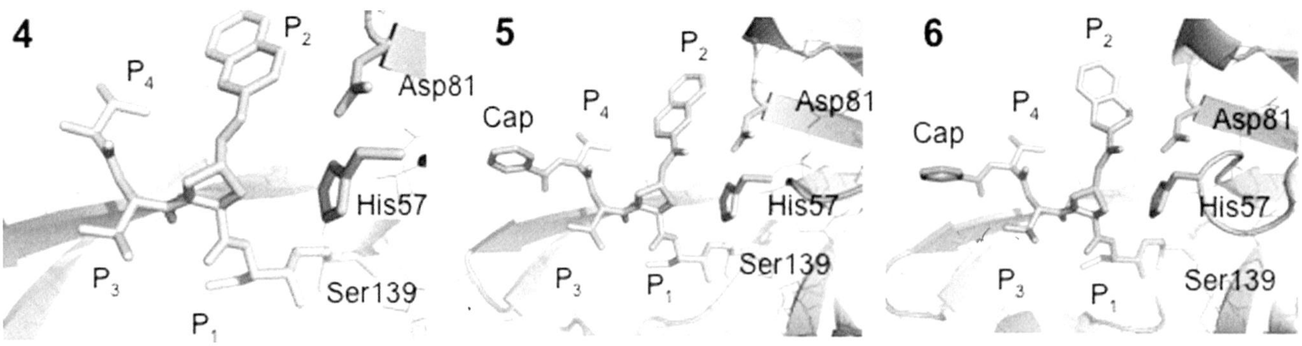

FIGURE 2 Crystal structure of inhibitors **4**, **5**, and **6**. The inhibitor and the catalytic triad (Ser139, His57, and Asp81) are shown as sticks. The protein is shown in lines as well as in ribbon representation. The naphthyl of the P_2 group in compounds **4** and **5** make the same contacts with the binding site; however, compound **5** is more potent, due to its rigid ester linker. The THIQ group linked as a carbamate in compound **6** is twisted and makes fewer optimal contacts and is therefore slightly weaker than compound **4**. The catalytic Ser139 makes a covalent interaction with the inhibitor aldehyde warhead. The His57 and Asp81 residues are also shown in a stick diagram. (The P_4 cap of compound **4** was not defined in the x-ray structure.)

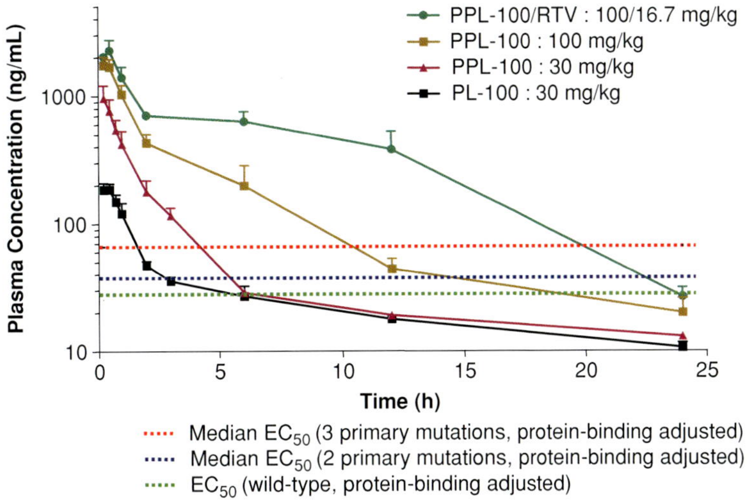

CHAPTER 2, FIGURE 1 Pharmacokinetic profiles of PL-100 and PPL-100 in rats in relation to cross-resistance patterns.

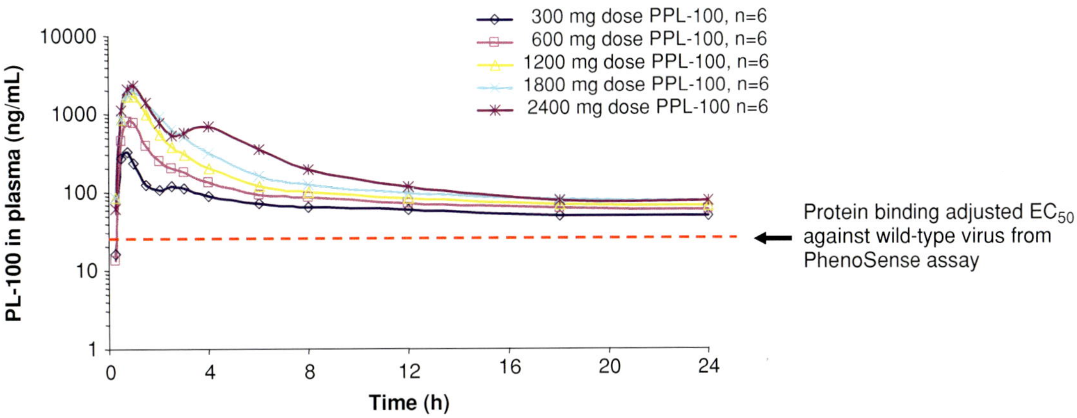

CHAPTER 2, FIGURE 2 Clinical PK profile of PL-100 in single-dose escalation studies in relation to its protein binding–adjusted antiviral activity.

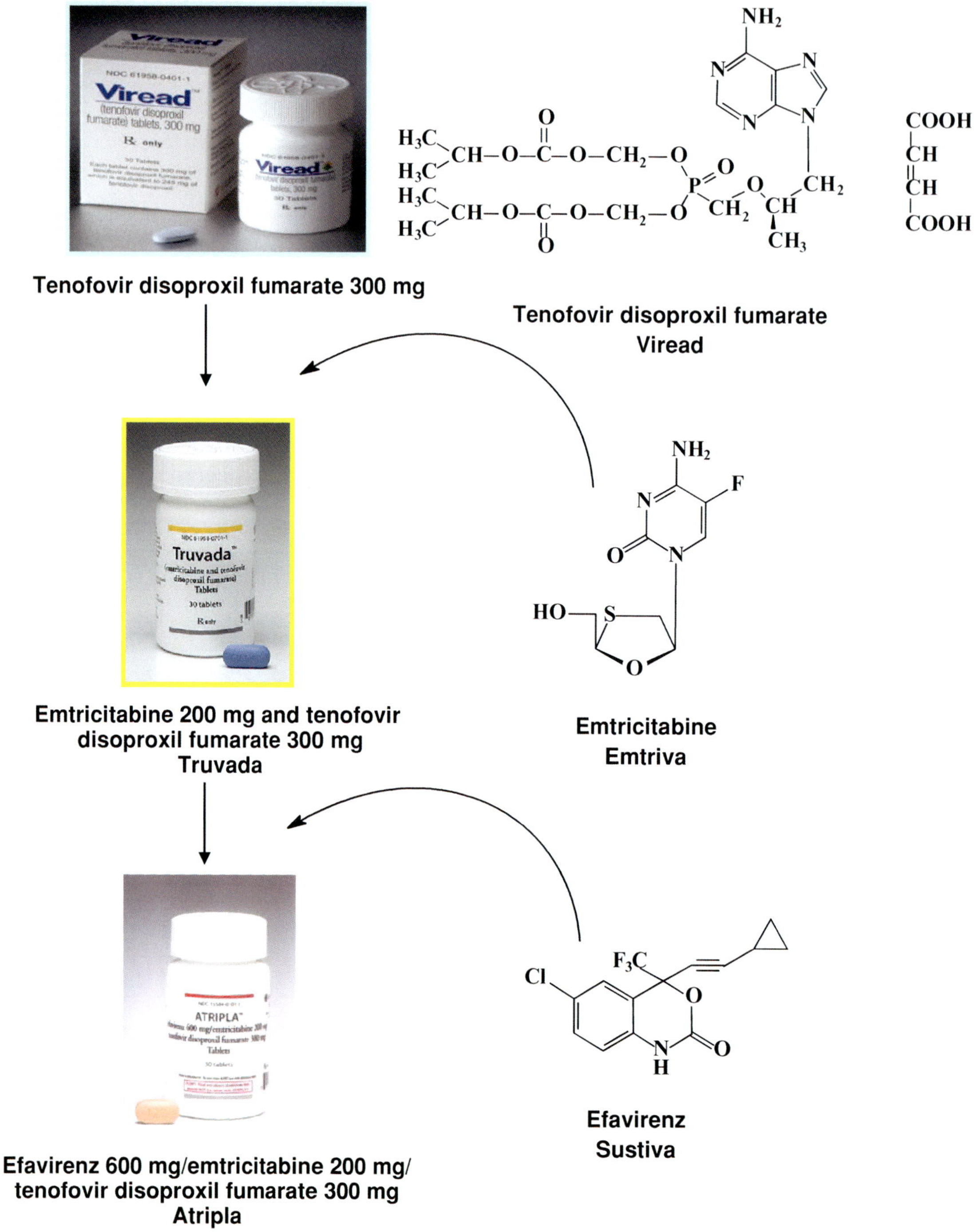

CHAPTER 7, FIGURE 5 Development of Atripla from Viread via Truvada.

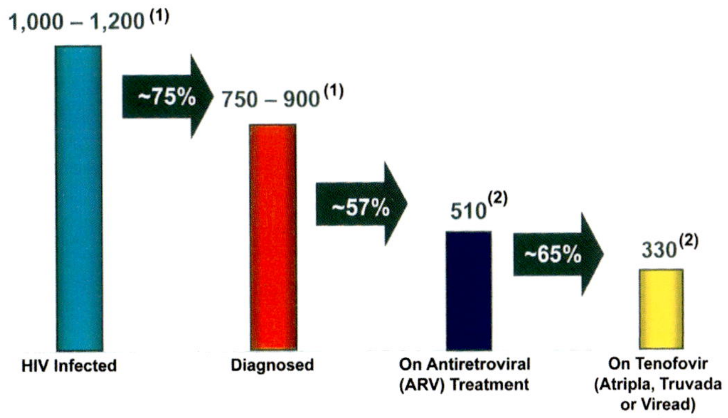

CHAPTER 7, FIGURE 7 U.S. HIV market dynamics (thousands of patients). Less than half of HIV-infected persons are currently on ARV therapy.

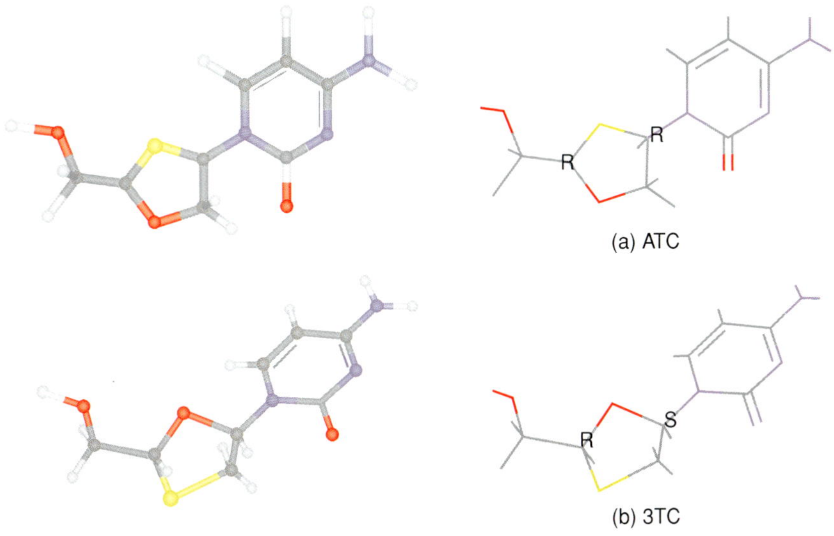

CHAPTER 8, FIGURE 1 Three-dimensional representation of ATC in comparison to 3TC.

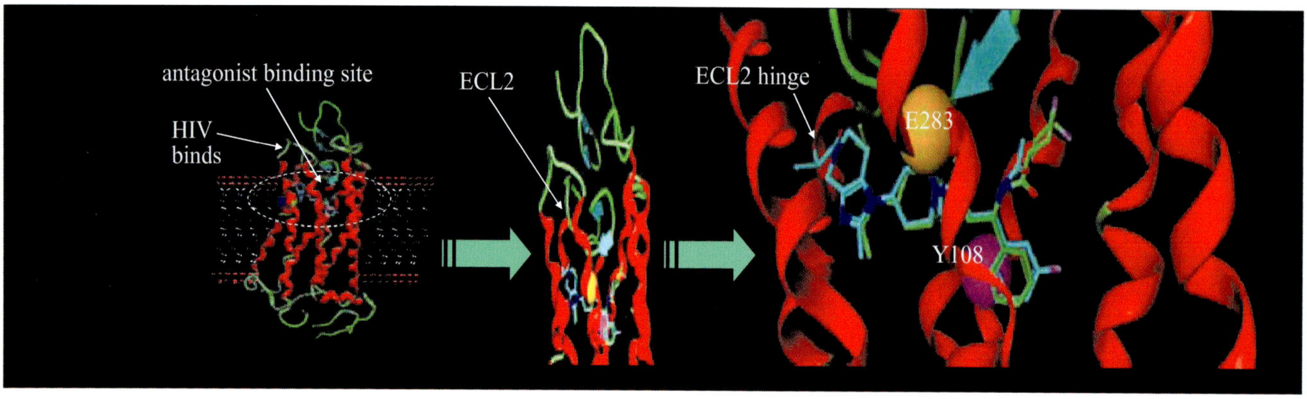

CHAPTER 9, FIGURE 3 Diagrammatic representation of CCR5 in the cytoplasmic membrane of an immune cell. Overlaps of PF-232798 (pale blue) and MVC (green) are highlighted. Interaction of the ionic interaction between the basic nitrogen of the antagonists and hydrophobic interaction of their phenyl moieties with the E283 and Y108 residues, respectively, in the transmembrane pocket are highlighted. All images generated using the computer modeling Pfizer software package FLOPS (flexes ligands optimizing property similarity) and Pfizer crystal structure database, as guided by assay data from site-directed alanine mutagenesis, where loss of functional binding was observed for E238A and Y108A mutants for maraviroc and PF-232798.

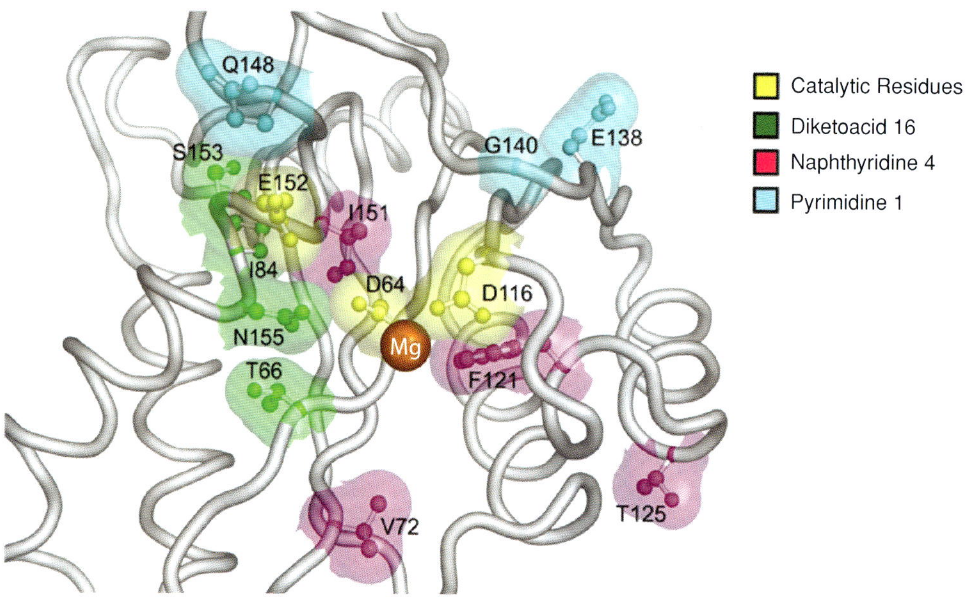

CHAPTER 12, FIGURE 6 Modeling depiction of x-ray data for an HIV integrase active site. Colored residues (magenta, cyan, green) indicate residues found in mutant viruses generated from extended serial passage of cells cultured with integrase inhibitors of different structural classes. Yellow: HIV integrase catalytic residues [28]. Green: amino acids mutated in response to prolonged incubation with a diketo acid inhibitor (compound **16**). Pink: amino acids mutated in response to prolonged incubation with a naphthyridine analog inhibitor (compound **4**). Light blue: amino acids mutated in response to prolonged incubation with a pyrimidine analog inhibitor (compound **1**).

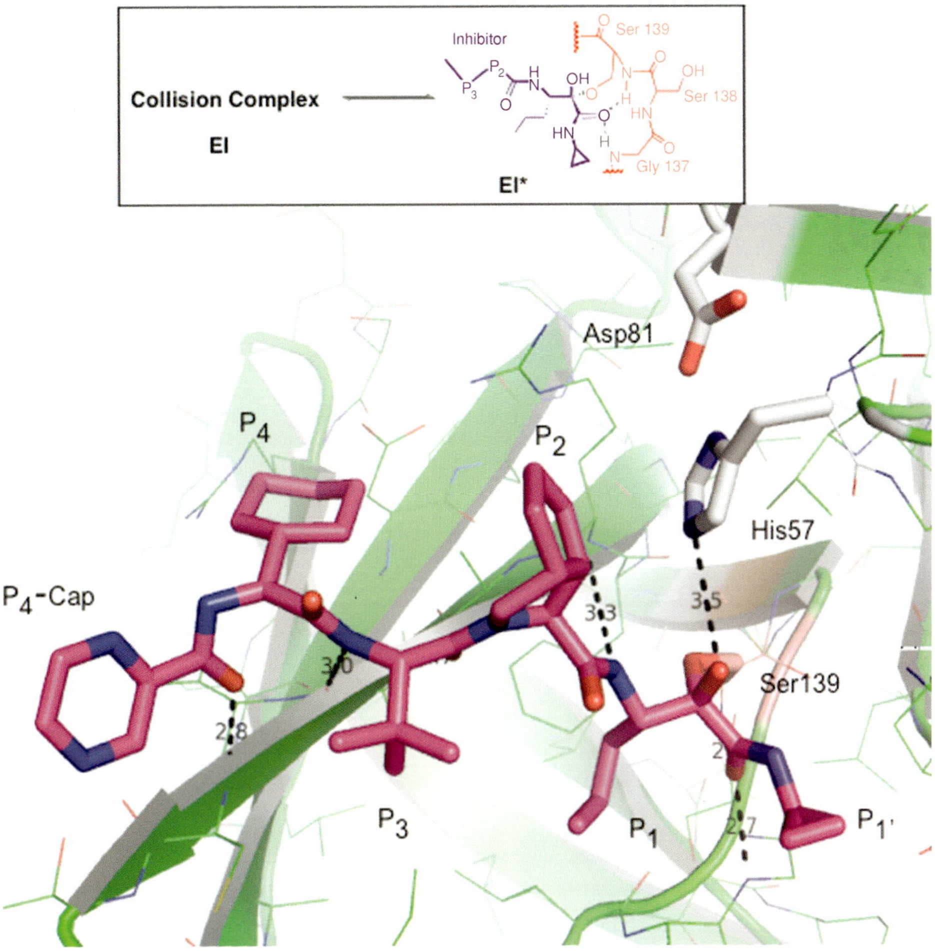

CHAPTER 15, FIGURE 3 Crystal structure of telaprevir complexed with NS3 protease and NS4A peptide cofactor. The inhibitor is shown in a stick diagram with the color scheme: C (purple), N (blue), and O (red). The active site triad (Ser139, His57, and Asp81) are also shown as sticks with C in gray. The rest of the protein is shown with C in green. The secondary structure of the protein is shown in a ribbon diagram. Telaprevir makes four inhibitor main-chain to protein main-chain hydrogen bonds. The side chains of the inhibitor fill the S4, S3, S2, S1, and S1′ binding pockets. The Ser139 residue makes a covalent interaction with the ketoamide warhead.

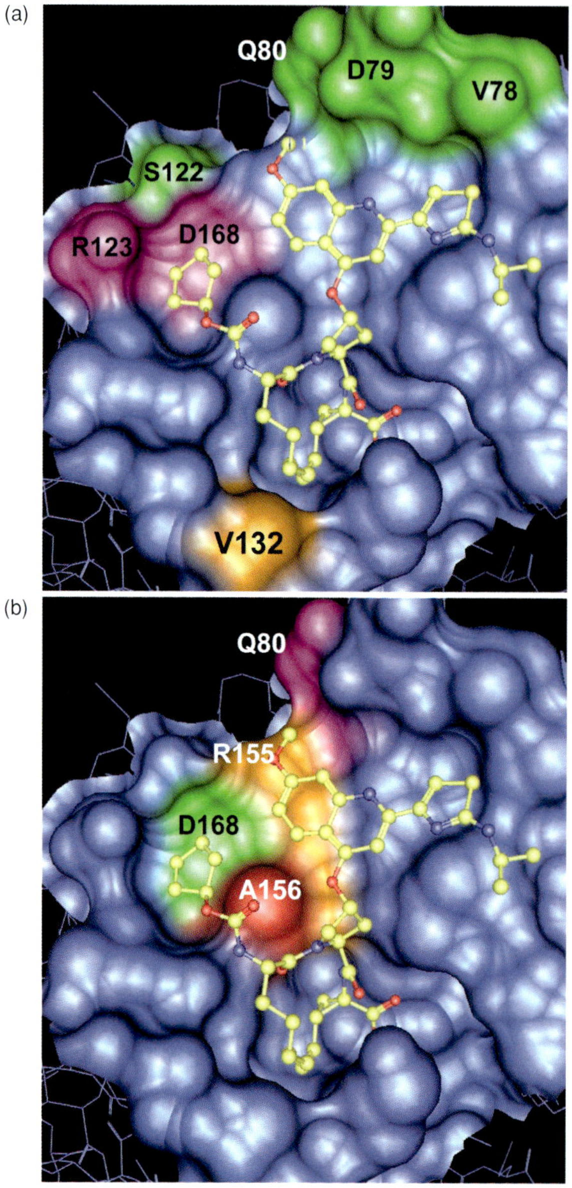

CHAPTER 16, FIGURE 1 BILN 2061 modeled into an NS3-NS4A active site, with surface shown for residues within 5 Å of the inhibitor. (a) Amino acids that differ from genotype 1 are highlighted. Amino acids that differ in genotype 2 are shown in green; those that differ in genotype 3 are shown in magenta; amino acid 132, that varies between subtypes, is shown in brown. (b) Amino acids that are substituted as a result of resistance mutations are highlighted.

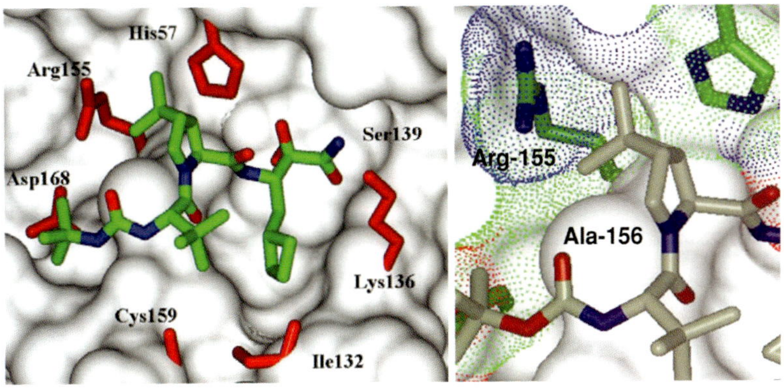

CHAPTER 17, FIGURE 16

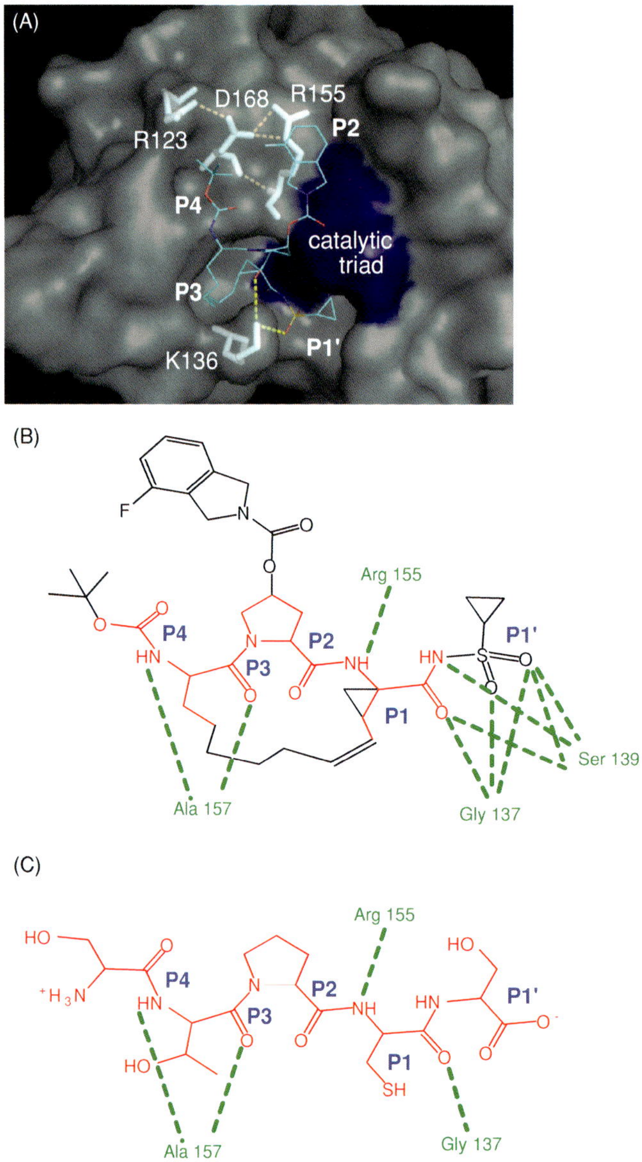

CHAPTER 18, FIGURE 1 Structural biology. (A) Crystal structure of danoprevir NS3/4A complex at 3.1 Å resolution showing P4, P3, P2, and P1′ sites (blue), catalytic triad (dark blue), and four residues that undergo conformational change upon danoprevir binding (white) and have polar interactions that are modulated by danoprevir binding (cyan). (B) Groups analogous to peptide sites P1′, P1, P2, P3, and P4 are indicated. Groups found in natural substrates of NS3/4A are shown in red. Polar contacts to NS3/4A are shown as thick green lines and the protein amino acid indicated. (C) Structure of the NS4B/5A junction of the HCV polyprotein that is cleaved by NS3/4A. Peptide sites P1′, P1, P2, P3, and P4, and scissile amide bond are indicated. Groups transferred directly to danoprevir are shown in red. Polar contacts to NS3/4A are shown as thick green lines and the protein amino acid indicated.

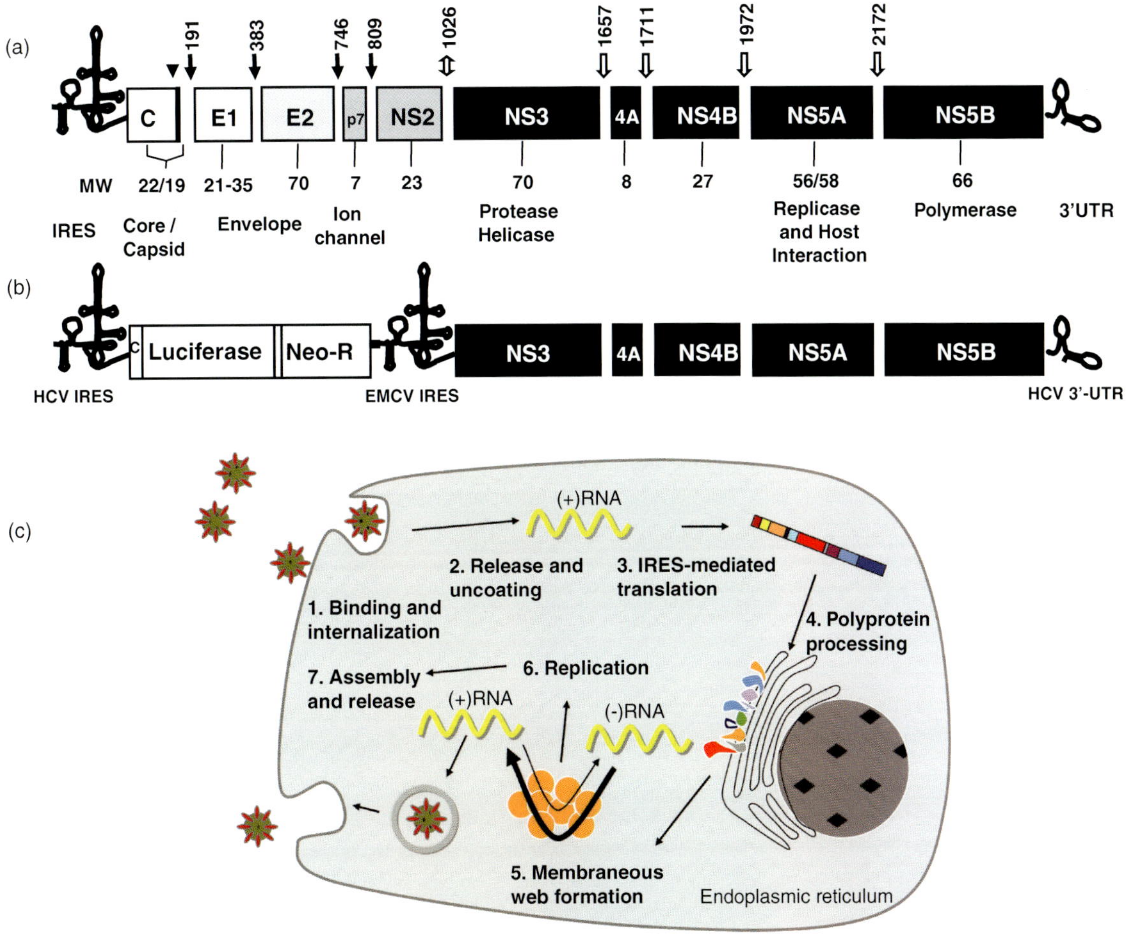

CHAPTER 20, FIGURE 1 (a) HCV genome organization; (b) HCV bicistronic replicon; (c) HCV life cycle. Solid arrows show cleavage sites for host signal peptidases, open arrows show cleavage sites for HCV NS3-4A protease, and the double arrow shows a cleavage site for NS2-3 protease. (Adapted from [11].)

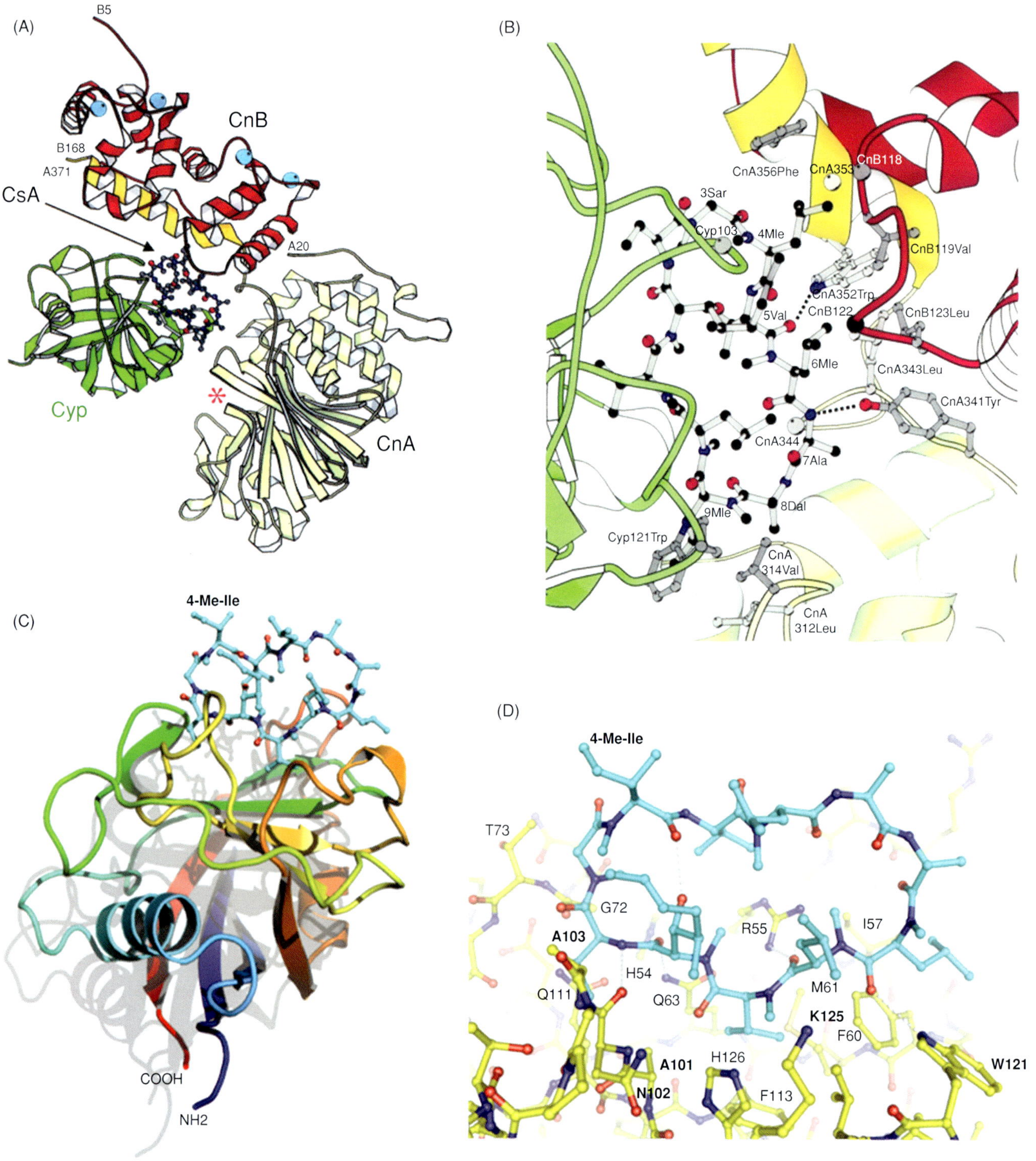

CHAPTER 22, FIGURE 2 Co-crystal structures of CypA/CsA/Cn and CypA/NIM811. (A) A ribbon diagram of the CypA/CsA/Cn ternary complex. The two subunits of Cn are shown in yellow (CnA) and red (CnB). CypA is in green. (B) Details of the interaction between CsA and Cn. (C) Ribbon diagram of the CypA/NIM811 complex. (D) Details of the interaction between NIM811 and CypA. [(A,B) from Jin [33], with permission; (C,D) from Kallen [34].]

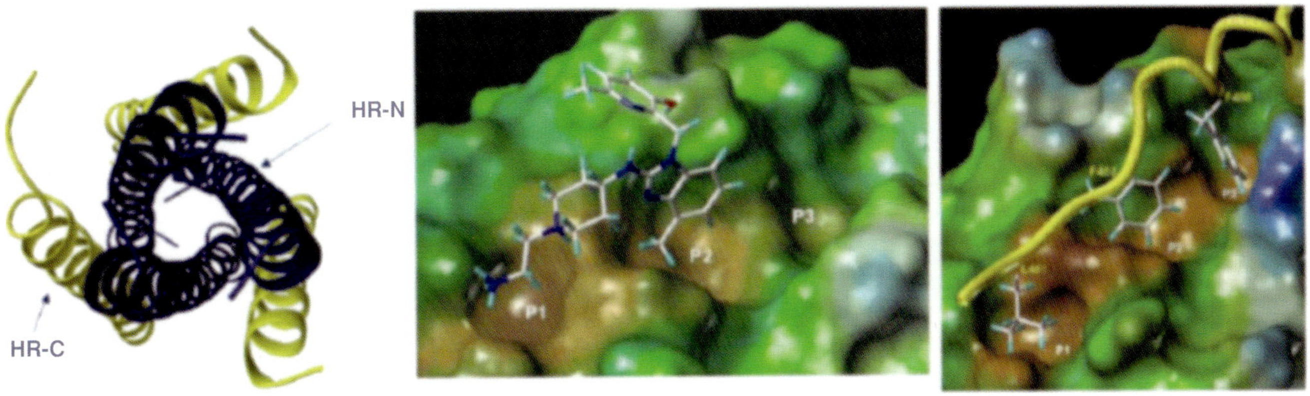

CHAPTER 24, FIGURE 4 1G2C x-ray structure of the RSV 6HB [36] (left). HR-N helices of the central inner trimeric coiled coil are presented in blue. The three HR-C helices, binding into three hydrophobic grooves each formed by two neighboring HR-N helices, are indicated in yellow. The binding of the natural substrate HR-C (right) and the binding of JNJ-2408068 (middle) to the hydrophobic pocket situated in the central trimeric coiled coil of the 6HB are compared.

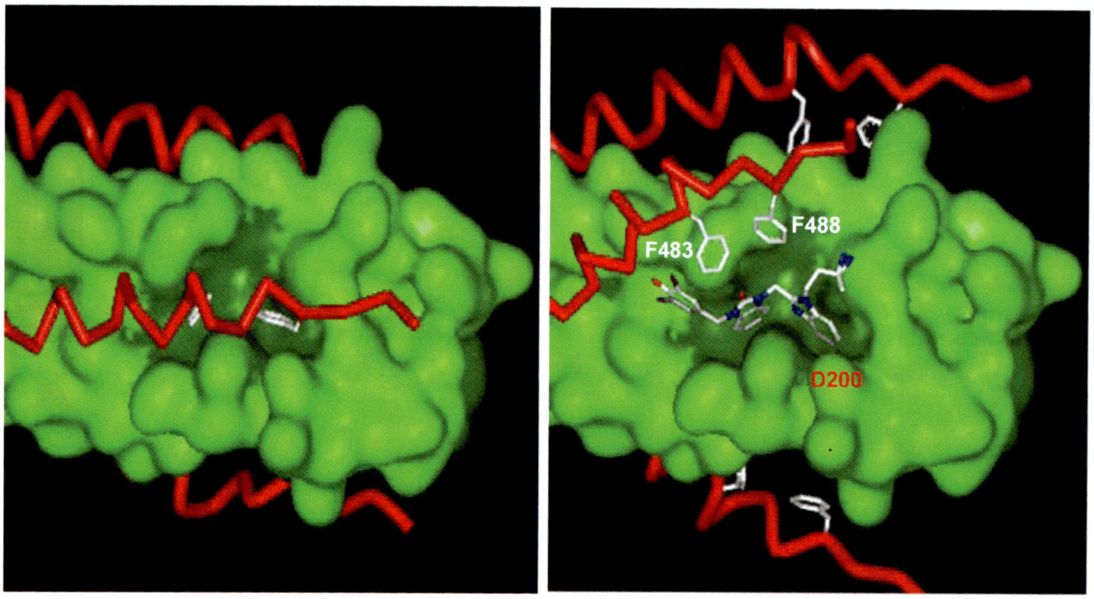

(A) (B)

CHAPTER 25, FIGURE 5 (A) Segment of the six-helix bundle of the RSV F protein in its fusogenic conformation with the assembled trimeric N-terminal heptad repeat (HR-N) depicted as a green surface showing Phe483 and Phe488 of the C-terminal heptad repeat (HR-C) projecting into the HR-N hydrophobic pocket. The peptide backbone of HR-C is shown as a red stick with the side-chain elements of residues Phe483 and Phe488 highlighted in white. These key amino acids reside in the HR-N hydrophobic pocket. (B) Model of the photoaffinity label **16** bound into the HR-N hydrophobic pocket with the orientation postulated based on known SAR and placing the diazirine moiety proximal to Tyr198. The peptide backbone of HR-C and Phe483 and Phe488 are depicted as displaced merely to accommodate **16** and are not intended to suggest specific mechanistic insight into the precise mode of action of this class of RSV fusion inhibitor. D200 is labeled in red.

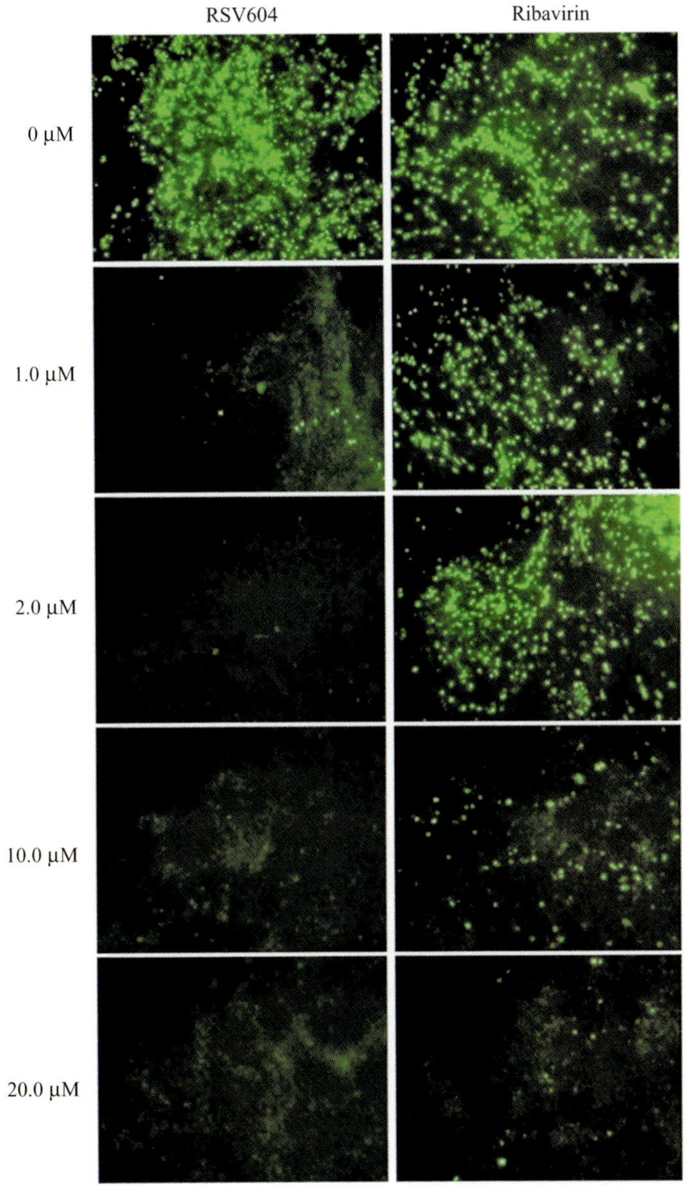

CHAPTER 26, FIGURE 8 Dose-dependent inhibition of RSV replication in an in vitro model of human ciliated epithelium. RSV replication was measured visually by the expression of fluorescent green protein from the virus genome [41]. The top two panels show control cultures in the absence of drug. Compound (RSV604, ribavirin) was added to the basolateral media concomitantly with the virus at the concentrations indicated.

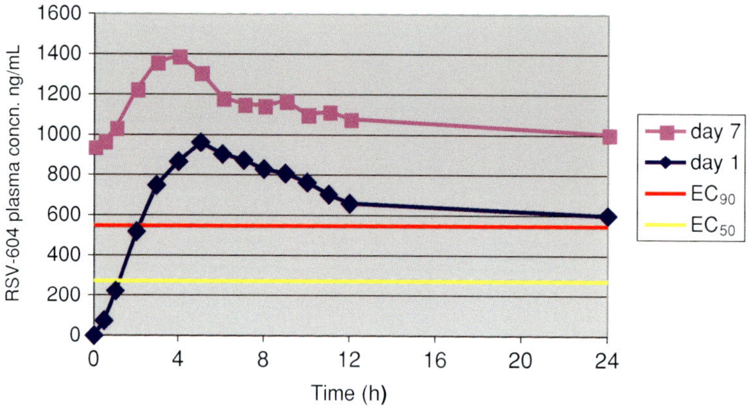

CHAPTER 26, FIGURE 10 RSV604 human PK data, where volunteers received 600 mg on day 1 followed by 450 mg on days 2 to 7.

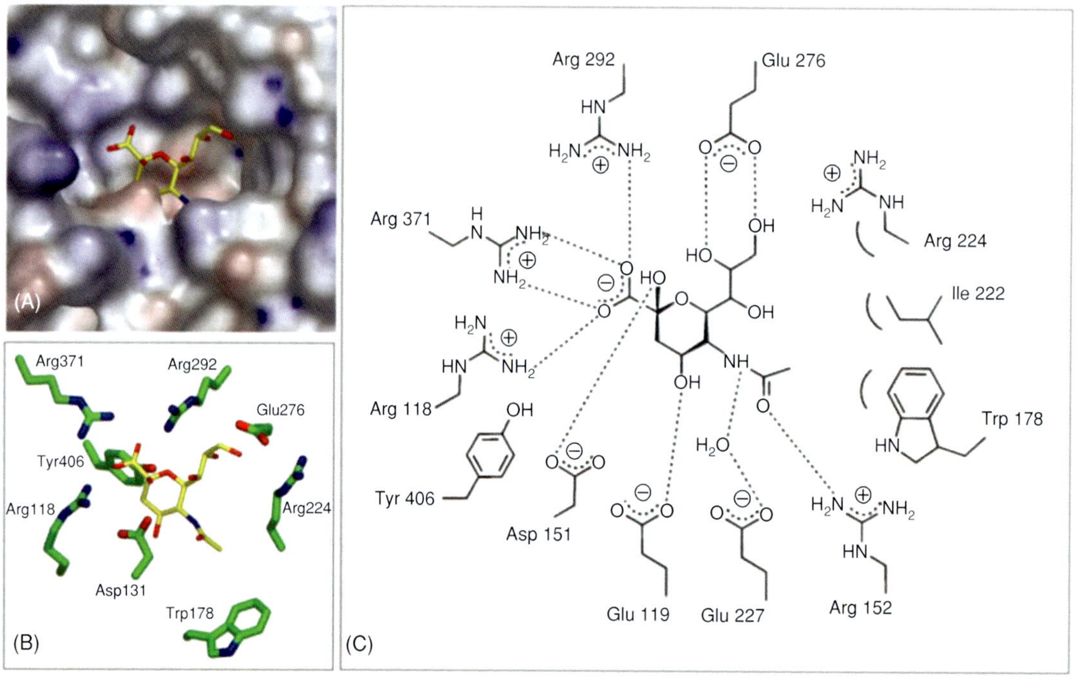

CHAPTER 27, FIGURE 2 Representations of the A/N2:α-Neu5Ac (**4**) complex (pdb 2BAT). (A) View of active site with protein surface colored by electrostatic potential (blue, positive; red, negative). α-Neu5Ac carbons in yellow. (B) Key active-site residues surrounding α-Neu5Ac. (C) Schematic representation of the A/N2 active site showing some key interactions of α-Neu5Ac with conserved residues. Conserved interacting active site residues include Arg118, Arg371, Arg292, Glu276, Arg152, and Glu227. Hydrophobic interactions are made between the C5 acetamido methyl group and Ile222 and Trp178. Tyr406 and Asp151 are involved in enzyme catalysis [25].

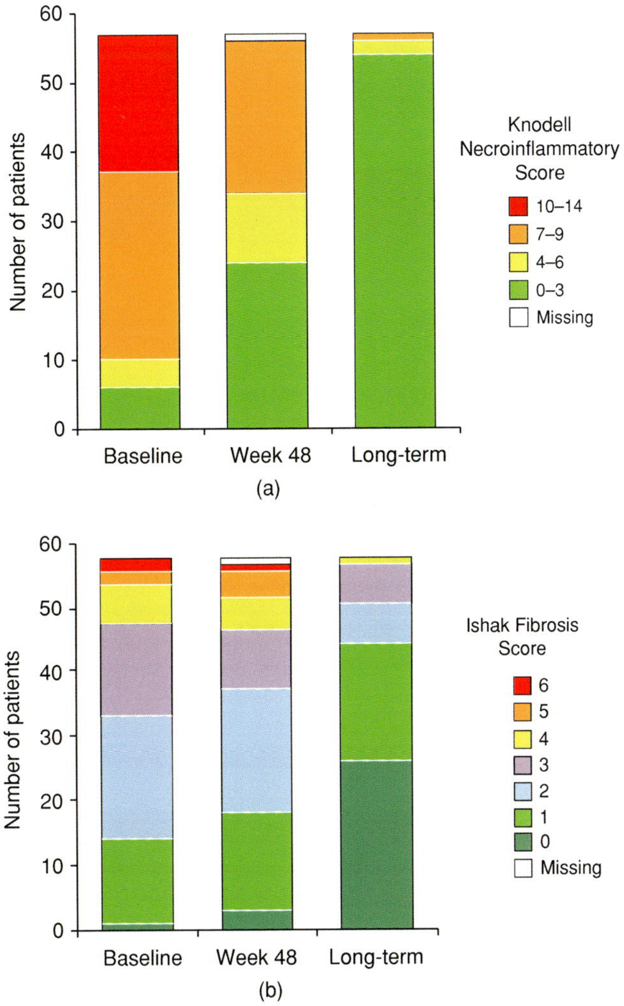

CHAPTER 28, FIGURE 6 Distribution of (a) Knodell necroinflammatory and (b) Ishak fibrosis scores at phase III baseline after 48 weeks of entecavir treatment and at the time of long-term biopsy [median 6 years of entecavir treatment (range 3 to 7 years)]. (Reprinted with permission from *Hepatology*.)

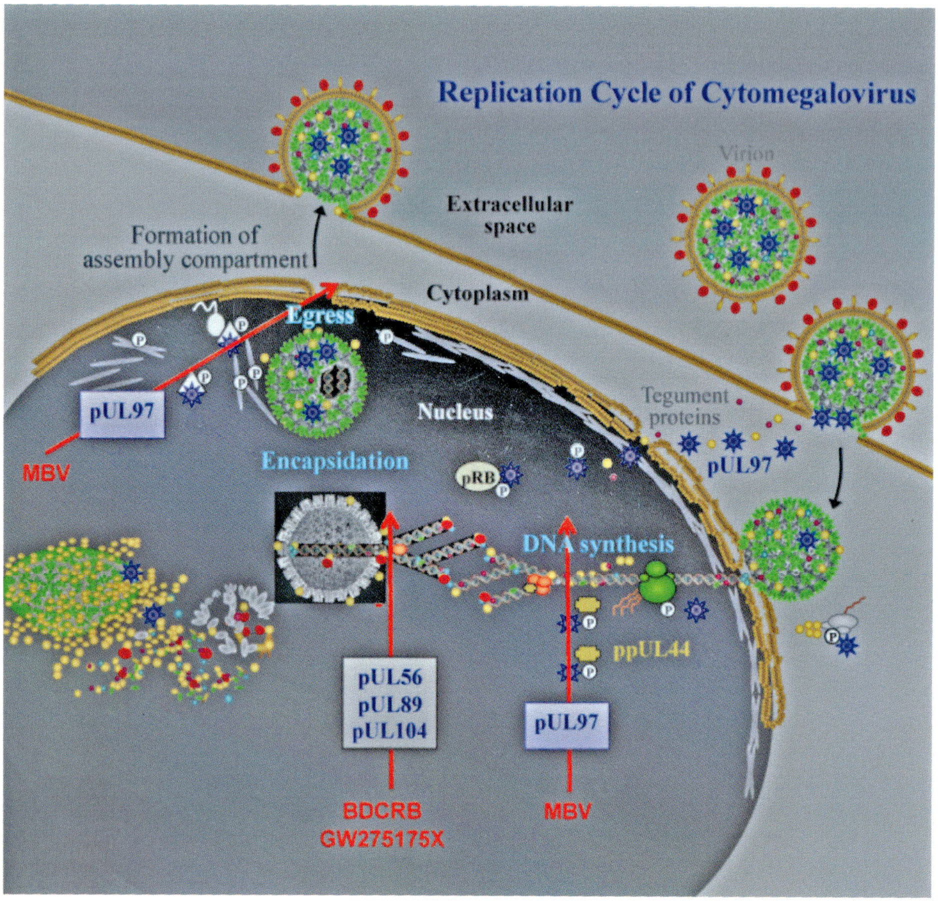

CHAPTER 29, FIGURE 2 Inhibition of human cytomegalovirus replication by benzimidazole nucleosides. Inhibition of key aspects of the replication cycle by maribavir (MBV), BDCRB, and GW275175X are illustrated by red arrows. HCMV proteins inhibited by or involved in the action of the compounds are shown in boxes attached to the arrows.

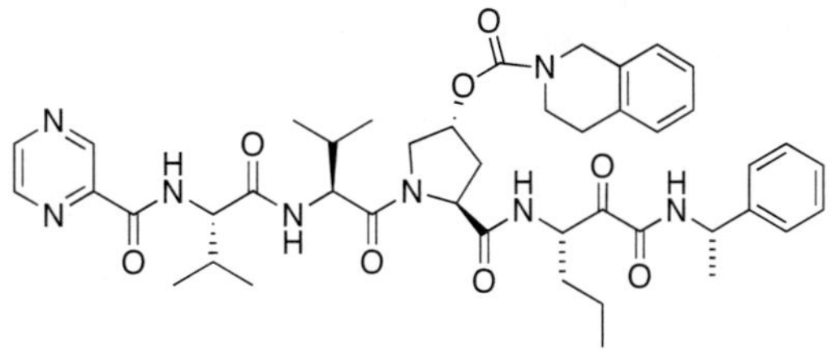

7
K_i = 0.22 μM
Replicon IC_{50} = 0.31 μM

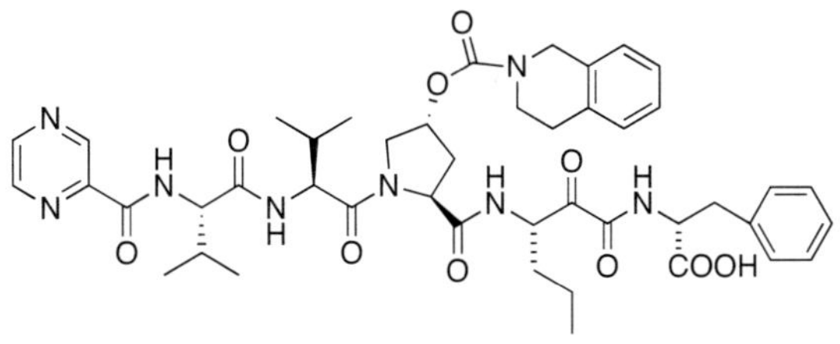

8
K_i = 0.026 μM
Replicon IC_{50} > 10 μM

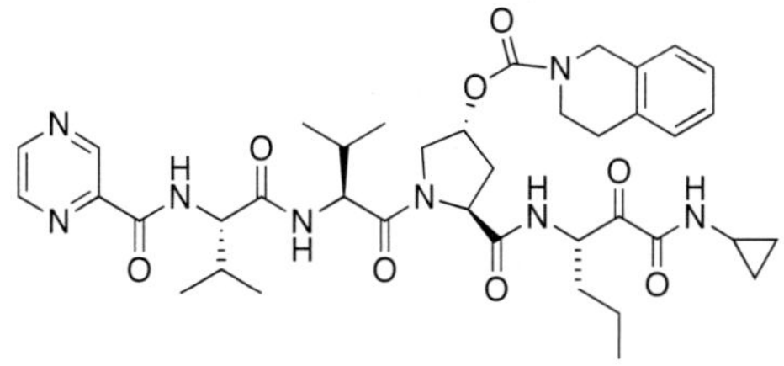

9
K_i = 0.42 μM
Replicon IC_{50} = 2.3 μM

SCHEME 3 Structures of ketoamide inhibitors **7**, **8**, and **9**.

that prevented cell membrane penetration. Small aliphatic groups such as cyclopropyl (**9**, Scheme 3) also displayed encouraging enzyme and cell potency.

Considerable effort and time was spent on the optimization of the THIQ carbamate proline α-ketoamide subclass, and over 300 compounds were prepared, leading to compounds with nanomolar potency in the replicon assay. However, most of these compounds displayed poor pharmacokinetic (PK) profiles, presumably because of their poor physicochemical properties due to the large size of the P2 residue, and low liver and plasma exposures upon a single oral dose administration in mice were observed. At this time, the P2 was revisited to investigate proline substitution other than 4-hydroxyproline-based [38]. Reexamination of the crystal structure of hydroxyproline-based inhibitor **10** led to the hypothesis that proline-based P2s bearing a 1-to-4 carbon substituent at the 3 position on the α face could result in displacement of a putative water molecule in the enzyme active site, thus leading to improved binding affinity [38]. To test this hypothesis, compound **11** was prepared and showed a K_i of 1.4 μM. Subsequent crystal structure examination disproved the water molecule displacement hypothesis, yet the reasonable activity of compound **11** led to further exploration of P2's having this substitution pattern. In addition, 3-alkyl proline-based inhibitors exhibited a PK profile that resulted in significantly improved liver exposure following a single oral dose administration in mice, providing further incentive for optimization, which eventually led to the discovery of telaprevir. Key compounds toward telaprevir are shown in Scheme 4. Extension of the methyl substituent to ethyl eventually led to the bicyclic ketone **14** (K_i = 40 nM). Reduction of the ketone moiety to the bicyclic carbocycle, coupled with further optimization at P1′, P1, P3, and P4, led to telaprevir [39]. Telaprevir was selected for advancement based on its potency and its good liver exposure in rodents.

BIOCHEMICAL AND BIOLOGICAL CHARACTERIZATION

The selection of telaprevir relied most heavily on the in vitro enzyme assays and 2-day replicon assay described below. Although the enzyme assays were designed to take advantage of our covalent warhead strategy, the discrete kinetics of inhibition were not used as an explicit design criterion. Instead, we relied on the 2-day replicon assay as the primary measure of in vitro efficacy. We expected that any benefit of slow-binding inhibition in the disruption of the highly regulated events involved in viral replication would be reflected in the observed potency in this assay.

Enzymatic Assays

The initial assay used to evaluate compounds as inhibitors of HCV protease was a spectrophotometric assay that followed the cleavage of *p*-nitroanilide (*p*NA) from the C-terminus of a hexapeptide substrate [25]. This assay provided significant throughput and the kinetic advantage of continuously monitoring product release. However, the *p*NA assay is limited by two factors: a high enzyme concentration that limits the overall sensitivity of the assay, and a high concentration of substrate (∼ 1 mM) that can limit the solubility of

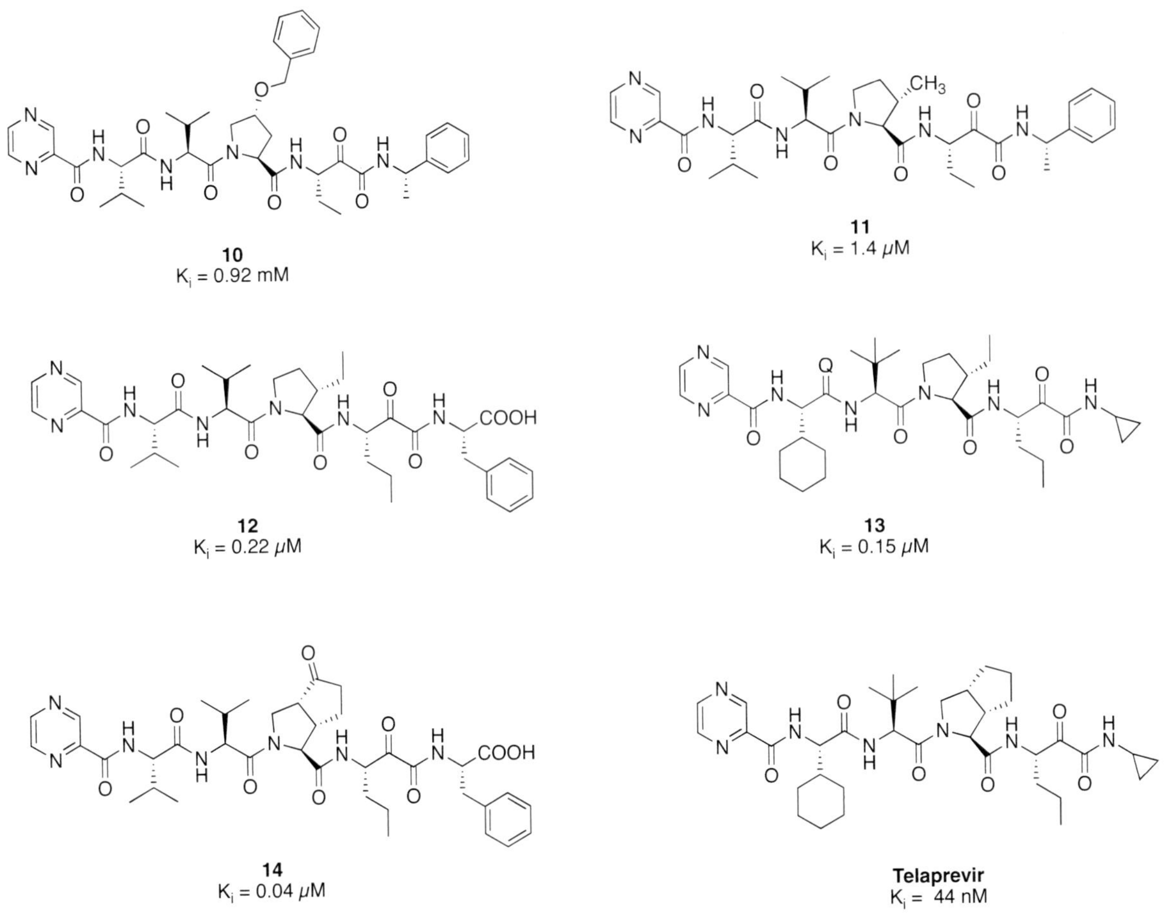

SCHEME 4 Inhibitor progression toward telaprevir.

compounds of interest. To combat these limitations, we moved to the high-performance liquid chromatography (HPLC)-based detection of products generated from the cleavage of an unlabeled peptide with high homology to a naturally occurring cleavage site within the HCV polypeptide [25]. The HPLC-based assay gave good sensitivity along with excellent data quality, and coupling the HPLC to a microplate-compatible autosampler allowed us to maintain sufficient throughput to use this assay as the primary assay for initial compound evaluation toward the selection of telaprevir.

Both the *p*NA assay and the HPLC assay utilize a 15-min incubation of enzyme and inhibitor prior to initiation of the reaction by the addition of substrate. This incubation period complements the covalent reversible warhead approach described above in that it allows the enzyme to react with the inhibitor in the absence of competing substrate, improving the sensitivity of the assay. The apparent inhibition constant of telaprevir in the HPLC assay is 44 nM [34].

As expected, telaprevir forms a covalent tetrahedral intermediate with the nucleophilic active-site serine of HCV protease, as shown in the crystal structure of telaprevir complexed with the NS3 protease catalytic domain and an NS4A peptide cofactor (Figure 3, unpublished results). This observation led us to examine the kinetic nature of the telaprevir inhibition of HCV protease using a continuous fluorescent depsipeptide cleavage assay [34,40]. Progress curve analysis suggests that telaprevir forms an initial, weakly bound complex with the HCV protease, which then rearranges to a more tightly bound form. Under steady-state conditions the inhibition constant for telaprevir inhibition of HCV protease (K_i^*) is 7 nM. Additionally, we found that telaprevir is a slowly dissociating inhibitor of the HCV protease; the half-life observed for the tightly bound complex is 58 min. The slow-binding nature of telaprevir inhibition may provide a therapeutic advantage over compounds of similar potency, which act at diffusion-controlled rates [41].

Inhibition of HCV Replication in Cellular Systems

Compounds that showed significant potency in the enzyme assays above were further evaluated in a 2-day replicon

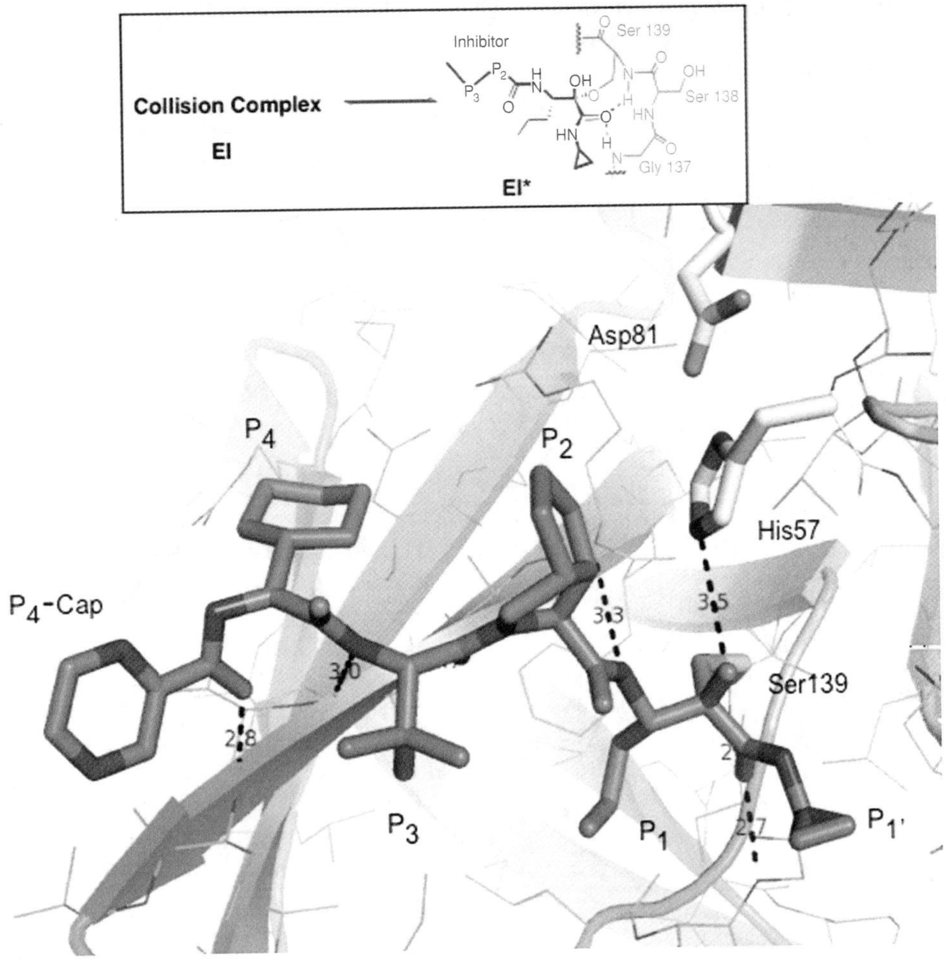

FIGURE 3 Crystal structure of telaprevir complexed with NS3 protease and NS4A peptide cofactor. The inhibitor is shown in a stick diagram with the color scheme: C (purple), N (blue), and O (red). The active site triad (Ser139, His57, and Asp81) are also shown as sticks with C in gray. The rest of the protein is shown with C in green. The secondary structure of the protein is shown in a ribbon diagram. Telaprevir makes four inhibitor main-chain to protein main-chain hydrogen bonds. The side chains of the inhibitor fill the S4, S3, S2, S1, and S1′ binding pockets. The Ser139 residue makes a covalent interaction with the ketoamide warhead. (*See insert for color representation of the figure.*)

assay [32,34]. Huh7 cells harboring a subgenomic replicon of the HCV subtype 1b Con1 strain were incubated with compound for 48 h, at which point the level of HCV RNA was quantitated using QRT-PCR. Telaprevir has an IC_{50} value of 354 nM in this assay; the CC_{50}, determined in parallel with the IC_{50}, was found to be 83 μM, yielding a selectivity index (CC_{50}/IC_{50}) of 230.

A more stringent replicon assay was used to evaluate telaprevir's ability to produce a multilog decrease in HCV RNA levels in vitro. Replicon cells were incubated with 7-μM telaprevir (20 × 2-day replicon IC_{50}) for 3, 6, or 9 days prior to HCV RNA quantitation. As reported previously [34], the number of HCV RNA copies per cell continued to drop with increasing incubation time, resulting in nearly a 4 log drop in RNA levels after 9 days of treatment. The observation of a multilog drop in RNA levels prompted us to test for rebound of HCV RNA levels following the removal of telaprevir from treated cells. Replicon cells were treated with 17.5-μM telaprevir (50 × 2-day replicon IC_{50}) for 13 days in the absence of selective pressure, resulting in a more than 5 log drop in HCV RNA levels. Telaprevir was then removed and G418 was added. G418 is an antibiotic that is used to select cells containing the replicon, which expresses *neo*, the neomycin phosphotransferase gene. Cells without *neo* are cells in which telaprevir has cleared the replicon; thus, they will die in the presence of G418. In this experiment, no growth was observed for 21 days post-telaprevir removal, indicating that telaprevir was able to clear the replicon RNA from the treated cells [34].

To obviate the possibility that the results from the subtype 1b subgenomic replicon assay were artifactual, we tested telaprevir in a subtype 1a infectious assay system using primary cells. Human fetal liver cells were maintained in hormonally defined media for 5 days. The cells were then treated with HCV genotype 1a containing serum for 24 h to establish infection, followed by treatment with telaprevir for 5 days. The IC_{50} for telaprevir in this assay was determined to be 280 nM, consistent with the inhibition observed in the 2-day replicon assay (354 nM) [34].

In Vitro Resistance

Direct antivirals such as protease inhibitors have the potential to generate resistance. Every day, 10^{12} HCV virions are produced. This observation, coupled with the fact that the HCV RNA polymerase has low replicative fidelity and has no proofreading ability, leads to the estimate that point mutations will arise at each position of the HCV genome every day [42]. As a result, quasispecies, or minor variant viral populations, can be the source of rapidly emerging resistance in HCV patients treated with direct antiviral therapies. In vitro studies using genotype 1b HCV replicon cell lines identified three mutations of the alanine 156 residue in the protease active site which conferred resistance to telaprevir. Substitution of the wild-type alanine residue with a serine (A156S) conferred lower levels of in vitro resistance (9.6-fold), while substitution with a valine (A156V), or a threonine residue (A156T) conferred high-level resistance ($>$ 62-fold) in the HCV replicon assay. The A156V/T variants, but not the A156S variant, had severely reduced in vitro replication capacity [43,44].

Telaprevir Activity in an In Vivo Model

In the absence of a reliable small-animal model of HCV infection, we developed an alternative method to demonstrate the ability of telaprevir to inhibit HCV protease after oral delivery in an in vivo setting [34]. Recombinant adenovirus was used to deliver a gene encoding the HCV protease fused to secreted alkaline phosphatase (SEAP) to SCID mice, with a known HCV cleavage site engineered between the two proteins. The adenovirus concentrated in the liver, allowing us to test for telaprevir activity in the target organ. Active HCV protease was able to cleave the fusion protein, releasing SEAP and allowing its detection in the serum [34]. No SEAP activity was observed in the absence of active HCV protease, as demonstrated via delivery of a gene encoding a fusion protein in which the active-site catalytic serine had been mutated to alanine [34].

Mice injected with the wild-type fusion protein adenovirus and treated via oral administration with either 10 or 20 mg/kg of telaprevir showed significant decreases in SEAP levels as compared to vehicle controls. This demonstrated the ability of telaprevir to inhibit HCV protease in the liver. Although this assay was a step removed from demonstrating activity against infected cells in vivo, it did provide evidence that telaprevir retains the expected inhibitory activity against HCV protease in the liver of a live animal.

Additionally, there was a dose-dependent increase in telaprevir exposure at 1 h post-dosing in both liver and plasma in this model. At the lowest dose tested (10 mg/kg), the level of telaprevir in the mouse liver 1 h after oral dosing corresponded to 5.68 μM, which was about sixfold higher than that in the plasma (0.94 μM), confirming the liver-targeting nature of this drug. This liver concentration at 1 h is about 16-fold higher than the 48-h IC_{50} of telaprevir in HCV replicon cells. At dosages higher than 10 mg/kg, the ratio of liver to plasma exposure of telaprevir at 1 h after dosing ranged from 11- to 16-fold. By 12 h, the levels of telaprevir in the mouse liver and plasma were significantly reduced, although still measurable in the liver.

SYNTHESIS

The retrosynthesis of telaprevir is depicted in Scheme 5. To enable a reliable and convergent synthesis of this tetrapeptide, we investigated a number of strategies and demonstrated that disconnecting first between P1 and P2 was optimal, generating tripeptide **15** and warhead precursor **16**. This approach allowed installation of the P1–P1′ fragment as the hydroxy amide **16** in the final stage, to avoid epimerization of the P1 norvaline side chain. Further disconnections, generating key synthetic bicyclic P2 scaffold **17** and commercially available *tert*-butyl glycine P3, cyclohexyl glycine P4, and 2-pyrazine carboxylic acid cap, offered the safest route to minimize epimerization of the three amino acid stereocenters during the synthesis.

Several synthetic routes were explored to gain access to the warhead piece **16**. The two most promising routes with the potential to minimize the number of synthetic steps and maintain enantiomeric purity are summarized in Scheme 6. The Passerini approach [45] (route **1A**) proceeded efficiently under mild conditions to generate a norvaline-based warhead precursor without enantiomeric erosion, which was further elaborated into hydroxyamide **16**.

An alternative approach (route **1B**) generates the key hydroxy acid **19** through a one-carbon homologation of Cbz-norvaline via cyanohydrin formation [46] and hydrolysis. Subsequent coupling and hydrogenation provided the desired P_1–P'_1 warhead precursor **16**. Route **1B** was favored on a large scale since it avoided the generation of volatile toxic materials (isonitrile **18** in route **1A**), and maintained the desired norvaline side-chain stereochemistry.

Bicycloproline **17** was the subject of intense synthetic efforts. The three more successful syntheses investigated are described herein. The first synthesis proceeded through bicyclic ketone **22**, for which a synthesis via tetracyclic diastereomers **21** generated from a cycloaddition cyclization of thiazolium ylide **20** with 2-cyclopentenone had been reported in the literature [47] (Scheme 7) with good overall yield on a 100-g scale. Chiral resolution of **22**, followed by

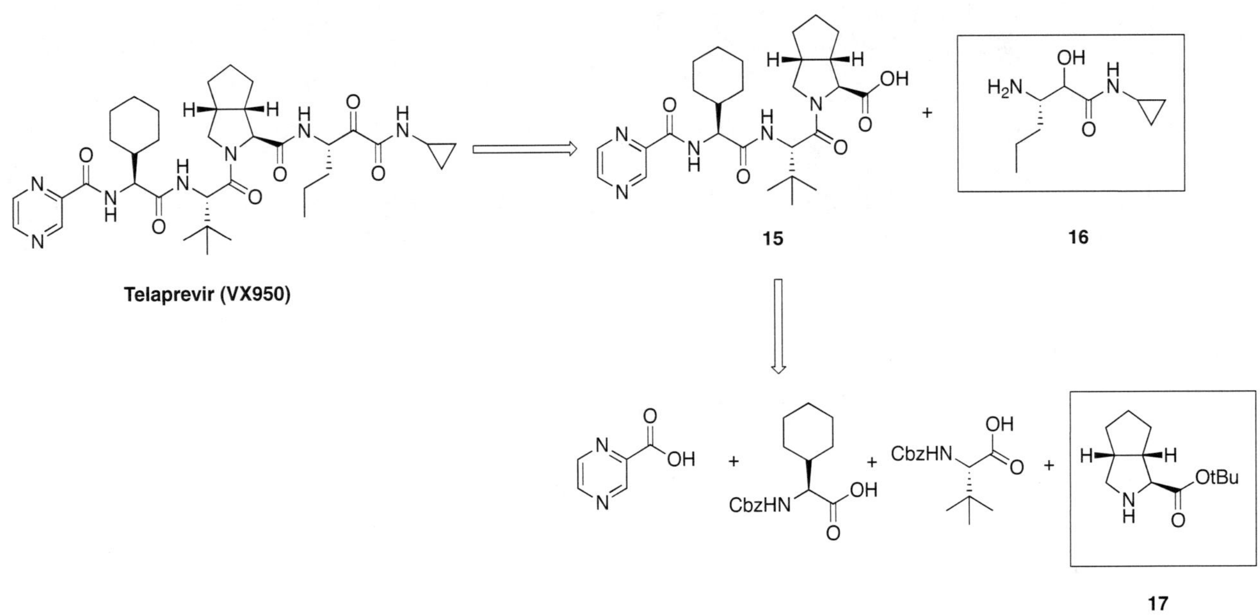

SCHEME 5 Retrosynthetic strategy for telaprevir.

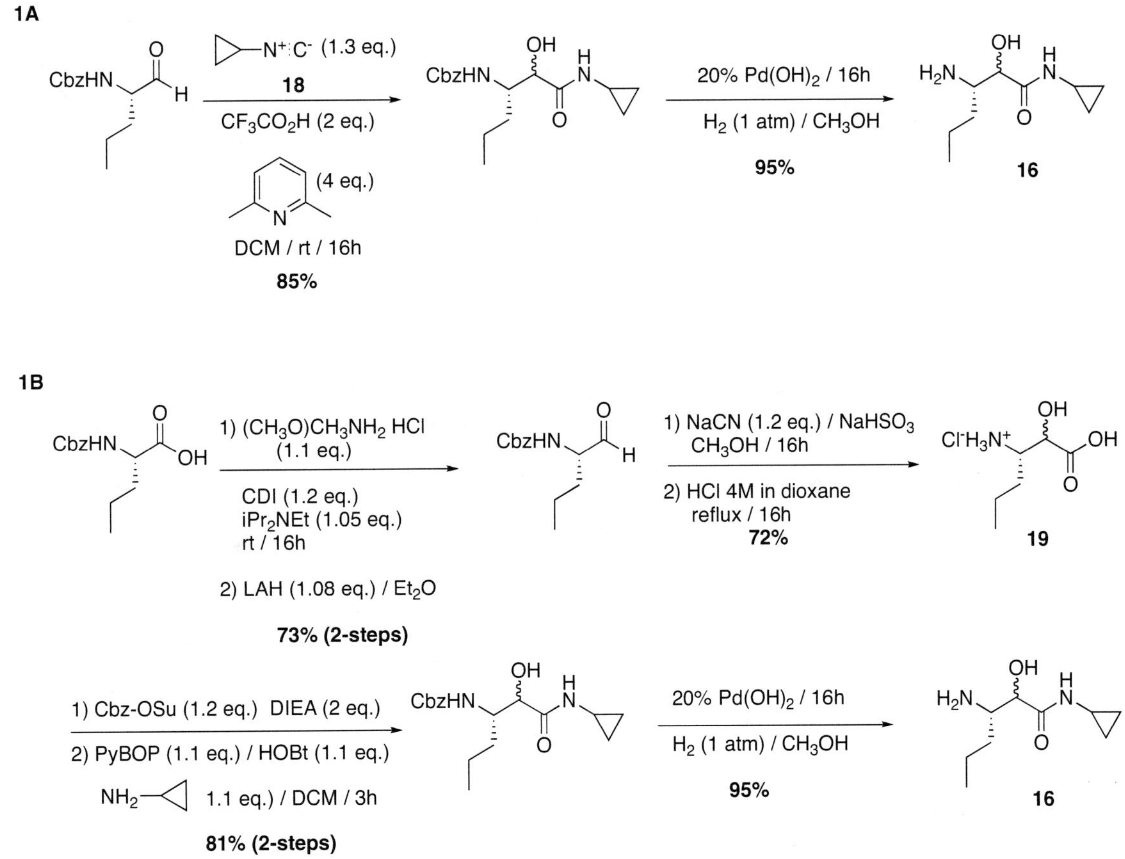

SCHEME 6 Synthetic strategies for the hydroxyamide warhead precursor.

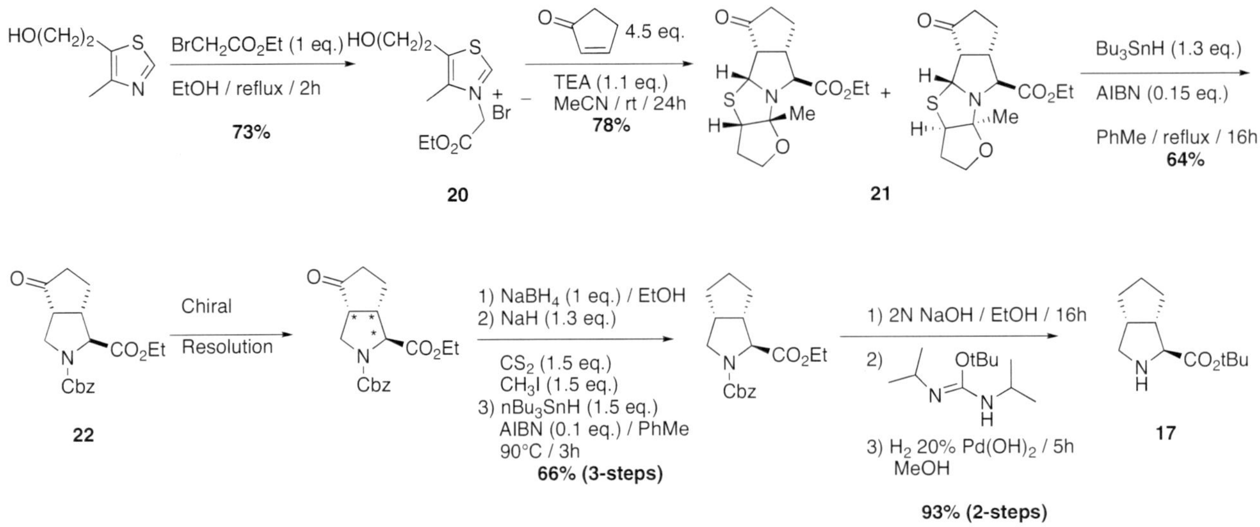

SCHEME 7 Initial synthesis of bicyclic proline P_2.

ring deoxygenation and protective group adjustments [39], provided the key P_2 bicyclic proline scaffold **17**.

The utility of this 10-step synthesis on a large scale was limited due to its length and its use of toxic tin reagents. An improved six-step synthesis [48,49] was developed to circumvent the chiral resolution step and enable the production of the first 100 kg of **17**. This synthesis proceeded through chiral Michael addition of camphor imine **23**, available in one step from (1*S*)-(−) camphor and *tert*-butyl glycine ester [50], to methyl cyclopentenecarboxylate **24** to afford Michael adduct **25** as a single diastereomer (Scheme 8). Imine hydrolysis and subsequent cyclization yielded the lactam ester **26**. Subsequent nitrogen protection, lactam reduction, and carbamate deprotection provided key bicyclic proline **17** in high yield.

A P_2 synthesis used for large-scale reactor production (> 100 kg) employs very cheap raw material 3-azabicyclo-[3.3.0]octane hydrochloride (**27**) as starting material, and avoids the somewhat expensive unnatural camphor chiral auxiliary and its recycling. This five-step novel synthesis is delineated in Scheme 9 [51]. The synthesis started with the Boc carbamate protection of 3-azabicyclo[3.3.0]nonane hydrochloride (**27**), delivering the required precursor **28** for α-carboxylation. 2-Lithiation followed by trapping of the anion with carbon dioxide under equilibrating conditions generated the desired racemate acid **29** with a high degree of diastereoselectivity. The resolution of racemic bicyclic P_2 amino acid mixture **29** via salt formation with an optically active base such as (*S*)-1,2,3,4-tetrahydro-1-naphthylammonium salt provided key bicyclic proline salt **30** in high yield and high enantiomeric purity. Salt neutralization and subsequent esterification provided bicyclic proline **17**.

With the key synthetic P_1–P'_1 **16** and P_2 scaffold **17** in hand, the total synthesis of telaprevir became a linear eight-step sequence [51] summarized in Scheme 10. The

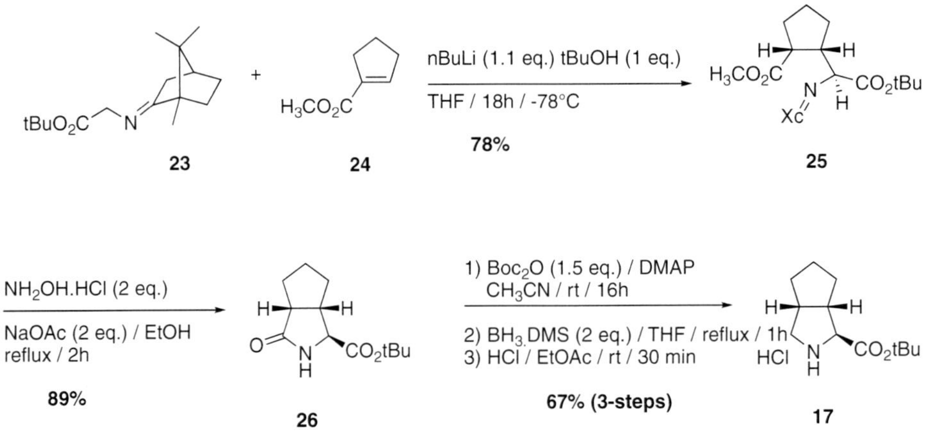

SCHEME 8 Improved synthesis of bicyclic proline P_2.

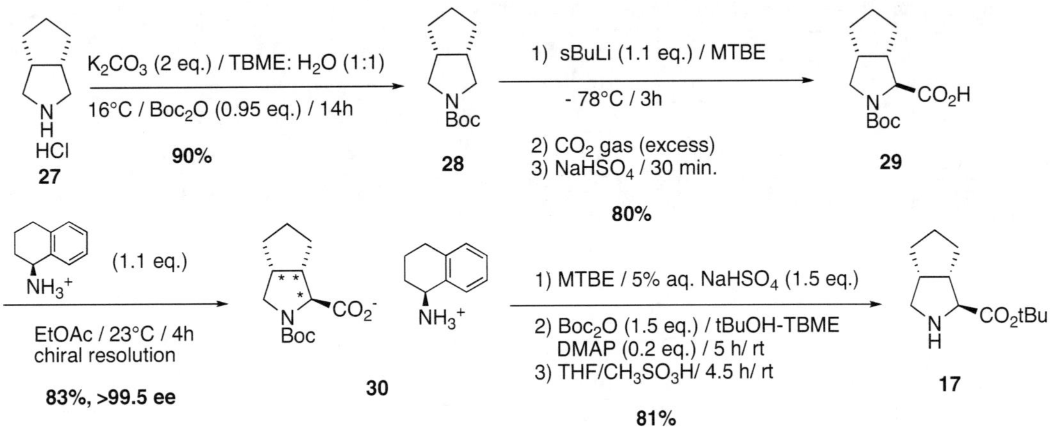

SCHEME 9 Large-scale synthesis of bicyclic proline P_2.

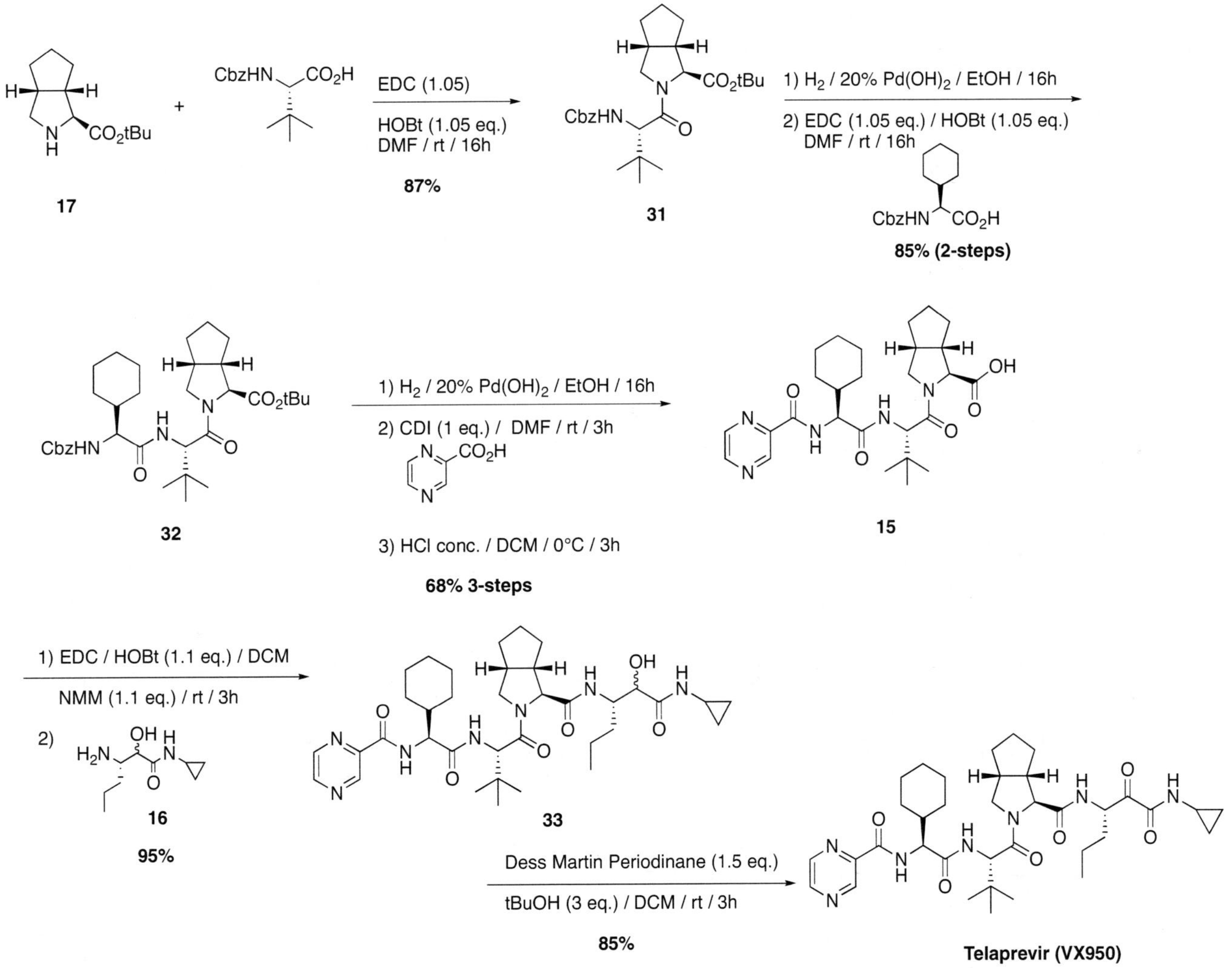

SCHEME 10 Total synthesis of telaprevir.

TABLE 1 Pharmacokinetic Parameters of Intravenously Administered VX-950 in Rats and Dogs[a]

Species	Dose (mg/kg)	$AUC_{0\text{-inf}}$ (μg·h/mL)	C_{max} (μg/mL)	Cl ($mL{\cdot}min^{-1}/kg^{-1}$)	$t_{1/2}$ (h)	V_{ss} (L/kg)
Rat[b]	0.95	0.30 ± 0.02	0.51 ± 0.06	53.7 ± 4.2	1.73 ± 0.06	5.81 ± 1.13
Dog[b]	3.5	1.47 ± 0.44	2.38 ± 0.82	41.8 ± 10.7	0.93 ± 0.14	1.84 ± 0.44

[a]VX-950 was intravenously dosed as a solution at the indicated dose in Sprague–Dawley rats or beagle dogs. The average ± S.D. values from three animals are shown.
[b]The rat samples were analyzed using the chiral LS-MS-MS method; the dog samples were separated by the nonchiral method.

elaboration of capped tripeptide intermediate **15** started with the coupling of Cbz-*tert*-butyl glycine with bicyclic proline ester **17** using standard conditions to provide dipeptide **31**. Protecting group removal followed by coupling of CBZ-protected cyclohexyl glycine delivered tripeptide **32**. CBZ-group deprotection of **32** and CDI-mediated coupling with 1,4-pyrazine carboxylic acid afforded, after ester hydrolysis, P_4-capped tripeptide acid precursor **15**. The key coupling between warhead precursor **16** and tripeptide **15** was conducted under standard conditions using *N*-methylmorpholine as a base to generate an epimeric mixture of hydroxyamide precursor **33**. In the final step, oxidation of **33** proceeded uneventfully using the Dess–Martin periodinane oxidant, to provide telaprevir in good yield.

PRECLINICAL AND HUMAN PHARMACOKINETICS

The pharmacokinetic profile of telaprevir in preclinical species has been published [34]. In general, because of their high molecular weight and low water solubility, the pharmacokinetics of peptidomimetics can be less than ideal. As shown in Table 1, telaprevir has moderate-to-high systemic clearance after intravenous dosing in rats and dogs. However, good volumes of distribution in both species suggest adequate tissue distribution. Good oral exposure was observed with telaprevir. Following oral administration as an amorphous suspension in a PVP-based formulation, bioavailabilities of 25% in rat and 40% in dog were observed (Table 2).

Hepatitis C is a disease of the liver, and most if not all of the HCV replication occurs in that organ. As stated above, one of our criteria for selection of an HCV protease inhibitor as a preclinical candidate was its ability to partition predominantly to the liver. Telaprevir performed especially well with regard to this parameter compared to other close analogs. For telaprevir, the average liver-to-plasma ratio was determined to be 35 in rats over an 8-h time course following administration of a single 30-mg/kg oral dose (Table 3). At this dose, the telaprevir exposure in the liver is about 14 μM, which is 30-fold above the 48-h IC_{50} in replicon cells. A similar liver distribution of telaprevir was observed in the mouse model described above. This observation was a key component in the decision to select telaprevir as a clinical candidate.

Human Pharmacokinetics The predicted exposure of telaprevir from patients dosed concomitantly with telaprevir, peginterferon, and ribavirin has been reported [52]. Telaprevir absorption was characterized by an initial slow phase followed by a second rapid phase. Absorption was delayed by 0.21 h. The population-predicted median $AUC_{0\text{-}8}$ value at steady state for telaprevir was 26.4 mg·h/mL. The median trough concentration of telaprevir predicted from the final population pharmacokinetic model was 2568 ng/mL.

PHASE I–II SAFETY AND EFFICACY STUDIES

Multiple recent clinical reviews of protease inhibitors in the clinic reflect the large degree of interest in the HCV-treating clinical community over the development of specifically targeted antiviral therapy for hepatitis C (STAT-C) inhibitors in general [53–57], and NS3 protease inhibitors in particular [58], in combination with peginterferon and ribavirin. This interest is due in part to the paradigm shift represented by the promising results in trials of STAT-Cs combined with peginterferon and ribavirin, compared to peginterferon and

TABLE 2 Pharmacokinetic Parameters for Orally Administered VX-950 in Rats and Dogs[a]

Species	Dose (mg/kg)	$AUC_{0\text{-inf}}$ (μg·h/mL)	C_{max} (μg/mL)	T_{max} (h)	$t_{1/2}$ (h)	Bioavailability (%)
Rat	40	3.34 ± 0.35	1.55 ± 0.66	0.42 ± 0.14	3.32 ± 1.71	25.0 ± 2.55
Dog	9.6	1.64 ± 0.89	1.08 ± 0.45	0.44 ± 0.13	3.14 ± 2.46	40.7 ± 22.1

[a]VX-950 was dosed orally as a solution in PVP K30 + 2% SLS + water at the indicated dose in Sprague–Dawley rats and beagle dogs. The average ± S.D. values from three animals are shown.

TABLE 3 Systemic Plasma and Liver Exposure of Orally Administered VX-950 in Rats[a]

Organ	AUC_{0-8} (μg·h/mL)	C_{max} (μg/mL)	C_{min} (μg/mL)	C_{avg} (μg/mL)
Liver[b]	78.5 ± 40.0	19.9 ± 10.5	3.30 ± 2.32	9.82 ± 5.00
Plasma	2.23 ± 1.53	0.49 ± 0.24	0.04 ± 0.03	0.28 ± 0.19
Liver/plasma ratio	35.1	40.6	82.5	35.1

[a]VX-950 was dosed orally as a solution in propylene glycol at 30 mg/kg in Fisher rats. The average ± S.D. values from three animals are shown.

[b]It is assumed that the density of liver tissue is 1 g/mL.

ribavirin alone. The results obtained with telaprevir in phase I and II clinical studies are summarized herein.

Phase I Studies

In the first phase 1b dose-finding study [59], 34 genotype 1 HCV-infected patients were treated with placebo, 450 or 750 mg of telaprevir every 8 h, or 1250 mg of telaprevir every 12 h for 14 days. In all telaprevir dose groups, a rapid first-phase decline in plasma HCV RNA was observed followed by a slower second-phase decline, which culminated in a continuous decline, plateau, or viral rebound in HCV RNA after 14 days of dosing. The 750-mg group achieved the highest drug trough plasma concentrations, and a median 4.4 $\log_{10}$ reduction in HCV RNA was observed; the viral load became undetectable in two patients after only 14 days of treatment. Viral rebound was seen in the 450- and 1250-mg telaprevir dose groups, and viral RNA sequencing performed once dosing was completed demonstrated the presence of variants with reduced sensitivity to telaprevir at four loci in the NS3 protease domain. In addition to the A156S/V/T variants that had been observed in vitro, amino acid changes at three additional sites (V36A/M, T54A, and R155K/T) conferring low-level resistance to telaprevir were observed [60]. Variants with double mutations were also evidenced at position 36/155 or 36/156. The V36M/R155K variant was more fit replicatively than V36M or R155K alone, and conferred high-level resistance to telaprevir. After the end of dosing, wild-type virus reappeared and the proportion of resistant variants diminished rapidly in all patients [60].

Because telaprevir-resistant variants are fully sensitive to inhibition by interferon and ribavirin [43] and the combination of telaprevir and interferon is additive to moderately synergistic in the HCV replicon system in vitro [61], two additional phase I studies focused on a combination treatment. Twenty treatment-naive patients with genotype 1 chronic HCV infection were treated with either 2 weeks of pegylated interferon α-2a (Peg-IFN, 180 μg weekly), telaprevir (TVR) monotherapy (1250-mg loading dose followed by 750 mg every 8 h), or interferon and telaprevir (Peg-IFN/TVR) combined therapy [62]. Both telaprevir alone and the telaprevir plus peginterferon combination were significantly more potent than peginterferon alone, decreasing plasma HCV RNA 4.0 and 5.5 $\log_{10}$ IU/mL, respectively, compared to 1.1 $\log_{10}$ with peginterferon alone.

In an additional phase I study, the triple combination of telaprevir plus peginterferon and ribavirin was evaluated in a single-arm open-label study design [52]. Twelve treatment-naive genotype 1 patients were given 28 days of telaprevir (a 1250-mg loading dose on day 1 followed by 750 mg every 8 h), peginterferon (180 μg weekly), and ribavirin (weight-based, 1000 to 1200 mg daily). Triple therapy was well tolerated and all patients achieved a rapid virological response (RVR) with undetectable virus at day 28 for all patients. These studies suggested that the antiviral potency of telaprevir in vivo could be increased by the addition of peginterferon and ribavirin, which inhibit viral variants selected by telaprevir. Consistent with preclinical in vitro results, all telaprevir-resistant variants remained sensitive to peginterferon/ribavirin treatment in the clinic [63].

Phase II PROVE1 and PROVE2 Studies

In two large phase II studies, treatment-naive patients in North America (PROVE1) and Europe (PROVE2) were assigned randomly to various telaprevir-containing regimens or to a control group. In PROVE1, which enrolled 250 HCV genotype 1–infected patients, the control group received standard doses of Peg-IFN and RBV for 48 weeks, plus telaprevir-matched placebo for the first 12 weeks (the PR48 group, 75 patients) [64]. Two groups received telaprevir (1250 mg on day 1 and 750 mg every 8 h thereafter) for 12 weeks as well as peginterferon and ribavirin for 24 weeks (the T12PR24 group, 79 patients) or 48 weeks (the T12PR48 group, 79 patients). SVR rates were significantly higher in the T12PR24 (61%, $p = 0.02$) and in the T12PR48 group (67%, $p = 0.002$) than in the PR48 group (41%). In PROVE2, patients in the control group (the PR48 group, 82 patients) received standard doses of peginterferon and ribavirin for 48 weeks, plus telaprevir-matched placebo for the first 12 weeks [65]. Two groups received telaprevir (1250 mg on day 1 and 750 mg every 8 h thereafter) for 12 weeks in combination with 12 weeks (the T12PR12 group, 82 patients) or 24 weeks (the T12PR24 group, 81 patients) of peginterferon and ribavirin. A third group (T12P12 group, 78 patients) received telaprevir plus peginterferon without ribavirin for 12 weeks. The SVR rate was significantly higher in the T12PR24 group (69%) than in the PR48 group (46%) ($p = 0.004$). The rate was 60% in the T12PR12 group as compared with 36% in the T12P12 group ($p = 0.003$), suggesting that ribavirin is an integral part of the treatment regimen.

In these two studies, the prevalence of telaprevir-resistance-associated mutations in patients with no prior exposure to telaprevir was characterized [66,67]. Only variants with amino acid changes at the four canonical codons (54, 36, 155, and 156) in HCV protease were observed. All patients receiving telaprevir regimens had an initial decrease in HCV RNA levels. Breakthroughs were defined as patients whose HCV RNA levels increased after an initial decline or who never became undetectable. The breakthrough rate in patients receiving telaprevir, peginterferon, and ribavirin was low: 7% in PROVE1 and 5% in PROVE2. Most breakthroughs that occurred were associated with variants conveying high-level resistance to telaprevir. Relapsers were defined as patients whose HCV RNA levels were undetectable at the end of treatment but became detectable during the 24-week post-treatment waiting period before they could reach an SVR. Most relapses were associated with variants conveying low-level resistance to telaprevir. The relapse rates were 2 and 6% in the 24- and 48-week treatment groups in PROVE1, and 30 and 14% in the 12- and 24-week triple therapy groups in PROVE2.

In both PROVE1 and PROVE2, adverse events with increased frequency in the telaprevir-based groups were pruritus, rash, and anemia, and the rate of discontinuation was higher in the telaprevir-based groups, with rash being the most common reason for discontinuation. In these trials, treatment with a telaprevir-based regimen significantly improved SVR rates in treatment-naive patients infected with genotype 1 HCV, albeit with higher rates of discontinuation because of adverse events.

PHASE III STUDIES

Three large phase III studies, designed to further evaluate the safety and efficacy of telaprevir-based regimens in treatment-naive and treatment-experienced patient populations, are ongoing. The first study (ADVANCE), in treatment-naive genotype 1–infected patients, is aimed at evaluating the treatment duration (8 vs. 12 weeks) of telaprevir in combination with peginterferon α-2a or 2b plus ribavirin, followed by 12 or 36 weeks of peginterferon and ribavirin, in a response-guided regimen. The second study (ILLUMINATE), also conducted in treatment-naive genotype 1–infected patients, is designed to assess the relative benefits of 24 or 48 weeks of total treatment in people who respond rapidly and in a sustained manner to a telaprevir-based treatment, using response-guided therapy. The third study (REALIZE) evaluates the safety and efficacy of treatment with telaprevir plus peginterferon and ribavirin compared to peginterferon and ribavirin only, with or without a 4-week lead-in course of peginterferon and ribavirin alone, in patients who did not respond to one or more prior courses of peginterferon and ribavirin. Final results from these phase III studies are expected by the end of 2010.

FUTURE DIRECTIONS

Short-term goals for future therapies include increasing the SVR rate, decreasing treatment duration, minimizing resistance while developing treatment strategies for patients in whom resistance may have emerged, and treating patients who have not achieved SVR with standard therapy. Additionally, the safety and efficacy of new treatment regimens must be evaluated in patients with historically low response rates, such as African Americans, patients with advanced cirrhosis, liver transplant patients, HIV/HCV coinfected patients, and patients with kidney failure.

The development of HIV drugs over the past decades suggests that first-generation protease inhibitors could be replaced in the long term by second- and third-generation inhibitors having improved potency and a higher barrier to resistance, and that new formulations and combinations with other classes of drugs already in development, such as HCV polymerase inhibitors, could potentially reduce pill burden. Although interferon-based therapy will remain the foundation of HCV treatments for years to come, the development of multiple STAT-C agents with complementary modes of action and additive potency raise the hope of interferon-free drug combination regimens for HCV patients in the future.

REFERENCES

[1] Purcell, R. H. The hepatitis C virus: overview. *Hepatology* **1997**, *26*(Suppl 1), 11S–14S.

[2] Strader, D. B., et al. Diagnosis, management, and treatment of hepatitis C. *Hepatology* **2004**, *39*, 1147–1171.

[3] Alter, H. J.; Seef, L. B. Recovery, persistence, and sequelae in hepatitis C infection: a perspective on long-term outcome. *Semin. Liver Dis.* **2000**, *20*, 17–35.

[4] Saito, I. T., et al. Hepatitis C virus infection is associated with the development of hepatocellular carcinoma. *Proc. Natl. Acad. Sci. USA* **1990**, *87*, 6547–6549.

[5] Kronenberger, B.; Zeuzem, S. Current and future treatment options for HCV. *Ann. Hepatol.* **2009**, *8*, 103–112.

[6] Nelson, D., et al. Hepatitis C virus: a critical appraisal of approaches to therapy. *Clin. Gastroenterol. Hepatol.* **2008**, *7*, 397–414.

[7] Neukam, K., et al. A review of current anti-HCV treatment regimens and possible future strategies. *Expert Opin. Pharmacother.* **2009**, *10*, 417–433.

[8] Zeuzem, S., et al. Expert opinion on the treatment of patients with chronic hepatitis C. *J. Viral Hepatol.* **2009**, *16*, 75–90.

[9] Manns, M. P., et al. Peginterferon alfa-2b plus ribavirin compared with interferon alfa-2b plus ribavirin for initial treatment of chronic hepatitis C: a randomised trial. *Lancet* **2001**, *358*, 958–965.

[10] Fried, M. W., et al. Peginterferon alfa-2a plus ribavirin for chronic hepatitis C virus infection. *N. Engl. J. Med.* **2002**, *347*, 975–982.

[11] McHutchison, J. G., et al. Peginterferon alfa-2b or alfa-2a with ribavirin for treatment of hepatitis C infection. *N. Engl. J. Med.* **2009**, *361*, 580–593.

[12] Lindenbach, B. D.; Rice, C. M. Unravelling hepatitis C virus replication: from genome to function. *Nature* **2005**, *436*, 933–938.

[13] Moradpour, D., et al. Membrane association of the RNA-dependent RNA polymerase is essential for hepatitis C virus RNA replication. *J. Virol.* **2004**, *78*, 13278–13284.

[14] Ma, H., et al. Inhibition of native hepatitis C virus replicase by nucleotide and non-nucleoside inhibitors. *Virology* **2005**, *332*, 8–15.

[15] Salonen, A.; Ahola, T.; Kaariainen, L. Viral RNA replication in association with cellular membranes. *Curr. Top. Microbiol. Immunol.* **2005**, *285*, 139–173.

[16] Failla, C.; Tomei, L.; De Francesco, R. Both NS3 and NS4A are required for proteolytic processing of hepatitis C virus nonstructural proteins. *J. Virol.* **1994**, *68*, 3753–3760.

[17] Bartenschlager, R., et al. Complex formation between the NS3 serine-type proteinase of the hepatitis C virus and NS4A and its importance for polyprotein maturation. *J. Virol.* **1995**, *69*, 7519–7528.

[18] Failla, C.; Tomei, L.; De Francesco, R. An amino-terminal domain of the hepatitis C virus NS3 protease is essential for interaction with NS4A. *J. Virol.* **1995**, *69*, 1769–1777.

[19] Lin, C.; Rice, C. M. The hepatitis C virus NS3 serine proteinase and NS4A cofactor: establishment of a cell-free trans-processing assay. *Proc. Natl. Acad. Sci. USA* **1995**, *92*, 7622–7626.

[20] Lin, C.; Thomson, J. A.; Rice, C. M. A central region in the hepatitis C virus NS4A protein allows formation of an active NS3-NS4A serine proteinase complex in vivo and in vitro. *J. Virol.* **1995**, *69*, 4373–4380.

[21] Tanji, Y., et al. Hepatitis C virus–encoded nonstructural protein NS4A has versatile functions in viral protein processing. *J. Virol.* **1995**, *69*, 1575–1581.

[22] Kim, J. L., et al. Crystal structure of the hepatitis C virus NS3 protease domain complexed with a synthetic NS4A cofactor peptide. *Cell* **1996**, *87*, 343–355.

[23] Love, R.A., et al. The crystal structure of hepatitis C virus proteinase reveals a trypsin-like fold and a structural zinc binding site. *Cell* **1996**, *87*, 331–342.

[24] Sali, D. L., et al. Serine protease of hepatitis C virus expressed in insect cells as the NS3/4a complex. *Biochemistry* **1998**, *37*, 3392–3401.

[25] Landro, J. A., et al. Mechanistic role of an NS4A peptide cofactor with the truncated NS3 protease of hepatitis C virus: elucidation of the NS4A stimulatory effect via kinetic analysis and inhibitor mapping. *Biochemistry* **1997**, *36*, 9340–9348.

[26] Lindenbach, B. D.; Rice, C. M. Flaviviridae: the viruses and their replication. In *Fields Virology*, 4th ed., Knipe, D. M., Howley, P. M., Griffin, D. E., Eds, Lippincott Williams & Wilkins, Philadelphia, 2001; pp. 991–1041.

[27] Lopez-Labrador, F. X. Hepatitis C virus NS3/4A protease inhibitors. *Recent Pat. Anti-infect. Drug Discov.* **2008**, *3*, 157–167.

[28] Gentile, I., et al. Telaprevir: a promising protease inhibitor for the treatment of hepatitis C virus infection. *Curr. Med. Chem.* **2009**, *16*, 1115–1121.

[29] Reesink, H. W.; Weegink, C. J. New hope for a cure for chronic hepatitis C. *J. Hepatol.* **2009**, *51*, 835–837.

[30] Reiser, M.; Timm, J. Serine protease inhibitors as anti-hepatitis C virus agents. *Expert Rev. Anti-infect. Ther.* **2009**, *7*, 537–547.

[31] Perni, R. B. NS3·4A protease as a target for interfering with hepatitis C virus replication. *Drug News Perspect.* **2000**, *13*, 69–77.

[32] Lohmann, V., et al. Replication of subgenomic hepatitis C virus RNAs in a hepatoma cell line. *Science* **1999**, *285*, 110–113.

[33] Lin, C., et al. Discovery and development of VX-950, a novel, covalent and reversible inhibitor of hepatitis C virus NS3·4A serine protease. *Infect. Disord. Drug Targets* **2006**, *6*, 3–16.

[34] Perni, R. B., et al. Preclinical profile of VX-950, a potent, selective, and orally bioavailable inhibitor of hepatitis C virus NS3-4A serine protease. *Antimicrob. Agents Chemother.* **2006**, *50*, 899–909.

[35] Leung, D.; Abbenante, G.; Farlie, D. P. Protease inhibitors: current status and future prospects. *J. Med. Chem.* **2000**, *43*, 305.

[36] Perni, R. B., et al. Inhibitors of hepatitis C virus NS3·4A protease: 1. Non-charged tetrapeptide variants. *Bioorg. Med. Chem. Lett.* **2003**, *13*, 4059–4063.

[37] Perni, R. B., et al. Inhibitors of hepatitis C virus NS3·4A protease: 2. Warhead SAR and optimization. *Bioorg. Med. Chem. Lett.* **2004**, *14*, 1441–1446.

[38] Perni, R. B., et al. Inhibitors of hepatitis C virus NS3·4A protease: 3: P2 proline variants. *Bioorg. Med. Chem. Lett.* **2004**, *14*, 1939–1942.

[39] Yip, Y., et al. Discovery of a novel bicycloproline P2 bearing peptidyl α-ketoamide LY514962 as HCV protease inhibitor. *Bioorg. Med. Chem. Lett.* **2004**, *14*, 251–256.

[40] Taliani, M., et al. A continuous assay of hepatitis C virus protease based on resonance energy transfer depsipeptide substrates. *Anal. Biochem.* **1996**, *240*, 60–67.

[41] Copeland, R. A.; Pompliano, D. L.; Meek, T. D. Drug–target residence time and its implications for lead optimization. *Nat. Rev. Drug Discov.* **2006**, *5*, 730–739.

[42] Neuman, A. U., et al. Hepatitis C viral dynamics in vivo and the antiviral efficacy of interferon-α therapy. *Science* **1998**, *282*, 103–107.

[43] Lin, C., et al. In vitro resistance studies of hepatitis C virus serine protease inhibitors, VX-950 and BILN 2061: structural

analysis indicates different resistance mechanisms. *J. Biol. Chem.* **2004**, *279*, 17508–17514.

[44] Lin, C., et al. In vitro studies of cross-resistance mutations against two hepatitis C virus serine protease inhibitors, VX-950 and BILN-2061. *J. Biol. Chem.* **2005**, *280*, 36784–36791.

[45] Doemling, A.; Ugi, I. Multicomponent reactions with isocyanides. *Angew. Chem. Int. Ed. Engl.* **2000**, *39*, 3168–3210.

[46] Harbeson, S. L., et al. Stereospecific synthesis of peptidyl α-keto amides as inhibitors of calpain. *J. Med. Chem.* **1994**, *37*, 2918–2929.

[47] Monn, J. A.; Valli, M. J. A concise, stereocontrolled thiazolium ylide approach to kainic acid. *J. Org. Chem.* **1994**, *59*, 2773–2778.

[48] Kanemasa, S.; Tatsukawa, A.; Wada, E. Highly diastereoselective michael addition of lithiated camphor imines of glycine esters to a,b-unsaturated esters: synthesis of optically pure 5-oxo-2,4-pyrrolidinedicarboxylates of unnatural stereochemistry. *J. Org. Chem*, **1991**, *56*, 2875–2883.

[49] Farmer, L. J., et al. Inhibitors of hepatitis C virus NS3·4A protease: P2 proline variants. *Lett. Drug Des. Discov.* **2005**, *2*, 497–502.

[50] Zhou, C.; Chen, D.; Jiang, Y. A convenient catalytic system of potassium carbonate and alkanol: the michael addition and carbonyl addition reactions of imine compounds. *Synth. Commun.* **1987**, *17*, 1377–1382.

[51] Tanoury, G. J.; Chen, M.; Cochran, J. E. Processes and intermediates. WO2007/022459A2.

[52] Lawitz, E., et al. Antiviral effects and safety of telaprevir, peginterferon-alfa-2a and ribavirin for 28 days in hepatitis C patients. *J. Hepatol.* **2008**, *49*, 163–169.

[53] Kwong, A. D., et al. Recent progress in the development of selected hepatitis C virus NS3·4A protease and NS5B polymerase inhibitors. *Curr. Opin. Pharmacol.* **2008**, *8*, 522–531.

[54] Asselah, T.; Benhamou, Y.; Marcellin, P. Protease and polymerase inhibitors for the treatment of hepatitis C. *Liver Int.* **2009**, *29*(Suppl. 1), 57–67.

[55] De Brujine, J., et al. New developments in the antiviral treatment of hepatitis C. *Vox Sang.* **2009**, *97*, 1–12.

[56] Pereira, A. A.; Jacobson, I. M. New and experimental therapies for HCV. *Nat. Rev. Gastroenterol. Hepatol.* **2009**, *6*, 403–411.

[57] Soriano, V.; Peters, M. G.; Zeuzem, S. New therapies for hepatitis C infection. *Clin. Infect. Dis.* **2009**, *48*, 313–320.

[58] Weisberg, I. S.; Jacobson, I. M. Telaprevir: hope on the horizon, getting closer. *Clin. Liver Dis.* **2009**, *13*, 441–452.

[59] Reesink, H. W., et al. Rapid decline of viral RNA in hepatitis C patients treated with VX-950: a phase 1b, placebo-controlled, randomized study. *Gastroenterology* **2006**, *131*, 997–1002.

[60] Sarrazin, C., et al. Dynamic hepatitis C virus genotypic and phenotypic changes in patients treated with the protease inhibitor telaprevir. *Gastroenterology* **2007**, *132*, 1767–1777.

[61] Lin, K., et al. VX-950, a novel hepatitis C virus (HCV) NS3-4A protease inhibitor, exhibits potent antiviral activities in HCV replicon cells. *Antimicrob. Agents Chemother.* **2006**, *50*, 1813–1822.

[62] Forestier, N. H., et al. Antiviral activity of telaprevir (VX-950) and peginterferon alfa-2a in patients with hepatitis C. *Hepatology* **2007**, *46*, 640–648.

[63] Kieffer, T. L., et al. Telaprevir and pegylated interferon-alpha-2a inhibit wild-type and resistant genotype 1 hepatitis C virus replication in patients. *Hepatology* **2007**, *46*, 631–639.

[64] McHutchison, J. G., et al. Telaprevir with peginterferon and ribavirin for chronic HCV genotype 1 infection. *N. Engl. J. Med.* **2009**, *360*, 1827–1838.

[65] Hézode, C., et al. Telaprevir and peginterferon with or without ribavirin for chronic HCV infection. *N. Engl. J. Med.* **2009**, *360*, 1839–1850.

[66] Bartels, D. J., et al. Natural prevalence of hepatitis C virus variants with decreased sensitivity to NS3·4A protease inhibitors in treatment-naive subjects. *J. Infect. Dis.* **2008**, *198*, 800–807.

[67] Kuntzen, T., et al. Naturally occurring dominant resistance mutations to hepatitis C virus protease and polymerase inhibitors in treatment-naive patients. *Hepatology* **2008**, *48*, 1769–1778.

16

DISCOVERY AND DEVELOPMENT OF BILN 2061 AND FOLLOW-UP BI 201335

MONTSE LLINÀS-BRUNET AND PETER W. WHITE
Boehringer Ingelheim (Canada), Ltd., Laval, Quebec, Canada

INTRODUCTION

The hepatitis C virus (HCV), the causative agent of non-A non-B hepatitis, was discovered 20 years ago. Researchers at Chiron reported in 1989 the discovery of HCV, a small-enveloped single-stranded RNA virus belonging to the Flaviviridae family [1]. The HCV genome consists of approximately 9600 bases, encoding a single polyprotein of approximately 3000 amino acids, flanked by conserved 5′ and 3′ untranslated regions (UTR). The viral polyprotein comprises four structural proteins followed by six nonstructural (NS) proteins. The bifunctional NS3 protein consists of an N-terminal protease domain and a C-terminal helicase [2]. The NS3 protease plays a critical role in the maturation of the viral polyprotein precursor, and it was recognized early on as a potential target for antiviral drugs. The absolute requirement of the NS3 protease for viral replication was demonstrated with mutations inactivating protease activity both in vitro and in vivo. Knockout of NS3 protease activity abolished replication of the subgenomic replicon in the Huh 7 human liver cell line [3]. In chimpanzees, no productive infection was observed after inoculation of HCV clones containing inactivating mutations [4]. For these reasons the NS3 protease became a preferred target for the design of direct-acting antivirals against the HCV virus.

A distinctive feature of the NS3 protease is its susceptibility to feedback inhibition by the N-terminal products released from the cleavage of its peptide substrates. A unique characteristic of these substrate-based inhibitors is the presence of a free carboxylic acid on the C-terminal P1 residue [5,6]. The finding that a carboxylic acid can establish crucial and unique interactions with the enzyme active site, while imparting selectivity with respect to other serine proteases has resulted in significant efforts on the development of noncovalent inhibitors. Hexapeptide **1** (Scheme 1) was used as a starting point for the inhibitor design [7]. However, this compound suffers from many drawbacks. It has weak affinity for the enzyme, is highly peptidic, and contains three carboxylic acids, which are detrimental for cell permeability. Moreover, compound **1** contains a cysteine as the P1 residue, the sulfhydryl group of which is chemically reactive [7].

TOWARD INHIBITORS WITH CELL-BASED POTENCY

We first improved potency of hexapeptide **1** and then optimized its biopharmaceutical properties. Two findings during early optimization led to a significant improvement in potency and resulted in inhibitors that showed activity in cell-based assays [3]. The first breakthrough came with the discovery of (1*R*,2*S*)-1-amino-2-vinylcyclopropane carboxylic acid (vinyl-ACCA) as a chemically stable replacement for the cysteine P1 residue [8]. Most important, this residue increased considerably the potency of inhibitors. The second significant finding was the realization that the addition of a 4*R*-benzyloxy-group on the P2 proline was beneficial for potency, culminating in the discovery of the 2-phenyl-4-oxoquinoline, which resulted in a greater than 10,000-fold improvement in activity [9]. Compound **2** [10,11]

Antiviral Drugs: From Basic Discovery Through Clinical Trials, First Edition. Edited by Wieslaw M. Kazmierski.

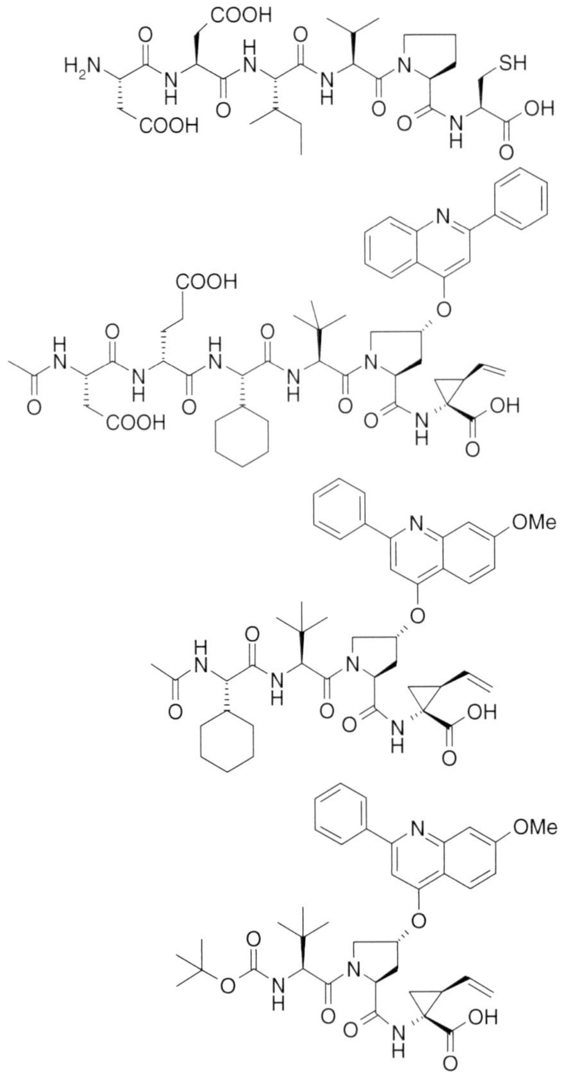

1 K_i = 79,000 nM

2 K_i = 0.074 nM
EC_{50} = 1,900 nM

3 IC_{50} = 1 nM
EC_{50} = 750 nM

4 IC_{50} = 29 nM
EC_{50} = 410 nM

SCHEME 1 Potent and specific peptidomimetic inhibitors of the NS3-NS4A protease.

(Scheme 1) is exquisitely potent and represents a 10^6-fold improvement over hexapeptide **1**.

Having made significant improvements in potency, our next step was to improve biopharmaceutical properties. N-terminal truncation provided potent tetrapeptide inhibitors that are less peptidic and in which two carboxylic acid residues have been eliminated. Tetrapeptide **3,** which also incorporates a more optimal quinoline moiety [12], is a very potent inhibitor but still has weak activity in the replicon. However, further truncation to carbamate **4** produced inhibitors with better cell culture activity. The somewhat rigid nature of the carbamate allows for proper positioning of the N-terminal alkyl group into the S4 binding pocket of the enzyme [12]. Tripeptide inhibitors of the NS3 protease displaying low-nanomolar and submicromolar potencies in the enzymatic and the cell-based replicon assays, respectively, had been identified.

The next step in the optimization of the tripeptide inhibitors came with the rigidification of the scaffold into the bound conformation. Extensive NMR studies [13,14], together with the x-ray structure of a tripeptide–protease complex, revealed the proximity of the P1 and P3 residues when these peptides are bound to the protease. In addition, the NMR conformation of the NS3-bound inhibitors was found to be different from that of its free state [15]. In the free state, the conformation of the P1 vinyl-ACCA residue was rotated by 180° as shown in Scheme 2. Therefore, a rigid macrocyclic scaffold that mimics the bound conformation was expected to have a small loss in entropy on binding to the enzyme and therefore to have a higher binding affinity. The resulting novel macrocyclic inhibitor **5** (Scheme 2) [16] is a potent and selective inhibitor of the NS3 protease (IC_{50} = 11 nM) also displaying good cell-based activity (EC_{50} = 76 nM).

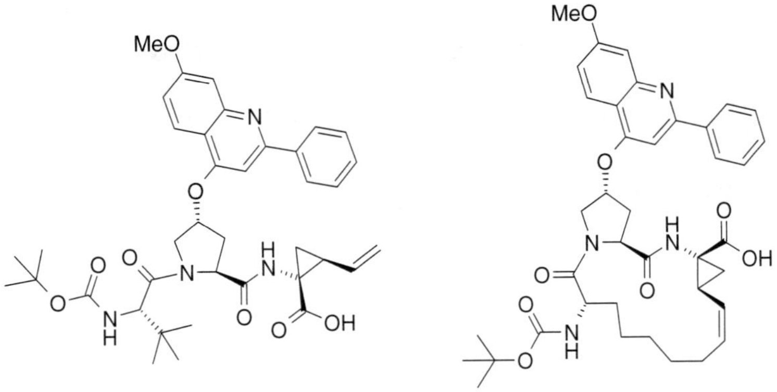

4 Free conformation

5 IC_{50} = 9 nM
EC_{50} = 76 nM

SCHEME 2 Rigidification into the bioactive conformation.

The crystal structure of compound **5** bound to the NS3-protease/NS4A-peptide complex [16] showed that the inhibitor binds in close proximity to the catalytic residues and that the C-terminal carboxylate binds similarly to the protease cleavage product [17], forming hydrogen bonds with the side chains of the catalytic triad residues His 57 and to a lesser extent Ser139 and also with the oxyanion hole. The cyclopropyl residue occupies the shallow S1 pocket, while the aliphatic bridge between the P1 and P3 sidechains binds within the S1–S3 channel and curves along the protease surface. In contrast, the large P2 residue lies on the enzyme surface above the active-site residues Asp81 and His57, partially shielding this region of the protease from solvent [16].

Studies of the tripeptide macrocyclic inhibitor series demonstrated that the 15-membered heterocycle is optimal [15]. The C-terminal carboxylic acid was maintained since it contributes considerably to the potency and specificity of the inhibitors. Therefore, subsequent structure–activity relationship (SAR) focused on two pharmacophores: the novel tricyclic substituent on the 4-*R*-hydroxyproline moiety and the left-hand-side carbamate group (capping group) in order to further improve the potency and biopharmaceutical properties of these inhibitors.

TABLE 1 SAR Leading to BILN 2061

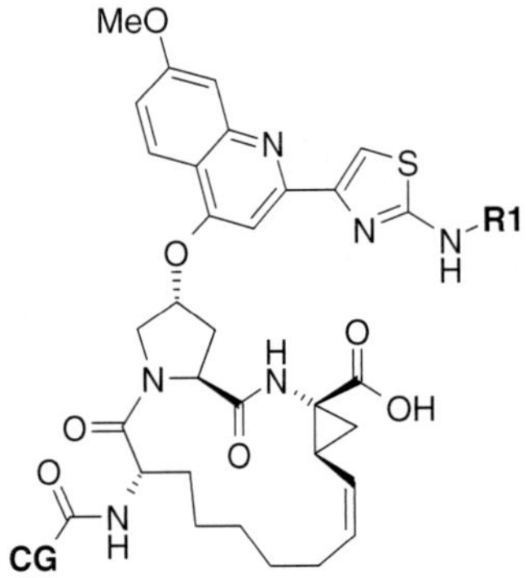

CG	R1	Compound	IC_{50} (nM)	EC_{50} (nM)
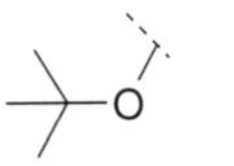	H	**6**	5.5	3.2
	Me	**7**	6.4	6.0
	COMe	**8**	4.8	4.5
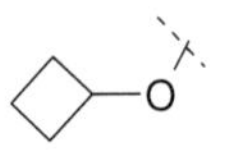	COMe	**9**	2.8	0.6
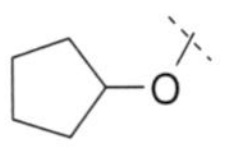	COMe	**10**	2.5	0.4
	H	**11**	3.5	1.6
	Me	**12**	2.5	0.8
	Et	**13**	2.9	1.0
	i-Pr	BILN2061	3.0	1.2

DISCOVERY OF BILN 2061

Replacement of the 2-phenyl ring on the P2 7-methoxyquinolinoxy moiety with different five-membered-ring aromatic heterocycles containing one, two, or three heteroatoms (O, N, and S) was very well tolerated [18]. Among the best heterocycles identified were the 2-amino-4-thiazolyl derivatives. Compounds **6, 7,** and **8** (Table 1) are low-nanomolar inhibitors of the NS3 protease in both enzymatic and cellular assays. The stability of the *tert*-butyl carbamate capping group found in these inhibitors was a concern since it is well documented that the *tert*-butyl carbamate is not stable under acidic conditions [19]. Early SAR studies conducted on a related series of acyclic inhibitors had identified carbamates arising from cyclic alcohols that are well tolerated and impart chemical stability [12]. Based on these studies, cyclobutyl (**9**) and cyclopentyl (**10**) carbamates were introduced in combination with the 2-(2-acetylamino-4-thiazolyl)quinoline present in compound **8**. Either cyclobutyl or cyclopentyl carbamate considerably improved replicon potency. Indeed, compounds **9** and **10** were about 10-fold more potent than

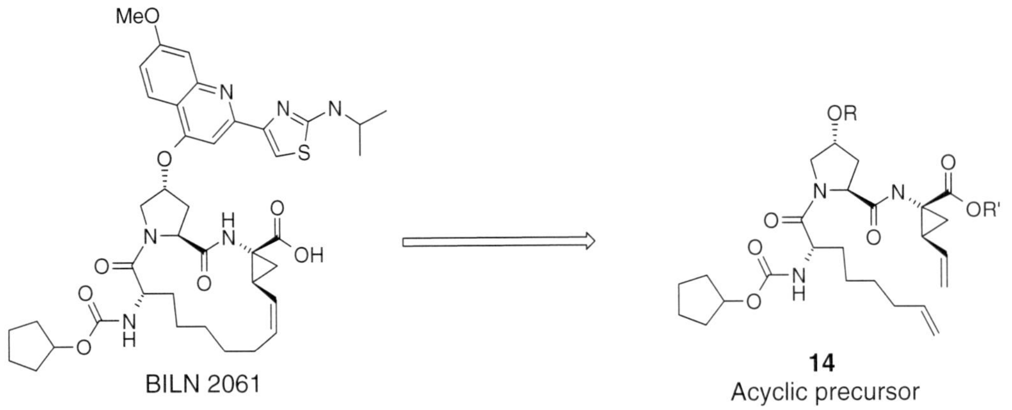

SCHEME 3 Approach to the synthesis of BILN 2061 by RCM macrocyclization.

analog **8** and are representative of a group of compounds with subnanomolar potency against the HCV replicon.

The combination of the cyclopentyl carbamate with other aminothiazole-containing derivatives (**10** to **13**, BILN 2061) led in all cases to a replicon potency improvement. Several compounds with low-nanomolar and subnanomolar activity were identified. Our next step was to evaluate the pharmacokinetic properties of these inhibitors in rats. Oral dosing of compounds **11** and **12** in rats did not result in significant plasma levels. However, dosing of compound **10** resulted in low but measurable plasma concentrations, although intravenous dosing revealed a short half-life for this compound. Higher plasma levels were observed for compound **13**, but the half-life was still short. Increasing the size of the alkyl group on the 2-aminothiazolyl derivative from ethyl to isopropyl generated BILN 2061, which showed an improved pharmacokinetic profile with a higher plasma exposure and longer half-life. Based on the excellent in vitro potency and adequate pharmacokinetic profile in rats, BILN 2061 was chosen for further evaluation.

SYNTHESIS OF BILN 2061

The key step in the synthesis of BILN 2061 was macrocyclization leading to the 15-membered ring. Several routes were contemplated for the formation of this macrocycle, and the ring-closing metathesis (RCM) of acyclic precursor **14** was chosen as the most promising (Scheme 3) [20]. Since the discovery of BILN 2061, several approaches to the synthesis have been reported, from an early medicinal chemistry synthesis [21] to a pilot-plant process [22,23]. The general analysis shown in Scheme 4 was employed for all the synthetic approaches. Retro-synthetic analysis led to disconnection of the two amide bond linkages and the oxoquinoline moiety on the proline, giving the four fragments (**15** to **18**)

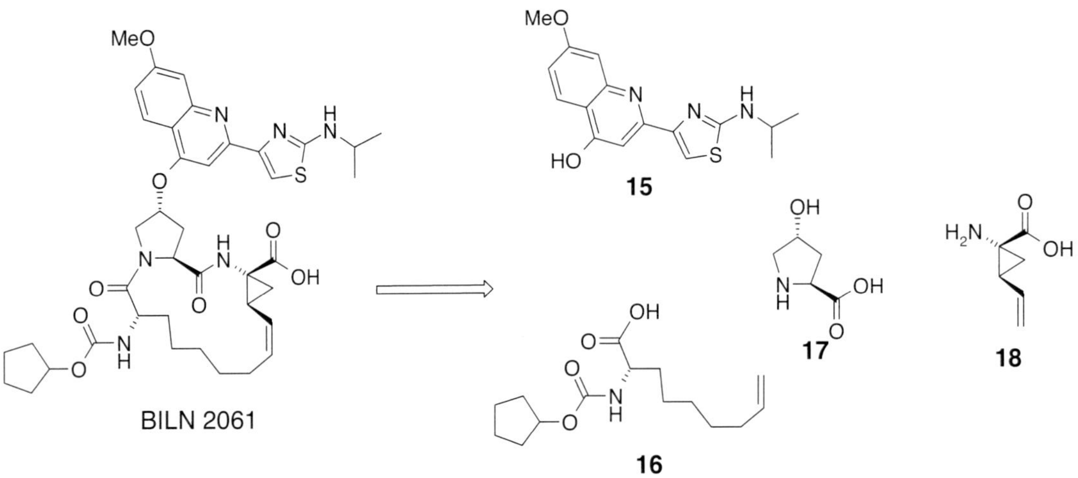

SCHEME 4 Retrosynthetic analysis for the synthesis of BILN 2061.

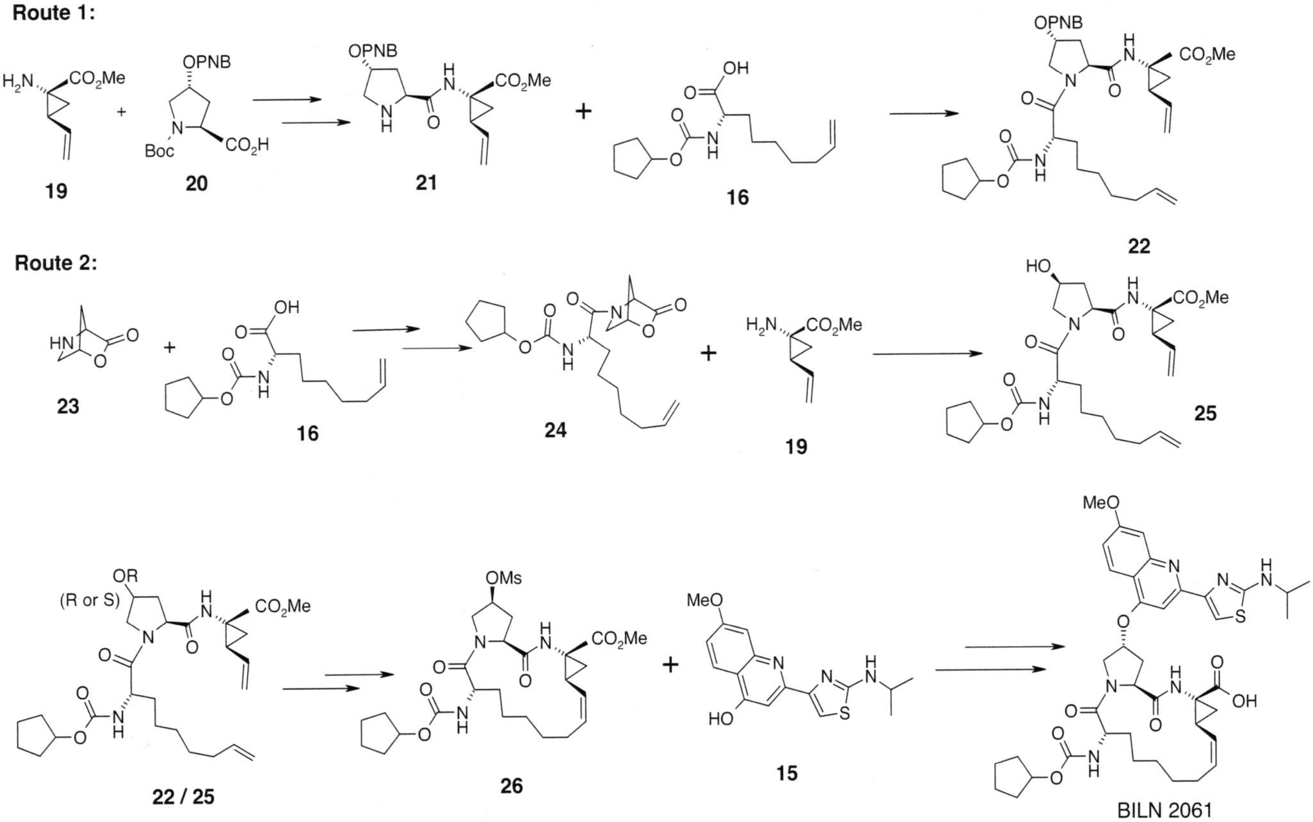

SCHEME 5 Synthesis of BILN 2061.

shown in Scheme 4. All reported syntheses of BILN 2061 are based on the preparation and assembly of these four fragments, and thus are very convergent. The main differences between the syntheses are in the way that these fragments were joined. Efficient syntheses were developed for the individual fragments **15**, **16**, and **18** [24–26], with **18** being the most difficult. However, the most challenging step in all cases was the RCM.

The two large-scale synthetic routes for the RCM precursor are depicted in Scheme 5. The initial assembly process, shown in route 1, was not very efficient, with the need for extensive protection and deprotection operations, as shown with intermediates **20** and **21** [*t*-butyl carbonate (Boc) and *p*-nitrobenzoate (PNB) groups]. In addition, attachment of costly vinylcyclopropane amino acid ester **19** also was carried out as the last step, which was undesirable [23]. Therefore, an assembly strategy that reduced the number of steps and improved the overall throughput and cost scenario was desired. Route 2, using lactone **23** as a starting material, gave a shorter and more efficient synthetic sequence [23]. This key intermediate provided three very favorable features. The correct proline C4 stereochemistry was introduced at a very early stage when no other amino acid was present in the substrate; it served as a protecting group in the first peptide coupling step and as an activating group in the second one. In addition, the lactone moiety was coupled without generating a molecular fragment and without the use of any peptide coupling reagent, which translated into a very atom-economical process. In this route the coupling with fragment **19** was also realized at a later stage in the synthesis.

Implementation of RCM macrocyclizations in an industrial setting is extremely problematic and very uncommon, since these reactions generally require high dilution and high catalyst loading (2 to 10 mol%) [27]. Therefore, a considerable effort was devoted to the ring-closing metathesis reaction. The first large-scale process reported [23], although allowing the synthesis of more than 100 kg, was still not very practical. The RCM reaction still required high catalyst load and long reaction times, and had to be performed at high dilution (0.01 M). The introduction of a Boc group on the P2–P1 amide as shown on Scheme 6 led to a remarkable improvement in the reaction by changing the initiation step. This reaction could be carried out at "acceptable" plant concentrations (>0.2 M) and low catalyst loadings (=0.1 mol%), making this the first example of a truly practical RCM macrocyclization [28]. In summary, by introducing a practical RCM macrocyclization reaction, a practical large-scale synthesis of BILN 2061 was developed.

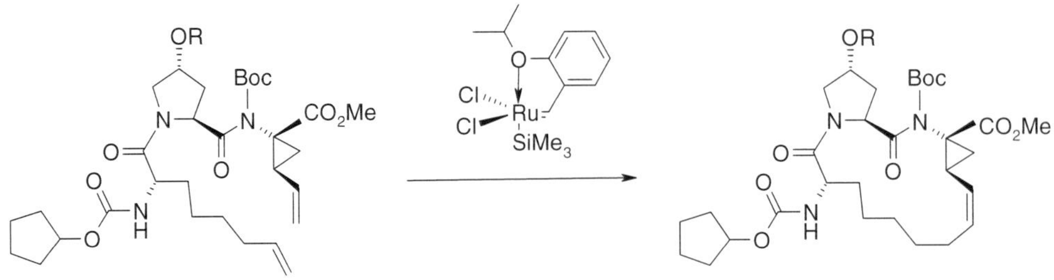

SCHEME 6 Improved RCM.

IN VITRO CHARACTERIZATION OF BILN 2061

BILN 2061 was optimized for potency against genotype 1 NS3 proteins, since this is the most prevalent genotype and also the most difficult to treat with standard pegylated interferon plus ribavirin therapy (pegIFN/RBV). It is a potent inhibitor of genotype 1 protease activity, as shown in Table 2 [29]. In the cell-based replicon assay, BILN 2061 has similar activity, with EC_{50} values very close to the enzymatic IC_{50} values [30]. It has weaker but still significant activity against genotype 2 and 3 NS3 [29]. More recently, BILN 2061 was tested against the genotype 2a JFH1 replicon and also a JFH1-based full virus replication assay [31]. The EC_{50} values observed are consistent with the result for genotype 2 purified enzymes. Although the active site of NS3 protease is fairly well conserved across genotypes, there are a small number of residues that differ in genotype 2 or 3 relative to genotype 1 (Fig. 1a). A mutagenesis study supported the idea that differences in inhibitor binding are due primarily to these active-site residues rather than other amino acid differences more remote from the bound inhibitor [29].

Several groups have reported in vitro resistance studies for BILN 2061 in the genotype 1b replicon. Substitutions at NS3 residues Arg155 (to glutamine), Ala156 (to threonine

TABLE 2 In Vitro Pharmacodynamics of BILN 2061

Assay	Result (nM)
GT 1a K_i	1.5
GT 1b K_i	1.6
GT 2ac K_i	86
GT 2b K_i	83
GT 3a K_i	90
Elastase IC_{50}	>30,000
Cathepsin B IC_{50}	>30,000
GT 1a replicon EC_{50}	4
GT 1b replicon EC_{50}	3
GT 2a JFH1 replicon EC_{50}	67
GT 2a JFH1 virus EC_{50}	120
Huh-7 CC_{50} (MTT)	33,000

Source: K_i values are from [29], JFH1 EC_{50} values are from [31], and other values are from [30].

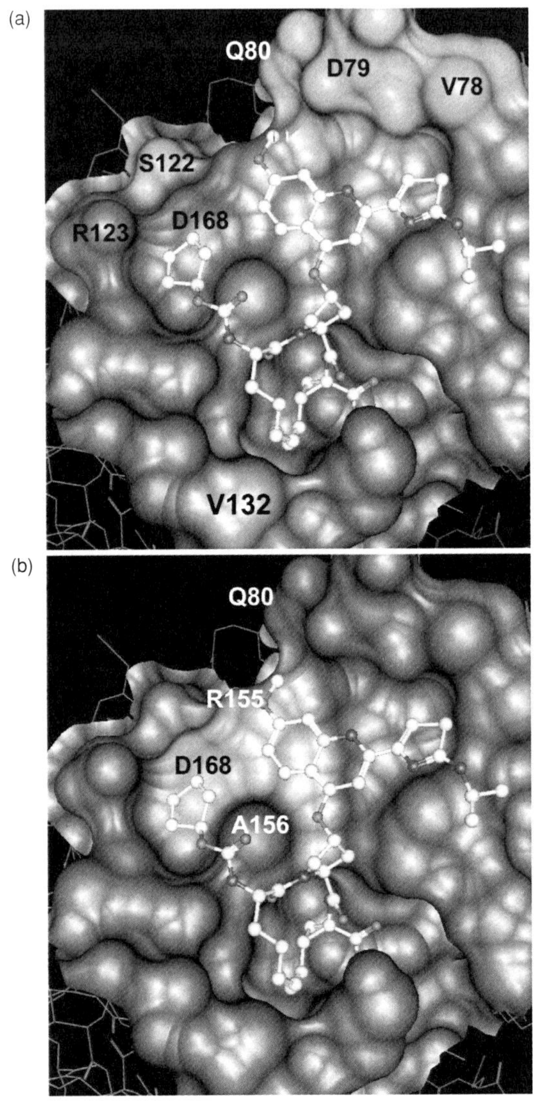

FIGURE 1 BILN 2061 modeled into an NS3-NS4A active site, with surface shown for residues within 5 Å of the inhibitor. (a) Amino acids that differ from genotype 1 are highlighted. Amino acids that differ in genotype 2 are shown in green; those that differ in genotype 3 are shown in magenta; amino acid 132, that varies between subtypes, is shown in brown. (b) Amino acids that are substituted as a result of resistance mutations are highlighted. (*See insert for color representation of the figure.*)

or valine), and Asp168 (to valine or alanine) were identified consistently. Shifts in EC_{50} ranged from 20- to 40-fold for R155Q to several hundredfold for D168V. Shifts of similar magnitude were observed in biochemical assays using purified NS3 proteins encoding these substitutions. Replicon studies also identified substitutions of Asp168 to glycine or Asn80 for arginine, but these caused a smaller shift in EC_{50}. All of these substitutions are located near the inhibitor binding site (Fig. 1b), and the changes observed can thus be rationalized by a combination of steric and local conformational effects [32–34]. As described below, the clinical significance for BILN 2061 of any of these substitutions remains unknown.

Little, if any, off-target activity was found for BILN 2061. We have previously shown that unlike compounds with electrophilic "warheads," C-terminal carboxylic acid inhibitors do not have significant activity against serine or cysteine proteases [7]. BILN 2061 was inactive against human leukocyte elastase, a serine protease with similar P3-P1 substrate residues selectivity and also against the cysteine protease cathepsin B (Table 2). BILN 2061 had little if any activity ($IC_{50} \geq 10$ μM) against a panel of proteases, other enzymes, and receptors [30]. A window of approximately 10,000-fold was observed between genotype 1 replicon activity and cytotoxicity (Table 2) [30].

The in vitro ADME profile of BILN 2061 was acceptable, with low rates of metabolism observed for hepatic microsomes from multiple species, including human. IC_{50} values against a panel of human cytochrome P450 enzymes were all greater thant 7 μM. It also had no significant activity at up to 10 μM in the isolated guinea pig papillary muscle assay and was negative in a battery of genotoxicity assays [30].

PRECLINICAL IN VIVO STUDIES WITH BILN 2061

Rat, dog, and rhesus monkey pharmacokinetics have been described [30] and key parameters are summarized in Table 3. Oral bioavailability was low to moderate, and consistent with in vitro results, clearance was low relative to hepatic blood flow in all three species. Liver concentrations in rats ranged from five- to 39-fold greater than plasma concentrations at different time points [30]. In mouse and rat general pharmacology assays, BILN 2061 had no physiologically relevant central nervous system, cardiovascular, pulmonary, renal, or gastrointestinal effects at doses from 10 to 300 mg/kg, which provided exposures which substantially exceeded the in vitro EC_{50} for the compound (25- to 6700-fold). Single- and repeat-dose toxicology studies also supported the initiation of clinical trials [30].

CLINICAL EVALUATION OF BILN 2061 (CILUPREVIR)

During clinical trials BILN 2061 received the generic name ciluprevir, however, we have continued to refer to it as BILN 2061 because this is how it is known most widely. BILN 2061 was first given to humans in a single rising dose trial to establish a safe and suitable dose range and dosing frequency for patients. Thirteen dose levels, ranging from 5 to 2400 mg, were administered as a solution in PEG-400 and ethanol [35]. Doses up to 2000 mg were well tolerated, but gastrointestinal adverse events were common at the 2400-mg dose. There were no significant laboratory findings at any dose. In general, C_{max} was observed at 2 to 4 h, followed by a biphasic decline yielding an elimination half-life of approximately 4 h. At the 200-mg dose the C_{max} was 1 μM and the $C_{12\,h}$ was 42 nM, 10- to 14-fold the genotype 1 replicon EC_{50} values. In the absence, at that time, of any data on the effectiveness of specific HCV antivirals, this dose was selected as the middle dose for administration to HCV patients. It was known that standard dosing of pegIFN/RBV yields a plasma concentration with a similar fold over the replicon EC_{50} value [36].

BILN 2061 was given to six different cohorts of HCV patients in four separate trials. All groups received four doses of BILN 2061 every 12 h for 2 days. The goal of these trials was to evaluate, for the first time in humans, the short-term effect of a specific HCV antiviral. The prospective criterion for success in all of these trials was to achieve an average 10-fold decline in HCV viral load after 2 days of treatment, significantly better than the average observed for patients who respond to standard pegIFN/RBV therapy [37].

TABLE 3 Selected Pharmacokinetic Parameters for BILN 2061[a]

	Oral Dosing (5 mg/kg)			Intravenous Dosing (2 mg/kg)		
Species (Sex: M/F)	C_{max} (ng/mL)	$AUC_{0\text{-}8}$ (ng·h/mL)	F (%)	Cl (mL·min/kg)	V_{ss} (L/kg)	$t_{1/2}$ (h)
Rat (M)	250	800	13	14.3	1.04	0.8
Rhesus (M)	300	900	7	5.5	0.45	7.0
Dog (M)	2,100	13,000	38	2.3	0.33	2.2
Dog (F)	4,000	24,300	32	1.1	0.24	4.7

[a]For experimental details, see [30].

TABLE 4 Summary of BILN 2061 Clinical Trial Data by Group

GT Dose Histology	1a/b 25 0-2	1a/b 200 0-2	1a/b 200 3-4	1a/b 200 5-6	1a/b 500 0-2	1a/b Placebo 0-6	2/3 500 0-2	2/3 Placebo 0-2
No. in group	9	8	8	8	8	10	8	2
No. TN/TE[a]	4/5	4/4	4/4	0/8	4/4	4/6	7/1	2/0
Maximum viral load reduction (no./group)[b]								
1 log copies/mL	9	8	8	8	8	0	4	0
2 log copies/mL	7	8	8	8	8	0	3	0
3 log copies/mL	3	3	4	6	7	0	0	0
Blocking efficiency (e)	98.88	99.91	99.89	99.78	99.92	N.D.[c]	N.D.	N.D.

[a]Number treatment-naive patients vs. treatment-experienced patients.
[b]Data from bDNA assay.
[c]N.D., not determined.

Distinguishing characteristics of the trial patients are given in Table 4. Five of the cohorts were patients infected with genotype 1. All these groups contained a mix of genotypes 1a and 1b as well as treatment-naive and treatment-experienced persons. Of these five groups, three had minimal liver fibrosis (Ishak 0-2), one had advanced fibrosis (Ishak 3-4), and one had compensated cirrhosis (Ishak 5-6) [36]. The sixth cohort studied was a mix of genotype 2- and 3-infected, treatment-naive or treatment-experienced patients with minimal liver fibrosis [38]. It is noteworthy that although only 49 HCV patients received BILN 2061 in these trials (12 of 61 patients in the trials received placebo), comparisons of antiviral effects were made for multiple doses and also for many of the important characteristics of the infection, such as genotype, patient prior-treatment status, and disease stage.

The effect of BILN 2061 dose was studied in three cohorts of genotype 1 patients with minimal fibrosis who were given four doses of 25, 200, or 500 mg [36]. The 200-mg dose was selected as described above. The 500-mg dose was judged to be the maximum well-tolerated dose (for administration over 2 days) based on the single-dose healthy volunteer study. The 25-mg dose level was chosen as one likely to have a minimal effect. No serious adverse events were observed, and no other safety concerns were raised by clinical observations or laboratory tests. The changes observed in viral load are shown in Figure 2a for the 200-mg group, and the number of patients in each group achieving 1, 2, or 3 log drops in viral load is shown in Table 3. Results exceeded expectations. The majority achieved a greater than 3 log decrease, and all but two in the 25-mg group achieved a greater than 2 log decrease. It is important to note that significant improvements have been made in the sensitivity of HCV viral load measurements since these trials were carried out in 2001. The Cobas Amplicor assay used for Figure 2a has a lower limit of quantification of 600 IU/mL (approximately 1500 copies/mL) and an upper limit of 500,000 IU/mL (2,125,000 copies/mL) [36]. The bDNA assay used for data in Table 4 and Figure 2a has a lower limit of quantification of 615 IU/mL and a much higher upper limit [38]. Current assays have no upper limit of quantification and a lower limit of quantification of 25 IU/mL (see below). Since for several patients at the 200- and 500-mg dose levels, viral loads went below the limit of quantification, viral load drops of greater than 3 logs would probably have been measured with current assays. A more sensitive but qualitative assay was used for all samples below the limit of quantification, and viral loads remained above the 10-IU/mL limit of detection for this assay in all samples obtained during this short trial [36].

For the 200- and 500-mg dose groups, plasma levels of BILN 2061 increased between the first and second days with $C_{\max}$ and $AUC_{0\text{-}8h}$ both roughly twofold higher at 200 mg and fourfold higher at 500 mg [36]. The day 1 $C_{\max}$ and AUC observed at 200 mg were also nearly double the values observed in the healthy volunteer single-dose trial. This increase in exposure for HCV patients has been reported for other HCV drugs in clinical trials, and may be a general phenomenon for patients with liver disease, although the cause of increased exposure has not yet been identified. No significant difference in the viral load decrease was observed in these two dose groups, perhaps because available assays could not quantify the largest changes in viral load rather than because of a true saturation of the drug effect. The antiviral effect of the 25-mg dose was clearly lower, although still more significant than expected a priori. For this dose, no observations were outside the range of quantification, and a PK–PD relationship was observed: The three patients who achieved greater than 3 log reductions in viral load had the highest plasma levels of BILN 2061.

Modeling of viral kinetics under treatment with BILN 2061 showed that doses of 500, 200, and 25 mg BILN 2061 had values of e (efficiency in blocking viral production) of 99.92, 99.91, and 98.9% (Table 4) [39]. For the 25-mg group, e values for different patients ranged from 90 to 99.9% and

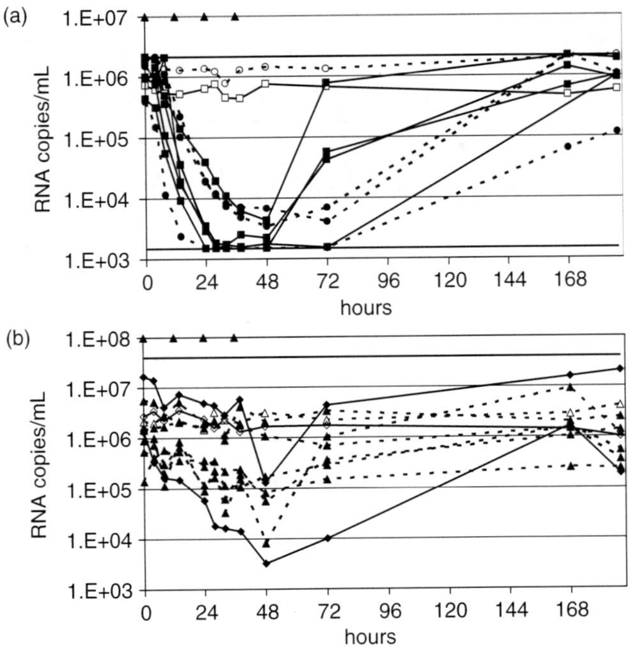

FIGURE 2 Antiviral effect of BILN 2061. (a) 200 mg given for 2 days to genotype 1 patients with no or minimal fibrosis. Viral loads were measured using the Cobas Amplicor assay and are expressed as RNA copies/mL. Upper and lower limits of quantification are indicated by straight lines. Data for treatment-naive patients are shown with circles and dashed lines. Data for treatment-experienced patients are shown with squares and solid lines. Data for two placebo patients are shown with open circles or squares, respectively. The four dosing time points are indicated by triangles. The last time point is graphed at approximately 190 h for ease of viewing, but samples were taken several days later. (b) 500 mg given for 2 days to genotype 2 and 3 patients. Viral loads were measured using the bDNA assay and are expressed as RNA copies/mL. The upper limit of quantification is indicated by a straight line. Data for genotype 2 patients are shown with diamonds and solid lines. Data for treatment genotype 3 patients are shown with triangles and dashed lines. Data for one genotype 2 patient and one genotype 3 patients who received placebo are shown as open diamonds and triangles, respectively. The four dosing time points are indicated by triangles at the top of the graph. The last time point is graphed at approximately 190 h for ease of viewing, but samples were taken several days later.

could be correlated with BILN 2061 exposure, whereas the very high values of *e*, experimental variation, and limits of the viral load assay prevented demonstration of any such relationship for the two higher doses. These *e* values can be compared to a value of 98% for 3 μg/kg peg-IFN-α2b (double the normal dose), demonstrating the superior antiviral efficacy of specific inhibitors of HCV protein function. Whether interferon has other effects (e.g., in removal of HCV-infected cells) which will be essential for curing patients remains to be demonstrated. It is clear from a number of recently disclosed trials that resistance to HCV-directed antivirals emerges rapidly, and the emergence of resistance is well controlled by pegIFN/RBV. No study of resistance mutations was carried out for these short trials, but based on the in vitro results described above, it is certain that resistance would have emerged in longer trials.

The two cohorts with advanced fibrosis and compensated cirrhosis received four 200-mg doses of BILN 2061. Despite having more advanced disease, viral load decreases for both groups were very similar to those for patients with minimal liver disease. Viral kinetic analysis detected a statistically significant but small decrease in *e* values for the cirrhosis group, 99.78 vs. 99.91. Plasma levels of BILN 2061 were higher in both of these groups than for patients with minimal disease, on both day 1 and day 2. Day 2 AUC values were 32 and 48%, and day 2 $C_{\max}$ values were 23 and 19% higher in the advanced fibrosis and cirrhosis groups, respectively, compared to patients with minimal liver damage [36].

HCV genotype 2 and 3 patients were evaluated in the final BILN 2061 trial [38]. Two and six patients with these respective genotypes received 500-mg doses of BILN 2061 (Table 4). Viral load decreases in this group (Table 4 and Fig. 2b) were notably smaller and more variable than for the genotype 1 cohorts, although there was no significant difference between genotype 2 and 3 patients. Although average plasma levels of BILN 2061 were very comparable to the genotype 1 patients who received 500 mg-doses, pharmacokinetic parameters were more variable in this group than in any of the genotype 1 groups, with CVs of 100% or more for most parameters, compared to approximately 50% for the other groups. Similar to what was observed for genotype 1 patients who received 25-mg doses, viral loads were quantifiable at all time points, and a correlation between BILN 2061 AUC and viral load change was observed. The two patients with the highest drug levels experienced the greatest decrease in viral load, and three patients with the lowest response had no significant response. NS3-NS4A enzymes were cloned from selected patients in this study, and differences in response could not be attributed to differences in in vitro potency of BILN 2061 against genotype 2 or 3 sequence variants [29,38]. However, as reported above, activity against genotype 2 and 3 NS3 was approximately 50-fold less than against genotype 1 NS3. BILN 2061 AUC (geometric mean) for the genotype 2 and 3 group was only ninefold higher than for the 25 mg-dose genotype 1 group on day 1 and only 21-fold higher on day 2. Thus, relative to drug potency, genotype 2 and 3 patients achieved a lower drug exposure than did genotype 1 patients in the 25-mg cohort. All of these results confirm the general idea on which development of BILN 2061 was based: that efficacy in patients could be predicted by in vitro potency and human pharmacokinetics. The moderate efficacy of BILN 2061 against genotypes 2 or 3 might still provide a useful boost in response to standard-of-care treatment with pegIFN/RBV.

CARDIOTOXICITY OF BILN 2061 IN RHESUS MONKEYS

A 4-week BILN 2061 toxicology study was performed in rhesus monkeys in preparation for longer-duration clinical trials. At the end of this study, one animal that had received 1000 mg/kg per day died suddenly of congestive heart failure. This animal and three other animals from the same group were found to have myocardial vacuolation by light microscopy. As a result, clinical development was put on hold. Follow-up studies on the patients and healthy volunteers who received BILN 2061 revealed no evidence of drug-induced cardiac abnormalities [40]. It is important to note that doses to monkeys which resulted in cardiotoxicity far exceeded those administered to humans.

Additional 4-week monkey studies were carried out to better understand the frequency and nature of this toxicity. In general, there were no significant in-life observations during these studies, and electrocardiograms remained normal. However, multiple animals in 500- or 1000-mg/kg per day groups were found to have myocardial vacuolation by light microscopy, ranging from minimal to severe. Further analysis by electron microscopy revealed that the vacuoles were swollen mitochondria. Vacuolation was rare and focal in minimal cases but severe and diffusely distributed in more severe cases. Even in severe cases, normal mitochondria could be found adjacent to swollen mitochondria in the same cell. Myocardial degeneration and necrosis were rarely observed, and inflammatory cell infiltration and evidence of fibrosis were generally absent [40].

A time-course study was carried out in which monkeys administered 1000 mg/kg per day BILN 2061 were necropsied after 1, 3, 14, or 28 days of drug exposure, or after a 10-week recovery period [40]. No cardiac abnormalities were observed in the day 1 necropsy, but focal vacuolation was observed in two and one animals at the day 3 and day 14 time points, respectively. At day 28, vacuolation was observed in five of six animals, ranging from minimal to severe. Consistent with the lack of cardiomyocyte necrosis, levels of cardiac troponin I and T remained in the normal range for all animals throughout the study. Six animals were necropsied after a 10-week recovery period, and their hearts were normal by both light and electron microscopy. Staining for evidence of lipofuscin, fibrosis, or calcification was also negative. In this study, heart function was monitored by electrocardiogram and echocardiogram at baseline and throughout the study. Electrocardiograms remained normal. Echocardiograms remained normal throughout the dosing period, except on day 28, when two of 12 animals were found to have a decreased ejection fraction. One animal was necropsied and was found to be the one in this group with severe vacuolation. The other was kept in the recovery group. At the end of the 10-week recovery period, its ejection fraction had returned to the normal range, and as mentioned above, light and electron microscopic evaluations suggested a complete recovery.

The cardiotoxicity induced by BILN 2061 appears to be unique in the literature, both in its progression and in the nature of the lesions observed. Neither blood tests nor functional measurements revealed any early-stage evidence of cardiotoxicity. Based on observations for two animals in the time-course study, it appeared to be reversible even when reaching a severe level that could be detected by echocardiography. However, as described for the first 4-week study, in rare cases animals with severe lesions were at risk of congestive heart failure [40]. Thus no biomarker for cardiotoxicity was identified which would provide the necessary assurance that trials of this drug could proceed safely. Further clinical evaluation of BILN 2061 was terminated, and Boehringer Ingelheim focused on identifying follow-up compounds devoid of cardiotoxicity.

BI 201335: PROOF-OF-PRINCIPLE CLINICAL TRIALS

Boehringer Ingelheim established a policy of performing thorough toxicological examination of all potential protease inhibitor candidates in several species, including rhesus monkeys, prior to the initiation of human trials. BI 201335 is a novel NS3-NS4A protease inhibitor with EC_{50} values of 6.5 and 3.1 nM against genotype 1a and 1b replicons, respectively. It underwent thorough toxicological examination prior to human trials. High exposures were achieved in monkey studies of up to 26 weeks' duration, and no signs of cardiotoxicity were observed at any dose. The structure and detailed preclinical profile for this compound were not disclosed at the time of writing, but a proof-of-principle trial in HCV patients was recently described [41]. In initial trials in healthy volunteers, BI 201335 demonstrated a steady-state half-life of 22 to 31 h (depending on dose), showing that significant drug levels could be maintained with once-daily (q.d.) dosing. In the first trial in patients, BI 201335 was administered for 4 weeks to subjects infected with genotype 1 virus, subtype 1a or 1b (approximately equal numbers per dose group). Four groups of treatment-naive patients received the compound for 2 weeks as monotherapy (doses for treatment-naive patients were 20, 48, 120, and 240 mg). This initial monotherapy treatment was selected to study the antiviral effect and the selection of resistance mutations under treatment pressure with BI 201335.

Monotherapy was followed by 2 weeks of combination therapy with standard doses of pegIFN/RBV. The 2-week period of triple combination following monotherapy was designed primarily to ensure the continuous presence of antiviral pressure during the BI 201335 washout period. There were two patients on placebo at each dose level. All treatment-experienced patients received active drug for 4 weeks in

TABLE 5 Summary of BI 201335 Clinical Trial Data by Group

Dose (mg, q.d.) Prior treatment	Placebo No	20 No	48 No	120 No	240 No	48 Yes	120 Yes	240 Yes
No. in group	8	6	7	7	6	6	7	6
Median maximum change in viral load ($\log_{10}$ IU/mL)[a]	−0.04	−2.9	−3.5	−3.7	−4.0	−5.0	−5.2	−5.3
No. achieving viral load < LLQ at day 28	0	1	2	2	3	3	4	5

[a]Viral loads were measured with the COBAS Taqman assay (Roche); lower limit of quantitation (LLQ) = 25 IU/mL.

combination with pegIFN/RBV; none were given BI 201335 monotherapy or placebo. They were treated with the three higher dose levels of 48, 120, or 240 mg. In both groups, at the end of BI 201335 dosing, patients continued on pegIFN/RBV for 44 additional weeks at the discretion of the investigator.

Significant decreases in viral load were observed in this trial (Table 5 and Fig. 3). Except for one person in the 20-mg group encoding an NS3 polymorphism at baseline (see below), all patients had a maximum viral load decrease of greater than 2 $\log_{10}$ IU/mL, which was the primary endpoint for the trial. In fact, at doses of 48 mg q.d. or higher, virtually all treatment-naive patients achieved a greater than 3 $\log_{10}$ reduction in viral load within 3 days of initiating monotherapy with BI 201335. This initial viral load decrease was qualitatively similar to what had previously been observed for BILN 2061, although recorded values are somewhat larger in part because of the more sensitive viral load assays now available.

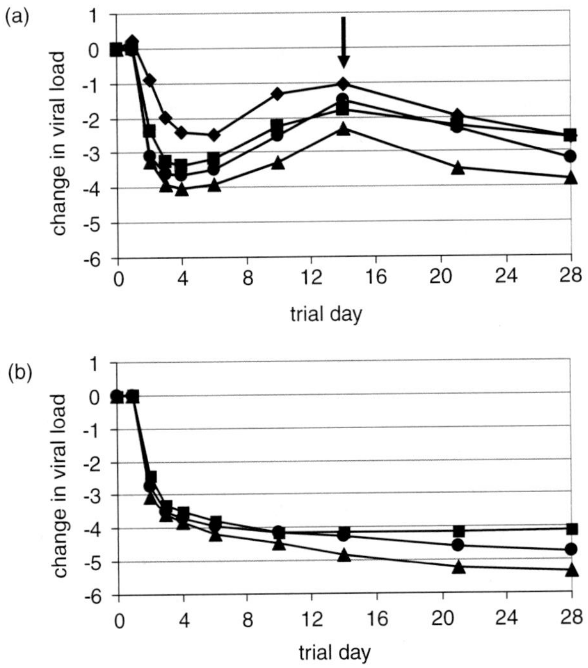

FIGURE 3 Antiviral effect of BI 201335. (a) Group mean data for treatment-naive genotype 1 patients given 20-mg (diamonds), 48-mg (squares), 120 mg (circles), or 240-mg (triangles) doses of BI 201335 once daily. The arrow indicates the point at which administration of pegIFN/RBV was initiated. (b) Group mean data for treatment-experienced genotype 1 patients given 48, 120, or 240 mg once daily in combination with pegIFN/RBV. The symbols are the same as in part (a). In both graphs data shown are mean changes (IU/mL) from baseline at each time point.

For patients on monotherapy, however, after reaching a minimum between days 2 and 4, viral load rebound was observed in most cases, and amino acid substitutions characteristic of resistance were observed. The predominant amino acid substitution depended on HCV genotype, with R155K being observed most frequently for genotype 1a and D168V for genotype 1b. Previous in vitro studies have suggested that R155K virus is more fit than D168V. The predominance of D168V rather than R155K on breakthrough for genotype 1b patients can be explained by the fact that for genotype 1b the R155K substitution requires a two-base mutation, whereas only a single-base mutation is needed for D168V. Population sequencing at baseline had revealed no amino acid substitutions expected to cause a shift in BI 201335 potency, except for the one patient in the 20-mg dose group who experienced a suboptimal response. Genotype 1b virus from this patient encoded a V170T substitution in NS3. This is a rare polymorphism, but an alanine substitution at this position is known to reduce the potency of other protease inhibitors [42]. An eightfold increase in BI 201335 EC_{50} relative to the subtype reference was measured for the V170T substitution.

The in vitro activity of BI 201335 against the proteases encoded by patient sequences was evaluated using chimeric replicons containing the patient NS3 protease sequence in the context of Con1 genotype 1b. Group average EC_{50} values at baseline for subtypes 1a and 1b were 10 ± 8 nM and 9 ± 4 nM, respectively. Both of the major resistance mutations caused significant shifts in EC_{50}; R155K EC_{50} values ranged from 1.8 to 6.5 μM and D168V EC_{50} values from 3.6 to 15 μM.

Results in treatment-experienced patients who received 4 weeks of triple combination therapy clearly demonstrated that the combination of BI 201335 with pegIFN/RBV is highly effective in reducing viral loads and suppressing the emergence of resistance. Virologic breakthrough was observed for only three of these 19 patients, two of whom were in the lowest-dose group of 48 mg, one in the 120-mg group. The resistance substitutions that were observed were the same as those described above for treatment-naive patients. In this small trial, treatment-experienced patients were not stratified further by degree of prior response, but in the 120-mg group four of seven patients were null responders in prior treatment ($< 0.5\ \log_{10}$ decrease in viral load), and three of these four had viral load below the limit of quantification at day 28. In the 240-mg group, five of six patients had unquantifiable viral loads at day 28, and no patient had a breakthrough.

No dose-dependent adverse events were observed, and only one serious adverse event (asthenia), which occurred in the 20-mg dose group. Most adverse events were minor and were not attributed by investigators to BI 201335. Dose-dependent increases in indirect (unconjugated) bilirubin were observed. In both the treatment-naive and treatment-experienced groups the increase in total bilirubin was significant only at the 240-mg dose level (at most two- to three-fold of the upper limit of normal), and reversed shortly after treatment with BI 201335 was completed. Dose-dependent increases in unconjugated bilirubin had been observed previously in trials in healthy volunteers and in monkey toxicology studies. This bilirubin increase was not associated with hemolysis or with elevations in liver enzymes or any other sign of liver toxicity. Hyperbilirubinemia may be explained by BI 201335 inhibiting of one or more steps of bilirubin elimination. During the 28-day trial in patients, significant decreases in aspartate and alanine aminotransferase liver enzymes were also measured (at day 14 for treatment-naive and day 28 for treatment-experienced patients), potentially indicative of improved liver function in these subjects.

After these strong preliminary results in short-term trials, BI 201335 is now being tested in larger phase II trials for both treatment-naive and treatment-experienced patients to evaluate the potential of this inhibitor to improve cure rates in hepatitis C genotype 1 infection when used in combination with pegIFN/RBV, or in the future with other direct-acting antivirals.

REFERENCES

[1] Choo, Q. L.; Kuo, G.; Weiner, A. J.; Overby, L. R.; Bradley, D. W.; Houghton, M. Isolation of a cDNA clone derived from a blood-borne non-A, non-B viral hepatitis genome. *Science* **1989**, *244*, 359–362.

[2] Gallinari, P.; Brennan, D.; Nardi, C.; Brunetti, M.; Tomei, L.; Steinkuhler, C.; De Francesco, R. Multiple enzymatic activities associated with recombinant NS3 protein of hepatitis C virus. *J. Virol.* **1998**, *72*, 6758–6769.

[3] Lohmann, V.; Korner, F.; Koch, J.; Herian, U.; Theilmann, L.; Bartenschlager, R. Replication of subgenomic hepatitis C virus RNAs in a hepatoma cell line. *Science* **1999**, *285*, 110–113.

[4] Kolykhalov, A. A.; Mihalik, K.; Feinstone, S. M.; Rice, C. M. Hepatitis C virus-encoded enzymatic activities and conserved RNA elements in the 3 nontranslated region are essential for virus replication in vivo. *J. Virol.* **2000**, *74*, 2046–2051.

[5] Llinas-Brunet, M.; Bailey, M.; Fazal, G.; Goulet, S.; Halmos, T.; Laplante, S.; Maurice, R.; Poirier, M.; Poupart, M. A.; Thibeault, D.; et al. Peptide-based inhibitors of the hepatitis C virus serine protease. *Bioorg. Med. Chem. Lett.* **1998**, *8*, 1713–1718.

[6] Steinkuhler, C.; Biasiol, G.; Brunetti, M.; Urbani, A.; Koch, U.; Cortese, R.; Pessi, A.; De Francesco, R. Product inhibition of the hepatitis C virus NS3 protease. *Biochemistry* **1998**, *37*, 8899–8905.

[7] Llinas-Brunet, M.; Bailey, M.; Deziel, R.; Fazal, G.; Gorys, V.; Goulet, S.; Halmos, T.; Maurice, R.; Poirier, M.; Poupart, M. A.; et al. Studies on the C-terminal of hexapeptide inhibitors of the hepatitis C virus serine protease. *Bioorg. Med. Chem. Lett.* **1998**, *8*, 2719–2724.

[8] Rancourt, J.; Cameron, D. R.; Gorys, V.; Lamarre, D.; Poirier, M.; Thibeault, D.; Llinas-Brunet, M. Peptide-based inhibitors of the hepatitis C virus NS3 protease: structure–activity relationship at the C-terminal position. *J. Med. Chem.* **2004**, *47*, 2511–2522.

[9] Goudreau, N.; Cameron, D. R.; Bonneau, P.; Gorys, V.; Plouffe, C.; Poirier, M.; Lamarre, D.; Llinas-Brunet, M. NMR structural characterization of peptide inhibitors bound to the hepatitis C virus NS3 protease: design of a new P2 substituent. *J. Med. Chem.* **2004**, *47*, 123–132.

[10] Llinas-Brunet, M.; Bailey, M.; Fazal, G.; Ghiro, E.; Gorys, V.; Goulet, S.; Halmos, T.; Maurice, R.; Poirier, M.; Poupart, M. A.; et al. Highly potent and selective peptide-based inhibitors of the hepatitis C virus serine protease: towards smaller inhibitors. *Bioorg. Med. Chem. Lett.* **2000**, *10*, 2267–2270.

[11] Pause, A.; Kukolj, G.; Bailey, M.; Brault, M.; Do, F.; Halmos, T.; Lagace, L.; Maurice, R.; Marquis, M.; McKercher, G.; et al. An NS3 serine protease inhibitor abrogates replication of subgenomic hepatitis C virus RNA. *J. Biol. Chem.* **2003**, *278*, 20374–20380.

[12] Llinas-Brunet, M.; Bailey, M. D.; Ghiro, E.; Gorys, V.; Halmos, T.; Poirier, M.; Rancourt, J.; Goudreau, N. A systematic approach to the optimization of substrate-based inhibitors of the hepatitis C virus NS3 protease: discovery of potent and specific tripeptide inhibitors. *J. Med. Chem.* **2004**, *47*, 6584–6594.

[13] LaPlante, S. R.; Cameron, D. R.; Aubry, N.; Lefebvre, S.; Kukolj, G.; Maurice, R.; Thibeault, D.; Lamarre, D.; Llinas-Brunet, M. Solution structure of substrate-based ligands when bound to hepatitis C virus NS3 protease domain. *J. Biol. Chem.* **1999**, *274*, 18618–18624.

[14] LaPlante, S. R.; Aubry, N.; Bonneau, P. R.; Kukolj, G.; Lamarre, D.; Lefebvre, S. Li, H.; Llinas-Brunet, M.; Plouffe, C.; Cameron, D. R. NMR line-broadening and transferred NOESY as a medicinal chemistry tool for studying inhibitors

of the hepatitis C virus NS3 protease domain. *Bioorg. Med. Chem. Lett.* **2000**, *10*, 2271–2274.

[15] Goudreau, N.; Brochu, C.; Cameron, D. R.; Duceppe, J. S.; Faucher, A. M.; Ferland, J. M.; Grand-Maitre, C.; Poirier, M.; Simoneau, B.; Tsantrizos, Y. S. Potent inhibitors of the hepatitis C virus NS3 protease: design and synthesis of macrocyclic substrate-based beta-strand mimics. *J. Org. Chem.* **2004**, *69*, 6185–6201.

[16] Tsantrizos, Y. S.; Bolger, G.; Bonneau, P.; Cameron, D. R.; Goudreau, N.; Kukolj, G.; LaPlante, S. R.; Llinas-Brunet, M.; Nar, H.; Lamarre, D. Macrocyclic inhibitors of the NS3 protease as potential therapeutic agents of hepatitis C virus infection. *Angew. Chem. Int. Ed. Engl.* **2003**, *42*, 1356–1360.

[17] Yao, N.; Reichert, P.; Taremi, S. S.; Prosise, W. W.; Weber, P. C. Molecular views of viral polyprotein processing revealed by the crystal structure of the hepatitis C virus bifunctional protease-helicase. *Structure* **1999**, *7*, 1353–1363.

[18] Llinas-Brunet, M. Bailey, M. D.; Bolger, G.; Brochu, C.; Faucher, A. M.; Ferland, J. M.; Garneau, M.; Ghiro, E.; Gorys, V.; Grand-Maitre, C.; et al. Structure–activity study on a novel series of macrocyclic inhibitors of the hepatitis C virus NS3 protease leading to the discovery of BILN 2061. *J. Med. Chem.* **2004**, *47*, 1605–1608.

[19] Greene, T. W.; Wuts, P. G. M. *Protective Groups in Organic Synthesis*. Wiley, New York, **1999**, 518.

[20] Grubbs, R. H. Olefin-metathesis catalysts for the preparation of molecules and materials (Nobel lecture). *Angew. Chem. Int.* **2006**, *45*, 3760–3765.

[21] Faucher, A. M.; Bailey, M. D.; Beaulieu, P. L.; Brochu, C.; Duceppe, J. S.; Ferland, J. M.; Ghiro, E.; Gorys, V.; Halmos, T.; Kawai, S. H.; et al. Synthesis of BILN 2061, an HCV NS3 protease inhibitor with proven antiviral effect in humans. *Org. Lett.* **2004**, *6*, 2901–2904.

[22] Nicola, T.; Brenner, M.; Donsbach, K.; Kreye, P. First scale-up to production scale of a ring closing metathesis reaction forming a 15-membered macrocycle as a precursor of an active pharmaceutical ingredient. *Org. Process Res. Dev.* **2005**, *9*, 513–515.

[23] Yee, N. K.; Farina, V.; Houpis, I. N.; Haddad, N.; Frutos, R. P.; Gallou, F.; Wang, X. J.; Wei, X.; Simpson, R. D.; Feng, X.; et al. Efficient large-scale synthesis of BILN 2061, a potent HCV protease inhibitor, by a convergent approach based on ring-closing metathesis. *J. Org. Chem.* **2006**, *71*, 7133–7145.

[24] Frutos, R. P.; Haddad, N.; Houpis, I. N.; Johnson, M.; Smith-Keenan, L. L.; Fuchs, V.; Yee, N. K.; Farina, V.; Faucher, A. M.; Brochu, C.; et al. Practical synthesis of 2-(2-isopropylaminothiazol-4-yl)-7-methoxy-1*H*-quinolin-4-one: key intermediate for the synthesis of potent HCV NS3 protease inhibitor BILN 2061. *Synthesis* **2006**, *2009*, 2563–2567.

[25] Wang, X. J.; Zhang, L.; Smith-Keenan, L. L.; Houpis, I. N.; Farina, V. Efficient synthesis of (*S*)-2-(cyclopentyloxycarbonyl)-amino-8-nonenoic acid: key building block for BILN 2061, an HCV NS3 protease inhibitor. *Org. Process Res. Dev.* **2007**, *11*, 60–63.

[26] Beaulieu, P. L.; Gillard, J.; Bailey, M. D.; Boucher, C.; Duceppe, J. S.; Simoneau, B.; Wang, X. J.; Zhang, L.; Grozinger, K.; Houpis, I.; et al. Synthesis of (1*R*,2*S*)-1-amino-2-vinylcyclopropanecarboxylic acid vinyl-ACCA) derivatives: key intermediates for the preparation of inhibitors of the hepatitis C virus NS3 protease. *J. Org. Chem.* **2005**, *70*, 5869–5879.

[27] Poirier, M.; Aubry, N.; Boucher, C.; Ferland, J. M.; Laplante, S.; Tsantrizos, Y. S. RCM of tripeptide dienes containing a chiral vinylcyclopropane moiety: impact of different Ru-based catalysts on the stereochemical integrity of the macrocyclic products. *J. Org. Chem.* **2005**, *70*, 10765–10773.

[28] Shu, C.; Zeng, X.; Hao, M. H.; Wei, X.; Yee, N. K.; Busacca, C. A.; Han, Z.; Farina, V.; Senanayake, C. H. RCM macrocyclization made practical: an efficient synthesis of HCV protease inhibitor BILN 2061. *Org. Lett.* **2008**, *10*, 1303–1306.

[29] Thibeault, D. Bousquet, C.; Gingras, R.; Lagace, L.; Maurice, R.; White, P. W.; Lamarre, D. Sensitivity of NS3 serine proteases from hepatitis C virus genotypes 2 and 3 to the inhibitor BILN 2061. *J. Virol.* **2004**, *78*, 7352–7359.

[30] Lamarre, D.; Anderson, P. C.; Bailey, M.; Beaulieu, P.; Bolger, G.; Bonneau, P.; Bos, M.; Cameron, D. R.; Cartier, M.; Cordingley, M. G.; et al. An NS3 protease inhibitor with antiviral effects in humans infected with hepatitis C virus. *Nature* **2003**, *426*, 186–189.

[31] Paulson, M. S.; Yang, H.; Shih, I. H.; Feng, J. Y.; Mabery, E. M.; Robinson, M. F.; Zhong, W.; Delaney, W. E. Comparison of HCV NS3 protease and NS5B polymerase inhibitor activity in 1a, 1b and 2a replicons and 2a infectious virus. *Antiviral Res.* **2009**, *83*, 135–142.

[32] Lagace, L.; Marquis, M.; Bousquet, C.; Do, F.; Gingras, R.; Lamarre, D.; Lamarre, L.; Maurice, R.; Pause, A.; Pellerin, C.; et al. BILN 2061 and beyond: pre-clinical evaluation of HCV subgenomic replicon resistance to a NS3 protease inhibitor. In *Framing the Knowledge of Viral Hepatitis*, Schinazi, R. F., Schiff, E. R., Eds., IHL Press, College Park, GA, **2006**, pp. 263–278.

[33] Lu, L.; Pilot-Matias, T. J.; Stewart, K. D.; Randolph, J. T.; Pithawalla, R.; He, W.; Huang, P. P.; Klein, L. L.; Mo, H.; Molla, A. Mutations conferring resistance to a potent hepatitis C virus serine protease inhibitor in vitro. *Antimicrob. Agents Chemother.* **2004**, *48*, 2260–2266.

[34] Lin, C. Lin, K.; Luong, Y. P.; Rao, B. G.; Wei, Y. Y.; Brennan, D. L.; Fulghum, J. R.; Hsiao, H. M.; Ma, S.; Maxwell, J. P.; et al. In vitro resistance studies of hepatitis C virus serine protease inhibitors, VX-950 and BILN 2061: structural analysis indicates different resistance mechanisms. *J. Biol. Chem.* **2004**, *279*, 17508–17514.

[35] Narjes, H. Yong, C. L.; Stahle, H.; Steinmann, G. Tolerability and pharmacokinetics of BILN 2061, a novel HCV serine protease inhibitor, after oral single doses of 5 to 2400 mg in healthy male subjects. *Hepatology* **2002**, *36*, 363A.

[36] Hinrichsen, H. Benhamou, Y.; Wedemeyer, H.; Reiser, M.; Sentjens, R. E.; Calleja, J. L.; Forns, X.; Erhardt, A.; Cronlein, J.; Chaves, R. L.; et al. Short-term antiviral efficacy of BILN

2061, a hepatitis C virus serine protease inhibitor, in hepatitis C genotype 1 patients. *Gastroenterology* **2004**, *127*, 1347–1355.

[37] Herrmann, E.; Lee, J. H.; Marinos, G.; Modi, M.; Zeuzem, S. Effect of ribavirin on hepatitis C viral kinetics in patients treated with pegylated interferon. *Hepatology* **2003**, *37*, 1351–1358.

[38] Reiser, M.; Hinrichsen, H.; Benhamou, Y.; Reesink, H. W.; Wedemeyer, H.; Avendano, C.; Riba, N.; Yong, C. L.; Nehmiz, G.; Steinmann, G. G. Antiviral efficacy of NS3-serine protease inhibitor BILN-2061 in patients with chronic genotype 2 and 3 hepatitis C. *Hepatology* **2005**, *41*, 832–835.

[39] Herrmann, E. Zeuzem, S.; Sarrazin, C.; Hinrichsen, H.; Benhamou, Y.; Manns, M. P.; Reiser, M.; Reesink, H.; Calleja, J. L.; Forns, X.; et al. Viral kinetics in patients with chronic hepatitis C treated with the serine protease inhibitor BILN 2061. *Antiviral Ther.* **2006**, *11*, 371–376.

[40] Stoltz, J. H.; Stern, J. O.; Huang, Q.; Seidler, R. W.; Pack, F. D.; Knight, B. L. A 28-day mechanistic time course study in the rhesus monkey with hepatitis C virus protease inhibitor BILN 2061. *Toxicol. Pathol.* **2011** (in press).

[41] Manns, M. P.; Bourlière, M.; Benhamou, Y.; Pol, S.; Bonacini, M.; Trepo, C.; Wright, D.; Berg, T.; Calleja, J. L.; White, P. W.; et al. Potency, safety and pharmacokinetics of the NS3/4A protease inhibitor BI 201335 in patients with chronic HCV genotype-1 infection. *J. Hepatol.* Published online December 9, 2010. doi:10.1016/j.hep.2010.08.040.

[42] Thompson, A. J.; McHutchison, J. G.; Antiviral resistance and specifically targeted therapy for HCV (STAT-C). *J. Viral Hepatitis*. **2009**, *16*, 377–387.

17

INTERVENTION OF HEPATITIS C REPLICATION THROUGH NS3-4A, THE PROTEASE INHIBITOR BOCEPREVIR

SRIKANTH VENKATRAMAN AND F. GEORGE NJOROGE

Schering Plough Research Institute, Kenilworth, New Jersey

INTRODUCTION

The primary reasons for liver transplantation in the United States are liver cirrhosis and hepatocelullar carcinoma caused by chronic HCV infections. The slow progression of the disease accompanied with minimal or no symptoms has made hepatitis C infections a primary health concern. About 3% of the world population is infected with HCV, making it a grave public concern [1–3]. The current gold standard for treatment of HCV infections is treating patients with pegylated interferon and antiviral ribavirin [4–8]. Approximately 40% of patients infected with genotype 1 respond to this therapy, achieving undetectable titers after treatment. Lack of effective treatments for interferon nonresponders and relapse patients necessitates discovery of new drug candidates. Recent efforts have been directed toward the inhibition of viral enzymes vital for HCV replication [9–17].

HCV virus is a positive strand virus which is transmitted primarily by blood transfusion and sharing of hypodermic needles by intravenous drug users. The virus internalizes into the hepatocytes, uncoats, and releases a single positive strand RNA of about 9000 kb. This RNA, with the help of the cell host proteins, produces a single polyprotein of about 3000 amino acids that contain all the proteins required for viral replication [18]. The encoded polypeptide C–E1–E2–P7–NS2–NS3–NS4A–NS4B–NS5A–NS5B undergoes a *cis* cleavage of the NS3–NS4A junction followed by a *trans* cleavage at the NS4A–NS4B and NS4B–NS5A and NS5A–NS5B site, catalyzed by NS3 serine protease to produce functional proteins for viral replication (Fig. 1) [19–22]. This central role played by HCV NS3 protease makes it an excellent target for therapeutic intervention. This has been a very active field with many groups actively involved in development of inhibitor to arrest this pivotal enzyme. Many novel compounds such as telaprevir, MK7009, ITMN-191, and TMC435350 have been identified and are currently undergoing clinical investigations [23–26].

The x-ray structure of HCV NS3 protease has been solved and the structure reveals a shallow active site located on the surface of the protein [27–31]. The catalytic triad histidine-57, aspartic acid-81, and serine-139 are located between two β-barrels. A 54-amino acid cofactor enhances the activity of the protease by reorganizing the active site after binding to the enzyme. Thus, in the absence of the cofactor, the activity of the enzyme is greatly diminished.

Cysteine is conserved as the P_1 amino acid in NS3 substrate in an all-*trans* cleavage event, and it is replaced by a threonine in a *cis* cleavage event. The P_1' is a small hydorphobic amino acid and the P_2, P_3, and P_4 are all hydrophobic in nature [32–34]. The P_5 and P_6 residues contain an acidic functionality with P_5 and P_6 being either aspartic or glutaminc acid.

We initially screened numerous compound libraries to identify a promising lead for the inhibition of HCV NS3 protease. None of these compounds inhibited NS3 enzyme appreciably, to provide a suitable starting point amenable for structural activity studies. We therefore resorted to a

Antiviral Drugs: From Basic Discovery Through Clinical Trials, First Edition. Edited by Wieslaw M. Kazmierski.

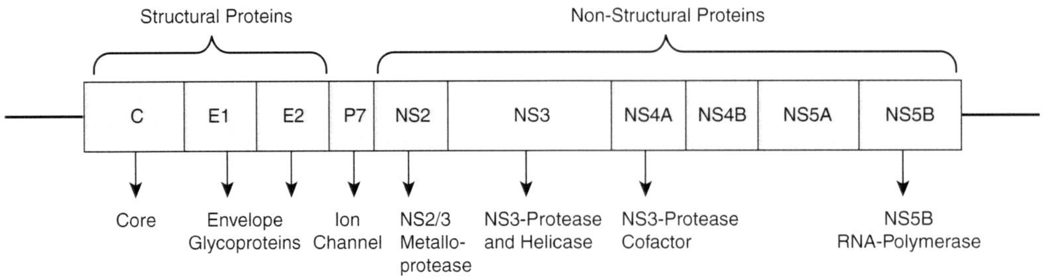

FIGURE 1 Schematic representation of HCV genome.

structure-based drug design and explored the introduction of electrophilic traps in the natural ligand of protease (Fig. 2). We evaluated incorporation of various functionalities such as keto-heterocycles, fluoroketone, and boronic acids as potential serine traps. Many of these analogs yielded compounds that inhibited HCV protease in the micromolar range. However, the introduction of a α-ketoamide moiety resulted in compound **7**, which demonstrated excellent inhibitory activity ($K_i^* = 1.9$ nM) [35] and a HNE/HCV (HNE = human neutrophil elastase) selectivity of 6.8. This was our first compound that exhibited inhibitory activity against the NS3 protease in the low-nanomolar region. Analysis of the x-ray structure of **7** bound to HCV protease revealed that serine-139 from the enzyme made a nucleophilic attack on the ketoamide carbonyl, and the oxygen of the amide occupied the oxyanion hole.

It was evident from the structure of **7** that the compound lacked many required druglike characteristics. Inhibitor **7** was peptidic, containing many amide bonds derived from natural amino acids that would be hydrolyzed readily by peptidases in the body. In addition, the molecular weight of **7** exceeded far beyond the desirable range (MW ~ 500 to 600 Da) to demonstrate acceptable oral pharmacokinetics. We therefore decided to investigate truncations of inhibitor **7** to evaluate the contributions of different moieties toward binding the compound to the enzyme.

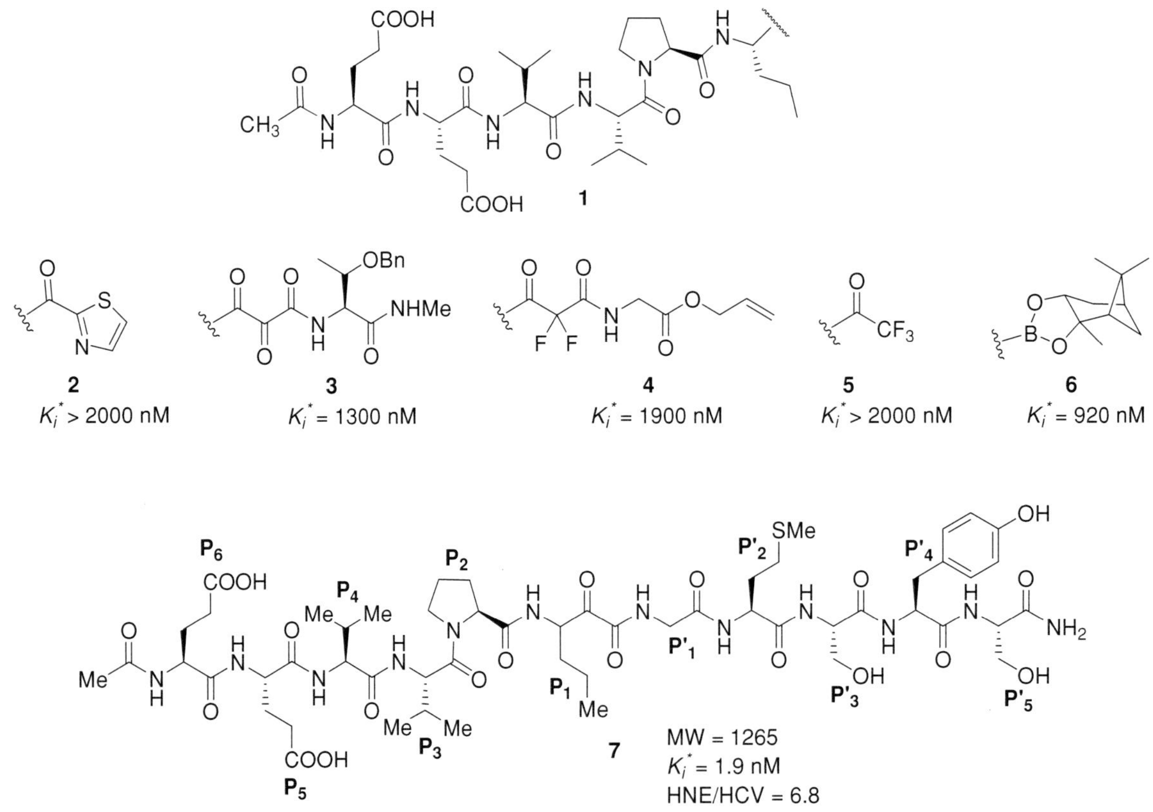

FIGURE 2

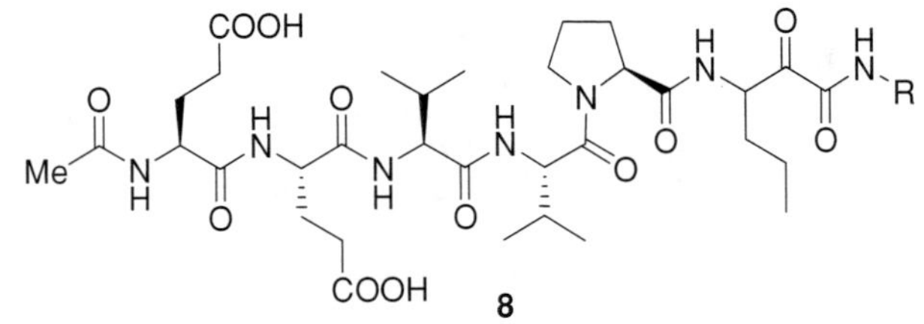

8

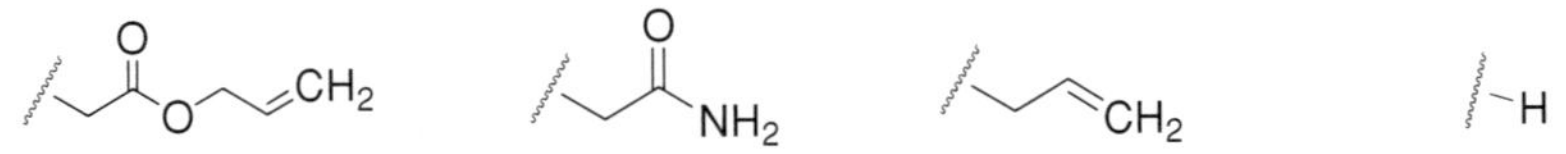

9 $K_i^* = 57$ nM | 10 $K_i^* = 270$ nM | 11 $K_i^* = 43$ nM | 12 $K_i^* = 760$ nM

FIGURE 3

Replacement of the P'_1–P'_5 segment of **7** with glycine allyl ester resulted in compound **9**, which demonstrated a K_i^* value of 57 nM; a 30-fold losses potency compared to **7** (Fig. 3). Similarly, replacement of the same segment with glycine amide resulted in inhibitor **10** ($K_i^* = 270$ nM) demonstrating a 142-fold loss in binding. We next investigated the effect of truncating the lead at the P_1 position. Thus, truncation of **7** at P_1 with allyl amide and primary amide resulted in compounds **11** ($K_i^* = 43$ nM) and **12** ($K_i^* = 760$ nM) with 23- and 400-fold losses in potency compared to **7**. Even though the results of these modifications resulted in diminished potency of the lead compound, they clearly demonstrated that truncations did not result in total loss in activity. Compounds spanning from P_6–P_1 such as **11** and **12** still demonstrated appreciable enzyme activity.

We next explored the effect of truncation at the P region of inhibitor **7**. Contemporaneous to our truncation studies, we also evaluated replacements of various amino acids in **7** with other natural and nonnatural amino acid residues. After significant structure–activity relationship (SAR) explorations, we identified that replacement of P_2 proline with leucine and P_3 valine group with cyclohexylglycine in lead compound **7** led to analogs of acceptable potency. SAR studies also identified the introduction of a P'_2 phenylglycine allowed significant improvement in enzyme inhibitory activity. These modifications allowed the truncation of undecapeptide inhibitors of type **7** at P_3, capping it with an isobutyl carbamate or a *tert*-butyl carbamate cap (Fig. 4).

Thus, P_2 leucine derivative **13** truncated at P'_1 with glycine demonstrated a binding $K_i^* = 6400$ nM. Truncation at P'_1 by introducing glycine benzyl ester resulted in compound **14** ($K_i^* = 8100$ nM) with enzyme activity similar to that of acid **13**. Incorporation of P'_2 phenylglycine resulted in derivatives **15** ($K_i^* = 120$ nM) and **16** ($K_i^* = 66$ nM) with much improved enzyme activity compared to P'_1 truncated analog. In an effort to understand the dramatic improvement in enzyme binding resulting from the introduction of P'_2 phenylglycine, x-ray structure of leucine derivative **16** bound to NS3 protease was solved. Analysis of the x-ray structure revealed the P'_1–P'_2 glycine–phenylglycine segment formed part of a "C-clamp" that overlapped over the amino butyl chain of lysine-136. The aromatic ring of P'_2 phenylglycine formed a

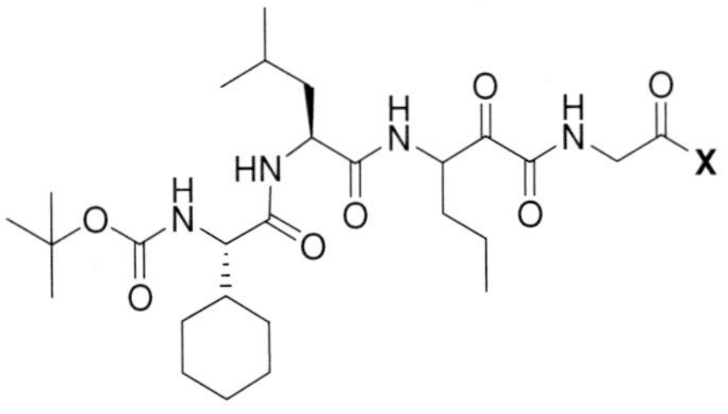

13; X = OH; $K_i^* = 6400$ nM;
14; X = OBn; $K_i^* = 8100$ nM;

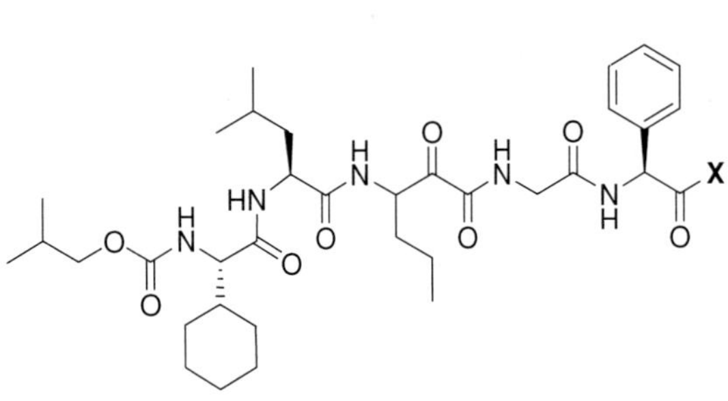

15; X = OH; $K_i^* = 120$ nM; HNE/HCV = 3
16; X = NH$_2$; $K_i^* = 66$ nM; HNE/HCV = 5

FIGURE 4

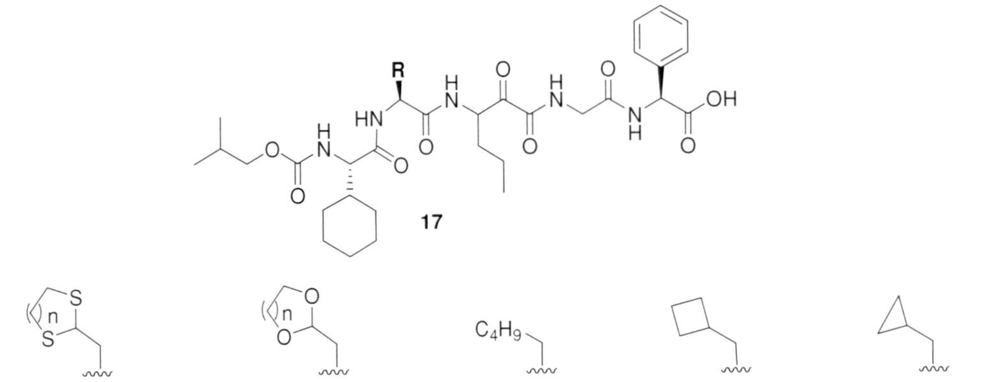

18; n=1 K_i^* = 90 nM
19; n=2 K_i^* = 250 nM

20; n=1 K_i^* = 300 nM
21; n=2 K_i^* = 430 nM

22
K_i^* = 300 nM

23
K_i^* = 140 nM

24
K_i^* = 50 nM

FIGURE 5

lipophilic interaction with the side chain of lysine. The amide nitrogen and the oxygen of phenylglycine formed a pair of hydrogen bonds to threonine-42.

Having identified that introducing P_2' phenylglycine resulted in significant improvement in enzyme activity ($K_i^* <$ 100 nM), we next evaluated the SAR of P_2 residue (Fig. 5) [36]. Various leucine mimics were synthesized and introduced into the inhibitor maintaining P_2' phenylglycine.

Introduction of five-membered dithioacetal-derived P_2 resulted in compound **18** ($K_i^* = 90$ nM), which was similar in potency to the P_2 leucine derivative **15**. The effect of expanding the ring size of the dithioacetal ring to a six-membered ring was evaluated. The six-membered analog **19** ($K_i^* = 250$ nM) was significantly less potent than the five-membered derivative **18**. Syntheses of five- and six-membered acetal derivatives resulted in compounds **20** ($K_i^* = 300$ nM) and **21** ($K_i^* = 430$ nM) that were much less potent than leucine derivative **15** and dithiane derivatives **18** and **19**. Incorporation of nonnatural amino acids containing alkyl side chains, such as pentyl glycine, cyclobutyl alanine, and cyclopropyl alanine, resulted in compounds with similar or improved activity compared to leucine derivative. The incorporation of pentyl glycine and cyclobutyl alanine resulted in compounds **22** ($K_i^* = 300$ nM) and **23** ($K_i^* = 140$ nM) with a partial loss in potency compared to leucine derivative **15**, whereas introduction of branched amino acid cyclopropyl alanine **24** ($K_i^* = 50$ nM) resulted in improved binding compared to leucine derivative **15**. Further SAR studies identified that replacement of P_1 norvaline of **24** with cyclopropyl alanine yielded derivative **25** with further improved activity ($K_i^* = 15$ nM, Fig. 6). The x-ray structures of cyclopropyl alanine derivative **25** bound to HCV NS3 protease revealed that the P_2 cyclopropyl alanine interacted with arginine-155 of the enzyme, augmenting enzyme-binding efficiency.

Having identified very potent inhibitors that bind to the active site of HCV NS3 protease, we next evaluated these inhibitors in a replicon-based cellular assay and for other drug characteristics. Investigation of analog **25** in the replicon-based cellular assay revealed that many of these inhibitors had poor cellular activity [37] ($EC_{90} > 5.0$ μM) even though they were very potent inhibitors in the enzyme assay. We reasoned that these compounds were still peptidic and did not penetrate the cell membrane efficiently and therefore wanted to depeptidize these analogs and improve their physiochemical properties. In an attempt to depeptidize these analogs, we synthesized macrocyclic inhibitors that mimicked the binding conformation of acyclic inhibitors (Fig. 7). Macrocyclization has been an effective tool in depeptidizing various peptidic inhibitors and have been demonstrated to mimic extended conformations of peptidic inhibitors [39]. Analysis of the x-ray structure of **25** bound to HCV protease revealed close proximity of S_2–S_4 pockets and the S_1–S_3 pockets. We therefore explored cyclic structures of inhibitors of type **25**.

Macrocyclization of P_2 *meta*-tyrosine and P_4 phenylacetic acid analog resulted in 17-membered compound **26** that demonstrated an enzyme binding $K_i^* = 110$ nM (Fig. 7) [40]. Increasing the ring size to 18- and 19-membered macrocycles resulted in compounds **27** ($K_i^* = 300$ nM) and **28**

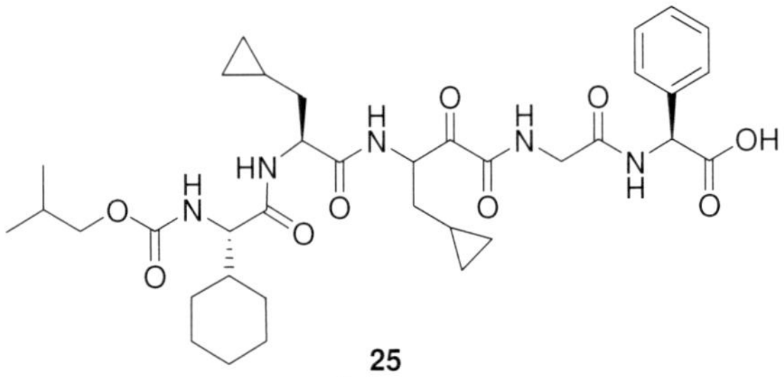

25
K_i^* = 15 nM
EC_{90} > 5.0 μM

FIGURE 6

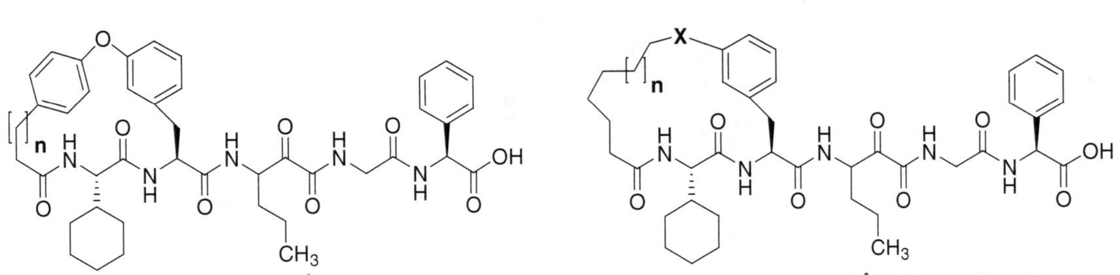

26: n = 1, $K_i^* = 110$ nM
27: n = 2, $K_i^* = 300$ nM
28: n = 3, $K_i^* = 160$ nM

29: n = 0; $K_i^* = 1200$ nM (X = O)
30: n = 1; $K_i^* = 160$ nM (X = O)
31: n = 1; $K_i^* = 250$ nM (X = CH_2)

FIGURE 7

($K_i^* = 160$ nM) with similar potency to the 17-membered analog **26**. Replacement of rigid P_4 phenylacetic acid linker with flexible hexanoic acid or heptanoic acid linker resulted in compounds **29** ($K_i^* = 1200$ nM) and **30** ($K_i^* = 160$ nM) [41]. Similarly, replacement of bridgehead oxygen with carbon in compound **29** led to inhibitors **31** ($K_i^* = 250$ nM) that was similar in potency to the oxygen analog **30**. X-ray structure of the biaryl macrocyclic inhibitor **26** bound to protease revealed that the P_2–P_4 macrocyclic portion of the molecule made close contact with the protein and the P_2 *meta*-tyrosine moiety made van der Waals interaction with arginine-155. The macrocyclic portion of the molecule made lipophilic contacts encircling the methyl group of alanine-156 of the enzyme, contributing to the binding desired.

Even though our attempts to depeptidize peptidic inhibitors using macrocyclization strategy yielded potent series of inhibitors, most of these compounds lacked activity in the cellular assay in the desirable range. We therefore decided to interrogate acyclic series of compounds further in the replicon-based cellular assay (Fig. 8). [38].

Inhibitor **25** derived from P_2 cyclopropyl alanine and P_2' phenylglycine acid demonstrated a potent inhibitory activity in enzyme-based assay ($K_i^* = 15$ nM); however, it had a poor cellular activity with an $EC_{90} > 5000$ nM. We reasoned that the poor cellular potency of **25** was probably due to the presence of P_2' carboxylic acid. We therefore replaced it with dimethyl amide to synthesize analog **32** ($K_i^* = 50$ nM; $EC_{90} > 5000$ nM). Evaluation of this analog in the cellular assay still demonstrated a poor cellular activity. We therefore decided to reduce the number of hydrogen-bond donors in the molecule by alkylating different amide nitrogens with methyl groups. Methylation of P_2–P_3 amide nitrogen of inhibitor **25** resulted in compound **33** ($K_i^* = 120$ nM; $EC_{90} > 5000$ nM), which still displayed a poor cellular activity. However, methylation of P_2–P_3 amide nitrogen of inhibitor **32** resulted in compound **34**, which demonstrated that $K_i^* = 60$ nM and $EC_{90} = 950$ nM. This was the first class of compounds that displayed submicromolar cellular activity. It became clear from these studies that for these classes of compounds to demonstrate potent cellular activity it was required to incorporate a secondary P_2 amide and have the P_2' carboxylic acid suitably modified with less polar functionality. Having identified the requirement of a secondary amide at P_2 to impart cellular activity, we investigated various modified proline derivatives at this position, maintaining phenylglycine dimethyl amide at P_2' [42].

Synthesis of 4-*tert*-butoxy-substituted proline analog yielded compound **35**, which had values of $K_i^* = 19$ nM and $EC_{90} = 2000$ nM. To further improve potency and expand the SAR, we explored the effect of 3,4-fused bicyclic proline analogs as potential P_2 residues (Fig. 9). Incorporation of of 3,4-cyclopentyl fused bicyclic proline P_2

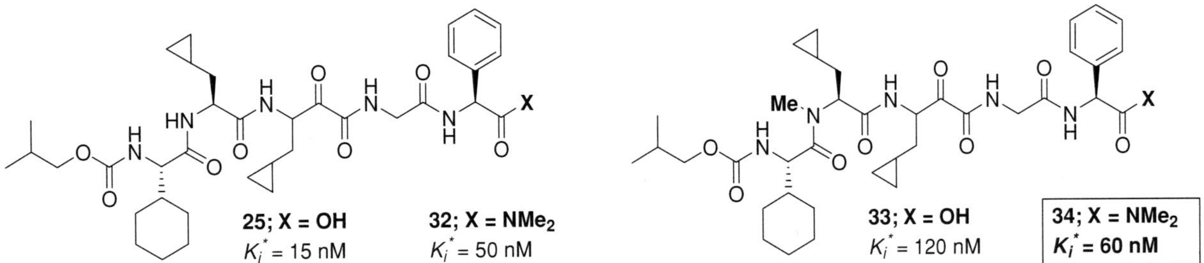

25; X = OH
$K_i^* = 15$ nM
$EC_{90} > 5000$ nM

32; X = NMe_2
$K_i^* = 50$ nM
$EC_{90} > 5000$ nM

33; X = OH
$K_i^* = 120$ nM
$EC_{90} > 5000$ nM

34; X = NMe_2
$K_i^* = 60$ nM
$EC_{90} = 950$ nM

FIGURE 8

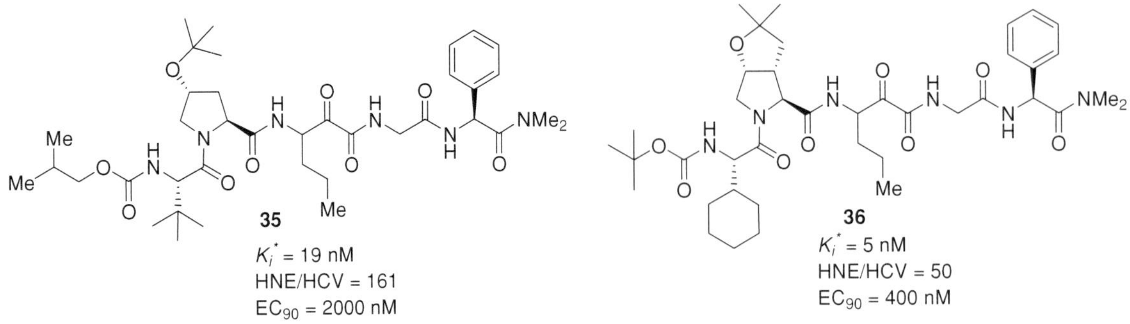

FIGURE 9

resulted in compound **36**, which demonstrated $K_i^* = 5$ nM and $EC_{90} = 400$ nM, fourfold more potent than **35** in the replicon cellular assay. This exercise clearly demonstrated that analogs with both potent binding and cellular activity could be achieved by incorporating modified bicyclic proline P_2 derivatives.

Having discovered that leucine is an excellent P_2 amino acid that yielded compounds with potent enzyme activities and proline as P_2 residue that imparted potent cellular activity, we envisioned combining these two moieties into a single bicyclic proline derivative. A review of the literature led to work by Zhang and Madalengoitia, who had described the synthesis and modeling studies of (1*R*,2*S*,5*S*)-6,6-dimethyl-3-azabicyclo[3.1.0]hexane-2-carboxylic acid, a bicyclic proline derivative that mimicked leucine [43,44]. We therefore decided to evaluate this amino acid as a potential P_2 group (Fig. 10).

The introduction of (1*R*,2*S*,5*S*)-6,6-dimethyl-3-azabicyclo[3.1.0]hexane-2-carboxylic acid at P_2 had a profound effect on the cellular activity of the synthesized inhibitors. Compound **37** derived from (*1R,2S,5S*)-6,6-dimethyl-3-azabicyclo[3.1.0]hexane-2-carboxylic acid P_2 and cylopropyl alanine P_1 moiety demonstrated an enzyme activity of $K_i^* = 1.4$ nM and a much improved replicon cellular activity: $EC_{90} = 90$ nM. There was a fourfold improvement in cellular activity compared to compounds derived from 3,4 fused furan analogs **36**. The replacement of P_3 cyclohexylglycine in **37** with *tert*-butylglycine resulted in compound **38** (Sch-6) which had values of $K_i^* = 3.8$ nM and $EC_{90} = 100$ nM. Having identified inhibitors with excellent binding and cellular activity, we evaluated these compounds in rats for its pharmacokinetic properties. As shown in Figure 10, compounds **37** and **38** both had suboptimal oral absorption demonstrating AUC = 0.23 and 0.35 μM·h when dosed in rats at 10 mg/kg. The bioavailabilities were also poor, ranging in the low single digits. From these studies it was clear that these compounds were poorly absorbed. X-ray crystal structure of Sch-6 (**38**) bound to the HCV NS3 protease was solved, which revealed that the dimethyl cyclopropyl moiety fused to the proline made van der Waals contact with alanine-156 and the methyl group interacted with arginine-155.

With knowledge of synthesizing potent inhibitors with excellent enzyme and cellular activities, we next devoted our efforts toward improving the pharmacokinetic parameters of these compounds. We revisited our depeptidization efforts retaining P_2 proline residues in an effort to improve oral pharmacokinetics. A series of P_2–P_4 and P_1–P_3 macrocyclic compounds were synthesized and evaluated in enzyme and cellular assays (Fig. 11).

Cyclization of 4-hydroxyproline P_2 to the 3-hydroxyphenyl acetic acid P_4 with a propyl linker resulted in

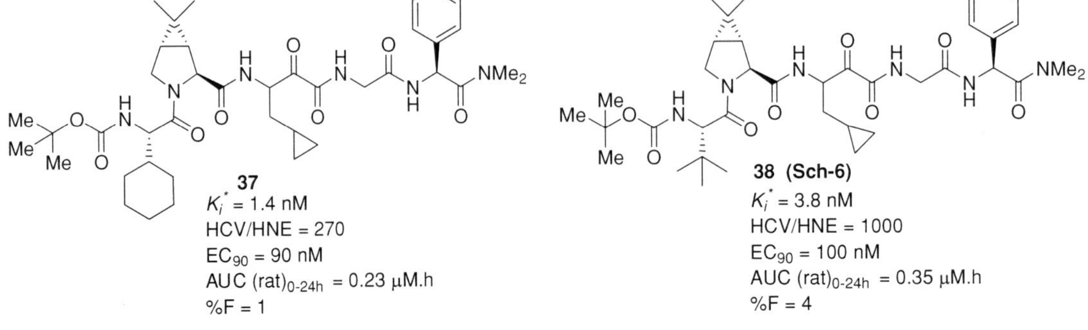

FIGURE 10

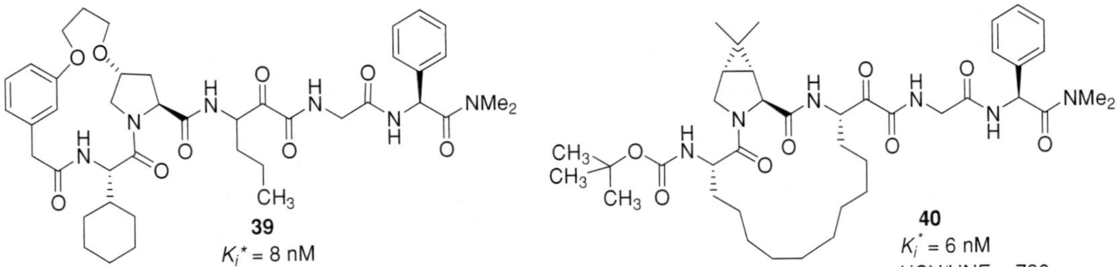

39
K_i^* = 8 nM
HCV/HNE = 46
EC_{90} = 1500 nM
AUC rat $_{0\text{-}24h}$ = 1.5 μM.h
%F = 3

40
K_i^* = 6 nM
HCV/HNE = 780
EC_{90} = 600 nM

FIGURE 11

16-membered P_2–P_4 macrocyclic analog **39** with $K_i^* = 8$ nM and $EC_{90} = 1500$ nM [45]. Inhibitor **39** was evaluated for oral pharmacokinetics (PK) in rats, which demonstrated an acceptable AUC = 1.5 μM·h with poor bioavailability (F = 3%) when dosed at 10 mg/kg. Synthesis of 17-membered macrocyclic inhibitor that linked P_1–P_3 residues with an aliphatic straight chain resulted in analog **40** ($K_i^* = 6.0$ nM, $EC_{90} = 600$ nM), similar in potency to the P_2–P_4 analog **39**. Our attempts to synthesize depeptidized analogs yielded potent compounds in the enzyme binding and cellular assay. However, all our attempts to improve pharmacokinetics and bioavailabilities resulted in limited success. The macrocyclic analogs we synthesized had a binding and pharmacokinetic profile similar to that of acyclic analogs. We therefore had to revise our strategy and generate molecules that retained desired binding and cellular activities while improving pharmacokinetics. Analysis of our lead inhibitors that spanned from P_3 to P_2' revealed that many of these analogs had molecular weights ranging between 750 and 850 Da. These analogs had many heteroatoms with multiple hydrogen-bond donors and acceptors. Moreover, these analogs were still peptidic containing many amide bonds. We therefore decided to truncate these analogs further by reducing the molecular weights and number of amide bonds to enable better absorption and distribution. We decided to incorporate individual ligands that made a greater contribution to overall binding. With this in mind we further explored truncation of P_3–P_2' analogs of type **38**.

The first truncation we evaluated was the removal of the P_2' dimethyl amide group in inhibitors of type **38**. As shown in Figure 12, removal of a single amide bond had a profound effect on PK, even though the truncated compounds were less potent in the enzyme-binding assay.

Replacement of P_2' phenylglycine dimethyl amide with benzyl amide resulted in compound **41**, which had an enzyme-binding activity of $K_i^* = 56$ nM and a much improved rat plasma exposure of 1.27 μM·h over 6 h. It was very reassuring to learn that removal of a single amide functionality allowed significant improvement in plasma levels in rats. Similarly, replacement of P_2' with (S)-α-methyl benzyl amine resulted in compound **42**, which had activity similar to that of the benzyl derivative **41**, but better PK, with $AUC_{0\text{-}6h}$ = 2.66 μM·h. We therefore decided to evaluate truncating our inhibitors at the P_1' position (Fig. 13).

Replacement of the glycine-phenyl glycine dimethyl amide segment of **38** with allyl amide resulted in inhibitor **44**, with a K_i^* value of 280 nM. Analysis of this compound in the rapid rat assay [46] for oral PK in rats indicated an $AUC_{0\text{-}6h}$ value of 26 μM·h. This was a clear indication that we were on the right track. We further explored the P_1' substitution by replacement of the glycine-phenylglycine segment with methyl amide to yield compound **45** ($K_i^* = 1500$ nM). Once again this compound demonstrated a good oral PK in rats, with $AUC_{0\text{-}6h}$ = 13.4 μM·h. We next evaluated the replacement of P_1' with a primary ketoamide moiety. Synthesis of this analog resulted in compound **46**, which demonstrated a binding of

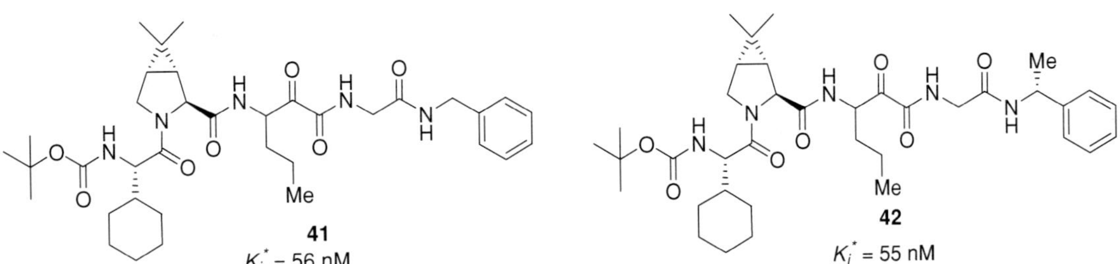

41
K_i^* = 56 nM
AUC (rat)$_{0\text{-}6h}$ = 1.27 μM.h

42
K_i^* = 55 nM
AUC (rat)$_{0\text{-}6h}$ = 2.66 μM.h

FIGURE 12

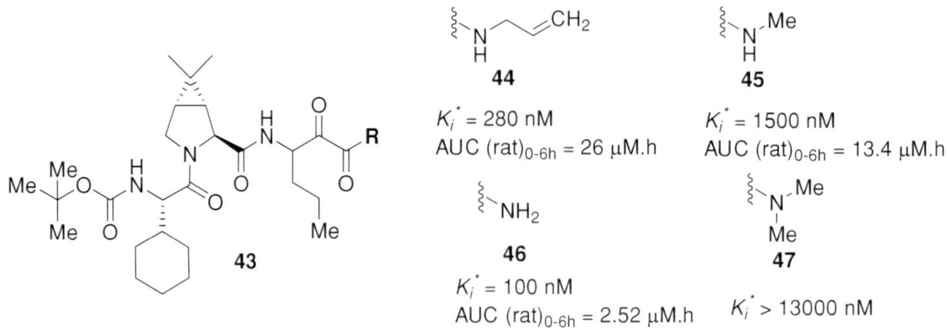

FIGURE 13

$K_i^* = 100$ nM and a good rat $AUC_{0\text{-}6h} = 2.52$ μM·h. This was one of our first truncated compounds which demonstrated good enzyme-binding activity and acceptable PK in rats. It also showed that when modified appropriately, we could achieve truncated compounds with good binding. Our attempts to introduce a secondary amide such as dimethyl amide at P_1' results in loss of potency, yielding inhibitors of type **47** displaying a K_i^*value $> 13{,}000$ nM. This clearly indicated that the hydrogen of the amide was required and was probably involved in hydrogen bonding with the protein, which contributed significantly to binding free energy.

Having identified that incorporation of a primary ketoamide resulted in compounds with good binding ($K_i^* =$ 100 nM) and acceptable plasma exposure, we next explored the potential to improve the enzyme potency by modifying P_1 norvaline residue. As outlined in Figure 14, we synthesized a variety of nonproteinogenic P_1 amino acids and incorporated them in our inhibitor.

Replacement of P_1 norvaline with (*S*)-2-aminobutyric acid resulted in compound **49** ($K_i^* = 740$ nM), a sevenfold loss in potency compared to the norvaline derivative **46**. Extension of carbon chain length resulted in butenyl glycine derivative **50** ($K_i^* = 150$ nM), which had activity similar to that of the norvaline derivative **46**. We next evaluated the effect of branching by incorporating methallyl glycine and isoleucine to yield inhibitors **51** ($K_i^* = 300$ nM) and **52** ($K_i^* = 400$ nM), respectively, which were less potent than the corresponding norvaline analog, clearly indicating that branching was detrimental to activity. The effect of introducing cyclic alanine amino acids at P_1 were evaluated by

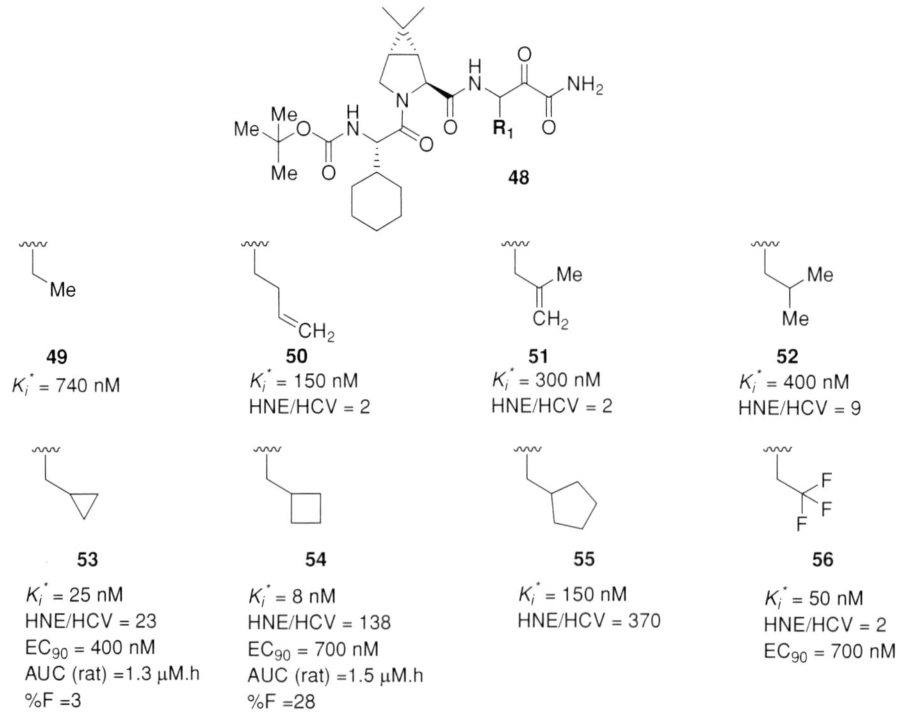

FIGURE 14

incorporating cyclopropyl alanine, cyclobutyl alanine, and cyclopentyl alanine. The cyclopropyl analog **53** ($K_i^* =$ 25 nM) demonstrated a fourfold-improved enzyme activity over that of the norvaline analog **46**. The compound demonstrated $EC_{90} = 400$ nM in the replicon-based cellular assay. The cyclobutyl alanine analog **54** had a further improved enzyme activity with a $K_i^* = 8$ nM and $EC_{90} = 700$ nM. Expansion of the cyclobutyl ring to a cyclopentyl ring resulted in analog **55** ($K_i^* = 150$ nM), which was less active than cylopropyl and cyclobutyl derivatives. It was clear from these studies that the S_1 pocket was narrow and the cyclobutyl ring was the maximum ring size that was tolerated, yielding compound with good potency. It was also interesting to observe that the HNE/HCV selectivity depended on the ring size of the group occupying the S_1 pocket. The larger the size of the ring, the more selective the compound was for HCV. The cyclopropyl analog had a HNE/HCV selectivity of 23, whereas the cyclobutyl derivative had a selectivity of 138 and the cyclopentyl derivative demonstrated a HNE/HCV selectivity of 370. The cyclopropyl analog **53** and cyclobutyl analog **54** were evaluated for oral PK in rats. It was gratifying to see that both analogs demonstrated appreciable PK, with the cyclopropyl derivative **53** demonstrating AUC = 1.3 μM·h with a bioavailability of 3% and the cyclobutyl analog **54** AUC = 1.5 μM·h with a bioavailability of 28%. From our SAR explorations we identified that cyclopropyl alanine and cyclobutyl alanine residues as excellent P_1 moieties that improved activity while demonstrating cellular potency and PK.

Our next efforts were to understand the effect of P_3 variations. We chose cyclopropyl and cyclobutyl alanine P_1 groups and evaluated the effect of varying the P_3 residue in the primary ketoamide series. The effects of these modifications are tabulated in Table 1.

TABLE 1

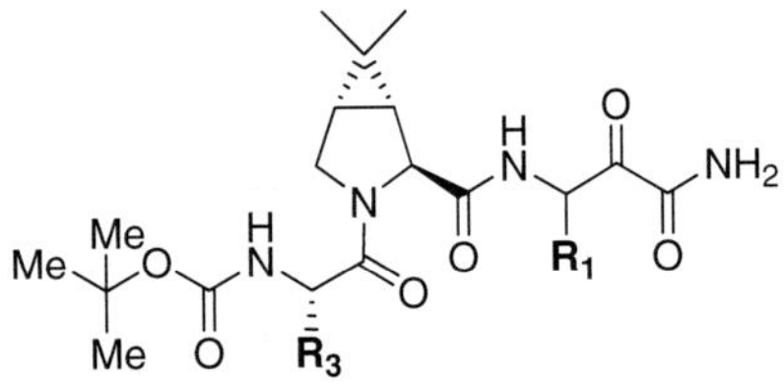

Compound	R_3	R_1	K_i^* (nM)	HNE/HCV	EC_{90} (nM)
57	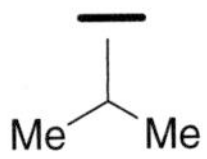	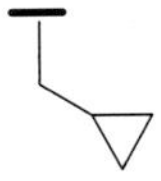	210	19	—
58	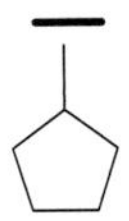	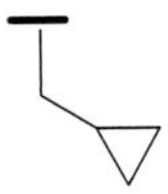	100	11	—
59	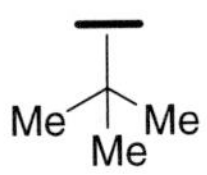	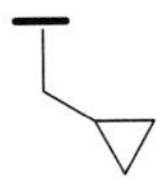	57	112	600
60	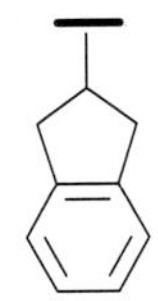	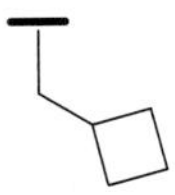	470	—	2000
61	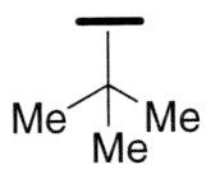	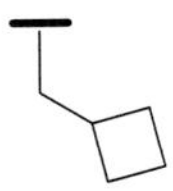	76	684	800
62	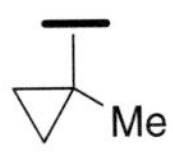	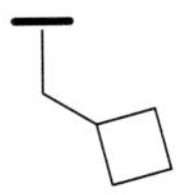	700	—	—
63	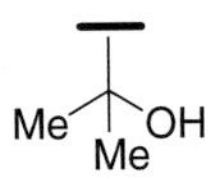	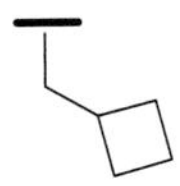	220	55	—

Replacement of cyclohexyl glycine of **53** with valine resulted in compound **57**, which demonstrated an enzyme-binding activity $K_i^* = 210$ nM, a tenfold loss in enzyme-binding activity compared to **53**. The side chain of valine was replaced with a cyclopentyl group, resulting in compound **58** ($K_i^* = 100$ nM), which improved binding by twofold compared to the valine derivative **57**. We next evaluated the effect of introducing 2-indanyl glycine by synthesizing compound **60** ($K_i^* = 470$ nM), which demonstrated a much diminished activity compared to **54**. We next evaluated the introduction of P_3 *tert*-butyl glycine. Replacement of P_3 cyclohexyl glycine of **53** with *tert*-butyl glycine resulted in analog **59**, which demonstrated an enzyme activity of $K_i^* = 57$ nM and $EC_{90} = 600$ nM. This modification resulted in a compound that was similar in potency to the cyclohexyl analog.

Introduction of P_3 *tert*-butyl glycine in the P_1 cyclobutyl series resulted in compound **61**, which demonstrated a binding activity ($K_i^* = 76$ nM) and cellular activity of $EC_{90} = 800$ nM. A comparison of the cyclobutyl and cyclopropyl analogs with P_3 *tert*-butyl glycine demonstrated that both these analogs had similar enzyme activities; however, the cyclobutyl analog **61** demonstrated much better HNE/HCV selectivity (684 compared to 112) compared to cyclopropyl analog. Our attempts to cyclize the two methyl groups of P_3 *tert*-butyl gylcine into a three-membered ring resulted in compound **62** ($K_i^* = 700$ nM), with a significant loss in binding. Similarly, our efforts to introduce a hydroxyl group at the P_3 *tert*-butyl glycine resulted in **63** ($K_i^* = 220$ nM), resulting in a fourfold loss in potency compared to the *tert*-butyl analog **61**.

From our structure–activity investigation of the P_3 and P_1 groups, we identified cyclobutyl alanine and cyclopropyl alanine as desirable P_1 residues that yielded compounds with good enzyme and cellular activities. Similarly, we discovered *tert*-butyl glycine as a preferred P_3 group that yielded compounds with improved HNE/HCV selectivity. We therefore retained these residues for further investigation of the SAR of the P_3 capping site (Table 2).

TABLE 2

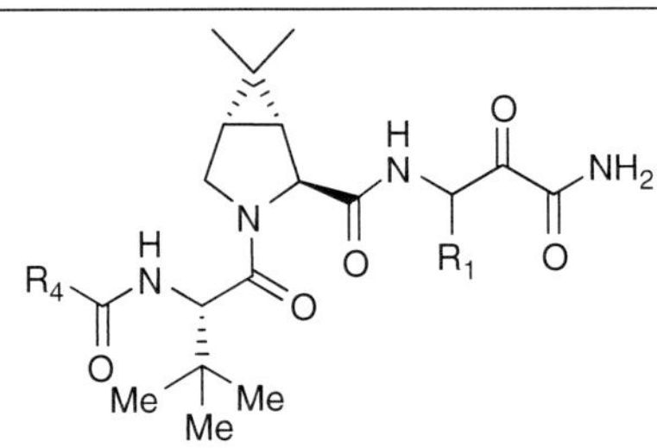

Compound	R_4	R_1	K_i^* (nM)	HNE/HCV	EC_{90} (nM)
64	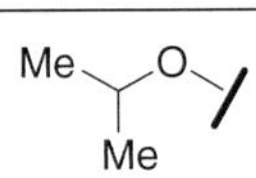	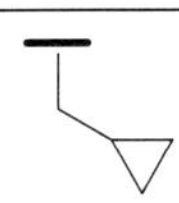	150	100	—
65	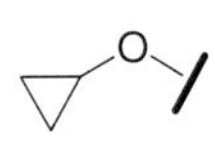	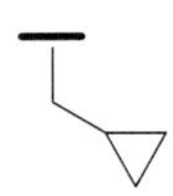	300	—	—
66	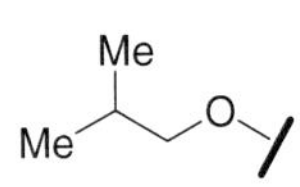	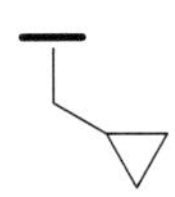	70	160	—
67	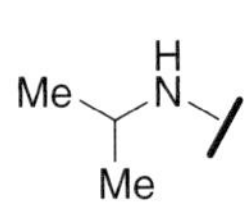	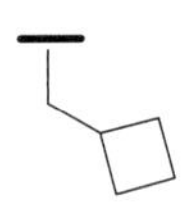	16	4200	730
68	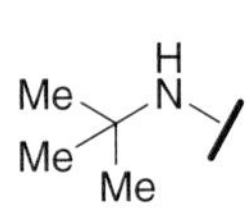	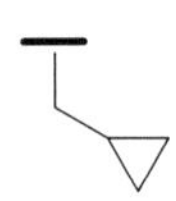	13	369	400
69	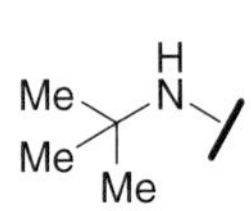	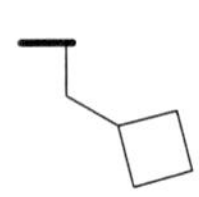	14	2200	350
70	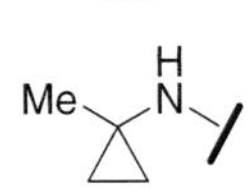	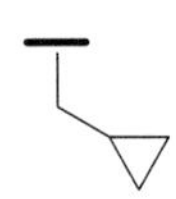	80	100	900

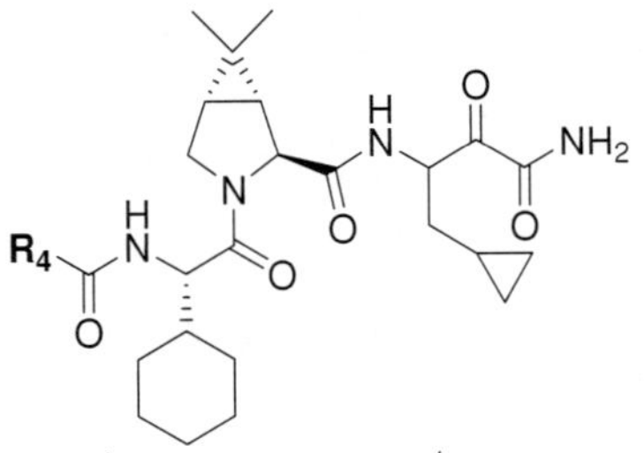

53; $R_4 = {}^tBuO$
$K_i^* = 25$ nM
HNE/HCV= 23

71; $R_4 = {}^tBuNH$
$K_i^* = 50$ nM
HNE/HCV= 38

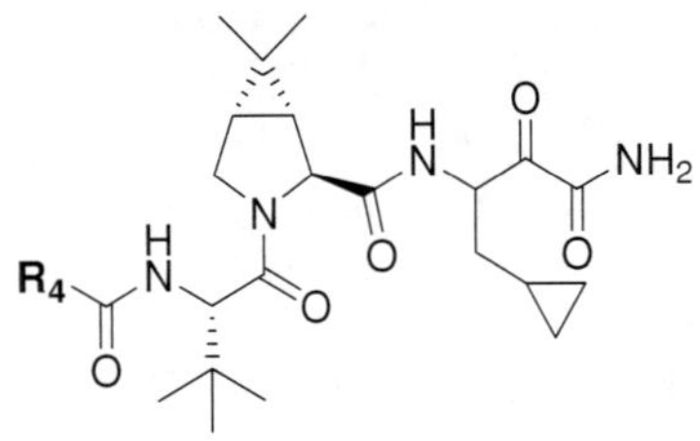

59; $R_4 = {}^tBuO$
$K_i^* = 57$ nM
HNE/HCV= 112

68; $R_4 = {}^tBuNH$
$K_i^* = 13$ nM
HNE/HCV= 369

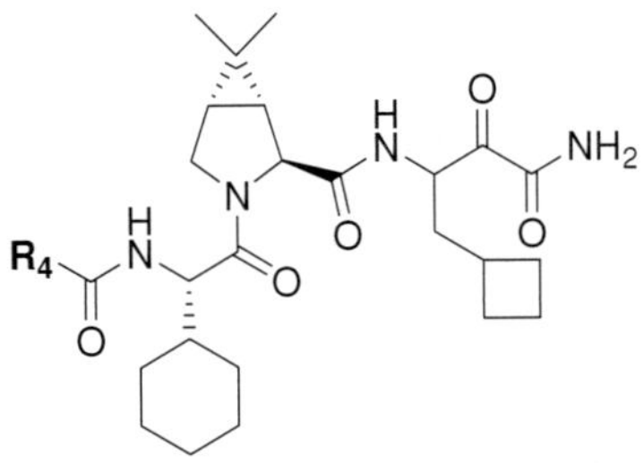

54; $R_4 = {}^tBuO$
$K_i^* = 8$ nM
HNE/HCV= 138

72; $R_4 = {}^tBuNH$
$K_i^* = 50$ nM
HNE/HCV= 90

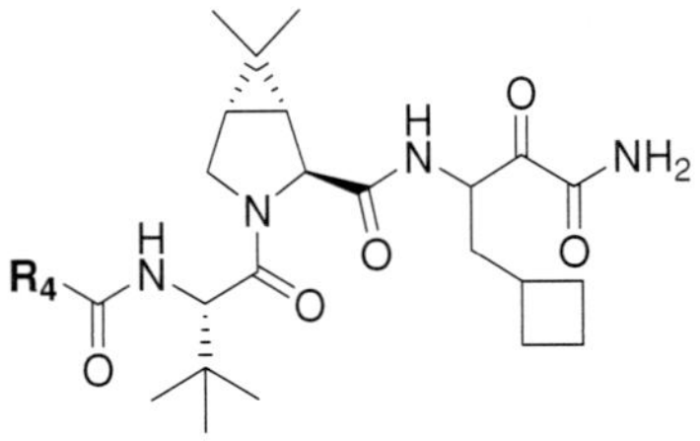

61; $R_4 = {}^tBuO$
$K_i^* = 76$ nM
HNE/HCV= 684

69; $R_4 = {}^tBuNH$
$K_i^* = 14$ nM
HNE/HCV= 2200

FIGURE 15

P_3 *tert*-butyl carbamate of inhibitors **59** and **61** were replaced with a wide variety of carbamates and ureas. Replacement of *tert*-butyl carbamate of **59** with isopropyl carbamate resulted in analog **64** ($K_i^* = 150$ nM and HNE/HCV $= 100$), threefold less active than the corresponding derivative **59**. Introduction of cyclopropyl carbamate resulted in a further twofold loss in potency, yielding analog **65** with an enzyme activity $K_i^* = 300$ nM. Extension of the cap from isopropyl to isobutyl carbamate resulted in inhibitor **66** ($K_i^* = 70$ nM), similar in potency to the derivative **59**. We next evaluated the effect of introducing urea derivatives as P_3 capping. This modification would replace hydrogen-bond acceptor oxygen with hydrogen-bond donor nitrogen on the P_3 cap. Replacement of Boc groups in inhibitors **61** with isopropyl urea resulted in analog **67** ($K_i^* = 16$ nM, HNE/HCV $= 4200$, $EC_{90} = 730$ nM). The incorporation of urea functionality improved the binding of cyclobutyl derivative sixfold. In addition, the HNE/HCV selectivity was further improved to 4200. With the knowledge that the introduction of a urea derivative improved the enzyme activity and HNE/HCV selectivity, we wanted to study the effect a *tert*-butyl urea group which would be an isosteric replacement for a Boc group. Incorporation of *tert*-butyl urea as the P_3 capping resulted in compounds **68** ($K_i^* = 13$ nM, HNE/HCV $= 369$, $EC_{90} = 400$ nM) and **69** ($K_i^* = 14$ nM, HNE/HCV $= 2200$, $EC_{90} = 350$ nM), with the cyclobutyl analog **69** demonstrating improved enzyme activity, HNE/HCV selectivity, and cellular activity compared to the corresponding Boc analog **61**. We next evaluated the constriction of *tert*-butyl urea in the form of a ring to synthesize methylated cyclopropyl urea analog **70** ($K_i^* = 80$ nM, HNE/HCV $= 100$, $EC_{90} = 900$ nM). This resulted in a loss of activity compared to the *tert*-butyl urea derivative **69**. With the acceptable profile of **69** (Sch 503034) [47,48], we evaluated this analog further in animal PK for its ADME properties.

SYNERGISTIC EFFECTS THAT INFLUENCE ENZYME BINDING AND HNE/HCV SELECTIVITY

In the process of investigating SAR toward identification of **69** (Sch 503034), we observed a number of synergies between P_1–P_3 moieties and P_3–P_3 capping moieties that influenced enzyme binding and HNE/HCV selectivity. These effects have been exemplified in Figure 15.

Synergistic Effect of P_3 with P_3 Capping Group on Enzyme Binding

As shown in Figure 15, the potency of these inhibitors depended on a combination of P_3 and P_3 capping residues. P_1 cyclopropyl derivative **53** ($K_i^* = 25$ nM, HNE/HCV $=$ 23, $EC_{90} = 400$ nM) and P_1 cyclobutyl alanine derivative **54** ($K_i^* = 8$ nM, HNE/HCV $= 138$, $EC_{90} = 700$ nM) that contained P_3 cyclohexyl glycine and P_3 capping *tert*-butyl carbamate demonstrated better enzyme activity than analogs **59** ($K_i^* = 57$ nM, HNE/HCV = 112, EC_{90} = 600 nM) and **61** ($K_i^* = 76$ nM, HNE/HCV = 684, EC_{90} = 800 nM), which contained a P_3 *tert*-butyl glycine. P_3 cyclohexyl glycine imparted better enzyme activity when the *tert*-butyl carbamate group was P_3 capping. In contrast, when P_3 capping was replaced with a *tert*-butyl urea, the P_3 *tert*-butyl glycine analogs **68** ($K_i^* = 13$ nM, HNE/HCV = 369) and **69** ($K_i^* = 14$ nM, HNE/HCV = 2200) demonstrated enzyme inhibition superior to those of the P_3 cyclohexyl glycine analogs **71** ($K_i^* = 50$ nM, HNE/HCV = 38) and **72** ($K_i^* = 50$ nM, HNE/HCV = 90).

Effect of P_3 and P_1 Substitution on HNE/HCV Selectivity

A closer examination of the HNE/HCV selectivity of inhibitors in Figure 15 also indicated that in all cases, compounds derived from P_1 cyclobutyl alanine demonstrated better HNE/HCV selectivity than that of P_1 cyclopropyl alanine derivatives. Moreover, in the series containing P_1 cyclobutyl alanine, P_3 *tert*-butyl glycine compound **69** (HNE/HCV = 2200) was more selective than P_3 cyclohexyl glycine derivative **72** (HNE/HCV = 90).

PHARMACOKINETICS OF BOCEPREVIR

Based on the desirable enzyme binding, the HNE/HCV selectivity and cellular activity of Sch 503034 (**69**), we evaluated its pharmacokinetic parameters in rats, dogs, monkeys, and mice. The pharmacokinetic parameters of boceprevir are shown in Table 3 [49]. As outlined in the table, the PK of inhibitor **69** depended on the species evaluated. The oral exposure of boceprevir was good in rat, mouse, and dog, whereas the exposure in monkeys was poor. It demonstrated an AUC = 1.5 μM·h in rats when dosed at 10 mg/kg with an oral bioavailability of 26% and a moderate $t_{1/2} = 4.2$ h. Dosing boceprevir in dogs at 3 mg/kg resulted in an oral AUC = 3.1 μM·h with an oral bioavailability of 30%. However, the compound demonstrated a suboptimal PK in monkeys with a poor oral exposure AUC = 0.12 μM·h at 3 mg/kg and a variable bioavailability of 4 to 11%. The compound also demonstrated short half-lives in dogs and monkeys, with $t_{1/2} = 1.1$ and 1.2 h, respectively.

TABLE 3 PK Properties of Boceprevir (Sch 503034, 69)

	Dose (mg/kg)		AUC (μM·h)			
Species	i.v.	p.o.	i.v.	p.o.	% Bioavailability	$t_{1/2}$ (h)
Rat	10	10	5.9	1.5	26	4.2
Dog	1.7	3	5.8	3.1	30	1.1
Monkey	3	3	2.9	0.12	4–11	1.2
Mouse	10	10	2.7	0.93	34	1.7

We also evaluated the absorption and distribution of boceprevir into the liver, which is the repository organ for hepatitis C virus. Evaluation of the distribution in rats demonstrated that it was well distributed into the liver with a liver/plasma ratio of 30-fold. This was very desirable since the compound was more available in the site of virus. Evaluation of absorption and elimination with radio-labeled compound demonstrated that it was moderately absorbed with 36% in rats and 23% in dogs.

Boceprevir was also evaluated for other drug safety parameters, such as hERG and CYP inhibition. It demonstrated no issues with CYP inhibition, with > 30 μM inhibition of CYP isoforms 2D6, 2C9, and 2C19. The compound demonstrated a moderate inhibition of CYP3A4 (coinc/prein > 30/8.6 μM).

SYNTHESIS OF BOCEPREVIR

Sch 503034 (**69**) was assembled in a convergent synthesis with the formation of two key fragments. The P_1 ketoamide segment **78** was synthesized starting from the ethyl (2-diphenylmethyleneamino)acetate (Scheme 1), whereas the nonproteinogenic P_2 was synthesized starting from the pyroglutamic acid derivative **79**.

Alkylation of glycine derivative **73** with potassium *tert*-butoxide and cyclobutylmethyl bromide resulted in cyclobutyl alanine ethyl ester **74**. Boc protection of amine **74** followed by hydrolysis of ethyl ester resulted in carboxylic acid **75**. The acid was converted to the Weinreb amide using *N,O*-dimethyl hydroxylamine and BOP reagent. The resulting amide was further reduced to the aldehyde **76** with $LiAlH_4$. Treatment of aldehyde **76** with acetone cyanohydrin resulted in cyanide transfer, which was hydrolyzed to the hydroxyamide **77** using basic hydrogen peroxide. Deprotection of the Boc group of **77** with 4 M HCl resulted in the amine segment **78**.

Synthesis of the P_2 segment was initiated with pyroglutamic acid derivative **79** (Scheme 2). Oxidation of **79** to α,β-unsaturated lactam **80** was accomplished by selenation with phenylselenium bromide, followed by oxidation of the intermediate selenide to selenoxide and subsequent elimination. The dimethylcyclopropyl group was installed by treatment of **80** with isopropyl phosphonium bromide and butyllithium. The resulting dimethylcyclopropyl lactam was reduced by refluxing with a solution of $LiAlH_4$ in THF to form benzyl-protected amino alcohol **81** in excellent yields. Deprotection of the *N*-benzyl group using catalytic hydrogenation followed by Boc protection yielded a Boc-protected prolinol intermediate, which was oxidized with Jones reagent to yield functionalized proline **82**. The P_2 amino acid **82** was

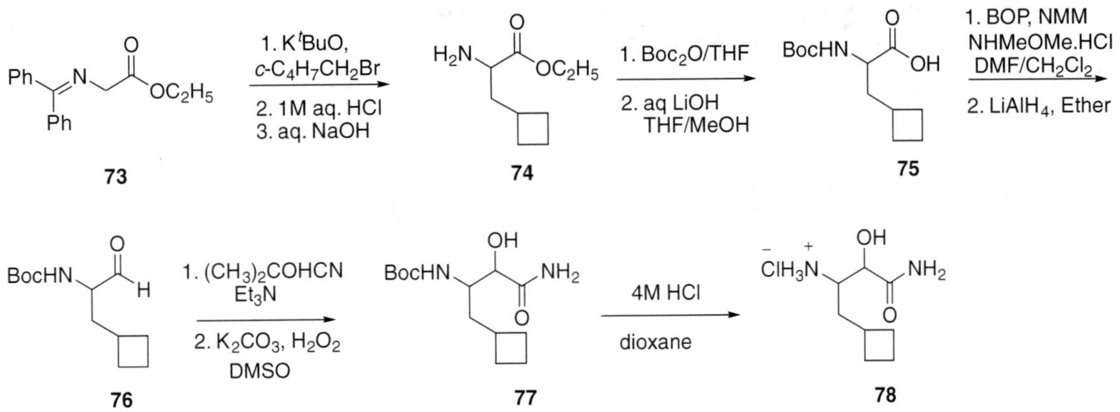

SCHEME 1 Synthesis of ketoamide segment.

coupled with P_3 *tert*-butyl glycine, using HATU to yield Boc-protected dipeptide. The Boc group of the resulting dipeptide was deprotected with methanolic HCl and treated with *tert*-butyl isocyanate to form *tert*-butyl urea P_3 capped compound **83**. The methyl ester of **83** was hydrolyzed with aqueous LiOH and the resulting acid was coupled with P_1 amine salt **78** using EDCI, HOBt, and NMM to yield the hydroxyamide precursor of boceprevir (**69**). Finally, the ketoamide functionality was installed by oxidizing the hydroxyamide derivative under Moffat conditions using EDCI, DMSO, and $Cl_2CHCOOH$ to form Sch 503034 (**69**).

X-RAY STRUCTURE OF BOCEPREVIR BOUND TO HCV-NS3 PROTEASE

The x-ray structure of boceprevir bound to HCV-NS3 protease was solved, and many salient features paramount for effective binding to the protease were identified (Fig. 16). Analysis of the x-ray structure revealed a shallow binding pocket that was occupied by inhibitor **69** [50]. The hydroxyl group of serine-139 made a nucleophilic attack on ketoamide reversibly trapping the inhibitor while the amide oxygen pointed toward the oxy-anion hole. The P_1 cyclobutyl alanine occupied the S_1 pocket, with the (*S*)-stereochemistry being preferred at the ketoamide center. The P_2 dimethylcyclopropyl fused proline moiety efficiently made contact with the S_2 pocket, with the two methyl groups interacting with protein residues arginine-155 and alanine-156. The dimethyl cyclopropanated proline adopts a bent conformation which makes an effective overlap with the methyl group of alanine-156. The *tert*-butyl groups of P_3 *tert*-butyl glycine and P_3 capping *tert*-butyl urea made efficient van der Waals contact with the shallow S_3 pocket and S_4 pockets, respectively. Thus, a series of efficient van der Waals interactions contributed to potent binding of the inhibitor to the protease.

In addition to lipophilic interactions, boceprevir made an array of hydrogen bonds with the protein backbone that contributed to enhanced enzyme binding and selectivity. A

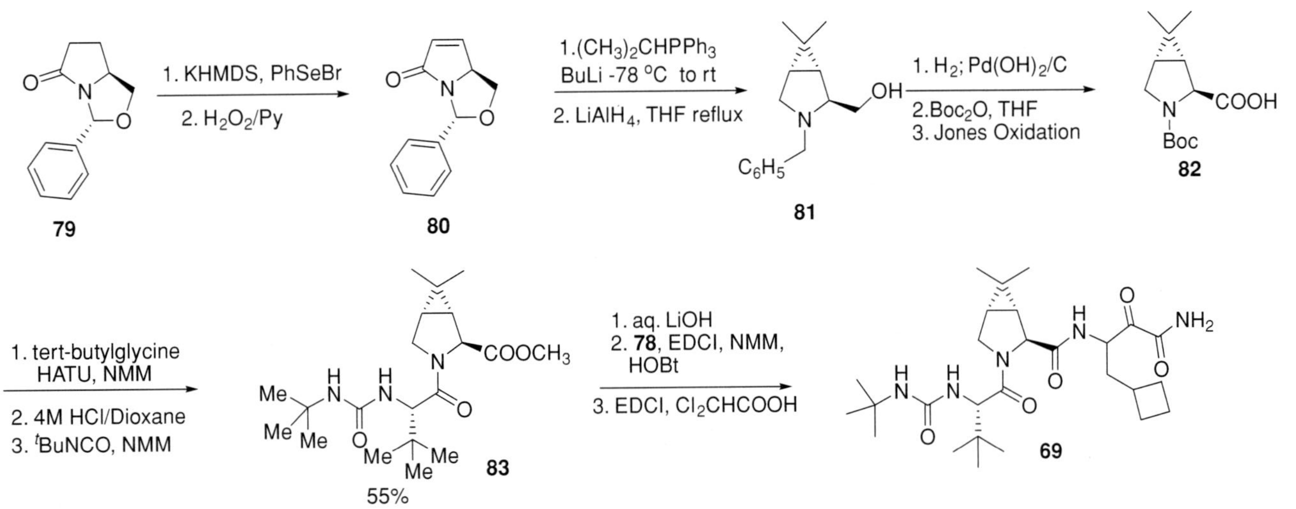

SCHEME 2 Synthesis of boceprevir.

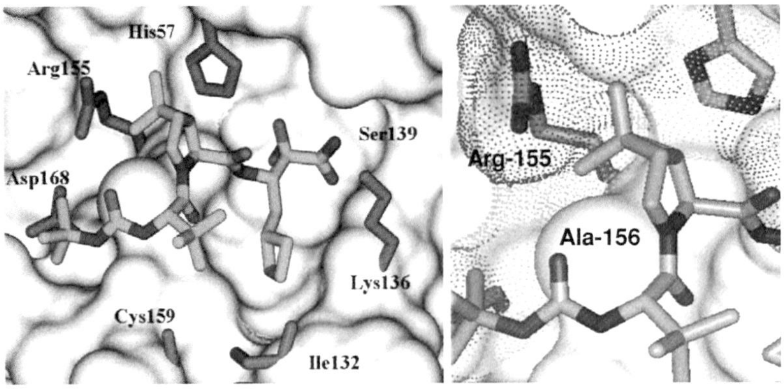

FIGURE 16 *See insert for color representation of the figure.*

schematic diagram of these mapped interactions is outlined in Figure 17.

Analysis of these hydrogen-bonding interactions revealed that the hydrogen of primary ketoamide formed a hydrogen bond with an oxygen of glutamine-41, whereas the oxygen of the primary amide accepted a hydrogen bond from residues glycine-137 and serine-139. The NH of the P_1 cyclobutyl alanine moiety is at a hydrogen-bonding distance to arginine-155, whereas the urea hydrogens donated a pair of hydrogen bonds to the oxygen of alanine-157. These interactions are specific, enhancing the effectiveness of binding of boceprevir to HCV protease.

A computational analysis was conducted to evaluate the contribution of various residues to the overall binding of the inhibitor to the enzyme. These calculations indicate that a substantial proportion of binding correlates well with the contact surface area. It was estimated that nearly 50% of the surface area of boceprevir made hydrophobic contact with the protease, which contributes to 10^5 orders in binding. The remaining potency gain was achieved with boceprevir, making hydrogen bonds to the protease and the covalent bond to serine-139.

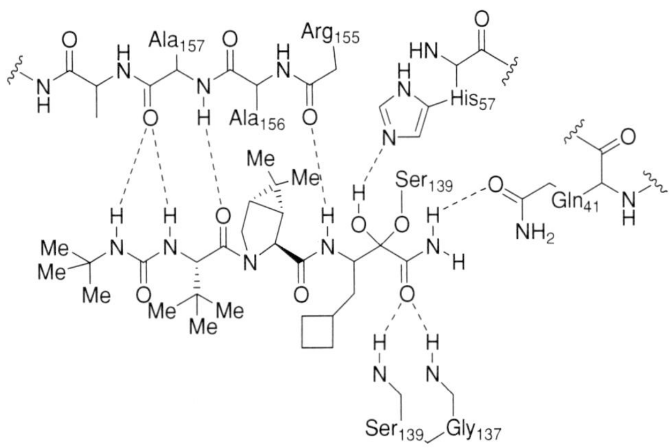

FIGURE 17

IN VITRO COMBINATION STUDIES OF BOCEPREVIR AND α-INTERFERON

The effect of combination of α-interferon with boceprevir was evaluated by treating different concentrations of **69** to a fixed dose of α-interferon in a 10 × 10 matrix, varying the concentration from EC_{50} to EC_{90}. Analysis of replicon RNA levels after 72 h at 90% suppression indicated that the effect of combination with α-interferon was additive [48].

Clinical studies of boceprevir. Boceprevir has completed initial Phase III clinical trials and the result is currently being reviwed by drug authorities as a potential treatment of HCV infections.

Resistance studies. Mutations conferring resistance to boceprevir have been identified and characterized by selection in the replicon cells [51,52]. T54A, A156S, A156T, and V170A were detected as the major resistance loci prevalent, in frequencies ranging from 12 to 31%.

CONCLUSIONS

Lack of success in identifying nonpeptic leads using a screening approach forced us to pursue a structure-based rational drug development strategy guided by the x-ray crystal structure of NS3 protease. An undecapeptide **7** incorporating a ketoamide as a serine trap was identified as an initial lead that had a molecular weight of 1265 Da. This inhibited the enzyme with a $K_i^* = 1.9$ nM. We undertook the daunting task of modifying this lead to identify boceprevir. Initially, we followed a truncation approach to reduce the molecular weight and determine the effect on enzyme binding of each amino acid replacement. Using a systematic study, we identified leucine and cyclopropyl alanine as excellent P_2 residues that yielded novel inhibitors with excellent enzyme inhibition. A conscious effort to truncate the molecule at P_3 limiting molecular weights in the desirable drug range was undertaken. The incorporation of a P_1'–P_2' glycine-phenylglycine segment yielded compounds such as

25, spanning from P_3 to P_2' with excellent enzyme activity. These compounds demonstrated an enzyme inhibition in the low nanomolar range, with molecular weights ranging between 700 and 800 Da.

We next evaluated these potent inhibitors for their activity in the replicon-based cellular assay and pharmacokinetics in animals. To our disappointment, most of these compounds showed poor cellular activity and oral PK. To address these issues we embarked on a depeptidization strategy of investigating a series of macrocyclic inhibitors and replacing amide bonds with peptide isosteres. A series of novel P_2 to P_4- and P_1–P_3-derived macrocycles spanning from P_3 to P_2' were synthesized and evaluated for their binding and cellular activity. None of these modifications resulted in compounds with desirable cellular potency and PK.

Concomitant to these investigations, we discovered that incorporation of a secondary amide at P_2 resulted in analogs that were active in the replicon cellular assay. This was a major discovery which allowed us to engineer novel compounds that were potent in both the enzyme-binding and cellular assay. A series of inhibitors containing modified proline derivatives were synthesized and incorporated in our series of inhibitors. A novel dimethylcyclopropyl-fused proline that mimicked leucine and cyclopropyl alanine were synthesized and incorporated in the inhibitors, resulting in compounds with excellent enzyme-binding and replicon activity. This led to the identification of Sch-6 (**38**), which demonstrated EC_{90} = 100 nM in the replicon cellular assay. However, an evaluation of these compounds for PK in animals demonstrated that these compounds had a suboptimal oral exposure. It was determined that these compounds were poorly absorbed and needed further modification to introduce druglike properties.

Our quest for compounds with oral PK mandated that we reduce the molecular weights of these inhibitors further or reduce the number of hydrogen-bond donors and acceptors. We revisited our truncation strategy and truncated Sch-6 at P_1 by incorporating a primary ketoamide. This resulted in compounds of type **38** that had acceptable binding and cellular activity and PK. Systematic modification of various residues at P_1, P_3, and P_3 capping identified cyclobutyl alanine, *tert*-butylglycine, and *tert*-butylurea as desired groups resulting in compound **69** (Sch 503034), which demonstrated a combination of good enzyme activity, cellular potency, HNE selectivity, and PK. In the course of these investigations we discovered novel synergies between P_1–P_3, P_3, and P_3 capping groups that influenced enzyme binding and HNE selectivity positively and detrimentally.

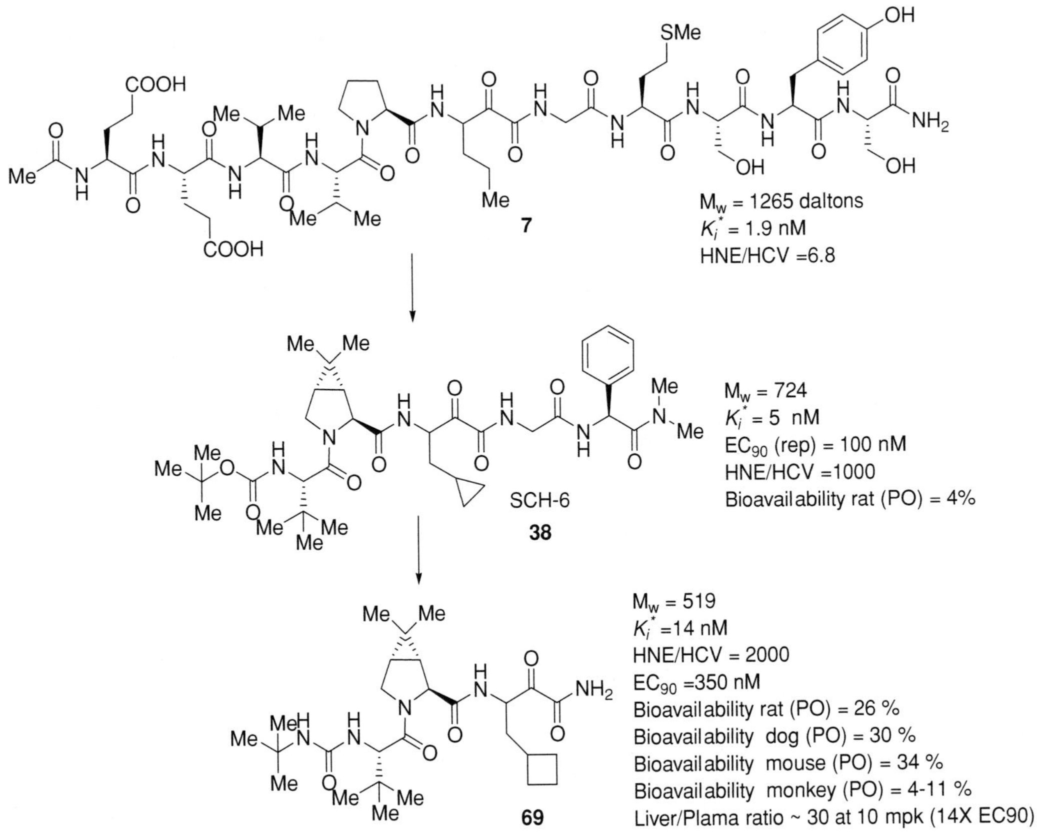

FIGURE 18

Our journey from the undecapeptide to boceprevir is summarized in Figure 18. The undecapeptide **7** was first modified to Sch-6 (**38**), which reduced the molecular weights from 1265 Da to 724 Da, imparting excellent enzyme-binding and cellular activity. However, these classes of compounds demonstrated poor PK in rats. We therefore investigated truncating these compounds, simultaneously modifying the P_1 and P_3 moiety to identify Sch 503034 (**69**) with a molecular weight of 519 Da and good enzyme and cellular activity. It also demonstrated acceptable PK in rat, mouse, and dog.

Boceprevir has completed initial Phase III clinical trials and the result is currently being reviewed by drug authorities as a potential treatment of HCV infections.

Acknowledgment

The authors would like to thank Andrew Prongay for kindly providing pictures of various x-ray structures.

REFERENCES

[1] World Health Organization. Fact sheet 164, Oct. 2000.

[2] Wasley, A., et al. Epidemiology of hepatitis C: geographic differences and temporal trends. *Semin. Liver Dis.* **2000**, *20*, 1–16.

[3] Brown, R. S., Jr., et al. Scope of worldwide hepatitis C problem. *Liver Transpl.* **2003**, *9* (11), S10–S13.

[4] McHutchison, J. G., et al. Interferon alfa-2b alone or in combination with ribavirin as initial treatment for chronic hepatitis C. *N. Engl. J. Med.* **1998**, *339*, 1485–1492.

[5] Davis, G. L., et al. Interferon alfa-2b alone or in combination with ribavirin for treatment of relapse of chronic hepatitis C. *N. Engl. J. Med.* **1998**, *339*, 1493–1499.

[6] Zeuzem, S., et al. Peginterferon alfa-2a in patients with chronic hepatitis C. *N. Engl. J. Med.* **2000**, *343*, 1666–1172.

[7] Heathcote, E. J., et al. Peginterferon alfa-2a in patients with chronic hepatitis C and cirrhosis. *N. Engl. J. Med.* **2000**, *343*, 1673–1680.

[8] Manns, M. P., et al. Peginterferon alfa-2b plus ribavirin compared with interferon alfa-2b plus ribavirin for initial treatment of chronic hepatitis C: a randomized trial. *Lancet* **2001**, *358*, 958–965.

[9] Lamarre, D., et al. An NS3 protease inhibitor with antiviral effects in humans infected with hepatitis C virus. *Nature* **2003**, *426*, 186–189.

[10] Labrador, L., et al. Hepatitis C virus NS3/4A protease inhibitors. *Recent Pat. Anti-infect. Drug Discov.* **2008**, *3*, 157–167.

[11] Thompson, A., et al. Directly acting antivirals for the treatment of patients with hepatitis C infection: a clinical development update addressing key future challenges. *J. Hepatol.* **2009**, *50*, 184–194.

[12] De Francesco, R., et al. Challenges and successes in developing new therapies for hepatitis C. *Nature* **2005**, *436*, 953–960.

[13] Tsantrizos, Y. S. Peptidomimetic therapeutic agents targeting the protease enzyme of the human immunodeficiency virus and hepatitis C virus. *Acc. Chem. Res.* **2008**, *41*, 1252–1263.

[14] Sheldon, J., et al. Novel protease and polymerase inhibitors for the treatment of hepatitis C virus infection. *Expert Opin. Invest. Drugs* **2007**, *16*, 1171–1181.

[15] Chen, K. X., et al. A review of HCV protease inhibitors. *Curr. Opin. Invest. Drugs* **2009**, *10*, 821–837.

[16] Brazil, M. Antiviral drugs: macrocyclic inhibitor for hepatitis C. *Nat. Rev. Drug Discov.* **2003**, *212*, 945.

[17] Tsantrizos, Y. S., et al. Macrocyclic inhibitors of the NS3 protease as potential therapeutic agents of hepatitis C virus infection. *Angew. Chem. Int. Ed.* **2003**, *42*, 1356.

[18] Kaito, M., et al. Hepatitis C virus particle detected by immunoelectron microscopic study. *J. Gen. Virol.* **1994**, *75*, 1755–1760.

[19] Bartenschlager, R. The NS3/4A proteinase of the hepatitis C virus: unravelling structure and function of an unusual enzyme and a prime target for antiviral therapy. *J. Viral. Hepatitis* **1999**, *6*, 165–181.

[20] Bartenschlager, R., et al. Nonstructural protein 3 of the hepatitis C virus encodes a serine-type proteinase required for cleavage at the NS3/4 and NS4/5 junctions. *J. Virol.* **1993**, *67*, 3835–3844.

[21] Reed, K. E., et al. Molecular characterization of hepatitis C virus. In *Hepatitis C Virus*, Reesink H. W., Ed., S. Karger, Basel, Switzerland, 1998, pp. 1–37.

[22] Lindenbach, B. D., et al. Unravelling hepatitis C virus replication from genome to function. *Nature* **2005**, *436*, 933–938.

[23] Perni, R. B., et al. Inhibitors of hepatitis C virus NS3·4A protease: 3. P_2 proline variants. *Bioorg. Med. Chem. Lett.* **2004**, *14*, 1939–1942.

[24] McCauley, J.A., et al. Discovery of vaniprevir (MK-7009), a macrocyclic hepatitis C verus NS3/4A protease inhibitor. *J. Med. Chem.* **2010**, *53*, 2443–2463.

[25] Seiwert, S. D., et al. Preclinical characteristics of the hepatitis C virus NS3/4A protease inhibitor ITMN-191 (R7227). *Animicrob. Agents Chemother.* **2008**, *52*, 4432–4441.

[26] Raboisson, P., et al. Structure–activity relationship study on a novel series of cyclopentane-containing macrocyclic inhibitors of the hepatitis C virus NS3/4A protease leading to the discovery of TMC435350. *Bioorg. Med. Chem. Lett.* **2008**, *18*, 4853–4858.

[27] Yan, Y., et al. Complex of NS3 protease and NS4A peptide of BK strain hepatitis C virus: a 2.2 Å resolution structure in a hexagonal crystal form. *Prot. Sci.* **1998**, *7*, 837–847.

[28] Love, R. A., et al. The crystal structure of hepatitis C virus NS3 proteinase reveals a trypsin-like fold and a structural zinc binding site. Cell **1996**, *87*, 331–342.

[29] Kim, J. L., et al. Hepatitis C virus NS3 RNA helicase domain with a bound oligonucleotide: the crystal structure provides insights into the mode of unwinding. *Structure* **1998**, *6*, 89–100.

[30] Kwong, A. D., et al. Hepatitis C virus NS3/4A protease. *Antiviral Res.* **1998**, *40*, 1–18.

[31] J. L. Kim, et al. Crystal structure of the hepatitis C virus NS3 protease domain complexed with a synthetic NS4A cofactor peptide. *Cell* **1996**, *87*, 343.

[32] Steinkuhler, C., et al. Activity of purified hepatitis C virus protease NS3 on peptide substrates. *J. Virol.* **1996**, *70*, 6694–6700.

[33] Urbani, A., et al. A substrate specificity of the hepatitis C virus serine protease NS3. *J. Biol. Chem.* **1997**, *272*, 9204–9209.

[34] Kolykhalov, A. A., et al. Specificity of the hepatitis C virus NS3 serine protease: effects of substitutions at the 3/4A, 4A/4B, 4B/5A, and 5A/5B cleavage sites on polyprotein processing. *J. Virol.* **1994**, *68*, 7525–7533.

[35] Zhang, R., et al. A continuous spectrophotometric assay for the hepatitis C virus serine protease. *Anal. Biochem.* **1999**, *270*, 268–275.

[36] Bogen, S. L., et al. Depeptidization efforts on P_3–P_2' α-ketoamide inhibitors of HCV NS3-4A serine protease: effect on HCV replicon activity. *Bioorg. Med. Chem. Letts.* **2006**, *16*, 1621–1627.

[37] Lohmann, V., et al. Replication of subgenomic hepatitis C virus RNAs in a hepatoma cell line. *Science* **1999**, *285*, 110–113.

[38] Bogen, S. L., et al. Hepatitis C virus NS3-4A serine protease inhibitors; Use of a P_2–P_1 cyclopropyl alanine combination for improved potency. *Bioorg. Med. Chem. Lett.* **2005**, *15*, 4515–4519.

[39] Tyndall, J. D. A., et al. Macrocycles mimic the extended peptide conformation recognized by aspartic, serine, cysteine, and metallo proteases. *Curr. Med. Chem.* **2001**, *8*, 893–907.

[40] Venkatraman, S., et al. Design and synthesis of depeptidized macrocyclic inhibitors of hepatitis C NS3-4A protease using structure-based drug design. *J. Med. Chem.* **2005**, *48*, 5088–5091.

[41] Chen, K. X., et al. Novel potent hepatitis C virus NS3 serine protease inhibitors derived from proline-based macrocycle. *J. Med. Chem.* **2006**, *49*, 995–1005.

[42] Bogen, S. L., et al. Discovery of SCH446211 (SCH6): A new ketoamide inhibitor of the HCV NS3 serine protease and HCV subgenomic RNA replication. *J. Med. Chem.* **2006**, *49*, 2750–2757.

[43] Mamai, A., et al. Poly-L-proline type-II peptide mimics based on the 3-azabicyclo[3.1.0]hexane system. *J. Org. Chem.* **2001**, *66*, 455–460.

[44] Zhang, R., et al. Design, synthesis and evaluation of poly-L-proline type-II peptide mimics based on the 3-azabicyclo[3.1.0]hexane system. *J. Org. Chem.* **1999**, *64*, 330–331.

[45] Arasappan, A., et al. Novel dipeptide macrocycles from 4-oxo, -thio, and -amino-substituted proline derivatives. *J. Org. Chem.* **2002**, *67*, 3923–3926.

[46] Cox, K. A., et al. A novel in vivo procedure for the rapid rat pharmacokinetic screening of discovery compounds in rat. *Drug Discov. Today* **1999**, *4*, 232–237.

[47] Venkatraman, S., et al. Discovery of (1*R*,5*S*)-*N*-[3-amino-1-(cyclobutylmethyl)-2-3-dioxopropyl]-3-[2(*S*)-[[[(1,1-dimethylethyl)-amino]carbonyl]amio]-3,3-dimethyl-1-oxobutyl]-6,6-dimethyl-3-azabicyclo[3.1.0]hexan-2(*S*)-carboxamide (Sch 503034), a selective, potent, orally bioavailable, hepatits C virus NS3 protease inhibitor: a potential therapeutic agent for the treatment of hepatitis C infection. *J. Med. Chem.* **2006**, *49*, 6074–6086.

[48] Malcolm, B., et al. Sch 503034, a mechanism-based inhibitor of hepatitis C virus NS3 protease, suppresses polyprotein maturation and enhances the antiviral activity of alpha interferon in replicon cells. *Antimicrob. Agents Chemother.* **2006**, *50* (3), 1013–1020.

[49] Cheng, K.-C., et al. Use of pre-clinical in vitro and in vivo pharmacokinetics for selection of potent hepatitis C protease inhibitor, boceprevir, for clinical development. *Lett. Drug Des. Discover.* **2009**, *6*, 312–318.

[50] Prongay, A., et al. Discovery of the HCV NS3/4A protease inhibitor (1*R*,5*S*)-*N*-[3-amino-1-(cyclobutylmethyl)-2,3-dioxopropyl]-3-[2(*S*)-[[[(1,1-dimethylethyl)amino]carbonyl] amino]-3,3-dimethyl-1-oxobutyl]-6,6-dimethyl-3-azabicyclo[3.1.0]hexan-2(*S*)-carboxamide (Sch 503034): key steps in structure-based optimization. *J. Med. Chem.* **2007**, *50*, 2310–2318.

[51] Tong, X., et al. Identification and analysis of fitness of resistance mutations against the HCV protease inhibitor Sch 503034. *Antiviral Res.* **2006**, *70*, 28–38.

[52] Tong, X., et al. Impact of naturally occurring variants of HCV protease on the binding of different classes of protease inhibitors. *Biochemistry* **2006**, *45*, 1353–1361.

18

DISCOVERY AND DEVELOPMENT OF THE HCV NS3/4A PROTEASE INHIBITOR DANOPREVIR (ITMN-191/RG7227)

SCOTT D. SEIWERT, KARL KOSSEN, LIN PAN, JYANWEI LIU, AND BRAD O. BUCKMAN

InterMune, Inc., Brisbane, California

INTRODUCTION

Chronic hepatitis C virus (HCV) infection afflicts more than 170 million people worldwide and is the leading cause of liver transplantation in the United States [1,2]. Standard of care (SoC) for this disease is weekly injection of pegylated interferon α and twice-daily oral administration of ribavirin. This regimen has significant side effects and achieves the clinically relevant endpoint of sustained virological response (SVR), defined as viral negativity 6 months following cessation of therapy, in only half of treated patients [3,4]. Poorer response rates are observed in certain subpopulations, including persons harboring genotype 1 virus or a high viral load, cirrhotic patients, and African Americans [3,4]. Thus, novel therapeutic approaches that have milder side effects and that enhance SVR rates compared with SoC are needed to better treat this prevalent and serious disease.

Direct antiviral agents (DAA) target essential HCV-encoded enzymes, including the protease activity of nonstructural protein 3/4A (NS3/4A) and the RNA-directed RNA polymerase activity of NS5B [5–7]. NS3 is a chymotrypsin-like serine protease that is activated by association with NS4A. Following translation of the HCV RNA genome into a polyprotein, the NS3/4A protease cleaves four sites to liberate five viral proteins essential for HCV replication. In addition, the proteolytic activity of NS3/4A recently has been shown to dampen cellular sensing of viral components, and in doing so reduce type 1 interferon production [8,9]. Thus, inhibitors of NS3/4A may disrupt two separate processes relevant for suppression of HCV.

NS3/4A protease inhibitors (PIs) have shown potent antiviral activity in early clinical trials, highlighting the significant potential of this class of compounds. In landmark studies, ciluprevir (BILN-2061) was found to reduce the average plasma concentration of genotype 1 HCV by approximately 3.0 $\log_{10}$ following twice-daily dosing of 200 mg for 2 days [10,11]. Despite robust and rapid antiviral activity that at the time was unprecedented, further clinical development of ciluprevir was discontinued due to severe cardiac toxicity in nonclinical species [12].

Subsequently, several other NS3/4A PIs have demonstrated robust antiviral activity as monotherapy in chronic HCV [13–17]. In combination with SoC for 14 to 28 days, these compounds drive viral loads below the limit of quantification or detection in a majority of patients [14,16,18,19]. Two linear/nonmacrocyclic mechanism-based covalent inhibitors administered three times a day, boceprevir (Sch 503034) [20,21] and telaprevir (VX-950) [22–24], are considered first-generation NS3/4A PIs. Both boceprevir and telaprevir substantially improve SVR when added to SoC and therefore demonstrate the significant clinical utility of NS3/4A PIs [23–25]. However, both compounds equally demonstrate that side effects associated with triple combination therapy can compromise clinical utility due to treatment discontinuation [23–25]. Moreover, the requirement for three times daily dosing with first-generation PIs may lead to patient noncompliance, which in turn may allow drug-resistant viral variants to develop. Second-generation PIs have attempted to address these issues in order to further improve treatment outcomes.

Antiviral Drugs: From Basic Discovery Through Clinical Trials, First Edition. Edited by Wieslaw M. Kazmierski.

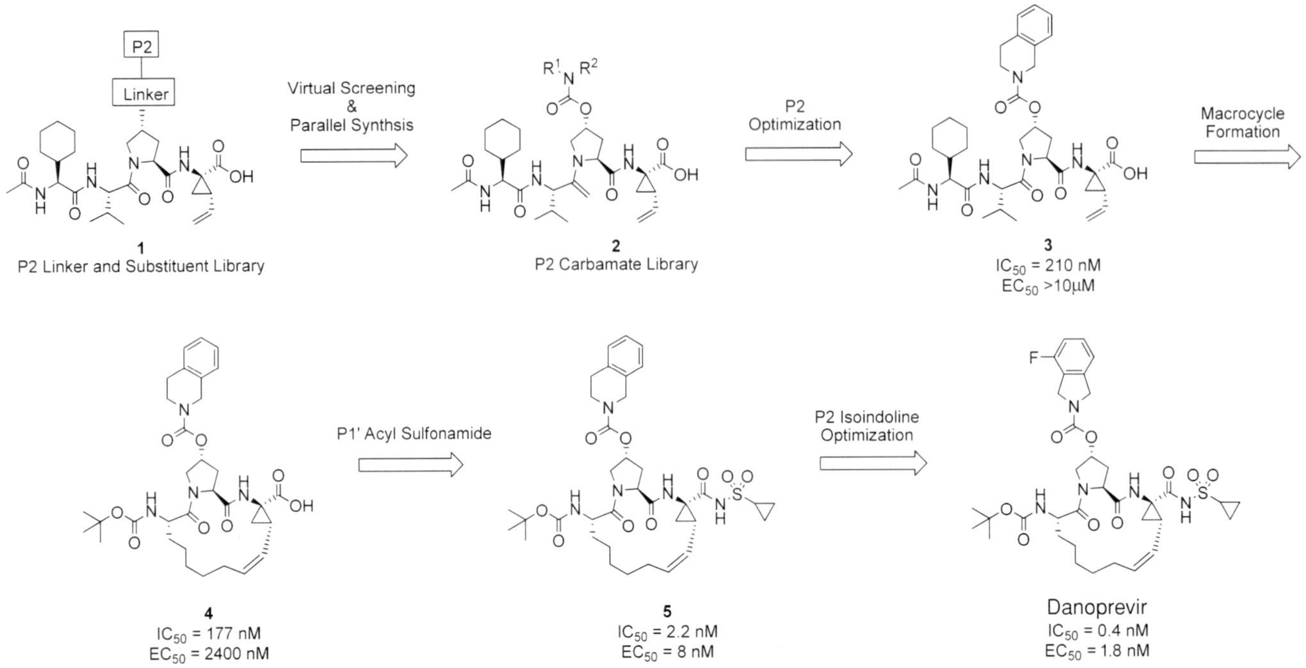

SCHEME 1 Significant compounds leading to the discovery of danoprevir.

The discovery campaign leading to danoprevir (RG7227/ITMN-191) focused on several fundamental principles to identify compounds with the potential for milder side effects and less frequent dosing relative to first-generation PIs. A premium was placed on maximizing potency and selectivity since more potent compounds require lower exposure to achieve a given pharmacological effect. Low exposure, combined with high selectivity, was hypothesized to translate into a superior safety profile. To further minimize side effects due to off-target effects, significant emphasis was placed on identifying compounds that, like statins [26–28], have preferential distribution to the liver. Since ribivirin and most NS5B polymerase inhibitors currently in development are administered twice daily, this dosing scheme was also viewed as desirable.

In this chapter we describe the data available for danoprevir, a compound discovered following the principles noted above. Clinical studies completed to date indicate that danoprevir has low systemic exposure, possesses a very favorable side-effect profile, and elicits a potent antiviral effect. The strategy used in the discovery of danoprevir parallels that of statins and suggests that this approach may be of general value in the discovery of liver-targeted therapies.

DISCOVERY

Initially, a virtual chemical library of approximately 500 molecules was designed and screened using a docking model developed from NS3 x-ray crystal structures and peptide-substrate binding motifs. Through this structure-based design approach, virtual tetrapeptide compound libraries were generated and scored in a docking model using NS3/4A protease domain. These libraries carried a P1–P1′ carboxylic acid group and a diverse collection of P2 linkers and P2 substituents to probe the lipophilic S2 protein surface region (**1**, Scheme 1). Based on initial potency data in a biochemical screening assay, tetrapeptides with P2 carbamates extending from a hydroxyproline were selected as targets, and a library of over 70 tetrapeptides with various P2 carbamates attached to proline was synthesized (**2,** Scheme 1). A clear trend in the structure–activity relationship (SAR) emerged in which an appropriately placed lipophilic P2 group, preferably a fused or pendent aromatic, provided a significant improvement in biochemical potency. Through several iterations of P2 optimization, P2 tetrahydroisoquinoline carbamates emerged as a promising lead (**3,** Scheme 1). This lead, although potent in the biochemical screening assay, showed no cellular potency in a replicon-based assay at its top concentration (10 μM).

Two strategies were pursued to increase the cellular potency of **3**: (1) the P4 amino acid residue was truncated, and (2) macrocyclization was used to rigidify the molecule. By linking P1 and P3 portions of **3** and truncating the P4 one residue at the same time, the 15-membered macrocyclic tripeptide mimetic **4** was obtained. This compound retained equivalent potency to its tetrapeptide predecessor in the enzyme assay, and more importantly, marked the first inhibitor

TABLE 1 Pharmacokinetics of Closely Related Analogs in Rat Following a 30-mg/kg Oral Dose

Compound	Replicon EC50 (nM)	P2	P1′	Liver $AUC_{0\text{-}24h}$ (ng·h/mL)	Plasma $AUC_{0\text{-}24h}$ (ng·h/mL)	LPR (AUC)
ITMN-381	4.5	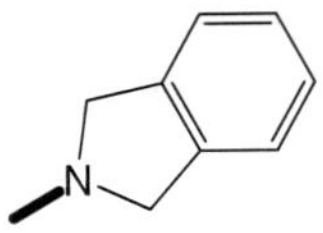	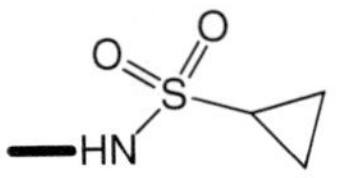	40.3	32.9	1.2
ITMN-119	9.2	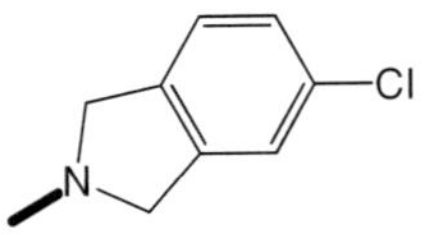	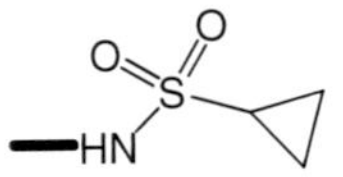	92.6	123.0	0.8
ITMN-408 (**5**, Scheme 1)	7.9	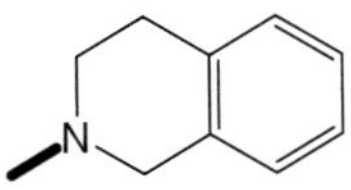	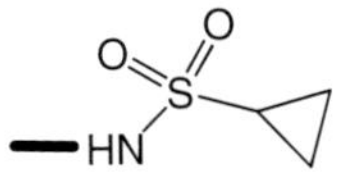	276.5	0.1	4608
ITMN-187	4.4	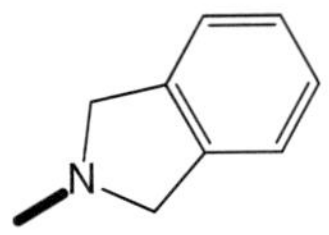	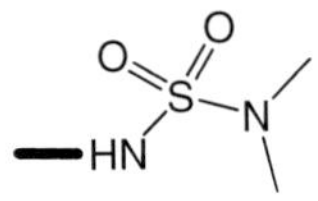	136.3	1.0	132
Danoprevir	1.8	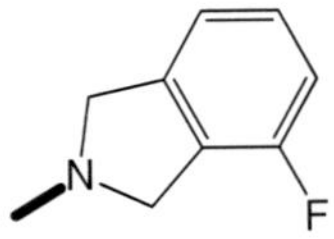	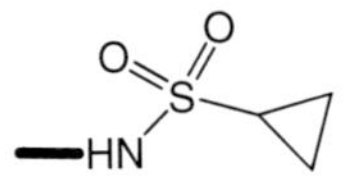	90.8	9.5	10

of this class to show antiviral activity in the replicon assay ($EC_{50} = 2400$ nM). These compounds were further optimized using a strategy to improve cellular permeability by replacing the P1–P1′ carboxylic acid with a bioisostere such as an acylsulfonamide [29]. Modification of the P1–P1′ carboxylic acid to an acylsulfonamide generated **5**, which showed excellent potency in cellular assays ($EC_{50} = 8$ nM).

Peptiodomimetic NS3/4A inhibitors in general, and macrocyclic compounds in particular, are large and non-"Lipinski"-like in character. These compounds are actively transported, and transporter interactions probably contribute significantly to their disposition in vivo. Perhaps because of this, classic in vitro ADME (absorption, distribution, metabolism, and excretion) profiling assays are generally not predictive of in vivo exposure. Consequently, in the danoprevir discovery campaign, such assays were deemphasized in favor of in vivo characterization. While high concentrations in the liver were desired, as this is the site of pharmacological effect, high circulating concentrations of an HCV inhibitor could potentially give rise to toxicity, so compounds were sought that displayed adequate exposure in the target organ but minimal exposure elsewhere. Initial data demonstrating these features were followed by a screening paradigm that filtered compounds for advancement based on rodent liver exposure, plasma exposure, and liver/plasma ratio (LPR).

Modifications in all key regions of **5** were examined systematically to evaluate their effects on plasma and liver pharmacokinetics in rat. Modifications examined included alternative macrocycles (saturated and heteroatom substitutions), various P2 urea and amide linkers, various P4 linker modifications, and various P2 tetrahydroisoquinoline replacements and substitutions. From initial data it was clearly evident that plasma concentration, liver concentration, and LPR varied widely in closely related analogs, making it impossible to use plasma concentration to predict whether the target organ enjoyed adequate exposure. Even small changes in the P2 and P1′ groups resulted in radically different exposure in liver and plasma, with LPRs ranging from 0.8 to approximately 4600 (Table 1 and see [30]). The significantly different exposure displayed by these analogs may reflect different affinities for uptake and efflux transporters as well as differences in their physiochemical properties.

More thorough profiling of the macrocyclic protease lead set revealed that a select group of these compounds dissociate very slowly from NS3/4A protease, leading to prolonged enzyme inhibition [31]. This characteristic was unexpected, as this series of compounds lacks the catalytic warhead found in first-generation protease inhibitors, which forms a covalent bond to the active-site serine and results in slowly reversible enzyme inhibition [22]. To more fully understand the inhibition kinetics, a biochemical assay was developed to characterize the dissociation rates. Structure–activity correlations using compounds lacking various features of the fully decorated macrocyclic core indicate that a single feature of a P1–P3 macrocycle was unlikely to be responsible for slow dissociation: compounds such as **5** show slow dissociation,

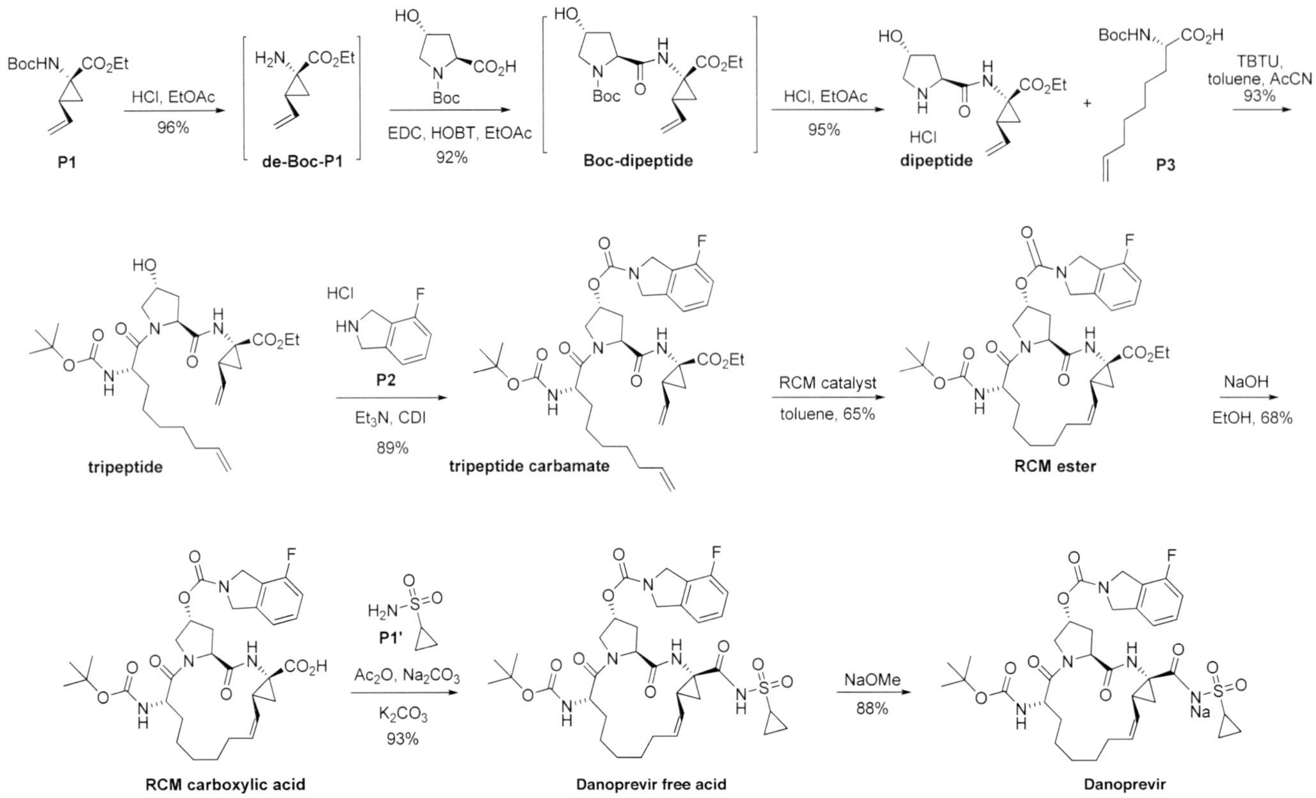

SCHEME 2 Danoprevir manufacturing process.

but analogs lacking P2, P4, the macrocyclic core, or the P1′ acylsulfonamide group display slow dissociation to lesser degrees or not at all. These observations are consistent with the fast dissociation rates reported for TMC-435350 [32] and ciluprevir [10] that lack P4 and P1′ groups, respectively. Slow dissociation from NS3/4A is a biochemical property that was considered desirable because it could potentially allow a pharmacodynamic effect after unbound drug is cleared. Thus, it was concluded that compounds with acyl sulfonamides such as **5** display more desirable NS3/4A inhibition kinetics than earlier prototype compounds lacking this functionality, P4 groups, the macrocyclic core, or carrying nonpreferable P2 groups.

An extensive effort, relying in part on screening potent, slowly dissociating compounds for exposure in rodent, led to the discovery of danoprevir (Scheme 1). Danoprevir features a 4-fluoro-substituted tetrahydroisoindoline P2 and an acyl sulfonamide in P1′. This compound's dissociation from NS3 is unexpectedly slow, it is over four-times more potent than **5** in the replicon cell assay, it displays a high degree of target specificity in biochemical and cell-based assays, and it displays high liver exposure relative to its potency and low exposure in plasma. Relative to compounds such as **5**, the plasma exposure of danoprevir in animals suggested that its exposure in humans could be monitored readily in the plasma compartment.

SYNTHESIS

The danoprevir manufacturing process is a nine-step linear synthesis with 24% overall yield at a 100-kg scale (Scheme 2). Retrosynthetically, danoprevir can be disconnected into five building blocks: P1, P2, P3, *N*-Boc hydroxyproline, and P1′. The synthesis proceeds through a ring-closing metathesis (RCM) reaction from a 17-membered open chain precursor. P1 is treated with HCl to remove the Boc protecting group. Without isolation the labile intermediate de-Boc-P1 is reacted with *N*-Boc-hydroxyproline to give the Boc-dipeptide, which is deprotected to provide crystalline dipeptide in 84% yield over three steps. P3 free amine, derived from the corresponding P3 dicyclohexylamine salt, is coupled with the dipeptide to afford the tripeptide, and it is subsequently reacted with P2 HCl salt in the presence of CDI to form the tripeptide carbamate in 89% isolated yield.

The tripeptide carbamate is subjected to a ring-closing metathesis reaction in toluene catalyzed by a ruthenium-based catalyst to give 65% isolated RCM ester.

Saponification of RCM ester yielded RCM carboxylic acid as a crystalline material in 68% yield. Activation of the RCM carboxylic acid by acetic anhydride followed by coupling reaction with P1′ produces danoprevir free acid in 93% yield. The sodium salt of danoprevir is obtained by treating a solution of the free acid in ethyl acetate with sodium methoxide and adding water to induce crystallization of the danoprevir salt in 80% yield.

STRUCTURAL BIOLOGY

Crystal structures of the NS3 protease domain in a complex with a 16-amino acid fragment of NS4A with and without danoprevir were determined through x-ray diffraction [33]. The danoprevir-bound structure identifies specific interactions that impart high affinity of danoprevir to NS3/4A (Fig. 1A). Danoprevir occupies the S1′–S4 portion of the substrate binding pocket with the P1′ cyclopropyl acyl sulfonamide filling both the serine protease active site and the adjacent P1′ pocket. The macrocycle fills a deep hydrophobic groove constituting the S1 through S3 substrate binding region and positions the P2 fluoroisoindolene carbamate and the P4 *tert*-butyl carbamate to interact with the S2 and S4 regions, respectively. Additionally, specific and extensive hydrogen-bonding interactions exist between residues of the active-site oxyanion hole and the P1′ acyl sulfonamide as well as the P1 amide and P4 N—H moieties and protein backbone carbonyls in the NS3/4A active site (Fig. 1B). Many but not all of these contacts are observed with natural substrates of NS3/4A (Fig. 1C). Comparison of the danoprevir-bound conformation of NS3/4A to the apo form reveals altered conformations of residues R123, D168 and R155, which define the P2 binding site, as well as K136. These structural alterations may relate to the slow dissociative property of danoprevir.

BIOCHEMICAL CHARACTERISTICS

Inhibition

A detailed kinetic characterization of the binding mechanism of danoprevir to NS3/4A has been reported [31]. Danoprevir appears to associate with NS3/4A in a two-step binding mechanism where an initial enzyme–inhibitor complex (EI) forms rapidly and converts slowly to a more stable form (EI^*). Microscopic rate constants within this mechanism were defined using a combination of enzyme inhibition assays and direct binding methods and together define the overall binding scheme (Fig. 2). Fitting biphasic reaction progress curves generates NS3 inactivation rate constants, which show a hyperbolic dependence on danoprevir concentration. This dependence provides values for the affinity of the initial complex (K_i = 100 nM), the rate constant for the conversion

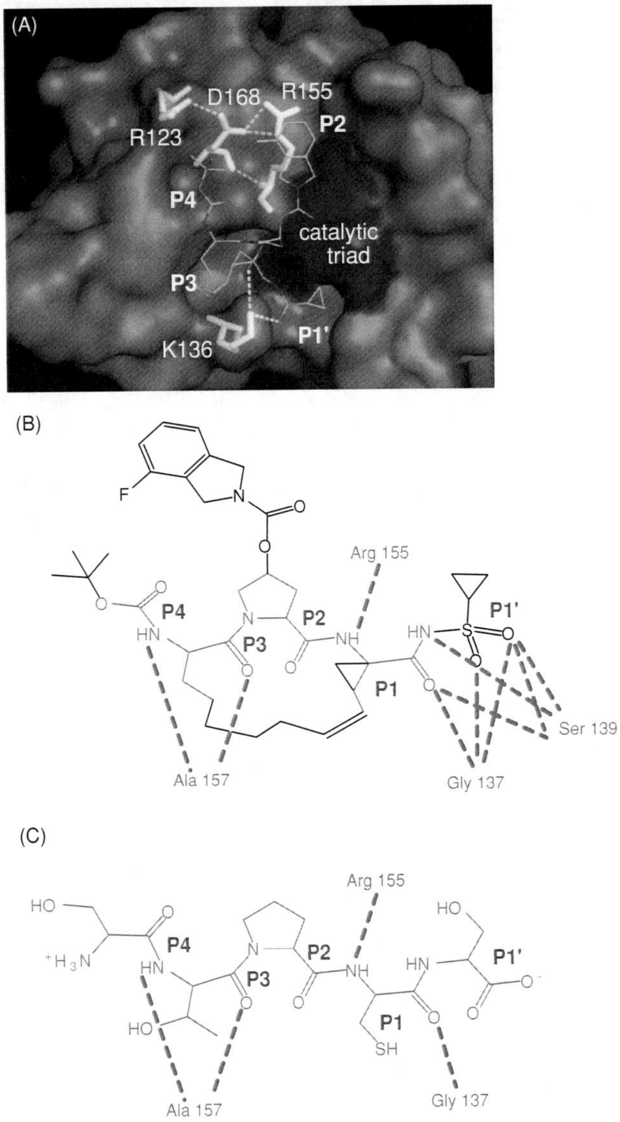

FIGURE 1 Structural biology. (A) Crystal structure of danoprevir·NS3/4A complex at 3.1 Å resolution showing P4, P3, P2, and P1′ sites (blue), catalytic triad (dark blue), and four residues that undergo conformational change upon danoprevir binding (white) and have polar interactions that are modulated by danoprevir binding (cyan). (B) Groups analogous to peptide sites P1′, P1, P2, P3, and P4 are indicated. Groups found in natural substrates of NS3/4A are shown in red. Polar contacts to NS3/4A are shown as thick green lines and the protein amino acid indicated. (C) Structure of the NS4B/5A junction of the HCV polyprotein that is cleaved by NS3/4A. Peptide sites P1′, P1, P2, P3, and P4, and scissile amide bond are indicated. Groups transferred directly to danoprevir are shown in red. Polar contacts to NS3/4A are shown as thick green lines and the protein amino acid indicated. (*See insert for color representation of the figure.*)

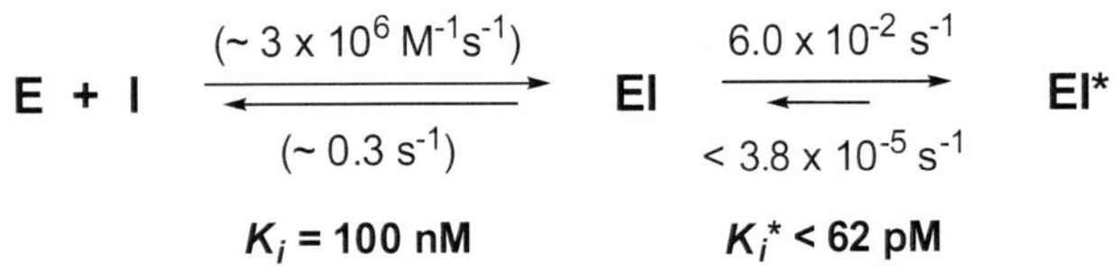

FIGURE 2 Kinetics of NS3/4A inhibition by danoprevir. Values for the rate and equilibrium constants associated with the proposed two-step binding mechanism are provided. Simulated rates are given in parentheses.

of EI to EI* ($k_3 = 6.2 \times 10^{-2}$ s^{-1}), and the conversion of EI* to EI ($k_4 < 3.8 \times 10^{-5}$ s^{-1}). This k_4 estimate implies that the NS3·danoprevir complex has a half-life of about 5 h if k_4 is assumed to be the rate-limiting step in dissociation. Additional experiments to determine the rate of danoprevir dissociation directly suggest that the EI* complex may be considerably more stable. Surface plasmon resonance and dilution experiments provide estimates of danoprevir dissociation rate constants of $< 2.1 \times 10^{-5}$ s^{-1} and $< 1.3 \times 10^{-6}$ s^{-1} ($t_{1/2} > 9$ h and > 6 days), respectively. However, the accuracy of these determinations are limited by the minimal dissociation or reactivation observed. Consequently, k_4 and K_i^* are conservatively reported as $< 3.8 \times 10^{-5}$ s^{-1} ($t_{1/2} >$ 5 h) and $<$ 62 pM, respectively, as determined by indirect kinetic methods (Fig. 2).

The exceptional potency of danoprevir due to its very slow dissociation from NS3/4A is an unexpected property that may have a potential benefit for both safety and efficacy. The ideal dosing scheme for a slowly dissociating drug reflects both its pharmacokinetics and the dissociative half-life of the drug–target complex. The concept of "ultimate physiological inhibition" has been coined to describe a situation where the pharmacological effect of a drug is limited by the synthesis of new target protein [34], and this concept is supported by experimental evidence [35,36]. Admittedly by this model, the assessment of the clinical impact of slow dissociation of an NS3/4A protease inhibitor is dependent on a reliable measure of viral protein turnover in infected human hepatocytes. Although a relevant measure of HCV protein synthesis has not been reported to our knowledge, the doubling time of HCV is about 22 h in cell culture [37] and 6 to 8 h in infected patients and chimpanzees [38,39]. If the time scale for viral protein turnover is similar, an appreciable contribution from slow dissociative behavior can be expected if the half-life of the inhibitor–protease complex is on the order of that displayed by danoprevir·NS3/4A. Thus, a slowly dissociating inhibitor such as danoprevir is expected to exert an antiviral effect even after unbound drug is cleared from the body. In a similar fashion, the HIV-1 protease inhibitors indinavir, saquinavir, and others dissociate slowly from the WT HIV-1 protease with half-lives of 10 to 100 min [40].

TABLE 2 Biochemical Specificity

	Number of Proteins Inhibited by 10 μM Drug[a]		
	Danoprevir	Ciluprevir	Telaprevir
Protease selectivity panel (53 proteins)	0	8[b]	9[c]
Broad ligand panel (26 proteins)	0	1[d]	0

[a]Proteins displaying = 50% inhibition at a drug concentration of 10 μM, suggesting an IC_{50} = 10 μM.
[b]Calpain-1, chymase, cathepsin G, cathepsin L2, cathepsin S, endothelin converting enzyme-1, factor Xa, HIV-1 protease.
[c]Chymase, chymotrypsin, cathepsin B, cathepsin E, cathepsin G, cathepsin L2, cathepsin S, neutrophil elastase 2, pancreatic elastase 1.
[d]hERG.

Off-Target Effects

As mentioned above, the side-effect profile of first-generation PIs reduces their utility in treatment by increasing treatment discontinuations [23,41–43]. In the discovery campaign of danoprevir, an early emphasis was placed on minimizing off-target activity. Chemical classes with progressively higher degrees of specificity were advanced. Thus, the specificity of danoprevir compares favorably with BILN-2061 and first-generation NS3/4A PIs (Table 2, see also [44]): None of a panel of 53 proteases or a panel of 23 ion channels and receptors is inhibited by more than 50% with 10 μM danoprevir, indicating an IC_{50} higher than 10 μM against every protease in this panel [45]. The high degree of selectivity displayed by danoprevir in biochemical assays is clearly evident in cell-based specificity assays as 50% cytotoxic concentrations (CC_{50} values) ranging from 75 to 340 μM in Huh7 cells and primary cultures of normal human hepatocytes, microvascular endothelial cells, human skeletal muscle myoblasts, human cardiac myocytes, human cardiac fibroblasts, human articular chondrocytes, human lung fibroblasts, and renal proximal tubule epithelial cells cultured under proliferating and nonproliferating conditions [45]. Biochemical and cellular specificity are more than 35,000- and 41,000-fold, respectively, and compare favorably to other experimental PIs which show much narrower specificity indices. Since ciluprevir and telaprevir display dissociation rates that are either substantially faster (ciluprevir, [10]) or relatively faster (telaprevir, [46]) than danoprevir, these data indicate that potency and specificity are not necessarily mutually exclusive for slowly dissociating noncovalent compounds such as danoprevir.

Genotypic Coverage

Biochemical potency was determined against full-length NS3/4A derived from clinical isolates representing all six

TABLE 3 Biochemical Potency of Danoprevir and Other NS3/4A Protease Inhibitors

	IC_{50} (nM)[a]				Fold Shift from K2040 Reference			
	Danoprevir	Telaprevir	Boceprevir	Ciluprevir	Danoprevir	Telaprevir	Boceprevir	Ciluprevir
1b-(K2040)	0.29 ± 0.07	130 ± 61	80 ± 15	0.73 ± 0.08	—	—	—	—
1a	0.20 ± 0.01	87 ± 5	80 ± 15	0.9 ± 0.2	0.69	0.67	1	1
1b	0.23 ± 0.01	98 ± 2	83 ± 6	0.8 ± 0.1	0.79	0.75	1	1
2b	1.6 ± 0.1	145 ± 5	76 ± 6	11 ± 1	5.5	1.1	1	15
3a	3.5 ± 0.5	1590 ± 22	230 ± 33	11.5 ± 0.8	12	12	3	16
4	0.24 ± 0.02	470 ± 16	170 ± 10	0.6 ± 0.1	0.83	3.6	2	0.8
5	0.35 ± 0.01	130 ± 58	70 ± 10	0.8 ± 0.2	1.2	1.0	0.9	1
6	0.45 ± 0.01	36.9 ± 0.8	54 ± 6	1.0 ± 0.2	1.6	0.28	0.7	1.4

[a]Values are reported as mean ± standard deviation based on a minimum of three independent experiments.

genotypes of HCV. Potency was measured under preequilibrium conditions that do not fully account for the contribution of slow dissociation to potency. Even so, these conditions provide an estimate of the relative effectiveness across different HCV genotypes. Given that clinical data exist for other NS3/4A inhibitors across multiple HCV genotypes, it is instructive to compare the performance of danoprevir to that of other compounds to model its potential performance against nongenotype 1 HCV in the clinic.

The IC_{50} of danoprevir, telaprevir, boceprevir, and ciluprevir against genotype 1a and 1b protein isolated from clinical samples is similar to their IC_{50} against the reference genotypes 1b protein (Table 3). Telaprevir and boceprevir also display similar potency against genotypes 1 and 2b NS3/4A, while the macrocyclic compounds ciluprevir and danoprevir lose potency against genotype 2b. All inhibitors except boceprevir show slightly more than a 10-fold loss of potency against NS3/4A derived from genotype 3a. Both macrocyclic inhibitors show undiminished activity against genotype 4 NS3/4A, whereas both linear tetrapetide inhibitors lose potency. All inhibitors show activity against genotype 5 or 6 NS3/4A.

Emerging clinical data describing compound activity across HCV genotypes suggests that biochemical inhibition data may be a useful indicator of clinical response. The clinical activity of telaprevir against genotype 1 and 2 HCV is similar, but markedly reduced activity against genotypes 3 and 4 is observed [41,47]. Clinical studies examining the antiviral efficacy of ciluprevir in a population comprised primarily of those harboring genotype 3 HCV indicate that short-term virologic response of ciluprevir monotherapy is marked, albeit reduced relative to its effect against genotype 1 HCV [12]. Consequently, provided that the same extrapolation holds for danoprevir, it is expected to be equally effective against genotype 1, 4, 5, and 6 HCV. Reduced activity against genotype 2 and 3 HCV is expected, so higher exposures would be required for efficacy in genotypes 2 and 3 compared to genotypes 1, 4, 5, and 6.

IN VITRO PHARMACOLOGY

Cellular Potency Against an HCV Subgenomic Replicon

The appreciable biochemical potency of danoprevir translates into significant antireplicon activity [45]. Against a genotype 1b (Con1) subgenomic HCV replicon, a 50% effective concentration (EC_{50}) was determined to be 1.8 nM. Calculation of the compound amount required for a 1 $\log_{10}$, 2 $\log_{10}$, or 3 $\log_{10}$ drop in replicon RNA (i.e., EC_{90}, EC_{99}, and $EC_{99.9}$) yielded 14, 160, and 1600 nM, respectively, indicating a standard, cooperative binding transition. A cell-based phenotyping assay provides an EC_{50} of 3.2 nM for a Con1 NS3/4A sequence; median danoprevir potency against multiple clinical isolates of subtype 1a NS3 ($n = 16$) and subtype 1b NS3 ($n = 24$) was 3.5 and 4.5 nM, respectively, showing that the compound inhibited multiple examples of genotype 1 NS3 with equal potency. The antiviral activity of danoprevir was also determined against con1 replicon following a 14-day exposure to replicon-bearing cells. Treatment with 45 nM danoprevir (~threefold its EC_{90}) reduced HCV replicon RNA levels below the RT-PCR detection limit and prevented selection of replicon containing cells in a 4-week follow-up period. Thus, the high potency of danoprevir in biochemical assays translated directly into high potency in cell-based assays.

Antiviral Activity in Combination with Peginterferon α-2a

As has been firmly established in the HIV PI field [48], early clinical development in HCV has indicated that NS3/4A PIs must be combined with other antiviral agents to suppress the emergence of PI-resistant HCV [49–52]. Except in a single case to be discussed below, combination regimens in HCV have employed one DAA in combination with SoC. Since the peginterferon component of SoC contributes to sustained virologic response by inducing direct antiviral effcts in infected hepatocytes, the antiviral effect of danoprevir was characterized in vitro in combination with peginterferon α-2a. In vitro dose–response curves for danoprevir and peginterferon α-2a indicate that the potency of each agent improves significantly when used in combination. Combination index (CI) values at fixed dose ratios are less than 1, indicating synergistic interaction. Antiviral synergy is confirmed by isobologram analysis based on Loewe additivity principles and by Bliss independence modeling of variable drug ratios. Thus, two orthogonal formal analyses indicate that danoprevir and peginterferon α-2a display significant antiviral synergy.

The combined antiviral effects of danoprevir and peginterferon α-2a were investigated following 14-day exposure of HCV replicon. When the minimum human plasma concentration of peginterferon α-2a is added to the lowest concentration of danoprevir tested (15 nM), replicon RNA levels are reduced below the limit of detection by RT-PCR, and no replicon-containing cells are selected in a 4-week follow-up period. When danoprevir is examined separately, 45 nM was required to eliminate HCV replicon RNA from cells. Thus, not only do these two agents display formal antiviral synergy, but peginterferon α-2a significantly enhances the ability of danoprevir to clear HCV replicon from Huh7 cells. These in vitro data provide a strong rationale for clinical study of danoprevir in combination with SoC.

Antiviral Activity in Combination with the NS5B Polymerase Inhibitor R7128

SoC has a significant side-effect profile, and these side effects are not diminished by the addition of a PI. Thus, while addition of a PI to SoC is attractive because of the improved efficacy afforded by this triple combination, it is anticipated that interferon-sparing regimens with safety profiles superior to SoC triple combination would be of great value. Such regimens may be particularly useful in patients with poor interferon response, in those who have failed therapy with SoC, and in patients for whom SoC is contraindicated. It is anticipated that multiple antiviral agents of distinct mechanism of action will be required in interferon-sparing regimens to suppress drug-resistant HCV variants [23,41,51–54]. DAA cocktails, and later fixed-dose combinations, have been essential in the treatment of HIV [55].

Combination of NS3/4A PIs with NS5B polymerase nucleoside inhibitors (NI) represents a particularly interesting approach. Each of these inhibitor classes is in advanced development in combination with SoC, and PI and polymerase nucleoside inhibitor combinations have been highly successful in HIV [56,57]. NS3/4A PIs have potent antiviral activity but a relatively low barrier to the development of drug resistant HCV variants [13,49,51,58]. NS5B NIs have somewhat less dramatic virological responses in HCV monotherapy but have a very high genetic barrier to viral escape [59–61]. In combination with SoC, both NS3/4A PIs and NS5B NIs drive the viral load below the detectable limit in a majority of patients after 28 days or less of therapy [14,16,18,19,53,62–64].

Tan et al. reported in vitro studies on the combination of danoprevir with the active moiety of the NS5B NI R7128, indicating that the combination would increase the barrier to viral escape in chronic HCV patients [65]. Very low concentrations of the R7128 active moiety ($1\times EC_{50}$) prevent formation of danoprevir-resistant colonies otherwise associated with danoprevir exposure. In separate studies, replicon clearance in 14-day assays was greatly enhanced when the two agents were combined. Finally, mathematical analysis of combined antiviral effects indicated additive to slightly synergistic interactions between these two inhibitor classes. Such in vitro findings support the clinical exploration of danoprevir/R7128 combination as an option for certain HCV patients, particularly those with baseline characteristics predicting refraction to SoC treatment, patients who have failed SoC, and patients with interferon contraindications.

NONCLINICAL PHARMACOKINETICS

Preferential exposure to the target organ is a strategy that was employed with great success in the development of statins, which target HMG-CoA reductase in the liver to reduce circulating cholesterol. Several of these compounds, including lovastatin, have very low oral bioavailability owing to significant first-pass clearance to the liver [26–28]. Low systemic exposure outside the liver is thought to be related to the differing side-effect profiles associated with various statins [26–28]. Since the site of pharmacological action for both statins and anti-HCV drugs is the liver, the statin experience can be used as a model. Consequently, the discovery paradigm leading to danoprevir targeted compounds displaying liver concentrations predictive of efficacy, but low plasma exposure to minimize any potential toxicities associated with circulating drug.

Pharmacokinetic parameters were obtained following administration at multiple oral dose levels to rats or cynomolgus monkeys by harvesting liver and sampling plasma at multiple time points (see Table 4 for a 30-mg/kg single dose). Importantly, the concentrations of danoprevir observed in the liver of both species at modest doses was significantly above the EC_{50} of danoprevir, although concentrations in rat are higher than those in monkey (Table 4). In rat at 30 mg/kg, the maximum liver concentration (C_{max}) and the 12-h post-dose liver concentration (C_{12h}) are sufficient in vitro to reduce HCV replicon RNA levels by 4.0 $\log_{10}$ and 3.2 $\log_{10}$, respectively, in 2-day assays and to clear HCV replicon from cells in 14-day antiviral assays (Table 4). In monkey liver tissue after the same dose, the C_{max} and C_{12h} are sufficient to reduce HCV replicon RNA by 3.1 $\log_{10}$ and 2.0 $\log_{10}$, respectively,

TABLE 4 Nonclinical Pharmacokinetic Performance of Danoprevir (30 mg/kg, p.o.)

		Pharmacokinetic Parameters			Replicon Response Supported[a] ($\log_{10}$ Reduction)		Elimination of HCV Replicon Supported[b]	
		AUC_{inf}[c] (μg·h/mL)	C_{max}[d] (μg/mL)	$C_{12\,h}$[d] (μg/mL)	C_{max}	C_{12h}	C_{max}	C_{12h}
Rat	Liver	90.8	12.7 ± 4.3	2.0 ± 1.3	4.0	3.2	Yes	Yes
	Plasma	9.50	1.1 ± 0.3	0.16 ± 0.12	2.9	2.1	Yes	Yes
	Liver/plasma ratio	10	11	12				
Primate	Liver	7.61	1.61	0.138	3.1	2.0	Yes	Yes
	Plasma	0.06	0.02	0.001	1.2	0.3	No	No
	Liver/plasma ratio	127	85	116				

[a]In vitro antiviral effect in a 2-day assay supported by in vivo concentration. Calculated based on an EC_{50} = 1.8 nM in the 48-h replicon reduction assay and a four-parameter logistic fit of inhibition data. Rounded to nearest 0.1 $\log_{10}$.
[b]Describes whether in vivo concentration exceeds concentration required for elimination of HCV replicon from Huh7 cells upon 14 days of exposure.
[c]Sacrifice of animal cohorts at various times prevented determination of average AUC_{inf}.
[d]Values are reported as mean ± standard deviation based on concentration in three rodents or concentration in two cynomolgus monkeys.

and would also result in HCV replicon clearance from cells in 14-day antiviral assays (Table 4). Plasma exposure in both species is significantly lower than liver exposure, suggesting that a majority of absorbed drug is subject to first-pass clearance to the liver. Thus, in nonclinical species danoprevir displays liver concentrations that if maintained in humans would be predictive of efficacy. As desired, plasma exposure in nonclinical species is low, minimizing the potential for systemic toxicities.

In rat, the LPR is roughly 10-, 11-, and 12-fold, based on total observed exposure (AUC_{inf}), C_{max}, and C_{12h}, respectively, while in monkey these ratios are 127-, 80-, and 40-fold, respectively (Table 4). These data indicate that the LPR differs in different nonclinical species. Interestingly, plotting AUC-based LPR from rat, monkey, and dog from several single- and multidose studies at various dose levels as a function of fractional plasma protein binding (PPB) provides a negative linear regression with $r^2 = 0.9$. Extrapolation to humans using human PPB suggests that liver exposure in humans would be 63 times the exposure observed in the plasma compartment. This type of analysis, together with human plasma exposure data from an early clinical study, was used to gauge whether liver exposure in humans at a specific dose would be adequate for virologic effect.

CLINICAL EXPERIENCE

Single Ascending Dose in Healthy Volunteers

Initial clinical experience with danoprevir was obtained in a single escalating dose study in healthy volunteers. Doses of 2, 100, 200, 400, 800, and 1600 mg were administered under fasted conditions. To investigate potential food effects, doses of 400 and 1600 mg were administered under high-fat fed conditions in a crossover design with their respective fasted doses. There were no serious adverse events or clinically significant laboratory or ECG abnormalities in this study [66]. All adverse events (AEs) reported by subjects receiving danoprevir were assessed by investigators as mild. AEs were similar between patients treated with placebo or danoprevir, with the exception of a higher frequency of mild and transient diarrhea and abdominal pain in the 1600-mg danoprevir dose groups. The PK of danoprevir was linear from 100 to 800 mg; a more than dose-proportional exposure increase was observed at 1600 mg. Coadministration with food delayed the time to maximal drug concentration (T_{max}), increased the expected trough and increased the area under the concentration–time curve ($AUC_{0-\infty}$). As with preclinical species, plasma exposure was low; a 400-mg dose under fed condition provided mean C_{max}, C_{12h}, and AUC_{inf} of 75 ng/mL, 0.3 ng/mL, and 122 ng·h/mL, respectively. Extrapolating liver exposure using predicted human LPR as calculated from plasma exposure and its relation to PPB evidenced in nonclinical species, the mean 12-h trough concentration in liver at this dose level would be approximately 12 times greater than the cell-based potency of the compound. These data provided a strong rationale for the study of danoprevir in chronic HCV.

Danoprevir Monotherapy in HCV Patients for 14 Days

To investigate the antiviral effect of danoprevir initially, treatment-naive, chronic HCV patients harboring genotype 1 were administered 100 or 200 mg of danoprevir every 8 h (q8h) or every 12 h (q12h) for 14 days. Prior null responders to SoC, those who had failed to achieve a ≥ 2 log10 reduction in HCV RNA at week 12 or undetectable HCV RNA at week 24 or beyond were administered 300 mg every 12 h. Danoprevir was safe and well tolerated in this study [13]. Adverse events were generally mild and transient and without association to treatment group or dose level. Danoprevir reduced HCV RNA in a dose-dependent manner in both q8h and q12h schedules; reductions occurred rapidly and were typically sustained through day 14. Maximal HCV RNA reductions approached 4 $\log_{10}$ IU/mL in both the 200-mg q12h and 200-mg q8h dosing cohorts. Comparison of the danoprevir AUC from hour 0 to trough on days 1 and 14 showed that danoprevir does not accumulate upon multiple dosing [67]. As designed in the discovery campaign and demonstrated in healthy volunteers, HCV patients displayed low plasma concentrations of danoprevir despite its robust virologic effect. At the highest dose tested (200 mg q8h), the mean day 1 $AUC_{0\text{-}24h}$, C_{max}, and C_{min} values were 500 ng·h/mL, 91 ng/mL, and 2.78 ng/mL, respectively. The corresponding mean maximum decline in HCV RNA was 3.9 $\log_{10}$ IU/mL. Other protease inhibitors, such as the macrocyclic inhibitor BILN-2061 and the first-generation protease inhibitor telaprevir, have plasma exposure at efficacious doses that, respectively, is 65 and 192 times higher than danoprevir at the highest dose tested in this study (Table 5). The higher plasma exposures of other PIs may be related to unwanted side effects and toxicities associated with their administration [11,23–25]. Thus, the uniquely low plasma exposure of danoprevir may, in part, reflect the favorable safety profile of danoprevir relative to these other compounds.

Viral Resistance During Monotherapy

Patients receiving danoprevir as monotherapy ($n = 40$) displayed continual decline ($n = 14$), plateau ($n = 12$), and breakthrough ($n = 14$) viral response patterns [51]. Genotype 1b patients experienced breakthrough less frequently than did genotype 1a patients. By population sequence analysis, all genotype 1a breakthrough patients carried a lysine substitution in place of the consensus arginine at position 155 (R155K). Interestingly, the genotype 1b patients who experienced viral breakthrough also carried R155K despite the requirement for two nucleotide substitutions for R155K in genotype 1b compared to the single nucleotide substitution required in genotype 1a. Despite the differing number of nucleotide substitutions required in the two subtypes, patients experiencing virologic rebound showed a similar median time between start of therapy and a viral load increase of 0.5 $\log_{10}$ IU/mL above nadir. Moreover, except for one patient, extensive clonal sequencing did not provide evidence for single nucleotide substitutions as intermediates of the doubly substituted codon required for R155K in subtype 1b. Thus, although the lower incidence of escape in subtype 1b compared to 1a may reflect a higher genetic barrier in this subtype, the similarly late emergence of R155K as the dominant sequence in most rebound patients, without evidence for intermediate transitions, suggests that this substitution is either selected from a small preexisting population or that potential intermediates are transient. Further data are required to discriminate between these two possibilities.

Structural studies indicate that R155 is engaged in an extensive set of polar interactions that forms the P2 binding site (Fig. 1, and see [33,45]). This site is engaged in the binding of all NS3/4A PIs currently in development [19,49–52,68]. Substitution of this amino acid, in particular R155K, was identified through in vitro selections for NS3/4A PI resistance [69]. The R155K substitution disrupts polar interactions required for appropriate constitution of the P2 site (Fig. 1, and see [33,70]) and reduces significantly the potency of all PIs reported to date. In all PI monotherapy studies reported , viral escape is associated with R155K to some degree but is usually restricted to subtype 1a [49,50]. Thus, association of R155K substitution with viral escape to danoprevir in subtype 1b is in marked contrast to other PIs, where viral breakthrough in this subtype is associated with substitution at position 156 (first-generation inhibitors, [49,71]) or 168 (macrocycles, [50]), as these substitutions require only a single nucleotide substitution in subtype 1b. The different resistance pathways in subtypes 1a and 1b for these other compounds may reflect the in vitro finding that compared to danoprevir, 168 and 156 substitutions have a more pronounced impact on the potency of other PIs [72].

Biochemical characterization of R155K-bearing NS3/4A demonstrated that danoprevir dissociates rapidly from the R155K variant. In dilution-recovery experiments, preformed complexes of danoprevir and R155K-bearing NS3/4A are rapidly reactivated upon dilution, indicating that R155K compromises the slow dissociative property of danoprevir [31]. Thus, the loss of cellular potency associated with this substitution (over 100-fold loss in con1 replicon) and its ultimate appearance in patients who experience virologic rebound during danoprevir monotherapy reflects an increased

TABLE 5 Plasma Exposure of Various NS3/4A PIs at Efficacious Doses

	Mean $AUC_{ss,0\text{-}24h}$[a] (ng·h/mL)	Ratio to 200 mg q12h Danoprevir AUC	Ratio to 200 mg q8h Danoprevir AUC
Danoprevir, 200 mg q12[b]	226		
Danoprevir, 200 mg q8[b]	413		
Telaprevir, 750 mg q8[c]	79,200[d]	350	192
Ciluprevir, 200 mg b.i.d.[e]	26,799	119	65

[a]Steady-state AUC over 24 h.
[b]Pharmacokinetic parameters reported by Rubino et al. [67].
[c]Pharmacokinetic parameters reported by Lawitz et al. [78].
[d]Median value.
[e]Pharmacokinetic parameters reported by Hinrichsen et al. [11].

rate of danoprevir dissociation compared to that observed with wild-type protein. In a similar fashion, the HIV-1 protease inhibitors indinavir, saquinavir, and others dissociate slowly from the WT HIV-1 protease with half-lives of 10 to 100 min [40] but rapidly from clinically observed resistant mutants [73,74].

Combination with SoC for 14 Days

The clinical experience with danoprevir monotherapy is consistent with other NS3/4A PIs in terms of the magnitude of virological effect provided and the occurrence of viral rebound in a subset of patients [19,49–52] . Thus, early clinical trials with single DAA in HCV bear out long accepted principles in HIV treatment: that effective therapy will require a combination of multiple compounds with differing mechanisms of action [56,57]. Given the well-characterized efficacy and safety profiles of SoC, a favored strategy in current drug development in HCV is the addition of a single DAA to SoC.

Zeuzem presented results of a phase Ib randomized double-blind placebo-controlled 14-day triple combination study in treatment-naive patients chronically infected with HCV genotype 1 [18]. As with danoprevir monotherapy, twice daily and three times daily regimens were explored, but at slightly higher doses. This study was designed to inform dose selection and study design of the danoprevir phase II program in combination with peginterferon α-2a (Pegasys) and ribavirin. After 14 days of triple combination therapy, the median reduction in HCV RNA from baseline exceeded 5 $\log_{10}$ IU/mL in five of the six cohorts and was 5.4 and 5.7 $\log_{10}$ IU/mL in the best-performing q12h and q8h cohorts, respectively (Fig. 3). Considering all cohorts, HCV RNA was below the limit of quantification after only 14 days of treatment in 71% (32/45) of patients who received treatment with danoprevir. Virological responses in optimal q12h cohorts were comparable to those observed for first-generation protease inhibitors when dosed q8h. Consistent with the favorable safety profile of danoprevir in monotherapy, triple therapy displayed an AE profile that was similar to that observed historically for SoC. No serious adverse events (SAEs) or grade 4 AEs were observed during treatment with danoprevir, and there were no discontinuations. Importantly, viral breakthrough was not observed in any patient in this study, suggesting that even at the lowest q12h dose tested, combination with SoC suppressed viral rebound regardless of HCV subtype. These data suggest that danoprevir can be dosed twice daily, making its administration compatible with ribavirin and with many other DAAs in development in chronic HCV.

Combination of Danoprevir and the NS5B Polymerase Inhibitor R7128 for 14 Days

Only approximately 50% of all patients treated with SoC achieve SVR, and the significant side-effect profile of both ribavirin and interferon components of SoC results in black-box warnings for these products. Although addition of a single DAA to SoC may improve efficacy, it does not address the suboptimal safety profile of SoC or obviate the need for subcutaneous injection of peginterferon. Optimal regimens would have milder side-effect profiles and greater convenience. Such regimens may be particularly beneficial in patients contraindicated for interferon and patients who have responded or are predicted to respond poorly to interferon. The combined use of PIs and NIs has been highly effective in HIV treatment [56,57] and represents an attractive all-oral therapeutic modality of interest in HCV with the potential for milder side effects.

R7128 is a NS5B NI that promotes multi-$\log_{10}$ reductions in circulating HCV RNA in short-duration monotherapy studies [75]. Unlike NS3/4A PI monotherapy, viral escape

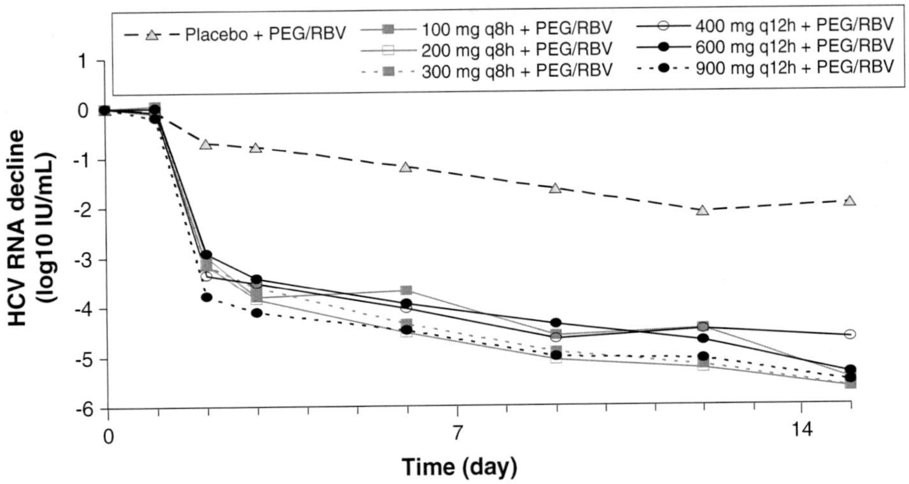

FIGURE 3 Virological response promoted by danoprevir in combination with peginterferon α-2a and ribavirin.

is not observed with R7128 monotherapy, suggesting that NS5B NIs have a high barrier to the development of drug-resistant forms [59,62–64,76]. As described previously, in vitro studies indicate that the active moiety of R7128 has a high barrier to resistance and that combination with danoprevir suppresses the emergence of danoprevir-resistant variants [59,60]. Both danoprevir and R7128 are safe and well tolerated when given alone and in combination with peginterferon α-2a (Pegasys) and ribavirin, and drive viral loads in a majority of patients below the level of quantification or detection within 28 days [18,62]. R7128 and danoprevir do not have overlapping routes of metabolism or elimination, and have a low likelihood of drug–drug interactions.

The rationale described above led to the combined use of danoprevir and R7128 in the first-ever clinical study of two DAAs in combination, the INFORM-1 study. Gane presented interim results from this study [77] describing results for 57 patients enrolled in a randomized double-blind ascending dose phase Ib trial. Patients receiving the combination of danoprevir and R7128 for 13 day, without pegylated interferon or ribavirin, experienced a median reduction in viral levels of 4.8 to 5.2 $\log_{10}$ IU/mL in the highest doses reported (Table 6). This level of viral suppression is similar to that observed when a DAA is used in triple combination with SoC. The addition of R7128 to R7227 resulted in sustained viral load reductions over the dosing period, with aproximately 63% of patients experiencing a decrease in viral levels below the quantification limit of the diagnostic assay (less than 40 IU/mL). Furthermore, viral loads in 25% of patients in the higher three dosage groups reported in this interim analysis were below the limit of detection (less than 15 IU/mL) after 13 days. Median viral load at the end of treatment ranged from 35 to 20 IU/mL in the higher three dosage cohorts reported. Twice-daily doses of danoprevir (600 and 900 mg b.i.d.) in combination with twice-daily doses of R7128 (1000 mg b.i.d.) in treatment-experienced and treatment-naive patients were not reported as of October 2009. No treatment-related SAEs, no dose reductions, and no discontinuations were reported. Pharmacokinetic analysis confirmed that there were no drug–drug interactions between the compounds. Thus, this study provides the first evidence that two DAAs can be safely combined for short durations. Although it remains to be determined if SVR can be achieved in the absence of peginterferon, INFORM-1 demonstrates that an all-oral regimen combining a NS5B NI and and NS3/4A PI can drive viral loads below the limit of detection in short-duration studies at the same frequency as reported for triple combination cocktails comprising a NS3/4A PI, peginterferon, and ribavirin [14,16,18,19].

CONCLUSIONS AND FUTURE PROSPECTS

Danoprevir was discovered through a rational design campaign that sought to identify potent compounds with high exposure in liver but low exposure in plasma. In humans, plasma exposure of danoprevir is very low compared to other NS3/4A PIs, while the efficacy and safety profiles of danoprevir dosed twice daily compare favorably to first-generation protease inhibitors dosed q8h. Danoprevir dosing is therefore compatible with both ribavirin and other direct-acting antiviral agents currently in development. As with other NS3/4A PIs, danoprevir monotherapy resulted in the emergence of a drug-resistant viral variant in a subset of patients. Combination with SoC enhances and sustains antiviral effects, suppresses the emergence of resistance variants, and further supports the continued development of twice-daily regimens. In the first-ever study combining two direct-acting antiviral agents in chronic HCV, danoprevir in combination with the NS5B nucleoside inhibitor R7128 showed dramatic efficacy in the absence of interferon, providing the first evidence that viral loads could become undetectable in a therapeutic regimen lacking interferon and its associated toxicities. Thus, while future work is clearly needed to fully define the optimal development path for danoprevir and define its long-term safety profile, data available to date suggest that the strategy to minimize plasma exposure of a potent, slowly dissociating compound is an effective approach for the discovery of safe and efficacious liver-targeted drugs.

TABLE 6 Interim INFORM-1 HCV RNA Results from Low-Dose 14-Day Cohorts[a]

Regimen (R7128 mg/ R7227 mg)	*n*	Baseline VL (IU/mL)	VL Change from Baseline (log10 IU/mL) Median (Range)	Day 14 VL (IU/mL) Median (Range)	Patients < LLOQ[b] *n* (%)	Patients < LLOD[c] *n* (%)
500/100	8	2.8×10^6	−3.9 (−5.0 to −2.9)	288 (<15 to 588)	1/8 (13%)	1/8 (13%)
500/200	8	8.3×10^6	−5.2 (−5.5 to −3.1)	35 (<15 to 701)	5/8 (63%)	2/8 (25%)
1000/100	7	2.2×10^6	−4.8 (−5.7 to −4.5)	20 (<15 to 173)	5/7 (71%)	2/7 (29%)
1000/200	8	2.2×10^6	−4.8 (−5.5 to −2.7)	22 (<15 to 660)	5/8 (63%)	2/8 (25%)

[a]Interum results as presented by Gane et al. [77].
[b]Lower limit of quantitation (LLOQ) = 40 IU/mL.
[c]Lower limit of detection (LLOD) = 15 IU/mL.

Acknowledgments

We would like to thank all members of the NS3/4A research teams of InterMune, Inc. and Array Biopharma, Inc., and the development teams of InterMune, Inc., Roche Pharmaceuticals, and Pharmasset, Inc. for their valuable contributions to the program and comments on this manuscript.

REFERENCES

[1] Shepard, C. W., et al. Global epidemiology of hepatitis C virus infection. *Lancet Infect. Dis.* **2005**, *5*, 558–567.

[2] NIH consensus statement on management of hepatitis C: 2002. NIH Consens. State. Sci. State. **2002**, *19*, 1–46.

[3] Manns, M. P., et al. Peginterferon alfa-2b plus ribavirin compared with interferon alfa-2b plus ribavirin for initial treatment of chronic hepatitis C: a randomised trial. *Lancet* **2001**, *358*, 958–965.

[4] Fried, M. W., et al. Peginterferon alfa-2a plus ribavirin for chronic hepatitis C virus infection. *N. Engl. J. Med.* **2002**, *347*, 975–982.

[5] Lemon, S. M., et al. "Strong reasons make strong actions": the antiviral efficacy of NS3/4A protease inhibitors. *Hepatology* **2005**, *41*, 671–674.

[6] Neukam, K., et al. A review of current anti-HCV treatment regimens and possible future strategies. *Expert Opin. Pharmacother.* **2009**, *10*, 417–433.

[7] Pawlotsky, J. M. Hepatitis C: it's a long way to new therapy, it's a long way to go. *Gastroenterology* **2004**, *127*, 1629–1632.

[8] Gale, M., Jr.; Foy, E. M. Evasion of intracellular host defense by hepatitis C virus. *Nature* **2005**, *436*, 939–945.

[9] Thimme, R., et al. A target on the move: innate and adaptive immune escape strategies of hepatitis C virus. *Antiviral Res.* **2006**, *69*, 129–141.

[10] Lamarre, D., et al. An NS3 protease inhibitor with antiviral effects in humans infected with hepatitis C virus. *Nature* **2003**, *426*, 186–189.

[11] Hinrichsen, H., et al. Short-term antiviral efficacy of BILN 2061, a hepatitis C virus serine protease inhibitor, in hepatitis C genotype 1 patients. *Gastroenterology* **2004**, *127*, 1347–1355.

[12] Reiser, M., et al. Antiviral efficacy of NS3-serine protease inhibitor BILN-2061 in patients with chronic genotype 2 and 3 hepatitis C. *Hepatology* **2005**, *41*, 832–835.

[13] Forestier, N., et al. Treatment of chronic hepatitis C virus (HCV) genotype 1 patients with the NS3/4A protease inhibitor ITMN-191 leads to rapid reductions in plasma HCV RNA: results of a phase 1b multiple ascending dose (MAD) study. *Hepatology* **2008**, *48*, 1132A.

[14] Manns, M., et al. Safety and antiviral activity of TMC436350 in treatment-naive genotype 1 HCV-infected patients. *Hepatology* **2008**, *48*, 1023A.

[15] Lawitz, E., et al. Safety, Tolerability and antiviral activity of MK-7009, a novel inhibitor of the hepatitis C virus NS3/4A protease, in patients with chronic HCV genotype 1 infection. *Hepatology* **2008**, *48*, 403A.

[16] Manns, M. P., et al. Safety and antiviral activity of BI 201335, a new HCV NS3 protease inhibitor, on combination therapy with peginterferon alfa-2a (P) and ribavirin (R) for 28 days in P + R treatment-experienced patients with chronic hepatitis C genotype 1 infection. *Hepatology* **2008**, *48*, 1151A–1152A.

[17] Reesink, H., et al. Safety and antiviral activity of Sch900518 administered as monotherapy and in combination with peginterferon alfa-2b to naive and treatment-experienced HCV-1 infected patients. *J. Hepatol.* **2009**, *50*(Suppl. 1), S35.

[18] Forestier, N., et al. Antiviral activity and safety of ITMN-191 in combination with peginterferon alfa-2a and ribavirin in patients with chronic hepatitis C virus (HCV). *J. Hepatol.* **2009**, *50*, S35.

[19] Manns, M. P., et al. MK-7009 significantly improves rapid viral response (RVR) in combination with pegylated interferon alfa-2a and ribavirin in patients with chronic hepatitis C (CHC) genotype 1 infection. *J. Hepatol.* **2009**, *50*(Suppl. 1), S384.

[20] Mederacke, I., et al. Boceprevir, an NS3 serine protease inhibitor of hepatitis C virus, for the treatment of HCV infection. *Curr. Opin. Invest. Drugs* **2009**, *10*, 181–189.

[21] Njoroge, F. G., et al. Challenges in modern drug discovery: a case study of boceprevir, an HCV protease inhibitor for the treatment of hepatitis C virus infection. *Acc. Chem. Res.* **2008**, *41*, 50–59.

[22] Perni, R. B., et al. Preclinical profile of VX-950, a potent, selective, and orally bioavailable inhibitor of hepatitis C virus NS3-4A serine protease. *Antimicrob. Agents Chemother.* **2006**, *50*, 899–909.

[23] McHutchison, J. G., et al. Telaprevir with peginterferon and ribavirin for chronic HCV genotype 1 infection. *N. Engl. J. Med.* **2009**, *360*, 1827–1838.

[24] Hezode, C., et al. Telaprevir and peginterferon with or without ribavirin for chronic HCV infection. *N. Engl. J. Med.* **2009**, *360*, 1839–1850.

[25] Kwo, P., et al. Final results: SVR 24 NS3 protease inhibitor boceprevir plus pegIFN alpha-2b/ribavirin HCV 1 in treatment naive patients. *J. Hepatol.* **2009**, *50*(Suppl. 1), S4.

[26] Evans, M.; Rees, A. The myotoxicity of statins. *Curr. Opin. Lipidol.* **2002**, *13*, 415–420.

[27] Evans, M.; Rees, A. Effects of HMG-CoA reductase inhibitors on skeletal muscle: Are all statins the same? *Drug Saf.* **2002**, *25*, 649–663.

[28] Igel, M., et al. Pharmacology of 3-hydroxy-3-methylglutaryl-coenzyme A reductase inhibitors (statins), including rosuvastatin and pitavastatin. *J. Clin. Pharmacol.* **2002**, *42*, 835–845.

[29] Johansson, A., et al. Acyl sulfonamides as potent protease inhibitors of the hepatitis C virus full-length NS3 (protease-helicase/NTPase): a comparative study of different C-terminals. *Bioorg. Med. Chem.* **2003**, *11*, 2551–2568.

[30] Rieger, R. A., et al. Pharmacokinetic analysis and liver concentrations of a series of macrocyclic peptidomimetic inhibitors

of HCV NS3/4A protease: identification of ITMN-191, a potent NS3/4A protease inhibitor with high liver exposure across multiple species. *Gastroenterology* **2006**, *130*, A-835.

[31] Rajagopalan, P. T. R., et al. Characterization of HCV NA3/4a protease inhibition by ITMN 191 reveals picomolar potency and slow dissociation: implications for the use of ITMN 191 in chronic HCV treatment. *Gastroenterology* **2007**, *132*, A-782.

[32] Lin, T., et al. Inhibitory activity of TMC435350 on HCV NS3/4A proteases from genotypes 1 to 6. *Hepatology* **2008**, *48*, 1166A.

[33] Condroski, K., et al. Structure-based design of novel isoindolene inhibitors of HCV NS3/4A protease and binding mode analysis of ITMN 191 by x-ray crystallography. *Gastroenterology* **2006**, *130*, A835.

[34] Lewandowicz, A., et al. Achieving the ultimate physiological goal in transition state analogue inhibitors for purine nucleoside phosphorylase. *J. Biol. Chem.* **2003**, *278*, 31465–31468.

[35] Tian, G. In vivo time-dependent inhibition of human steroid 5 alpha-reductase by finasteride. *J. Pharm. Sci.* **1996**, *85*, 106–111.

[36] Bull, H. G., et al. Mechanism-based inhibition of human steroid 5a-reductase by finasteride: enzyme-catalyzed formation of NADP-dihydrofinasteride, a potent bisubstrate analog inhibitor. *J. Am. Chem. Soc.* **1996**, *118*, 2359–2365.

[37] Zhong, J., et al. Robust hepatitis C virus infection in vitro. *Proc. Natl. Acad. Sci. USA* **2005**, *102*, 9294–9299.

[38] Neumann, A. U., et al. Hepatitis C viral dynamics in vivo and the antiviral efficacy of interferon-alpha therapy. *Science* **1998**, *282*, 103–107.

[39] Tanaka, J., et al. Early dynamics of hepatitis C virus in the circulation of chimpanzees with experimental infection. *Intervirology* **2005**, *48*, 120–123.

[40] Dierynck, I., et al. Binding kinetics of darunavir to human immunodeficiency virus type 1 protease explain the potent antiviral activity and high genetic barrier. *J. Virol.* **2007**, *81*, 13845–13851.

[41] Foster, G. R., et al. Activity of telaprevir alone or in combination with peginterferon alfa-2a and ribavirin in treatment naive genotype 2 and 3 hepatitis-C patients: interim results of study C209. *J. Hepatol.* **2009**, *50*(Suppl. 1), S22.

[42] Hoofnagle, J. H. A step forward in therapy for hepatitis C. *N. Engl. J. Med.* **2009**, *360*, 1899–1901.

[43] Thompson, A., et al. Directly acting antivirals for the treatment of patients with hepatitis C infection: a clinical development update addressing key future challenges. *J. Hepatol.* **2009**, *50*, 184–194.

[44] Chen, K. X., et al. Second generation highly potent and selective inhibitors of the hepatitis C virus NS3 serine protein. *J. Am. Chem. Soc.* **2009**, *52*, 1370–1379.

[45] Seiwert, S. D., et al. Preclinical characteristics of the hepatitis C virus NS3/4A protease inhibitor ITMN-191 (R7227). *Antimicrob. Agents Chemother.* **2008**, *52*, 4432–4441.

[46] Perni, R. B., et al. VX-950: The discovery of an inhibitor of the hepatitis C NS3/4A protease and a potential hepatitis C virus therapeutic. *Hepatology* **2003**, *38*, 130A.

[47] Benhamou, Y., et al. Results of a proof of concept study (C210) of telaprevir monotherapy and in combination with peginterferon alfa-2a and ribavirin in treatment-naive genotype 4 HCV patients. *J. Hepatol.* **2009**, *50*(Suppl. 1), S6.

[48] Bierman, W. F., et al. HIV monotherapy with ritonavir-boosted protease inhibitors: a systematic review. *AIDS* **2009**, *23*, 279–291.

[49] Sarrazin, C., et al. Dynamic hepatitis C virus genotypic and phenotypic changes in patients treated with the protease inhibitor telaprevir. *Gastroenterology* **2007**, *132*, 1767–1777.

[50] Kukolj, G., et al. BI 201335, a potent HCV NS3 protease inhibitor, in treatment-naive and -experienced chronic HCV genotype-1 infection: genotypic and phenotypic analysis of the NS3 protease domain. *J. Hepatol.* **2009**, *50*, S347.

[51] Sarrazin, C., et al. Incidence of virologic escape observed during ITMN-191 (R7227) monotherapy is genotype dependent, associated with a specific NS3 substitution, and suppressed upon combination with peginterferon alfa-2a/ribavirin. *J. Hepatol.* **2009**, *50*(Suppl, 1), S345.

[52] Manns, M., et al. Opera-1 Trial: interim analysis of safety and antiviral activity of TMC435 in treatment-naive genotype 1 HCV patients. *J. Hepatol.* **2009**, *50*(Suppl. 1), S7.

[53] Forestier, N., et al. Antiviral activity of telaprevir (VX-950) and peginterferon alfa-2a in patients with hepatitis C. *Hepatology* **2007**, *46*, 640–648.

[54] Kieffer, T. L., et al. Telaprevir and pegylated interferon-alpha-2a inhibit wild-type and resistant genotype 1 hepatitis C virus replication in patients. *Hepatology* **2007**, *46*, 631–639.

[55] Nijhuis, M., et al. Antiviral resistance and impact on viral replication capacity: evolution of viruses under antiviral pressure occurs in three phases. *Handb. Exp. Pharmacol.* **2009**, *189*, 299–320.

[56] De Clercq, E. The design of drugs for HIV and HCV. *Nat. Rev. Drug Discov.* **2007**, *6*, 1001–1018.

[57] De Clercq, E. Anti-HIV drugs: 25 compounds approved within 25 years after the discovery of HIV. *Int. J. Antimicrob. Agents* **2009**, *33*, 307–320.

[58] Reesink, H. W., et al. Rapid decline of viral RNA in hepatitis C patients treated with VX-950: a phase Ib, placebo-controlled, randomized study. *Gastroenterology* **2006**, *131*, 997–1002.

[59] Le Pogam, S., et al. No evidence of R7128 drug resistance after up to 4 weeks treatment of genotype 1, 2, and 3 hepatitis C virus infected individuals. *J. Hepatol.* **2009**, *50*(Suppl. 1), S348.

[60] Le Pogam, S., et al. Existence of hepatitis C virus NS5B variants naturally resistant to non-nucleoside, but not to nucleoside, polymerase inhibitors among untreated patients. *J. Antimicrob. Chemother.* **2008**, *61*, 1205–1216.

[61] McCown, M. F., et al. The hepatitis C virus replicon presents a higher barrier to resistance to nucleoside analogs than to nonnucleoside polymerase or protease inhibitors. *Antimicrob. Agents Chemother.* **2008**, *52*, 1604–1612.

[62] Lalezari, J., et al. Potent antiviral activity of the HCV nucleoside polymerase inhibitor, R7128, in combination with peg-IFN α-2a and ribavirin. *J. Hepatol.* **2008**, *48*, S29.

[63] Gane, E. J., et al. Antiviral activity of the HCV nucleoside polymerase inhibitor R7128 in HCV genotype 2 and 3 prior non-responders: results of R7128 1500mg BID with PEG-IFN and ribavirin for 28 days. *Hepatology* **2008**, 48.

[64] Pockros, P. J., et al. Robust synergistic antiviral effect of R1626 in combination with peginterferon alfa-2a 940KD), with or without ribavirin: interim analysis of results of phase 2A study. *Hepatology* **2007**, *46*, 311A.

[65] Tan, H., et al. Combination of the NS3/4A protease inhibitor ITMN-191 (R7227) with the active moiety of the NS5B inhibitors R1626 or R7128 enhances replicon clearance and reduces the emergence of drug resistant variants. *Hepatology* **2008**, *48*, 1153A.

[66] Bradford, W. Z., et al. A Phase 1 study of the safety, tolerability, and pharmacokinetics of single ascending oral doses of the NS3/4A protease inhibitor ITMN-191 in healthy subjects. *Hepatology* **2008**, *48*, 1146A.

[67] Rubino, C., et al. Pharmacokinetic–pharmacodynamic (PK-PD) relationships for ITMN-191 in a phase 1 multiple ascending dose trial in patients with genotype 1 chronic hepatitis C (CHC) infection. *Hepatology* **2008**, *48*, 1140A.

[68] Susser, S., et al. Detection of resistant variants in the hepatitis C virus NS3 protease gene by clonal sequencing at long term follow-up in patients treated with boceprevir. *J. Hepatol.* **2009**, *50*, S7.

[69] Lu, L., et al. Mutations conferring resistance to a potent hepatitis C virus serine protease inhibitor in vitro. *Antimicrob. Agents Chemother.* **2004**, *48*, 2260–2266.

[70] Zhou, Y., et al. Phenotypic and structural analyses of hepatitis C virus NS3 protease Arg155 variants: sensitivity to telaprevir (VX-950) and interferon alpha. *J. Biol. Chem.* **2007**, *282*, 22619–22628.

[71] McCown, M. F., et al. GT-1a or GT-1b subtype-specific resistance profiles for hepatitis C virus inhibitors telaprevir and HCV-796. *Antimicrob. Agents Chemother.* **2009**, *53*, 2129–2132.

[72] He, Y., et al. Relative replication capacity and selective advantage profiles of protease inhibitor-resistant hepatitis C virus (HCV) NS3 protease mutants in the HCV genotype 1b replicon system. *Antimicrob. Agents Chemother.* **2008**, *52*, 1101–1110.

[73] Maschera, B., et al. Human immunodeficiency virus: mutations in the viral protease that confer resistance to saquinavir increase the dissociation rate constant of the protease–saquinavir complex. *J. Biol. Chem.* **1996**, *271*, 33231–33235.

[74] Shuman, C. F., et al. Elucidation of HIV-1 protease resistance by characterization of interaction kinetics between inhibitors and enzyme variants. *Antiviral Res.* **2003**, *58*, 235–242.

[75] Reddy, R., et al. Antiviral activity, pharmacokinetics, safety, and tolerability of R7128, a novel nucleoside HCV RNA polymerase inhibitor, following multiple, ascending, oral doses in patients with HCV genotype 1 infection who have failed prior interferon therapy. *Hepatology* **2007**, *46*, 862A–863A.

[76] Brown, N. A. Progress towards improving antiviral therapy for hepatitis C with hepatitis C virus polymerase inhibitors: I. Nucleoside analogues. *Expert Opin. Invest. Drugs* **2009**, *18*, 709–725.

[77] Gane, E. J., et al. First-in-man demonstration of potent antiviral activity with a nucleoside polymerase (R7128) and protease (R7227/ITMN-191) inhibitor combination in HCV: safety, pharmacokinetics, and virologic results from INFORM-1. *J. Hepatol.* **2009**, *50*(Suppl. 1), S380.

[78] Lawitz, E., et al. Antiviral effects and safety of telaprevir, peginterferon alfa-2a, and ribavirin for 28 days in hepatitis C patients. *J. Hepatol.* **2008**, *49*, 163–169.

19

DISCOVERY AND DEVELOPMENT OF THE HCV PROTEASE INHIBITOR TMC435

Pierre Raboisson, Gregory Fanning, Herman de Kock, Åsa Rosenquist, René Verloes, and Kenneth Simmen

Tibotec BVBA, Beerse, Belgium, and Tibotec Pharmaceuticals, Ltd., Little Island, County Cork, Ireland

INTRODUCTION

Hepatitis C virus (HCV) is a positive-stranded RNA virus of the Flaviviridae family causing serious liver, disease, including cirrhosis, hepatocellular carcinoma, and liver failure [1]. As a result, HCV is currently the most common underlying cause for liver transplantation [1,2]. An estimated 170 to 200 million people worldwide are chronically infected by HCV, and in the absence of a vaccine currently available to prevent hepatitis C, about 3 to 4 million people are newly infected each year [3,4]. The current standard of care therapy, pegylated interferon-α (pegIFNα), in combination with ribavirin, given for 48 weeks is characterized by a limited efficacy, especially in patients infected with genotypes 1 and 4, and is often associated with side effects leading to treatment discontinuation [5–7]. It has been shown that antiviral drugs that specifically inhibit the function of viral proteins can efficiently suppress HCV-RNA levels and may increase cure rates, possibly with shortened treatment duration [8–10]. Consequently, there is an ongoing effort to identify more effective, orally active, and well-tolerated therapies. Initial efforts to develop HCV antiviral agents have focused on inhibition of essential virally encoded enzymes such as the RNA-dependent RNA polymerase (RdRp) NS5B and NS3/4A protease [11–15]. NS3/4A proteins have been identified as potent inhibitors of cytokine gene expression, suggesting an important role for HCV proteases in counteracting host cell antiviral response [16]. Consequently, multiple agents targeting these enzymes are currently under clinical development [17].

The HCV trypsin-like NS3/4A serine protease is formed by the noncovalent association of NS3 with its cofactor NS4A. This heterodimeric complex is responsible for the proteolytic cleavage of the viral polyprotein, an essential step in viral replication. Proteases have proven to be very amenable targets for antiviral drug discovery, making NS3/4A a target of choice in the development of novel anti-HCV agents [18]. Although the identification of NS3/4A inhibitors using high-throughput screening techniques were unsuccessful, it was observed that N-terminal cleavage products of NS3/4A are inhibitors of the enzyme itself, which aided the development of novel inhibitors [19,20]. Preliminary SAR studies facilitated the identification of nanomolar substrate-based hexapeptide inhibitors [19,21]. Druglike properties of these initial poorly permeable polypeptides [22] were improved by (1) decreasing the peptidic character, which was achieved by successive N-terminal truncations, and (2) replacing the cysteine in P1 by a vinylcyclopropylamino acid bioisostere [22]. These modifications, combined with an improved quinoline-substituted P2 fragment, led to the discovery of potent and selective tripeptide inhibitors [21]. Further improvement of pharmaceutical properties was achieved by the design of macrocyclic β-strand mimic scaffolds, culminating in discovery of the potent, highly selective, and orally bioavailable drug BILN 2061 (Fig. 1) [23].

Oral administration of BILN 2061 to patients with HCV genotype 1 resulted in a substantial reduction in viral RNA levels (2 to 3 $\log_{10}$ after 2 days). Although this established proof-of-concept for HCV NS3/4A protease inhibitors as therapeutic agents [24], BILN 2061 was associated with

Antiviral Drugs: From Basic Discovery Through Clinical Trials, First Edition. Edited by Wieslaw M. Kazmierski.

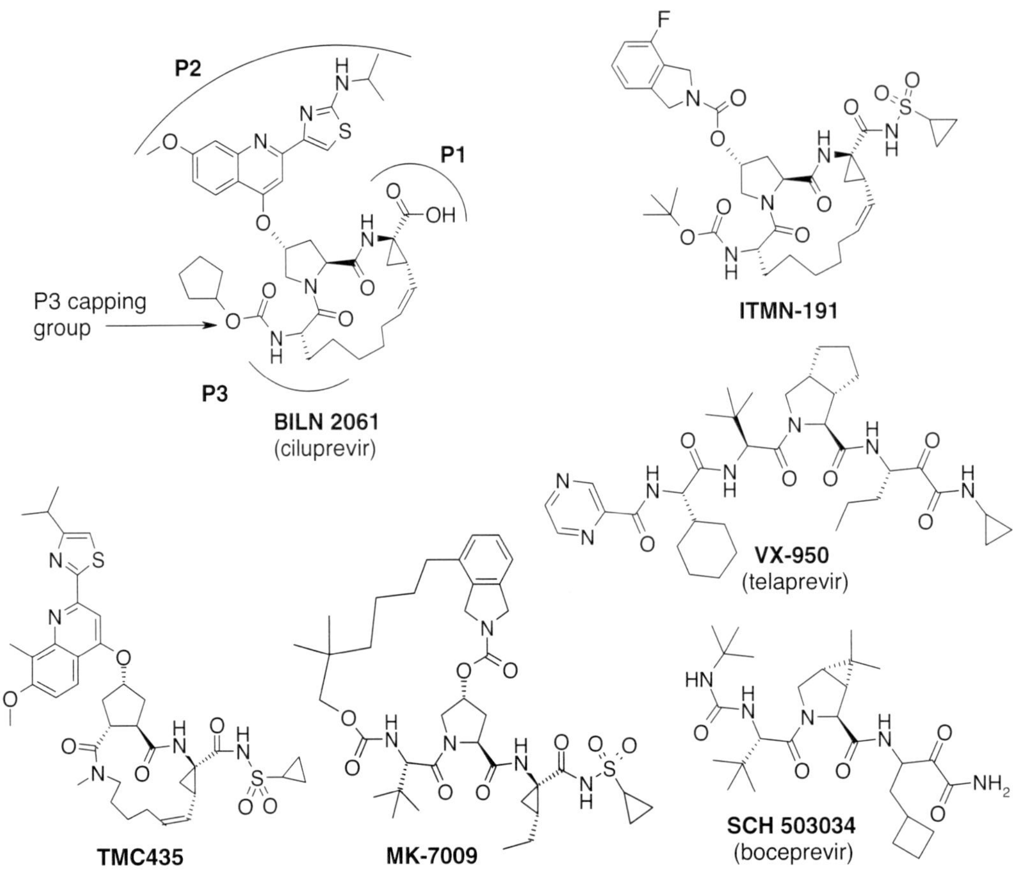

FIGURE 1 Structure of reference HCV protease inhibitors.

cardiotoxic effects in primates [25]. While the mechanism by which BILN 2061 exerted cardiotoxic effects remains unclear, it is assumed that the toxicity observed with the pioneer drug was compound specific. Multiple drug discovery programs have resulted in a number of other novel noncovalent macrocyclic NS3/4A agents (e.g., TMC435, ITMN-191, MK-7009) with anti-HCV activity in patients [17,26]. These compounds belong to a different chemical class than that of the α-ketoamide electrophilic trap containing the inhibitors telaprevir and boceprevir, the most advanced HCV antivirals in clinical development [8,27].

DISCOVERY

Medivir (Huddinge, Sweden) scientists demonstrated that replacement of the central P2 *N*-acyl-(*4R*)-hydroxyproline of compound **1** [25] with a trisubstituted cyclopentane dicarbonyl moiety resulted in a novel series of potent HCV NS3/4A protease inhibitors, exemplified by compound **2**, which had an NS3-K_i value of 22 nM [28] (Fig. 2). Further research by Tibotec (County Cork, Ireland) in collaboration with Medivir was initiated to perform a parallel exploration of the SAR in five different macrocyclic series, as characterized by their central P2 scaffold (Fig. 3). These NS3/4A inhibitors were characterized by a further reduction in peptidic nature compared to the tripeptide BILN 2061 [23]. Removal of the P3 amino moiety and its capping group resulted

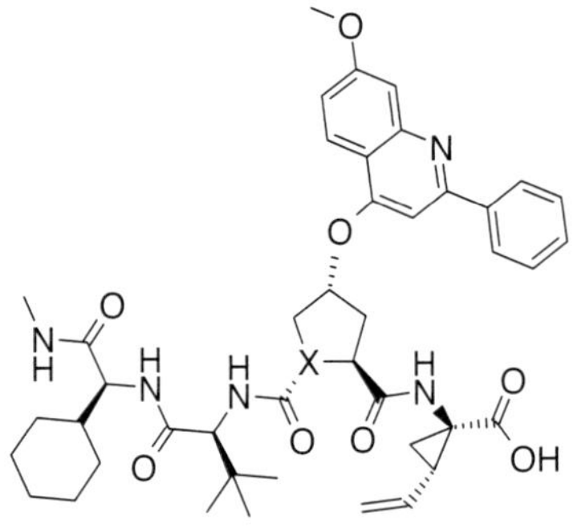

1, (X = N)
2, (X = CH)

FIGURE 2 Bioisosteric replacement of the P2 [*N*-acyl-(*4R*)-hydroxyproline] with a trisubstituted cyclopentane dicarbonyl moiety. (From [28].)

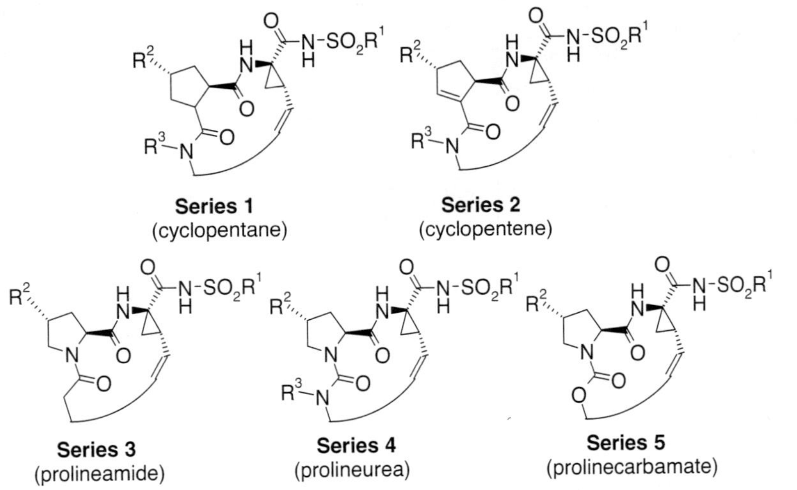

FIGURE 3 The five lead series optimized in parallel by tibotec and medivir.

in dipeptide macrocyclic structures (series 1 to 5, Fig. 3). Previous structural studies have indicated that the rigid carbamate functionality of the P3 capping group is responsible for the positioning of the N-terminal alkyl group into the shallow S4 binding pocket of the enzyme [29] and that the amino and carbonyl groups of the P3 residue are involved in hydrogen bonding with the protein backbone [29–31]. Predictably, removal of the P3 amino moiety and its capping group leads to an important loss of potency (compare compound **4** with compound **3** (Fig. 4) [32]. Similar results were observed for the four other lead series depicted in Figure 3 [33–35]. This loss of potency could be counterbalanced in all five lead series by introducing an acyl sulfonamide group [33–35].

Hence, nanomolar inhibitors depicted by compounds **5** to **9** in Figure 4 were obtained and were chosen as lead candidates for further optimization. Each of the lead candidates **5** to **9** suffered from different series-specific drawbacks, limiting

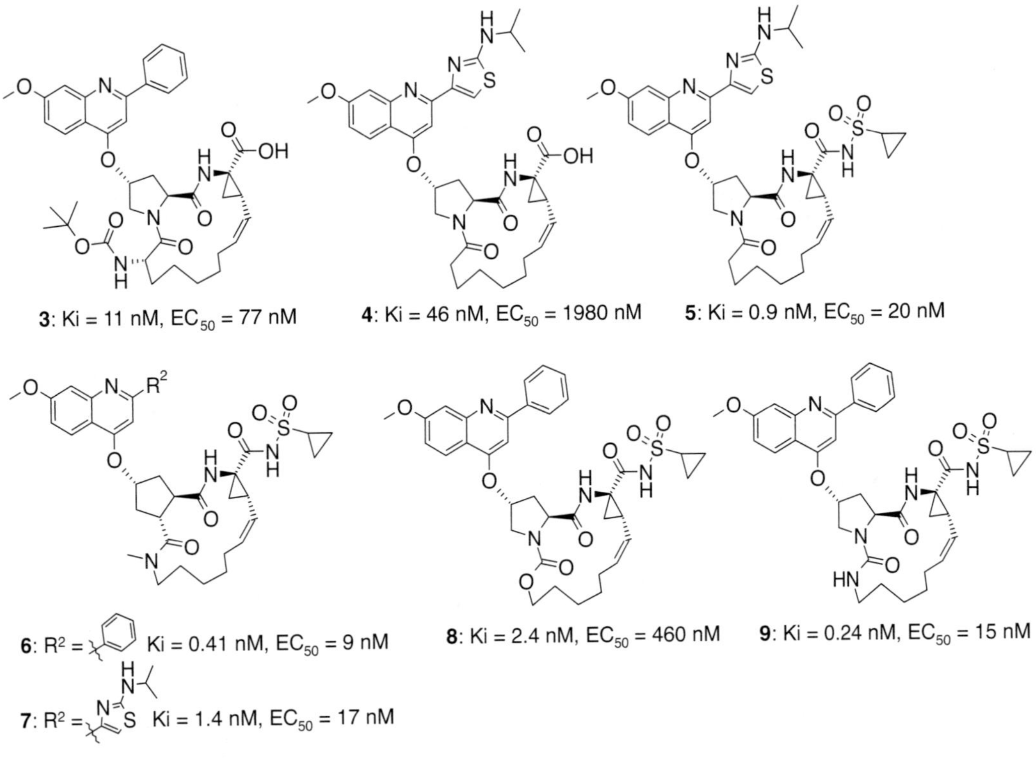

FIGURE 4 Lead compounds identified at the early stage of the program.

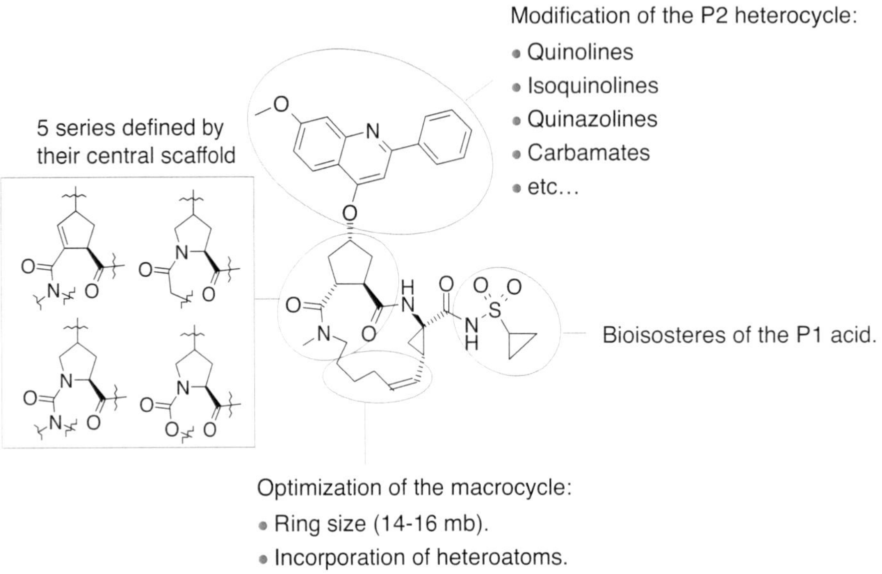

FIGURE 5 Lead optimization strategy.

their potential as clinical entities. For example, the lead proline amide compound **5** exhibited low metabolic stability in human liver microsome preparations. After 15 min, 91.5% of compound **5** was metabolized compared with 28.5% of BILN 2061 [34]. Although the lead cyclopentane compound **6** showed promising in vitro Caco-2 permeability [apical-to-basolateral apparent permeability coefficient (P_{app}) = 3.8 × 10^{-6} cm/s], and medium intrinsic clearance in both human and rat liver microsomes (Cl_{int} = 46 μL·min/mg) [32,33], the rat pharmacokinetic (PK) profile was characterized by a low oral bioavailability (F = 2.5%) associated with a high plasma clearance (2.79 L·h/kg), due to intensive bile elimination. One hour after intravenous administration of 1 mg/kg of compound **5**, 95% of the product was found unchanged in the bile [32,33]. Moreover, the lead prolinecarbamate compound **8** was found poorly permeable in Caco-2 cells, which is in line with its limited potency in the replicon model and the high shift between the enzymatic and replicon activity [35]. Finally, with the exception of compound **6**, none of the lead compounds **4** to **9** exhibited single-digit nanomolar potency in the genotype 1b cell-based replicon assay, a minimum requirement for our target compound profile.

To maximize the chance of identifying a compound with the properties desired, the five series shown in Figure 3 were optimized in parallel following the strategy summarized in Figure 5. This approach enabled a systematic exploration of P1, P2, and truncated P3 moieties. Structural information on the macrocyclic inhibitor **3** (Fig. 4) bound to the active site of the NS3 protease guided the design of new inhibitors [36]. The P1 carboxylate oxygen atoms of **3** were shown to bind in the oxyanion hole of NS3, establishing interactions with various residues, including G137, S139, and H57 [36]. Therefore, P1 SAR analysis is limited to substitution of the sulfonamide moiety with acid bioisosteres. Binding of the macrocyclic inhibitor **3** to NS3/4A induces conformational changes of the R155 and D168 side chains, leading to the formation of a salt bridge between these residues and facilitating the interaction of the guanidine group of the R155 side chain with the P2 methoxy quinoline heterocycle [36]. Similar interactions can be achieved by replacing the quinoline with other aromatic ring systems (e.g., isoquinolines, quinazolines, aryl carbamates). Finally, optimization of the macrocycle ring size and introduction of heteroatoms in the hydrocarbon tether led to the identification of very active compounds **10** to **14** (Fig. 6), which showed significant structural diversity, and to TMC435 [Fig. 1; half maximal effective concentration in the replicon model (EC_{50}) = 8 nM] [32,34,35,37–39].

Although each class of compounds had its own characteristics, some beneficial modifications were identified. For example, the introduction of a methyl group in position 8 of the quinoline heterocycle led to derivatives (e.g., compounds **11**, **13**, and **14** and TMC435) that were more potent in the replicon assay and metabolically more stable in human liver microsomes than were the 8-unsubstituted parent compounds [32,34,38]. Similar observations were made for the quinazoline derivatives (e.g., compound **12**) [39]. Interestingly, the P3-NH-capping group moiety of the metabolically stable compound BILN 2061 (Fig. 1) is known to constrain the inhibitor in a β-strand mimic conformation [23,25]. Removal of the P3-NH-capping group led to compounds **4** and **5** (Fig. 4) [34]. These compounds were metabolically unstable in human liver microsome preparations, which might be attributed to the more flexible scaffold generated by P3 truncation [34]. For the cyclopentanes (series 1, Fig. 3) and

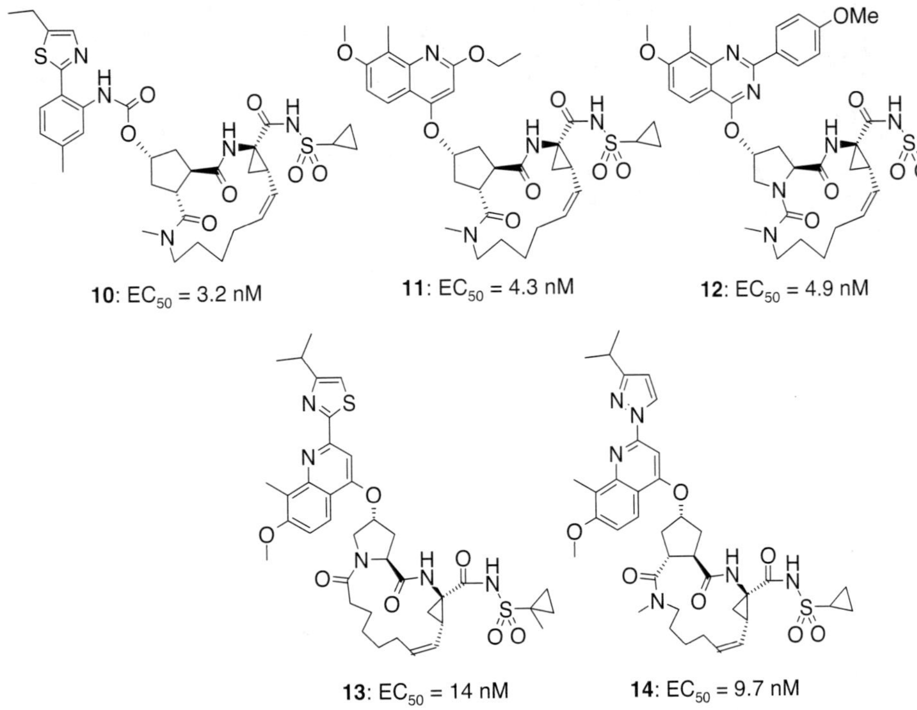

FIGURE 6 Diversity set of compounds obtained after lead optimization.

prolineamides (series 3, Fig. 3), the metabolic stability could be improved by reducing the size of the macrocyclic ring to 14 member atoms (compared with the 15-member ring of BILN 2061), without affecting the activity of these inhibitors [32,34]. Eventually, very active compounds [e.g., compounds **13** and **14** (Fig. 6) and TMC435] that were metabolically stable in human liver microsome preparations and permeable in Caco-2 cells, were selected for in vivo PK parameter measurements [32,34].

PRECLINICAL CHARACTERIZATION

From Table 1 it can be seen that of the compounds tested, TMC435 had the best pharmacokinetic (PK) profile, with a mean time to maximum plasma concentration (T_{max}) of 3.0 h following oral dosing, indicating a medium rate of absorption, and data from intravenous administration suggesting slow clearance (0.505 L·h/kg) and a low volume of distribution (0.49 L·kg) [32]. Data from oral administration showed

TABLE 1 Mean Plasma and Tissue Levels and Basic Pharmacokinetic Parameters of Macrocycle Compounds 13 and 14 and TMC435[a]

		Compound		
	Property[b]	**13**	TMC435	**14**
Intravenous (2 mg/kg, $n = 2$)	Cl (L·h/kg)	—	0.505	2.5
	Vd_{ss} (L/kg)	—	0.49	4.6
	AUC (μM·h)	—	5.21	1.05
Oral (10 mg/kg, $n = 2$)	AUC (μM·h)	1.0	2.79	1.30
	C_{max} (μM)	0.23	0.73	0.31
	T_{max} (h)	0.75	3.0	1.5
	$t_{1/2}$ (h)	6.0	2.8	2.2
	F (%)	—	11	25
	Liver/plasma ratio	126	32	44

[a]Results following a single intravenous administration of 2 mg/kg in 20% hydroxypropyl-β-cyclodextrine or oral administration of 10 mg/kg in 50% PEG-400 containing 2.5% of vitamin E-TPGS in the male Sprague–Dawley rat.
[b]AUC, area under the plasma concentration–time curve; Cl, clearance; C_{max}, maximum plasma concentration; F, percentage of dose reaching systemic circulation; T_{max}, time to maximum plasma concentration; $t_{1/2}$, plasma half-life; Vd_{ss}, volume of distribution at steady state.

TABLE 2 Oral Pharmacokinetic Properties of TMC435 in Rat ($n = 3$)[a]

Dose (mg/kg)	C_{max} (μg/mL)	T_{max} (h)	$AUC_{0\text{-}inf}$ (μg·h/ml)	$t_{1/2}$ (h)	F (%)
40	1.4	2.0	7.8	2.6	44

[a]Vehicle: poly(ethylene glycol) 400/D-α-tocopheryl poly(ethylene glycol)-1000 succinate. Properties as in Table 1.

that the liver concentration was 32 times higher than that of the plasma, which was seen as an important factor given that the viral replication of HCV is reported to occur primarily in hepatocytes.

The plasma PK and tissue distribution of TMC435 (40 mg/kg) in Sprague–Dawley rats (Table 2) revealed an extensive distribution of the compound to the liver and gastrointestinal tract (small and large intestines), with tissue/plasma ratios above 35 [40]. Both the plasma exposure at 8 h postdosing and the liver exposure 31 h after oral administration were found to exceed the replicon EC_{99} value. The concentration in kidney, adrenal gland, lung, spleen, heart, and thymus was similar to the plasma concentration (ratios ranging between 0.5 and 1.3), whereas levels measured in the thyroid gland and brain were detectable but considerably lower than plasma levels [40]. In dogs, TMC435 had a better PK profile than in rats. Dog PK was characterized by complete absorption ($F = 100\%$) after oral administration of 6.5 mg/kg, high values of C_{max} (4.72 μM) and AUC (14,986 ng·h/mL) and a long half-life ($t_{1/2} = 5.1$ h) [32].

TMC435 was found inactive in a battery of genotoxicity assays and had an in vivo safety pharmacology (central nervous system, cardiovascular, and pulmonary functions) profile that provided a strong basis for continued development. To further assess the potential of TMC435, the in vitro activity of TMC435 alone or in combination with different classes of HCV inhibitors was studied. Biochemically, TMC435 displayed potent inhibition of HCV NS3/4A protease with K_i values of 0.5 and 0.4 nM for subtypes 1a (H77) and 1b (Con1) enzymes, respectively [40]. The compound was over 1000 times less active against 20 human proteases, including human leukocyte elastase, trypsin, and chymotrypsin, indicating specificity of TMC435 for the HCV NS3/4A protease (Tables 3 and 4) [40].

In a subgenomic genotype 1b (G1b) replicon assay, an EC_{50} value of 8 nM was determined for TMC435 with a selectivity index of over 2000 against the human cell lines analyzed [40]. Although TMC435 was found to be bound extensively to plasma proteins (>99%), a limited 1.4- to 1.8-fold shift in EC_{50} values was observed upon addition of human α_1-acid glycoprotein (AAG), human serum albumin (HSA), or human serum (HS) in the replicon assay, suggesting a limited effect of functional protein binding on the antiviral activity of TMC435 (EC_{50} at 40% HS = 11.2 nM) [40]. TMC435 is also a potent inhibitor of NS3/4A protease from genotypes 2 to 6, with IC_{50} values below 13 nM for all HCV NS3/4A enzymes tested, with the exception of genotype 3a protease (37 nM) [41]. Furthermore, TMC435 showed no antiviral effect against a panel of DNA and RNA viruses up to the highest concentration tested (10 or 100 μM), including closely related Flaviviridae viruses such as bovine viral diarrhea virus and yellow fever virus, further supporting the specificity of this drug candidate [40].

Recent studies have shown that mutant viral species resistant to HCV NS3/4A protease inhibitors can emerge both in vitro and in patients [42–45], as summarized in Figure 7. In vitro selection experiments using TMC435 performed in three replicon cell lines (two G1b and one G1a) showed that 85% of the 75 replicon cell colonies analyzed using population sequencing contained a mutation at NS3 position 168 [44]. In other replicon colonies, mutations were detected at NS3 positions 80 and 156. Mutations at these positions

TABLE 3 Inhibitory Activity of TMC435 (10 μM) vs. a Panel of Human Proteases Reported as a Percentage of Inhibition[a]

Name	Family	% Inhibition at 10 μM
Tryptase	serine	0.0
Chymotrypsin	serine	6.8
Tissue plasminogen activator	serine	36.6
Kallikrein	serine	18.4
Chymase	serine	−18.1
Proteinase 3	serine	−11.3
Factor VIIa	serine	8.5
Urokinase	serine	−17.0
Streptokinase	serine	4.6
Factor Xa	serine	10.4

[a]All data were generated using standard assays based on fluorescence resonance energy transfer.

TABLE 4 Inhibitory Activity of TMC435 vs. a Panel of Human Proteases Reported as Half Maximal Inhibitory Concentration (IC_{50})[a]

Name	Family	IC_{50} (μM)
Leukocyte-elastase	serine	1.5
Plasmin	serine	5.8
Thrombin	serine	5.6
Trypsin	serine	5.7
Cathepsin G	serine	3.8
Cathepsin S	cysteine	0.8
Cathepsin L	cysteine	>20
Cathepsin B	cysteine	>20
Cathepsin E	aspartic	>20
Cathepsin D	aspartic	>20

[a]All data were generated using standard assays based on fluorescence resonance energy transfer.

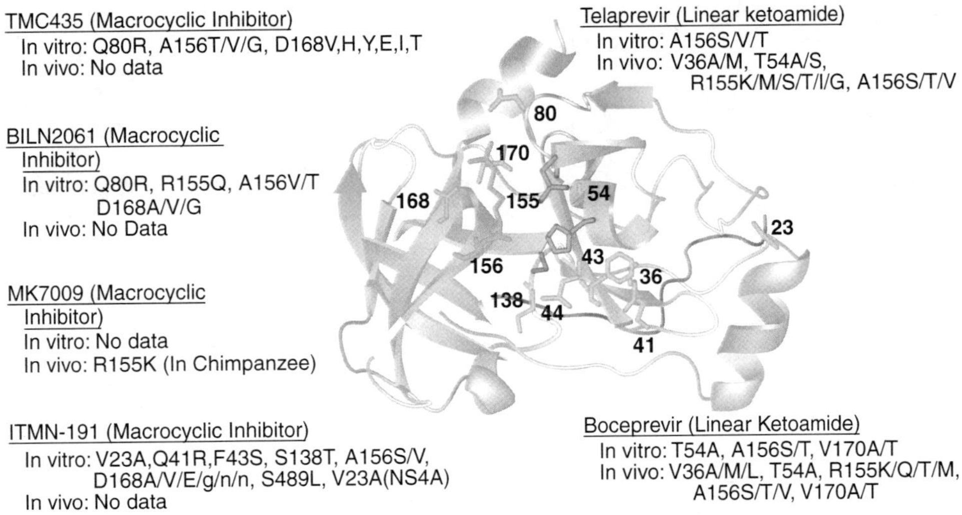

FIGURE 7 Mutations identified in vitro and in vivo with reference HCV NS3/4A protease inhibitors.

were observed after in vivo or in vitro exposure to other protease inhibitors (Fig. 7) [43–45].

Sustained virological response (SVR) rates are likely to be improved in the future by combining specifically targeted antiviral drugs with IFNα and ribavirin [45,46]. In vitro combination studies using a replicon assay have shown that the anti-HCV activity of TMC435 was additive with ribavirin, whereas a clear synergism was observed with IFNα, the polymerase nucleoside inhibitor NM-107, and the polymerase non-nucleoside inhibitor HCV-796 [40]. Additionally, the combination of TMC435 with IFNα reduced the emergence of drug-resistant replicon colonies [40]. No evidence for changes in cytotoxicity (CC_{50}) was observed upon combination [40]. Based on the overall profile described above, TMC435 was selected for early drug development.

SYNTHESIS

The synthesis of TMC435 used at the lead optimization stage is outlined in Scheme 1 [32,47]. Lactone acid **15** was submitted to a tandem of coupling reactions, first with the *N*-methylhex-5-enamine **16** then with the P1 amino acid **17**, to provide intermediate compound **18**. A Mitsunobu coupling reaction [48] between **18** and 4-hydroxy-2-(4-isopropylthiazol-2-yl)-7-methoxy-8-methylquinoline provided the open derivative **19** [32,47], which by using the Hoveyda–Grubbs first-generation catalyst for ring-closing olefin metathesis [49,50], was converted to the *cis*-macrocyclic ester **20**. Hydrolysis of the ethyl ester **20**, followed by activation of the resulting acid **21** with carbonyldiimidazole (CDI), afforded the corresponding oxazolidinone **22** [32,47]. Finally, intermediate **22** was readily opened with cyclopropyl sulfonamide in the presence of 1,8-diazabicyclo[5.4.0]undec-7-ene (DBU) to give TMC435 [32,47].

Process chemistry, outlined in Scheme 2, was performed to provide cyclopentane intermediate **30** in a high enough yield and purity suitable for large-scale industrial production of TMC435 [51]. Esterification of 1,2,3,4-butanetetracarboxylic acid **23**, followed by ring closure in the presence of sodium methoxide, afforded the target ketone **25** in 83% overall yield as a *trans*-racemic mixture [51]. The racemic lactone **27** was obtained via a tandem of reactions involving a hydrogenation of the ketone **25**, followed by a lactonization of **26** in the presence of ethyl chloroformate [51]. Esterification of **27** with benzyl alcohol, followed by the opening of the so-formed lactone **28**, led to a racemic diester intermediate which could be separated on Chiralpak AD to give **29** in 49% isolated yield [51]. Finally, hydrogenolysis of the benzyl group of **29** provided the monoacid intermediate **30**, a key intermediate for the large-scale production of TMC435 [51].

CLINICAL STUDIES

The PK and safety of TMC435 were assessed in study TMC435350-C101, a randomized double-blind placebo-controlled phase I trial in 49 healthy volunteers. In addition, this study also assessed, in an open-label non-placebo-controlled manner, the antiviral activity of TMC435 in 6 genotype 1 hepatitis C patients. The PK results following administration of single doses of TMC435 (50 to 600 mg; $n = 6$ for each dose) showed a median T_{max} of 5 h (50 and 100 mg) or 6 h (200, 300, 450, and 600 mg) with a range of 4 to 6 h

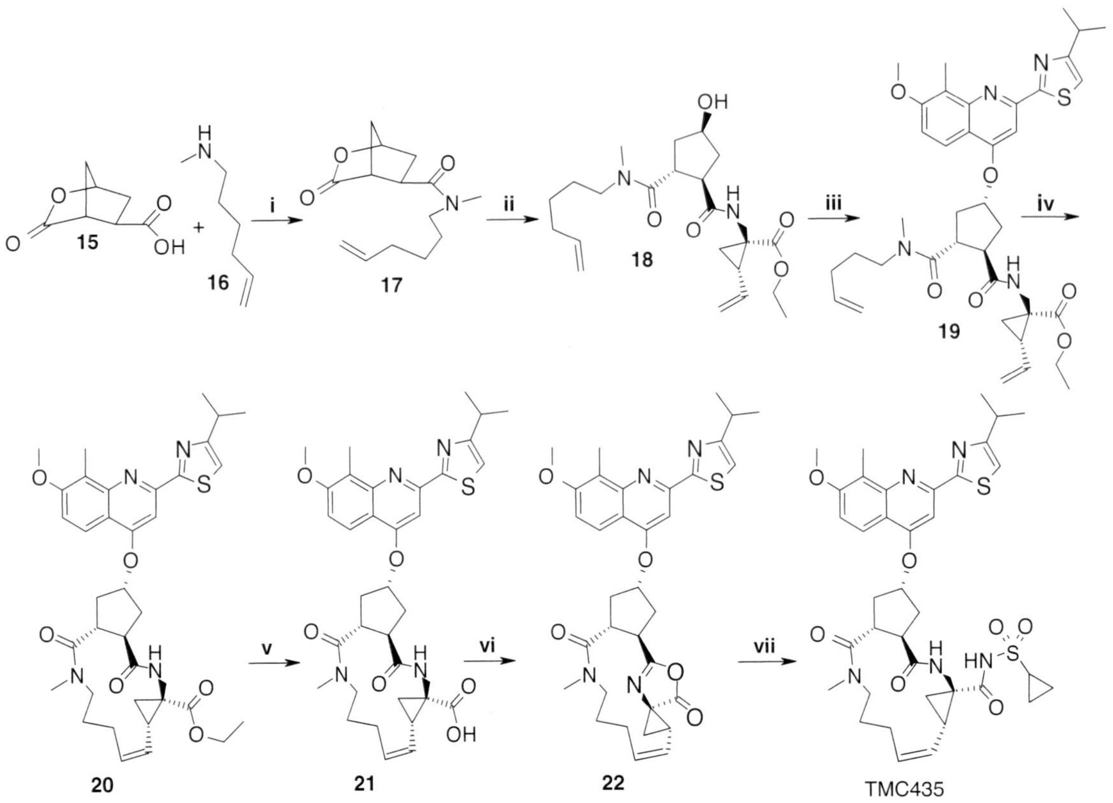

SCHEME 1 Reactions and conditions: (i) HATU [2-(7-aza-1*H*-benzotriazole-1-yl)-1,1,3,3-tetramethyluronium hexafluorophosphate], diisopropylethylamine, DMF (dimethylformamide), 0°C to room temperature; (ii) (a) LiOH, THF (tetrahydrofuran)/methanol/water, 0°C; (b) (1*R*,2*S*)-1-amino-2-vinylcyclopropane carboxylic acid ethyl ester hydrochloride, HATU, diisopropylethylamine, DMF, 0°C to room temperature; (iii) 4-hydroxy-2-(4-isopropylthiazol-2-yl)-7-methoxy-8-methylquinoline, PPh_3 (triphenylphosphine), DIAD (diisopropyl azodicarboxylate), THF, −15°C to room temperature; (iv) Hoveyda–Grubbs first-generation catalyst, dichloroethane, 70°C; (v) LiOH, THF/methanol/water, room temperature; (vi) CDI, THF, reflux; (vii) cyclopropylsulfonamide, DBU, THF, 50°C.

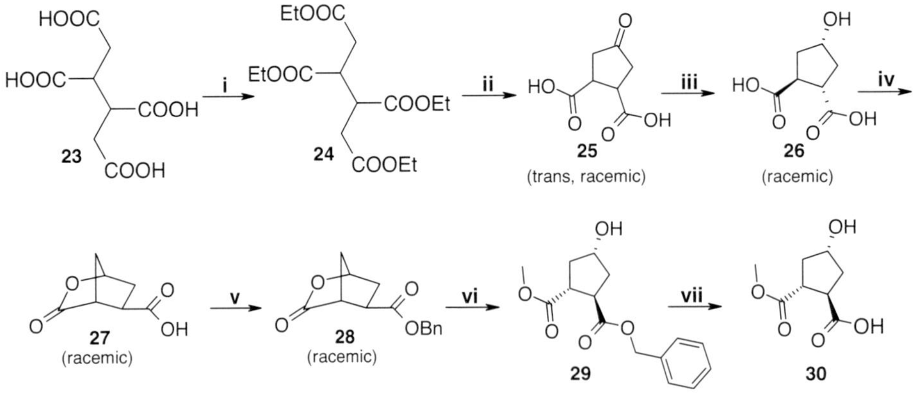

SCHEME 2 Reactions and conditions: (i) H_2SO_4, ethanol, toluene, reflux, 91%; (ii) (a) sodium methoxide, methanol, room temperature; (b) HCl, H_2O, reflux, 91%; (iii) (a) H_2, Rh/C, NaOH, H_2O, 60°C; (b) 4-methyl-2-pentanone, acetone, H_2SO_4, 50 to 22°C, 66%; (iv) triethylamine, ethylchloroformate, THF, 0–5 to 22°C, 48%; (v) benzyl alcohol, DMAP (dimethylaminopyridine), EDCI [1-ethyl-3-(3-dimethylaminopropyl)carbodiimide], ethyl acetate, room temperature, 88%; (vi) (a) methanol, Amberlyst 15, room temperature, 94%; (b) Chiralpak AD separation, 49%; (vii) H_2, 10% Pd/C, THF, quantitative.

TABLE 5 PK of Multiple Ascending Doses of TMC435 in Healthy Volunteers and HCV-Infected Patients

Pharmacokinetics of Multiple-Dose TMC435 [mean ± S.D., T_{max}: median (range)]	100 mg TMC435 ($n = 4$)	200 mg TMC435 ($n = 5$)	400 mg TMC435 ($n = 6$)	200 mg TMC435 ($n = 6$, HCV+)
Day 1				
T_{max} (h)	5.0 (3.0–6.0)	4.0 (3.0–6.0)	6.0 (4.0–8.0)	6.0 (4.0–8.0)
C_{max} (μg/mL)	0.68 ± 0.17	2.30 ± 0.92	7.09 ± 1.35	4.07 ± 1.48
AUC_{24h} (μg·h/mL)	6.35 ± 1.61	24.6 ± 7.33	75.7 ± 15.5	56.4 ± 22.5
Day 5				
C_{min} (μg/mL)	0.09 ± 0.03	1.40 ± 0.79	7.80 ± 4.02	5.74 ± 4.09
C_{max} (μg/mL)	0.76 ± 0.21	6.17 ± 2.86	19.40 ± 6.25	11.50 ± 5.34
T_{max} (h)	4.0 (4.0–6.0)	4.0 (4.0–8.0)	4.0 (3.0–6.0)	4.0 (4.0–8.0)
AUC_{24h} (μg·h/mL)	7.62 ± 1.91	79.70 ± 37.23	332.00 ± 120.00	206.0 ± 114.00
Ratio AUC_{24h}: day 5/day 1 (%)	120.1 ± 5.272	316.0 ± 101.2	431.8 ± 82.59	344.8 ± 67.16

for all but the 50-mg dose (range 3 to 6 h). The mean terminal half-life was approximately 10 h at the 50- and 100-mg doses (the accuracy of these measurements at the higher-dose levels was limited). The TMC435 exposure increased more than proportionally to the dose, and additional PK analyses showed that there was no difference in the oral bioavailability of 200 mg TMC435 when administered in a fed or fasted state.

The safety, tolerability, and PK profile was also studied in a 5-day multiple ascending-dose panel [100 mg once daily (q.d.), 200 mg q.d., 200 mg twice daily (b.i.d.), or 400 mg q.d.] in healthy volunteers. TMC435 exposure increased more than proportionally to the dose, both in comparing the AUC for the 100- and 200-mg, and the 200- and 400-mg q.d. dose (Table 5). The dose-disproportional PK may be explained partially by an apparent prolonged absorption, which becomes more evident at higher doses. Steady state was attained on day 3 for the 100-mg q.d. regimen, but for both higher doses the 5-day evaluation period was insufficient to reach steady state. In a later study (TMC435350-C104) designed to evaluate the PK of TMC435 delivered as a capsule, steady state for a 200-mg q.d. regimen was attained within 7 days.

In study TMC435350-C101, the trough concentrations (C_{min}) of TMC435 achieved for all doses were considerably in excess of EC_{50} concentrations determined for the genotype 1b in vitro replicon system (8 nM or 6 ng/mL) [51]. No serious adverse events or adverse events leading to discontinuation were reported in healthy volunteers (Table 6). In the multiple-dose part of the trial, 3/4 (75.0%), 4/5 (80.0%), and 4/6 (66.7%) subjects reported at least one adverse event during TMC435 100, 200, and 400 mg q.d. administration, respectively. There was no apparent dose relationship between any of the adverse events reported in more than one subject in any of the dose groups, and no adverse events considered to be possibly (or probably) related to TMC435

TABLE 6 Summary of Adverse Events (AEs) by Body System and Preferred Term (Regardless of Severity) Observed During the Multiple Ascending Dose of TMC435 in Healthy Volunteers

	100 mg q.d.		200 mg q.d.		200 mg b.i.d.		400 mg q.d.	
	TMC 435 ($n = 4$)	Placebo ($n = 2$)	TMC 435 ($n = 5$)	Placebo ($n = 2$)	TMC 435 ($n = 6$)	Placebo ($n = 3$)	TMC 435 ($n = 6$)	Placebo ($n = 3$)
AEs reported in >1 subject in any group, n (%)								
Headache	1 (25)	0	3 (60)	1 (50)	0	0	0	0
Photosensitivity reaction	0	0	0	0	3 (50)	0	0	0
Diarrhea	0	0	0	0	2 (33)	0	0	0
Abdominal pain, upper	0	0	0	0	2 (33)	0	0	0
Abdominal distension	1 (25)	0	0	0	1 (17)	0	0	0
AEs reported in >1 subject at least possibly related to TMC435, n (%)								
Photosensitivity reaction	0	0	0	0	3 (50)	0	0	0
Diarrhea	0	0	0	0	2 (33)	0	0	0
Abdominal pain upper	0	0	0	0	2 (33)	0	0	0

were reported in any of the once-daily dose groups. In the 200-mg b.i.d. group, transient mild photosensitivity (short-lasting facial redness) was observed in three of the six healthy volunteers receiving TMC435, and resolved spontaneously. Photosensitivity has not led to discontinuation in any patient during clinical development of TMC435. A dose of 200 mg q.d. was selected for proof-of-concept assessment of antiviral activity and to evaluate PK and safety in hepatitis C patients.

Six patients with HCV genotype 1 who had not responded to ($n = 4$), or relapsed during ($n = 2$), previous IFN-based therapy were enrolled in study TMC435350-C101 (Table 7). The median plasma HCV-RNA level was 6.75 $\log_{10}$ IU/mL (range 6.47 to 7.03 $\log_{10}$ IU/mL) at baseline. Four hepatitis C patients were infected with genotype 1a and two with genotype 1b as assessed by NS5B-based sequence analysis.

In patients receiving 200 mg q.d. TMC435, a PK profile was seen similar in shape to that seen in healthy volunteers. The mean exposure to drug was higher in the six patients compared with healthy volunteers following a dose of 200 mg q.d., resulting in exposures between those observed for the 200- and 400-mg q.d. dose in healthy volunteers (Fig. 8). The mean plasma trough levels observed in patients in study TMC435-C101 were over 900 times the replicon (1b) EC_{50} value (Table 5).

Serum HCV-RNA levels declined rapidly in all six patients with a reduction of more than 3 $\log_{10}$ IU/mL in plasma HCV-RNA compared with baseline. The first-phase viral decay was steep, as anticipated for this class of compounds, and was complete by 72 h. The median HCV-RNA load decrease at day 3 (first phase) was 3.46 $\log_{10}$, and on day 6, 24 h after administration of the last dose, the decrease ranged from 2.91 $\log_{10}$ to 4.05 $\log_{10}$ (Fig. 9). Using these data, a viral kinetics model described by Neuman et al. estimated the mean turnover of infected cells to be 0.24 day (day 1), the half-life of infected cells to be 2.8 days ($t_{1/2}$), the clearance of virus to be 0.26/h, and half-life of free virus to be 2.66 h consistent with the literature [52]. An in vivo potency (ε) value of 0.9993 was calculated, positioning this drug among the most potent of its class, with a potential advantage of a once-a-day dosing regimen. HCV-RNA levels in the 3 days following the last dose remained relatively constant, changing less than 0.5 $\log_{10}$ in all patients, suggesting continued suppression of viral replication.

There was no indication of differences in antiviral activity of TMC435 between patients infected with genotype 1a or 1b virus, previous nonresponders or relapsers, or patients presenting with hemophilia. HCV-RNA levels returned to pretreatment levels between 2 and 4 weeks after the final dose. While the safety profile observed in this study supports further exploration of the 200-mg q.d. dose, the high plasma exposure of TMC435 potentially allows for lower doses without limiting antiviral activity. Based on PK modeling, trough plasma and liver concentrations of TMC435 at steady state were estimated to exceed the protein-binding-corrected ($\times$ 2) replicon EC_{50} value by more than 15- and 500-fold, respectively, following a dose of 25 mg q.d.

A phase IIa double-blind randomized placebo-controlled study [OPERA-1 (TMC435350-C201)] in genotype-1-HCV-infected subjects was designed to study the antiviral activity, safety, and PK of repeated doses of TMC435, with or without standard IFNα-2a and ribavirin. At the time of this writing, the results of a 4-week analysis of safety and antiviral activity data for TMC435 in treatment-naive hepatitis C patients (cohorts 1 and 2) and patients who had failed previous IFN-based therapy (cohort 4) was available. These interim results are summarized below.

Treatment-naive patients were randomized to receive either 7 days of monotherapy with once-daily TMC435 25 mg ($n = 9$), 75 mg ($n = 10$), or 200 mg ($n = 9$) followed by 21 days of combination therapy with TMC435 (at the randomized dose), pegIFNα-2a, and ribavirin; 28 days of combination therapy with TMC435 25 mg ($n = 9$), 75 mg ($n = 9$), or 200 mg ($n = 9$), pegIFNα-2a and ribavirin; or placebo ($n = 19$) administered as monotherapy for 7 days, then with pegIFNα-2a and ribavirin for 21 days or with pegIFNα-2a and ribavirin for 28 days. Patients who had failed previous treatment were randomized to receive 28 days of combination therapy with TMC435 75 mg ($n = 9$), 150 mg ($n = 9$), 200 mg ($n = 10$), or placebo ($n = 9$), pegIFNα-2a, and ribavirin. After the 28 days of combined therapy, all patients continued on PegIFNα-2a/ribavirin alone for up to 48 weeks.

In the treatment-naive patients, a dose relationship in antiviral activity was observed during 7 days of monotherapy across the 25-, 75-, and 200-mg doses of TMC435 (mean reductions in HCV-RNA of 2.63, 3.43, and 4.13 $\log_{10}$ IU/mL, respectively). After a further 21 days of combination treatment with TMC435, the mean reduction in viral load drop had increased to 4.26, 4.48, and 4.60 $\log_{10}$ IU/mL, respectively. For naive patients who had received 28 days of combination treatment with TMC435, the mean reductions in HCV-RNA viral load were slightly greater (ranging from 4.74 to 5.44 $\log_{10}$ IU/mL), with results for the 75- and 200-mg dose groups showing a similar viral decline.

In treatment-naive patients receiving 28 days of combination therapy with TMC435, HCV-RNA levels in all patients randomized to the TMC435 75- and 200-mg dose groups were below the lower limit of quantification (<25 IU/mL) at day 28. Furthermore, at day 28, 88.9 and 70.0% of patients in the TMC435 75- and 200-mg dose groups, respectively, achieved undetectable HCV-RNA (<10 IU/mL).

In patients who had received an initial 7 days of monotherapy, five patients had viral breakthroughs during the four-week treatment period (two patients each in the 25- and 75-mg groups and one patient in the 200-mg group), while no viral breakthrough was observed in patients who received 28 days of combination treatment. At day 28, 6/9 (66.7%) of patients in the 25-mg group, and all of the patients in

TABLE 7 Baseline Demographics of the Study Subjects

Parameter	Single Ascending Dose			Multiple Ascending Doses					
	TMC435 50, 200, 450 mg/placebo ($n = 9$)	TMC435 11, 300, 600 mg/placebo ($n = 9$)	Total ($n = 18$)	TMC435 100 mg q.d./placebo ($n = 6$)	TMC435 200 mg q.d./placebo ($n = 7$)	TMC435 200 mg b.i.d./placebo ($n = 9$)	TMC435 400 mg q.d./placebo ($n = 9$)	Total ($n = 31$)	HCV + TNC435 200 mg q.d. ($n = 6$)
Age, years Median (range)	37.0 (21 to 55)	38.0 (23 to 55)	37.5 (21 to 55)	40.5 (22 to 53)	25.0 (23 to 51)	38.0 (25 to 54)	24.0 (20 to 44)	27.0 (20 to 54)	56.5 (32 to 67)
BMI, kg/m^2 Median (range)	24.7 (19 to 30)	24.4 (21 to 28)	24.5 (19 to 30)	22.5 (19 to 27)	26.0 (21 to 30)	24.3 (22 to 29)	22.1 (19 to 27)	23.6; (19 to 30)	23.3 (21 to 27)
Gender, *n*									
Male	8	9	17	3	7	8	8	26	6
Female	1	0	1	3	0	1	1	5	0
Ethnic origin, *n*									
Caucasian/white	8	7	15	6	7	9	8	30	6
Oriental/Asian	0	1	1	0	0	0	1	1	
Black	0	1	1	0	0	0	0	0	
Other	1	0	1	0	0	0	0	0	

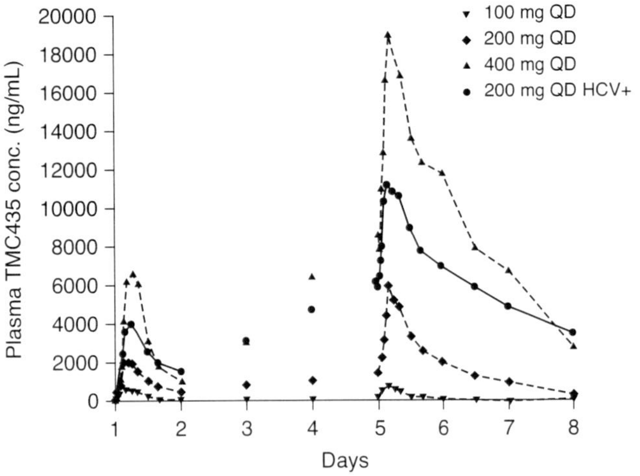

FIGURE 8 Mean PK profiles for multiple ascending-dose study of TMC435 in healthy volunteers and hepatitis C patients.

the 75- and 200-mg groups, had HCV-RNA levels below the lower limit of quantification (<25 IU/mL) with 3/9 (33.3%), 8/9 (88.9%), and 7/10 (70.0%) patients in the 25-, 75-, and 200-mg groups, respectively, had undetectable HCV-RNA (<10 IU/mL).

In the 37 patients who had failed previous IFN-based therapy, at the end of 28 days of combination therapy with TMC435, mean decreases in plasma HCV-RNA from baseline were 4.3, 5.5, and 5.3 $\log_{10}$ IU/mL in patients receiving 75, 150, and 200 mg TMC435, respectively, compared with 1.5 $\log_{10}$ IU/mL in the placebo group. Overall, 4/9 (44.4%),

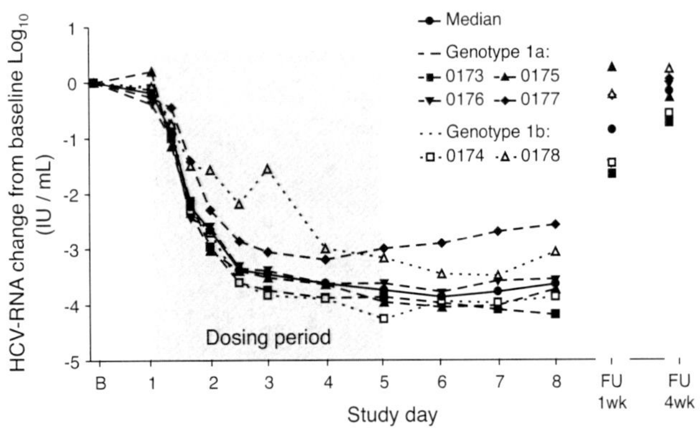

FIGURE 9 HCV-RNA viral load change from baseline for panel 7 of study TMC435350-C101. HCV-RNA levels were determined in plasma using the Cobas Taqman HCV/HPS assay v2.0 (at Covance) with a dynamic range of 30 to 200,000,000 IU/mL and with a lower limit of quantification of 25 IU/mL and a lower limit of detection of approximately 10 IU/mL. Samples were taken at screening, on day −1, on day 1 (every 8 h, including pre-dose), on day 2 (every 12 h, including pre-dose), on days 3 to 5 (pre-dose), and at 24, 48, and 72 h after the last dose to coincide with sampling for PK measurements. Viral load was determined at 10 to 14 days and 30 to 35 days after the last drug intake.

7/9 (77.8%), and 7/10 (70.0%) patients receiving 75, 150, and 200 mg TMC435, respectively, and no patients in the placebo group achieved HCV-RNA below the lower limit of quantification. Three viral breakthroughs were observed exclusively in patients with HCV genotype 1b: two in the 75-mg group and one in the 150-mg group.

In all three cohorts, there were no TMC435-related treatment discontinuations or serious adverse events. In both treatment-naive patients and patients who had failed previous IFN-based treatment AST and ALT values improved during therapy with TMC435. Mild-to-moderate increases in bilirubin (total, direct and indirect) were observed in some patients in all three cohorts, mainly in those receiving the 200-mg dose. There were no clinically relevant changes in other laboratory parameters, ECGs, or vital signs in any of the cohorts. The most common adverse events reported in treatment-naive patients were headache, fatigue, influenza-like illness, and nausea. In patients who had failed previous treatment, the most common adverse events reported were headache, influenza-like illness, dyspnea, and nausea. There were no reports of photosensitivity during treatment in any of the treatment groups. Given the positive proof-of-concept data from this study, further clinical trials are ongoing to assess the safety and efficacy of TMC435 in combination with IFNα/ribavirin in longer treatment regimens.

FUTURE DEVELOPMENT

Future development of TMC435 will follow the rapidly evolving treatment paradigm for hepatitis C and will involve drug combinations to improve SVR rates in different patient populations. At this point, the pipeline for potential anti-HCV drugs is strong, and three- and four-drug combinations can be envisaged to cure patients of HCV infection. Proof-of-concept data for combining HCV NS3/4A protease inhibitors with pegylated IFNα and ribavirin are very encouraging, with SVRs of 69% realized in phase II studies for naive patients [53]. The challenge for protease inhibitors including TMC435 is to optimize SVR rates in combination with standard of care while shortening treatment duration. Given its safety profile, once-daily dosing regimen, combination potential, and antiviral potency, the NS3/4A protease inhibitor TMC435 is a promising addition to the growing arsenal of direct antiviral drugs against HCV. Further assessment of TMC435 will be undertaken in the overall clinical development program, including the dose-finding study, which will be begun shortly.

REFERENCES

[1] Liang, T. J.; Heller, T. *Gastroenterology* **2004**, *127*, S62.
[2] Brown, R. S. *Nature* **2005**, *436*, 973–978.
[3] Shepard, C. W.; Alter, M. J. *Lancet* **2005**, *5*(8), 524.

[4] Salmon-Ceron, D.; Lewden, C.; Morlat, P.; Fvilacqua, S. B.; Jougla, E.; Bonnet, F.; Fripret, L. H.; Costagliola, D.; May, T.; Chêne, G. *J. Hepatol.* **2005**, *42*, 799–805.

[5] Fried, M. W.; Shiffman, M. L.; Reddy, K. R.; Smith, C.; Marinos, G.; Goncales, F. L., Jr.; Haussinger, D.; Diago, M.; Carosi, G.; Dhumeaux, D.; et al. *N. Engl. J. Med.* **2002**, *347* (13), 975.

[6] Manns, M. P.; McHutchison, J. G.; Gordon, S. C.; Rustgi, V. K.; Shiffman, M.; Reindollar, R.; Goodman, Z. D.; Koury, K.; Ling, M.-H.; Albrecht, J. K. (International Hepatitis Interventional Therapy Group). *Lancet* **2001**, *358*(9286), 958.

[7] Soriano, V.; Miralles, C.; Berdún, M. A.; Losada, E.; Aguirrebengoa, K.; Ocampo, A.; Arazo, P.; Cervantes, M.; de los Santos, I.; San Joaquín, I.; et al. *Antiviral. Ther.* **2007**, *12*(4), 469.

[8] Lawitz, E.; Rodriguez-Torres, M.; Muir, A. J.; Kieffer, T. L.; McNair, L.; Khunvichai, A.; McHutchison, J. G. Antiviral effects and safety of telaprevir, peginterferon alfa-2a, and ribavirin for 28 days in hepatitis C patients. *J. Hepatol.* **2008**, *49*, 163–169.

[9] Sarrazin, C.; Rouzier, R.; Wagner, F.; Forestier, N.; Larrey, D.; Gupta, S. K.; Hussain, M.; Shah, A.; Cutler, D.; Zhang, J.; Zeuzem, S. *Gastroenterology* **2007**, *132*, 1270.

[10] McHutchison, J. G.; Everson, G. T.; Gordon, S. C.; Jacobson, I. M.; Sulkowski, M.; Kauffman, R.; McNair, L.; Alam, J.; Muir, A. J. (PROVE1 Study Team). *N. Engl. J. Med.* **2009**, *360*, 1827.

[11] De Francesco, R.; Tomei, L.; Altamura, S.; Summa, V.; Migliaccio, G. *Antiviral Res.* **2003**, *58*, 1.

[12] Griffith, R. C.; Lou, L.; Roberts, C. D.; Schm, U. *Annu. Rep. Med. Chem.* **2005**, *39*, 223.

[13] Ni, Z.-J.; Wagman, A. S. *Curr. Opin. Drug Discov. Dev.* **2004**, *7*, 446.

[14] Goudreau, N.; Llinàs-Brunet, M. *Expert Opin. Invest. Drugs* **2005**, *14*, 1129.

[15] Lamarre, D.; Anderson, P. C.; Bailey, M.; Beaulieu, P.; Bolger, G.; Bonneau, P.; Bos, M.; Cameron, D. R.; Cartier, M.; Cordingley, M. G.; et al. *Nature* **2003**, *426*, 186.

[16] Kaukinen, P.; Sillanpaa, M.; Kotenko, S.; Lin, R.; Hiscott, J.; Melen, K.; Julkunen, I. *Virol. J.* **2006**, *3*, 66.

[17] López-Labrador, F. X. *Recent Pat. Antiinfect. Drug Discov.* **2008**, *3*, 157–167.

[18] Failla, C.; Tomei, L., De Francesco, R. *J. Virol.* **1994**, *68*, 3753.

[19] Llinàs-Brunet, M.; Bailey, M.; Fazal, G.; Goulet, S.; Halmos, T.; LaPante, S.; Maurice, R.; Poirier, M.; Poupart, M.-A.; Thibeault, D.; et al. *Bioorg. Med. Chem. Lett.* **1998**, *8*, 1713.

[20] Steinkühler, C.; Biasiol, G.; Brunetti, M.; Urbani, A.; Koch, U.; Cortese, R.; Pessi, A.; De Francesco, R. *Biochemistry* **1998**, *37*, 8899.

[21] Llinàs-Brunet, M.; Bailey, M. D.; Ghiro, E.; Gorys, V.; Halmos, T.; Poirier, M.; Rancourt, J.; Goudreau, N. *J. Med. Chem.* **2004**, *47*, 6584.

[22] Lipinski, C. A.; Lombardo, F.; Domony, B. W.; Feeney, P. J. *Adv. Drug Deliv. Rev.* **1997**, *23*, 3.

[23] Llinàs-Brunet, M.; Bailey, M. D.; Bolger, G.; Brochu, C.; Faucher, A.-M.; Ferland, J. M.; Garneau, M.; Ghiro, E.; Gorys, V.; et al. *J. Med. Chem.* **2004**, *47*, 1605.

[24] Lamarre, D.; Anderson, P.; Bailey, M.; Beaulieu, P.; Bolger, G.; Bonneau, P.; Bös. M.; Cameron, D.; Cartier, M.; Cordingley, M.; et al. *Nature* **2003**, *426*, 186.

[25] Llinàs-Brunet, M.; Bailey, M. D.; Ghiro, E.; Gorys, V.; Halmos, T.; Poirier, M.; Rancourt, J.; Goudreau, N. *J. Med. Chem.* **2004**, *47*, 6584.

[26] Manns, M. P.; Foster, G. R.; Rockstroh, J. K.; Zeuzem, S.; Zoulim, F.; Houghton, M. *Nat. Rev. Drug Discov.* **2007**, *6*, 991–1000.

[27] Kwo, P.; Lawitz, E.; McCone, J.; Schiff, E.; Vierling, J.; Pound, D.; Davis, M.; Galati, J.; Gordon, S.; Ravendhran, N.; et al. Interim results from HCV SPRINT-1: RVR/EVR from phase 2 study of boceprevir plus pegintron (peginterferon alfa-2b)/ribavirin in treatment-naive subjects with genotype-1 CHC. *J. Hepatol.* **2008**, *48*, S372.

[28] Johansson, P.-O.; Bäck, M.; Kvarnström, I.; Vrang, L.; Hamelink, E.; Hallberg, A.; Rosenquist, Å.; Samuelsson, B. Potent inhibitors of the hepatitis C virus NS3 protease: use of a novel P2 cyclopentane-derived template. *Bioorg. Med. Chem.* **2006**, *14*, 5136–5151.

[29] Tsantrizos, Y. S.; Bolger, G.; Bonneau, P.; Cameron, D. R.; Goudreau, N.; Kukolj, G.; LaPlante, S. R.; Llinàs-Brunet, M.; Nar, H.; Lamarre, D. *Angew. Chem. Int. Ed.* **2003**, *42*, 1356.

[30] Goudreau, N.; Cameron, D. R.; Bonneau, P.; Gorys, V.; Plouffe, C.; Poirier, M.; Lamarre, D.; Llinàs-Brunet, M. *J. Med. Chem.* **2004**, *47*, 123–132.

[31] Perni, R. B.; Britt, S. D.; Court, J. C.; Courtney, L. F.; Deininger, D. D.; Farmer, L. J.; Gates, C. A.; Harbeson, S. L.; Kim, J. L.; Landro, J. A.; et al. *Bioorg. Med. Chem. Lett.* **2003**, *13*, 4059–4063.

[32] Raboisson, P.; Lin, T.-I; de Kock, H.; Vendeville, S.; Van de Vreken, W.; McGowan, D.; Tahri, A.; Hu, L.; Lenz, O.; Delouvroy, F.; et al. *Bioorg. Med. Chem. Lett.* **2008**, *18*, 5095–5100.

[33] Bäck, M.; Johansson, P.-O.; Wångsell, F.; Thorstensson, F.; Kvarnström, I.; Ayesa Alvarez, S.; Wähling, H.; Pelcman, M.; Jansson, K.; Lindström, S.; et al. Novel potent macrocyclic inhibitors of the hepatitis C virus NS3 protease: use of cyclopentane and cyclopentene P2-motifs. *Bioorg. Med. Chem.* **2007**, *15*, 7184–7202.

[34] Raboisson, P.; de Kock, H.; Rosenquist, Å.; Nilsson, M.; Salvador-Oden, L.; Lin, T.-I; Roue, N.; Ivanov, V.; Wähling, H.; Wickström, K.; et al. *Bioorg. Med. Chem. Lett.* **2008**, *18*, 4853–4858.

[35] Vendeville, S.; Nilsson, M.; Antonov, D.; Classon, B.; Ayesa, S.; Ivanov, V.; Johansson, P.-O.; Kahnberg, P.; Eneroth, A.; Wikström, K.; et al. *Bioorg. Med. Chem. Lett.* **2008**, *18*, 6189–6193.

[36] Tsantrizos, Y. S.; Bolger, G.; Bonneau, P.; Cameron, D. R.; Goudreau, N.; Kukolj, G.; LaPlante, S. R.; Llinàs-Brunet, M.; Nar, H.; Lamarre, D. *Angew. Chem. Int. Ed.* **2003**, *42*, 1356–1360.

[37] Raboisson, P. J.-M. B.; De Kock, H. A.; Simmen, K. A.; Joensson, C. E. D.; Nilsson, K. M.; Rosenquist, Å. A. K.; Samuelsson, B. B.; Antonov, D.; Salvador, O. L.; Ayesa, A. S.; Classon, B. O. Preparation of macrocyclic inhibitors of hepatitis C virus. WO2007014922A1, 2007.

[38] Raboisson, P. J.-M. B.; DeKock, H. A.; McGowan, D. C.; Van de Vreken, W.; Hu, L.; Tahri, A.; Vendeville, S. M. H. Preparation of macrocyclic peptides as inhibitors of hepatitis C virus. WO2008059046A1, 2008.

[39] Raboisson, P. J.-M. B.; De Kock, H. A.; Hu, L.; Simmen, K. A.; Lindquist, K. C.; Lindstroem, M. S.; Belfrage, A. K. G. L.; Waehling, H. J.; Nilsson, K. M.; Samuelsson, B. B.; et al. Preparation of macrocyclic inhibitors of hepatitis C virus. WO2007014927A2, 2007.

[40] Lin, T.-I.; Lenz, O.; Fanning, G.; Verbinnen, T.; Delouvroy, F.; Scholliers, A.; Vermeiren, K.; Rosenquist, Å.; Edlund, M.; Samuelsson, B.; et al. In vitro activity and pre-clinical profile of TMC435350, a potent HCV protease inhibitor. *Antimicrob. Agents Chemother.* **2009**, *53*, 1377–1385.

[41] Lin, T.-I.; Devogelaere, B.; Lenz, O.; Nyanguile, O.; van der Helm, E.; Vermeiren, K.; Vandercruyssen, G.; Cleiren, E.; Lindberg, J.; Edlund, M.; et al. Inhibitory activity of TMC435350 on HCV NS3/4A proteases from genotypes 1 to 6. *Hepatology* **2008**, *48*, 1166A.

[42] Middleton, T.; He, Y.; Pilot-Matias, T.; Tripathi, R.; Lim, H. B.; Roth, A.; Chen, C. M.; Koev, G.; Ng, T. I.; Krishnan, P.; et al. A replicon-based shuttle vector system for assessing the phenotype of HCV NS5B polymerase genes isolated from patient populations. *J. Virol. Methods* **2007**, *145*, 137–145.

[43] He, Y.; King, M. S.; Kempf, D. J.; Lu, L.; Lim, H. B.; Krishnan, P.; Kati, W.; Middleton, T.; Molla, A. Relative replication capacity and selective advantage profiles of protease inhibitor-resistant hepatitis C virus (HCV) NS3 protease mutants in the HCV genotype 1b replicon system. *Antimicrob. Agents Chemother.* **2008**, *52*, 1101–1110.

[44] Lenz, O. Progress in the development of HCV protease inhibitors. HCV Resistance Workshop, Boston, June 5–6, 2008.

[45] Koev, G.; Kati, W. The emerging field of HCV drug resistance. *Expert. Opin. Invest. Drugs* **2008**, *17*, 303–319.

[46] Manns, M. P.; Foster, G. R.; Rockstroh, J. K.; Zeuzem, S.; Zoulim, F.; Houghton, M. The way forward in HCV treatment: finding the right path. *Nat. Rev. Drug Discov.* **2007**, *6*, 991–1000.

[47] Raboisson, P. J.-M. B.; De Kock, H. A.; Hu, L.; Vendeville, S. M. H.; Tahri, A.; Surleraux, D. L. N. G.; Simmen, K. A.; Nilsson, K. M.; Samuelsson, B. B.; Rosenquist, Å. A. K.; et al. Preparation of macrocyclic inhibitors of hepatitis C virus. WO2007014926A1, 2007.

[48] Mitsunobu, O. The use of diethyl azodicarboxylate and triphenylphosphine in synthesis and transformation of natural products. *Synthesis* **1981**, 1–28.

[49] Harrity, J. P. A.; La, D. S.; Visser, M. S.; Hoveyda, A. H. Chromenes through metal-catalyzed reactions of styrenyl ethers: mechanism and utility in synthesis. *J. Am. Chem. Soc.* **1998**, *120*, 2343–2351.

[50] Kingsbury, J. S.; Harrity, J. P. A.; Bonitatebus, P. J.; Hoveyda, A. H. A recyclable Ru-based metathesis catalyst. *J. Am. Chem. Soc.* **1999**, *121*, 791–799.

[51] Horvath, A.; Depre, D. P. M.; Ormerod, D. J. Processes and intermediates for preparing a macrocyclic HCV protease inhibitor. WO2008092955A1, 2008.

[52] Neumann, A. U.; Lam, N. P.; Dahari, H.; Gretch, D. R.; Wiley, T. E.; Layden, T. J.; Perelson, A. S. Hepatitis C viral dynamics in vivo and the antiviral efficacy of interferon-α therapy. *Science* **1998**, *282*, 103–107.

[53] Hézode, C.; Forestier, N.; Dusheiko, G.; Ferenci, P.; Pol, S.; Goeser, T.; Bronowicki, J. P.; Bourlière, M.; Gharakhanian, S.; Bengtsson, L.; et al. (PROVE2 Study Team). Telaprevir and peginterferon with or without ribavirin for chronic HCV infection. *N. Engl. J. Med.* **2009** Apr 30; *360*(18), 1839–1850.

20

DISCOVERY AND CLINICAL EVALUATION OF THE NUCLEOSIDE ANALOG BALAPIRAVIR (R1626) FOR THE TREATMENT OF HCV INFECTION

KLAUS KLUMPP AND DAVID B. SMITH

Roche Palo Alto Llc, Palo Alto, California

INTRODUCTION

Hepatitis C virus (HCV) infection is associated with significant morbidity and mortality, but available options for therapy and cure are very limited and associated with suboptimal safety, tolerability, and efficacy in a large proportion of patients [1–5]. There is an urgent need to develop new, more effective, and better tolerated therapies for the treatment of HCV infection. Interferon α and ribavirin are both nonspecific, broad-spectrum agents which affect multiple cell functions as well as virus replication. Intensive research activities have therefore focused on two areas: (1) to generate a better understanding of the molecular mechanisms of HCV replication and host interactions, and (2) to deliver more specific drugs that target key mechanisms of the HCV replication cycle in a more selective fashion and with higher potency.

Hepatitis C Virus Replication

HCV is a spherical, enveloped, positive-strand RNA virus and is the type member of the genus *Hepacivirus* within the family Flaviviridae [6]. The HCV genome consists of a single stranded RNA molecule of approximately 9600 nucleotides. This RNA contains a single, large open reading frame that encodes a polyprotein of approximately 3000 amino acid residues. Individual viral proteins are released by proteolytic cleavage of the polyprotein, a process that requires both host and viral protease enzymes. The N-terminus of the polyprotein contains the structural protein core, E1 and E2, a central region contains two proteins, p7 and NS2, which are believed to be important for viral budding and release, and a C-terminal region forms the nonstructural proteins (NS3, NS4A, NS4B, NS5A, and NS5B) (Fig. 1a) [7]. An important milestone in establishing tools for drug discovery was the demonstration that a bicistronic RNA construct, called a *replicon*, carrying the HCV nonstructural proteins and an antibiotic resistance selection marker, could replicate autonomously in a human hepatoma cell line (Huh7) and be maintained in cell culture under selective pressure [8]. The HCV replicon system has proven to be clearly predictive of clinical antiviral efficacy for drug candidates targeting the nonstructural protein NS3 protease, NS5A, and NS5B, the HCV polymerase [9]. The structural proteins have been replaced by a new fusion protein that consists of the N-terminus of the core protein for efficient translation initiation, a reporter gene such as luciferase, and a neomycin resistance gene to allow for the selection of replicon carrying cells with G418 antibiotic (Fig. 1b) [10]. The RNA packaged into HCV virions is positive strand, which means that after cell entry, the RNA functions as a messenger RNA. The 5′-untranslated region (UTR) constitutes an internal ribosomal entry site (IRES), which directs the assembly of ribosomes and initiation of protein synthesis (translation) immediately following the cell entry of HCV particles. The newly generated viral nonstructural proteins assemble into endoplasmic reticulum (ER) membrane-associated HCV replicase complexes, which carry out new RNA synthesis within infected cells (Fig. 1c) [11–17].

Antiviral Drugs: From Basic Discovery Through Clinical Trials, First Edition. Edited by Wieslaw M. Kazmierski.

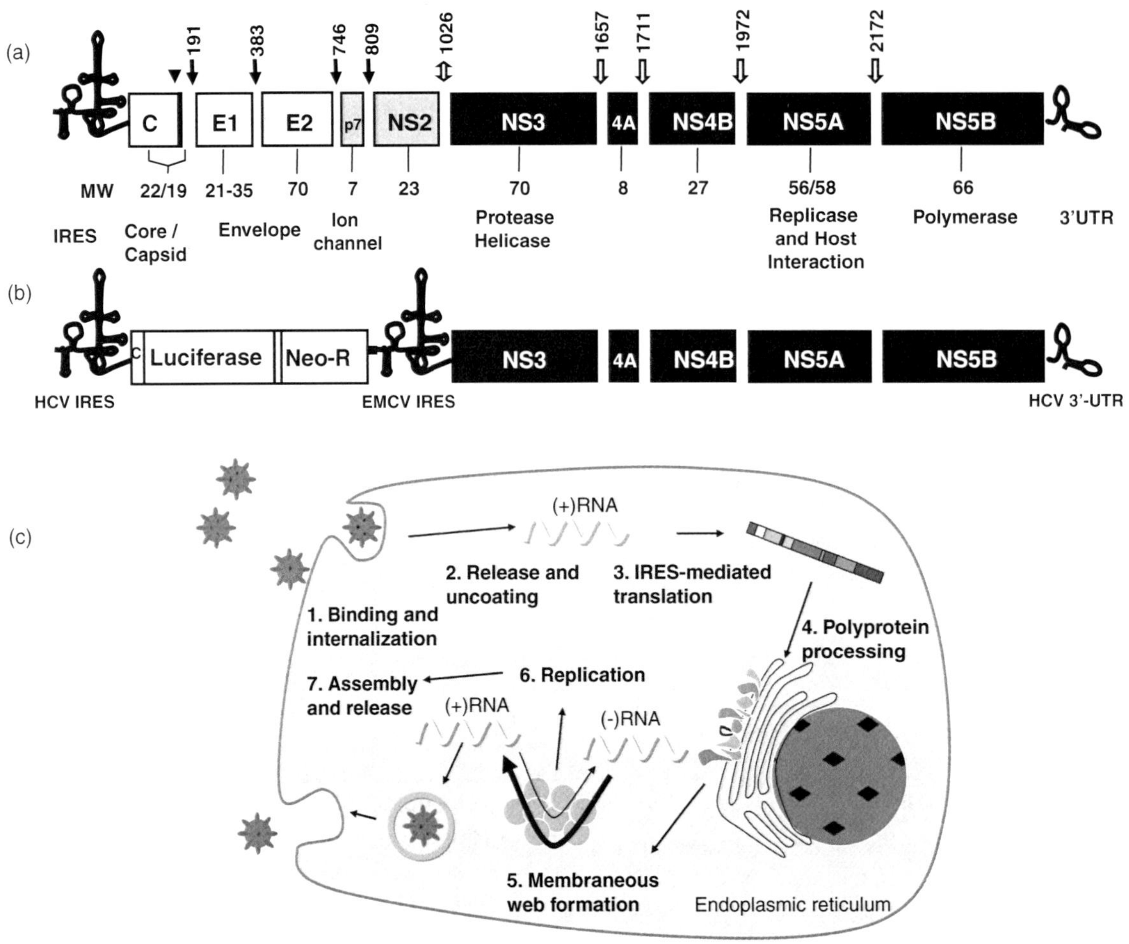

FIGURE 1 (a) HCV genome organization; (b) HCV bicistronic replicon; (c) HCV life cycle. Solid arrows show cleavage sites for host signal peptidases, open arrows show cleavage sites for HCV NS3-4A protease, and the double arrow shows a cleavage site for NS2-3 protease. (Adapted from [11].) (*See insert for color representation of the figure.*)

A remarkable feature of HCV is its high genetic diversity. Based on NS5B sequence comparison, six distinct genotypes and a large number of subtypes are apparent. Virus isolates from different genotypes differ in 30 to 35% of nucleotides on average across the genome, whereas those from different subtypes differ in 20 to 25%. This extent of sequence difference between genotypes approaches that of serologically and genetically distinct viruses within the genus *Flavivirus* [18,19]. This remarkable sequence diversity represents a formidable challenge to the design of small-molecule replication inhibitors that could bind with high affinity to viral targets across the different HCV genotypes and subtypes. The highest sequence variability is found within the envelope protein sequences and NS5A, whereas the 5′-UTR (IRES) is the most highly conserved region of the genome. Also, within infected subjects the sequence variability of HCV is substantial. The RNA-dependent RNA polymerase NS5B introduces nucleotide sequence changes at a rate of approximately one change per 1 to 10 genomes about 10^4 nucleotides in length, and HCV-infected subjects generate an estimated 10^{12} virus particles per day [20]. Therefore, all possible single and double amino acid mutations across the viral proteins can be expected to be generated daily at low frequency. The virus populations in HCV-infected subjects are thus highly heterogeneous in sequence, forming a "quasispecies," where at any moment in time one or a few sequences will be dominant. The sequence diversity among individual virus particles generated daily in this quasispecies allows rapid adaptation to changes in selection pressure and rapid drug resistance selection and thus constitutes a considerable challenge to antiviral drug discovery.

Antiviral Drug Resistance

The high sequence diversity of the HCV quasispecies allows the virus to adapt to the presence of antiviral drugs. Exposure to HCV protease inhibitors or non-nucleoside polymerase inhibitors in monotherapy leads to the rapid selection of virus variants that can replicate in the presence of the drugs [21–26]. For potent antiviral drugs with a low genetic barrier to resistance, therefore, a typical clinical resistance profile is characterized by an initial steep viral load reduction as the replication of the dominant sensitive virus is abolished, followed by a rebound in viral load as the drug-resistant virus variants continue replicating and multiply from a minority species to eventually become the dominant virus in the quasispecies.

Drug-resistant virus variants can also be generated de novo under drug pressure. This process requires ongoing virus replication in the presence of the drug and can occur when the antiviral drug exposure is suboptimal and does not achieve complete inhibition of viral replication. The clinical barrier to resistance describes the likelihood for a drug-resistant virus variant to emerge during antiviral treatment. The barrier to resistance is a function of the frequency of naturally occurring drug-resistant virus variants at baseline, the replication capacity of resistant virus variants, the resistance fold shift associated with the resistance mutation, and the exposure to the active drug at the end of the dosing interval relative to the intrinsic antiviral potency of the drug. The latter is often expressed as the inhibitory quotient, $IQ = C_{min}/\text{adjusted } EC_{50}$. Thus, antiviral drugs with lower intrinsic antiviral potency (EC_{50}) can achieve high clinical efficacy if they reach high exposure, whereas antiviral agents with high intrinsic antiviral potency in vitro may be associated with low clinical efficacy and a low barrier to resistance if they only achieve suboptimal exposure [27]. In addition to intrinsic potency, exposure, and absence of naturally resistant virus variants at baseline, other factors can also contribute to the barrier to resistance; most important, these are the replication capacity of drug-resistant variants (fitness) and the relative impact of resistance mutations on the intrinsic inhibitory potency of the drug (resistance fold shift). Compounds with high intrinsic potency that achieve high exposure relative to their antiviral potency and for which naturally occurring drug-resistant variants are rare in the quasispecies therefore have an increased likelihood of achieving a high barrier to resistance, especially if resistance mutations substantially reduce virus replication fitness. Also, if the fold shift of resistance mutations on antiviral potency is low, drugs at a standard or slightly higher dose may achieve sufficiently high exposure to effectively prevent replication of such virus variants.

Nucleoside Analogs

Nucleoside analogs have been developed successfully for the treatment of viral diseases and constitute the standard of care for the treatment of human immunodeficiency virus (HIV), hepatitis B virus (HBV), and herpesviruses. Most nucleoside analogs are metabolized by virus-infected target cells to their 5′-triphosphate derivatives, which are selective substrates for the viral polymerases and cause chain termination after incorporation. To achieve antiviral potency and selectivity, it is therefore minimally required that (1) antiviral nucleoside analogs are substrates for cellular kinases to generate the corresponding 5′-triphosphates, (2) the nucleosides and phosphate derivatives are not converted to inactive metabolites by cellular enzymes, (3) the nucleoside triphosphate analogs are efficient substrates for the viral polymerases, and (4) the nucleoside triphosphate analogs are inefficient substrates for cellular polymerases. As all four aspects require optimization, historically the selection and discovery of antiviral nucleoside analogs has generally been performed in cell-based antiviral assay systems.

DISCOVERY OF R1479 (4′-AZIDOCYTIDINE) AS A POTENT INHIBITOR OF HCV REPLICATION

The HCV replicon system was used to screen a library of nucleoside analogs, a subset of the Roche compound library, as well as commercially available compounds. Nucleosides from this screening activity were classified into four groups, based on their effect on HCV replicon reporter gene expression, cell viability, and cell proliferation, as shown in Table 1. The majority of nucleosides tested did not inhibit HCV replication in the Huh7 cell-based replicon system. Examples of such compounds include 4′-azidouridine (**1**) and 4′-ethynylcytidine (**2**). Such compounds may be intrinsically inactive as HCV replication inhibitors, may not be phosphorylated, or may be metabolically unstable. A second group of compounds was cytotoxic and thus reduced HCV reporter gene activity nonspecifically. 4′-Cyanocytidine (**3**), 5-fluorouridine (**4**) and 7-deazaadenosine (Tubercidin) (**5**) were examples of compounds that were cytotoxic to HCV replicon cells. A third group of nucleosides inhibited HCV reporter gene expression without apparent cytotoxicity. These compounds were, however, cytostatic; that is, they inhibited cell proliferation, measured as an inhibition of incorporation of tritiated thymidine into cellular DNA. 2′-Deoxy-4′-azidoadenosine (**6**) and 2′-deoxy-2′-fluorocytidine (**7**) were examples of potently cytostatic compounds. Importantly, the maintenance of HCV RNA in the replicon system is dependent on cell proliferation. Cytostatic agents therefore reduce HCV RNA levels nonspecifically in this system [29]. The replicon system is therefore not suitable for assessing cytostatic compounds, and careful assessment in other systems of HCV replication, such as recombinant enzyme systems or animal models, would be required to determine if such compounds have specific HCV replication inhibition components. The fourth group of compounds contained nucleoside analogs that specifically inhibited HCV replication in the replicon system without affecting cell viability or cell proliferation. 4′-Azidocytidine (R1479) (**8**) was an example

TABLE 1 Nucleoside Library Screen in HCV Replicon cells[a]

	HCV Replicon Inhibition[b] IC_{50} < 20 μM	Cytotoxic[c] CC_{50} < 20 μM	Cytostatic[d] IC_{50} < 20 μM	Fraction of the Library (%)	Examples
Group A (inactive)	–	N.D.	N.D.	>95%	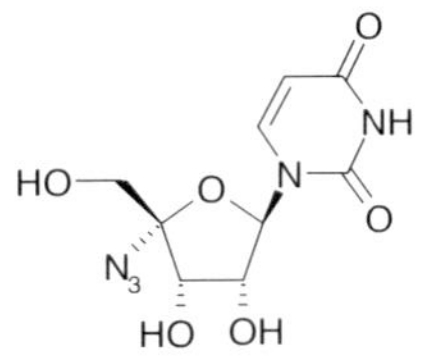 **1** 4′-azido-uridine 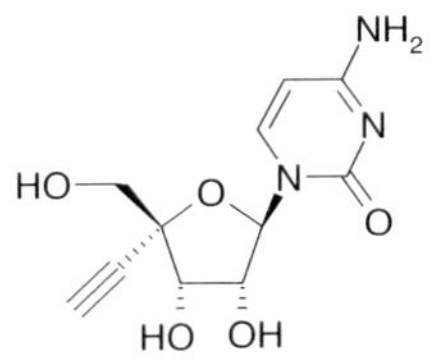 **2** 4′-ethynyl-cytidine
Group B (cytotoxic)	+	+	N.D.	<1%	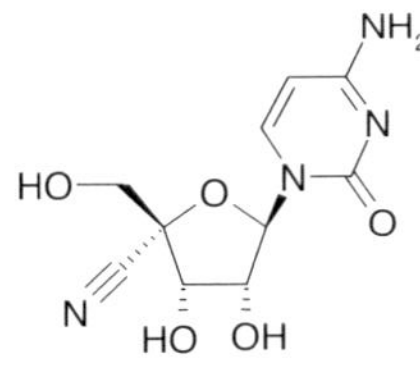 **3** 4′-cyano-cytidine 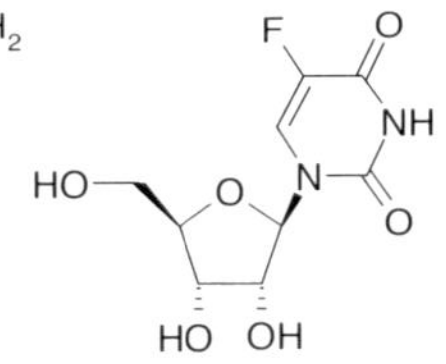 **4** 5-fluoro-uridine 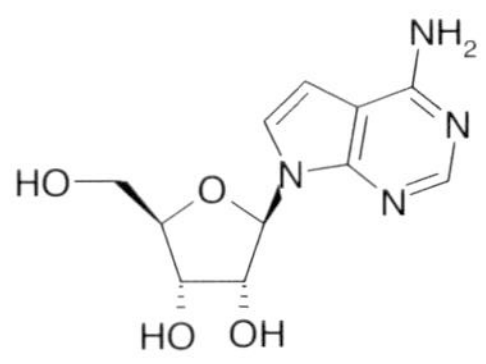 **5** 7-deaza-adenosine
Group C (cytostatic)	+	–	+	~4%	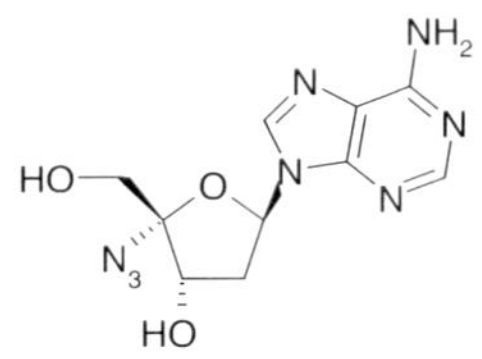 **6** 2′-deoxy-4′-azido-adenosine 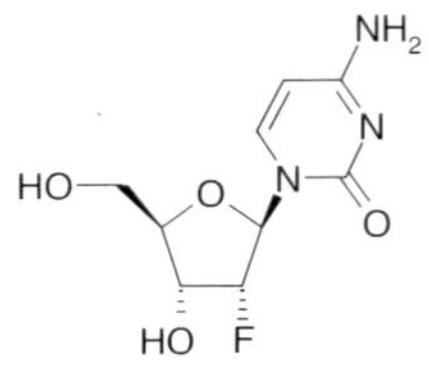 **3** 2′-deoxy-2′-fluoro-cytidine
Group D (specific HCV replication inhibition)	+	–	–	0.25%	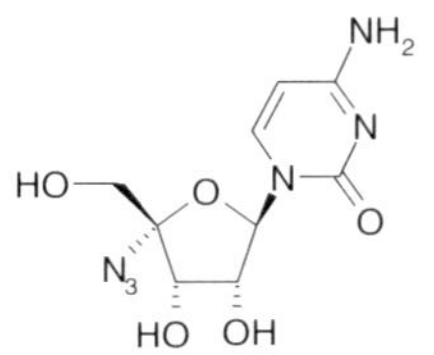 **8** 4′-azido-cytidine

[a]GT-1b Con1 HCV replicon assay was performed as described [28]; N.D., not determined.
[b]HCV replication inhibition was measured as the reduction of HCV replicon expressed luciferase activity.
[c]Cell viability measured using WST-1 (Roche Diagnostics).
[d]Cell proliferation measured tritiated thymidine incorporation SPA assay (GE Healthcare).

of this group of compounds and was chosen for further characterization [28,30]. A number of substitutions at the 4′-position were tested, including ethyl, ethoxy, hydroxymethyl, ethynyl, propynyl, and vinyl. These derivatives of (**8**) were inactive in the HCV replicon system (group A), whereas the 4′-cyano and 4′-allyl derivatives were cytotoxic (group B) [30]. Also, all uridine analogs tested in this series of compounds were inactive in the HCV replicon system. For a number of compounds, including 4′-azidouridine and 4′-azidoadenosine, this lack of potency was determined to be based on a lack of phosphorylation in HCV replicon cells to form the nucleoside monophosphate derivatives [31,32].

Mechanism of Action

R1479 is an efficient substrate for human deoxycytidine kinase and is further phosphorylated to the corresponding 5′-triphosphate, R1479-TP, in human target cells [33]. R1479-TP is a substrate of HCV polymerase (NS5B). In a nucleophilic substitution reaction with the 3′-hydroxyl group of the nascent RNA as the nucleophile and the β-γ-pyrophosphate of R1479-TP as a leaving group, R1479-MP gets incorporated into nascent HCV RNA molecules. This incorporation occurs in a template sequence-dependent manner, by base pairing of R1479 through its cytosine base to guanosine residues on the template RNA. R1479-TP is thus a specific, competitive inhibitor of CMP incorporation by NS5B, but a noncompetitive inhibitor of incorporation of the other nucleotide substrates [28]. The K_i for R1479-TP inhibition of CMP incorporation was determined as 40 ± 25 nM. This value was about twofold lower than the K_m for CTP (81 ± 25 nM) determined under the same conditions, indicating a favorable K_i/K_m ratio and efficient inhibition of NS5B by R1479-TP. Incorporation of R1479-MP into nascent HCV RNA results in inhibition of further RNA chain extension [28]. Therefore, despite the presence of a 3′-hydroxyl group, R1479 can function as a nonobligatory chain terminator. Although a crystal structure of NS5B bound to R1479 has not been solved to date, the incorporation of R1479-MP into HCV RNA may lead to a misalignment of the R1479-3′-hydroxyl group and the α-phosphate of the incoming next NTP in the NS5B active site. R1479-TP is a highly efficient substrate of NS5B during the initiation of RNA synthesis. R1479-TP was incorporated by NS5B with an efficiency (k_{cat}/K_m) at transcription initiation 3.3-fold higher than 3′-deoxy-CTP and only 4.3-fold lower than the natural substrate CTP [33]. HCV replication occurs in membrane-associated replication complexes that are part of a membranous web structure induced by HCV. The HCV replicase contains the HCV nonstructural proteins HCV RNA and probably a number of cellular protein cofactors. The membrane-associated replicase is shielded from the cytoplasm to such an extent that replicase activity is not affected by exposure of membrane fractions to extensive treatment with either proteinase K or RNAse [14,15]. The native HCV replicase was, however, fully sensitive to inhibition by R1479-triphosphate, similar to results obtained with recombinant NS5B, suggesting full access of nucleoside triphosphate, and specifically R1479-TP, to the NS5B active site in the context of the HCV replicase complex [28].

ANTIVIRAL POTENCY AND SAR

R1479 inhibited HCV RNA replication in the genotype 1b (Con1) replicon system with a mean IC_{50} value of 1.3 μM without showing cytotoxicity ($CC_{50} > 2$ mM) or cytostatic properties [28]. Similar antiviral potency was observed in the HCV replicon system, when measured either as an inhibition of luciferase reporter gene expression or by quantitative RT-PCR. Similar potencies were also observed when comparing permanent HCV replicon cell lines to the transient replicon system [28,34]. Importantly, antiviral potency was also similar across 58 NS5B clinical isolates (15 genotype 1b and 43 genotype 1a) in the HCV replicon NS5B phenotyping assay [25]. All 58 clinical isolates were similarly sensitive to inhibition by R1479 in the transient replicon with phenotypic EC_{50} values within the 2.5-fold variability of the assay [25]. These data are consistent with a high sequence conservation of the NS5B active site. Indeed, R1479-TP showed potent inhibitory activity across representative NS5B enzymes from all six HCV genotypes, a significant difference compared to non-nucleoside inhibitors of HCV polymerase, which show more strain-, subtype-, and genotype-specific inhibition patterns [35]. In vitro combination of R1479 with other antiviral agents provided favorable data in support of clinical studies in combination with interferon α, ribavirin, other nucleoside and non-nucleoside inhibitors of HCV polymerase, and HCV protease inhibitors. In particular, R1479 showed synergistic antiviral potency with interferon α and ribavirin in the HCV replicon system and additive effects with nucleoside analogs PSI-6130 (2′-*C*-methyl-2′-fluorocytidine) and NM107 (2′-*C*-methylcytidine), palm binding and thumb-binding non-nucleoside analogs, and BILN 2061, a protease inhibitor [36]. Interestingly, in contrast to BILN 2061, a synergistic effect was apparent in the HCV replicon system when R1479 was combined with another HCV protease inhibitor, ITMN-191 [37].

In Vitro Resistance Selection to R1479

Prolonged incubation of HCV replicon cells with 6 μM R1479 (approximately five times IC_{50}) led to a continuous decrease in HCV RNA and eventually resulted in HCV RNA clearance within 15 days of incubation [28]. A comparison of resistance selection of HCV replicon variants resistant to R1479 in vitro with non-nucleoside polymerase inhibitors and protease inhibitors demonstrated a higher barrier to resistance selection with the nucleoside analog R1479 [38], such that the selection of resistant replicons required long-term culture and passaging at slowly increasing drug concentrations. After such long-term passaging in vitro in the presence of increasing concentrations of R1479, starting at IC_{50} concentration of drug, replicon variants containing point mutations S96T and S96T in combination with N142T were detected after 37 passages of HCV replicon cells [34]. Replicons containing the S96T point mutation or the S96T/N142T double mutation in the coding sequence of NS5B showed a low level of resistance to inhibition by R1479 (4.2- and 5.3-fold increased IC_{50}, respectively). The R1479-resistant replicons did not show cross-resistance with other antiviral agents, including interferon α, ribavirin, and 2′-*C*-methylnucleoside analogs [34]. Conversely, replicon cell lines resistant to inhibition by other antiviral agents were as sensitive as wild-type replicons to inhibition by R1479, suggesting no apparent cross-resistance with current antiviral agents targeting HCV replication. Positions S96 and N142 are distant from the nucleoside binding site on HCV polymerase. The molecular mechanism on how mutations at these positions affect the inhibitory potency of R1479 remains to be determined.

R1479 SAR

A series of substitutions at the 4′-position of either uridine or cytidine were explored and compared to 4′-azidocytidine (R1479). Among the substitutions tested, ethyl, ethoxy, hydroxymethyl, ethynyl, propynyl, and vinyl at the 4′-position provided primarily nucleosides without appreciable antiviral potency or cytotoxicity in the HCV replicon system [30]. 4′-Cyanocytidine and 4′-allyluridine were cytotoxic in replicon cells. Interestingly, none of the uridine analogs were active in this series. In particular, 4′-azidouridine, the analog of R1479, was not active in the replicon cells, and 4′-cyanouridine was not cytotoxic, while its cytidine analog, 4′-cyanocytidine, was cytotoxic. These results are consistent with lack of phosphorylation of uridine analogs in the replicon cells [32]. Interestingly, a different result was obtained with the pair of 4′-allylnucleosides. 4′-Allylcytidine was not active and not cytotoxic, whereas 4′-allyluridine was cytotoxic, suggesting that this compound may cause cytotoxicity through a different mechanism then that of 4′-cyanocytidine, or that 4′-allyluridine is a substrate of a kinase that did not phosphorylate the other uridine analogs of this series [30]. A number of analogs of R1479 were made to explore 2′- and 3′-modifications in addition to the 4′-azido moiety. The available results suggest that the 3′-hydroxy group may be important for antiviral activity in HCV replicon cells. 3′-Deoxy-4′-azidocytidine was inactive, similar to 3′-deoxycytidine and the other three 3′-deoxy-NTPs [39,40]. When the 3′-hydroxyl group was inverted to form 4′-azidoxylocytidine, weak cytotoxicity and probable nonspecific inhibition of HCV replicon were observed [40]. Modifications at the 2′-position have generated more interesting results to date. It was found initially that 2′-*C*-methyl modification could confer good antiviral potency in the HCV replicon system and selectivity against inhibition of cell proliferation [41–43]. 2′-Methylcytidine was indeed advanced into clinical development but eventually abandoned, due to an unfavorable safety profile in humans. Interestingly, the combination of the 2′-*C*-methyl modification and the 4′-azido moiety resulted in an inactive cytidine analog, suggesting that the conformational or structural effects of having both modifications present on a cytidine backbone was not tolerated by either cellular kinases or the HCV polymerase [40]. Unexpectedly, removal of the 2′-hydroxyl moiety from the 2′-position of the typical ribose scaffold resulted in highly potent inhibitors of HCV replication. In particular, 4′-azidoarabinocytidine (RO-9187) and 4′-azido-2′-fluoroarabinocytidine (RO-0622) inhibited HCV replication in the replicon system with EC_{50} values of 171 and 24 nM, respectively [33,40,44]. Further exploration of ribose modifications and combinations thereof at the 2′,3′, and 4′-positions are ongoing.

PRODRUGS OF R1479 AND SELECTION OF R1626

Physicochemical Properties and Pharmacokinetic Profile of R1479

Physicochemical properties of R1479 are similar to those of other ribonucleoside analogs, with typical high polarity and water solubility [45]. The hemisulfate salt of R1479 ($C_{19}H_{12}N_6O_5 \cdot 0.5\ H_2SO_4$) is a white-to-tan crystalline powder with pK_a values of 3.95 and 12.12, and a log $P_{O/W}$ (octanol/water partition coefficient) of −1.5 at pH 6.5. The aqueous solubility of R1479 is thus pH dependent, with 12 mg/mL at pH 6.5. Solubility in dimethylsulfoxide is >100 mg/mL. The Biopharmaceutical Classification of the compound is class III (high solubility, low permeability). Consistent with these properties, R1479 exhibited low permeability in Caco-2 cell monolayers (0.9×10^{-6} cm/s) and variable oral bioavailability across species, ranging from 22% in cynomolgus monkeys to 92% in dogs at 10 mg/kg (Table 2) [45].

Plasma exposure in humans after oral administration of R1479 was found to be low and limited by absorption. Measurement of urine excretion allowed an estimation of 6 to 18% oral absorption in humans [45]. However, R1479 showed high metabolic stability, low clearance, and long plasma half-life across species. Further efforts were therefore focused on designing a prodrug of R1479 that could effectively deliver R1479 to systemic circulation after oral administration.

Prodrugs of R1479

Several approaches were investigated in order to increase absorption of R1479. One approach was to mask the polarity of the molecule by introducing mono-, di- and triesters at the 2′-,

TABLE 2 Mean Plasma Pharmacokinetic Parameters of R1479[a]

Species (*n*)	Dose (mg/kg)	Route	C_{max} (μ g/mL)	$AUC_{0\text{-}t}$ (μ g·h/mL)	AUC_{inf} (μ g·h/mL)	Plasma *Cl* (L·h/kg)	% Hepatic (% Renal) Blood Flow	Vd_{ss} (L/kg)	*F* (%)	$t_{1/2}$ (h)
Mouse (5)	10	i.v.	18.4	$25.9_{(48h)}$	26.3	0.380	7.0(9.7)	2.70	—	$9.1_{(10-48h)}$
Rat (4)	10	i.v.	9.15	$37.5_{(48h)}$	43.3	0.233	7.1(10.5)	4.67	—	$18.4_{(7-48h)}$
Dog (6)	10	i.v.	14.3	$218_{(168h)}$	244	0.043	2.3(3.3)	2.58	—	$50.6_{(10-168h)}$
Monkey (6)	10	i.v.	17.1	$29.2_{(72h)}$	29.4	0.344	13.2(20.7)	2.39	—	$14.8_{(10-72h)}$
Rabbit (3)	10	i.v.	13.5	$56.1_{(48h)}$	58.8	0.170	4.0(8.9)	1.92	—	$13.3_{(10-48h)}$
Micropig (3)	10	i.v.	23.2	$25.9_{(96h)}$	26.8	0.376	—	1.15	—	$9.71_{(5-32h)}$
Mouse (5)	10	p.o.	2.50	$17.8_{(48h)}$	17.9	—	—	—	68	$6.8_{(10-48h)}$
Rat (5)	10	p.o.	1.47	$32.0_{(48h)}$	38.5	—	—	—	89	$17.6_{(2-48h)}$
Dog (6)	10	p.o.	11.2	$204_{(168h)}$	221	—	—	—	92	$48.0_{(10-168h)}$
Monkey (6)	10	p.o.	0.534	$6.20_{(48h)}$	6.35	—	—	—	22	$10.2_{(10-48h)}$
Rabbit (3)	10	p.o.	3.78	$33.0_{(24h)}$	36.7	—	—	—	62	$16.5_{(10-48h)}$
Micropig (2)	10	p.o.	0.634	$9.73_{(48h)}$	10.1	—	—	—	36	$9.65_{(5-48h)}$

[a]Doses and concentrations are expressed as the R1479 free base. All doses were administered as solutions in saline. *n*, number of animals for each time point; i.v., intravenous; p.o., oral; *Cl*, clearance; Vd_{ss}, volume of distribution at steady state; $t_{1/2}$, half-life, values in parentheses indicate portions of the curves used to calculate half-life; $AUC_{0\text{-}t}$, AUC values from time 0 to the last time point with measurable plasma concentrations of R1479; AUC_{inf}, AUC values from time 0 to infinity. *Cl* and Vd_{ss} are calculated using AUC_{inf} where possible. *F* (%) was calculated from the ratio of AUC_{inf} after the p.o. dose to that after the same i.v. dose in the same study only.

3′-, and 5′-ribose positions. This also included exploration of modifications at the cytidine base, by introducing lipophilic amides at the N4 position. A number of synthetically accessible monoesters, diesters, and triesters were synthesized, as were cytidine amide derivates and tetraacyl compounds (Fig. 2). Increasing lipophilicity of R1479 was aimed at increasing the efficiency of transcellular uptake after oral administration [45].

A second approach to improving the oral bioavailability of R1479 was to target transporters such as PepT1, known to shuttle highly polar cargo attached to amino acid moieties. This strategy was utilized with success in the cases of acyclovir, gancyclovir, and most recently, NM107, leading to the orally dosed prodrugs Valtrex, Valcyte, and Valopicitabine, respectively [46–48]. Following these examples, several 5′-amino acid derivatives of 4′-azidocytidine were prepared (Fig. 3).

N-acylcarbamate derivatives have also been employed successfully for the targeted delivery of nucleosides [49]. This approach followed a strategy similar to that which previously resulted in the discovery of capecitabine [Xeloda; N^4-(pentyloxy)carbonyl-5′-deoxy-5-fluorocytidine]. The *N*-acylcarbamate capecitabine is efficiently absorbed after oral administration and reaches the portal vein intact. In the liver, capecitabine is sequentially converted first to 5′-deoxy-5-fluorocytidine (5′-DFCR) and then to 5′-deoxy-5-fluorouridine (5′-DFUR). 5′-DFUR is itself a prodrug of 5-FU, which is formed from 5′-DFUR by deribosylation, catalyzed by thymidine phosphorylase. 5-FU is preferentially formed in tumor cells due to an overexpression of

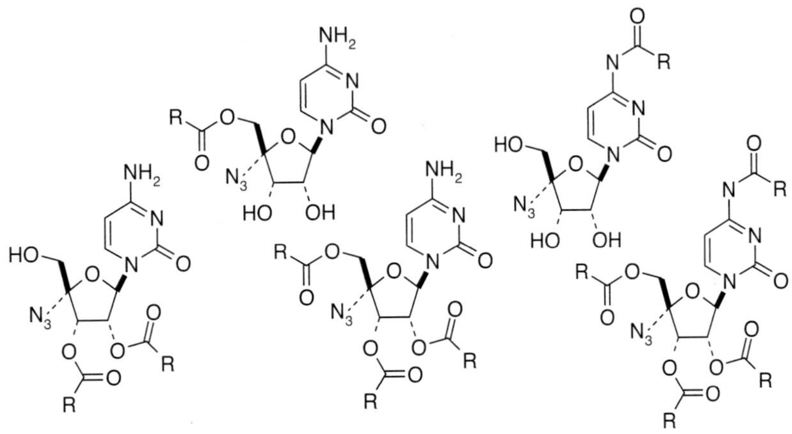

FIGURE 2 R1479 esters and amides.

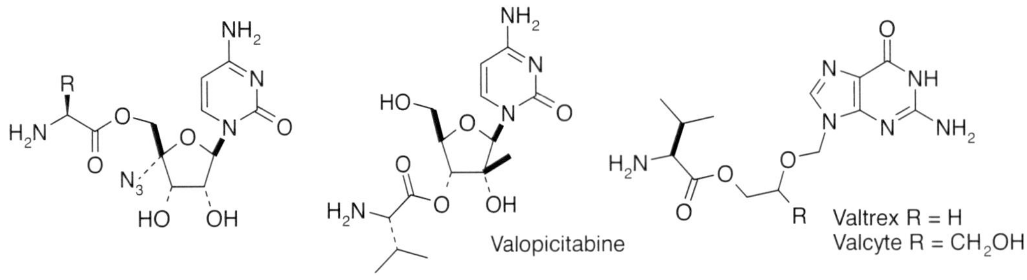

FIGURE 3 Amino acid ester approach with literature examples.

the final anabolizing enzyme, thymidine phosphorylase, in neoplastic tissues (Fig. 4). Given the intrinsic stability of R1479, which is not subject to cytidine deamination, N^4-acylcarbamate derivatives of R1479 were evaluated for absorption and release of R1479 in the liver.

R1479 PRODRUG SYNTHESIS

To assess the potential of these various strategies to provide increased plasma exposure of the parent nucleoside R1479, synthetic routes for each class of prodrug needed to be developed. These efforts relied on the availability of 4′-azidocytidine as well as the related 4′-azidouridine. The medicinal chemistry syntheses of 4′-azidouridine and 4′-azidocytidine (R1479) begin with uridine and have been described [30]. For large-scale synthesis of R1479 and advanced studies including clinical work, an alternative process chemistry route was developed [50]. In the following section we describe the general medicinal chemistry approaches used successfully to access R1479 prodrugs at the 100-mg level.

The synthesis of 5′-substituted analogs began with 4′-azidouridine and is shown in Scheme 1. After protection of the 2′- and 3′-hydroxyls as the acetonide, installation of the 5′-acyl group was conducted, either using standard diimide coupling chemistry from the carboxylic acid (used primarily for amino acid analogs) or through direct reaction with a carboxylic acid chloride. The uridine was converted to the cytidine following a protocol developed by Reese and co-workers [51]. Simple deprotection using warm aqueous acetic acid then furnished the desired 5′-acyl analogs. Triesters were also obtained using 4′-azidouridine as the starting material (Scheme 2). The compound was readily acylated at 2′, 3′, and 5′ to provide the triacyl uridine. Conversion to the triacyl cytidine could then be accomplished following the Reese protocol.

Most other analogs were prepared using 4′-azidocytidine as the starting material. 2′- and 3′-diesters utilized an initial selective protection of the 5′-hydroxyl as the *t*-butyldimethylsilyl ether (Scheme 3). Following this, the acyl groups were installed by reaction of the free hydroxyl groups under standard conditions using either the acid chloride or anhydride. This introduced an unwanted acyl group onto the cytidine nitrogen. The undesired acyl group was removed with high selectivity following treatment of the compound with zinc bromide in a mixture of methanol and chloroform at reflux [52]. Finally, the desired 2′- and 3′-diacyl derivatives of R1479 were obtained by trifluoroacetic acid mediated removal of the 5′-silyl protection.

Tetraacyl analogs of R1479 were prepared following a similar strategy, but without the need for protection. 4′-Azidocytidine could be per-acylated readily using excess acid chloride or anhydride directly to afford the tetraacyl derivatives (Scheme 4). Along with the tetraacyl derivatives, the *N*-acyl derivatives were among the most easily obtained, being available in an efficient one-pot protocol as shown in Scheme 5 [53]. Exposure of 4′-azidocytidine to trimethylsilyl chloride in pyridine resulted in transient in situ protection

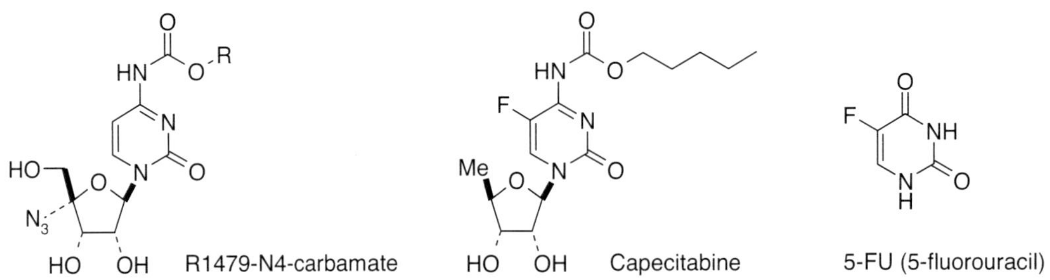

FIGURE 4 *N*-Acyl carbamate derivatives of 4′-azidocytidine (R1479) and capecitabine.

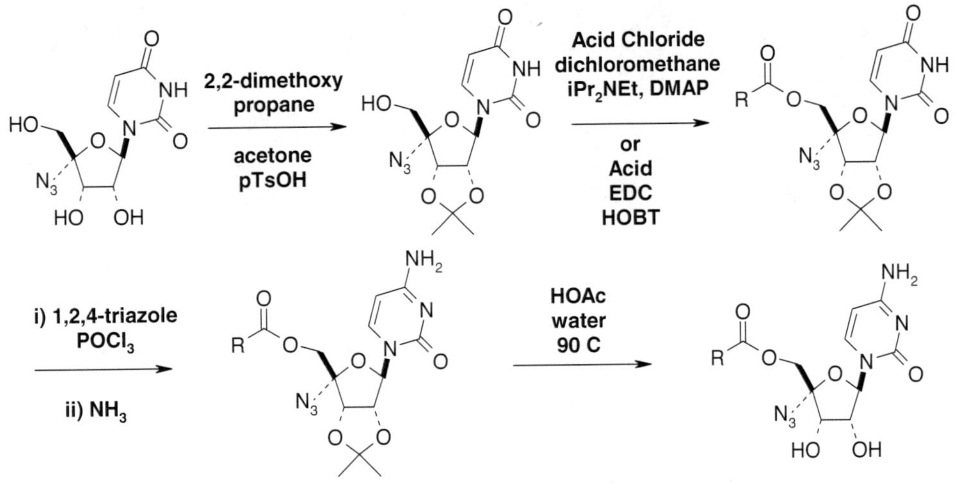

SCHEME 1

of the 2′-, 3′-, and 5′-hydroxyls. Under these conditions, the cytidine amino group remains free to be functionalized as an amide or carbamate derivate. Following workup of the reactions, which included the addition of *n*-butylammonium fluoride, the *N*-acyl cytidine derivatives were obtained directly.

NONCLINICAL PHARMACOKINETICS: SELECTION OF R1479 PRODRUG CANDIDATES

The purpose of R1479 prodrugs was to enhance absorption through increased GI absorption, thus to provide increased systemic exposure to R1479 and, consequently, increased

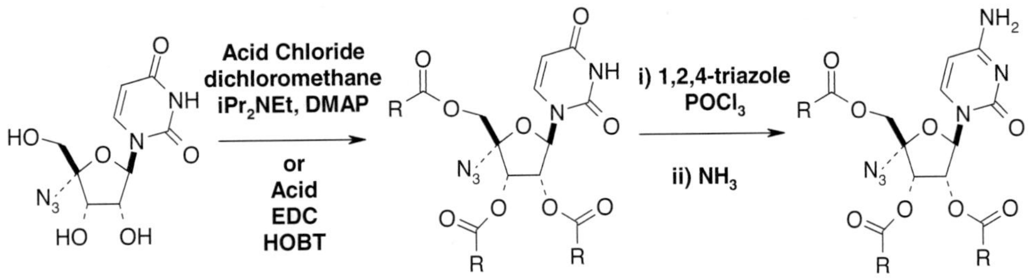

SCHEME 2

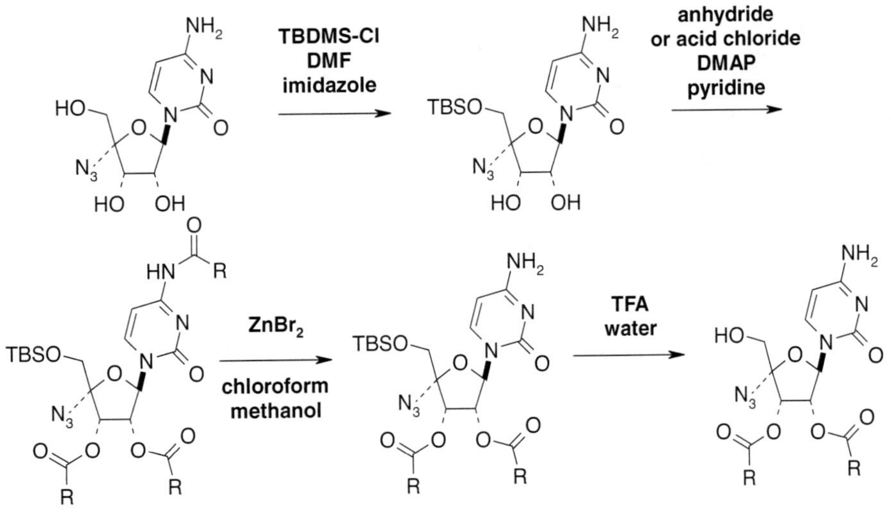

SCHEME 3

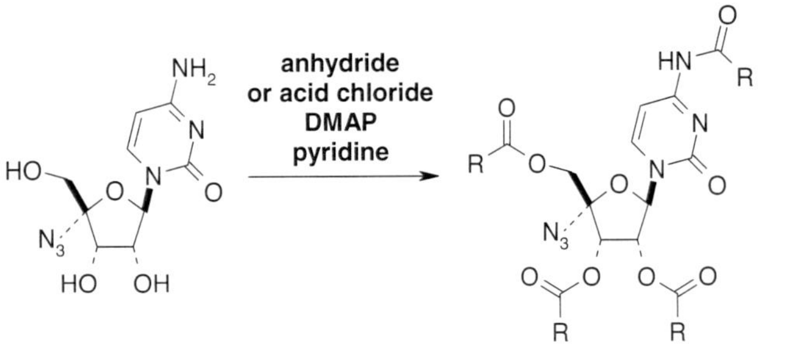

SCHEME 4

R1479-TP concentration in the liver. More than 100 R1479 prodrugs were synthesized for this purpose. All prodrugs were initially assessed for in vitro stability in simulated gastric fluid (SGF, pH 1.2) and simulated intestinal fluid (SIF, pH 7.5). Chemical stability of prodrugs in these media increases the likelihood of prodrugs passing through the upper GI tract and reaching the site of absorption intact. All 5′-monoesters, 2′,3′-diesters, and 2′,3′,5′-triesters showed acceptable stability profiles and were thus included for further characterization. N^4-amides showed good solution stability at pH 7.5 but poor stability at acidic pH. In contrast, the N^4-acylcarbamates showed good chemical solution stability in both SIF and SGF. The second major step for the assessment of candidate potential to achieve increased oral bioavailability was to assess permeability through a Caco-2 cell layer. The Caco-2 cell line is an immortalized human epithelial cell line, which is widely used to predict the absorption rate of candidate drug compounds across the intestinal epithelial cell barrier. The assay requires that drug absorption rates be determined after Caco-2 cells have formed a closed cell monolayer. Table 3 shows a representative set of prodrugs characterized in the Caco-2 permeability assay [54].

As described earlier, the intrinsic permeability of R1479 was low at 0.9×10^{-6} cm/s in the Caco-2 assay. In contrast, a number of R1479 prodrugs showed significantly improved in vitro permeability compared to R1479. In all prodrug classes, increases in permeability seemed to correlate roughly with increases in measured log *P*. From available compounds with acceptable chemical stability and cell permeability enhancement properties, approximately 30 compounds were selected for pharmacokinetic studies in cynomolgus monkeys. Prodrugs were dosed orally at 5 mg/kg and compared to R1479. Our target in this assay was to achieve at least a threefold increase in R1479 exposure by prodrug administration, as measured by AUC. Representative data from our screening of these compounds are presented in Table 3 [54]. Notably, and in contrast to the enhanced absorption seen using this strategy with other nucleosides, the amino acid ester approach failed to provide increased exposure when applied to R1479. These results suggested that the amino acid esters were probably not recognized by the PepT1 transporter protein. The more lipophilic 5′-monoesters showed excellent absorption and subsequent cleavage to R1479 in plasma, with the 12-carbon chain laurate ester proving to be one of the better examples, suggesting that increasing lipophilicity had been successful in this subseries. These results demonstrated that 5′-monoesters could substantially increase the oral bioavailability of R1479.

TABLE 3 Caco-2 Permeability, Log *P*, and DMPK Data for Representative R1479 Prodrugs

Table Entry	Compound	Log $P_{O/W}$	Caco-2 Permeability (10^{-6} cm/s)	R1479 Exposure $AUC_{0\text{-}24h}$ (μ g·h/mL)
1	R1479	−1.5	0.9	2.84
2	5′-Octanoate	3.32	6.0	5.68
3	5′-Laurate	4.98	11.6	10.63
4	5′-Valinate	−0.27	0.1	2.37
5	5′-Isoleucinate	0.23	0.1	2.38
6	2′,3′-Diisobutyrate	2.32	2.5	10.91
7	2′,3′-Dipentanoate	3.65	5.0	12.96
8	Triacetate	0.67	0.1	3.34
9	Triisobutyrate	2.45	15.0	10.50
10	Tripropionate	2.14	3.5	9.50
11	Tripivalate	4.75	9.0	1.64

In contrast, most of the *N*-acylcarbamates failed to deliver R1479 to plasma, and instead resulted in actual decreases of R1479 exposure (data not shown). Not unexpectedly, significant levels of *N*-acylcarbamate prodrugs were found in

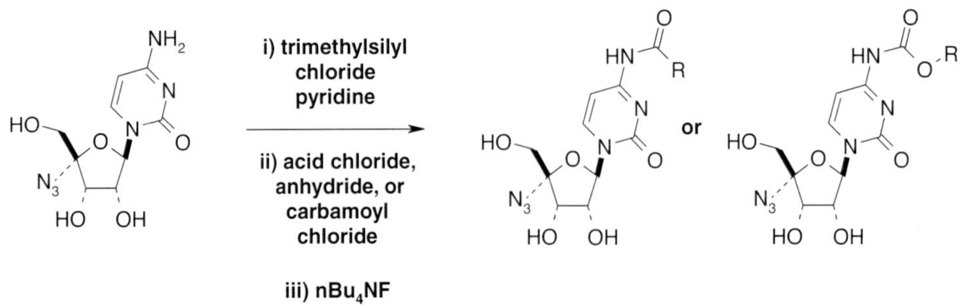

SCHEME 5

plasma, suggesting that metabolic conversion of the carbamates to release R1479 was rate limiting in this series. The *N*-heptylcarbamate was an exception, with an approximately twofold R1479 exposure compared to dosing R1479 alone. Further investigation into the SAR of the enzymatic cytidine carbamate conversion may provide guidance for further improvements in this series of prodrugs. Most 2′,3′-diesters showed significant improvements in R1479 exposure after oral administration to cynomolgus monkeys, with AUC increases between 2.3- and 4.6-fold. The dipentanoate provided the highest exposure, again suggesting a correlation between increased lipophilicity and bioavailability. Finally, several 2′,3′,5′-triesters provided increased R1479 exposures in this assay. Taken together, data on this series of R1479 prodrugs are consistent with a correlation of log *P*, Caco-2 permeability, and R1479 bioavailability.

Most compounds with log *P* greater than about 2 showed good Caco-2 permeability and usually displayed greater than twofold enhancement in R1479 exposure relative to dosing R1479 itself. In contrast, examples such as 5′-valinate, 5′-isoleucinate, and triacetate showed log $P < 1$, poor Caco-2 permeability, and low R1479 exposure. Within a given class of prodrug, increased lipophilicity tended to correlate with increased exposure; for example, the 5′-laurate, 2′,3′-dipentanoate, and the triisobutyrate all provided a greater than threefold increase in R1479 exposure. The tripivalate was an exception to this trend. Even with a high log *P* value and good Caco-2 permeability, this compound actually displayed reduced R1479 exposure upon dosing, probably due to increased stability toward hydrolysis for this highly sterically hindered triester. To investigate dose proportionality and performance further, at higher oral doses, a number of compounds were selected for more detailed pharmacokinetic studies in cynomolgus monkeys. Table 4 shows data obtained with the 5′-laurate, 2′,3′-diisobutyrate, 2′,3′-dipentanoate, and triisobutyrate esters of R1479. These compounds combined good physicochemical properties, chemical stability, permeability, and oral bioavailability and were accessible through reasonable chemical routes. All four of these prodrugs delivered more than 3.7-fold enhancement of R1479 exposure compared to dosing R1479 orally at all three dose levels. The triisobutyrate consistently provided the best performance in this series and increased AUC by 14- and 10-fold at the 30- and 300-mg/kg dose levels, respectively. The hydrochloride salt of the triisobutyrate derivative of R1479 became balapiravir (R1626).

SYNTHESIS AND CHARACTERIZATION OF BALAPIRAVIR

Balapiravir is the hydrochloride salt of the triisobutyrate ester of 4′-azidocytidine. The compound is a white crystalline solid with a melting point of 148°C [55]. The compound has a measured log *P* of 2.45 and an aqueous solubility of 10 mg/mL. Solubility of the free base of balapiravir is 0.19 mg/mL. In stability studies conducted using simulated gastric fluid (pH 1.2) the compound showed a T_{90} value of 4.6 h at 37°C. In simulated intestinal fluid, T_{90} was 11.1 h under similar conditions. In a pH stability profile, the compound was most stable at about pH 5 [55]. Using the Caco-2 model, balapiravir demonstrated a high permeability of 15×10^{-6} cm/s.

TABLE 4 Dose-Ranging Studies with Selected R1479 Prodrugs in Cynomolgus Monkeys

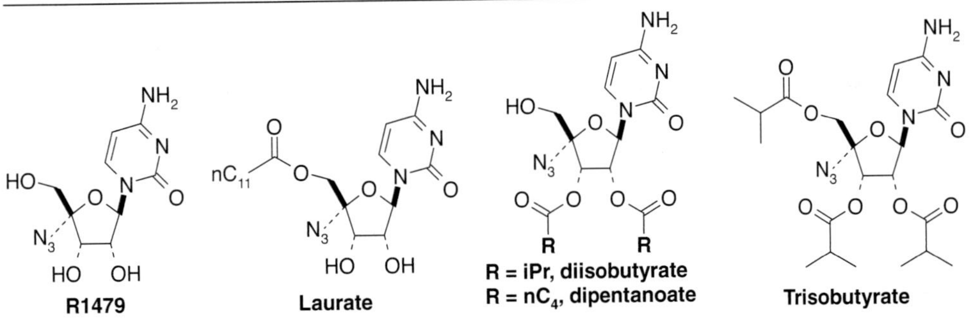

Compound	Exposure of R1479 Following Prodrug Dosing in Cynomolgus Monkey ($AUC_{0\text{-}24h}$, µg·h/mL) 5 mg/kg	30 mg/kg	300 mg/kg
R1479	2.84	4.4	21.6
Laurate	10.63	27.0	169.5
Diisobutyrate	10.91	16.6	169.5
Dipentanoate	12.96	20.1	206.5
Triisobutyrate	10.50	61.5	219.8

TABLE 5 R1479 Exposure in Rat, Dog, and Monkey After Oral Administration of Balapiravir

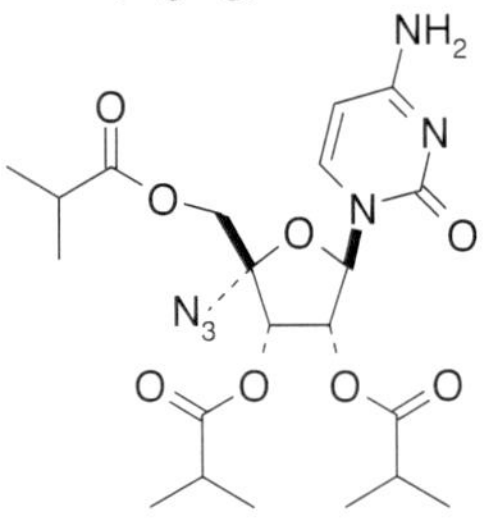

Dose (mg/kg)	Exposure of R1479 Following Dosing of Balapiravir ($AUC_{0\text{-}24h}$, μg·h/mL)		
	Rat	Dog	Cynomolgus Monkey
30	46	127.5	61.5
100	150.5	237.1	103.3
300	390.0	375.35	219.8

This represented a >15-fold improvement in permeability over the parent nucleoside R1479 as measured in the same assay. Initially, sufficient compound was available using the medicinal chemistry route, as shown in Scheme 5. For advanced studies including clinical work, an alternative process chemistry route was eventually developed [50,56,57].

With sufficient quantities of balapiravir available, further dose-proportionality studies were conducted in multiple species. As shown in Table 5, oral administration of balapiravir provided excellent exposure and dose proportionality of R1479 in rat, dog, and cynomolgus monkey.

BALAPIRAVIR CLINICAL DEVELOPMENT

Pharmacokinetics

Balapiravir also provided a robust delivery system for R1479 in humans. In a single ascending-dose phase I study in healthy volunteers, it was demonstrated that R1479 exposures increased linearly and nearly dose proportionally after oral administration of balapiravir [58]. Single doses between 500 mg and 12 g were found to be safe and well tolerated in this study. Mean C_{max} values ranged from 2.96 μg/mL (10.5 μM) after a single 500-mg dose to 46.4 μg/ml (165 μM) after a 12-g dose (Fig. 5, Table 6). In contrast, when R1479 was dosed orally, a mean C_{max} value of 2.5 μg/mL (8.89 μM) was reached with a single 7200-mg dose. Therefore, an approximate 10-fold enhancement in R1479 exposure of was observed with balapiravir in humans, an improvement similar to that observed in cynomolgus monkeys for oral administration of balapiravir as compared to R1479. Renal clearance of R1479 (7.3 to 9.9 L/h) was similar to a mean glomerular filtration rate (GFR) of approximately 9 L/h in healthy subjects. There was therefore no evidence for reabsorption or active secretion of R1479. The conversion of the triester balapiravir to the free nucleoside R1479 was very efficient, with only negligible levels of prodrug (< 1%) observed in urine. These observations were also consistent with very low plasma stability of balapiravir and efficient conversion to R1479 in vitro.

Exposures of R1479 achieved upon multiple-day dosing of Balapiravir in HCV-infected persons are summarized in Table 7. Plasma exposures of R1479 increased linearly up to 4500 mg b.i.d. and reached trough concentrations in excess of the mean human serum adjusted in vitro HCV replicon EC_{50} in dose groups receiving 1500 mg b.i.d. or higher.

The inhibition quotient was calculated, defined as plasma R1479 C_{min} divided by the HCV replicon EC_{50} of R1479 determined in the presence of human serum. As expected for nucleoside analogs, the effect of human serum on inhibition potency of R1479 in the replicon system was small. The mean serum-adjusted Con-1 replicon EC_{50} value was 2.68 ± 0.42 μM, approximately twofold above the value determined in the absence of human serum (1.28 μM). This difference was not determined to be significant. R1479 pharmacokinetics

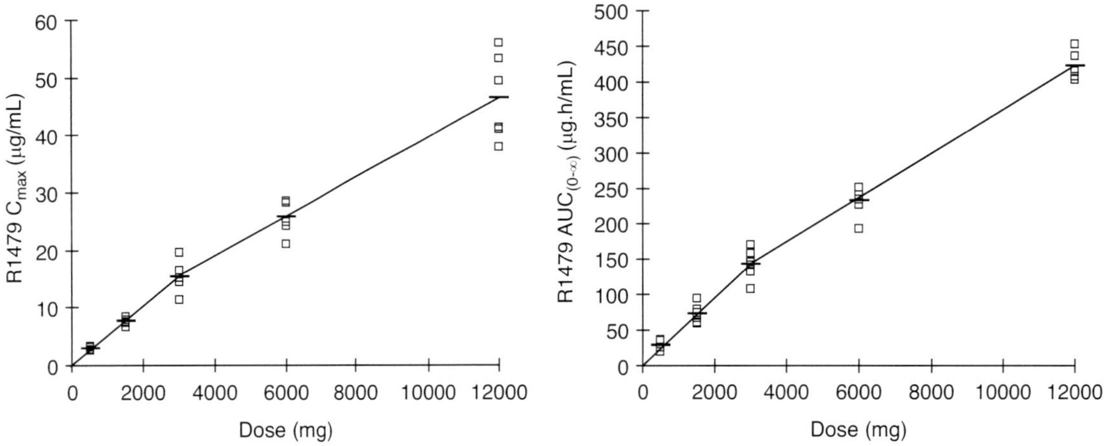

FIGURE 5 Dose proportionality for R1479 after administration of single oral doses of balapiravir in healthy volunteers. (From [58].)

TABLE 6 Summary of R1479 Pharmacokinetics Following Single-Dose Administration of Balapiravir in Healthy Volunteers [Mean (% CV)]

	Group 1 500 mg $n = 6$	Group 2 1500 mg $n = 6$	Group 3 3000 mg $n = 6$	Group 4 6000 mg $n = 6$	Group 5 12000 mg $n = 6$
C_{max} (μg/mL)	2.96 (9)	7.70 (9)	15.4 (18)	25.8 (11)	46.4 (16)
T_{max} (h)	2.7 (31)	3.5 (39)	4.0 (32)	4.7 (32)	5.5 (22)
$AUC_{0-\infty}$ (μg·h/mL)	29.5 (22)	72.6 (18)	143 (15)	232 (9)	422 (5)
$t_{1/2}$ (h)	28.3 (12)	28.4 (16)	26.5 (15)	23.4 (16)	18.9 (9)
Ae (0–72 h) (%)[a]	64.9 (15)	66.1 (10)	72.8 (18)	64.3 (19)	58.0 (20)
Cl (L/h)	7.3 (30)	8.6 (20)	9.4 (23)	9.9 (22)	9.7 (22)

Source: [58].
[a]Cumulative urinary excretion: percent of dose (equivalent) excreted in urine from 0 to 72 h.

were also determined when balapiravir was dosed in combination with pegylated interferon α-2a (PEG) and ribavirin (RBV). The results from the population PK analysis of study PV18369/B showed that R1479 plasma concentrations were similar when balapiravir was dosed in monotherapy or in combination with PEG and RBV (Table 8) [61]. These results suggested no pharmacokinetic interaction between balapiravir, ribavirin, and pegylated interferon α.

Antiviral Efficacy of Balapiravir in HCV-Infected Persons

Monotherapy Balapiravir showed dose- and time-dependent reductions in plasma HCV RNA when dosed as monotherapy for 14 days in treatment-naive HCV genotype 1–infected persons (Table 9) [59,60]. No difference in response in persons infected with HCV subtypes 1a and 1b was observed, consistent with broad in vitro potency of R1479-triphosphate against all HCV genotypes. Dosing of 500 mg b.i.d. balapiravir was associated with only a borderline antiviral effect, with plasma HCV RNA (viral load) reductions after 14 days of dosing, ranging between 0.01 and 0.71 $\log_{10}$ IU/mL, using Roche Cobas Amplicor HCV Monitor test version 2.0. Viral load differences within 0.5 $\log_{10}$ IU/mL were considered within the variability of the assay. Three subjects in the 500-mg b.i.d. dose group never achieved viral load reductions above 0.5 $\log_{10}$ during the 14-day dosing period, and were therefore considered nonresponders to 500 mg b.i.d. balapiravir. Three subjects showed viral load rebound, defined as viral load reduction of 0.5 $\log_{10}$ or greater followed by a 0.5 $\log_{10}$ or greater increase in HCV RNA before the end of treatment. Phenotyping and sequencing, including clonal sequence analysis, of samples from these six subjects, showed no evidence for selection of R1626 resistant virus variants [59,60]. Considering the small changes in viral load (<0.71 log), these results were therefore nonspecific outliers of the Amplicor HCV Monitor test and are consistent with only a very weak antiviral effect of balapiravir at the 500 mg b.i.d. dose in monotherapy.

No nonresponders or subjects with viral load rebound were observed in any of the other monotherapy dose groups. Dosing of the nucleoside analog Balapiravir for 14 days in monotherapy was therefore not associated with resistance selection. These results are substantially different from those observed with inhibitors of HCV protease or non-nucleoside

TABLE 7 Summary of R1479 Pharmacokinetics After 14 Days of Administration of Balapiravir in HCV-Infected Persons (Mean ± S.D.)

	Group 1 500 mg b.i.d. $n = 9$	Group 2 1500 mg b.i.d. $n = 9$	Group 3 3000 mg b.i.d. $n = 8$	Group 4 4500 mg b.i.d. $n = 8$
C_{max} (μg/mL)	3.7 ± 0.6	9.8 ± 1.3	17 ± 3.4	25 ± 3.1
t_{max} (h)	2.9 ± 1.1	3.6 ± 0.9	4.5 ± 1.3	3.8 ± 1.3
AUC_{0-12h} (μg·h/mL)	24 ± 4.3	67 ± 8.4	116 ± 21	175 ± 26
$t_{1/2}$ (h)	26 ± 4.2	23 ± 6.4	21 ± 5.4	20 ± 1.7
C_{min} (μg/mL) (μM)	0.86 ± 0.26 (3.1 ± 0.92)	2.61 ± 0.53 (9.3 ± 1.9)	3.78 ± 1.63 (13 ± 5.6)	5.98 ± 1.49 (21 ± 5.3)
Inhibition quotient[a]	1.2	3.5	4.9	7.8

Source: [59,60].
[a]C_{min} divided by HCV replicon EC_{50}, determined using the 2209 replicon cell line (Con1, genotype 1b) in the presence of 40% human serum [28].

TABLE 8 Summary of R1479 Population Pharmacokinetics Analysis after 14 Days of Administration of Balapiravir in HCV-Infected Persons (Mean ± S.D.)

	Balapiravir Monotherapy 1500 mg b.i.d.	Balapiravir Combination Therapy 1500 mg b.i.d.
C_{max} (μg/mL)	9.9	9.4
$AUC_{0\text{-}12h}$ (μg·h/mL)	69	63
C_{min} (μg/mL)	2.7	2.5

Source: [61].

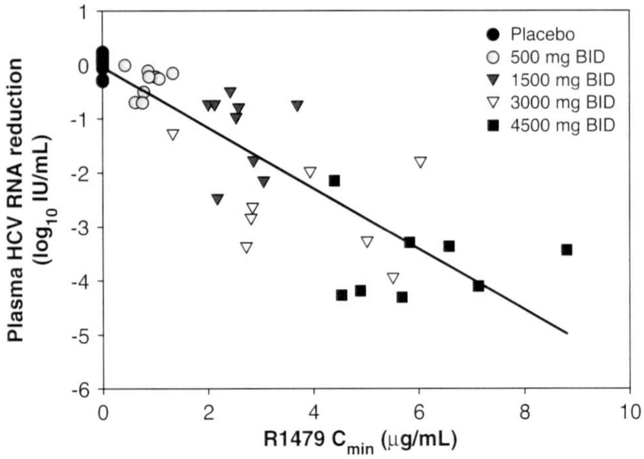

FIGURE 6 Correlation between HCV viral load reduction and R1479 C_{min}.

inhibitors of HCV polymerase, where viral load rebound was frequently observed in monotherapy studies of longer than 3-day durations [60]. Considering the quasispecies nature of HCV, the nucleotide substitution–mutation rate of HCV replication and the volume of daily virus production, the strong antiviral effect and absence of resistance selection in monotherapy were remarkable, but consistent with the high in vitro barrier to resistance of balapiravir as compared to protease and non-nucleoside polymerase inhibitors [25,38]. Balapiravir showed a clear dose-dependent increase in antiviral potency up to 4500 mg b.i.d. All subjects in the 4500-mg b.i.d. dose group experienced more than 2 $\log_{10}$ viral load reduction at week 2, and more than half had the viral load reduced more than 4 $\log_{10}$. All subjects with viral load reductions of more than 4 $\log_{10}$ had HCV RNA levels below 50 IU/ml. Taken together, the 4500-mg b.i.d. dosage group achieved a high mean (median) viral load reduction of 3.7 (4.1) $\log_{10}$ IU/mL. Five subjects in this dosage group had the viral load reduced below the level of detection (<50 IU/mL) [59,60]. Exposure of R1479 within dosage groups showed relatively low variability, and there was a good correlation between exposure (measured as C_{max}, $AUC_{0\text{-}12h}$, or C_{min}) and antiviral effect (measured as plasma HCV RNA reduction) [59,60]. All three PK parameters gave similarly good correlations with viral load reduction, and the results obtained with C_{min} are shown in Figure 6 [59,60].

The extrapolation of these data suggested that the maximal antiviral potency of balapiravir had not yet been reached at the 4500-mg dose. A further increase in potency may therefore be expected with nucleoside analogs that provide a higher intrinsic potency (triphosphate incorporation efficiency by HCV polymerase or phosphorylation efficiency in the target cells) compared to R1479 [33].

Combination Therapy Balapiravir showed significant synergy in vitro in the HCV replicon system when combined with interferon α or ribavirin [33]. Although the molecular basis of the in vitro synergistic effect has not yet been determined, it is of interest to note that a larger-than-expected enhancement of antiviral potency was observed in HCV-infected persons who received balapiravir in combination with PEG and RBV [61]. When balapiravir (1500 mg b.i.d.) was combined with pegylated interferon α-2a (PEG) for the treatment of HCV genotype 1 infection in treatment-naive persons, mean (median) plasma viral load declined 3.1 (3.1) log from baseline by week 2. In comparison, balapiravir monotherapy (1500 mg b.i.d.) resulted in only a 1.2 (0.8) log decline from baseline. Although PEG alone was not administered in this study, historical data suggest that approximately a 0.4 to 0.5 log decline may be expected from PEG monotherapy at week 2 [61,62]. Therefore, when combining balapiravir 1500 mg b.i.d. with PEG, only approximately a 1.7 log reduction in viral load was expected at week 2 (Table 10). The molecular basis for this larger-than-expected effect of balapiravir in combination with PEG is unknown, but does warrant further study. Ribavirin also has a larger impact in combination with

TABLE 9 Viral Load Reduction After 14 Days of Monotherapy with Balapiravir in Treatment-Naive Genotype 1–Infected Persons

R1626 Dose (mg b.i.d.)	n	> 1 $\log_{10}$	> 2 $\log_{10}$	> 3 $\log_{10}$	> 4 $\log_{10}$	Mean	Median	Range
500	9	0	0	0	0	0.32	0.22	0.01–0.71
1500	9	1 (11%)	2 (22%)	0	0	1.2	0.8	0.49–2.46
3000	8	3 (38%)	2 (25%)	3 (38%)	0	2.6	2.7	1.27–3.93
4500	9	0	1 (11%)	3 (33%)	5 (56%)	3.7	4.1	2.15–4.39

Source: [59,60].

TABLE 10 Viral Load Reduction After 14 Days of Monotherapy with Balapiravir or Combination Therapy of Balapiravir with PEG and/or RBV in Treatment-Naive Genotype 1–Infected Persons

	R1626 1500 mg b.i.d. Monotherapy	R1626 1500 mg b.i.d. + PEG	R1626 1500 mg b.i.d. + PEG + RBV	PEG	PEG + RBV (SoC)
Viral load reduction at week 2 ($\log_{10}$ IU/mL) mean (median; range)	1.2 (0.8; 0.49–2.46)	3.1 (3.1; 0.0–5.5)	4.6 (4.7; 2.5–6.6)	0.5[a]	1.6 (1.1; 0.1–3.8)
Additive effect[b]	1.2	1.7	2.8	0.5	0.5[c]

Source: [61].
[a]Estimated, based on [62].
[b]Adding monotherapy effects from the combination therapy components observed at week 2; monotherapy of PEG based on [62].
[c]Lack of effect of RBV on plasma HCV RNA at week 2 [63,64].

PEG than is expected from the PEG and RBV monotherapy results, and the molecular basis for that interaction also remains to be determined. The largest antiviral effect was observed when balapiravir was combined with PEG and RBV in triple combination. The PEG + RBV combination arm in study PV18369/B resulted in a mean (median) viral load reduction of 1.6 (1.1) log by week 2 [61]. Considering the 1.2 (0.8) log reduction observed with balapiravir monotherapy, an approximate 2.8 (1.9) log viral load reduction was expected from the triple combination (Table 10). Instead, 4.6 (4.7) log reduction of plasma HCV RNA was observed in this triple combination, representing an additional 1.8 (2.8) log above expectations [61]. These results also suggest a significant effect of RBV in triple combination with R1626 and PEG as early as week 2 of treatment, despite the fact that steady-state plasma concentrations of RBV are reached only after 4 weeks of dosing. Of the subjects in the balapiravir + PEG + RBV TRIPLE1500 arm, 52% achieved HCV RNA levels < 50 IU/mL and 42% achieved levels < 15 IU/mL at week 2, while 81 and 71% achieved these levels at week 4 (RVR) (Table 11). Consistent with the high barrier to resistance of the three study drugs (balapiravir, PEG, and RBV), there was no evidence for the selection of drug-resistant HCV variants in this phase IIa study (PV18369/B), based on phenotyping and sequencing, including clonal sequence analyses [61].

It is important to note that the assessment of virological response in this study (PV18369/B) was affected at and beyond week 4 of treatment by a substantial proportion of subjects with protocol-defined dose modifications and temporal discontinuations of balapiravir, PEG, and/or RBV as a result of laboratory abnormalities [65]. Although the combination was generally well tolerated, decreases in red and white blood cells and platelets were more pronounced in patients receiving balapiravir combinations than in those receiving the PEG + RBV combination. Of the subjects in the balapiravir + PEG + RBV triple arm, 90% had dose modifications and 39% discontinued balapiravir before the end of the 4-week dosing period, in the majority of cases as a result of grade 4 neutropenia [61,65]. The interpretation of virologic data at week 4 and beyond is therefore complicated. After a further dose-finding phase IIb study exploring various doses of balapiravir and PEG in combination with RBV, it was eventually decided to discontinue further development of balapiravir for the treatment of HCV infection and to focus on other antiviral candidates in development for this indication.

CONCLUSIONS

Balapiravir has demonstrated potent antiviral activity and a high barrier to resistance in HCV-infected persons. The antiviral performance of balapiravir, including plasma exposure requirements for activity, prodrug conversion, metabolic stability of R1479, and synergy with PEG and RBV, was

TABLE 11 Virological Response Rates with Balapiravir in Combination Therapy[a]

	R1626 1500 mg b.i.d + PEG for 4 Weeks, Followed by PEG + RBV for 44 Weeks	R1626 3000 mg b.i.d. + PEG for 4 Weeks, Followed by PEG + RBV for 44 Weeks	R1626 1500 mg b.i.d. + PEG + RBV for 4 Weeks, Followed by PEG + RBV for 44 Weeks	PEG + RBV for 48 Weeks
Week 2 (RVR2)	14% (3/21)	50% (16/32)	42% (13/31)	5% (1/20)
Week 4 (RVR4)	29% (6/21)	69% (22/32)	74% (23/31)	5% (1/20)
Week 48 (EOT)	52% (11/21)	66% (21/32)	81% (25/31)	60% (12/20)
Week 72 (SVR)	24% (5/21)	53% (17/32)	58% (18/31)	50% (10/20)

[a]Virological response defined as reduction of plasma HCV RNA to < 15 IU/mL, as determined by the Roche Cobas Taqman assay [61].

well predicted from nonclinical data. The lipophilic prodrug balapiravir effectively delivered R1479 to systemic circulation after oral administration. The available nonclinical and clinical data for balapiravir clearly indicate opportunities for achieving improved performance with future nucleoside analogs for this and other indications. To date, the possibility of designing more potent analogs of R1479 has already been demonstrated [33,40,44]. Learning from delineating the molecular mechanisms that may have led to the observation of unexpected laboratory abnormalities with balapiravir will also contribute to the design of safer, more potent generations of nucleoside analogs.

REFERENCES

[1] Fried, M. W., et al. Peginterferon alfa-2a plus ribavirin for chronic hepatitis C virus infection. *N. Engl. J. Med.* **2002**, *347*, 975–982.

[2] Manns, M. P., et al. Peginterferon alfa-2b plus ribavirin compared with interferon alfa-2b plus ribavirin for initial treatment of chronic hepatitis C: a randomised trial. *Lancet* **2001**, *358*, 958–965.

[3] Chung, R. T., et al. Peginterferon Alfa-2a plus ribavirin versus interferon alfa-2a plus ribavirin for chronic hepatitis C in HIV-coinfected persons. *N. Engl. J. Med.* **2004**, *351*, 451–459.

[4] Pawlotsky, J. M. Treating hepatitis C in "difficult-to-treat" patients. *N. Engl. J. Med.* **2004**, *351*, 422–423.

[5] Torriani, F. J., et al. Alfa-2a plus ribavirin for chronic hepatitis C virus infection in HIV-infected patients. *N. Engl. J. Med.* **2004**, *351*, 438–450.

[6] Lindenbach, B. D.; Thiel, H.-J.; Rice, C. M. Flaviviridae: the viruses and their replication. In *Fields Virology*, 5th ed., Knipe, D. M., Howley, P. M., Eds., Lippincott Williams & Wilkins, Philadelphia, **2007**, pp 1101–1153.

[7] Lemon, S. M.; Walker, C. M.; Alter, M. J.; Yi, M. Hepatitis C Virus. In *Fields Virology*, 5th ed., Knipe, D. M., Howley, P. M., Eds.; Lippincott Williams & Wilkins, Philadelphia, **2007**, pp. 1253–1305.

[8] Lohmann, V., et al. Replication of subgenomic hepatitis C virus RNAs in a hepatoma cell line. *Science* **1999**, *285*, 110–113.

[9] Khromykh, A. A.; Westaway, E. G. Subgenomic replicons of the flavivirus Kunjin: construction and applications. *J. Virol.* **1997**, *71*, 1497–1505.

[10] Vrolijk, J. M., et al. A replicon-based bioassay for the measurement of interferons in patients with chronic hepatitis C. *J. Virol. Methods* **2003**, *110*, 201–209.

[11] Moradpour, D.; Penin, F.; Rice, C. M. Replication of hepatitis C virus. *Nat. Rev. Microbiol.* **2007**, *5*, 453–463.

[12] Gosert, R., et al. Identification of the hepatitis C virus RNA replication complex in Huh-7 cells harboring subgenomic replicons. *J. Virol.* **2003**, *77*, 5487–5492.

[13] Rouille, Y., et al. Subcellular localization of hepatitis C virus structural proteins in a cell culture system that efficiently replicates the virus. *J. Virol.* **2006**, *80*, 2832–2841.

[14] Miyanari, Y., et al. Hepatitis C virus non-structural proteins in the probable membranous compartment function in viral genome replication. *J. Biol. Chem.* **2003**, *278*, 50301–50308.

[15] Quinkert, D.; Bartenschlager, R.; Lohmann, V. Quantitative analysis of the hepatitis C virus replication complex. *J. Virol.* **2005**, *79*, 13594–13605.

[16] Ma, Y., et al. NS3 helicase domains involved in infectious intracellular hepatitis C virus particle assembly. *J. Virol.* **2008**, *82*, 7624–7639.

[17] Roingeard, P., et al. Hepatitis C virus budding at lipid droplet-associated ER membrane visualized by 3D electron microscopy. *Histochem. Cell Biol.* **2008**, *130*, 561–566.

[18] Bukh, J.; Miller, R. H.; Purcell, R. H. Genetic heterogeneity of hepatitis C virus: quasispecies and genotypes. *Semin. Liver Dis.* **1995**, *15*, 41–63.

[19] Simmonds, P. Genetic diversity and evolution of hepatitis C virus—15 years on. *J. Gen. Virol.* **2004**, *85*, 3173–3188.

[20] Neumann, A. U., et al. Hepatitis C viral dynamics in vivo and the antiviral efficacy of interferon-alpha therapy. *Science* **1998**, *282*, 103–107.

[21] Bartels, D. J., et al. Natural prevalence of hepatitis C virus variants with decreased sensitivity to NS3.4A protease inhibitors in treatment-naive subjects. *J. Infect. Dis.* **2008**, *198*, 800–807.

[22] Curry, S.; Qiu, P.; Tong, X. Analysis of HCV resistance mutations during combination therapy with protease inhibitor boceprevir and PEG-IFN alpha-2b using TaqMan mismatch amplification mutation assay. *J. Virol. Methods* **2008**, *153*, 156–162.

[23] Kim, A. Y., et al. Temporal dynamics of a predominant protease inhibitor-resistance mutation in a treatment-naive, hepatitis C virus-infected individual. *J. Infect. Dis.* **2009**, *199*, 737–741.

[24] Kuntzen, T., et al. Naturally occurring dominant resistance mutations to hepatitis C virus protease and polymerase inhibitors in treatment-naive patients. *Hepatology* **2008**, *48*, 1769–1778.

[25] Le Pogam, S., et al. Existence of hepatitis C virus NS5B variants naturally resistant to non-nucleoside, but not to nucleoside, polymerase inhibitors among untreated patients. *J. Antimicrob. Chemother.* **2008**, *61*, 1205–1216.

[26] Thompson, A. J.; McHutchison, J. G. Antiviral resistance and specifically targeted therapy for HCV (STAT-C). *J. Viral Hepatitis* **2009**, *16*, 377–387.

[27] Sweeney, Z. K.; Klumpp, K. Improving non-nucleoside reverse transcriptase inhibitors for first-line treatment of HIV infection: the development pipeline and recent clinical data. *Curr. Opin. Drug Discov. Dev.* **2008**, *11*, 458–470.

[28] Klumpp, K., et al. The novel nucleoside analog R1479 (4′-azidocytidine) is a potent inhibitor of NS5B-dependent RNA synthesis and hepatitis C virus replication in cell culture. *J. Biol. Chem.* **2006**, *281*, 3793–3799.

[29] Pietschmann, T., et al. Characterization of cell lines carrying self-replicating hepatitis C virus RNAs. *J. Virol.* **2001**, *75*, 1252–1264.

[30] Smith, D. B., et al. Design, synthesis, and antiviral properties of 4′-substituted ribonucleosides as inhibitors of hepatitis C virus replication: the discovery of R1479. *Bioorg. Med. Chem. Lett.* **2007**, *17*, 2570–2576.

[31] Perrone, P., et al. First example of phosphoramidate approach applied to a 4′-substituted purine nucleoside (4′-azidoadenosine): conversion of an inactive nucleoside to a submicromolar compound versus hepatitis C virus. *J. Med. Chem.* **2007**, *50*, 5463–5470.

[32] Perrone, P., et al. Application of the phosphoramidate ProTide approach to 4′-azidouridine confers sub-micromolar potency versus hepatitis C virus on an inactive nucleoside. *J. Med. Chem.* **2007**, *50*, 1840–1849.

[33] Klumpp, K., et al. 2′-Deoxy-4′-azido nucleoside analogs are highly potent inhibitors of hepatitis C virus replication despite the lack of 2′-alpha-hydroxyl groups. *J. Biol. Chem.* **2008**, *283*, 2167–2175.

[34] Le Pogam, S., et al. In vitro selected Con1 subgenomic replicons resistant to 2′-C-methyl-cytidine or to R1479 show lack of cross resistance. *Virology* **2006**, *351*, 349–359.

[35] Leveque, V., et al. R1626 (prodrug of R1479) demonstrates potent antiviral activity across HCV genotypes 1–6 in vitro. 43rd Annual Meeting of the European Association for the Study of the Liver (EASL), Milan, Italy, Apr. 23–27, 2008.

[36] Jiang, W.-R., et al. In vitro antiviral interactions of a novel HCV inhibitor R1479 with interferon alpha-2A, ribavirin and other HCV inhibitors. *Hepatology* **2006**, *44*, 533A.

[37] Seiwert, S.; Tan, H.; Blatt, L. M. Additive to synergistic antiviral effects of an NS3/4A protease inhibitor (ITMN-191) and an NS5B RNA-dependent RNA polymerase inhibitor (R1479) in a HCV replicon system. 42nd Annual Meeting of the European Association for the Study of the Liver (EASL), Barcelona, Spain, Apr. 11–15, 2007.

[38] McCown, M. F., et al. The hepatitis C virus replicon presents a higher barrier to resistance to nucleoside analogs than to nonnucleoside polymerase or protease inhibitors. *Antimicrob. Agents Chemother.* **2008**, *52*, 1604–1612.

[39] Shim, J., et al. Canonical 3′-deoxyribonucleotides as a chain terminator for HCV NS5B RNA-dependent RNA polymerase. *Antiviral Res.* **2003**, *58*, 243–251.

[40] Smith, D. B., et al. The design, synthesis, and antiviral activity of 4′-azidocytidine analogues against hepatitis C virus replication: the discovery of 4′-azidoarabinocytidine. *J. Med. Chem.* **2009**, *52*, 219–223.

[41] Eldrup, A. B., et al. Structure–activity relationship of purine ribonucleosides for inhibition of hepatitis C virus RNA-dependent RNA polymerase. *J. Med. Chem.* **2004**, *47*, 2283–2295.

[42] Eldrup, A. B., et al. Structure–activity relationship of heterobase-modified 2′-C-methyl ribonucleosides as inhibitors of hepatitis C virus RNA replication. *J. Med. Chem.* **2004**, *47*, 5284–5297.

[43] Migliaccio, G., et al. Characterization of resistance to non-obligate chain-terminating ribonucleoside analogs that inhibit hepatitis C virus replication in vitro. *J. Biol. Chem.* **2003**, *278*, 49164–49170.

[44] Smith, D. B., et al. The design, synthesis, and antiviral activity of monofluoro and difluoro analogues of 4′-azidocytidine against hepatitis C virus replication: the discovery of 4′-azido-2′-deoxy-2′-fluorocytidine and 4′-azido-2′-dideoxy-2′,2′-difluorocytidine. *J. Med. Chem.* **2009**, *52*, 2971–2978.

[45] Li, F.; Maag, H.; Alfredson, T. Prodrugs of nucleoside analogues for improved oral absorption and tissue targeting. *J. Pharm. Sci.* **2008**, *97*, 1109–1134.

[46] Antman, M. D.; Gudmundsson, O. S. Valacyclovir: a prodrug of acyclovir. *Biotechnol. Pharm. Aspects* **2007**, *5*(Pt. 2, Prodrugs: Challenges and Rewards), 669–676.

[47] Maag, H. Valganciclovir: a prodrug of ganciclovir. *Biotechnol. Pharm. Aspects* **2007**, *5*(Pt. 2, Prodrugs: Challenges and Rewards), 677–686.

[48] Pierra, C., et al. Synthesis and pharmacokinetics of valopicitabine (NM283), an efficient prodrug of the potent anti-HCV agent 2′-C-methylcytidine. *J. Med. Chem.* **2006**, *49*, 6614–6620.

[49] Shitsuka, H.; Shimma, N. Capecitabine preclinical studies: from discovery to translational research. *Modified Nucleosides* **2008**, 587–600.

[50] Connolly, T. J., et al. Processes for preparing 4′-azido nucleoside derivatives. U.S. Patent Application US20050038240 A1, **2005**.

[51] Divakar, K. J.; Reese, C. B. 4-1,2,4-Triazol-1-yl)- and 4-(3-nitro-1,2,4-triazol-1-yl)-1-(beta-D-2.3.5-tri-*O*-acetylarabinofuranosyl)pyrimidin-2(1*H*)-ones: valuable intermediates in the synthesis of derivatives of 1-(beta-D-arabinofuranosyl)cytosine (ara-C). *J. Chem. Soc. Perkin Trans. 1* **1982**, *5*, 1171–1176.

[52] Kierzek, R., et al. Selective N-deacylation of N,O-protected nucleosides by zinc bromide. *Tetrahedron Lett.* **1981**, *22*, 3761–3764.

[53] Zhu, X.-F.; Williams, H. J. J.; Scott, A. I. An improved transient method for the synthesis of N-benzoylated nucleosides. *Synth. Commun.* **2003**, *33*, 1233–1243.

[54] Alfredson, T., et al. Design and evaluation of novel HCV polymerase inhibitor prodrugs with enhanced oral bioavailability. AAPS Annual Meeting, San Antonio, TX, 2006.

[55] Brandl, M., et al. Physicochemical properties of the nucleoside prodrug R1626 leading to high oral bioavailability. *Drug Dev. Ind. Pharm.* **2008**, *34*, 683–691.

[56] Harrington, P. J.; Hildbrand, S.; Sarma, K. Process for preparation of 4′-azido cytidine derivatives. U.S. Patent Application US20080161550 A1, 2008.

[57] Sarma, K. Selective O-Acylation of Nucleosides. U.S. Patent US7439344 B2, 2008.

[58] Robson, R., et al. Safety, tolerability and pharmacokinetics of R1626, a novel nucleoside analog targeting HCV polymerase: results from a phase 1 single dose escalation trial in healthy subjects. ASCPT Annual Meeting, Anaheim, CA, Mar. 21–24, 2007.

[59] Roberts, S., et al. Results of a phase 1B, multiple dose study of R1626, a novel nucleoside analog targeting HCV polymerase in chronic HCV genotype 1 patients. *Hepatology* **2006**, *44*, 692A.

[60] Roberts, S. K., et al. Robust antiviral activity of R1626, a novel nucleoside analog: a randomized, placebo-controlled study in patients with chronic hepatitis C. *Hepatology* **2008**, *48*, 398–406.

[61] Pockros, P. J., et al. R1626 plus peginterferon alfa-2a provides potent suppression of hepatitis C virus RNA and significant antiviral synergy in combination with ribavirin. *Hepatology* **2008**, *48*, 385–397.

[62] Herrmann, E., et al. Effect of ribavirin on hepatitis C viral kinetics in patients treated with pegylated interferon. *Hepatology* **2003**, *37*, 1351–1358.

[63] Lee, J. H., et al. Effect of ribavirin on virus load and quasispecies distribution in patients infected with hepatitis C virus. *J. Hepatol.* **1998**, *29*, 29–35.

[64] Pawlotsky, J. M., et al. Antiviral action of ribavirin in chronic hepatitis C. *Gastroenterology* **2004**, *126*, 703–714.

[65] Pockros, P., et al. High relapse rate seen at week 72 for patients treated with R1626 combination therapy. *Hepatology* **2008**, *48*, 1349–1350.

21

DISCOVERY AND DEVELOPMENT OF PSI-6130/RG7128

PHILLIP A. FURMAN, MICHAEL J. OTTO, AND MICHAEL J. SOFIA
Pharmasset, Inc., Princeton, New Jersey

INTRODUCTION

Hepatitis C virus (HCV) is a single-stranded positive-sense RNA virus and a member of the hepacivirus genus in the Flaviviridae family. Acute infection with HCV progresses into chronic infection in approximately 80% of infected patients. Chronic HCV infection is a major cause of liver cirrhosis and hepatocellular carcinoma. There are approximately170 million cases of chronic hepatitis C infections worldwide [1], with 5 million people in Europe and 4 million people in the United States chronically infected. The current treatment for chronic hepatitis C is pegylated interferon α (IFN-α) in combination with ribavirin. This regimen results in a sustained antiviral response (SVR) in approximately 40 to 60% of patients treated [2,3]. However, SVRs in genotype 1–infected patients, the predominant genotype infecting patients in Western countries, is much lower than for patients infected with other genotypes. Moreover, dose-limiting and sometimes severe side effects, such as flulike symptoms, fatigue, hemolytic anemia, and depression, may cause patients to discontinue treatment. The suboptimal SVR rate, combined with the a high prevalence of undesirable side effects of interferon and ribavirin has prompted focused efforts to develop antiviral therapies that specifically target HCV. As our knowledge of the replication cycle of HCV and the proteins involved increases, new opportunities for the discovery and development of antiviral therapies are evolving.

The life cycle of the HCV (Fig. 1) can generally be described by a series of steps, which include virus binding and endocytosis into the host cell, fusion and uncoating of the virion, translation and polyprotein processing, replication of the viral RNA, virion assembly, and finally, transport and release of a new viral particle [4]. To enable the virus replication process, the HCV genome codes for seven essential nonstructural proteins. Each of these nonstructural proteins is a potential target for direct-acting antiviral agents. One of these targets, the NS5B RNA-dependent RNA polymerase (RdRp), is particularly attractive for the development of a nucleoside direct-acting antiviral.

HCV forms a membrane-associated replication complex that is composed of the viral NS5B RNA-dependent RNA polymerase, other viral proteins, viral RNA, and altered cellular membranes. The NS5B enzyme is the key element of this replication complex. NS5B, in concert with other nonstructural viral proteins, is responsible for replicating the viral RNA chain. Viral RNA replication begins with the synthesis of minus-strand RNA using plus-strand genomic RNA as template. This is followed by subsequent rounds of minus- and plus-strand RNA synthesis. NS5B catalyzes the addition of nucleoside monophosphate building blocks to a growing RNA chain that is a complementary copy of the existing RNA template strand. NS5B is known to be devoid of a proofreading mechanism. Consequently, HCV RNA replication is a highly error-prone process, resulting in a high mutation rate. Because of the high mutation rate, drug-resistant variants would be expected to arise rapidly.

Since NS5B is required for HCV replication, it presents an attractive therapeutic target. Significant efforts have been devoted to the discovery and development of compounds that target the HCV RdRp. A number of companies have focused their drug discovery research on identifying compounds either as allosteric inhibitors or nucleoside analog inhibitors of HCV replication. Nucleoside analogs have long been the cornerstone of therapy for the treatment of a number of viral

Antiviral Drugs: From Basic Discovery Through Clinical Trials, First Edition. Edited by Wieslaw M. Kazmierski.

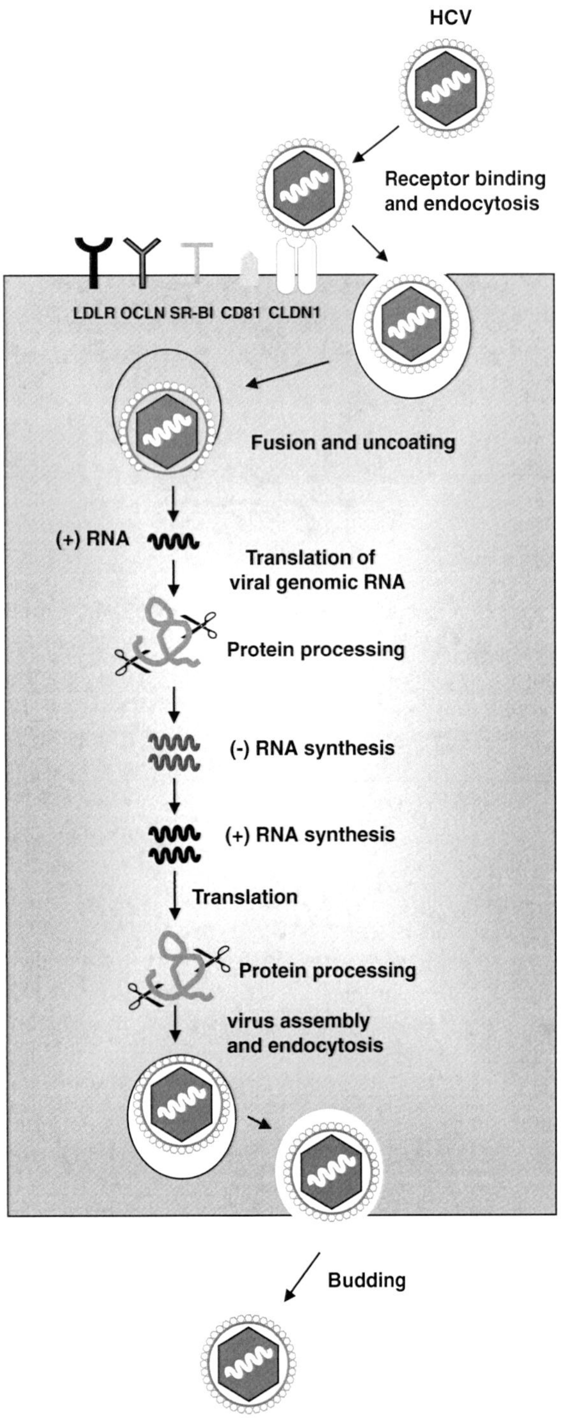

FIGURE 1 Replication cycle of hepatitis C virus.

diseases. The attractiveness of nucleosides as direct-acting antiviral drugs has been demonstrated clearly by their development for the treatment of HIV, HBV, and herpes virus, among other viral diseases [5]. This attractiveness also results from a well-known development path and a large body of knowledge available about associated toxicological signals related to nucleoside-based drugs.

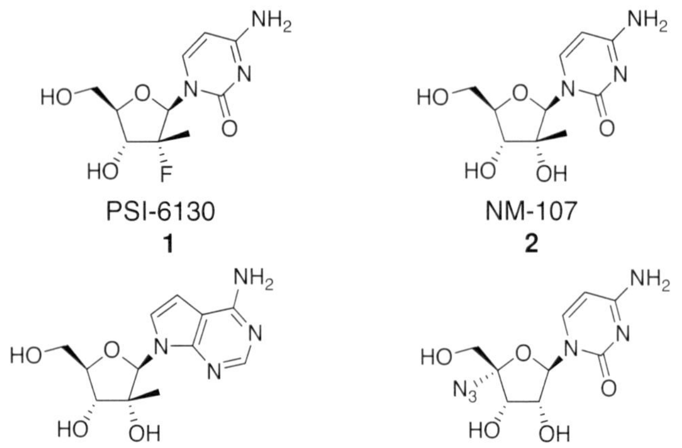

FIGURE 2

Because the HCV NS5B is an RNA-dependent RNA polymerase, it requires ribonucleoside triphosphates for the synthesis of its RNA genome. Unlike deoxyribonucleoside analogs, where there is an extensive structure–activity relationship (SAR), there is very little SAR surrounding ribonucleoside analogs. Nevertheless, in recent years specific nucleoside analog inhibitors of HCV have been identified, and two general classes of nucleosides have progressed to the clinical stage of development. These classes include the 2′-*C*-methyl chemotype represented by NM107 [6], PSI-6130 [7], MK0608 [8], and PSI-7851 [9] and the 4′-azido class of nucleosides represented by R1479 [10] (Fig. 2). To date the 4′-azido class of agents has been associated with hematological toxicity in the clinical setting [11]. NM107 and R1479 have not progressed clinically, due to significant toxicological problems [11,12]. Currently, only the 2′-F-2′-*C*-methyl nucleoside class remains in clinical development for the treatment of HCV.

STRUCTURE–ACTIVITY RELATIONSHIP OF HCV NUCLEOSIDE ANALOG INHIBITORS

The 2′-*F*-2′-*C*-methyl class of nucleosides represented by PSI-6130 and its prodrug derivative RG7128 is unique among nucleosides identified as inhibitors of HCV. The combination of a 2′-β-*C*-methyl and 2′-α-F substituent has a profound impact on the overall potency and safety profile of this class of nucleosides relative to other nucleoside inhibitors of HCV. In particular, the combination of a 2′-F and a 2′-methyl group produced an unexpected activity and in vitro safety profile relative to related 2′-substituted variations. It was shown that 2′-deoxycytidine nucleosides substituted with a fluorine atom at the 2′-position in either the α or β position or both, as in the case of gemcitibine, show nonspecific low-micromolar

TABLE 1 Comparison of 2′-Substituted Nucleosides

Compound	HCV Activity Replicon EC_{90} (μM)	Cytotoxicity (CC_{50}, μM)			
		CloneA	HepG2	BxPC3	CEM
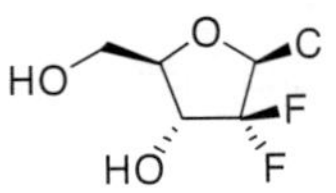	<1	<0.1	<1	<1	<1
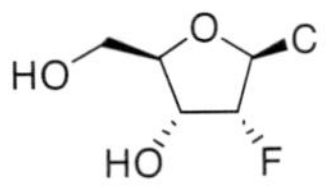	5.66	>100	400	10	6
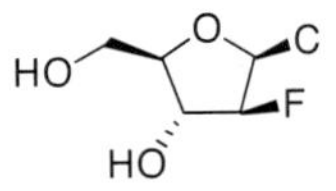	<1	<50	200	5	5
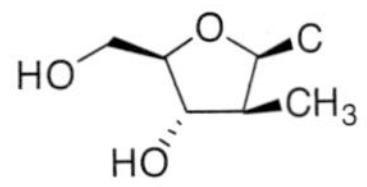	9.73	10.47	40	<1	<1
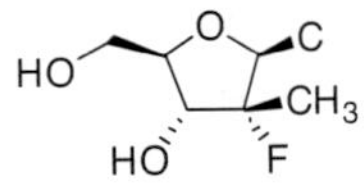 **PSI-6130**	4.5	>100	>1000	>1000	>1000

inhibitory activity toward HCV in the subgenomic replicon assay (Table 1) [13]. However, further investigation showed these fluorine-substituted nucleosides to be substantially cytotoxic when assayed against a panel of cell lines. In addition, in the case of the deoxycytidine nucleoside containing a 2′-β-methyl substitution, HCV inhibitory activity is observed, but again, this compound was shown to be cytotoxic at levels at which its activity is demonstrated. However, when the fluorine and methyl substitutions are combined at 2′ with the α-F and β-methyl configuration, one obtains a compound (β-D-2′-Deoxy-2′-fluoro-2′-*C*-methylcytidine; PSI-6130) that is a potent and specific inhibitor of HCV and demonstrates no cytotoxicity in vitro. The finding that one can combine two moieties, which each alone imparts a cytotoxic character to the molecule, and produce a compound that has a clean overall cytotoxicity profile demonstrates the unique characteristics of the 2′-F-2′-*C*-methyl substitution [14].

The uniqueness of the 2′-F-2′-*C*-methyl-substituted nucleoside PSI-6130 is also evident when comparing it to other nucleosides reported to be inhibitors of HCV RNA synthesis. A comparison with the 2′-*C*-methyl ribose nucleosides NM107 and MK0608 shows that PSI-6130 is about fivefold more potent than its direct 2′-hydroxyl analog NM107 and equipotent to the adenosine derivative MK0608 (Table 2). Equally striking is that PSI-6130 has a more favorable cytotoxicity profile than either of the other 2′-*C*-methyl derivatives. Similarly, when compared to the 4′-azido nucleoside R1479, PSI-6130 demonstrates improved potency and a preferred cytotoxicity profile [15].

Further understanding of the characteristics associated with the 2′-*C*-methyl-2′-F class of nucleosides was developed through an extensive structure–activity analysis. This analysis varied the nature of the substituents at 3′ and 4′ and the nature of the nuclear base in addition to the

TABLE 2 Comparison of Nucleoside Inhibitors for HCV

Compound	HCV Activity Replicon EC90 (μM)	Cytotoxicity (CC50, μM)				
		CloneA	Huh7	HepG2	CEM	PBM
PSI-6130 (2′-F, 2′-C-Me-C)	4.6 ± 2.0	>100	>100	>100	>100	>100
NM107 (2′-C-Me-C)	21.9 ± 4.3	>100	>100	>100	29.4	24.5
MK0608 (2′-C-Me-A)	2.1 ± 0.27	30.5	50.2	31.2	>100	>100
R1479 (4′-N_3-C)	17.5 ± 7.6	>100	>100	>100	5	

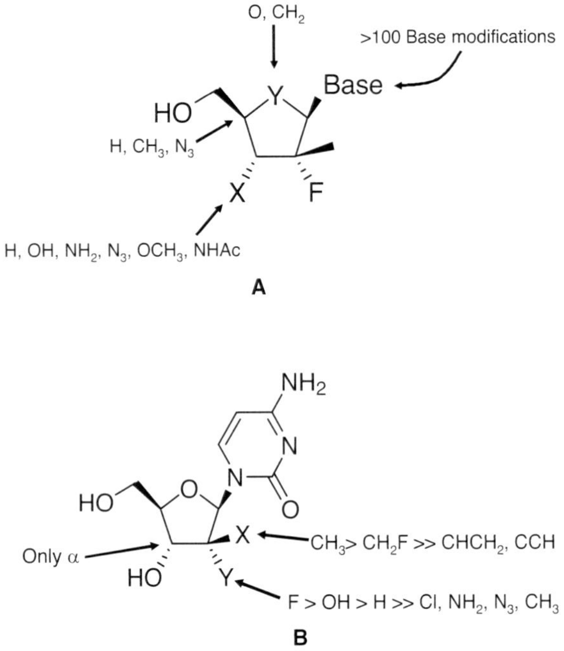

FIGURE 3

preparation of a carbocyclic version of the ribose moiety, replacing the ring oxygen with carbon (Fig. 3A). Since it was demonstrated that no substitution at the 3′-position other than α-hydroxy was tolerated, a 3′-hydroxyl group, is therefore critical for activity. In addition, no 4′-substitutions were shown to be compatible with the 2′-*C*-methyl-2′-F substitution and the ribose ring oxygen could not be replaced with a carbon atom [15,16]. Replacing the cytidine base of PSI-6130 with modified pyrimidine bases afforded no nucleoside analog with HCV inhibitory activity that was superior to PSI-6130. Replacement of the cytidine base with a purine led to compounds that were at best 20-fold less active than PSI-6130 [17].

Structure–activity relationship (SAR) exploration at the 2′-position, while maintaining the rest of the structure of PSI-6130 intact, further highlighted the uniqueness of the 2′-*C*-methyl-2′-F class of nucleosides (Fig. 3B). It was shown that one can replace the 2′-*C*-methyl substituent with a CH_2F group, but addition of any additional steric character (ethyl, ethynyl) is not tolerated. In the α position, F is the preferred substituent; however, as shown with NM107, hydroxyl is only slightly less active, but other substitutions (Cl, NH_2, N_3, CH_3) are not compatible with activity for HCV [15]. Based on the SAR data, it is clear that the 2′-*C*-methyl-2′-F class of nucleosides maintains little flexibility regarding substituent modifications to support potent HCV inhibitory activity. This finding clearly sets this class of nucleosides apart from its 2′-*C*-methyl ribose cousin, which seems to tolerate a number of modifications, at least at the base moiety.

ANTIVIRAL ACTIVITY, SPECIFICITY, AND SELECTIVITY OF PSI-6130

For many years HCV drug discovery was hampered by the lack of cell-based HCV assay systems to test compounds. The development of the HCV replicon was a milestone in HCV research and HCV antiviral drug discovery. Prior to development of the HCV replicon, surrogate viruses such as bovine diarrhea virus (BVDV) or yellow fever virus (YFV) were used to screen for compounds that might be active against HCV. Instead of using a surrogate virus for assaying compounds for anti-HCV activity, PSI-6130 was tested using a subgenomic or a full-length HCV replicon. EC_{90} values of 4.6 ± 2.0 μM and 1.6 ± 0.6 μM were obtained for PSI-6130 with the subgenomic [14] and full-length [14] replicon, respectively. Interestingly, when PSI-6130 was tested for activity using other members of the Flaviviridae family, including BVDV, little or no antiviral activity was observed [14]. This modest activity or lack of activity against other members of the flavivirus family, as well as HIV and HBV, suggests that PSI-6130, unlike 2′-*C*-MeC and 2′-*C*-MeA, is a specific inhibitor of HCV. The lack of significant antiviral activity seen with other flaviviruses could be due either to an inability of certain cells e.g., MDBK cells to phosphorylate PSI-6130, or alternatively, the RdRp of these viruses might be less susceptible to inhibition by the 5′-triphosphate of PSI-6130. Since the differential activity of PSI-6130 extends to a number of flaviviruses in different cell lines, it is more likely a result of target sensitivity brought about by the dual substitution of methyl and fluorine at the 2′ position than a result of levels of phosphorylation.

Studies performed to assess the cytotoxicity of PSI-6130 using several different cell types, including human bone marrow progenitor cells, indicated that no cytotoxicity or mitochondrial toxicity was associated with PSI-6130 at physiologically relevant concentrations [14].

MECHANISM OF ACTION OF PSI-6130

Activation Pathway of PSI-6130

For nucleoside analogs to be active, they must first be phosphorylated to an active 5′-triphosphate. Figure 4 summarizes the metabolic pathway of PSI-6130. The first step in the activation of PSI-6130 involves the phosphorylation of the compound to the 5′-monophosphate (PSI-6130-MP) by cellular deoxycytidine kinase [18]. Subsequent phosphorylation to the corresponding 5′-di- (PSI-6130-DP) and triphosphate (PSI-6130-TP) is catalyzed by UMP-CMP kinase (YMPK) and nucleoside diphosphate kinase (NDPK), respectively [18]. Cell metabolism studies in which cells were incubated with [^{3}H]PSI-6130 revealed that in addition to the presence of the mono-, di-, and triphosphates of PSI-6130, the

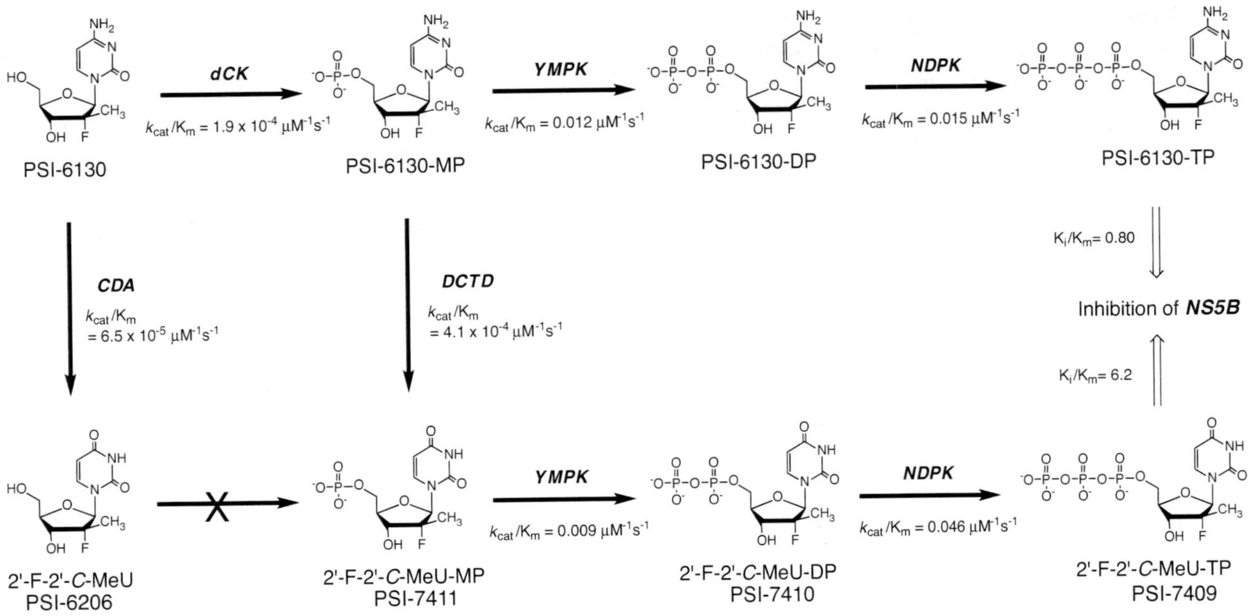

FIGURE 4 Intracellular metabolic pathway of PSI-6130.

mono-, di-, and triphosphates of the uridine metabolite were also formed in cells [18–20]. Although PSI-6130 can be deaminated to the corresponding uridine congener, the uridine analog is inactive in the replicon assay because it cannot be phosphorylated to the corresponding 5′-monophosphate and subsequently to the active triphosphate [19]. Instead, it was found that the pathway to the uridine triphosphate involved deamination of PSI-6130-MP to the uridine monophosphate congener by deoxycytidylate deaminase [19]. Subsequent phosphorylation to the corresponding di- and triphosphate was catalyzed by YMPK and NDPK, respectively.

The intracellular stability of PSI-6130-TP and the uridine congener was determined in primary human hepatocytes [20]. Following the removal of extracellular PSI-6130, the level of PSI-6130-TP remained constant for up to 1 h, whereupon PSI-6130-TP levels decreased following single-phase exponential decay kinetics. A mean half-life of 4.7 ± 0.6 h was determined for PSI-6130-TP. In contrast, the triphosphate of the uridine congener reached steady state 1 to 2 h after removal of PSI-6130 and remained at steady-state for approximately 6 h. Compared with PSI-6130-TP, the half-life for the uridine triphosphate was longer (mean half-life = 38.1 ± 16.1 h).

Inhibition of the HCV NS5B RNA–Dependent RNA Polymerase

The inhibition of HCV RNA dependent RNA–polymerase (RdRp) activity by PSI-6130-TP and the uridine triphosphate congener were studied in vitro using membrane-associated subcellular fractions containing replication complexes (replicase assay) or purified NS5B [18–20]. Both triphosphates were potent inhibitors of HCV RNA synthesis. PSI-6130-TP inhibited HCV RNA synthesis in the HCV replicase assay with a mean IC_{50} value of 0.34 μM, whereas the uridine triphosphate congener inhibited the replicase with a mean IC_{50} of 1.19 μM [20]. In two separate studies using purified NS5B, K_i values were determined for PSI-6130-TP and the uridine triphosphate congener using a heteropolymeric template derived from either the 3′-end of the minus strand of the HCV genome or the minus strand of the HCV internal ribosomal entry site [18–20]. The K_i value for PSI-6130-TP and the uridine triphosphate were 0.023 and 0.141 μM, respectively, when the 3′-end of the minus strand of the HCV genome was used as a template [20]. Using the minus strand of the HCV internal ribosomal entry site as template, the K_i value for PSI-6130-TP was determined to be 0.059 ± 0.011 μM and for the uridine triphosphate 0.42 ± 0.04 μM [18,19]. Studies to further elucidate the molecular mechanism of action of inhibition of the HCV RdRp demonstrated that both PSI-6130 and the uridine congener were incorporated into an elongating RNA chain by the enzyme [18,20]. Incorporation into the growing RNA chain prevented further elongation. Consequently, both molecules are considered to be nonobligate chain terminators.

RESISTANCE

In replicon cells, nucleoside analog inhibitors of HCV with the 2′-C-modification, including NM107, MK-0608, and 2-*C*-methyladenosine, selected the NS5B S282T mutation which resides within the active site of the polymerase [21,22]. In replicon assays, the presence of this mutation resulted in as much as a 20- to 100-fold reduction in sensitivity to these compounds [21,22]. However, the S282T mutation provoked only a 2.4- to 6-fold loss of activity for PSI-6130 in the replicon assay [23]. In vitro resistance selection studies performed by Ali et al. [23] demonstrated that PSI-6130 selected for the S282T mutation. However, this selection required long-term passage in the presence of PSI-6130 and that the emergence of the S282T mutation be accompanied by a number of co-selected mutations. Replicons containing the S282T mutation have a significant reduction in their replication fitness and certain combinations of the co-selected mutations appear to somewhat enhance the replication fitness of a S282T-containing mutant replicon. The ability of PSI-6130-TP and the uridine triphosphate to inhibit NS5B is reduced 7.5- fold and 23.7-fold, respectively, when the S282T mutation is present [19]. These results suggest that the presence of the 2′fluoro substitution, in conjunction with the 2′-methyl moiety on the ribose, may alter the interaction of PSI-6130-TP with wild-type polymerase and polymerase containing the S282T mutation, such that the loss of activity conferred by this mutation is modest (3- to 7.5-fold) compared to that of the uridine triphosphate congener (~20-fold) and other 2′-*C*-methyl analogs.

PRODRUG STRATEGY

With the unique and surprising characteristics of the 2′-F - 2′-*C*-methyl class of nucleosides and the clear superiority of PSI-6130 relative to other nucleosides being developed for the treatment of HCV, PSI-6130 was advanced into phase I clinical development. However, it was shown that when PSI-6130 was dosed orally, a certain percentage of it was metabolized to the inactive uridine derivative [19]. Biochemical studies revealed that PSI-6130 was deaminated to the uridine congener by human cytidine deaminase [19]. To compound the issue, the oral bioavailability of PSI-6130 was determined to be less than 25%. The low bioavailability in conjunction with the production of an inactive metabolite posed significant challenges for achieving sufficient therapeutic levels of active drug. To overcome these challenges, it was hypothesized that a prodrug approach would deliver greater exposure of the parent nucleoside and reduce the metabolism to the inactive uridine metabolite.

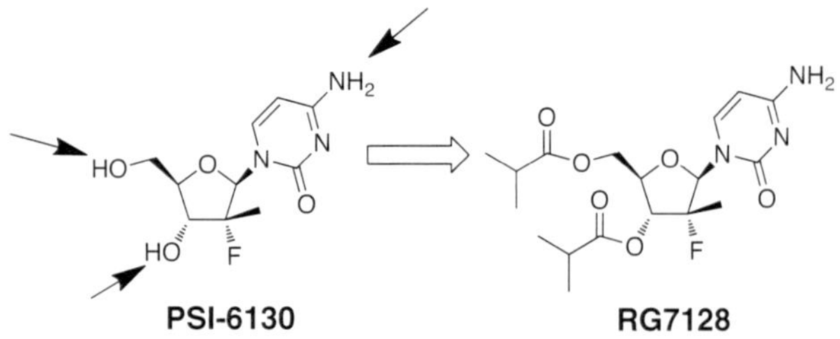

FIGURE 5

Identification of a suitable prodrug for PSI-6130 required the development of a compound that maintained stability in the gastrointestinal tract, was efficiently absorbed, and was released as the parent drug once the prodrug reached the systemic circulation. For PSI-6130 there were three sites on the molecule onto which a prodrug moiety could be attached (Fig. 5): the 3′- and 5′-hydroxyl groups and the N^4 amino group on the cytidine base. A variety of prodrug derivatives were investigated, including esters and carbonates at the 3′- and/or 5′-hydroxyl and amides, carbonates, or ureas at the N^4 amino group of the base. The 3′- and/or 5′-ester or carbonate prodrugs provided the best overall prodrug profile (Table 3). Ultimately, the 3′,5′-diisobutyrate ester prodrug of PSI-6130, RG7128, demonstrated the characteristics desired for the prodrug approach. RG7128 was subsequently advanced into clinical evaluation for the treatment of HCV.

Synthesis of the 2′-F- 2′-C-methyl-nucleoside and Prodrug

The synthesis of a 2′-*C*-methyl-2′-F nucleoside posed substantial challenges, especially as it related to the preparation of sufficient quantities of compound to support preclinical and clinical development efforts. For this class of nucleosides, the challenge was twofold. The first challenge focused on the introduction of the unique 2′-β-methyl-2′-α-F functional array, and the second focused on introduction of the base in the preferred β-configuration. The original medicinal chemistry synthesis (Scheme 1) started with a preconstructed

TABLE 3 Comparison of Properties of Prodrug R7128 to Parent Nucleoside PSI-6130[a]

Compound	EC_{90} (μM), CloneA	CC_{50} (μM)	Stability SGF (pH 1.2), $t_{1/2}$ (h), 37°C	Stability SIF (pH 7.4), $t_{1/2}$ (h) 37°C	Caco2 Papp $\times 10^{-6}$ (cm/s)	Rat PK 10 mg/kg $AUC_{0\text{-}24}$ (μg/mL·h) and C_{max} (μg/mL)
PSI-6130	3.03	>100	>20	>20	0.21	AUC(parent) = 2.97, $C_{max} = 0.6$
R7128	2.5	>100	25	36	6.4	AUC(parent) = 16.17, $C_{max} = 1.86$

[a]SGF, simulated gastric fluid; SIF, simulated intestinal fluid.

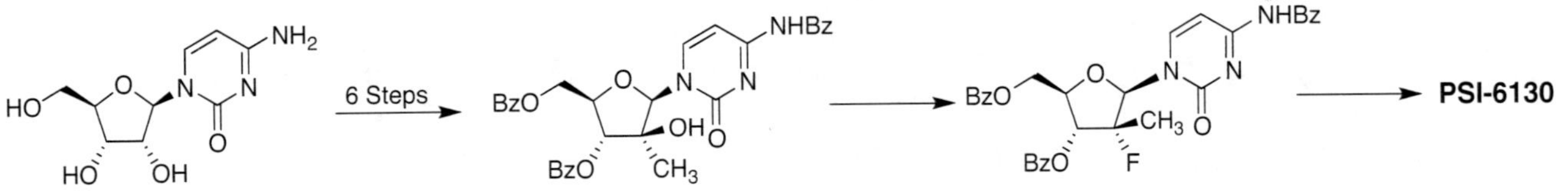

SCHEME 1

β-nucleoside, cytidine, and introduced the 2′-substituents first by oxidation of the 2′-hydroxyl group to the ketone and methylation to produce the intermediate 2′-β-hydroxy-2′-α-*C*-methylcytidine nucleoside [7]. The key step was then accomplished using DAST fluorination to introduce the 2′-α-F group through stereochemical inversion. However, this approach suffered from a very low-yielding DAST fluorination step, the significant formation of several side products, a difficult chromatography, and an overall yield of 3%. A rework of the synthesis was required to improve overall yield, eliminate costly chromatography steps, and improve stereochemical efficiency.

Ultimately, the approach taken envisioned preparation of a chiral ribonolactone onto which was appended the cytidine base via a Verbruggen-like coupling on the activated lactol (Scheme 2) [24]. The lactone was prepared from isopropylidene protected D-glyceraldehyde from which the desired chirality of the lactone was translated. This aldehyde was converted to the chiral diol intermediate without the use of chiral oxidizing agents. Regio- and stereoselective introduction of the key fluorine group was accomplished via opening of a cyclic sulfate with a nucleophilic fluoride reagent. Subsequent acid mediated lactonization and protection gave the desired lactone (Scheme 3).

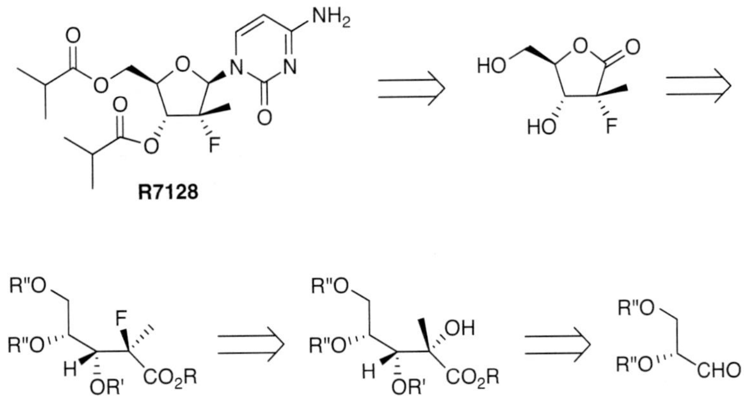

SCHEME 2

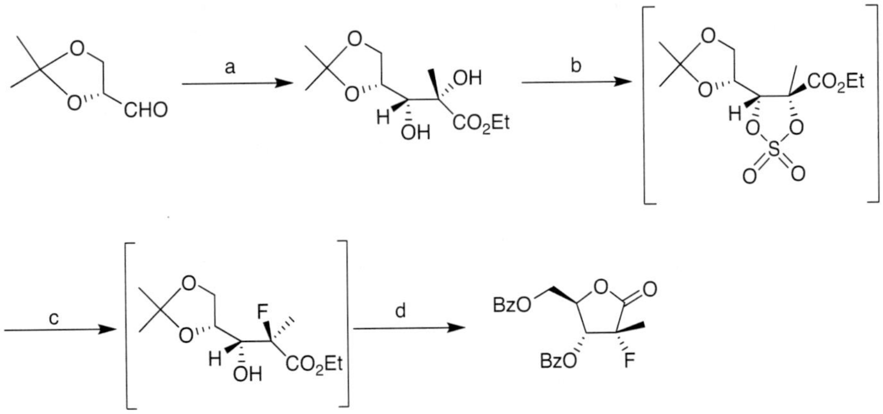

SCHEME 3 Reagents: (a) (i) $Ph_3PC(Me)CO_2Et$, DCM, −40°C, (ii) $KMnO_4$, acetone, 0°C; (b) (i) $SOCl_2$,TEA, DCM/0°C, (ii) aquous NaOCl, TEMPO $NaHCO_3$, MeCN, 0°C; (c) (i) TEAF, dioxane, 100°C, (ii) concentrated HCl, dioxane, room temp; (d) (i) EtOH, concentrated HCl, room temprature, (ii) Benzoyl chloride, pyridine, room temprature.

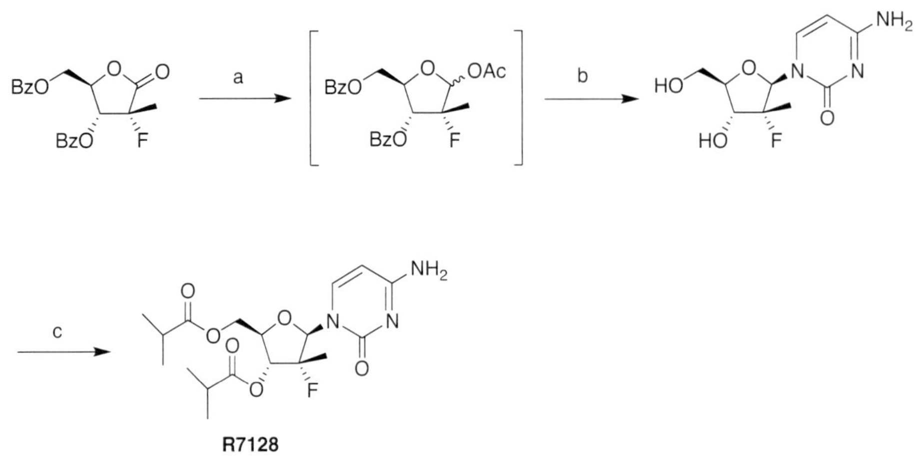

SCHEME 4 Reagents: (a) (i) Li(*O*-*t*Bu)$_3$AlH, THF, −20°C, (ii) Ac_2O, DMAP, −20°C; (b) (i) *N*-benzoyl-*O*-TMS cytosine, $SnCl_4$, PhCl, 65°C, (ii) NH_3, MeOH, room temperature; (c) isobutyryl chloride, DMAP, THF, DEA, 0°C.

With the chiral lactone in hand, the next significant hurdle was to couple the nucleobase to the ribonolactone. This was accomplished by reduction to the lactol and coupling a protected cytosine base with the activated lactol using $SnCl_4$ to give a highly favorable 4 : 1 β/α anomeric ratio. Deprotection and bisacylation gave R7128 the diisobutyryl ester prodrug of PSI-6130 (Scheme 4) [24,25]. This approach provided R7128 in 20% overall yield without the use of chromatographic steps and was sufficient to provide kilogram quantities to support clinical development efforts.

RG7128 CLINICAL STUDIES

RG7128 has been studied in a single ascending-dose protocol, a 14-day multiple ascending-dose monotherapy protocol, and a 28-day combination with interferon and ribavirin protocol in a total of 108 individuals. In all studies to date, RG7128 was well tolerated, with no drug-related discontinuations. Adverse events with RG7128 were generally mild to moderate and were not significantly different from those with placebo.

Multiple Ascending Dose Studies in HCV Genotype 1–Infected Subjects

A 14-day monotherapy study was conducted in 40 HCV genotype 1–infected patients who had previously failed an interferon-based therapeutic regimen. Once daily (q.d.) doses of 750 or 1500 mg, and twice-daily (b.i.d.) doses of 750 or 1500 mg were tested. All regimens resulted in significant reductions in HCV RNA in a dose-dependent manner. Table 4 shows the mean $\log_{10}$ decline in plasma HCV RNA in all RG7128 treatment groups. The decline occurred in a dose-dependent manner and reached nadir values at day 15, suggesting the potential for further viral suppression with continued therapy and a low potential for escape mutations during early dosing. The decrease in HCV RNA from baseline in the highest cohort, 1500 mg b.i.d., ranged from −1.2 to −4.2 $\log_{10}$ IU/mL. One subject's HCV RNA was suppressed below the limit of detection, 15 IU/mL [26,27].

Sequence analysis of patient samples was performed using both populations sequencing as well as clonal analysis. No mutations were identified that could be associated with a resistant phenotype. In particular, no NS5B S282T variants previously identified by in vitro replicon selection to have reduced susceptibility to PSI-6130 and RG7128 were detected [28].

28-Day Combination Study with R7128 Added to Pegasys and Copegus in HCV genotype 1–Infected Treatment-Naive Subjects

A 28-day study comparing BID dosing of RG7128 at 500, 1000, and 1500 mg added onto standard of care (Pegasys and Copegus) to standard of care (SoC) alone was conducted

TABLE 4 Mean Plasma HCV RNA ($\log_{10}$ Copies/mL) Change from Baseline

	Placebo	750 mg q.d.	1500 mg q.d.	750 mg b.i.d.	1500 mg b.i.d.
Number of subjects	8	8	8	9	7
Mean $\log_{10}$ change on day 15	−0.19	−0.90	−1.48	−2.12	−2.67
Range	0.1 to − 0.4	−0.3 to − 1.4	−0.8 to − 2.3	−1.7 to − 3.5	−1.2 to − 4.2

TABLE 5 Antiviral Effects of R7128 After 28 Days of Therapy

	SoC[a]	500 mg b.i.d. + SoC	1000 mg b.i.d. + SoC	1500 mg b.i.d. + SoC
Number of subjects	15	20	25	20
Mean Log_{10} change on day 29	−2.85	−3.86	5.05	−5.09
Percent subjects with HCV RNA <15 IU	20	32	92	89

[a]SoC, Pegasys + Copegus.

in treatment-naive HCV genotype 1 subjects. All doses were well tolerated, with no dose-defining adverse events reported. Adverse events at all doses of RG7128 were similar to those reported for interferon and ribavirin alone. The effects on mean HCV RNA levels are shown in Table 5. The antiviral effects were essentially identical at the two higher doses, and substantially less at the 500-mg dose level. Maximum reductions were seen at both the 1000- and 1500-mg dosage levels, with mean HCV RNA dropping by approximately 5 $\log_{10}$. More important, after 28 days of RG7128 plus SoC, 30, 88, and 85% in the 500-, 1000-, and 1500-mg b.i.d. groups, respectively, had reached RVR (rapid virological response), defined as the proportion of patients with HCV RNA below the limit of detection after 28 days of treatment) vs. 20% of the SoC patients [29].

A phenotypic and sequence assessment of resistance selection to RG7128 was performed as part of this combination study. Phenotypic and sequence analysis were performed on NS5B clinical isolates to monitor for the development of viral resistance in vivo. Sequence analysis of the entire NS5B coding region from all baseline samples showed no preexisting resistance mutation S282T and no common amino acid substitution across the patients treated with RG7128 that could be a predictor of response to treatment. Phenotypic characterization of the NS5B clinical isolates obtained from these patients showed that susceptibility to RG7128 and to interferon was similar before and at the end of treatment. These data show the lack of selection of resistance to RG7128 in HCV genotype 1 after 4 weeks of treatment with RG7128 in combination with SoC [30].

28-Day Combination Study with RG7128 Added to SoC in HCV Genotype 2 or 3–Infected Subjects Who Had Failed Previous Interferon-Based Treatment

A 28-day study comparing b.i.d. dosing of RG7128 at 1500 mg added to SoC with SoC alone was conducted in HCV genotype 2 or 3 subjects who were nonresponders to prior interferon-based treatment. As was observed in genotype 1 subjects, 1500 mg b.i.d. was well tolerated with no dose-defining adverse events reported. Adverse events in both groups were similar and similar to those commonly reported for interferon and ribavirin alone. Following 28 days of therapy, the combination of RG7128 plus SoC resulted in a 5.03 $\log_{10}$ decrease from baseline in plasma HCV RNA, vs. a 3.26 $\log_{10}$ decrease from baseline in patients who received SoC alone. Higher rates of RVR were seen in the RG7128 1500 mg b.i.d. plus SoC treatment group vs. SoC only group, with 40% (2 of 5) of SoC patients achieving RVR vs. 90% (18 of 20) in the RG7128 1500 mg b.i.d. plus SoC group [31].

As with HCV genotype 1–infected subjects, a phenotypic and sequence assessment of resistance selection to RG7128 was performed as part of this combination study in HCV genotype 2 and 3–infected subjects. Sequence analysis of the entire NS5B coding region from all baseline samples showed no preexisting resistance mutation S282T and no common amino acid substitution across the patients treated with RG7128 that could be a predictor of response to treatment. Phenotypic characterization of the NS5B clinical isolates obtained from these patients showed that susceptibility to RG7128 and to interferon was similar before and at the end of treatment. These data show the lack of selection of resistance to RG7128 in HCV genotype 2 or 3 after 4 weeks of treatment with RG7128 in combination with SoC [30].

REFERENCES

[1] Marcellin, P.; Boyer, N. Transition of care between paediatric and adult gastroenterology: chronic viral hepatitis. *Best Pract. Res. Clin. Gastroenterol.* **2003**, *17*, 259–275.

[2] McHutchison, J. G.; Fried, M. W. Current therapy for hepatitis C: pegylated interferon and ribavirin. *Clin. Liver Dis.* **2003**, *7* (1); 149–161.

[3] Manns, M. P.; McHutchison, J. G.; Gordon, S. C.; Rustgi, V. K.; Shiffman, M.; Reindollar, R.; Goodman, Z. D.; Koury, K.; Ling, M.; Albrecht, J. K. Peginterferon alfa-2b plus ribavirin compared with interferon alfa-2b plus ribavirin for initial treatment of chronic hepatitis C: a randomized trial. *Lancet* **2001**; *358*, 958–965.

[4] Linddenbach, B. D.; Rice, C. M. Unravelling hepatitis C virus replication from genome to function. *Nature* **2005**; *436*, 933–938.

[5] De Clerq, E. Recent highlights in the development of new antiviral drugs. *Curr. Opin. Microbiol.* **2005**, *8*, 552–560.

[6] Pierra, C.; Amador, A.; Benzaria, S.; Cretton-Scott, E.; D'Amours, M.; Mao, J.; Mathieu, S.; Moussa, A.; Bridges,

E. G.; Standring, D. N.; et al. Synthesis and pharmacokinetics of valopicitabine (NM283), an efficient prodrug of the potent anit-HCV agent 2′-D-methylcytidine. *J. Med. Chem.* **2006**; *49* (22), 6614–6620.

[7] Clark, J. L.; Hollecker, L.; Mason, J. C.; Stuyver, L. J.; Tharnish, P. M.; Lostia, S.; McBrayer, T. R.; Schinazi, R.; Watanabe, K. A.; Otto, M. J.; et al. Design, synthesis, and antiviral activity of 2′-deoxy-2′-fluoro-2′-*C*-methylcytidine, a potent inhibitor of hepatitis C virus replication. *J. Med. Chem.* **2005**, *48*, 5504–5508.

[8] Carroll, S. S.; Tomassini, J. E.; Bosserman, M.; Getty, K.; Stahlhut, M. W.; Eldrup, A. B.; Bhat, B.; Simcoe, A. L.; LaFemina, R.; Rutkowski, C. A.; et al. Inhibition of hepatitis C virus RNA replication by 2′-modified nucleoside analogs. *J. Biol. Chem.* **2003**, *278*, 11979–11984.

[9] Furman, P. A.; Wang, P.; Niu, C.; Bao, D.; Symonds, W.; Nagarathnam, D.; Steuer, H. M.; Rachakonda, S.; Ross, B. S.; Otto, M. J.; Sofia, M. J. PSI-7851: A novel liver-targeting nucleotide prodrug for the treatment of hepatitis C. 59th Annual Meeting of the American Association for the Study of Liver Diseases, Boston, Oct. 31–Nov. 4, **2008**.

[10] Klumpp, K.; Leveque, V.; Le Pogam, S.; Ma, H.; Jian, W.-R.; Kang, H.; Granycome, C.; Singer, M.; Laxton, C.; Hang, J. Q.; et al. The novel nucleoside analog R1479 (4′-azidocytidine) is a potent inhibitor of NS5B-dependent RNA synthesis and hepatitis C virus replication in cell culture. *J. Biol. Chem.* **2006**, *281*, 3793–3799.

[11] Nelson, D.; Pockors, P.; Godofsky, E.; Rodriguez-Torres, M.; Everson, G.; Fried, M.; Ghalib, R.; Harrison, S.; Nyberg, L.; Shiffman, M.; Chan, A. High end-of-treatment response (84%) after 4 weeks of R1626, peginterferon alfa-2A (40 kDa) and ribavirin. 43rd Annual Meeting of the European Association for the Study of the Liver, Milan, Italy, Apr. 23–27, **2008**.

[12] Afdahl, N.; Godofsky, E.; Dienstag, J.; Rustgi, V. K.; Schick, L.; McEniry, D.; Zhou, X.-J.; Chao, G.; Fang, C.; Fielman, B.; et al. Final phase I/II trial results for NM283, a new polymerase inhibitor for hepatitis C: antiviral efficacy and tolerance in patients with HCV-1 Infection, including previous interferon failures. 55th Annual Meeting of the American Association for the Study of Liver Diseases, Boston, Oct. 29–Nov. 2, **2004**.

[13] Stuyver, L. J.; McBrayer, T. R.; Whitaker, T.; Tharnish, P. M.; Ramesh, M.; Lostia, S.; Cartee, L.; Shi, J.; Hobbs, A.; Schinazi, R. F., et al. Inhibition of the subgenomic hepatitis C virus replicon in Huh-7 cells by 2′-deoxy-2′-fluorocytidine. *Antimicrob. Agents Chemother.* **2004**, *48*, 651–654.

[14] Stuyver, L. J.; McBrayer, T. R.; Tharnish, P. M.; Clark, J.; Hollecker, L.; Lostia, S.; Nachman, T.; Grier, J.; Bennett, M. A.; Xie, M-Y.; et al. Inhibition of hepatitis C replicon RNA synthesis by β-D-2′-deoxy-2′-fluoro-2′-*C*-methylcytidine: a specific inhibitor of hepatitis C virus replication. *Antiviral Chem. Chemother.* **2006**, *17*, 79–87.

[15] Sofia, M. J.; Du, J.; Wang, P.; Chun, K.; Rachakonda, S.; Ross, B.; Steuer, H.; Espiritu, C.; Murakami, E.; Bao, H.; et al. Structure activity relationships of 2′-*C*-methyl modified nucleosides as anti-HCV agents. 238th American Chemical Society National Meeting, Washington, DC, Aug. 16–19, **2009**. Abstract MEDI101.

[16] Liu, J.; Du, J.; Wang, P.; Nagarathnam, D.; Mosley, R.; Espiritu, C.; Bao, H.; Murakami, E.; Furman, P. A.; Otto, M. J.; Sofia, M. J. Preparation of 4-amino-1-((1R,2*S*,3*R*,4*R*)-2-fluoro-3-hydroxy-4-hydroxymethyl-2-methylcyclopentyl)pyrimidin-2(1*H*)-one: a carbocyclic analog of the potent HCV NS5B-polymerase inhibitor PSI-6130. 238th American Chemical Society National Meeting, Washington, DC, Aug. 16–19, **2009**. Abstract MEDI107.

[17] Wang, P.; Sofia, M. J.; Chun, B.-K.; Du, J.; Rachakonda, S.; Steuer, H.; Murakami, E.; Bao, H.; Nagarathnam, D.; Otto, M. J.; Furman, P. A. D-2′-Deoxy-2′-fluoro-2′-*C*-methylribofuranosyl nucleosides: effect of base modifications on anti-hepatitis C virus activity. 238th American Chemical Society National Meeting, Washington, DC, Aug. 16–19, **2009**. Abstract MEDI100.

[18] Murakami, E.; Niu, C.; Bao, H.; Ramesh, M.; McBrayer, T. R.; Whitaker, T.; Steuer, H. M.M.; Schinazi, R. F.; Stuyver, L. J.; Obikhod, A.; et al. Mechanism of action of β-D-2′-deoxy-2′-fluoro-2′-*C*-methylcytidine and inhibition of hepatitis C virus NS5B RNA polymerase. *Antimicrob. Agents Chemother.* **2007**; *52* (2), 503–509.

[19] Murakami, E.; Niu, C.; Bao, H.; Steuer, H.; Whitaker, T.; Nachman, T.; Sofia, M. J.; Wang, P.; Otto, M. J.; Furman, P. A. The mechanism of action of β-D-2′-deoxy-2′-fluoro-2′-*C*-methylcytidine involves a second metabolic pathway leading to β-D-2′-deoxy-2′-fluoro-2′-*C*-methyluridine 5′-triphosphate, a potent inhibitor of the hepatitis C virus RNA-dependent RNA polymerase. *Antimicrob. Agents Chemother.* **2008**, *52*, 458–464.

[20] Ma, H.; Jiang, W. R.; Robledo, N.; Leveque, V.; Ali, S.; Lara-Jaime, T.; Masjedizadeh, M.; Smith, D. B.; Cammack, N.; Klumpp, K.; Symons, J. Characterization of the metabolic activation of hepatitis C virus nucleoside inhibitor beta-D-2-deoxy-2-fluoro-2-*C*-methylcytidine (PSI-6130) and identification of a novel active 5-triphosphate species. *J. Biol. Chem.* **2007**, *282*, 29812–29820.

[21] Thompson, A. J. V.; McHutchison, J. G. Antiviral resistance and specifically targeted therapy for HCV (STAT-C). *J. Viral Hepatitis* **2009**, *16*, 377–387.

[22] Olsen, D. B.; Eldrup, A. B.; Bartholomew, L.; Bhat, B.; Bosserman, M. R.; Ceccacci, A.; Colwell, L. F.; Fay, J. F.; Flores, O. A.; Getty, K. L.; et al. A 7-deaza-adenosine analog is a potent and selective inhibitor of hepatitis C virus replication with excellent pharmacokinetic properties. *Antimicrob. Agents Chemother.* **2004**; *48* (10), 3944–3953.

[23] Ali, S.; Leveque, V.; Le Pogam, S.; Ma, H.; Philipp, F.; Inocencio, N.; Smith, M.; Alker, A.; Kang, H.; Najera, I.; et al. Selected replicon variants with low-level in vitro resistance to the hepatitis C virus NS5B polymerase inhibitor PSI-6130 lack cross-resistance with R1479. *Antimicrob. Agents Chemother.* **2008**, *52* (12), 4356–4369.

[24] Wang, P.; Chun, B.-K.; Rachakonda, S.; Du, J.; Khan, N.; Shi, J.; Stec, W.; Cleary, D.; Ross, B.; Sofia, M. J. An efficient and diasterioselective synthesis of PSI-6130: a clinically efficacious inhibitor of HCV NS5B polymerase. *J. Org. Chem.* **2009**; *74*, 6819–6824.

[25] Chun, B.-K.; Clark, J.; Sarma, K.; Wang, P. U.S. Patent Application. US2007/0197463 A1.

[26] Reddy, R.; Rodriguez-Torres, M.; Gane, E.; Robson, R.; Lalezari, J.; Everson, G. T.; DeJesus, E.; McHutchison, J. G.; Vargas, H. E.; Beard A.; et al. Antiviral activity, pharmacokinetics, safety, and tolerability of R7128, a novel nucleoside HCV RNA polymerase inhibitor, following multiple, ascending, oral doses in patients with HCV genotype 1 infection who have failed prior interferon therapy. 58th Annual Meeting of the American Association for the Study of Liver Diseases; Boston, Nov. 2–6, 2007.

[27] McHutchison, J. G.; Reddy, R.; Rodriguez-Torres, M.; Gane, E.; Robson, R.; Lalezari, J.; Everson, G. T.; DeJesus, E.; Vargus, H. E.; Beard, A.; et al. Potent antiviral activity of the nucleoside HCV inhibitor, R7128, in prior IFN non-responders. Frontiers in Drug Development in Viral Hepatitis (HEP-DART), Lahaina, Dec. 9–13, **2007**.

[28] Le Pogam, S.; Seshaadri, A.; Kosaka, A.; Hu, S.; Beard, A.; Symons, J.; Cammack, N.; Nanera, I. Lack of viral resistance after 14-day monotherapy treatment with R7128 in treatment-experienced patients infected with HCV genotype 1. EASL Conference on Hepatits B and C Resistance to Antiviral Therapies, Paris, Feb. 14–16, **2008**.

[29] Lalezari, J.; Gane, E.; Rodriguez-Torres, M.; DeJesus, E.; Nelson, D.; Everson, G.; Jacobson, I.; Reddy, R.; Hill, G. Z.; Beard, A.; et al. Potent antiviral activity of the HCV nucleoside polymerase inhibitor, R7128, in combination with PEG-IFN alfa-2a and ribavirin. 43rd Annual Meeting of the European Association for the Study of the Liver, Milan, Italy, Apr. 23–27, **2008**.

[30] Le Pogam, S.; Kang, H.; Seshaadri, A.; Kosaks, A.; Hu, S.; Ewing, A.; Yan, J.-M.; Beard, A.; Symons, J.; Cammack, N.; Najera, I. No evidence of R7128 drug resistance after up to 4 weeks treatment of GT 1, 2, and 3 hepatitis C virus infected individuals. 44th Annual Meeting of the European Association for the Study of the Liver, Copenhagen, Denmark, Apr. 22–26, **2009**.

[31] Gane, E. J.; Rodriguez-Torres, M.; Nelson, D. R.; Jacobson, I. M.; McHutchison, J. G.; Jeffers, L.; Beared, A.; Walker, S.; Shulman, N.; Symonds, W.; et al. Antiviral activity of the HCV nucleoside polymerase inhibitor R7128 in HCV genotype 2 and 3 prior non-responders: results of 7128 1500 mg BID with PEG-IFN and ribavirin for 28 days. 59th Annual Meeting of the American Association for the Study of Liver Diseases, San Francisco, Oct. 21–Nov. 4, **2008**.

22

DISCOVERY OF CYCLOPHILIN INHIBITOR NIM811 AS A NOVEL THERAPEUTIC AGENT FOR HCV

KAI LIN

Novartis Institutes for BioMedical Research, Inc., Cambridge, Massachusetts

INTRODUCTION

Over 170 million people, or about 3% of the world population, are infected with hepatitis C virus (HCV), which results in a significant global health burden. Up to 80% of patients will develop chronic liver diseases, which may eventually progress to cirrhosis, liver failure, or hepatocellular carcinoma. Chronic HCV infection is the leading cause of liver cancer and liver transplant in the United States, Europe, and Japan. Unfortunately, the current standard of care for HCV infection, pegylated interferon α (PEG IFN-α) in combination with ribavirin, is suboptimal. Less than 50% of patients infected with genotype 1 virus, the most widely distributed HCV genotype, can be treated successfully. Moreover, many patients cannot receive or tolerate the 24 to 48 weeks of interferon-based therapy, due to contraindication or side effects. Interferon is associated with flu-like symptoms (fever and fatigue), hematologic complications (leukopenia, thrombocytopenia), and neuropsychiatric issues (depression, insomnia). Ribavirin causes hemolytic anemia and is teratogenic. Consequently, the majority of HCV patients are not being treated with the current standard of care. More effective and better tolerated therapies are greatly needed.

HCV is a 9.6-kb, positive-sense, single-stranded RNA virus. It encodes a large single open reading frame corresponding to a polyprotein precursor of about 3000 amino acids, which is proteolytically processed by cellular signal peptidases and viral proteases into 10 individual proteins, in the order C–E1–E2–p7–NS2–NS3–NS4A–NS4B–NS5A–NS5B. Drug discovery efforts have been focused mainly on two viral proteins, the NS3-4A serine protease and the NS5B RNA-dependent RNA polymerase, not only because they are essential for viral replication but also because they have well-defined enzymatic functions and are considered highly druggable targets. Significant progress has been made over the last 10 years in identifying potent and selective inhibitors of NS3 and NS5B, which are described in other chapters of this book. The most advanced NS3 and NS5B inhibitors have shown promising antiviral efficacy in HCV patients and are currently in clinical development. On the other hand, it has also become apparent that such an approach may not be sufficient, as resistance can develop quickly both in vitro and in patients, compromising the effectiveness of these viral-specific inhibitors. This is because HCV, an RNA virus, has a low-fidelity polymerase, resulting in an error-prone replication of viral genome. Combined with the fact that HCV also has a high replication rate and typically a high viral load in patients, resistant virus with specific mutations in the targeted regions of viral genes can be selected and accumulated rapidly during antiviral therapy. To address this issue, an alternative and complementary strategy is to target host factors that are also required for viral replication. It is postulated that a host factor inhibitor may have the advantage of creating a higher genetic barrier to resistance and can be used in combination with viral-specific inhibitors. NIM811, a cyclophilin inhibitor with anti-HCV activity, represents such an approach.

Cyclophilins are a family of highly conserved cellular proteins with peptidyl-prolyl *cis-trans* isomerase (PPIase) activity. There are at least 16 human cyclophilins localized in various subcellular compartments with different

Antiviral Drugs: From Basic Discovery Through Clinical Trials, First Edition. Edited by Wieslaw M. Kazmierski.

functions [1]. Cyclophilin A (CypA) was first reported by Handschumacher et al. as the cytosolic-binding protein for cyclosporin A (CsA) [2], a potent immunosuppressive drug to prevent graft rejection in patients receiving organ transplant. It was later confirmed to be the same protein as a PPIase that had previously been identified [3–5]. The immunosuppressive activity of CsA is mediated through its binding to CypA but is independent of the PPIase function of CypA, as CsA is still capable of interacting with enzymatically inactive CypA and inhibiting calcineurin [6]. The other cyclophilins have different subcellular localization and are involved in different cellular processes. For example, CypB and CypC have N-terminal signal peptide sequences that anchor them to the ER, and both can be secreted. CypD is localized in the mitochondria and regulates mitochondria transition pore. CypE is in the nucleus and regulates mRNA splicing.

Besides immunosuppressive function, CsA also has anti-inflammatory activity and has been used for the treatment of psoriasis and ulcerative colitis. While investigating the ability of CsA to suppress inflammation associated with viral hepatitis in HCV patients, Inoue et al. surprisingly found that the combination of CsA and IFN-α2b resulted in a significantly improved antiviral response than IFN-α2b alone [7]. In a controlled trial comparing patients treated with a standard dose of IFN-α2b (10 MU daily for 4 weeks followed by three times weekly for 20 weeks) alone vs. patients receiving an additional 200 mg/day of CsA in four divided doses for the first 4 weeks followed by 100 mg/day in four divided doses for 20 weeks, the sustained virological response rate was significantly ($p = 0.01$) higher in the CsA plus IFN-α2b combination group (42/76) than in the IFN-α2b monotherapy group (14/44). The difference was even more remarkable in patients with genotype 1 virus and viral load of $>$ 100,000 copies/mL, 16/38 in the combination group vs. 1/21 in the monotherapy group ($p = 0.006$). The side effects of the two groups were similar.

Although it had been reported previously that CsA has inhibitory activities against a number of viruses, such as HIV, HSV, VSV, and HBV [8–14], it was not clear whether CsA had any direct antiviral effect on HCV or simply enhanced the activity of IFN-α through an unknown mechanism. Using a newly developed HCV replicon cell culture system, Watashi et al. first demonstrated that CsA suppressed HCV replication directly in vitro [15]. Interestingly, another calcineurin inhibitor (FK-506), whose immunosuppressive activity is mediated by FKBP rather than cyclophilin, did not inhibit HCV, suggesting that the anti-HCV activity of CsA is mediated by cyclophilin but not calcineurin. In addition, the effect of CsA was not related to IFN-α-induced signal transduction pathway as the levels of 2′,5′-oligoadenylate (2′,5′-OAS) and double-stranded RNA-dependent protein kinase (PKR) were not affected. These findings were confirmed by Nakagawa et al. in an independent study using a different HCV replicon cell line [16].

Although it was very interesting to discover the anti-HCV activity of CsA, there are obvious concerns about using such a highly immunosuppressive drug to treat a chronic infection. Therefore, it is important to understand the mechanism of the antiviral effect of CsA and determine whether it can be separated from the immunosuppressive function of the compound. Fortunately, following the initial discovery of CsA, a number of different cyclosporin analogs have been identified over years of research at Sandoz (merged with Ciba-Geigy in 1996 to form Novartis). Some of these compounds have very different properties in terms of cyclophilin binding and immunosuppression and were selected to examine for their activity in inhibiting HCV replication in the in vitro replicon system. As shown in Table 1, there was a very good correlation between the HCV-inhibitory activity of these compounds and their cyclophilin-binding activity, but not with the immunosuppressive function [17].

The more direct evidence confirming the role of cyclophilins in HCV replication came from the siRNA experiment: siRNAs specifically knocking down the level of individual cyclophilins in the replicon cells led to a strong inhibition of HCV replication [15,16]. However, there has been some discrepancy on which cyclophilins are involved. Watashi et al. reported that CypB but not CypA was required

TABLE 1 The HCV-Inhibitory Activities of Various Cyclosporin Analogs Correlated with Their Cyclophilin-Binding Affinities but Not Immunosuppressive Activities

		Fold Increase of EC_{50} Over CsA		
Compound	HCV Replicon EC_{50} (μM)	Replicon Inhibition	CypA Binding	Immuno-suppression
[MeIle[4]]Cs (NIM811)	0.10	0.22	0.59	> 1700
[*O*-Acetyl-D-MeSer[3]]Cs	0.14	0.31	0.75	2.4
[MeVal[4]]Cs	0.15	0.33	0.54	> 2500
CsA	0.45	1	1	1
[D-Lys[8]]Cs	2.07	4.60	2.6	150
[MeAla[10]]Cs	8.48	18.84	26	15
[*O*-Acetyl-MeBmt[1]]Cs	>10	> 22	> 97	270

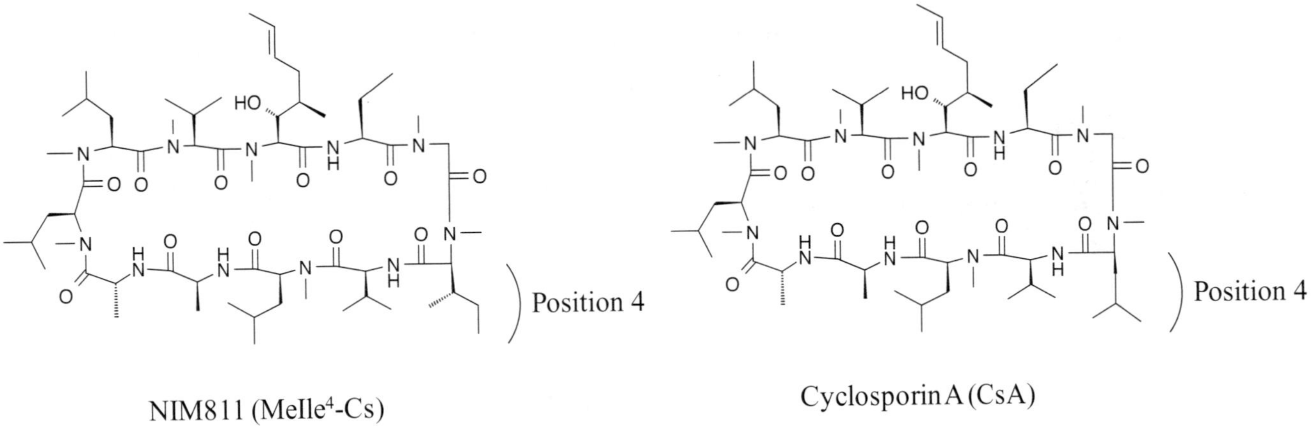

FIGURE 1

for HCV replication through its interaction with NS5B [18]. This finding was confirmed by Heck et al., who demonstrated further that CypB stimulated RNA synthesis by NS5B in vitro but that the PPIase activity of CypB was not required for this function [19]. In contrast, Yang et al. suggested that CypA was the main mediator of HCV replication [20], and furthermore, Liu et al. and Chatterji et al. reported that the PPIase activity of CypA was essential [21,22]. Drug resistance analysis revealed that mutations in both NS5A and NS5B may contribute resistance to CsA in vitro [23,24]. Moreover, Honoulle et al. observed a direct interaction between domain 2 of NS5A and both CypA and CypB and showed that NS5A domain 2 was a substrate of both CypA and CypB PPIases [25]. So it remains to be confirmed whether the anti-HCV activity of cyclophilin inhibitors is mediated primarily by CypA or CypB or both, and whether NS5A or NS5B or both are involved. Different cellular systems and assay conditions used by various groups could have contributed to the different findings in these studies. It is quite possible that multiple cyclophilins are involved in HCV replication [26,27] and that both NS5A and NS5B may interact directly or indirectly with cyclophilins, since they are both present in the HCV replication complex.

DISCOVERY

The discovery of NIM811 ([MeIle[4]]Cs) was an accident. In 1985, prompted by the finding of high immunosuppressive activity with [D-Ser[8]]Cs, Traber et al. at then Sandoz Pharma made an attempt to prepare [D-Thr[8]]Cs by adding D-threonine to the fermentation medium of *Tolypocladium niveum*, the fungus strain producing cyclosporin A (CsA). Surprisingly, although the desired compound was not synthesized, a novel cyclosporin analog was obtained as a minor product in the fermentation, which was later designated SDZ-NIM811 [28]. Subsequent structural elucidation revealed that the only difference between NIM811 and CsA was that the methylleucine group at position 4 of CsA was replaced by a methylisoleucine in NIM811 (Fig. 1). Interestingly, it turned out that such a small chemical modification in the compound causes a significant change in its biological activity.

It has been well established that CsA exerts its immunosuppressive function primarily through its interaction with CypA. The CsA–CypA complex binds to calcium and calmodulin-dependent phosphatase calcineurin (Cn) [29], which inhibits dephosphorylation and nuclear translocation of the nuclear factor of activated T-cell (NFAT) and thus blocks T-cell receptor-mediated cytokine transcription and T-cell activation [30,31]. The key interactions among CsA, CypA, and Cn are illustrated in their co-crystal structure shown in Fig. 2A and B [32,33]. While the methyl leucine group at position 4 (MeLeu[4]) of CsA does not play any role in its binding to CypA, it is critical for the interaction of CsA with the two subunits of calcineurin (CnA and CnB). Specifically, the side chain of MeLeu[4] of CsA fits into a hydrophobic pocket defined by the aromatic rings of Trp[352] and Phe[356] of CnA and the backbones and Cβ atoms of Ser[353] of CnA and Met[118] and Val[119] of CnB. The change of MeLeu[4] to MeIle[4] in NIM811 does not affect its binding to cyclophilin, as illustrated in the co-crystal structure of NIM811-CypA shown in Figure 1C and D [34]. In fact, NIM811 exhibits two- to fivefold higher binding affinity to various cyclophilins than to CsA, as shown in Table 2 [35]. However, the change of MeLeu[4] at the recognition site of calcineurin to MeIle[4] essentially blocks the binding of the compound to calcineurin and abolishes its ability to induce calcineurin-mediated immunosuppression [9,35]. In a two-way murine mixed-lymphocyte reaction assay, NIM811 was inactive at 1.2 μg/mL, while the IC_{50} of CsA was 0.008 μg/mL. In addition, NIM811 failed to inhibit the activation of IL-2 promoter in a reporter-based assay at up to 10 μg/mL, whereas the IC_{50} of CsA was 0.003 μg/mL. The lack of immunosuppressive activity with NIM811 has also been demonstrated in several animal models [36].

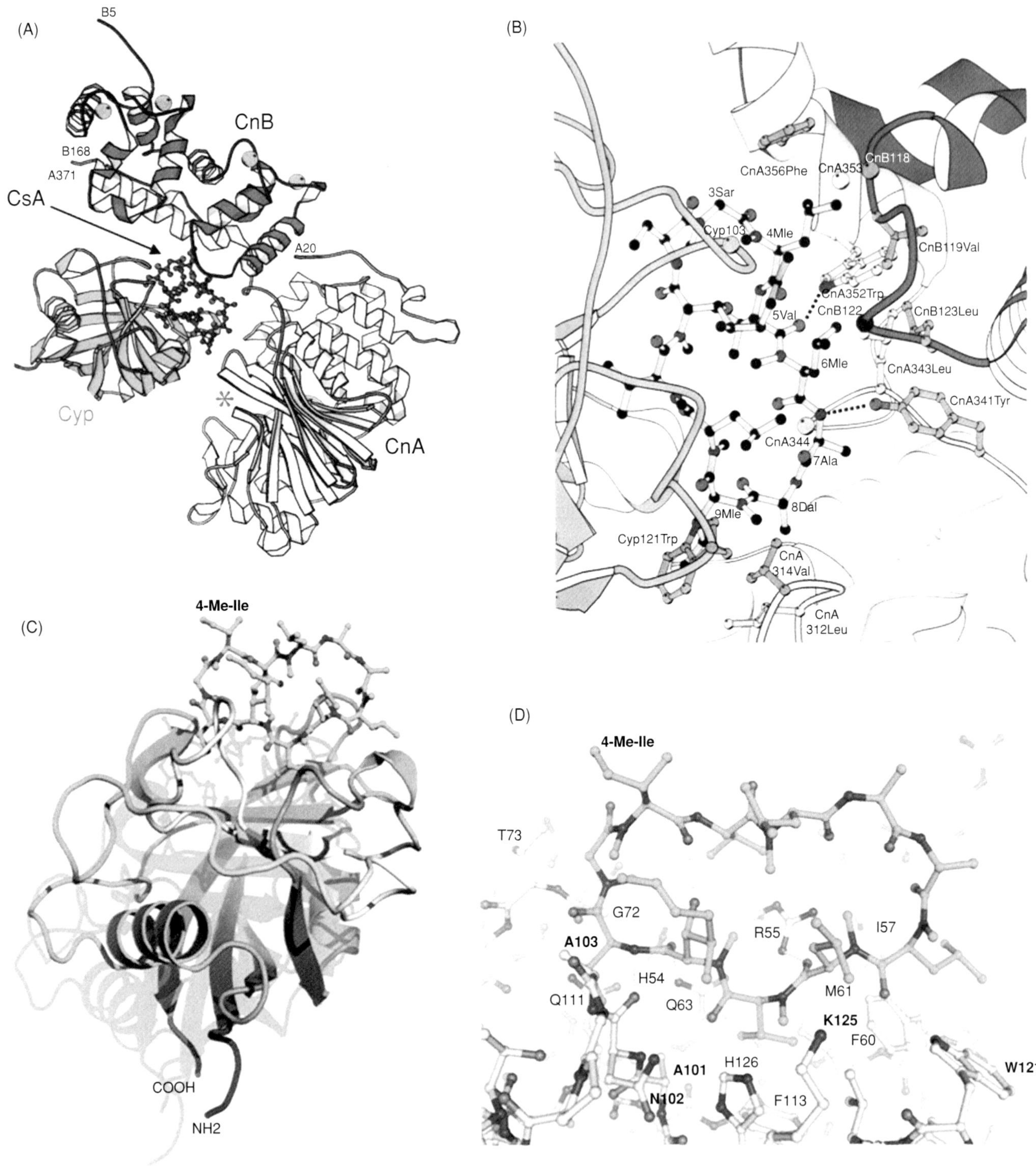

FIGURE 2 Co-crystal structures of CypA/CsA/Cn and CypA/NIM811. (A) A ribbon diagram of the CypA/CsA/Cn ternary complex. The two subunits of Cn are shown in yellow (CnA) and red (CnB). CypA is in green. (B) Details of the interaction between CsA and Cn. (C) Ribbon diagram of the CypA/NIM811 complex. (D) Details of the interaction between NIM811 and CypA. [(A,B) from Jin [33], with permission; (C,D) from Kallen [34].] (*See insert for color representation of the figure.*)

TABLE 2 Binding Affinity (nM) of NIM811 and CsA to Various Cyclophilins as Determined by Surface Plasmon Resonance

Compound	CypA	CypB	CypC
NIM811	6.14	2.23	10.8
CsA	24.7	7.96	52.6

Source: [35].

NIM811 was initially considered as a potential candidate for HIV-1 therapy. It potently inhibited a number of laboratory strains and clinical isolates of HIV-1 in primary T4 lymphocytes and monocytes with IC_{50}s of 0.011 to 0.057 μg/mL [36]. The mechanism of NIM811 against HIV-1 has also been well characterized. The $p24^{gag}$ protein of HIV-1 binds specifically to CypA, which not only is required for viral replication and but also gets incorporated into the virions [37–39]. NIM811 blocks the interaction of HIV-1 Gag and CypA and interferes with viral replication through both inhibiting the translocation of pre-integration complexes into the nucleus and reducing infectious viral particles [9,40]. NIM811 is orally bioavailable and has a pharmacokinetic profile similar to that of CsA in mouse, rat, dog, and monkey [36]. Moreover, the compound appears to differentiae from CsA in terms of nephrotoxicity potential, possibly due to the lack of calcineurin inhibition.

Following the discovery of anti-HCV activity of CsA, NIM811 was immediately considered as an attractive drug development candidate because of its lack of calcineurin-mediated immunosuppressive activity and a favorable pharmacokinetics profile. The anti-HCV activity of the compound was first confirmed and characterized in vitro. NIM811 showed a concentration-dependent inhibition of HCV replication with EC_{50} values of 0.1 to 0.6 μM in various replicon clones following a 48-h treatment [17]. At 1 μM, NIM811 was able to reduce HCV RNA by > 3 $\log_{10}$ after treating the replicon cells for 9 days. It was equipotent against both genotype 1a and 1b HCV. The compound was also highly active against the genotype 2a JFH-1 infectious virus with an EC_{50} of 0.05 μM after 72 h. Consistent with its moderate protein-binding activity (87.8 to 89.3%), there was about a fivefold increase of replicon EC_{50} with NIM811 in the presence of 40% human serum. NIM811 also showed in vivo efficacy in the HCV replicon mouse model [41] when given orally at 100 mg/kg per day for 7 days (unpublished data).

Like other potential novel therapeutic agents being developed for HCV, NIM811 is expected first to be combined with the current standard of care in HCV patients. Therefore, the combination of NIM811 and IFN-α was evaluated in vitro using the HCV replicon system. In the standard 48-h HCV replicon assay, the combination was much more effective in inhibiting HCV replication than either agent alone, without any significant increase of cytotoxicity [17]. The effect of combination was determined to be additive as analyzed in a mathematic model based on the Bliss Independence model, MacSynergy [42]. In another experiment where HCV replicon cells were treated for 9 days, as shown in Figure 3, 5 IU/mL IFN-α or 0.5 μM NIM811 each resulted in a 1.2 $\log_{10}$ reduction of HCV RNA; in contrast, the combination of the two led to a 2.7 $\log_{10}$ viral RNA reduction, which was much more effective than either agent alone. Moreover, while 20 IU/mL IFN-α alone resulted in a 1.5 $\log_{10}$ reduction of HCV RNA after 9 days, the addition of 0.5 μM NIM811 resulted in a 3.7 $\log_{10}$ viral RNA reduction, which was greater than what can be achieved with a much higher concentration (100 IU/mL) of IFN-α alone (2.7 $\log_{10}$). These results exemplify the significant advantage of combination therapy in enhancing the antiviral efficacy and provide the rationale to further explore the combination of NIM811 with IFN-α in order to improve treatment response over the current standard of care.

An often-hypothesized advantage of targeting host factors is that such an inhibitor may be less prone to resistance,

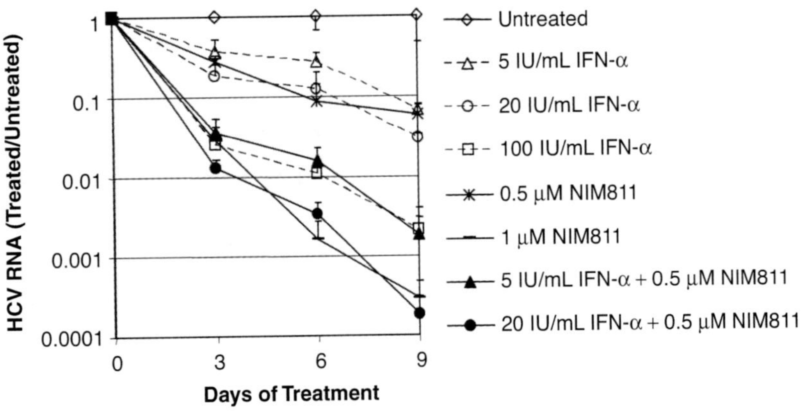

FIGURE 3 Combination of NIM811 with IFN-α-facilitated multilog HCV RNA reduction in vitro. HCV replicon cells were treated with various concentrations of NIM811 alone, IFN-α alone, or the two in combination for 3, 6, or 9 days. The level of remaining HCV RNA in compound-treated cells was compared to that of untreated cells at the same time point. (From [17], with permission.)

which is highly relevant for an RNA virus such as HCV. The RNA-dependent RNA polymerase of HCV that is responsible for the synthesis of both (+) and (−) strands of viral RNA lacks the proofreading function and has an error rate of about 10^{-4} or one mutation per genome per replication cycle. In addition, the virus replicates robustly ($10^{10\text{-}12}$ virions per day) and typically maintains a very high viral load ($>10^6$ mL^{-1} or 3×10^9 $3L^{-1}$ plasma) in patients. As a result, there is a huge population of viral quasispecies in every infected patient. In other words, mutations at every position of the 9.6-kb viral genome, except for those that are replication incompetent, are probably preexisting even before the start of antiviral therapy. While on treatment with a specific inhibitor of HCV, mutant viruses that are resistant to the compound would then have a selective growth advantage over wild-type virus and can accumulate rapidly and render the treatment ineffective. Indeed, it has been shown both in vitro and in patients that resistance can develop quickly against HCV protease or polymerase inhibitors, particularly when used as monotherapy. Since these inhibitors all bind to defined pockets on viral enzymes, specific mutations at the binding sites may arise during therapy, which can disrupt the binding of the inhibitors and lead to resistance. Unfortunately, for all the protease and polymerase inhibitors reported to date, resistance can be converted by a single mutation in the viral target genes.

In contrast, it is postulated that inhibitors targeting host factors could present a higher genetic barrier to resistance since they do not bind directly to the viral targets. To confirm this hypothesis, the likelihood or frequency of developing resistance with NIM811 and viral-specific inhibitors was compared in vitro using the replicon cells. HCV replicon cells were seeded at a low density on tissue culture plates and treated with various concentrations of inhibitors for about 3 weeks when resistant replicon started to appear as individual colonies. The number of colonies reflects the frequency of resistance. As shown in Figure 4, for all the HCV inhibitors tested, there was an inverse correlation

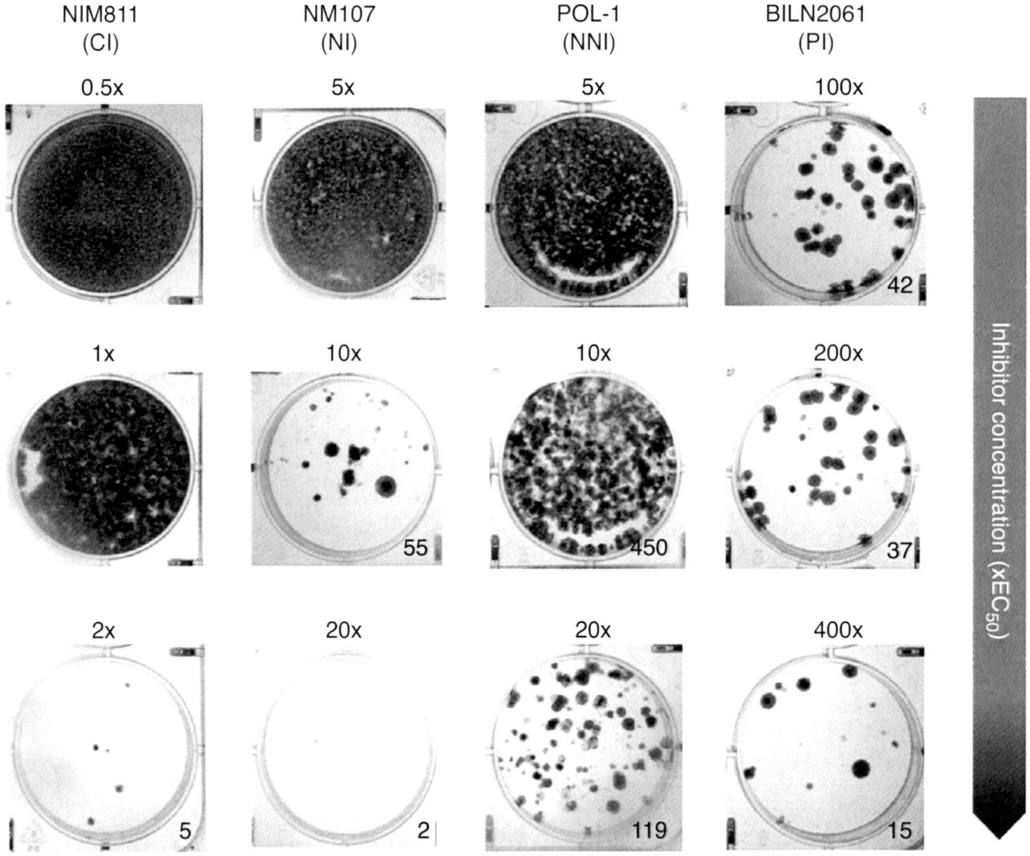

FIGURE 4 Comparison of resistance frequency of NIM811 vs. HCV protease and polymerase inhibitors. NIM811 is a cyclophilin inhibitor (CI); NM107 is a nucleoside inhibitor of NS5B polymerase (NI) [43]; POL-1 is a non-nucleoside inhibitor of NS5B polymerase (NNI) [44,48]; and BILN-2061 is a NS3 protease inhibitor (PI) [45]. HCV replicon cells were treated with various concentrations of these compounds (expressed as multiples of their respective EC_{50}s and labeled on top of each well) in the presence of G418. Resistance colonies appeared after 3 weeks of treatment. The numbers of colonies are labeled at the bottom right corner of each well unless there are too many to count.

between the concentration of the compound and the number of colonies, (i.e., the higher the concentration of the inhibitor, the lower the frequency of resistance). However, compared to the potency in inhibiting HCV replication (i.e., EC_{50}), there appeared to be a greater difference in the ability to block resistance for inhibitors of different mechanisms. For example, the resistance frequency against a nucleoside NS5B inhibitor NM107 [43] was lower than those of a non-nucleoside NS5B inhibitor (POL-1 [44]) at the same multiple (20×) of EC_{50} and a NS3 protease inhibitor (BILN2061 [45]) at a higher multiple (400×) of EC_{50}. This is likely because the resistant mutation associated with NM107 occurs at the active site of the polymerase (S282T) and causes significant fitness loss of the virus. Most notably, NIM811 was even more effective in blocking the emergence of resistance at a lower multiple (2×) of its EC_{50} than the nucleoside inhibitor (20×), which supports the notion that inhibitors targeting host factors may be less prone to resistance than inhibitors targeting viral genes. In addition, the mutations associated with NIM811 resistance also appeared to cause significant loss of fitness, as subsequent efforts to grow and expand these colonies had turned out to be slow and unsuccessful.

In a separate effort to generate a NIM811-resistant clone that can be maintained, it took more than 50 cell passages and six months to culture the replicon cells with gradually increasing concentrations of cyclosporin and NIM811 to 10 μM (~ 20 × EC_{50}) of NIM811. In contrast, resistant clones against viral protease or polymerase inhibitors usually can be selected within six cell passages and 3 weeks. The difficulty in developing resistance against NIM811 may be in part due to the fact that multiple cyclophilins are involved in the viral life cycle, which can all be inhibited by NIM811. The mechanism of resistance against NIM811 was shown to be mediated by viral rather than cellular changes, as transfection of viral RNA extracted from resistant clones conferred resistance on naive cells, while transfection of wild-type viral RNA to "cured" resistance cells did not [46]. Interestingly, mutations in several viral genes, including NS5A, NS5B, and NS3, have been reported to be associated with resistance against NIM811, CsA, or other cyclophilin inhibitors [20,23,24,46,47]. However, when introducing these mutations individually back to the wild-type replicon, the single mutation can only induce a low level (tow- to five-fold) of resistance. It appears that multiple mutations need to be acquired to reduce the susceptibility of cyclophilin inhibitors significantly, by > 10-fold, which explains the difficulty in selecting a resistant clone. In contrast, for all the viral protease or polymerase inhibitors reported to date, a single mutation is sufficient to confer a high level (typically, hundreds of folds) of resistance. In other words, NIM811, which targets a host factor, presents a much higher genetic barrier than those of viral specific inhibitors.

Although resistant mutations have been identified in several viral genes for cyclophilin inhibitors, the positions of these mutations (such as D320E in NS5A [46] and I432V in NS5B [23]) are different from those associated with viral specific inhibitors, suggesting that the mechanisms of resistance are different. This was confirmed by the cross-resistance analysis using a panel of HCV inhibitors and the resistant replicon clones selected with these inhibitors [48]. It was demonstrated that the NIM811-resistant HCV replicon cell line was fully susceptible to NS3 protease and NS5B polymerase inhibitors, while HCV replicon cell lines that were resistant to protease and polymerase inhibitors remained fully sensitive to NIM811. The lack of cross-resistance suggests that (1) NIM811 can be used to treat patients who have developed resistance against viral protease or polymerase inhibitors; (2) NIM811 can be used in combination with viral protease or polymerase inhibitors in treatment-naive patients to help prevent the emergence of resistance.

To confirm the second hypothesis, the abilities of the compounds alone or in combination to suppress resistance were compared in vitro by measuring the frequency of viral resistant colonies. One such example is shown in Figure 5, where NIM811 was combined with LDI133, an indole-based non-nucleoside inhibitor targeting allosteric binding site 1 of NS5B [49]. Two relatively low concentrations (0.1 and 0.2 μM) of NIM811 were used in the study to demonstrate the effect of combination. Even though NIM811 on its own can barely suppress HCV replication at these suboptimal concentrations, it was very effective in preventing the emergence of resistance with LDI133. For example, while 0.5 μM of LDI133 resulted in almost a full plate of resistant replicon cells, the addition of 0.2 μM of NIM811 completely blocked the emergence of resistance. The same effect can be achieved with the combination of only 0.1 μM of NIM811 and 1 μM of LDI133, which by itself resulted in 134 resistant colonies. Similar results were obtained with the combinations of NIM811 with NS3 protease inhibitors or nucleoside NS5B polymerase inhibitors. These findings strongly support the strategy of combining inhibitors of host and viral targets not only to maximize antiviral activity but also to suppress the emergence of resistance.

SYNTHESIS

Cyclosporin A (CsA) is the main component of ≥ 25 natural cyclosporins produced by the fungus *Tolypocladium niveum* [50]. It is one of the most widely used immunosuppressive drugs (Neoral or Sandimmun) and can be manufactured efficiently on a large scale through fermentation. The enzyme responsible for the biosynthesis of cyclosporin was later determined to be a single polypeptide with a molecular mass of about 1.4 MDa [51], cyclosporin synthetase [52], whose discovery enabled the synthesis of dozens of new cyclosporin analogs in vitro. NIM811 ([MeIle^4]Cs) was initially identified as a minor product when D-threonine was

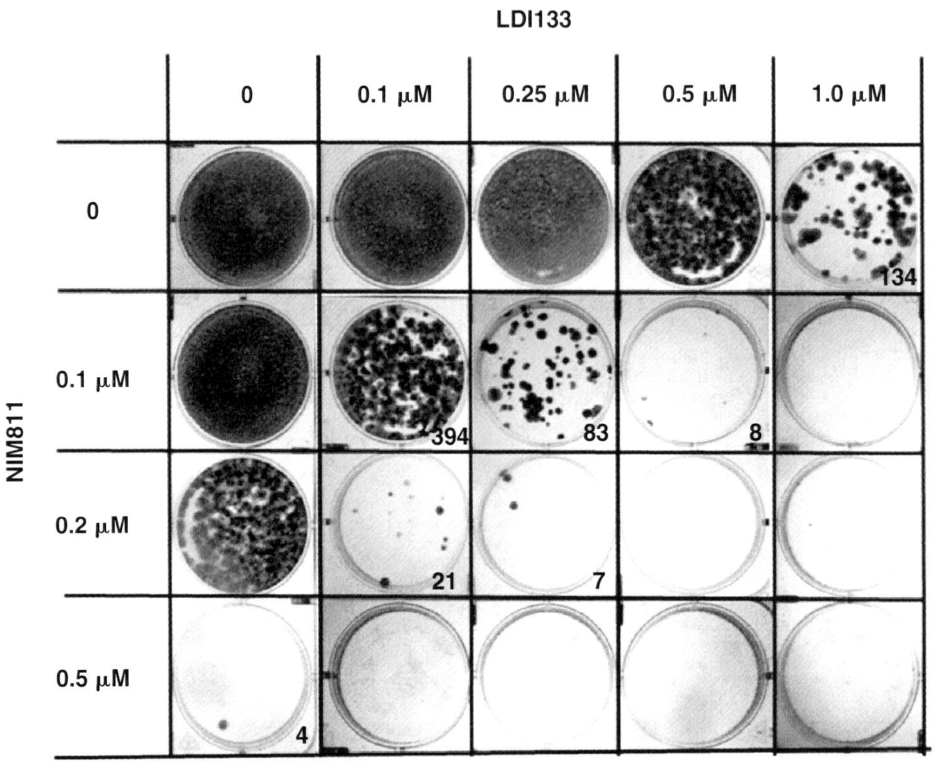

FIGURE 5 Combination of NIM811 with an HCV NS5B polymerase inhibitor suppressed the emergence of resistance. HCV replicon cells were treated with various concentrations of NIM811 and LDI133 [49], a non-nucleoside NS5B polymerase inhibitor, either alone or in combination. Resistance colonies were formed after 3 weeks of treatment. The numbers of colonies are labeled at the bottom right corner of each well unless there are too many to count (or there is no colony).

added to the fermentation medium of *T. niveum* [28]. A gram quantity of the compound at 98% purity was obtained through repeated column chromatography, which enabled its structural elucidation. The only difference between NIM811 and CsA is that the MeLeu at position 4 of CsA is replaced by MeIle in NIM811. Because MeLeu is the building block at four positions (4, 6, 9, and 10) of CsA, it is not possible to direct the exchange of one of these four MeLeu specifically. Surprisingly, when Ile was added to the in vitro biosynthesis mixture of cyclosporin, [MeIle^4]Cs was formed as the major product, indicating that cyclosporin synthetase has a higher affinity for Ile at position 4. However, neither the fermentation conditions nor the in vitro biosynthesis method appeared to be feasible for large-scale synthesis of the compound for drug development. A significant breakthrough was achieved through genetic manipulation of the cyclosporin-producing strain [53], which subsequently enabled efficient production of NIM811 through large-scale fermentation at high titers.

PHASE I SAFETY AND EFFICACY

NIM811 is orally bioavailable with a pharmacokinetics profile similar to that of CsA in mouse, rat, dog, and monkey [36]. A number of preclinical animal toxicology studies had also been conducted, which supported advancing the compound in human studies. The pharmacokinetics, safety, and tolerability of NIM811 were first evaluated in a single ascending-dose study in healthy volunteers [54]. The compound was administered orally to 40 healthy volunteers divided into five sequential dose groups (50, 150, 400, 800, and 1600 mg), with six active and two placebo subjects in each group. NIM811 was well tolerated at all doses. There was no serious adverse event or drug-related adverse event in either lab results or clinical evaluation. NIM811 was absorbed rapidly, with peak concentrations (C_{max}) occurring in blood at 1.5 h at all doses and a terminal elimination half-life ($t_{1/2}$) of about 12 to 20 h. Drug exposure (C_{max} or AUC) increased with dose but was slightly underproportional. Intersubject variability was low (< 30%).

The compound was then investigated in a double-blind placebo-controlled study in HCV-infected patients. Multiple ascending doses (25 and 75 mg q.d.; 100, 200, 400, and 600 mg b.i.d.) of NIM811 were given orally as monotherapy to treatment-naive or treatment-experienced HCV genotype 1–infected patients for 14 days. There was no significant change in C_{max} and only slightly higher AUC at day 13 than at day 1. The pharmacokinetics of NIM811 were comparable between HCV-infected patients and healthy subjects. All doses were well tolerated, and there was no serious adverse event. The most common adverse event was mild to moderate headache, 16% in drug-treated groups vs. 5.3% in placebo. Mild, clinically nonsignificant elevations of bilirubin and declines in platelet counts were observed in the 400- and 600-mg b.i.d. groups. Although significant antiviral efficacy was not achieved with NIM811 monotherapy at up to 600 mg b.i.d., interestingly, a significant reduction of ALT was observed with NIM811 at $\geq$ 100 mg b.i.d., suggesting a potential benefit of biochemical response with the compound even in the absence of virological response.

Considering the effect of the combination observed in vitro [17] as well as clinical experience with the combination of CsA and IFN-α [7], rather than increasing the dose of NIM811 further as a monotherapy, the compound was investigated in combination with interferon α in HCV genotype 1-infected patients who had relapsed in prior interferon therapy. Twenty patients were randomized to receive 600 mg NIM811 b.i.d. orally or matching placebo for 14 days and 180 μg PEG-IFNα-2a on study days 1 and 7. The mean reduction in HCV viral load was 2.78 $\log_{10}$ in the NIM811 + PEG-IFNα-2a group, compared to only 0.58 $\log_{10}$ reduction in the PEG-IFNα-2a alone group ($p < 0.0001$). Also, the mean ALT decreased from 78.4 IU/L at baseline to 26.3 IU/L by day 14 in the combination group, whereas it was unchanged at 66.0 IU/L in the PEG- IFNα-2a alone group. The main safety finding was a decrease in mean platelet count from 209,000 counts/mL on day 0 to 104,000 counts/mL on day 14 in the combination group, vs. 176 to 139,000 counts/mL in the PEG- IFNα-2a only group. There was also a statistically but not clinically significant increase in serum bilirubin. There was no serious adverse event in either group. In summary, proof-of-concept efficacy has been established for NIM811, which warrants further development of the compound as a novel therapeutic agent for HCV.

FUTURE DIRECTIONS

In the past few years cyclophilin inhibitors have emerged as an important new class of HCV drug candidates. Besides NIM811, two other cyclophilin inhibitors, DEBIO-025 and SCY-635, have also demonstrated proof-of-concept efficacy in hepatitis C patients [55–57]. The initial development of these compounds will probably continue focusing on the combination with the current standard of care (i.e., pegylated interferon α and ribavirin). Although the long-term benefit and safety of cyclophilin inhibitors remain to be investigated in further clinical trials, preliminary data with the combination of NIM811 and interferon α suggests that it may provide a significant improvement over current therapy.

Similarly, inhibitors of viral targets (NS3, NS5B, and NS5A) are also being investigated in combination with interferon and ribavirin, mainly because resistance can emerge quickly with these inhibitors as monotherapy, and interferon is thought to be necessary to help suppress the selection of resistant virus. Although such a strategy has resulted in improved antiviral response over the current standard of care, it does not address the tolerability issues associated with interferon and ribavirin. The combination of inhibitors of two viral targets, such as NS3 and NS5B, has been reported recently [58] and probably will be pursued eagerly. However, considering that only one mutation is needed to confer resistance against each drug of viral targets, it remains to be determined whether such an approach could create a high-enough barrier to resistance and will be sufficient to replace interferon. In this regard, a host factor inhibitor such as NIM811 could provide the much needed ammunition, as it appears to have a higher genetic barrier to resistance than do viral targeted inhibitors, and the combination of the two could constitute the most effective regimen in the absence of interferon.

A potential challenge for host factor inhibitors is to identify a therapeutically effective dose that does not interfere with the normal function of the host target, which may lead to unwanted side effects. Although NIM811 may not be as potent as some of the viral targeted inhibitors with nanomolar EC_{50} in inhibiting HCV replication, it appears to be more "potent" in blocking the emergence of resistance. In vitro data suggest that even a suboptimal dose of NIM811 can be very effective in helping suppress the emergence of resistance when combined with inhibitors of viral targets, which represents a potential development path of the compound but requires innovative study design and regulatory approval. In conclusion, the two-pronged approach of targeting both viral and host factors may provide the best opportunity not only to maximize antiviral efficacy but also to suppress the emergence of resistance.

REFERENCES

[1] Wang, P.; Heitman, J. The cyclophilins. *Genome Biol.* **2005**, *6*(7), 226.

[2] Handschumacher, R. E.; Harding, M. W.; Rice, J.; Drugge, R. J.; Speicher, D. W. Cyclophilin: a specific cytosolic binding protein for cyclosporin A. *Science* **1984**, *226*(4674), 544–547.

[3] Fischer, G.; Bang, H.; Mech, C. Determination of enzymatic catalysis for the *cis-trans*-isomerization of peptide binding in proline-containing peptides.] *Biomed. Biochim. Acta* **1984**, *43*(10), 1101–1111.

[4] Fischer, G.; Wittmann-Liebold, B.; Lang, K.; Kiefhaber, T.; Schmid, F. X. Cyclophilin and peptidyl-prolyl *cis-trans* isomerase are probably identical proteins. *Nature* **1989**, *337*(6206), 476–478.

[5] Takahashi, N.; Hayano, T.; Suzuki, M. Peptidyl-prolyl *cis-trans* isomerase is the cyclosporin A–binding protein cyclophilin. *Nature* **1989**, *337*(6206), 473–475.

[6] Zydowsky, L. D.; Etzkorn, F. A.; Chang, H. Y.; Ferguson, S. B.; Stolz, L. A.; Ho, S. I.; Walsh, C. T. Active site mutants of human cyclophilin A separate peptidyl-prolyl isomerase activity from cyclosporin A binding and calcineurin inhibition. *Protein Sci.* **1992**, *1*(9), 1092–1099.

[7] Inoue, K.; Sekiyama, K.; Yamada, M.; Watanabe, T.; Yasuda, H.; Yoshiba, M. Combined interferon alpha2b and cyclosporin A in the treatment of chronic hepatitis C: controlled trial. *J. Gastroenterol.* **2003**, *38*(6), 567–572.

[8] Rosenwirth, B.; Billich, A.; Datema, R.; Donatsch, P.; Hammerschmid, F.; Harrison, R.; Hiestand, P.; Jaksche, H.; Mayer, P.; Peichl, P. Inhibition of human immunodeficiency virus type 1 replication by SDZ NIM 811, a nonimmunosuppressive cyclosporine analog. *Antimicrob. Agents Chemother.* **1994**, *38*(8), 1763–1772.

[9] Billich, A.; Hammerschmid, F.; Peichl, P.; Wenger, R.; Zenke, G.; Quesniaux, V.; Rosenwirth, B. Mode of action of SDZ NIM 811, a nonimmunosuppressive cyclosporin A analog with activity against human immunodeficiency virus (HIV) type 1: interference with HIV protein–cyclophilin A interactions. *J. Virol.* **1995**, *69*(4), 2451–2461.

[10] Damaso, C. R.; Keller, S. J. Cyclosporin A inhibits vaccinia virus replication in vitro. *Arch. Virol.* **1994**, *134*(3–4), 303–319.

[11] Karpas, A.; Lowdell, M.; Jacobson, S. K.; Hill, F. Inhibition of human immunodeficiency virus and growth of infected T cells by the immunosuppressive drugs cyclosporin A and FK 506. *Proc. Natl. Acad. Sci. USA* **1992**, *89*(17), 8351–8355.

[12] Vahlne, A.; Larsson, P. A.; Horal, P.; Ahlmen, J.; Svennerholm, B.; Gronowitz, J. S.; Olofsson, S. Inhibition of herpes simplex virus production in vitro by cyclosporin A. *Arch. Virol.* **1992**, *122*(1–2), 61–75.

[13] Bose, S.; Mathur, M.; Bates, P.; Joshi, N.; Banerjee, A. K. Requirement for cyclophilin A for the replication of vesicular stomatitis virus New Jersey serotype. *J. Gen. Virol.* **2003**, *84*(Pt. 7), 1687–1699.

[14] Bouchard, M. J.; Puro, R. J.; Wang, L.; Schneider, R. J. Activation and inhibition of cellular calcium and tyrosine kinase signaling pathways identify targets of the HBx protein involved in hepatitis B virus replication. *J. Virol.* **2003**, *77*(14), 7713–7719.

[15] Watashi, K.; Hijikata, M.; Hosaka, M.; Yamaji, M.; Shimotohno, K. Cyclosporin A suppresses replication of hepatitis C virus genome in cultured hepatocytes. *Hepatology* **2003**, *38*(5), 1282–1288.

[16] Nakagawa, M.; Sakamoto, N.; Enomoto, N.; Tanabe, Y.; Kanazawa, N.; Koyama, T.; Kurosaki, M.; Maekawa, S.; Yamashiro, T.; Chen, C. H.; et al. Specific inhibition of hepatitis C virus replication by cyclosporin A. *Biochem. Biophys. Res. Commun.* **2004**, *313*(1), 42–47.

[17] Ma, S.; Boerner, J. E.; TiongYip, C.; Weidmann, B.; Ryder, N. S.; Cooreman, M. P.; Lin, K. NIM811, a cyclophilin inhibitor, exhibits potent in vitro activity against hepatitis C virus alone or in combination with alpha interferon. *Antimicrob. Agents Chemother.* **2006**, *50*(9), 2976–2982.

[18] Watashi, K.; Ishii, N.; Hijikata, M.; Inoue, D.; Murata, T.; Miyanari, Y.; Shimotohno, K. Cyclophilin B is a functional regulator of hepatitis C virus RNA polymerase. *Mol. Cell* **2005**, *19*(1), 111–122.

[19] Heck, J. A.; Meng, X.; Frick, D. N. Cyclophilin B stimulates RNA synthesis by the HCV RNA dependent RNA polymerase. *Biochem. Pharmacol.* **2009**, *77*(7), 1173–1180.

[20] Yang, F.; Robotham, J. M.; Nelson, H. B.; Irsigler, A.; Kenworthy, R.; Tang, H. Cyclophilin A is an essential cofactor for hepatitis C virus infection and the principal mediator of cyclosporine resistance in vitro. *J. Virol.* **2008**, *82*(11), 5269–5278.

[21] Chatterji, U.; Bobardt, M.; Selvarajah, S.; Yang, F.; Tang, H.; Sakamoto, N.; Vuagniaux, G.; Parkinson, T.; Gallay, P. The isomerase active site of cyclophilin a is critical for HCV replication. *J. Biol. Chem.* **2009**, *284*(25), 16998–17005.

[22] Liu, Z.; Yang, F.; Robotham, J. M.; Tang, H. A Critical role of cyclophilin A and its prolyl-peptidyl isomerase activity in the structure and function of the HCV replication complex. *J. Virol.* **2009**, *83*(13), 6554–6555.

[23] Robida, J. M.; Nelson, H. B.; Liu, Z.; Tang, H. Characterization of hepatitis C virus subgenomic replicon resistance to cyclosporine in vitro. *J. Virol.* **2007**, *81*(11), 5829–5840.

[24] Fernandes, F.; Poole, D. S.; Hoover, S.; Middleton, R.; Andrei, A. C.; Gerstner, J.; Striker, R. Sensitivity of hepatitis C virus to cyclosporine A depends on nonstructural proteins NS5A and NS5B. *Hepatology* **2007**, *46*(4), 1026–1033.

[25] Hanoulle, X.; Badillo, A.; Wieruszeski, J. M.; Verdegem, D.; Landrieu, I.; Bartenschlager, R.; Penin, F.; Lippens, G. Hepatitis C virus NS5A protein is a substrate for the peptidyl-prolyl *cis/trans* isomerase activity of cyclophilins A and B. *J. Biol. Chem.* **2009**, *284*(20), 13589–13601.

[26] Nakagawa, M.; Sakamoto, N.; Tanabe, Y.; Koyama, T.; Itsui, Y.; Takeda, Y.; Chen, C. H.; Kakinuma, S.; Oooka, S.; Maekawa, S.; et al. Suppression of hepatitis C virus replication by cyclosporin A is mediated by blockade of cyclophilins. *Gastroenterology* **2005**, *129*(3), 1031–1041.

[27] Wiedmann, B.; Puyang, X.; Brown, A.; Gaither, A.; Baryza, J.; Boerner, J. E.; Poulin, D.; Ma, S.; Shen, X.; Tao, J.; et al. Roles of cyclophilins in HCV replication and mode of action of the cyclophilin inhibitor NIM811. 14th International Symposium on Hepatitis C Virus and Related Viruses, 2007.

[28] Traber, R.; Kobel, H.; Loosli, H. R.; Senn, H.; Rosenwirth, B.; Lawen, A. [Melle([4])]cyclosporin, a novel natural cyclosporine with anti-HIV activity: structural elucidation, biosynthesis. *Antiviral Chem. Chemother.* **1994**, *5*(5), 331–339.

[29] Liu, J.; Farmer, J. D., Jr.; Lane, W. S.; Friedman, J.; Weissman, I.; Schreiber, S. L. Calcineurin is a common target of cyclophilin–cyclosporin A and FKBP-FK506 complexes. *Cell* **1991**, *66*(4), 807–815.

[30] Jain, J.; McCaffrey, P. G.; Miner, Z.; Kerppola, T. K.; Lambert, J. N.; Verdine, G. L.; Curran, T.; Rao, A. The T-cell transcription factor NFATp is a substrate for calcineurin and interacts with Fos and Jun. *Nature* **1993**, *365*(6444), 352–355.

[31] McCaffrey, P. G.; Luo, C.; Kerppola, T. K.; Jain, J.; Badalian, T. M.; Ho, A. M.; Burgeon, E.; Lane, W. S.; Lambert, J. N.; Curran, T. Isolation of the cyclosporin-sensitive T cell transcription factor NFATp. *Science* **1993**, *262*(5134), 750–754.

[32] Huai, Q.; Kim, H. Y.; Liu, Y.; Zhao, Y.; Mondragon, A.; Liu, J. O.; Ke, H. Crystal structure of calcineurin–cyclophilin–cyclosporin shows common but distinct recognition of immunophilin–drug complexes. *Proc. Natl. Acad. Sci. USA* **2002**, *99*(19), 12037–12042.

[33] Jin, L.; Harrison, S. C. Crystal structure of human calcineurin complexed with cyclosporin A and human cyclophilin. *Proc. Natl. Acad. Sci. USA* **2002**, *99*(21), 13522–13526.

[34] Kallen, J.; Mikol, V.; Taylor, P.; Walkinshaw, M. D. X-ray structures and analysis of 11 cyclosporin derivatives complexed with cyclophilin A. *J. Mol. Biol.* **1998**, *283*(2), 435–449.

[35] Lee, L. V.; Vickers, C. S.; Wiedmann, B.; Fujimoto, R.; Whitehead, L.; Lin, K.; Ryder, N. S.; Compton, T.; Evans, T. G.; Deng, G. Investigation of mechanism of action of NIM811 by surface plasma resonance, fluorescence polarization, and calcineurin assays. 48th Interscience Conference on Antimicrobial Agents and Chemotherapy, 2008.

[36] Rosenwirth, B.; Billich, A.; Datema, R.; Donatsch, P.; Hammerschmid, F.; Harrison, R.; Hiestand, P.; Jaksche, H.; Mayer, P.; Peichl, P. Inhibition of human immunodeficiency virus type 1 replication by SDZ NIM 811, a nonimmunosuppressive cyclosporine analog. *Antimicrob. Agents Chemother.* **1994**, *38*(8), 1763–1772.

[37] Franke, E. K.; Yuan, H. E.; Luban, J. Specific incorporation of cyclophilin A into HIV-1 virions. *Nature* **1994**, *372*(6504), 359–362.

[38] Luban, J.; Bossolt, K. L.; Franke, E. K.; Kalpana, G. V.; Goff, S. P. Human immunodeficiency virus type 1 Gag protein binds to cyclophilins A and B. *Cell* **1993**, *73*(6), 1067–1078.

[39] Thali, M.; Bukovsky, A.; Kondo, E.; Rosenwirth, B.; Walsh, C. T.; Sodroski, J.; Gottlinger, H. G. Functional association of cyclophilin A with HIV-1 virions. *Nature* **1994**, *372*(6504), 363–365.

[40] Mlynar, E.; Bevec, D.; Billich, A.; Rosenwirth, B.; Steinkasserer, A. The non-immunosuppressive cyclosporin A analogue SDZ NIM 811 inhibits cyclophilin A incorporation into virions and virus replication in human immunodeficiency virus type 1-infected primary and growth-arrested T cells. *J. Gen. Virol.* **1997**, *78*(Pt. 4), 825–835.

[41] Zhu, Q.; Oei, Y.; Mendel, D. B.; Garrett, E. N.; Patawaran, M. B.; Hollenbach, P. W.; Aukerman, S. L.; Weiner, A. J. Novel robust hepatitis C virus mouse efficacy model. *Antimicrob. Agents Chemother.* **2006**, *50*(10), 3260–3268.

[42] Prichard, M. N.; Shipman, C., Jr. A three-dimensional model to analyze drug–drug interactions. *Antiviral Res.* **1990**, *14*(4–5), 181–205.

[43] Pierra, C.; Amador, A.; Benzaria, S.; Cretton-Scott, E.; D'Amours, M.; Mao, J.; Mathieu, S.; Moussa, A.; Bridges, E. G.; Standring, D. N.; et al. Synthesis and pharmacokinetics of valopicitabine (NM283), an efficient prodrug of the potent anti-HCV agent 2′-C-methylcytidine. *J. Med. Chem.* **2006**, *49*(22), 6614–6620.

[44] Chan, L.; Pereira, O.; Reddy, T. J.; Das, S. K.; Poisson, C.; Courchesne, M.; Proulx, M.; Siddiqui, A.; Yannopoulos, C. G.; Nguyen-Ba, N.; et al. Discovery of thiophene-2-carboxylic acids as potent inhibitors of HCV NS5B polymerase and HCV subgenomic RNA replication: 2. tertiary amides. *Bioorg. Med. Chem. Lett.* **2004**, *14*(3), 797–800.

[45] Lamarre, D.; Anderson, P. C.; Bailey, M.; Beaulieu, P.; Bolger, G.; Bonneau, P.; Bos, M.; Cameron, D. R.; Cartier, M.; Cordingley, M. G.; et al. An NS3 protease inhibitor with antiviral effects in humans infected with hepatitis C virus. *Nature* **2003**, *426*(6963), 186–189.

[46] Wiedmann, B.; Puyang, X.; Poulin, D.; Mathy, J. E.; Ma, S.; Anderson, L. J.; Fujimoto, R.; Compton, T.; Lin, K. Characterization of mechanism of resistance to cyclophilin inhibitors in HCV replicon. 15th International Symposium on Hepatitis C Virus and Related Viruses, 2008.

[47] Coelmont, L.; Paeshuyse, J.; Kaptein, S.; Vliegen, I.; Kaul, A.; De, C. E.; Rosenwirth, B.; Crabbe, R.; Bartenschlager, R.; Dumont, J. M.; Neyts, J. The cyclophilin inhibitor Debio-025 is a potent inhibitor of hepatitis C virus replication in vitro and has a unique resistance profile. 14th International Symposium on Hepatitis C Virus and Related Viruses, 2007.

[48] Mathy, J. E.; Ma, S.; Compton, T.; Lin, K. Combinations of cyclophilin inhibitor NIM811 with hepatitis C virus NS3-4A protease or NS5B polymerase inhibitors enhance antiviral activity and suppress the emergence of resistance. *Antimicrob. Agents Chemother.* **2008**, *52*(9), 3267–3275.

[49] Sivaraja, M.; Pouliot, J.; Zhang, J.; Mathy, J. E.; Chenail, G.; Ma, S.; Deng, G.; Chopra, R.; Latour, D.; Fung, K.; et al. In vitro biochemical and virological characterization of GL60667 (LDI133), a potent nonnucleoside inhibitor of the HCV NS5B polymerase. 15th International Symposium on Hepatitis C Virus and Related Viruses, 2008.

[50] Traber, R.; Hofmann, H.; Loosli, H. R.; Ponelle, M.; Von Wartburg, A. Neue Cyclosporine aus *Tolypocladium inflatum*: Die Cyclosporine K-Z. *Helv. Chim. Acta* **1987**, *70*, 13–36.

[51] Schmidt, B.; Riesner, D.; Lawen, A.; Kleinkauf, H. Cyclosporin synthetase is a 1.4 MDa multienzyme polypeptide: re-evaluation of the molecular mass of various peptide synthetases. *FEBS Lett.* **1992**, *307*(3), 355–360.

[52] Lawen, A.; Zocher, R. Cyclosporin synthetase. The most complex peptide synthesizing multienzyme polypeptide so far described. *J. Biol. Chem.* **1990**, *265*(19), 11355–11360.

[53] Weber, G.; Schorgendorfer, K.; Schneider-Scherzer, E.; Leitner, E. The peptide synthetase catalyzing cyclosporine production in *Tolypocladium niveum* is encoded by a giant 45.8-kilobase open reading frame. *Curr. Genet.* **1994**, *26*(2), 120–125.

[54] Ke, J.; Lawitz E.; Rozier, R.; Marbury, T.; Nguyen, T.; Serra, D.; Dole, K.; Praestgaard, J.; Huang, M.; Evans, T. Safety and tolerability of NIM811, a novel cyclophilin inhibitor for HCV, following single and multiple acending doses in healthy volunteers and HCV-infected patients. 44th Annual Meeting of the European Association for the Study of the Liver. 2009.

[55] Flisiak, R.; Horban, A.; Gallay, P.; Bobardt, M.; Selvarajah, S.; Wiercinska-Drapalo, A.; Siwak, E.; Cielniak, I.; Higersberger, J.; Kierkus, J.; et al. The cyclophilin inhibitor Debio-025 shows potent anti-hepatitis C effect in patients coinfected with hepatitis C and human immunodeficiency virus. *Hepatology* **2008**, *47*(3), 817–826.

[56] Flisiak, R.; Feinman, S. V.; Jablkowski, M.; Horban, A.; Kryczka, W.; Pawlowska, M.; Heathcote, J. E.; Mazzella, G.; Vandelli, C.; Nicolas-Metral, V.; et al. The cyclophilin inhibitor Debio 025 combined with PEG IFNalpha2a significantly reduces viral load in treatment-naive hepatitis C patients. *Hepatology* **2009**, *49*(5), 1460–1468.

[57] Hopkins, S.; Heuman, D.; Gavis, E.; Lalezari, J.; Glutzer, E.; DiMassimo, B.; Rusnak, P.; Wring, S.; Smitley, C.; Ribeill, Y. Safety, plasma pharmacokinetics, and anti-viral activity of SCY-635 in adult patients with chronic hepatitis C virus infection. 44th Annual Meeting of the European Association for the Study of the Liver, 2009.

[58] Gane, E. J.; Roberts, S. K.; Stedman, C.; Angus, P. W.; Ritchie, B.; Elston, R.; Ipe, D.; Baher, L.; Morcos, P.; Najera, I.; et al. First-in-man demonstration of potent antiviral activity with a nucleoside polymerase (R7128) and protease (R7227/ITMN-191) inhibitor combination in HCV: safety, pharmacokinetics, and virologic results from INFORM-1. 44th Annual Meeting of the European Association for the Study of the Liver, 2009.

23

HCV VIRAL ENTRY INHIBITORS

FLOSSIE WONG-STAAL, GUOHONG LIU, AND JEFFREY MCKELVY
iTherX Pharmaceuticals, Inc., San Diego, California

INTRODUCTION

Hepatitis C virus (HCV) is a major cause of acute hepatitis and chronic liver disease. With 170 million people infected worldwide, HCV has become a major threat to human health and one of the most difficult challenges for pharmaceutical and medical researchers. There is no vaccine available for HCV. The current standard of care is the combination therapy of pegylated interferon and ribavirin, which is limited by low efficacy and undesirable toxicity. A large percentage of patients are infected with the genotype 1 HCV, which responds only partially, if at all, to the standard therapy. Liver cirrhosis and hepatocellular carcinoma associated with HCV infection are the leading indications for liver transplantation. Therefore, novel therapies against HCV infection are in great need [1].

The process of HCV infection and replication in host liver cells is only partially understood. The virus first attaches and enters the host cell via the specific interactions between viral envelope proteins and host-cell receptors. Following the endocytosis-mediated entry, the viral genome is released and processed in the cytoplasm. Genome replication and protein translation are initiated to produce viral components. The endoplasmic reticulum is the major site for virion assembly. The mature virion is eventually released into the extracellular space to infect neighboring cells. Theoretically, targeting any of the key steps in this infection process should prevent the generation of active HCV. Indeed, targeting the viral polymerase or protease to reduce viral replication has been a major strategy being pursued by many pharmaceutical companies for developing novel HCV therapeutics, and positive clinical outcomes have been reported. In contrast, although blocking viral entry is well recognized as a valid antiviral strategy, much less effort has been put on this approach, due to limited knowledge of the HCV entry mechanism. However, recent advances in HCV biology have provided novel information in this area, including the identification of several cellular receptors that may be exploited as therapeutic targets.

The HCV virion is composed of a positive-sense RNA genome encased in the viral capsid, surrounded by an envelope comprising the glycoproteins E1 and E2. It is now recognized that HCV viral entry is a complex process involving the sequential engagement of the envelope proteins with a series of cell receptors [2]. To enter into target cells, the virus first docks and attaches to the host-cell surface, probably via interaction with glycosaminoglycans. Attachment is followed by sequential specific interactions between the envelope glycoproteins with multiple HCV receptors, including SR-B1, CD81, CLDN1, and Occludin [3,4], culminating in a pH-dependent endocytosis step. The nature of the spatial and temporal interactions of the virus with these diverse receptors is still being unraveled.

Due to the lack of an efficient in vitro infection system until recently, several surrogate systems have been developed to study virus entry. These include direct E1E2 binding [5,6], viruslike particles (VLPs) [7,8], and HCV pseudoparticles (HCVpp) [9,10]. HCVpp, which utilizes the unmodified HCV envelope proteins to package retroviral particles, including HIV-1, most closely mimics native infection and can be neutralized by patient sera as well as monoclonal antibodies against HCV E2 protein [11–13]. Primary hepatocytes and human hepatoma cells are the major targets of HCVpp infection in vitro. Recently, a cell culture system that

Antiviral Drugs: From Basic Discovery Through Clinical Trials, First Edition. Edited by Wieslaw M. Kazmierski.

supports the production and propagation of infectious HCV in cell culture (HCVcc) has been developed [14–16]. The original infectious clone JFH-1 was derived from a genotype 2a virus. However, chimeric viruses containing the structural genes from other HCV genomes and the replicative genes of JFH-1 are also infectious in culture. These systems are very useful in validating the activity of entry inhibitors in a virus context.

Here we review several HCV entry inhibitors that are in development, with more detailed description of the programs at our company, iTherX Phramaceuticals, Inc. (henceforth referred to as iTherX). Diverse approaches targeting the viral envelope as well as various host proteins are being pursued. The results so far are encouraging for the feasibility of inhibiting viral entry as a novel HCV therapeutic strategy.

CLINICAL-STAGE COMPOUND ITX5061 TARGETS THE HOST-CELL RECEPTOR SRB1

We at iTherX are currently developing a clinical stage small-molecule compound, ITX5061, repurposed as an anti-HCV viral entry inhibitor. This first-in-class HCV entry inhibitor specifically targets the host-cell receptor SR-B1 (scavenger receptor B1). SR-B1 is expressed predominantly in the liver and steroidogenic tissues, where it mediates the selective uptake of cholesterol from ligands such as high-density lipoprotein (HDL). Interaction of the HCV envelope protein E2 with SR-B1 occurs via hypervariable region 1 located within the N-terminal region of the E2 glycoprotein, and this interaction is probably critical for HCV infection of hepatocytes. Anti-SR-B1 antibodies and small interfering RNA silencing of SR-B1 expression decrease HCV infection. ITX5061 is an aryl ketoamide of the general structure shown in Figure 1.

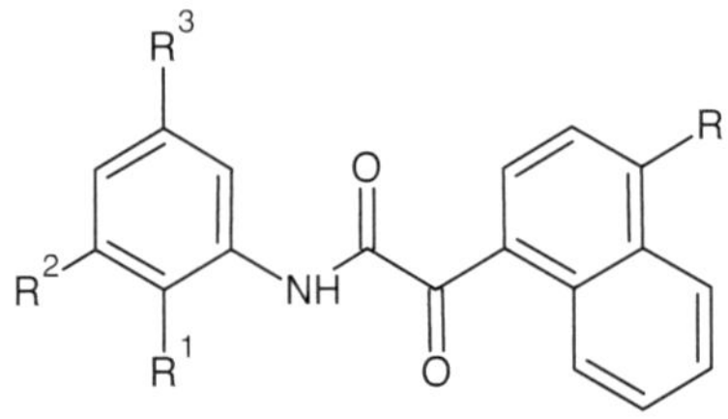

FIGURE 1

It was observed earlier that ITX5061 raised HDL levels in mice and in human subjects but not in mice with a knockout in the SR-B1 gene (Alan Tall, personal communication). ITX5061 was then assessed for its ability to inhibit HCV infection in a cell-based assay using infectious genotype 2a virus carrying a Renilla luciferase gene (HCV2aChLuc) or a chimeric infectious clone of genotypes 1a and 2a (HCV1a/2a ChRluc) (Fig. 2). ITX5061 inhibited both viruses with EC_{50} values of 0.05 to 0.5 nM and EC_{90} values of 15.0 to 5.0 nM. The compound had no effect on viral RNA replication (data not shown). In addition, cellular toxicity on Huh7 cells or primary hepatocytes was not observed up to 10 μM of ITX5061 (data not shown). ITX5061 was acquired from the company Kemia. Another compound, ITX4520, which was discovered internally at iTherX (see below), was five- to 10-fold less active in these assays.

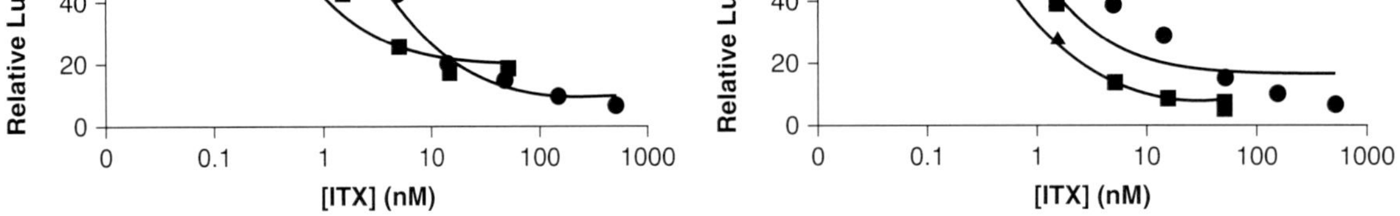

FIGURE 2 ITX HCV entry inhibitors show similar inhibition for HCV bearing structural proteins of genotype 1a (a) and 2a (b). The HCV 2a/2a (J6JFH) chimera was constructed by inserting Renilla Luciferase, FMDV 2A protease, Ubiquitin monomer sequence between 5′ NTR of HCV2a(JFH) and the open reading frame of core protein (HCV2aJb). The HCV1a/2a chimeric infectious clone contained sequences for the structural proteins derived from HCV genotype 1a H77 strain and the nonstructural proteins, 3′ NTR infected by either chimeric virus with increasing amounts of ITX5061 or ITX4520. Three days post-infection, the supernatant was removed and the cells were washed with PBS and then lysed for the luciferase assay.

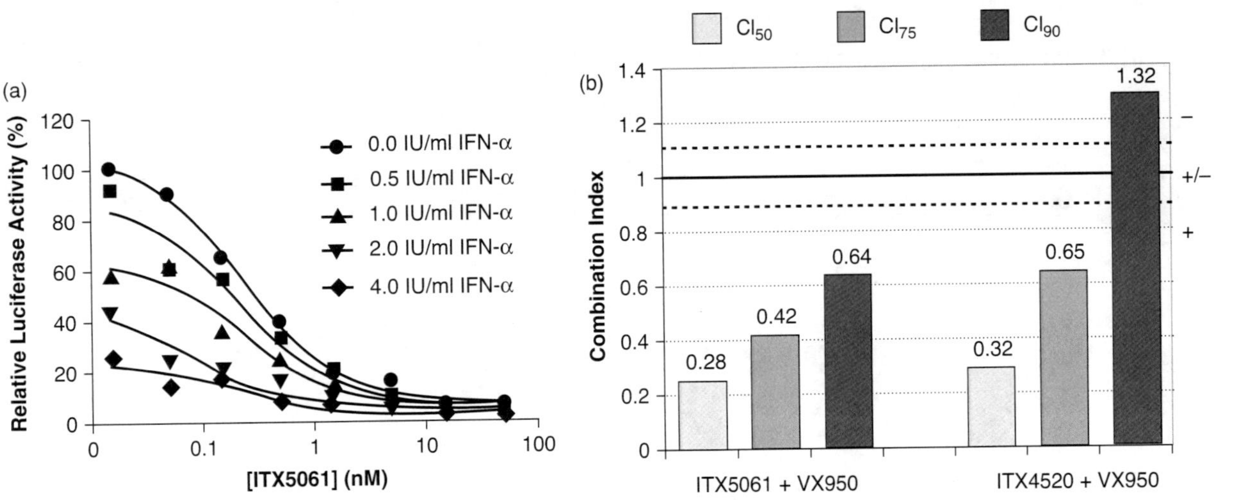

FIGURE 3 Combinatory effects of ITX compounds with interferon or protease inhibitor. Huh7 cells were infected with HCV1a/2a chimera in the presence of various concentrations of (a) ITX5061 in combination with various concentration of IFN-α for 72 h. (b) ITX5061 or ITX4520 in combination with various concentration of the HCV protease (VX950). Viral replication was measured byluciferase assay. The combination indices (CI) in (b) were determined with Calcusyn (Biosoft) at the EC_{50}, EC_{75}, and EC_{90} value of each compound. By convention a CI of < 0.9 was considered synergistic, a CI of ≥ 0.9 or ≤ 1.1 was considered additive, and a CI of >1.1 was deemed antagonistic. Numerical values above the bars are mean CI. +, synergy; ±, additivity; –, antagonism.

In vitro studies also demonstrated that ITX5061 acts additively or synergistically to IFN and to a HCV protease inhibitor (VX950) (Fig. 3). In addition, ITX5061 has no diminished activity against an HCV NS3 mutant (A156S) that is highly resistant to VX-950 (Fig. 4). These results confirm that since ITX5061 acts via a mechanism distinct from those of other HCV drugs, its addition should be beneficial to existing regimens, and no cross-resistance would be expected.

Several lines of evidence indicate that ITX5061 targets the SR-B1 receptor. An E2 mutant HCV2aCh virus, which is reported to have reduced dependency on SR-B1 and increased binding to CD81 [17,18], showed greater resistance to ITX5061 relative to the wild-type virus (Fig. 5). We also showed selective binding of a radiolabeled ITX5061 analog to SR-B1 expressing CHO cells (data not shown) and inhibition of soluble E2 to SR-B1 expressing CHO cells by ITX5061 (A. Syder et al., submitted).

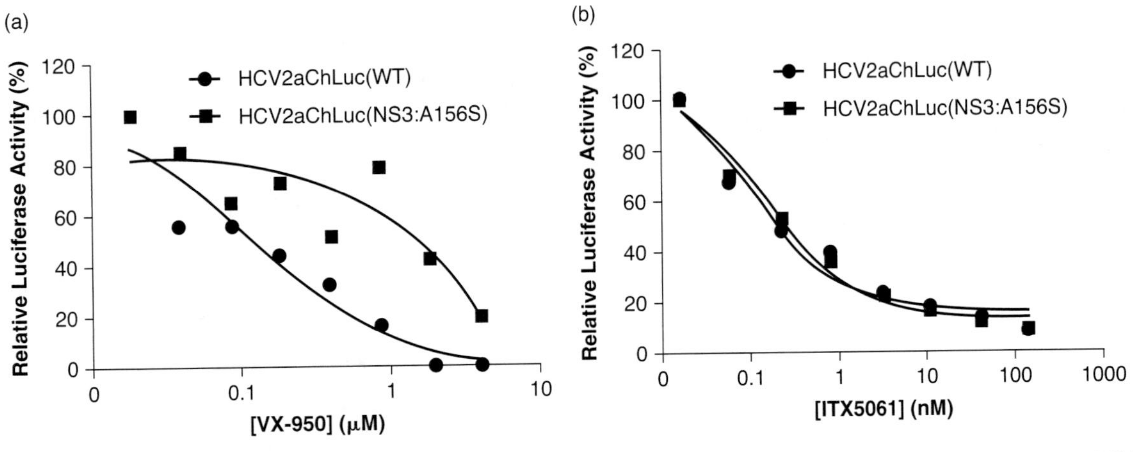

FIGURE 4 A protease mutant virus that is resistant to VX950 is sensitive to ITX5061 inhibition. The parental type and mutant (NS3:A156S) of HCV2aCh were inoculated onto Huh7 cells in the presence of (a) IFN-α as a control or (b) ITX5061 and further incubated for 3 days. Intracellular luciferase activity was measured 3 days post-infection.

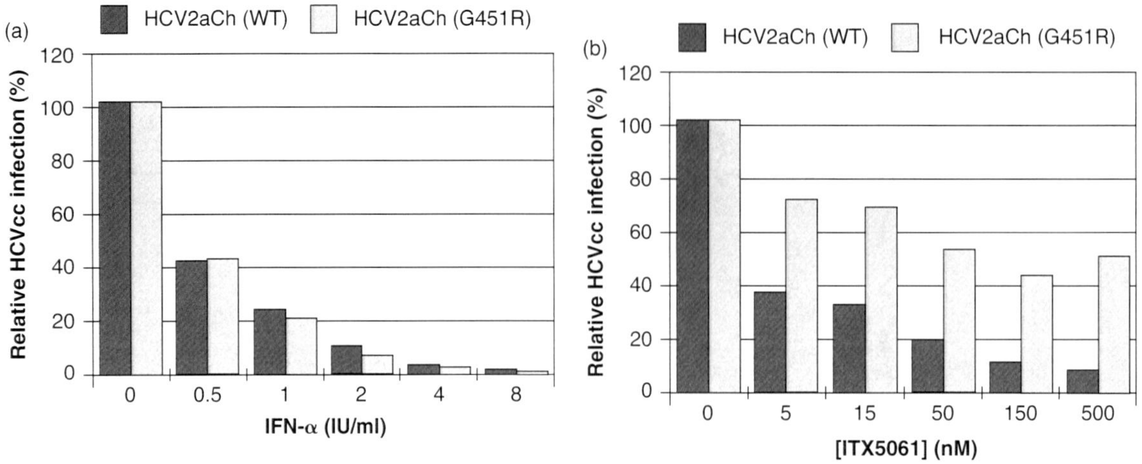

FIGURE 5 A E2 mutant virus that is less dependent of SR-B1 receptor showed greater resistance to ITX5061 relative to wild-type virus. (a) Taqman assay for viral RNA copies with wild-type HCV2aCh or HCV2aCH)E2: G451R) mutant virus in the presence of various concentrations of IFN-α (b) Immunofluorescence staining for viral infection with wild-type or HCV2aCh (G451R) mutant virus in the presence of various concentrations of ITX5061. Values were expressed relative samples with no inhibitors added.

PHARMACOKINETIC AND TOXICITY PROFILES OF ITX5061

Animal studies have shown that ITX5061 is absorbed extensively following oral administration and is eliminated primarily by hepatic metabolism, probably via the cytochrome P450 enzyme isoforms CYP3A4 and CYP3A5. The metabolites are excreted mainly via the biliary tract into feces. Nonclinical in vivo safety pharmacology studies and genotoxicity studies produced no clinically significant findings. Nonclinical 28- and 90-day toxicology studies in both rats and monkeys have been completed, as have chronic toxicity studies (6 months in rats and 9 months in monkeys). No adverse event levels determined in these studies provide significant safety margins for human studies (Table 1).

Notable observations included increases in HDL-cholesterol (HDL-C) levels (probably due to modulation of SR-B1), elevations in unconjugated (direct) bilirubin levels (due to inhibition of uridine 5′-diphosphoglucuronosyl transferase 1A1, UGT1A1), and adrenal gland hyperplasia/hypertrophy. Decreased red blood cell and hemoglobin levels and hepatobiliary findings of mild elevations in hepatic transaminases (both species) and bile duct hyperplasia and centrilobular hepatocellular hypertrophy (rats only) were observed at much higher doses. Embryo–fetal developmental toxicology studies were also performed in two species (rats and rabbits). In the rat study, a reduction in mean fetal weights and fetal skeletal variations or malformations was observed. In the rabbit study, dose-related increases in postimplantation fetal loss, hydrocephaly, and reduced ossification of the skull were exhibited. As a precaution, participants in clinical studies with ITX5061 must use highly effective means of contraception.

TABLE 1 NOAEL Values for Toxicology Studies

Duration and Species	NOAEL (mg/kg/day)
28-day rat	30
28-day monkey	35
90-day rat	>30
90-day monkey	>30
Chronic rat (6 months)	30
Chronic monkey (9 months)	100/75[a]

[a]On day 56, dosing was decreased in the highest dose group from 100 to 75 mg/kg per day to increase tolerability. Dosing was maintained at 75 mg/kg per day through the remainder of the study.

ITX5061 has now been studied in 95 subjects in phase I and 190 patients in phase II (other disease indications than HCV). Overall, ITX5061 has been well tolerated in these early clinical trials. During phase I studies, ITX5061 (doses up to 640 mg/day) was administered to 95 healthy volunteers in single- and repeat-dose studies for up to 12 days. In phase II studies, 190 patients have been randomized to receive ITX5061 once daily. In study ITX5061-C05, a randomized placebo-controlled study, 97 patients with rheumatoid arthritis received 150 mg (n = 50) or 300 mg (n = 47) ITX5061 for up to 12 weeks. In study ITX5061-C06, a randomized placebo-controlled study, 78 patients with dyslipidemia received 150 mg (n = 38) or 300 mg (n = 40) ITX5061 for up to 6 weeks. In study ITX5061-C08, an open-label study, 15 patients with pemphigus vulgaris received 300 mg ITX5061 for up to 12 weeks.

Clinical studies conducted to date have identified no other significant safety issues associated with once-daily dose levels up to, and including, 300 mg of ITX5061. We plan to initiate a phase IIa study to further evaluate the safety, tolerability, and potential antiviral effects of ITX5061 monotherapy in HCV-infected patients. The study will be performed as a double-blind placebo-controlled study at three once-daily oral doses (20, 50, 100 mg; six patients each group) over 4 weeks. The 4-week duration was chosen based on viral dynamics considerations. Entry inhibitors do not have an immediate impact on virus production from infected cells, but rather, decrease the pool of infected target cells by blocking new infections. Therefore, the kinetics of reduction in viral load in the plasma may depend in part on the rate of turnover of infected hepatocytes, which can vary from days to weeks [19,20]. In addition to safety monitoring and pharmacokinetic measurements in this patient population, changes in viral load will be assessed by viral RNA PCR. Doses in the current HCV study are lower than doses previously used in patients and will be evaluated for shorter dosing periods (28 days). Hence, risk is not likely to be increased in this patient population.

BACKUP COMPOUNDS FOR SR-B1 INHIBITION

iTherX has a pipeline of proprietary, preclinical-stage compounds that also inhibit SR-B1 activity. Many of these are structurally distinct from ITX5061 and were first identified as hits from a screen using the HCVpp cell culture system, and then confirmed in the HCVcc chimeric 2a/2a or 1a/2a cell culture systems (both are luciferase-based assays). The compounds that efficiently inhibit viral infectivity (IC_{50} < 10 nM, IC_{90} < 150 nM) were identified as initial lead compounds and subjected to further in vitro and in vivo characterizations. These include cell viability assays in Huh7 cells and primary hepatocytes, metabolic stability (in vitro microsomal assays and in vivo PK studies), oral bioavailability, and preliminary toxicity. Only compounds with low clearance rates and significant oral bioavailability

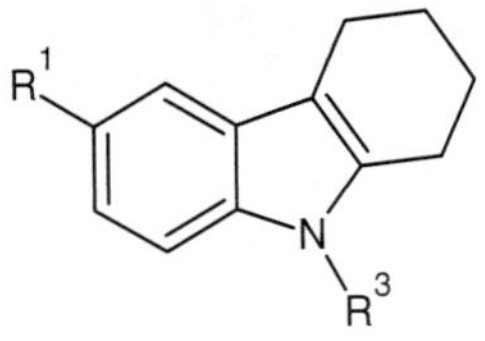

FIGURE 6

($\%F > 40\%$ in rats) will be carried on for downstream evaluations. Chemistry efforts were also devoted to the synthesis of improved analogs in potency and stability: for example, by protecting the identified metabolically active groups.

ITX4520, a lead compound for HCV entry inhibition, was identified following this screening strategy. ITX4520 is a tetrahydrocarbazole of the general structure shown in Figure 6. ITX4520 showed efficacious inhibition of HCVcc infection ($IC_{50} \sim 1.5$ nM) and a desirable therapeutic index (>1000). This compound exhibits high in vitro metabolic stability ($t_{1/2} \sim 60$ min) in hepatic microsomes extracted from different species (human, rat, or dog) (Table 2). Most important, the compound showed a low clearance rate and good bioavailability in PK studies conducted in rat and dog (Table 3). ITX4520 is currently under evaluation for in vivo toxicity in rat and dog. Preliminary in vitro tests indicate that this compound does not induce genotoxicity in Ames tests. Off-target toxicity assays to detect possible cross-reactivity with up to about 170 receptors/enzymes did not indicate significant effects (>50% inhibition at 10 μM) (Table 2).

ITX4520 is structurally unrelated to ITX5061, but also appears to target the SR-B1 receptor according to the criteria described above for ITX5061. Therefore, we consider this compound to be a backup for ITX5061, which is at the clinical evaluation stage.

TABLE 2 ITX4520 In Vitro Preclinical Properties

Chemistry	c$\log P$	6.55
	psa	69
Efficacy (EC_{50})	HCVpp	0.5 μM
	HCVcc2A	1.5 nM
	HCVcc1A	
CC_{50}	Huh7 cells	100 μM
In vitro metabolic stability	Rat microsome ($t_{1/2}$)	60 min
	Dog microsome ($t_{1/2}$)	60 min
	Human microsome ($t_{1/2}$)	60 min
	CYP450 3A4 (IC_{50})	4 μM
	CYP450 2C9 (IC_{50})	0.7 μM
	CYP450 2D6 (IC_{50})	1 μM
In vitro protein binding	Human albumin column	98%
Genotoxicity	Ames test	Negative at 10 μM
Off-target toxicity	Receptor/enzyme cross-reactivity	None

TABLE 3 ITX4520 In Vivo PK

		$AUC_{(0\text{-}t)}$ (μg/L·h)	$AUC_{(0\text{-}\infty)}$ (μg/L·h)	$MRT_{(0\text{-}\infty)}$ (h)	$t_{1/2}$ (h)	T_{max} (h)	Vz (L/kg)	Clz (L/h/kg)	C_{max} (μg/L)	F (%)
Sprague–Dowley Rats	i.v. (2 mg/kg)	1,184	1,195	0.95	1.5	0.08	3.65	1.68	2,988	
(male)	p.o. (20 mg/kg)	12,299	12,364	3.94	3.41	2	NA	NA	2,948	103
Beagle dogs	i.v. (2 mg/kg)	1,745	1,757	0.71	1.1	0.08	1.81	1.14	3,875	
(male)	p.o. (20 mg/kg)	2,908	2,961	4.18	5.46	2	NA	NA	903	34

CELGOSIVIR TARGETS CELLULAR α-GLUCOSIDEASE I

Celgosivir (MX-3253; Fig. 7) is a small-molecule compound developed by Migenix. It is a 6-*O*-butanoyl derivative of castanospermine, a substance derived from the Australian chestnut or black bean. Celgosivir targets host-cell α-glucosidase I to affect the early stages of viral glycoprotein processing, resulting in the production of aberrant viral structural proteins. Therefore, Celgosivir is expected to have broad antiviral acitivity and indeed is being evaluated in both HIV and HCV patients.

Although the compound does not inhibit HCV entry directly, it inhibits the production of infective virions and thus differentiates itself from replication inhibitors and can be loosely regarded as inhibiting subsequent rounds of virus entry. In preclinical studies, celgosivir has demonstrated strong synergy with interferon-α with and without ribavirin.

Celgosivir is rapidly converted to castanospermine in the body. Castanospermine is also active in inhibiting HCV at similar potency as celgosivir, based on in vitro potency tests. The metabolite castanospermine can be detected in serum within 5 min after drug administration. T_{max} is about 1 h, and $t_{\frac{1}{2}}$ is 19 to 23 h. The drug showed dose proportionality in the range 10 to 400 mg. Renal clearance is the major route of elimination.

As celgosivir was designed initially for HIV treatment, the early clinical safety data were obtained from healthy volunteer and HIV patients in five phase I clinical studies and two phase II studies. Data were evaluated from 500 HIV-positive patients and 51 healthy volunteers. A total of 274 patients or volunteers were exposed to at least 400 mg of celgosivir. In one phase I study, patients were dosed with celgosivir as high as 600 mg per day (300 mg/day; twice a day). At least 59 and 32 patients received 400 mg of celgosivir for 12 and 24 weeks, respectively. The drug is considered to be well tolerated in these patient populations. The gastrointestinal system was the target for most reported adverse events (AEs). MIGENIX believes that HCV will be more sensitive to celgosivir treatment than HIV because of the different intracellular sites for viral assembly and budding, and the more pivotal role that proper glycosylation plays in the release of HCV virus from the cell. Thus, phase II clinical trials were initiated to test safety and efficacy in HCV patients.

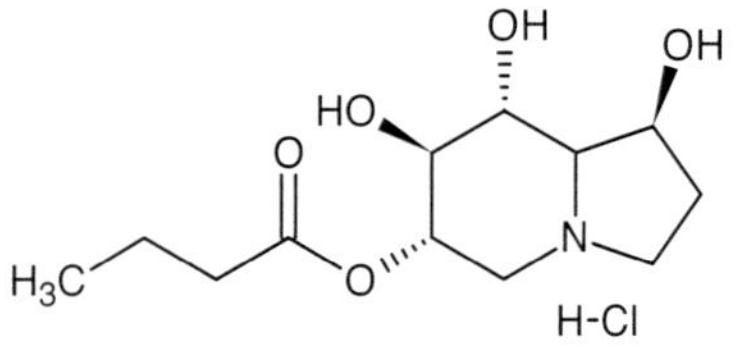

FIGURE 7

The phase IIa study is celgosivir monotherapy to test safety and tolerability in treatment-naive HCV patients. The study has been completed and demonstrated that celgosivir was well tolerated with some evidence of antiviral activity in treatment-naive chronic HCV patients [21]. The open-label phase II dose-ranging trial included 43 patients with genotype 1 HCV who were treatment-naive or interferon-intolerant. Participants were randomly assigned to one of three celgosivir monotherapy arms: (1) 200 mg once daily (q.d.), (2) 400 mg q.d., (3) 200 mg twice daily (b.i.d.). Among the 35 patients who completed 12 weeks of therapy, two (5%) had peak HCV viral load reductions of at least 1 log (1.0 log and 2.6 log) during treatment. The conclusion is that celgosivir used as monotherapy was well tolerated in all dosage groups and showed a modest antiviral effect.

A phase IIb combination therapy was then initiated in nonresponders to evaluate safety and efficacy. In a randomized double-blind multicenter study, HCV genotype 1 treatment-experienced patients with prior nonresponse or partial response to a combination of peglylated interferon (P) and ribavirin (R). Patients were randomized to one of three treatment groups: PRC group: P + R + Celgosivir 400 mg; PC group: P + Celgosivir 400 mg; and PR group: P + R standard of care. The results demonstrated that combination therapy was well tolerated and resulted in no significant adverse events. Some increased viral load reduction was observed in the PRC group compared to the PR group.

Another phase IIb viral kinetics study in treatment-naive patients was intitiated to evaluate celgosivir in combination with Peginterferon α-2b and ribavirin in treatment-naive patients with chronic hepatitis C. Preliminary 4-week interim results indicate that celgosivir has no negative effects on the tolerability, pharmacokinetics, and viral kinetics when combined with the standard of care drugs, but also no added benefits. Recently, Migenix announced a plan to add a

TABLE 4 Summary of Celgosivir Clinical trials

Clinical Stage	Subjects	Groups	Results
Phase I	Healthy volunteers and HIV patients	Various doses and durations	Well tolerated, no SAE
Phase IIa	Treatment-naive HCV patients	Monotherapy for 12 weeks 200 mg q.d. 400 mg q.d. 200 mg b.i.d.	Well tolerated, moderate efficacy
Phase IIb	Nonresponder HCV patients	Combination therapy for 12 weeks (celgosivir 400 mg), q.d. PRC PC PR	Well tolerated EVR of 42% PRC compared to 10% PR Mean VLR of 1.63 log PRC compared to 0.92 log PR Patients with 90% VLR are 66% PRC compared to 40% PR EVR in 57% of null responders (PRC)
	Treatment-naive HCV patients	Combination therapy for 12 weeks, q.d. PR PRC (400 mg C) PRC (600 mg C) (new arm)	Interim results (two arms only: PR and PRC 400 mg celgosivir for 4 weeks): Well tolerated Similar efficacy between groups

600-mg celgosivir combination therapy arm to this study. The approved protocol amendment also allows the flexibility to increase the total number of patients in the study from 20 to up to 50.

OTHER HCV ENTRY INHIBITORS IN EARLY DEVELOPMENT

1. REPLICor Inc. is developing a series of amphipathic phosphorothioate oligonucleotides (PS-ONs) with broad antiviral activities. These polymers feature hydrophilic and hydrophobic sides which mimic the amphipathic α-helices of the fusion proteins in type I viruses, such as HIV gp41, HSVgB, VSVG, and influenza HA. Therefore, these polymers can target to the amphipathic α-helical hinge domains of fusion proteins on these enveloped viruses and thereby inhibit the postbinding cell fusion/entry step. Long ($>$ 30 base) PS-Ons have been reported to inhibit HCV infection in both HCVcc and HCVpp systems with IC50 in the low-nanomolar range. A current lead under development is REP9AC, which has been shown to inhibit HCV, HBV, and HSV, and so on. Pharmacokinetic studies showed that REP9AC has a short residence time in the blood ($t_{1/2} < 1$ h) and tends to accumulate in the liver. The projected half-life in humans is more than 28 days. PS-ONs have been shown to be generally safe based on several clinical trials for other disease indications, such as Mipomersen for hypercholesterolemia by ISIS in Phase II, and Genasense for cancer by GENTA in phase III. REP9AC also exhibits an acceptable toxicity profile. This drug is still in preclinical development.
2. PRO206 is an orally available small molecule developed by Progenics Pharmaceuticals, Inc. PRO206 was reported to be a potent and selective inhibitor of HCV entry. The mechanism of action for this molecule is not reported. PRO206 also demonstrated high oral bioavailability and a prolonged pharmacokinetic half-life in animals. However, Progenics recently announced abandoning the development of PRO206 in favor of earlier backup compounds.
3. SP10 and SP30, being developed by Samaritan Pharmaceuticals, Inc., are orally bioavailable small-molecule HCV entry inhibitors. These molecules apparently target the host cell, but the mechanism has not been revealed.
4. HuMax-HepC antibody developed by Genmab A/S (a biotechnology company in Denmark) is a human antibody originally isolated from a patient who suffered from mild chronic hepatitis due to HCV infection. In preclinical studies, HuMax-HepC is broadly cross-reactive with several HCV genotypes, including 1a, 1b, 2a, 3a, and 4a. HuMax-HepC binds to a conformational epitope of the envelope protein (E2) and potently inhibits the binding of HCV-E2 to target cells. In May 2007, Genmab announced that HuMax-HepC antibody prevented HCV infection in a mouse model. Mice with a compromised immune system were transplanted with human liver cells (hepatocytes) and exposed to a mixture of patient-derived HCV of different genotypes. Replication of HCV was not observed in five of six mice (83%) treated with HuMax-HepC,

indicating that HuMax-HepC completely prevented HCV infection. The sixth mouse was infected with HCV, but the virus was subsequently cleared. In comparison, five of six mice that received a control antibody developed and sustained a robust HCV infection.

5. *Other potential antibody therapies.* In theory, any known coreceptor for HCV can potentially be targeted by antibody therapeutics. CD81 has long been recognized as an essential HCV receptor for entry, and efforts have been made to develop specific small-molecule inhibitors or antibodies against this receptor [22,23]. However, none of these efforts have led to a clinical trial. One concern of targeting CD81 is its ubiquitous expression in human cells and tissues. This can lead to issues of general toxicity as well as pharmacokinetics. It remains to be seen if antibodies against SR-B1 or CLDN1 would be pursued for HCV therapy.

   Utilization of neutralizing antibodies, such as those induced by vaccination of viral glycoproteins E1E2, has been attempted to prevent HCV infection [24,25]. The results are variable and sometimes conflicting, although this strategy is still pursued by some investigators. In addition, neutralizing monoclonal antibodies derived from patients have been shown to target the E2 envelope protein. Two such antibodies were able to inhibit or reduce HCV infection of human liver in a chimeric mouse model [26]. Crucell has licensed this technology from Stanford University for further development.

FUTURE DIRECTIONS

Recent development of tools and assay systems for studying HCV has greatly facilitated our understanding of its biology as well as efforts for drug development against this virus. While most drugs in development are directed at the replicative enzymes of the virus, inhibition of virus entry has been proven in principle for other viruses and remains an attractive alternative. Knowledge of the temporal and spatial molecular mechanisms of HCV viral attachment and internalization to host cells will no doubt help the design and identification of agents that specifically and efficaciously block these first steps of viral infection.

In theory, HCV viral entry inhibitors prevent infection of new target cells, but will not have an immediate effect on reducing virus production from infected cells. This feature should be taken into consideration in the design of proof-of-concept studies. For example, their efficacy in reducing viral load may not be manifest in the first few days before significant turnover of the infected cell pool has taken place. At the same time, they may show greater synergy in combination therapy with replication inhibitors, due to distinct mechanisms and nonoverlapping resistance profiles. Another potential issue with entry inhibitors is whether cell–cell transmission may bypass some of the coreceptors discussed above. Recent data suggest that SR-B1 is functionally obligatory for cell–cell transmission as well (J. McKeating, personal communication). In any event, combination therapy also makes sense for enhancing the efficacy via inhibiting both direct viral–cell infection and cell–cell transmission.

An additional potential clinical application of HCV viral entry inhibitors is to prevent HCV reinfection in liver transplant patients, where a high reinfection rate is observed. Once clinical validation is obtained for this class, entry inhibitors will be an essential component of the optimal combination therapy for HCV patients.

REFERENCES

[1] Manns, M. P., et al. The way forward in HCV treatment: finding the right path. *Nat. Rev. Drug Discov.* **2007**, *6*, 991–1000.

[2] Timpe, J. M.; McKeating, J. A. Hepatitis C virus entry: possible targets for therapy. *Gut* **2008**, *57*, 1728–1737.

[3] Ploss, A., et al. Human occludin is a hepatitis C virus entry factor required for infection of mouse cells. *Nature* **2009**, *457*, 882–886.

[4] von Hahn, T.; Rice, C. M. Hepatitis C virus entry. *J. Biol. Chem.* **2008**, *283*, 3689–3693.

[5] Pileri, P., et al. Binding of hepatitis C virus to CD81. *Science* **1998**, *282*, 938–941.

[6] Flint, M., et al. Characterization of hepatitis C virus E2 glycoprotein interaction with a putative cellular receptor, CD81. *J. Virol.* **1999**, *73*, 6235–6244.

[7] Baumert, T. F., et al. Hepatitis C virus structural proteins assemble into viruslike particles in insect cells. *J. Virol.* **1998**, *72*, 3827–3836.

[8] Wellnitz, S., et al. Binding of hepatitis C virus-like particles derived from infectious clone H77C to defined human cell lines. *J. Virol.* **2002**, *76*, 1181–1193.

[9] Bartosch, B.; Dubuisson, J.; Cosset, F. L. Infectious hepatitis C virus pseudo-particles containing functional E1-E2 envelope protein complexes. *J. Exp. Med.* **2003**, *197*, 633–642.

[10] Hsu, M., et al. Hepatitis C virus glycoproteins mediate pH-dependent cell entry of pseudotyped retroviral particles. *Proc. Natl. Acad. Sci. USA* **2003**, *100*, 7271–7276.

[11] Bartosch, B., et al. In vitro assay for neutralizing antibody to hepatitis C virus: evidence for broadly conserved neutralization epitopes. *Proc. Natl. Acad. Sci. USA* **2003**, *100*, 14199–14204.

[12] Logvinoff, C., et al. Neutralizing antibody response during acute and chronic hepatitis C virus infection. *Proc. Natl. Acad. Sci. USA* **2004**, *101*, 10149–10154.

[13] Meunier, J. C., et al. Evidence for cross-genotype neutralization of hepatitis C virus pseudo-particles and enhancement of infectivity by apolipoprotein C1. *Proc. Natl. Acad. Sci. USA* **2005**, *102*, 4560–4565.

[14] Lindenbach, B. D., et al. Complete replication of hepatitis C virus in cell culture. *Science* **2005**, *309*, 623–626.

[15] Wakita, T., et al. Production of infectious hepatitis C virus in tissue culture from a cloned viral genome. *Nat. Med.* **2005**, *11*, 791–796.

[16] Zhong, J., et al. Robust hepatitis C virus infection in vitro. *Proc. Natl. Acad. Sci. USA* **2005**, *102*, 9294–9299.

[17] Grove, J., et al. Identification of a residue in hepatitis C virus E2 glycoprotein that determines scavenger receptor BI and CD81 receptor dependency and sensitivity to neutralizing antibodies. *J. Virol.* **2008**, *82*, 12020–12029.

[18] Zhong, J., et al. Persistent hepatitis C virus infection in vitro: coevolution of virus and host. *J. Virol.* **2006**, *80*, 11082–11093.

[19] Perelson, A. S., et al. New kinetic models for the hepatitis C virus. *Hepatology* **2005**, *42*, 749–754.

[20] Shudo, E.; Ribeiro, R. M.; Perelson, A. S. Modeling HCV kinetics under therapy using PK and PD information. *Expert Opin. Drug Metab. Toxicol.* **2009**, *5*, 321–332.

[21] Kaita, K., et al. Ph II proof of concept study of celgosivir in combination with peginteferon and ribavirin in chronic hepatitis C genotype-1 non-responder patients. *J. Hepat.* **2007**, *46*, 556–557.

[22] Catanese, M. T., et al. High-avidity monoclonal antibodies against the human scavenger class B type I receptor efficiently block hepatitis C virus infection in the presence of high-density lipoprotein. *J. Virol.* **2007**, *81*, 8063–8071.

[23] Liu C., Dong H. Novel antiviral small molecules that block hepatitis C virus cellular entry through the CD81 receptor. 14th International Symposium on Hepatitis C and Related Viruses, 2007, 0–59.

[24] Law, M., et al. Broadly neutralizing antibodies protect against hepatitis C virus quasispecies challenge. *Nat. Med.* **2008**, *14*, 25–27.

[25] Leroux-Roels, G., et al. A candidate vaccine based on the hepatitis C E1 protein: tolerability and immunogenicity in healthy volunteers. *Vaccine* **2004**, *22*, 3080–3086.

[26] Eren R., et al. Preclinical evaluation of two neutralizing human monoclonal antibodies against hepatitis C virus (HCV): a potential treatment to prevent hcv reinfection in liver transplant patients. *J. Virol.* **2006**, *80*, 2654–2664.

PART III

RESPIRATORY SYNCYTIAL VIRUS INHIBITORS

24

DISCOVERY OF THE RSV INHIBITOR TMC353121

JEAN-FRANÇOIS BONFANTI
Janssen R&D, Janssen-Cilag, Johnson & Johnson, Val de Reuil, France

GABRIELA ISPAS AND FRANS VAN VELSEN
Tibotec BVBA, Beerse, Belgium

WIESLAWA OLSZEWSKA
Imperial College, London, UK

TOM GEVERS AND DIRK ROYMANS
Tibotec BVBA, Beerse, Belgium

INTRODUCTION

Human respiratory syncytial virus (RSV) was first isolated in 1957 and has since emerged as an important human respiratory pathogen [1–6]. Generally, infection is restricted to the upper respiratory tract and not associated with long-term pathology, but progression to a more severe lower respiratory tract infection is not uncommon. Thus, the virus is the main causative agent of lower respiratory tract infections, such as bronchiolitis and pneumonia in infants and young children [5–8]. Infants born prematurely, infants under 6 weeks old, or infants with bronchopulmonary dysplasia, congenital heart disease, or immunodeficiency are especially at risk for developing severe disease [9–11]. Moreover, severe RSV infections in the first year of life are a risk factor for asthma development [12–14]. Although virtually all children are infected with RSV at least once before the age of 2, reinfection is common [6,15,16]. In healthy adults, infection usually causes symptoms similar to the common cold, but in hospitalized elderly or severely immunocompromized patients with RSV pneumonia, mortality rates can reach 20 and 70%, respectively [17,18].

Despite extensive efforts, development of an anti-RSV vaccine has proven to be particularly challenging and has not been successful to date [19–21]. Therefore, prophylactic options are limited to passive immunization with the humanized monoclonal antibody Synagis. However, administration of Synagis is restricted to at-risk infants under the age of 2. For therapeutic intervention, the antiviral drug ribavirin is the only option, but its use is limited, due to its problematic mode of aerosolic administration, limited efficacy, and teratogenicity. Hence, effective therapeutic options are needed for treatment of the at-risk population, including adults and the elderly. Screening compound libraries in cellular antiviral assays produced several small-molecule inhibitors of RSV; however, most of them have failed in the pharmaceutical research and development process, and few are still in the clinic today [22–26]. In contrast, the development of next-generation antibodies, mainly targeting the attachment and fusion protein of RSV, has seen significant progress.

RSV is an enveloped virus with negative-sense single-stranded RNA that belongs to the family *Paramyxoviridae*, subfamily *Pneumovirinae*. For enveloped viruses the fusion process is crucial to gain access to the host cells, and the fusion or F protein of RSV plays a pivotal role in this process [27,28]. Before fusion, the F protein forms a homotrimer that is cleaved into two polypeptides, F_1 and F_2, held together by a disulfide bridge. F_1 contains an N-terminal

Antiviral Drugs: From Basic Discovery Through Clinical Trials, First Edition. Edited by Wieslaw M. Kazmierski.

hydrophobic fusion peptide and two heptad-repeat domains, N-terminal HR-N and C-terminal HR-C, separated by an intervening globular domain [29]. Once fusion is initiated, the F protein undergoes refolding, in which a trimeric coiled-coil structure of three HR-N heptad repeats is formed and the N-terminal fusion peptide is projected into the membrane of the target cell [30,31]. Then the three HR-C heptad repeats collapse irreversibly in the hydrophobic grooves of this trimeric coiled-coil structure, resulting in a stable trimer of hairpins, the six-helix bundle (6HB). Eventually, viral and cell membranes are brought into close proximity for membrane fusion and subsequent viral entry. RSV fusion inhibitors have been shown to bind target sites that become available during F-protein refolding, and as such, disturb the natural refolding process [32–35]. It has been suggested that the hydrophobic pockets in each of the three grooves of the central coiled oil are the drug target sites [36,37].

DISCOVERY

Our discovery of RSV inhibitors at Johnson & Johnson started in the 1990s with a screening campaign using a cellular assay. Among different potential hits, an antihistaminic series was selected for further evaluation. An extensive hit-to-lead program confirmed the significance of this benzimidazole family. A few modifications on the scaffolds ("head part" and "left-hand side") allowed the synthesis of the first submicromolar active RSV inhibitors (compound **2**, Figure 1). This new lead compound was then optimized to afford a first preclinical candidate, JNJ-2408068 (Fig. 1) [23]. The last optimization step, the introduction of hydroxyl and methyl groups on the "head part" and a second methyl group on the benzimidazole core heterocycle, resulted in a 3 log increase in antiviral activity.

JNJ-2408068 is a small-molecule antiviral with a high potency (picomolar activity) and a low cytotoxicity in a wide range of cells. Unfortunately, it showed long tissue retention times in several species (rat, dog, and monkey), which was a cause for concern for a first-in-human selection. Subsequent research efforts were therefore focused on how to reduce tissue retention while keeping the high RSV-inhibition potency [38]. Pharmacokinetic (PK) studies on different substructures of the lead benzimidazole derivative indicated that the most basic part of the compound (the aminoethylpiperidine moiety, highlighted in boldface type in Fig. 2) was probably responsible for the long elimination half-life from different tissues. Whereas S2 and S3 were rapidly eliminated from lung tissues, S1 had an elimination rate similar to that of JNJ-2408068.

Therefore, the program was focused on this part of the molecule in two different subseries: modulation of the aminoethyl group (keeping the piperidine) and modulation of the entire aminoethylpiperidine moiety. In the two subseries,

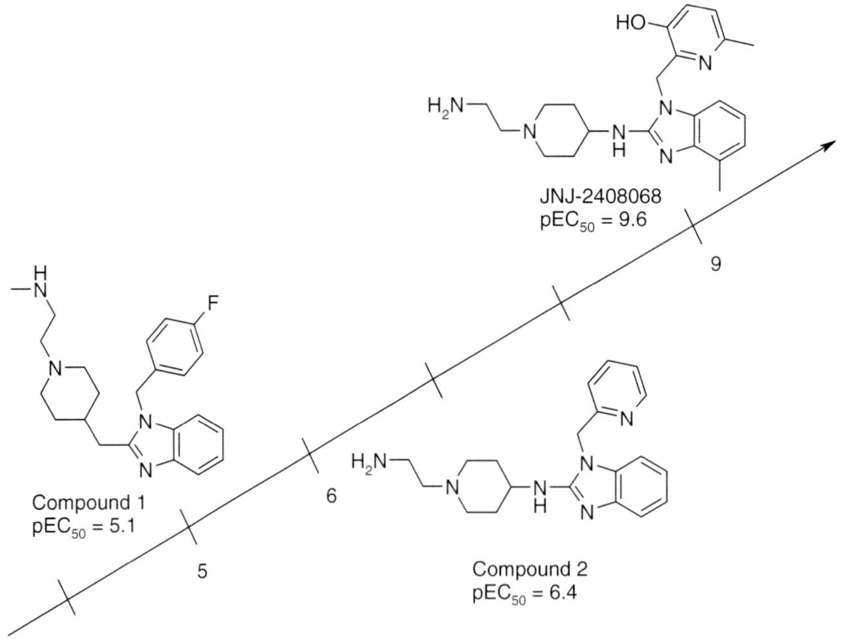

FIGURE 1 Discovery of JNJ-2408068 starting from an antihistaminic series. A tetrazolium-based colorimetric method was used to determine pEC_{50} values [$pEC_{50} = -\log_{10} EC_{50}$ (M)] reflecting antiviral activities as described. Briefly, compounds were tested in 96-well plates to evaluate their effects on virus- and mock-infected cells. Cells were infected with 100 median tissue culture infectious doses (TCID50) of virus. After 2 h of incubation at 37°C in a 5% CO_2 atmosphere, a suspension (4×10^5 cells/mL) of susceptible cells was added to all wells in a volume of 50 μL, and cultures were incubated further at 37°C for 4 to 7 days post-virus exposure. The viability of mock- and virus-infected cells was quantitated spectrophotometrically using the MTT method. (From [23].)

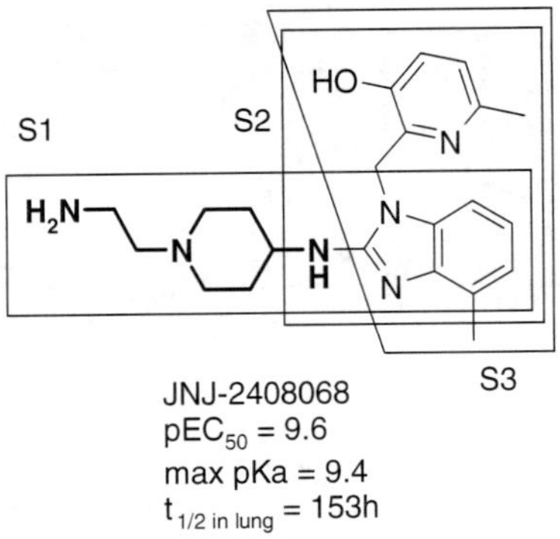

FIGURE 2 Disconnection of JNJ-2408068 in three substructures to identify the moiety responsible for tissue retention.

new compounds with improved PK profiles in terms of tissue retention were found (Fig. 3). These lower tissue retentions seem to be associated with the reduction of the basicity of the "left-hand side" of the molecules. Unfortunately, the new inhibitors were also less potent against RSV. Further optimization of these compounds was therefore needed.

The optimization strategy was based on a molecular modeling approach. Time-of-addition experiments had demonstrated that the substituted benzimidazole derivatives act at the beginning and at the end of the RSV replication cycle. At the beginning they prevent entry of the virus into uninfected cells (virus–cell fusion), while inhibiting the fusion of infected cells with uninfected cells (syncytium formation) at the end of the replication cycle [23]. This finding was supported by the isolation of resistance mutations in the fusion protein of the virus, which helped in identifying a putative binding site in the core domain of the protein [33,36], more precisely in a cavity on the surface of the central HR-N coiled coil. A published x-ray structure of the RSV 6HB (accession number: 1G2C) [36], was used to elaborate a model (Fig. 4).

After removal of the HR-C peptides, a binding pocket made by the contact of two HR-N peptides could be defined in the groove. This pocket is the most important locus for interaction between HR-N and HR-C peptides during 6HB formation. The most interesting solution after docking of JNJ-2408068 in this binding pocket is given in Figure 4 (left part). JNJ-2408068 binds in two subpockets, P1 and P2, and the hydroxyl group of the "head part" makes a hydrogen bond with a salt bridge. A comparison of the binding of the natural substrate HR-C with the binding of JNJ-2408068 shows that the latter leaves subpocket P3 free (Fig. 4). Replacement of the basic P1-binding "left-hand side" during the optimization of PK properties might have been the cause of the reduction observed in the binding affinity of the new inhibitors with the target F protein. It was postulated that the introduction of suitable substituents on the benzimidazole core heterocycle in the new inhibitors to reach the P3 subpocket might compensate the reduction in binding affinity.

To fit in the model, the new substituent should be anchored in position 6 of the benzimidazole scaffold. A phenethyl group with a methyl in the *meta* position of the phenyl ring

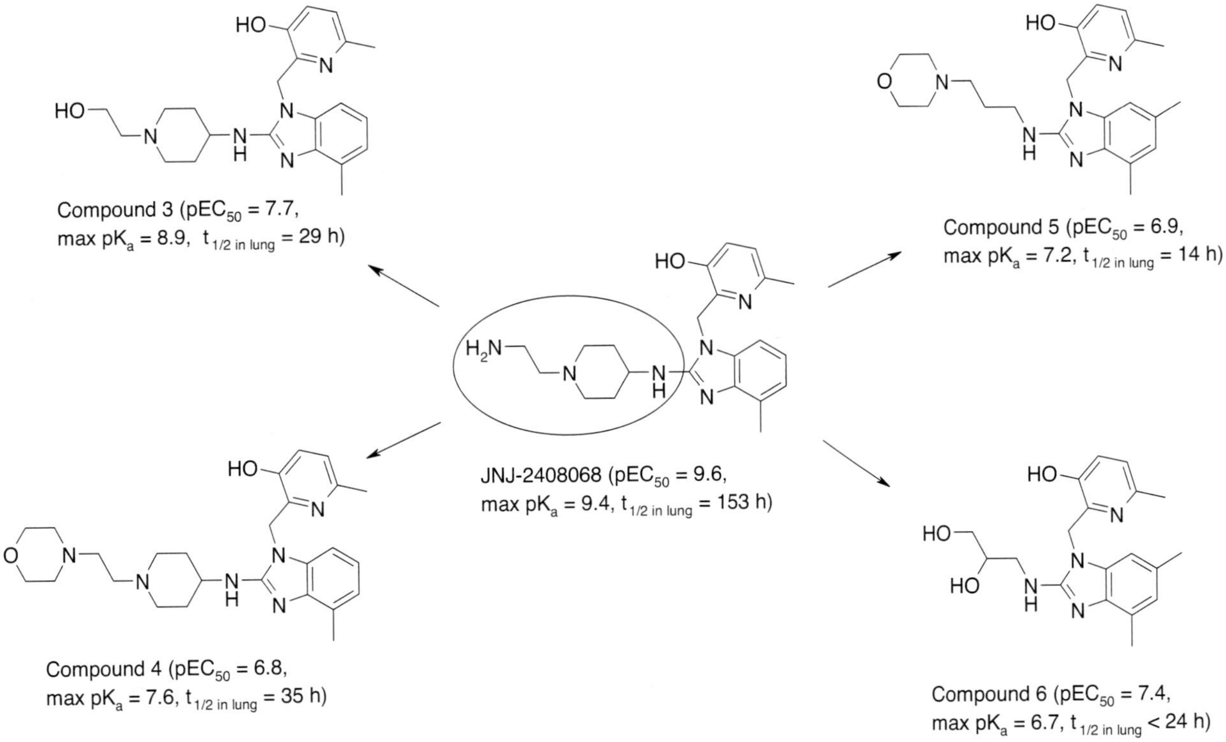

FIGURE 3 Identification of new RSV inhibitors with improved PK profiles in terms of tissue retention.

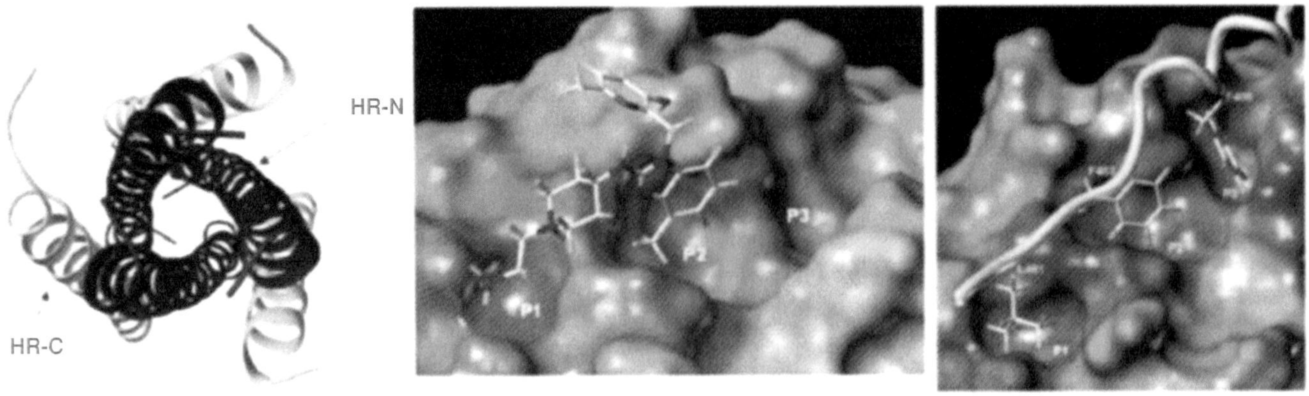

FIGURE 4 1G2C x-ray structure of the RSV 6HB [36] (left). HR-N helices of the central inner trimeric coiled coil are presented in blue. The three HR-C helices, binding into three hydrophobic grooves each formed by two neighboring HR-N helices, are indicated in yellow. The binding of the natural substrate HR-C (right) and the binding of JNJ-2408068 (middle) to the hydrophobic pocket situated in the central trimeric coiled coil of the 6HB are compared. (*See insert for color representation of the figure.*)

proved to be the best choice. To validate the model, an analog of JNJ-2408068 incorporating this new substituent was synthesized (compound **7**, Fig. 5). Its high in vitro anti-RSV activity demonstrated that this modulation on the scaffold was allowed, but it was obvious that the substituent would require further optimization. For chemical feasibility reasons, optimization was performed in the *N*-methyl piperidine series. The addition of the newly discovered phenethyl substituent on the scaffold already gave a much more potent compound (compound **9**, $pEC_{50} = 7.7$, in comparison to compound **8**, $pEC_{50} = 6.4$ in Fig. 6). Replacement of the methylene linked to the phenyl ring with an amino group and the addition of a second methyl group in the *meta* position afforded compound **10** (Fig. 6), the most potent inhibitor in this series.

This optimized substituent was then combined with the "left-hand sides" that had better PK profiles in terms of tissue retention. The hydroxyethyl-piperidine substituent (compound **11**, Table 1) led to a 1 log increase of activity but was not favorable for the PK profile ($t_{1/2}$ = 85 h instead of 29 h for compound **3**). With the dihydroxylpropyl chain, the potency was seriously reduced (compound **12**, Table 1, $pEC_{50} = 7.5$). The most promising result was obtained with the morpholinopropyl moiety, which allowed combining improved activity and favorable tissue retention (compound **13**, Table 1, $pEC_{50} = 9$, $t_{1/2}$ = 13.7 h). Starting from compound **13**, the optimization was completed with the introduction of a hydroxyl chain on the newly designed "right-hand-side" group, leading to the identification of TMC353121 as a clinical candidate (Fig. 7) [26].

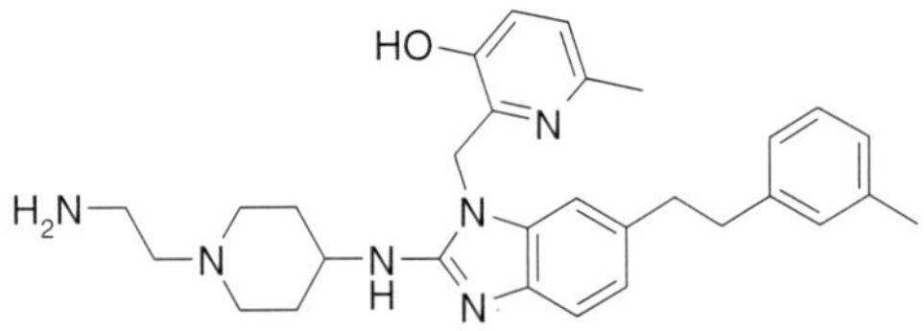

compound 7 $pEC_{50} = 9$

FIGURE 5 Structure of the compound synthesized to validate the P3 subpocket model.

SYNTHESIS

The synthesis of TMC353121 is described in Scheme 1. The number of steps was quite high, but the overall yield was reasonable (14%). The key step was the introduction of the hydroxylpyridine "head part" **f** on intermediate **e**, leading to the formation of two isomers **h** and **g** in the same proportion. Intermediate **e** was obtained in five steps starting from 3,4-diaminobenzoic acid **a**. Esterification, followed by a cyclization with urea in xylene at high temperature and, finally, $POCl_3$-mediated chlorination, gave the corresponding chlorobenzimidazole derivative **b**. The synthesis of intermediate **e** was performed with the reduction of the ethyl-ester group before the melting reaction with morpholinopropylamine, to prevent the formation of the unwanted amide. The desired isomer **h** was then oxidized to form the aldehyde group necessary for the final reductive amination reaction, affording TMC353121.

MECHANISM OF ACTION

To confirm the mechanism of action of TMC353121, time-of-addition and in vitro resistance selection assays were performed. In time-of-addition experiments, the compound behaved similarly to our first preclinical candidate, JNJ-2408068 [23], as well as two other demonstrated RSV-fusion

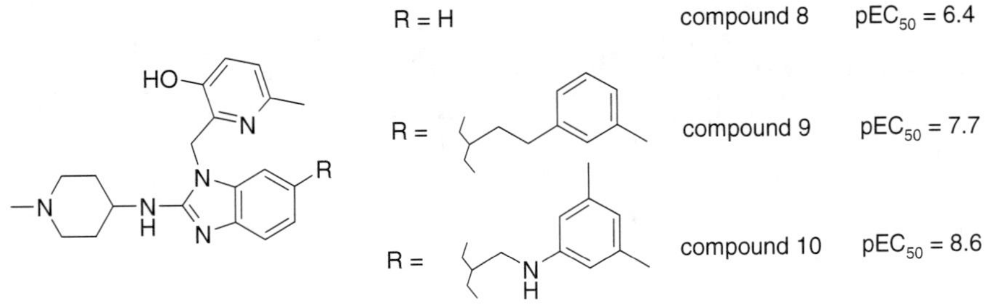

FIGURE 6 Optimization of the phenethyl substituent in the *N*-methylpiperidine series.

inhibitors (Fig. 8). TMC353121 was also found to inhibit RSV both early and very late in the viral replication cycle by preventing virus–cell fusion and syncytium formation, respectively.

As observed with JNJ-2408068, resistance mutations raised in vitro against TMC353121 appeared only in the F protein (Table 2), suggesting that this protein is the sole target of TMC353121. The mutations observed appeared in the same F_1 polypeptide regions as described previously for other small-molecule 6HB inhibitors of RSV [23,25,33]. Whereas K394R and S398L are situated in the cysteine-rich region of the globular loop region which intervenes with HR-N and HR-C, D486N is present in the HR-C region, which interacts with the HR-N hydrophobic pocket upon 6HB formation.

HR-N- and HR-C-derived peptide-binding experiments confirmed our model, which predicted that the compound will bind in the hydrophobic pockets present in the HR-N central trimeric coiled coil [38]. These experiments were confirmed by the crystal structure of TMC353121 bound to its 6HB target site [38]. The crystal structure shows that additional interactions with HR-C are crucial for proper binding of TMC353121. The latter observation is interesting because it may elucidate the function of the D486N mutation, and it is in agreement with an earlier hypothesis [38,39] that explains the mechanism of action of inhibitors targeting the hydrophobic pockets. 6HB-formation can be envisioned as the closing of a zipper. Interactions of the HR-C amino acid residues with the HR-N hydrophobic pockets at the N-terminal end of the 6HB are known to be crucial for providing stability to the 6HB. One possibility for the mechanism of action of TMC353121 is that the binding of the compound in this region could prevent the closing of the zipper at the N-terminal end, leading to inhibition of fusion. In addition, our model showed that the dimensions of the hydrophobic pockets are

TABLE 1 Combination of the Optimized Substituent with the Left-Hand Sides That Had Better Profiles in Terms of Tissue Retention

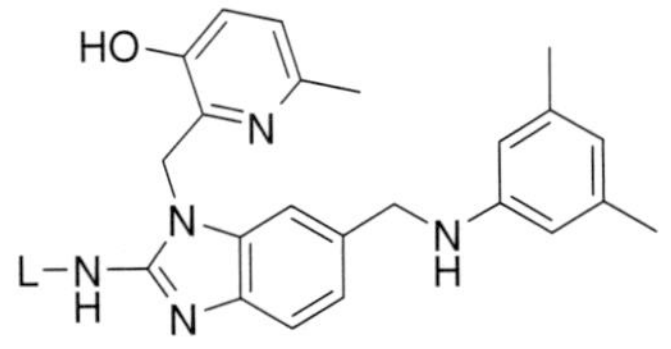

Compound	L	pEC_{50}	$t_{1/2\ (24\text{-}96h)}$ in lung (h)
11	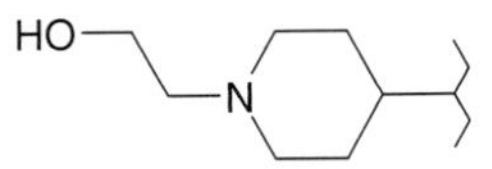	8.8	84.9
12	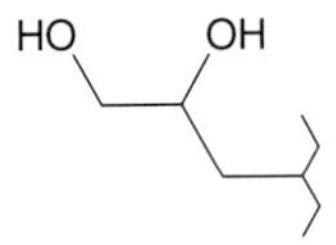	7.5	Not determined
13	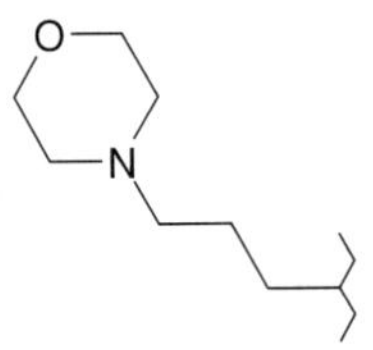	9	13.7

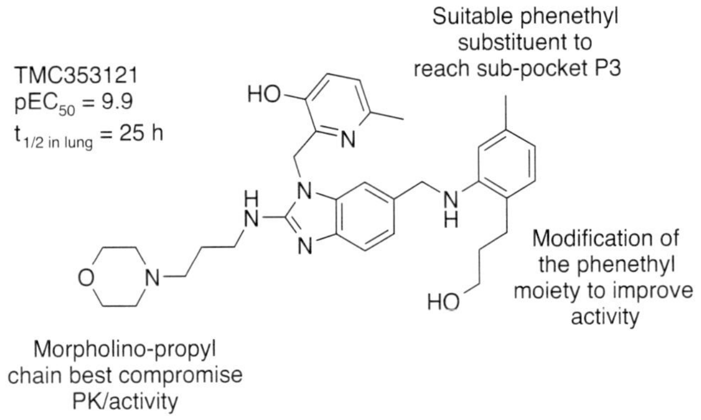

FIGURE 7 Discovery of TMC353121.

relatively shallow, and it was therefore considered surprising that the binding of TMC353121 to these HR-N pockets alone would result in such a potent antiviral effect. The peptide binding experiment and the binding mode of TMC353121 indeed confirmed that the compound does not find to just HR-N pockets [38]. An alternative possibility is therefore more likely. The HR-C residues (including D486N) that normally interact with the HR-N hydrophobic pockets seem to act as a cover, "sandwiching" the inhibitor between the hydrophobic pockets and the HR-C peptides. This disturbance in native 6HB formation could be sufficient for fusion inhibition, since it may dramatically change the stability of the 6HB. Mutation of D486N could influence the interactions with TMC353121, altering the susceptibility for the virus. The appearance of the K394R and S398L mutations could result in an altered stability of the prefusion conformation of the F protein, decreasing the energy required to trigger the fusion process [40].

EFFICACY IN ANIMAL SPECIES

Cotton Rat Efficacy Studies

The cotton rat model was used to demonstrate the in vivo efficacy of TMC353121. The animals are semipermissive for RSV infection, that is, the amount of virus recovered from the lungs is directly proportional to the amount of challenge virus, suggesting limited replication of the virus [41]. Cotton rat experiments were carried out using mainly prophylactic, but also therapeutic, drug administration schedules. Efficacy of TMC353121 was measured at maximal pulmonary RSV titer [i.e., ~10^6 infectious viruses/mL bronchoalveolar lavage fluid (BALF)], which is reached 4 days after the viral challenge. Lungs were flushed with physiological water and the infectious virus titer in the BALF was determined. Efficacy of TMC353121 in cotton rats was determined by administering the compound intravenously (Table 3) or via alternative administration routes, as indicated in Table 4.

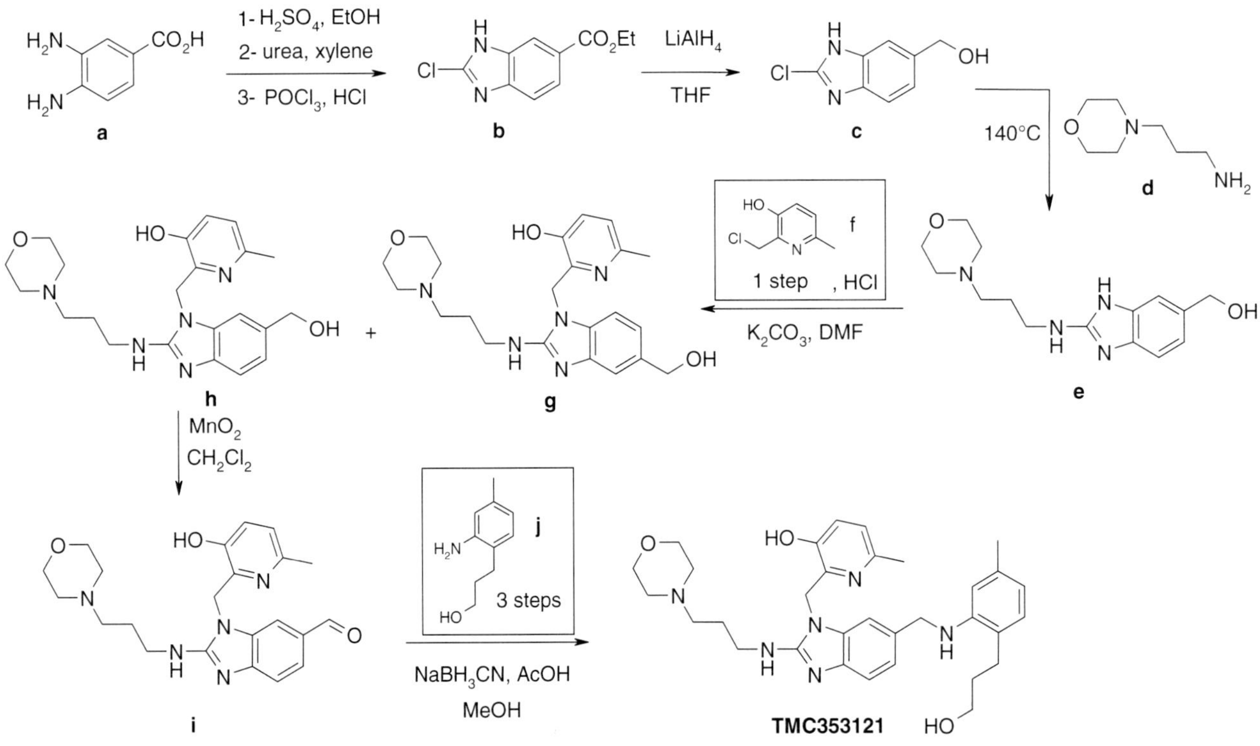

SCHEME 1 Synthesis of TMC353121.

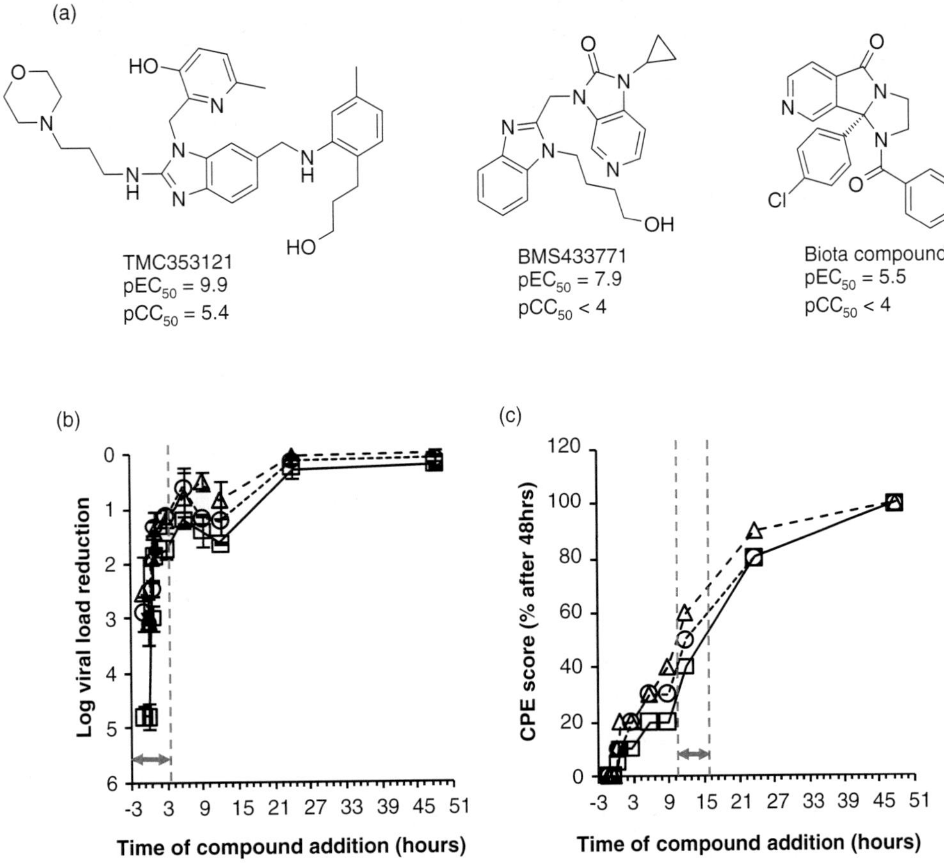

FIGURE 8 Time of addition profiling of 6HB inhibitors. (a) Structures of the fusion inhibitors, together with their in vitro anti-RSV activity [$pEC_{50} = -\log_{10} EC_{50}$ (M)] and cytotoxicity [$pCC_{50} = -\log_{10} CC_{50}$ (M)], that were included in the test panel. (b and c) TMC353121 (open squares, solid full line) and BMS433771 (open circles, dotted line) at a concentration of 100 × EC_{50} [20 × EC_{50} for the Biota compound (open triangles, dashed line)] were added in a time-of-addition experiment to the infected cells as indicated on the *x*-axis. Time point: 1 h represents a 1-h preincubation of compound and virus before infection. Gray arrows indicate the period of the replication cycle in which the compounds are able to block viral replication as demonstrated by (b) plaque assay or (c) to prevent 50% syncytium formation. Values are presented as the mean ± S.E.M. in part (b). Part (c) shows one representative result of three independent experiments.

Single-dose intravenous administration of TMC353121 (10 mg/kg) at different time points before and after RSV infection suggest that the presence of the compound is required around the time of virus challenge (e.g., 5 min) to achieve a maximal antiviral effect. To prevent replication, a sufficient level of TMC353121 has to be present during the fusion stage of the replication cycle. In fact, efficacy of TMC353121 decreased as a function of time between compound administration and virus challenge, in both prophylactic and therapeutic treatment regimens, reflecting the limited window of RSV replication in this model. When TMC353121 was administered intravenously, orally, or via inhalation, a dose–response relationship was observed, and the anti-RSV potential of this compound was confirmed.

TABLE 2 In Vitro Resistance Mutations in the RSV F Protein vs. TMC353121[a]

	S398L	K394R/S398L	D486N
TMC353121	194	62,125	2,474

[a]Resistance mutations selected against TMC353121 are indicated. Numbers represent the fold change of the compound's EC_{50} compared to the activity against wild-type virus.

BALB/c Efficacy Studies

The BALB/c mouse model [43] was used as a second model to demonstrate the in vivo anti-RSV efficacy of intravenously injected TMC353121. Similar to the cotton rat model, the BALB/c mouse is a semipermissive model, with maximal RSV replication at day 4 post-challenge. In this model, Long strain RSV inoculation will cause a lung disease similar to a mild pneumonia [44]. The loss in body weight is considered a clinical sign of disease and correlates with the dose of virus administered. In addition to monitoring the viral load, the

TABLE 3 Efficacy of TMC353121 (Aqueous Solution) on Viral Replication in Cotton Rats When Given at Various Time Points Before and After Viral Challenge

Administration of TMC353121			Viral Load Drop in BALF	
Route	Timing[a]	Dose (mg/kg)	Median Log Reduction[b]	p Value[c]
i.v.	−96 h	10	0.2	0.004
i.v.	−72 h	10	0.4	0.058
i.v.	−48 h	10	0.3	0.141
i.v.	−24 h	10	0.5	0.058
i.v.	−1 h	10	0.9	0.002
i.v.	−5 min	10	1.2	0.009
i.v.	+3 h	10	0.4	0.002
i.v.	+24 h	10	0.2	0.009

[a]When TMC353121 was administered before (−) or after (+) virus challenge.
[b]The median log reduction in BALF was calculated vs. a untreated control.
[c]The p-values were calculated using the Wilcoxon–Mann–Whitney test.

BALB/c mouse model was also used by us to measure indicators of lung inflammation as primary biomarkers, to score histopathology, and to follow BAL cell infiltration. BALB/c mice were infected by nasal instillation of 2×10^6 pfu RSV (A2 strain). RSV antiviral activity of TMC353121 was assessed using prophylactic and therapeutic dosing schedules (Table 5). Antiviral efficacy of TMC353121 was measured 4 days after virus inoculation.

TABLE 4 Efficacy of TMC353121 (Aqueous Solution) on Viral Replication in Cotton Rats When Given Via Various Administration Routes

Administration of TMC353121			Viral Load Drop in BALF	
Route	Timing[a]	Dose	Median Log Reduction[b]	p Value[c]
i.v.	−5 min	2 mg/kg	0.4	0.013
i.v.	−5 min	10 mg/kg	1.2	0.009
Inh.[d]	−1 h	0.25 mg/mL[e]	0.6	0.002
Inh.[d]	−1 h	1.25 mg/mL[e]	1.1	0.002
Inh.[d]	−1 h	5 mg/mL[e]	1.5	0.002
p.o.	−2 h	10 mg/kg	0.6	0.139
p.o.	−2 h	40 mg/kg	0.9	0.004

[a]When TMC353121 was administered before (−) virus challenge.
[b]The median log reduction in BALF was calculated versus untreated control.
[c]The p values were calculated using the Wilcoxon–Mann–Whitney test.
[d]The inhalation treatment duration is 1 h. A rough calculation of the dosage per kilogram body weight of drug delivered to the rats by aerosol was made using the following formula: estimated dose = aerosol concentration of drug × minutes of treatment × respiratory volume per min/kg for rats × pulmonary retention fraction [42].
[e]Inhalation doses are expressed as mg/mL (i.e., the concentration of the solution in the reservoir of the nebulizer).

TMC353121 administration, including single or multiple dosing before or following RSV infection, showed antiviral efficacy against RSV infection (Table 5). In addition,

TABLE 5 Summary of Studies on the Efficacy of TMC353121 on Viral Replication in BALB/c Mice

Administration of TMC353121			Viral Load Drop in Lung	
Study	Dose (mg/kg)	Timing[a]	Median Log Reduction[b]	p Value[c]
Study 1: multiple dose	10	Px (d − 5 to d0); Tx (d + 1)	0.9	0.008
	10	Px (d0)	0.4	0.090
	10	Px (d0), Tx (d + 1 to d + 3)	1.5	0.002
Study 2: multiple dose	10	Px (d0), Tx (d + 1 to d + 4)	0.8	0.041
	10	Tx (d + 1 to d + 4)	0.7	0.041
	10	Tx (d + 2 to d + 4)	1.0	0.040
	10	Tx (d + 3 to d + 4)	0.1	0.300
Study 3: single dose	2.5	−1 h	0.8	0.018
	5	−1 h	0.7	0.018
	10	−1 h	1.0	0.035
Study 4: single dose	0.25	−1 h	0.6	0.100
	1	−1 h	0.3	0.110
	2.5	−1 h	0.6	0.015
	10	−1 h	0.6	0.015
Study 5: single dose	0.025	−1 h	0.3	0.840
	0.25	−1 h	1.8	0.055
	2.5	−1 h	1.6	0.150

[a]Px, prophylactic; Tx, therapeutic; d, day; d0, day of RSV challenge.
[b]The median log reduction in lung was calculated vs. an untreated control.
[c]The p-values were calculated using the Wilcoxon–Mann–Whitney test.

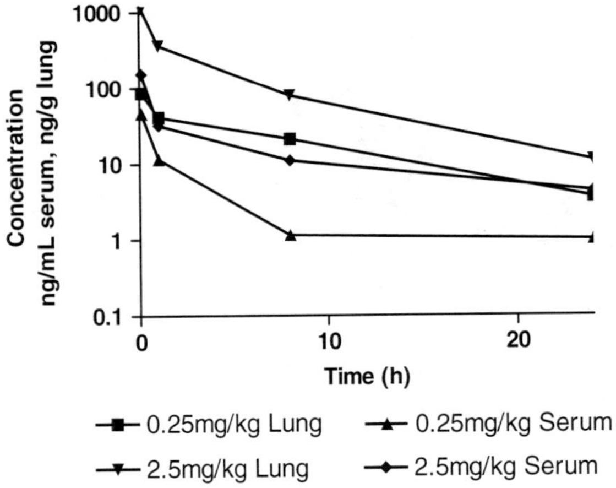

FIGURE 9 Kinetics of TMC353121 in BALB/c mice lung and serum. Two different doses were analyzed: 0.25 and 2.5 mg/kg, showing a similar PK profile, indicating dose-proportional kinetics. Drug was cleared, very rapidly from serum and lung in the first hour after intravenous bolus administration, and reached levels slightly above detection level at 24 h after administration.

repeated administration of TMC353121 starting 2 days after virus inoculation also demonstrated a significant reduction of viral load (study 2, Table 5). These results indicate that TMC353121 is efficacious in inhibiting viral replication of RSV in both prophylactic and therapeutic regimens in BALB/c mice.

For pharmacokinetic analysis, blood and lung samples were taken at several time points after intravenous bolus administration of TMC353121. The PK profile of TMC353121 in BALB/c mice shows that the compound is cleared rapidly from blood and lungs. TMC353121 shows a plasma level–time curve that follows a multicompartment model (Fig. 9).

No in vivo data on TMC353121 metabolism are available for BALB/c mice. However, in rat, unchanged TMC353121 was the major circulating compound after i.v. dosing. Antiviral activity of TMC353121 was associated with limited cell infiltration into the lung and with reduced lung inflammation. When infected mice were treated with a 10-mg/kg dose, a significant reduction of RSV viral load was measured and no lung inflammation was observed, similar to noninfected controls. In contrast, RSV-challenged and untreated mice showed a pronounced inflammation and cellular infiltration in peribronchiolar, perivascular, and alveolar space (Fig. 10). These effects were found to be dose dependent (Fig. 11; Table 5, study 5).

For TMC353121-treated mice, the lung damage caused by RSV infection was reduced compared to the control. Notably, two different doses: 2.5 and 0.25 mg/kg, showed similar viral log reduction (Table 5, step 5) but different lung histopathology results, with minimum lung inflammation at the higher dose of 2.5 mg/kg and pronounced lung inflammation at the 0.25-mg/kg dose. Hence, TMC353121 treatment of infected mice induced a 10-fold reduction in viral load with the absence of lung inflammation, resulting in a lung histopathology similar to that of uninfected mice. Correlation of the RSV viral load reduction with a protective effect on lung inflammation indicates a possible benefit for rapid eradication of clinical symptoms associated with RSV infection in humans and possible implication for a therapeutic application of RSV antivirals.

CONCLUSIONS

A combination of medicinal chemistry, molecular modeling, pharmacokinetic, and biological observations allowed us to discover the new morpholinopropyl-containing benzimidazole RSV fusion inhibitor TMC353121. The compound showed picomolar anti-RSV activity in vitro. Its viral-fusion-related mechanism of action has been assessed using time-of-addition experiments and by the isolation of resistant mutations on the F protein. Peptide binding experiments, together with the crystal structure of TMC353121 bound to its target site, provided clues for the molecular mode of action of the

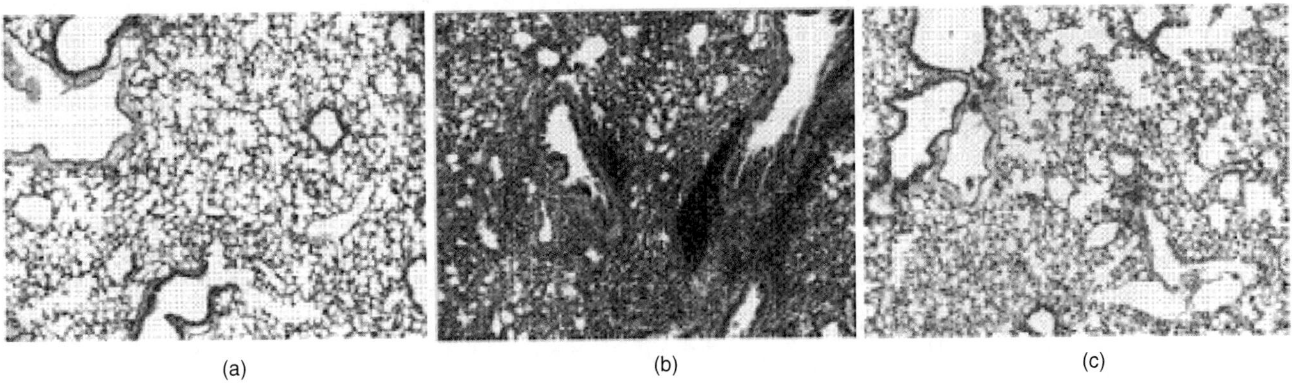

FIGURE 10 Lung infiltrate is reduced significantly in TMC353121-treated RSV-infected animals. H&E staining of lung sections. (a) Noninfected lung; (b) RSV-infected lung 5 days after infection; (c) TMC353121-treated and RSV-infected lung 5 days after infection.

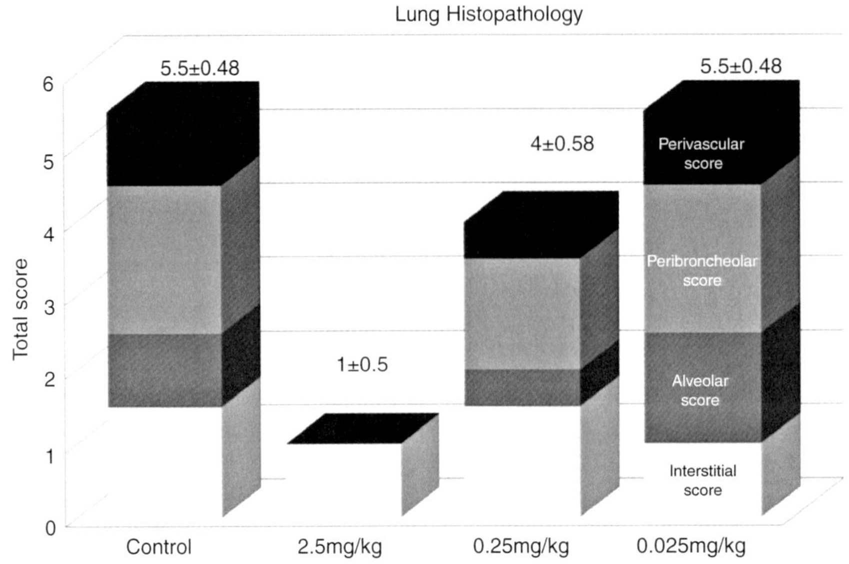

FIGURE 11 Total histopathologic score in BALB/c mice for different TMC353121 doses. Lung sections were stained with H&E to assess cell infiltrate and their localization. Lungs were evaluated for inflammatory infiltrates and graded according to a scheme similar to that described by Ponnuraj et al. [45]. Each group consisted of two mice. Three lung sections (upper, medium, and lower horizontal segments) were evaluated per lung.

compound. In vivo activity in the cotton rat model by different routes of administration was demonstrated. Experiments in a second animal model, the BALB-c mouse, indicated that TMC353121 is efficacious in inhibiting viral replication of RSV, both prophylactically and therapeutically. Interestingly, a reduction in lung damage caused by RSV infection was observed in TMC353121-treated mice compared to the control. Currently, TMC353121 is undergoing further evaluation.

Acknowledgments

The authors would like to thank K. Andries, E. Arnoult, M. De Meulder, F. Doublet, J. Fortin, P. Geluykens, J. Guillemont, A. Howe, P. Janssens, A. Koul, C. Meyer, P. Muller, D. Nauwelaers, M.-C. Rouan, H. Szel, E. Van Beirendonck, J. Van den Berg, M. Van Ginderen, B. Van Kerckhoven, P. Van Remoortere, M. Vanstockem, N. Verheyen, R. Verloes, A. Volny-Luraghi, L. Vranckx, and R. Willebrords for their contributions to the discovery and development of TMC353121, and Luc Geeraert for editing the manuscript.

REFERENCES

[1] Chanock, R.; Roizman, B.; Myers, R. Recovery from infants with respiratory illness of a virus related to chimpanzee coryza agent (CCA): I. Isolation, properties and characterization. *Am. J. Hyg.* **1957**, *66*(3), 281–290.

[2] Chanock, R.; Finberg, L. Recovery from infants with respiratory illness of a virus related to chimpanzee coryza agent (CCA): II. Epidemiologic aspects of infection in infants and young children. *Am. J. Hyg.* **1957**, *66*(3), 291–300.

[3] Ottolini, M. G.; Hemming, V. G. Prevention and treatment recommendations for respiratory syncytial virus infection: background and clinical experience 40 years after discovery. *Drugs* **1997**, *54*(6), 867–884.

[4] Simoes, E. A. F. Respiratory syncytial virus infection: pathogenesis, treatment and prevention. *Curr. Opin. Infect. Dis.* **1997**, *10*(3), 213–220.

[5] Simoes, E. A. F. Respiratory syncytial virus infection. *Lancet* **1999**, *354*(9181), 847–852.

[6] Hall, C. B.; Weinberg, G. A.; Iwane, M. K.; Blumkin, A. K.; Edwards, K. M.; Staat, M. A.; Auinger, P.; Griffin, M. R.; Poehling, K. A.; Erdman, D.; et al. The burden of respiratory syncytial virus infection in young children. *N. Engl. J. Med.* **2009**, *360*(6), 588–598.

[7] Shay, D. K; Holman, R. C.; Newman, R. D.; Liu, L. L.; Stout, J. W.; Anderson, L. J. Bronchiolitis-associated hospitalizations among US children, 1980–1996. *JAMA* **1999**, *282*(15), 1440–1446.

[8] Leader, S.; Kohlhase, K. Respiratory syncytial virus-coded pediatric hospitalizations, 1997 to 1999. *Pediatr. Infect. Dis. J.* **2002**, *21*(7), 629–632.

[9] Weisman, L. E. Populations at risk for developing respiratory syncytial virus and risk factors for respiratory syncytial virus severity: infants with predisposing conditions. *Pediatr. Infect. Dis. J.* **2003**, *22*(2 Suppl.), S33–S37.

[10] Hall, C. B.; Powell, K. R.; MacDonald, N. E.; Gala, C. L.; Menegus, M. E.; Suffin, S. C.; Cohen, H. J. Respiratory syncytial virus infection in children with immunocompromised immune function. *N. Engl. J. Med.* **1986**, *315*(2), 77–81.

[11] Feltes, T. F.; Sondheimer, H. M. Palivizumab and the prevention of respiratory syncytial virus illness in pediatric patients with congenital heart disease. *Expert Opin. Biol. Ther.* **2007**, *7*(9), 1471–1480.

[12] Mejias, A.; Chavez-Bueno, S.; Rios, A. M.; Fonseca-Aten, M.; Gomez, A. M.; Jafri, H. S.; Ramilo, O. Asthma and respiratory syncytial virus: new opportunities for therapeutic intervention. *Ann. Pediatr.* **2004**, *61*(3), 252–260.

[13] Sigurs, N.; Gustafsson, P. M.; Bjarnason, R.; Lundberg, F.; Schmidt, S.; Sigurbergsson, F.; Kjellman, B. Severe respiratory syncytial virus bronchiolitis in infancy and asthma and allergy at age 13. *Am. J. Respir. Crit. Care Med.* **2005**, *171*(2), 137–141.

[14] Hansbro, N. G.; Horvat, J. C.; Wark, P. A.; Hansbro, P. M. Understanding the mechanisms of viral induced asthma: new therapeutic directions. *Pharmacol. Ther.* **2008**, *117*(3), 313–353.

[15] Walsh, E. E.; Peterson, D. R.; Falsey, A. R. Risk factors for severe respiratory syncytial virus infection in elderly persons. *J. Infect. Dis.* **2004**, *189*(2), 233–238.

[16] Falsey, A. R.; Hennessey, P. A.; Formica, M. A.; Cox, C.; Walsh, E. E. Respiratory syncytial virus infection in elderly and high-risk adults. *N. Engl. J. Med.* **2005**, *352*(17), 1749–1759.

[17] Thompson, W. W.; Shay, D. K.; Weintraub, E.; Brammer, L.; Cox, N.; Anderson, L. J.; Fukuda, K. Mortality associated with influenza and respiratory syncytial virus in the United States. *JAMA* **2003**, *289*(2), 179–186.

[18] Falsey, A. R.; Walsh, E. E. Respiratory syncytial virus infection in adults. *Clin. Microbiol. Rev.* **2000**, *13*(3), 371–384.

[19] Schmidt, A. C. Progress in respiratory virus vaccine development. *Semin. Respir. Crit. Care Med.* **2007**, *28*(2), 243–252.

[20] Van Drunen Littel-van den Hurk, S.; Mapletoft, J. W.; Arsic, N.; Kovacs-Nolan, J. Immunopathology of hRSV infection: prospects for developing vaccines without this complication. *Rev. Med. Virol.* **2007**, *17*(1), 5–34.

[21] Piedra, P. A. Clinical experience with respiratory syncytial virus vaccines. *Pediatr. Infect. Dis. J.* **2003**, *22*(2 Suppl.), S94–S99.

[22] Nikitenko, A. A.; Raifeld, Y. E.; Wang, T. Z. The discovery of RFI-641 as a potent and selective inhibitor of the respiratory syncytial virus. *Bioorg. Med. Chem. Lett.* **2001**, *11*(8), 1041–1044.

[23] Andries, K.; Moeremans, M.; Gevers, T.; Willebrords, R.; Sommen, C.; Lacrampe, J.; Janssens, F.; Wyde, P. R. Substituted benzimidazoles with nanomolar activity against respiratory syncytial virus. *Antiviral Res.* **2003**, *60*(3), 209–219.

[24] Douglas, J. L.; Panis, M. L.; Ho, E.; Lin, K. Y.; Krawczyk, S. H.; Grant, D. M.; Cai, R.; Swaminathan, S.; Cihlar, T. Inhibition of respiratory syncytial virus fusion by the small molecule VP-14637 via specific interactions with F protein. *J. Virol.* **2003**, *77*(9), 5054–5064.

[25] Cianci, C.; Yu, K. L.; Combrink, K.; Sin, N.; Pearce, B.; Wang, A.; Civiello, R.; Voss, S.; Luo, G.; Kadow, K.; et al. Orally active fusion inhibitor of respiratory syncytial virus. *Antimicrob. Agents Chemother.* **2004**, *48*(2), 413–422.

[26] Bonfanti, J. F.; Meyer, C.; Doublet, F.; Fortin, J.; Muller, P.; Queguiner, L.; Gevers, T.; Janssens, P.; Szel, H.; Willebrords, R.; et al. Selection of a respiratory syncytial virus fusion inhibitor clinical candidate: 2. Discovery of a morpholinopropylaminobenzimidazole derivative (TMC353121). *J. Med. Chem.* **2008**, *51*(4), 875–896.

[27] Kielian, M.; Rey, F. A. Virus membrane-fusion proteins: more than one way to make a hairpin. *Nat. Rev. Microbiol.* **2006**, *4*(1), 67–76.

[28] Colman, P. M.; Lawrence, M. C. The structural biology of type I viral membrane fusion. *Nat. Rev. Mol. Cell. Biol.* **2003**, *4*(4), 309–319.

[29] Lamb, R. A.; Jardetzky, T. S. Structural basis of viral invasion: lessons from paramyxovirus F. *Curr. Opin. Struct. Biol.* **2007**, *17*(4), 427–436.

[30] Yin, H. S.; Wen, X.; Paterson, R. G.; Lamb, R. A.; Jardetzky, T. S. Structure of the parainfluenza virus 5 F protein in its metastable, prefusion conformation. *Nature* **2006**, *439*(7072), 38–44.

[31] Chan, D. C.; Kim, P. S. HIV entry and its inhibition. *Cell* **1998**, *93*(5), 681–684.

[32] Cianci, C.; Langley, D. R.; Dischino, D. D.; Sun, Y.; Yu, K. L.; Stanley, A.; Roach, J.; Li, Z.; Dalterio, R.; Colonno, R.; et al. Targeting a binding pocket within the trimer-of-hairpins: small-molecule inhibition of viral fusion. *Proc. Natl. Acad. Sci. USA* **2004**, *101*(42), 15046–15051.

[33] Douglas, J. L.; Panis, M. L.; Ho, E.; Lin, K. Y.; Krawczyk, S. H.; Grant, D. M.; Cai, R.; Swaminathan, S.; Chen, X.; Cihlar, T. Small molecules VP-14637 and JNJ-2408068 inhibit respiratory syncytial virus fusion by similar mechanisms. *Antimicrob. Agents Chemother.* **2005**, *49*(6), 2460–2466.

[34] Morton, C. J.; Cameron, R.; Lawrence, L. J.; Lin, B.; Lowe, M.; Luttick, A.; Mason, A.; McKimm-Breschkin, J.; Parker, M. W.; Ryan, J.; et al. Structural characterization of respiratory syncytial virus fusion inhibitor escape mutants: homology model of the F protein and a syncytium formation assay. *Virology* **2003**, *311*(2), 275–288.

[35] Johnson, S.; Oliver, C.; Prince, G. A.; Hemming, V. G.; Pfarr, D. S.; Wang, S. C.; Dormitzer, M.; O'Grady, J.; Koenig, S.; Tamura, J. K.; et al. Development of a humanized monoclonal antibody (MEDI-493) with potent in vitro and in vivo activity against respiratory syncytial virus. *J. Infect. Dis.* **1997**, *176*(5), 1215–1224.

[36] Zhao, X.; Singh, M.; Malashkevich, V. N.; Kim, P. S. Structural characterization of the human respiratory syncytial virus fusion protein core. *Proc. Natl. Acad. Sci. USA* **2000**, *97*(26), 14172–14177.

[37] Chan D. C.; Chutkowski, C. T.; Kim P. S. Evidence that a prominent cavity in the coiled coil of HIV type 1 gp41 is an attractive drug target. *Proc. Natl. Acad. Sci. USA* **1998**, *95*(26), 15613–15617.

[38] Roymans, D.; De Bondt, H. L.; Arnoult, E.; Geluykens, P.; Gevers, T.; Van Ginderen, M.; Verheyen, N.; Kim, H.; Willebrords, R.; Bonfanti, J.-F.; Bruinzeel, W.; Cummings, M. D.; van Vlijmen, H.; Andries, K. Binding of a potent small-molecule inhibitor of six-helix bundle formation requires

interactions with both heptad-repeats of the RSV fusion protein. *Proc. Natl. Acad. Sci. USA*. **2010**, *107*(1), 308–313.

[39] Bonfanti, J. F.; Doublet, F.; Fortin, J.; Lacrampe, J.; Guillemont, J.; Muller, P.; Queguiner, L.; Arnoult, E.; Gevers, T.; Janssens, P.; et al. Selection of a respiratory syncytial virus fusion inhibitor clinical candidate: 1. improving the pharmacokinetic profile using the structure–property relationship. *J. Med. Chem.* **2007**, *50*(19), 4572–4584.

[40] Prussia, A. J.; Plemper, R. K.; Snyder, J. P. Measles virus entry inhibitors: a structural proposal for mechanism of action and the development of resistance. *Biochemistry* **2008**, *47*(51), 13573–13583.

[41] Prince, G. A.; Jenson, A. B.; Horswood, R. L.; Camargo, E.; Chanock, R. M. The pathogenesis of respiratory syncytial virus infection in cotton rats. *Am. J. Pathol.* **1978**, *93*(3), 771–791.

[42] Wyde, P. R.; Wilson, L. Z.; Petrella, R.; Gilbert, B. E. Efficacy of high dose short duration ribavirin aerosol in the treatment of RSV infected cotton rats and influenza B infected mice. *Antiviral Res.* **1987**, *7*(4), 211–220.

[43] Openshaw, P. J. M.; Tregoning, J. S. Immune responses and disease enhancement during respiratory syncytial virus infection. Clin. Microbiol. Rev. **2005**, *18*(3), 541–555.

[44] Taylor, G.; Stott, E. J.; Hughes, M.; Collins, A. P. Respiratory syncytial virus infection in mice. *Infect. Immun.* **1984**, *43*(2), 649–655.

[45] Ponnuraj, E. M.; Hayward, A. R.; Raj, A.; Wilson, H.; Simoes, E. A. Increased replication of respiratory syncytial virus (RSV) in pulmonary infiltrates is associated with enhanced histopathological disease in bonnet monkeys (*Macaca radiata*) pre-immunized with a formalin-inactivated RSV vaccine. *J. Gen. Virol.* **2001**, *82*(11), 2663–2674.

25

DISCOVERY AND DEVELOPMENT OF ORALLY ACTIVE RSV FUSION INHIBITORS

NICHOLAS A. MEANWELL, CHRISTOPHER W. CIANCI, AND MARK R. KRYSTAL

Bristol-Myers Squibb Company Research and Development, Wallingford, Connecticut

INTRODUCTION

Respiratory syncytial virus (RSV) belongs to the pneumovirus subfamily within the Paramyxovirus family of viruses. RSV has long been recognized as the foremost cause of virus-induced lower respiratory tract disease in infants and young children [1–3]. In essence, every child will develop an RSV infection during the first two years of his or her life, but recurrent infections are frequent. RSV is especially serious in premature infants and in children with bronchopulmonary dysplasia (BPD) or congenital heart disease [4–6]. However, a recent study showed that in children 5 years of age and younger, individuals from these high-risk groups were a minority of the patients hospitalized for RSV infection or treated in outpatient settings [7]. Thus, the current strategy of prevention with the prophylactic monoclonal antibody palivizumab (Synagis) [8] or the recently discontinued investigational monoclonal agent motavizumab (Numax) [9] has only a limited effect on the total burden of RSV infection in young children. Clearly, the best approach for this population would be the development of a safe and effective vaccine [10].

Potential complications from RSV infection in young children have also been well documented. For example, RSV was the most common virus identified in the middle ear fluid of children diagnosed with acute otitis media [11–13], while a prodromal RSV infection has also been associated with childhood asthma and other long-term conditions involving pulmonary dysfunction [14–18]. What may not have been appreciated until recently is the toll inflicted by RSV infection on the adult and elderly population [19,20]. It has been estimated that 1 to 2.5 million healthy elderly and between 540,000 and 1.35 million high-risk adults in the United States are infected with RSV annually. RSV accounts for 2 to 5% of community-acquired pneumonias during the year (5 to 15% in the winter months) in community-dwelling elderly adults [19], while 3 to 7% of healthy elderly and 4 to 10% of high-risk adults are infected with RSV annually [20]. The incidence of RSV infection in adults hospitalized with acute cardiopulmonary disease was estimated at 9 to 10%, while in long-term care facilities the annual incidence is estimated at 5 to 10% [19–22]. RSV infection is particularly problematic in immunosuppressed adults with, for example, fatality rates as high as 50 to 100% in bone marrow transplant patients [5,23,24]. An analysis of RSV-associated deaths between 1990 and 1999 suggested that mortality rates are much higher in elderly persons than in other age groups, to the extent that more than 78% of RSV-associated deaths occurred among persons aged 65 years or older [25]. Within the adult population, the diagnosis of RSV infection can also be problematic since it frequently manifests as a flu-like illness that is often misdiagnosed as influenza [25]. This highlights the need for effective diagnostic tests that can be used routinely in hospitals and in both long-term care and point-of-care facilities. Most of the diagnostic tests available commercially were developed for use in children, and since the RSV titers in infected adults are significantly lower (at least 3 $\log_{10}$ pfu/mL) than in young children [26], many of these tests, especially those employing detection through immunoflourescence or enzyme immune assays, are relatively insensitive for detecting RSV in adults. Although nucleic

Antiviral Drugs: From Basic Discovery Through Clinical Trials, First Edition. Edited by Wieslaw M. Kazmierski.

acid–based diagnostic tests perform more effectively, there remains a compelling need for improved diagnostics for the adult and elderly populations [27,28].

STRATEGY FOR DISCOVERING INHIBITORS OF RSV

A high-throughput cell protection screen was used to evaluate the Bristol-Myers Squibb proprietary library of compounds in order to identify specific inhibitors of RSV by their ability to abrogate viral-induced cytopathic effects (CPE) in tissue culture. Both cell viability and cytotoxicity were assessed using a standard protocol that monitors mitochondrial metabolism [29]. This exercise was successful in that it revealed a series of low-molecular-weight benzimidazole derivatives that demonstrated excellent potency and specificity toward RSV inhibition and were appealing starting points for a medicinal chemistry campaign [30]. These compounds, represented by prototypes **1** and **2** (Fig. 1) were originally prepared in the mid-1960s by an Italian academic group for evaluation as potential analgesic or antiarrhythmic agents [31,32]. However, they had been sampled in an extensive series of high-throughput screening campaigns at Bristol-Myers Squibb without revealing significant biological activity. Compounds **1** and **2** inhibited RSV replication at submicromolar concentrations, with EC_{50} values of 470 and 220 nM, respectively, and demonstrated excellent therapeutic indexes, with CC_{50} values of 216 and 83 μM, respectively [30]. For the purpose of comparison, under identical conditions ribavirin demonstrated an EC_{50} value of 2.7 μM and a CC_{50} value of 34 μM, reflecting a low therapeutic index of 12 [30]. Compounds **1** and **2** were active toward both A and B subtypes of RSV, yet had no activity against Sendai, parainfluenza-3, influenza, vesicular stomatitis, human immunodeficiency, or herpes simplex viruses. Preliminary mode-of-action experiments indicated that these compounds inhibited fusion between RSV and host-cell membranes. This is an essential step in virus entry and is a proven antiviral mechanism in combating RSV infection since the approved drug palivizumab (Synagis), a monoclonal antibody targeted to the F protein, inhibits RSV-induced virus–cell membrane fusion [33]. Virus fusion as a mechanism for therapeutic intervention has been explored for a number of other viruses, including HIV, where clinical proof-of-principle has been exemplified by the peptidic inhibitor enfuvirtide, marketed as Fuzeon [34].

With a promising lead structure in hand and some insight into structure–activity relationships (SARs) from closely related compounds in the corporate collection [31,32], a medicinal chemistry campaign was initiated that sought to define the fundamentals of the pharmacophore, increase potency, and refine the chemotype into molecules with physical and pharmacokinetic properties compatible with oral dosing. Although it was anticipated that all aspects of the structure of the lead molecules would ultimately be examined, attention was focused initially on defining the basic structure–activity relationships (SARs) associated with the diethylamine-containing side chain of **1** and **2** [35]. This survey proved to be quite informative, revealing a remarkable tolerance for a wide range of functionality at the side-chain terminus that was compatible with potent antiviral activity. The synopsis of the key SAR summarized in Table 1

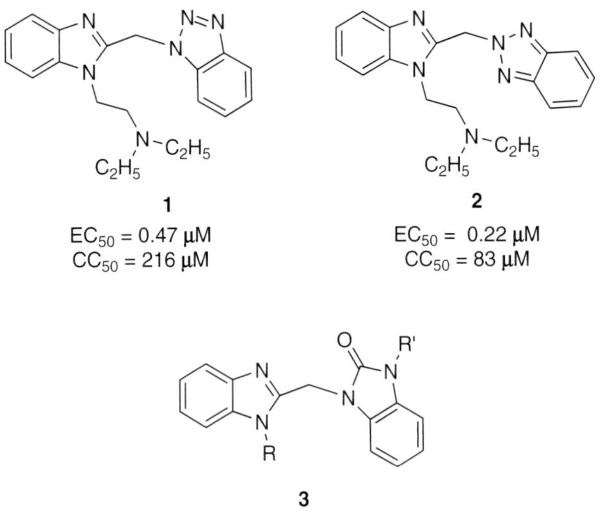

FIGURE 1

TABLE 1 Synopsis of SAR Surrounding the Side Chain of 1

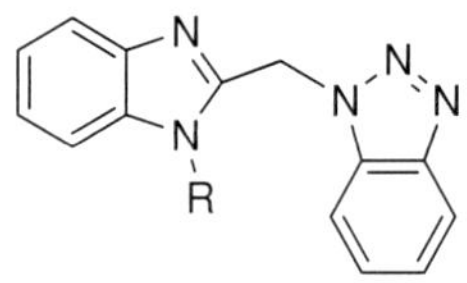

Entry Number	R	EC_{50} (μM)	CC_{50} (μM)
1	$CH_2CH_2N(CH_3)_2$	0.14	234
2	$CH_2CH_2N(CH_3)_3{}^{+}I^{-}$	0.87	42
3	$CH_2CH_2NHCH_3$	0.21	74
4	$CH_2CH_2NH_2$	3.3	
5	$CH_2CH_2N(i\text{-Pr})_2$	6.7	42.3
6	$CH_2CH_2CH(CH_3)_2$	0.1	40
7	$CH_2CH(CH_3)_2$	>15	15.5
8	$CH(CH_3)_2$	15	129
9	$CH_2CH_2CH_2CH(CH_3)_2$	0.19	24
10	$CH_2CH_2CH_2CH_3$	0.066	12
11	$CH_2CH_2SCH_3$	0.3	166
12	$CH_2CH_2SOCH_3$	0.43	56.4
13	$CH_2CH_2SO_2CH_3$	0.25	337
14	$CH_2CH_2CO_2H$	18.1	184
15	$CH_2CH_2CONH_2$	2.1	4.28
16	$CH_2CH_2CH(OH)CH_3$	0.12	>309
17	CH_2CH_2Ph	0.77	2.6

illustrates that basic, acidic, polar, and simple alkyl and phenyl moieties at the side-chain terminus are associated with potent RSV inhibitory activity. The key requirement was that side-chain branching or functional group deployment be at least two atoms way from the core heterocycle [35]. These observations provided confidence that structural variation of the side chain would provide a useful opportunity to modulate physical properties and address metabolism and pharmacokinetic issues as they arose.

With a basic understanding of side-chain SAR in hand, the role of the benzotriazole moiety was examined in the next phase of the survey. Small amounts of the 2-substitued benzotriazoles analogous to **2** were typically obtained along with the 1-substituted isomers, and these were shown to possess antiviral activity essentially equipotent to the 1-substituted compounds, suggesting a potential for structural modification of this element. The benzimidazol-2-one heterocycle was selected as the initial basis for this phase of the campaign, based on synthetic accessibility, and the ability to readily control the introduction of functionality in a regiospecific fashion [36]. Selection of this heterocycle proved to be quite propitious since compounds derived from **3** provided key insights into SAR and were generally found to be potent RSV inhibitors. As a consequence, the benzimidazol-2-one moiety was adopted as the basic structural theme for the program that ultimately led to the selection of a candidate compound for clinical evaluation. The second nitrogen atom of the benzimidazol-2-one heterocycle proved to be particularly useful, providing a synthetically readily accessible substituent vector not available to the benzotriazole moiety, an opportunity that was exploited extensively [37]. The structural simplicity, synthetic accessibility, and compatibility with a wide range of chemistries made the isoamyl moiety discovered with the benzotriazole series (Table 1, entry 6) the side chain of choice for the initial studies, a survey of which is summarized in Table 2. This series of compounds generally demonstrated improved activity compared to the benzotriazole prototypes, with both polar and lipophilic substituents providing potent RSV inhibitors. The benzimidazole side chain was subsequently probed in the context of several 3-substituted benzimidazol-2-one elements, revealing general concordance with the SAR established for the 1-substituted benzotriazole series while fully maintaining the theme of potent antiviral activity. The key compounds prepared in this series are compiled in Table 3.

While these structure–activity studies were being conducted, two animal models of RSV infection, the BALB/c mouse and the cotton rat, were established in-house to assess the in vivo antiviral properties of promising compounds [38–45]. Although proof-of-concept in an animal model was an objective, there is a poor understanding of the relevance of these models to human infection [46–48]. However, the demonstration of antiviral activity in animal models of infection was deemed necessary for further development of

TABLE 2 SAR Associated with the Benzimidazol-2-one 3-Substituent

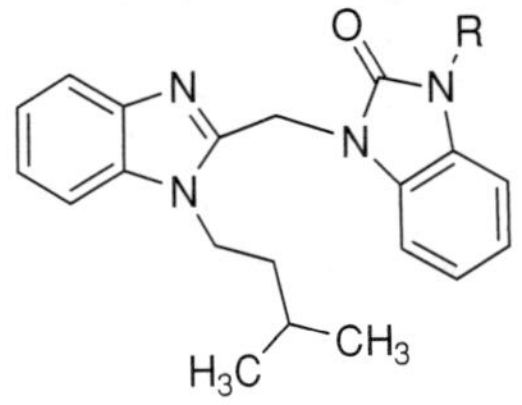

Entry Number	R	EC_{50} (nM)	CC_{50} (μM)
1	H	57	61.0
2	CH_2CH_3	11	18.6
3	$CH_2CH{=}CH_2$	16	12.8
4	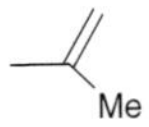	4	25.0
5	CH_2CN	28	46.8
6	$(CH_2)_3CN$	40	59.6
7	$(CH_2)_4CN$	35	15.0
8	$(CH_2)_5CN$	25	13.4
9	$CH_2{-}4{-}C_6H_4{-}OH$	18	59.9
10	$CH_2{-}4{-}C_6H_4{-}CN$	12	5.6
11	$CH_2{-}4{-}C_6H_4{-}SO_2CH_3$	9	7.5
12	$CONH_2$	50	133
13	CONHEt	52	18.7
14	CONHPh	41	21.6
15	$CONHCH_2Ph$	86	6.4
16	SO_2CH_3	7	16
17	$SO_2CH(CH_3)_2$	65	16.9
18	$SO_2N(CH_3)_2$	62	27.1

TABLE 3 Benzimidazole Substituent SAR

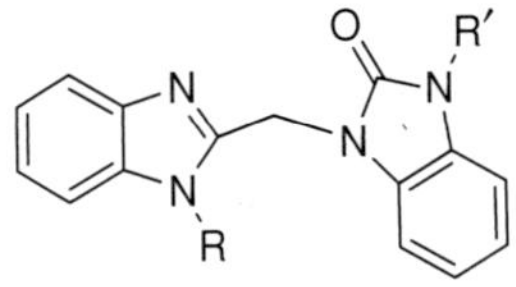

Entry Number	R	R′	EC_{50} (nM)	CC_{50} (μM)
1	$(CH_2)_2CH(CH_3)_2$	2-propenyl	4	25
2	$(CH_2)_2CH(CH_3)_2$	ethyl	11	18.6
3	$(CH_2)_2COCH_3$	2-propenyl	5	244.7
4	$(CH_2)_2CH(OH)CH_3$	2-propenyl	28	171.6
5	$(CH_2)_2OH$	ethyl	229	64.1
6	$(CH_2)_3OH$	ethyl	10	179.4
7	$(CH_2)_4OH$	ethyl	14	154
8	$(CH_2)_4OH$	2-propenyl	4	170.9
9	$(CH_2)_6OH$	2-propenyl	114	> 247.2
10	$(CH_2)_2CN$	2-propenyl	15	79.6
11	$(CH_2)_3CN$	2-propenyl	5	13.1
12	$(CH_2)_4CN$	2-propenyl	27	192.8
13	$(CH_2)_5CN$	2-propenyl	13	12.3
14	$(CH_2)_6CN$	2-propenyl	6	36.0/ > 241.8
15	$(CH_2)_3SO_2CH_3$	2-propenyl	30	123.3

the program, an aspect of the program that initially proved to be quite challenging. Many of the early compounds evaluated failed to demonstrate a significant antiviral effect in either model, despite examination of a wide range of dosing regimens that encompassed oral, intraperitoneal, and subcutaneous administration. Consequently, a decision was made to explore the potential to evaluate compounds delivered topically to lung tissue, and a collaboration was established with Philip Wyde in the Department of Molecular Virology and Microbiology at Baylor College of Medicine in Houston, Texas. The efficacy of small particle aerosol (SPA) delivery of antiviral agents had been demonstrated in models of both RSV and influenza in the cotton rat and mouse [49,50]. However, this approach imposed a significant demand on the physical properties of molecules to be evaluated, with an aqueous solubility of 10 mg/mL or greater targeted. In addition, compound requirements were typically high because it was necessary to conduct experiments in which animals were exposed to continuous SPA treatment for four consecutive days. The standard experimental protocol consumed approximately 600 mL of drug-containing solution for each 21-h period of aerosolization, and drug concentrations of up to 2 mg/mL were anticipated based on prior experience [49,50]. To identify compounds suitable for SPA delivery, the introduction of polar structural elements that would confer the required aqueous solubility on both the benzimidazole side chain and the benizimidzol-2-one 3-subsitituent was explored [51]. Fortunately, the pharmacophore for potent RSV inhibition was tolerant of the introduction of both basic and acidic moieties to either heterocycle, provided that these elements were deployed several atoms remote from the core [51]. Although basic amine derivatives were examined and provided potent RSV inhibitors, a series of mono- and diacidic compounds offered not only excellent antiviral properties but also reliably high levels of aqueous solubility when formulated as their salts. Consequently, this chemotype became the focus with which proof-of-concept was established in an animal model [51]. A broad range of acidic moieties were probed, encompassing carboxylic, sulfonic, and phosphonic acids, in addition to several carboxylic acid isosteres [51]. Representative compounds are compiled in Figure 2 and Table 4, from which several compounds were selected for evaluation in the in vivo experiment [51]. The four representative compounds depicted in Figure 2 demonstrated antiviral activity in the cotton rat, measured as a reduction in lung viral titers after sacrifice of the animals at day 4 post-inoculation, the peak of viral replication in this model. The phosphonic acid **4** reduced lung viral titers by 2.0 $\log_{10}$ compared to the control at a concentration of 2 mg/mL in the SPA solution, but lower concentrations of 0.01, 0.05, and 0.2 mg/mL were ineffective. The oxadiazolone **5** demonstrated identical efficacy to **4**, but at the lower concentration of 0.5 mg/mL in the aerosol solution, while the aspartic acid derivative **6** reduced lung viral titers by 1.5 $\log_{10}$ at a concentration of 2.0 mg/mL. Finally, from this series, the sulfonic acid **7** was associated with a 1.85 $\log_{10}$ reduction in viral titers at a concentration of 1.6 mg/mL. The efficacy of these four compounds was comparable to that observed with ribavirin, used as a control, which reduced viral titers by 1.6 $\log_{10}$ after intraperitoneal administration at a dose of 90 mg/kg b.i.d. [51].

Having established the efficacy of RSV fusion inhibitors in vivo following topical delivery, attention was redirected toward the original objective of identifying compounds with activity following oral dosing. Using the BALB/c mouse model, the oxadiazolone **5** reproducibly demonstrated efficacy, reducing viral titers by a modest but statistically significant 0.84 $\log_{10}$ and 0.93 $\log_{10}$ in successive experiments following subcutaneous dosing of 120 mg/kg. This was a key milestone for the program since it established that this class of RSV inhibitor had the potential to interfere with viral replication in the lung following systemic delivery. The amino ester **8** was subsequently selected for evaluation in this model, with the recognition that metabolism to the corresponding carboxylic acid **9** would very likely occur in vivo. However, since both compounds demonstrated potent RSV inhibition in cell culture with EC_{50}s of 15 and 196 nM, respectively, this was not viewed as an impediment to success. Subcutaneous administration of **8** at a dose of 50 mg/kg b.i.d. to infected mice reproducibly produced about a 1.0 $\log_{10}$ decrease in lung viral titers [51]. More important, oral administration of **8** at the same dose resulted in a positive effect, measured as an 0.89 $\log_{10}$ reduction in viral titers. The acid **9** was indeed detected in the plasma of infected mice, and oral administration of this compound at 50 mg/kg b.i.d. resulted in a small but statistically insignificant reduction in viral titers, and reduced efficacy, which presumably reflects the lower potency or, possibly, lower exposure in vivo [51]. To address the metabolic lability of **8**, the dimethylamide analog **10** was prepared, and although the potency of this compound was comparable to the acid **9**, $EC_{50} = 250$ nM, it showed good efficacy in the BALB/c mouse model following oral dosing at both 50 and 15 mg/kg b.i.d., producing 1.32 $\log_{10}$ and 0.82 $\log_{10}$ reductions in viral titers, respectively.

The amide moiety of **10** fulfilled the objective of increasing metabolic stability toward cleavage to the acid **9** in mouse and human liver microsomes, but the compound was extensively metabolized under these conditions. The major metabolic pathways were identified as demethylation of both the dimethylamine side chain and the amide moiety in addition to hydroxylation of both heterocyclic rings. This observation provided a clear focus for structural optimization, and with a reasonable understanding of the SAR associated with the substituents appended to both heterocycles, attention was focused initially on the effect of reducing the electron density of the benzimidazol-2-one ring by the introduction of a nitrogen atom. A survey of the four possible azabenzimidazol-2-one isomers was conducted in the context of a butyronitrile side chain attached to the benzimidazole, with structural

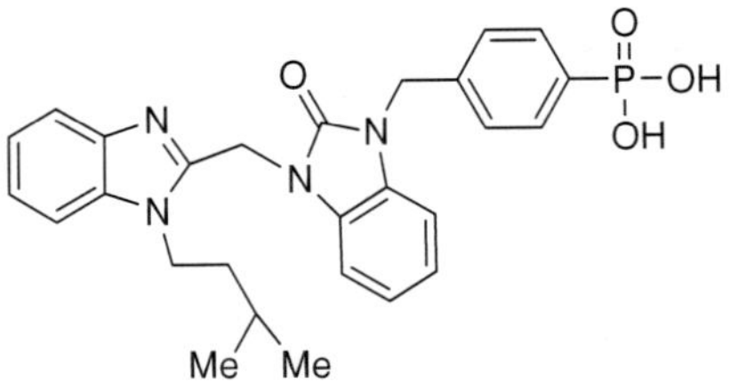

4
EC_{50} = 27 nM
CC_{50} = >175 μM

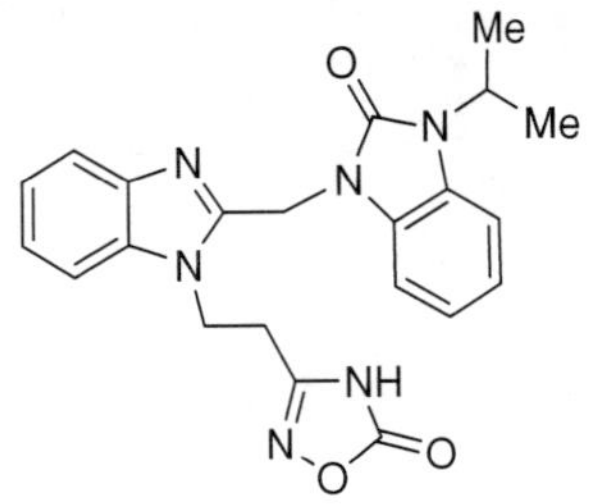

5
EC_{50} = 21 nM
CC_{50} = 75.5 μM

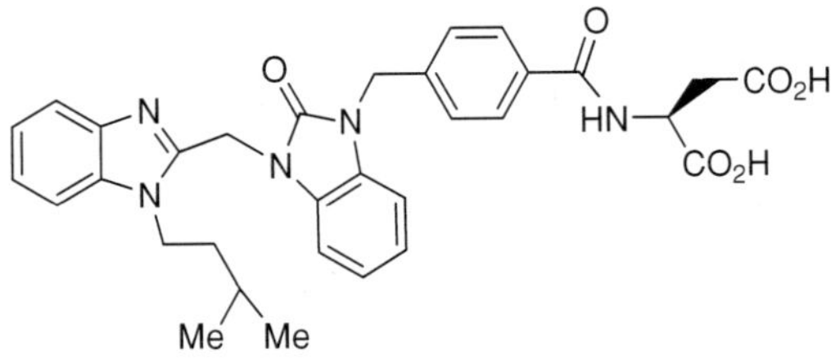

6
EC_{50} = 5 nM
CC_{50} = >144 μM

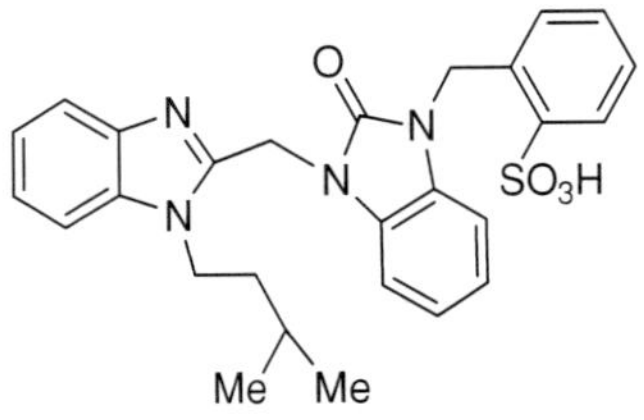

7
EC_{50} = 7 nM
CC_{50} = >19 μM

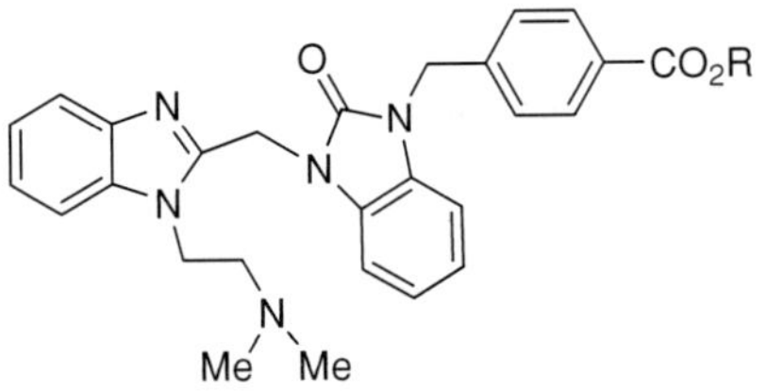

8: R = Me
EC_{50} = 15 nM
CC_{50} = 24 μM
HLM $T_{1/2}$ = 0.55 min

9: R = H

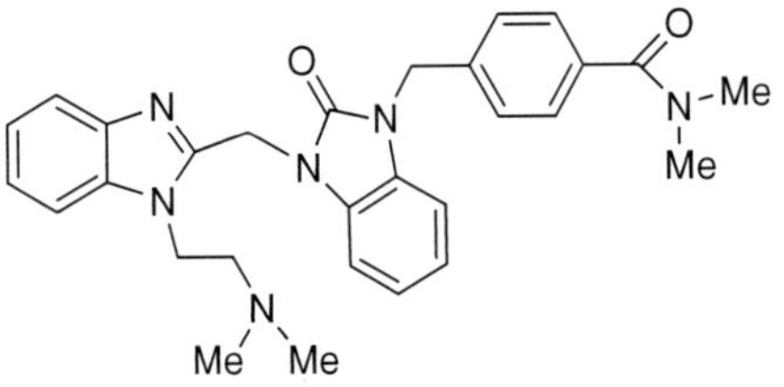

10
EC_{50} = 250 nM
CC_{50} = 39 μM
HLM $T_{1/2}$ = 1.8 min

FIGURE 2 Water-soluble compounds with activity in the cotton rat following topical exposure.

variation of the azabenzimidazole substituent examined to confirm trends [52]. The results of this survey, which are compiled in Table 5, provided a clear understanding of the requirements for potent RSV inhibition, revealing that 6- and 7-azabenzimidazol-2-ones are comparable to the identically substituted benzimidazol-2-one analogs, while the 4- and 5-isomers offer inferior antiviral properties [52]. Consequently, the 6- and 7-azabenzimidazol-2-ones became the focus of further optimization efforts, with considerable bias toward the 6-isomer since synthetic access to this topology was generally more facile. Small lipophilic elements were installed as the azabenzimidazol-2-one N-substituent, selected based on the anticipation of increased metabolic stability and leading to a tight focus on cyclopropyl, cyclobutyl, CHF_2, and CH_2CF_3 across the two series. A somewhat broader variation of the benzimidazole side chain was examined, and compounds were triaged based on antiviral potency, stability in human liver microsomal (HLM) preparations, and permeability across a confluent layer of Caco-2 cells. A half-life in HLM of >30 min was considered to extrapolate to intermediate clearance in humans, and a permeability coefficient of >100 nm/s predicted good absorption, with target parameters based on the performance of standard reference agents. The data for key compounds are compiled in Table 6 and reveal the optimal combination of substituents to address the three key parameters used to triage compounds. This process narrowed the candidates of interest to the five compounds, **11** to **15**, depicted in Figure 3 that possessed in vitro profiles predictive of exposure in vivo. However, although the sulfone-containing compounds **13** to **15** offered superior metabolic stability, their Caco-2 permeability was lower than that predictive of absorption, reflected in the observation

TABLE 4 Antiviral Activity Associated with RSV Inhibitors Incorporating Acidic Side Chains

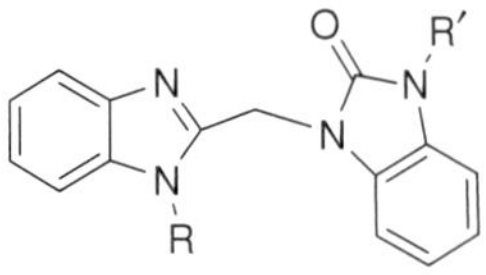

Entry Number	R	R′	EC_{50} (nM)	CC_{50} (μM)
1	$(CH_2)_2CH(CH_3)_2$	CH_2CO_2H	163	194.3′
2	$(CH_2)_2CH(CH_3)_2$	$CH_2CH_2CO_2H$	15	102
3	$(CH_2)_2CH(CH_3)_2$	$CH_2CH_2CH_2CO_2H$	75	138.2
4	$(CH_2)_2CH(CH_3)_2$	$CH_2CH_2CH_2CH_2CO_2H$	8	16.5
5	$(CH_2)_2CH(CH_3)_2$	$CH_2CH_2CH_2CH_2CH_2CO_2H$	15	16.5
6	$(CH_2)_2CH(CH_3)_2$	$CH_2CH_2CH_2CH_2CN_4H$	15	14.9
7	$(CH_2)_2CH(CH_3)_2$	$CH_2CH_2CH_2CH_2CH_2CN_4H$	13	90.0
8	$(CH_2)_2CH(CH_3)_2$	$CH_2CH_2CH_2SO_3H$	38	114.5/>209
9	$(CH_2)_2CH(CH_3)_2$	$CH_2CH_2CH_2CH_2SO_3H$	52	2.9
10	$(CH_2)_2CH(CH_3)_2$	CH_2-4-C_6H_4-CO_2H	11	27.3
11	$(CH_2)_2CH(CH_3)_2$	CH_2-3-C_6H_4-CO_2H	10	10.7
12	$(CH_2)_2CH(CH_3)_2$	CH_2-4-C_6H_4-CH_2-PO_3H_2	51	2.8
13	CH_2CN_4H	2-propenyl	8437	181/>227
14	$CH_2CH_2(CN_4H)$	2-propenyl	8	> 249
15	$CH_2CH_2CH_2(CN_4H)$	2-propenyl	14	> 0.33

of poor bioavailability in the rat and monkey. Ultimately, BMS-433771 (**12**) was selected for development, and the full profile of this compound is compiled in Tables 7 and 8.

TABLE 5 Azabenzimidazol-2-one-Based Inhibitors of RSV

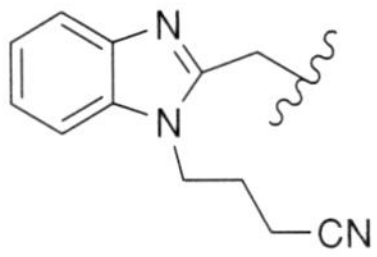

Ring System	R	EC_{50} (nM)	CC_{50} (μM)
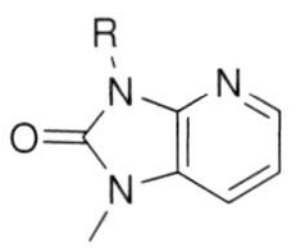	2-propenyl	202	149.8
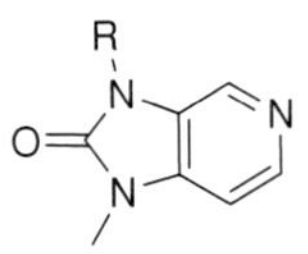	H	5710	263.9
	CH_2-4-C_6H_4-SO_2CH_3	75	40.9
	CH_2-4-C_6H_4-CN	622	36.8
	SO_2iPr	237	>228
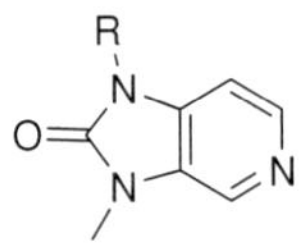	2-propenyl	6	236.6
	CH_2-4-C_6H_4-SO_2CH_3	<2.3	1.98
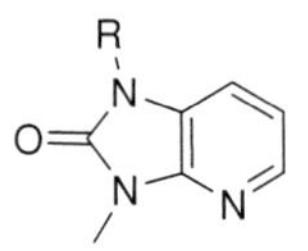	2-propenyl	3	>216

PRECLINICAL PROFILE OF BMS-433771

In Vitro Studies

BMS-433771 (**12**) was found to be a potent in vitro inhibitor of RSV replication in tissue culture that protected HEp-2 cells from RSV A Long strain–induced CPE with an EC_{50} of 12 nM [30]. However, cell protection assays are an indirect means of examining virus titers since they measure the apparent health of an infected cell through analysis of mitochondrial function. To examine viral replication directly, a virus-specific radiolabeling experiment was used. This assay measured virus-specific protein synthesis directly, and BMS-433771 (**12**) was shown to inhibit the Long strain of RSV with an EC_{50} value of 13 nM. Therefore, cell protection by BMS-433771 (**12**) was directly comparable to inhibition of new RSV protein expression. BMS-433771 (**12**) maintained excellent potency against multiple laboratory and clinical isolates of both group A and B viruses, with a median EC_{50} value in the protein synthesis assay of 20.4 nM [30]. The compound is a highly selective inhibitor of RSV replication, as it was inactive against all other viruses tested, including Sendai, parainfluenza-3, influenza, vesicular stomatitis, human immunodeficiency viruses and human rhinovirus [30].

The collective results from studies using the original lead compound, several prototypes, and BMS-433771 (**12**) suggested that the mechanism of action underlying the antiviral activity of this chemotype was inhibition of virus and host-cell membrane fusion [30]. Time-of-addition experiments showed that BMS-433771 (**12**) acts at an early stage in the virus replication cycle, and reversibility studies determined

TABLE 6 In Vitro Antiviral Activity, Metabolic Stability, and Caco-2 cell Permeability of Azabenzimidazol-2-one-Based RSV Inhibitors

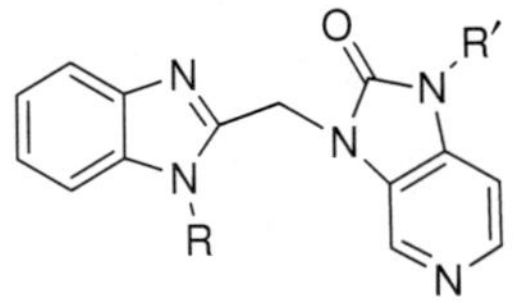

Entry Number	R	R′	EC_{50} (nM)	CC_{50} (μM)	HLM $t_{1/2}$ (min)	Caco-2 Cell Permeability (nm/s)
1	$(CH_2)_3CN$	*i*-Pr	4	> 55.6	7.4	169
2	$(CH_2)_3CN$	*t*-Bu	3	> 86.8	4.0	214
3	$(CH_2)_3CN$	*c*-Bu	16	> 258.8	4.6	168
4	$(CH_2)_3CN$	CH_2CF_3	15	> 195	12.3	197
5	$(CH_2)_3OH$	*c*-Pr	43	245.0	18	115
6	$(CH_2)_5OH$	*c*-Pr	13	> 229.5	18	96
7	$(CH_2)_3SO_2CH_3$	*c*-Pr	5	> 227	77	27
8	$(CH_2)_3SO_2CH_3$	*c*-Bu	21	> 227	5.3	
9	$(CH_2)_3SO_2C_2H_5$	*c*-Pr	6	> 227	37	34
10	$(CH_2)_4F$	*c*-Pr	10	158.4	11	247
11	$(CH_2)_4F$	CH_2CF_3	15	189.9	17	245
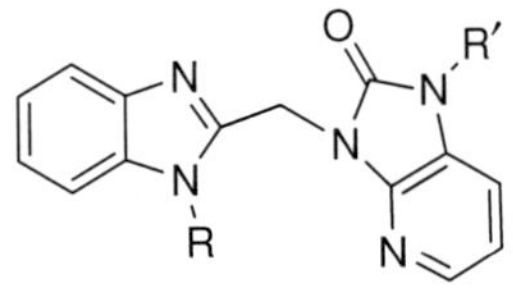						
12	$(CH_2)_3CN$	2-propenyl	3	> 216	11	230
13	$(CH_2)_3CN$	*c*-Pr	29	> 181	45	166
14	$(CH_2)_3CN$	CHF_2	11	> 205	84	188
15	$(CH_2)_4OH$	*c*-Pr	10	> 211	34	130
16	$(CH_2)_3SO_2CH_3$	*c*-Pr	9	> 230	> 100	39

that inhibition occurred at a step that remained susceptible to antibody neutralization. These observations clearly indicated that the inhibitory activity was occurring prior to virus penetration. However, it was also shown that the compound could act at a late stage in the infection cycle when added subsequent to the establishment of a productive infection *via* inhibition of syncytia formation. Taken together, these data were consistent with inhibition of fusion as the mechanism of action for BMS-433771 (**12**).

Additional evidence in support of fusion inhibition by BMS-433771 (**12**) was the finding that viruses isolated from cell culture exhibiting resistance to the compound had single amino acid changes in the F1 subunit of the F protein. Using a reverse genetics approach, it was shown that one of these changes, a single lysine to arginine change at amino acid position 394 within the F1 subunit, was responsible for resistance to BMS-433771 (**12**) [30]. To demonstrate direct binding of this series to the RSV fusion protein, the diazirine **16** was prepared as a radiolabeled photoaffinity reagent (Fig. 4) [55]. Irradiation of this probe with ultraviolet light in the presence of virus induced specific cross-linking with the F1 subunit of the RSV fusion protein (FP), a critical element in the fusion process [56]. This polypeptide contains a hydrophobic, fusogenic amino terminus that is hypothesized to insert into the target cellular membrane during the fusion process [57].

TABLE 7 In Vitro Antiviral Profile of BMS-433771 (12)

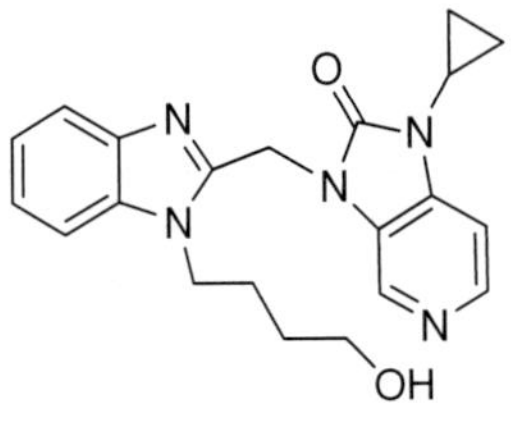

RSV EC_{50}	10 nM
CC_{50}	>218 μM
Average EC_{50} toward RSV A and B clinical isolates	20 nM
EC_{50} for inhibition of parainfluenza-3 virus, Sendai virus, VSV, influenza, human rhinovirus, poliovirus, HIV, HCMV, HSV, BVDV	>25 μM

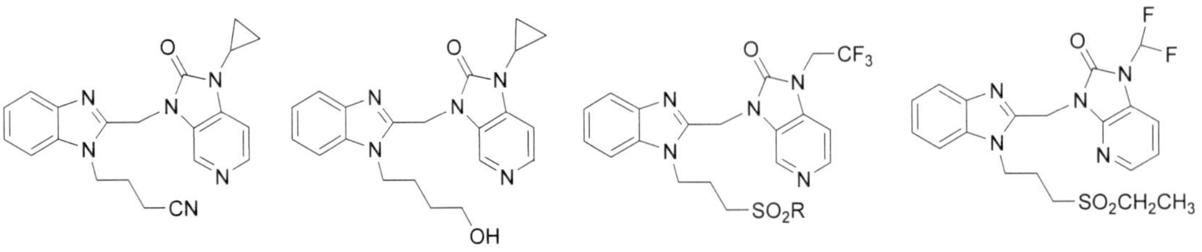

11
EC_{50} = 0.010 μM
CC_{50} = 236 μM
HLM $T_{1/2}$ = 38 min
Caco-2: 181 nM/s

12
EC_{50} = 0.010 μM
CC_{50} = >218 μM
HLM $T_{1/2}$ = 36 min
Caco-2: 143 nM/s

13
R = CH_3
EC_{50} = 0.012 μM
CC_{50} = 236 μM
HLM $T_{1/2}$ = 87 min
Caco-2: 33 nM/s

14
R = CH_2CH_3
EC_{50} = 0.004 μM
CC_{50} = 236 μM
HLM $T_{1/2}$ = 36 min
Caco-2: 92 nM/s

15
EC_{50} = 0.006 μM
CC_{50} = 236 μM
HLM $T_{1/2}$ = 55 min
Caco-2: 59 nM/s

FIGURE 3 The five final candidates.

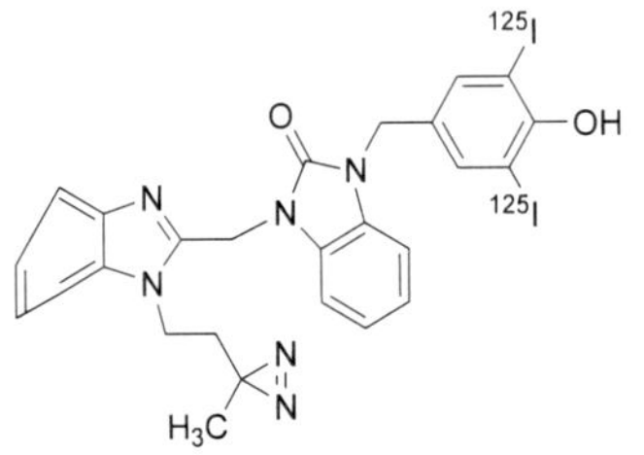

16

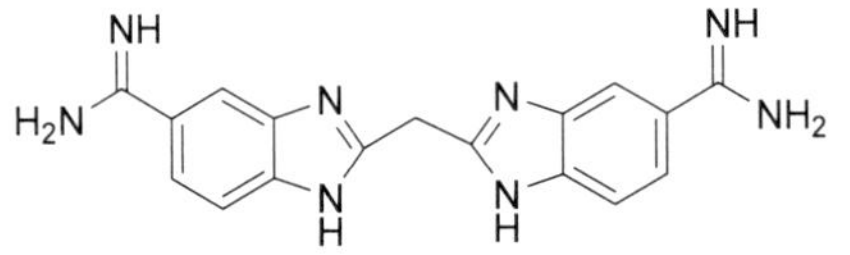

17 (BABIM)

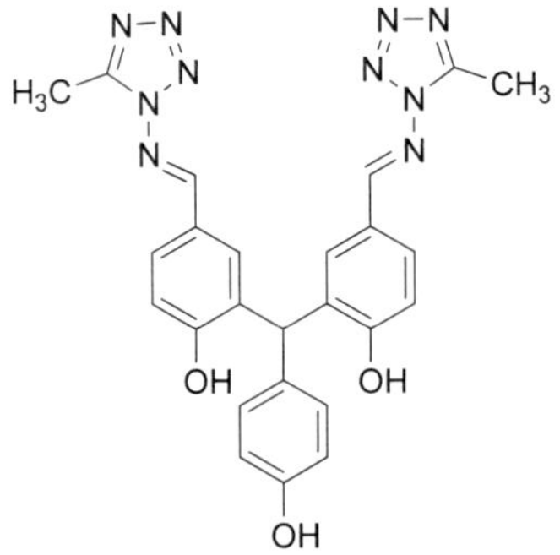

18 (VP-14637)

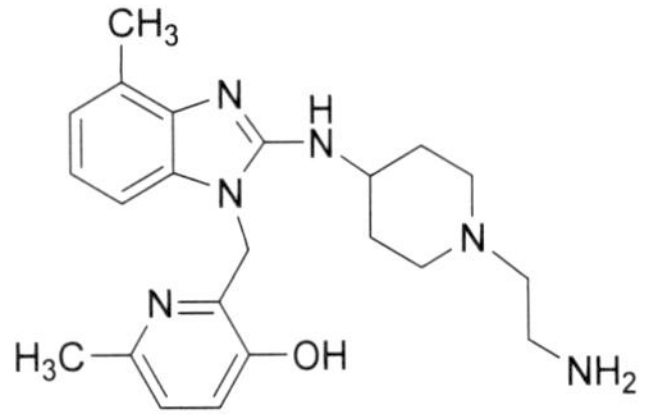

19 (JNJ-2408068)

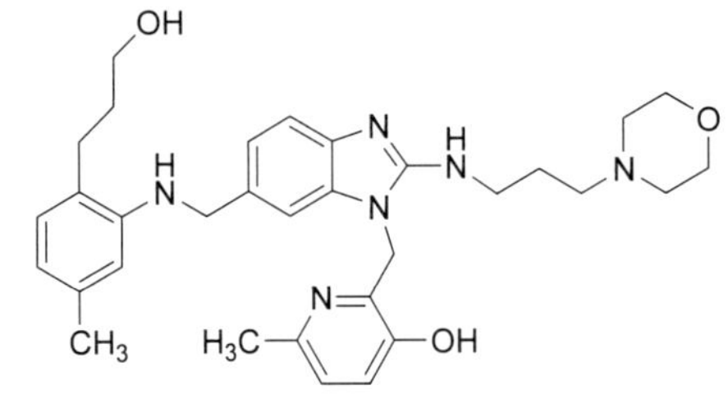

20 (TMC-353121)

FIGURE 4 Inhibitors of RSV fusion.

TABLE 8 In Vivo Profile of BMS-433771 (12)

	Mouse	Rat	Dog	Monkey
i.v. dose (mg/kg)	2	1	1	1
Cl (mL/min/kg)	99	61	12	7.3
Cl class	High	High	Intermediate	Intermediate
Vd_{ss} (L/kg)	0.65	0.57	1.3	2.9
Terminal $t_{1/2}$ (min)	4.9	8.9	271	618
p.o. dose (mg/kg)	10	5	5	5
F (%)	32	13	72	42
C_{max} (μg/mL)	1.9	0.19	3.5	0.99
Apparent terminal $t_{1/2}$ (min)	8.2	Cannot be determined	291	683

Adjacent to the fusion peptide is an N-terminal heptad repeat (HR-N), while a complementary C-terminal heptad repeat (HR-C) region is located proximal to the F1 transmembrane spanning domain [58,59].

Peptide mapping of the F1 photoaffinity-labeled site revealed that the attachment point was within the HR-N sequence [56]. Further studies using a trimeric assembly of a synthetic HR-N peptide allowed for direct peptide sequencing and localized the labeling site of the affinity probe primarily to Y198, a residue found to line a previously identified hydrophobic cavity formed when the N-terminal heptad repeats assemble into the trimeric complex [59]. Somewhat presciently, it was speculated that this binding pocket, located inside the deep groove of the HR-N57 heptad repeat trimer, had the potential to accommodate small-molecule inhibitors that might interfere with the function of the RSV F protein [59]. Two key aromatic residues from the C-terminal heptad repeat, Phe483 and Phe488, along with Ile492, are accommodated within this cavity in an interaction thought to be important in the formation of the six-helix bundle (Fig. 5A). Computer-based modeling studies based on intimate knowledge of the SAR placed BMS-433771 (**12**) and related compounds in this cavity in a fashion such that the two heterocyclic ring systems occupied the precise positions filled by Phe483, Phe488, and Ile492 [56]. This binding pose oriented the photoreactive diazirine of the photoaffinity probe toward Y198 in the HR-N cavity.

In Vivo Studies

Mice dosed orally with BMS-433771 (**12**) prior to challenge with an inoculation of RSV exhibited reduced viral titers in the lungs [53]. Intriguingly, a single dose of BMS-433771 (**12**) administered prophylactically provided efficacy equivalent to that observed when multiple doses of drug were administered postinfection, provided that the drug was administered prior to RSV inoculation. Dose titration studies established a dose–response relationship and demonstrated substantial inhibition with doses as low as 5 mg/kg [53]. That the viral titer reduction in the animal model was specific was proven by using RSV selected to be resistant to this class of fusion inhibitor. BMS-433771 (**12**) exhibited no significant antiviral activity toward the resistant virus in the mouse model. This established that the mechanism of inhibition in vivo was most likely via inhibition of viral-induced membrane fusion. Curiously, when treatment was initiated in a therapeutic regimen, an experiment in which compound was dosed after RSV inoculation, no specific inhibition was observed. This phenomenon has also been observed with other RSV fusion inhibitors and may be an indication of the limitations of this animal model [54]. BMS-433771 (**12**) was also evaluated for prophylactic efficacy against RSV in the cotton rat model of infection. Once again, a single oral dose administered 1 h prior to intratracheal inoculation with virus was able to reduce viral lung titers or titers obtained from lung lavage [53]. A dose–response relationship was observed, with doses approaching 50 mg/kg required to obtain greater than a 1 $\log_{10}$ reduction in titer. Thus, BMS-433771 (**12**) demonstrated efficacy in two separate rodent models of RSV infection.

The preclinical pharmacokinetic properties of BMS-433771 (**12**) in four animal species are presented in Table 8, and additional profiling data are summarized in Table 9. The oral bioavailability ranged from 13 to 72%, with the highest bioavailability observed in dogs, and the high volume of distribution suggested that the compound readily entered tissues from the blood. Total body clearance varied, ranging from 99 mL/min/kg in mice to 7.3 mL·min/kg in monkeys, yielding an apparent half-life that ranged from 0.08 h in mice to 10 h in monkeys (Table 8). Allometric scaling predicted a favorable half-life of 8 h in humans, and a human dose of 500 mg b.i.d. assuming 50% bioavailability. Protein binding ranged from 63% in dog plasma to 92% in human plasma, with a blood-to-plasma ratio of 0.84 in the human samples. The permeability of BMS-433771 (**12**) across a confluent layer of human bronchial epithelial cells was high, indicative of good lung penetration.

SYNTHESIS OF BMS-433771

The nomination of BMS-433771 (**12**) as a clinical candidate necessitated the development of significant quantities of material to support toxicological studies and the early clinical program. The synthetic approach utilized by the discovery group to map out the SAR and the reported process route to access BMS-433771 (**12**) are based on a similar

TABLE 9 In Vitro Properties Associated with BMS-433771 (12)

Property	Value
Human plasma protein binding	92%
Caco-2 permeability at pH 6.5	143 nm/s
Calu-3 permeability from blood to airway	82 nm/s at 1 μg/mL
Log *P*	1.9
Solubility of crystalline free base	0.09 mg/mL at pH 6.3
Solubility of bis-HCl salt	545 mg/mL at pH 0.9
pK_a	3.4 (benzimidazole) 5.7 (azabenzimidazolone)
Melting point of free base	196.4°C
Ames microbial mutagenicity study with *Salmonella typhimurium* tester strains TA98 and TA100	Not mutagenic up to 5000 μg/plate

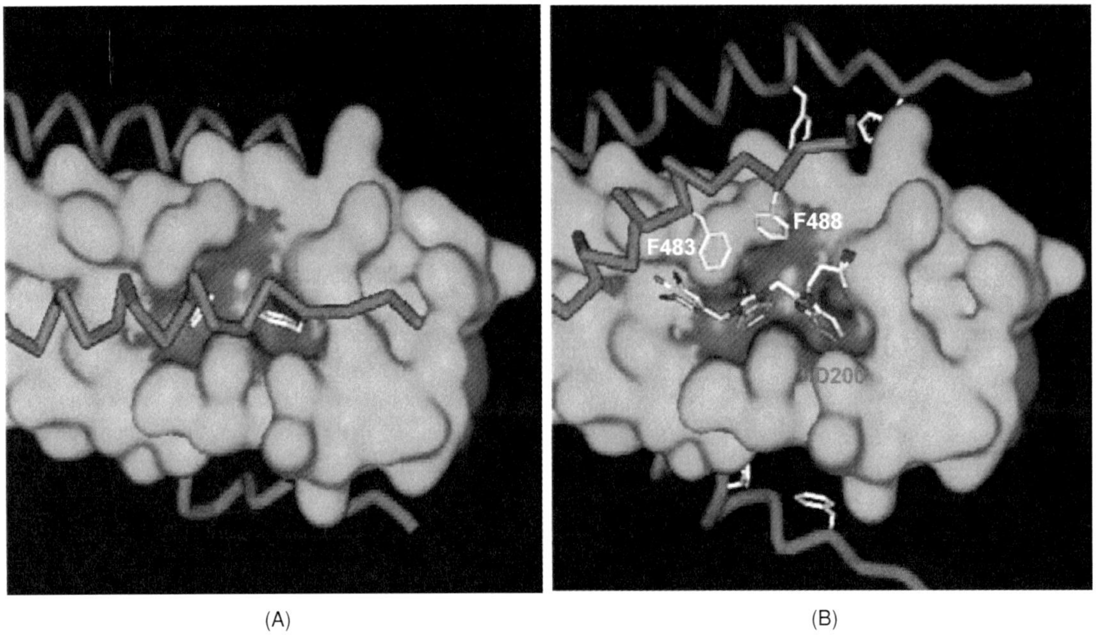

FIGURE 5 (A) Segment of the six-helix bundle of the RSV F protein in its fusogenic conformation with the assembled trimeric N-terminal heptad repeat (HR-N) depicted as a green surface showing Phe483 and Phe488 of the C-terminal heptad repeat (HR-C) projecting into the HR-N hydrophobic pocket. The peptide backbone of HR-C is shown as a red stick with the side-chain elements of residues Phe483 and Phe488 highlighted in white. These key amino acids reside in the HR-N hydrophobic pocket. (B) Model of the photoaffinity label **16** bound into the HR-N hydrophobic pocket with the orientation postulated based on known SAR and placing the diazirine moiety proximal to Tyr198. The peptide backbone of HR-C and Phe483 and Phe488 are depicted as displaced merely to accommodate **16** and are not intended to suggest specific mechanistic insight into the precise mode of action of this class of RSV fusion inhibitor. D200 is labeled in red. (*See insert for color representation of the figure.*)

retrosynthetic approach, with optimization of the process approach to accommodate practical aspects associated with reagents, conditions and availability of starting materials (Fig. 6) [60]. The azabenzimidazol-2-one moiety was prepared by heating 4-methoxy-3-nitropyridine with cyclopropylamine in the presence of di-*iso*-propylethylamine (Hunig's base) in EtOH at reflux for 3 h to effect an S_NAr displacement of MeOH that afforded the product in > 90% yield. Hydrogenation of the NO_2 moiety under palladium on charcoal catalysis followed by exposure of the diamine to carbonyldiimidazole provided the substituted azabenzimidazolone in 70% overall yield. The benzimidazole fragment was obtained from 2-hydroxymethylbenzimidazole by alkylation with 4-iodobutyl pivalate in acetone using KOH as the base at 50°C for 2.5 h. Conversion of the alcohol to the chloride was accomplished using the Vilsmeier reagent in DMF, with the product isolable as the HCl salt in > 95% yield; however, to avoid exposure to a mutagenic alkylating agent, this material was telescoped directly into the subsequent coupling reaction. Coupling of the chloride and the azabenzimidazol-2-one was achieved optimally in a mixture of dimethylacetamide (DMA) and DMF using KOH as the base under carefully controlled conditions designed to avoid pivaloate cleavage. The product was isolated by adding a 2.8 M solution of ammonium chloride to the organic phase followed by seeding with a small amount of the product, affording crystalline pivaloate in 86% yield over the two steps. This material was straightforwardly cleaved to the alcohol using 2 equivalents of NaOH in EtOH heated at 70°C, which provided crystalline BMS-433771 in 85 to 90% yield. This process was used to prepare the kilogram quantities of BMS-433771 (**12**) required for preclinical toxicology evaluation and early clinical studies [60]. Data from toxicological studies conducted in three animal species suggested a promising safety profile, with no observations that would preclude the initiation of human studies.

SAR EVOLUTION POST BMS-433771

The proposed mode of binding of RSV fusion inhibitors to the hydrophobic pockets created by the association of the three N-terminal heptad repeats of the F protein suggested that the introduction of substituents at C7 of the benzimidazole heterocycle would be poorly tolerated while there would be some tolerance for substitution at C4 (Fig. 5B). In contrast, C5 and C6 were predicted to accommodate only small substituents with both sites proximal to Asp200 and readily providing vectorial access to this residue. A synopsis of the survey conducted to explore this aspect of SAR

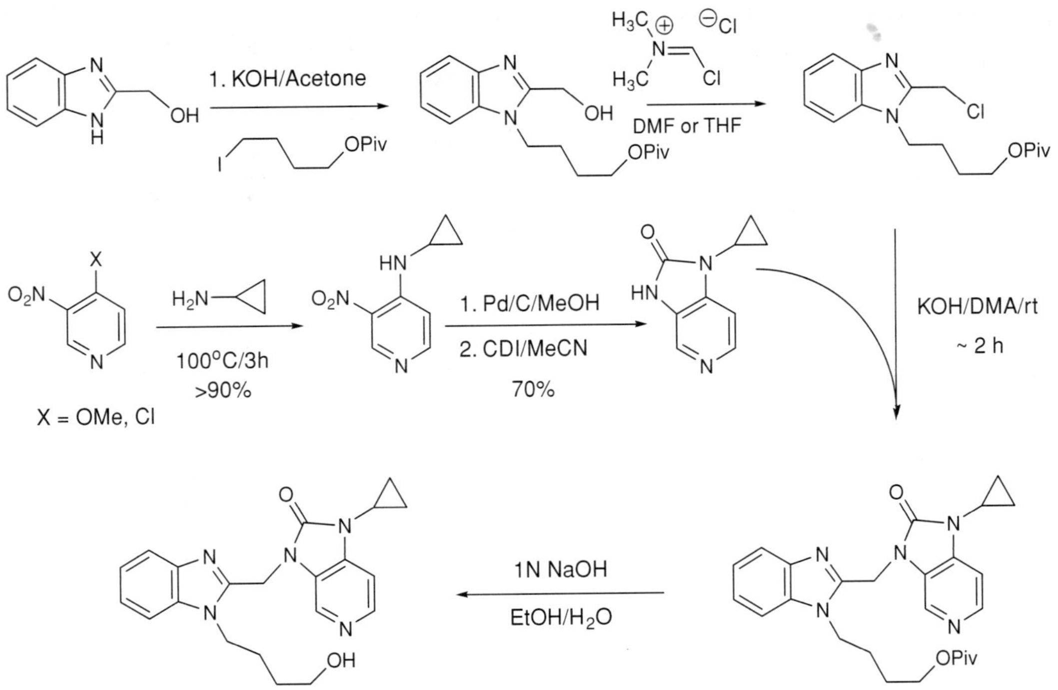

FIGURE 6 Synthesis of BMS-433771 (**12**).

is presented in Table 10 [61]. The data are consistent with the predictions of the computer-aided modeling hypothesis, with substituents at C7 uniformly poorly active while C4 was more accommodating, although substitution reduced antiviral activity compared to the parent [61]. At C6, a CH_2NH_2 substituent afforded good potency (Table 10, entry 4) but the homolog (Table 10, entry 4) was poorly active, while the analogous alcohol was similarly potent (Table 10, entry 6). In contrast, a carboxylic acid or carboxamide at C6 provided compounds essentially inactive (Table 10, entries 7 and 8). At C5, both a CH_2NH_2 and CH_2OH substituent exhibited good potency, while the carboxylic acid was inactive and the carboxamide offered intermediate potency (Table 10, entries 9 to 12). This prompted a deeper survey of C5 substitution, summarized in part in Table 10, entries 16 to 24, that provided SAR data consistent with an intimate interaction between this substituent and Asp200. Steric bulk on the benzylic CH_2 or the primary amine or homologation of the amine moiety in either direction eroded antiviral activity. Amidines and hydroxyamidines were equally well tolerated, the latter reinforcing the observation with the CH_2OH substituent that overt basicity is not a requirement for potent antiviral activity, an observation that presumably reflects a productive hydrogen-bonding interaction [61]. The potent RSV inhibitory activity associated with the 5-CH_2NH_2 derivative was unmasked most effectively when presented to the K394R virus developed to be resistant to BMS-433771 (**12**) (EC_{50} > 20 μM). The 5-CH_2NH_2 derivative half-maximally inhibited replication of the resistant virus at a concentration of 20 nM, which is over 1000-fold more potent than BMS-433771 (**12**). These results opened up a new avenue of structural modification with the potential to provide compounds with a higher genetic barrier to resistance.

Recognition of the importance of a basic amine or amidine moiety at C5 of BMS-433771 (**12**) and related compounds [62,63] provides an interesting coalescence of structural overlap with *bis*-(5-amidino-2-benzimidazolyl) methane (BABIM, **17**), a potent and broad-spectrum trypsin-like serine protease inhibitor that has been characterized as an inhibitor of RSV fusion [64–68]. The two heterocycles of BABIM (**17**) and their topological relationship are very similar to the benzotriazole **2**, a shape accommodated by the hydrophobic binding pocket formed in the RSV HR-N trimer after assembly. Although lacking the side chain found in **2**, BMS-433771 (**12**) and all of the other potent RSV fusion inhibitors described in this chapter, the presence of an amidine moiety in BABIM (**17**) capable of interacting with Asp200 would be anticipated to provide a productive and important compensating interaction. In our hands, the antiviral potency of BABIM (**17**) is somewhat modest, with EC_{50} = 100 nM toward the Long A strain of RSV, but point mutations in virus developed to be resistant to this compound revealed a F140I change that showed cross-resistance to BMS-433771 (**12**), suggesting a common mode of action [30,61]. In addition, several additional and structurally diverse inhibitors of RSV fusion have been described in the recent literature, including VP-14637 (**18**), JNJ-2408068 (R1750591, **19**), and TMC-353121 (**20**), which appear to function by interacting with

TABLE 10 Effect of Benzimidazole Substitution on Antiviral Activity

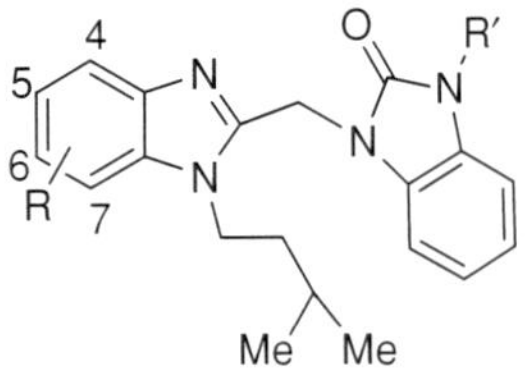

Entry Number	R	R′	EC_{50} (μM)	CC_{50} (μM)
1	7-CH_2NH_2	*i*-Pr	192	11.0
2	7-CH_2OH	*i*-Pr	246	246
3	7-CO_2CH_3	*i*-Pr	230	25.3
4	6-CH_2NH_2	*i*-Pr	0.095	28.1
5	6-$CH_2CH_2NH_2$	*i*-Pr	7.11	57.0
6	6-CH_2OH	*i*-Pr	0.134	81.6
7	6-CO_2H	*i*-Pr	238	125
8	6-$CONH_2$	*i*-Pr	123	49.9
9	5-CH_2NH_2	*i*-Pr	0.002	3.92
10	5-CH_2OH	*i*-Pr	0.050	31.6
11	5-CO_2H	*i*-Pr	238	17.3
12	5-$CONH_2$	*i*-Pr	0.166	23.4
13	4-CH_2NH_2	*i*-Pr	0.715	7.00
14	4-CH_2OH	*i*-Pr	0.82	22.0
15	4-CO_2CH_3	*i*-Pr	230	49.2

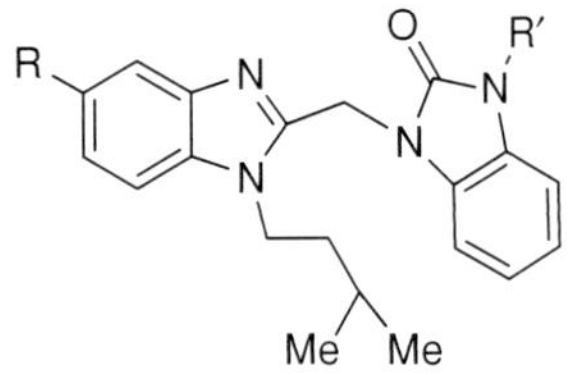

16	5-NH_2	*i*-Pr	0.125	32.2
17	5-$CH_2CH_2NH_2$	*i*-Pr	0.002	3.92
18	5-CH_2NHCH_3	*i*-Pr	0.057	1.48
19	5-$CH_2N(CH_3)_2$	*i*-Pr	183	5.65
20	5-$CH_2NH{\cdot}CO{\cdot}CH_3$	*i*-Pr	0.631	178
21	5-$C(CH_3)_2NH_2$	*i*-Pr	0.694	3.27
22	5-C(NH)NH_2	2-propenyl	0.004	10.8
23	5-C(NOH)NH_2	2-propenyl	0.005	3.47
24	5-C(NOH)NH_2	*i*-Pr	0.111	9.14

the N-terminal heptad repeat trimer [69–76]. However, only TMC-353121 (**20**) demonstrates antiviral activity in vivo following oral administration to cotton rats, although oral bioavailability in Sprague-Dawley rats was modest at 14% and the compound was slowly absorbed [73,74]. The other RSV fusion inhibitors have demonstrated antiviral activity in vivo only after topical administration [75,76].

FINAL COMMENTS

We have described the discovery and optimization of a series of RSV fusion inhibitors into compounds with potent and selective antiviral activity in cell culture and in two animal models of infection following oral dosing. BMS-433771 (**12**) and its close analogs were the first fusion inhibitors to demonstrate oral bioavailability. Unfortunately, further development of BMS-433771 (**12**) leading to clinical evaluation was not pursued, a consequence of a realignment of Bristol-Myers Squibb's business interests.

Acknowledgments

As with all contemporary drug discovery efforts, the success of this program was dependent on the contributions of an effective interdisciplinary team, and we would like to acknowledge the following colleagues: Kuo-Long Yu, Ny Sin, Xiangdong Alan Wang, Jan W. Thuring, Keith D. Combrink, H. Belgin Gulgeze, Bradley C. Pearce, Zhiwei Yin, Rita L. Civeillo, Ashok K. Trehan, and Brian L. Venables, all members of the Department of Chemistry; Yaxiong Sun and David R. Langley in the Department of Computer-Aided Drug Design; Zheng Yang and Lisa Zadjura in the Department of Metabolism and Pharmacokinetics; and Junius Clarke, Eugene Genovesi, Kathleen F. Kadow, Lucinda Lamb, Ivette Medina, Stacey Voss, Julia Roach, Zhufang Li, and Guangxiang Luo in the Department of Infectious Disease. We also wish to thank J. J. Kim Wright and Richard J. Colonno for their leadership and support throughout this work.

REFERENCES

[1] Chanock, R.; Roizman, B.; Myers, R. Recovery from infants with respiratory illness of a virus related to chimpanzee coryza agent (CCA). *Am. J. Hyg.* **1957**, *66*, 281–290.

[2] Glezen, W. P., et al. Risk of primary infection and reinfection with respiratory syncytial virus. *Am. J. Dis. Child* **1986**, *140*, 543 546.

[3] Holberg, C. J., et al. Risk factors for respiratory syncytial virus-associated lower respiratory illnesses in the first year of life. *Am. J. Epidemiol.* **1991**, *133*, 1135–1151.

[4] Mills, J. Management of respiratory syncytial virus infections. *Adv. Exp. Med. Biol.* **1996**, *394*, 163–174.

[5] Garcia, R., et al. Nosocomial respiratory syncytial virus infections: prevention and control in bone marrow transplant patients. *Infect. Control Hosp. Epidemiol.* **1997**, *18*, 412–416.

[6] Murry, A. R.; Dowell, S. F. Respiratory syncytial virus: not just for kids. *Hosp. Pract.* **1997**, Jul. 15; 87–88.

[7] Hall, C. B., et al. The burden of respiratory syncytial virus infection in young children. *N. Engl. J .Med.* **2009**, *360*, 588–598.

[8] Georgescu, G.; Chemaly, R. F. Palivizumab: Where to from here? *Expert Opin. Biol. Ther.* **2009**, *9*, 139–147.

[9] Madaan, A. Motaviizumab; humanized anti-RSV monoclonal antibody prevention of RSV infection. *Drugs Future* **2008**, *33*, 203–205.

[10] Power, U. F. Respiratory syncytial virus (RSV) vaccines: two steps back for one leap forward. *J. Clin. Virol.* **2008**, *41*, 38–44.

[11] Moyse, E., et al. Viral RNA in middle ear mucosa and exudates in patients with chronic otitis media with effusion. *Arch. Otolaryngol. Head Neck Surg.* **2000**, *126*, 1105–1110.

[12] Heikkinen, T.; Thint, M.; Chonmaitree, T. Prevalence of various respiratory viruses in the middle ear during acute otitis media. *N. Engl. J. Med.* **1999**, *340*, 260–264.

[13] Chonmaitree, T., et al. Viral upper respiratory tract infection and otitis media complication in young children. *Clin. Infect. Dis.* **2008**, *46*, 815–823.

[14] Sigurs N. Epidemiologic and clinical evidence of a respiratory syncytial virus-reactive airway disease link. *Am. J. Respir. Crit. Care Med.* **2001**, *163*, S2–S6.

[15] Stensballe, L. G., et al. Respiratory syncytial virus neutralizing antibodies in cord blood, respiratory syncytial virus hospitalization, and recurrent wheeze. *J. Allergy Clin. Immunol.* **2009**, *123*, 398–340.

[16] Faber, T. E.; Kimpen, J. L.; Bont, L. J. Respiratory syncytial virus bronchiolitis: prevention and treatment. *Expert Opin. Pharmacother.* **2008**, *9*, 2451–2458.

[17] Ramaswamy, M.; Groskreutz, D. J.; Look, D. C. Recognizing the importance of respiratory syncytial virus in chronic obstructive pulmonary disease. *COPD* **2009**, *6*, 64–75.

[18] Mohapatra, S. S.; Boyapalle, S. Epidemiologic, experimental, and clinical links between respiratory syncytial virus infection and asthma. *Clin. Microbiol. Rev.* **2008**, *21*, 495–504.

[19] Falsey, A. R.; Walsh, E. E. Respiratory syncytial virus infection in adults. *Clin. Microbiol. Rev.* **2000**, *13*, 371–384.

[20] Falsey, A. R., et al. Respiratory syncytial virus infection in elderly and high-risk adults. *N. Engl. J. Med.* **2005**, *352*, 1749–1759.

[21] Murata, Y.; Falsey, A. R. Respiratory syncytial virus infection in adults. *Antiviral Ther.* **2007**, *12*, 659–670.

[22] Murata, Y. Respiratory syncytial virus infection in adults. *Curr. Opin. Pulm. Med.* **2008**, *14*, 235–240.

[23] Englund, J. A., et al. Respiratory syncytial virus infection in immunocompromised adults. *Ann. Intern. Med.* **1988**, *109*, 203–208.

[24] Harrington, R. D., et al. An outbreak of respiratory syncytial virus in a bone marrow transplant center. *J. Infect. Dis.* **1992**, *165*, 987–993.

[25] Thompson, W. W., et al. Mortality associated with influenza and respiratory syncytial virus in the United States. *J. Amer. Med. Assoc.* **2003**, *289*, 179–186.

[26] Osterweil, D.; Norman, D. An outbreak of an influenza-like illness in a nursing home. *J. Am. Geriatr. Soc.* **1990**, *38*, 659–662.

[27] Hall, W. J.; Hall, C. B.; Speers, D. M. Respiratory syncytial virus infection in adults: clinical, virologic, and serial pulmonary function studies. *Ann. Intern. Med.* **1978**, *88*, 203–205.

[28] Falsey, A. R. Respiratory syncytial virus infection in adults. *Semin. Respir. Crit. Care Med.* **2007**, *28*, 171–181.

[29] Pauwels, R., et al. Rapid and automated tetrazolium-based colorimetric assay for the detection of anti-HIV compounds. *J. Virol. Methods* **1988**, *20*, 309–321.

[30] Cianci, C., et al. Orally active fusion inhibitor of respiratory syncytial virus. *Antimicrob. Agents Chemother.* **2004**, *48*, 413–422.

[31] Pagani, F.; Sparatore, F. Benzotriazolylalkyl benzimidazoles and their dialkylaminoalkyl derivatives. *Boll. Chim. Farm.* **1965**, *104*, 427–431.

[32] Paglietti, G.; Boido, V.; Sparatore, F. Dialkylaminoalkylbenzimidazoles of pharmacological interest: IV. *Farm. Ed. Sci.* **1975**, *30*, 505–511.

[33] Johnson, S., et al. Development of a humanized monoclonal antibody (MEDI-493) with potent in vitro and in vivo activity against respiratory syncytial virus. *J. Infect. Dis.* **1997**, *176*, 1215–1224.

[34] Kilby, J. M., et al. Potent suppression of HIV-1 replication in humans by T-20, a peptide inhibitor of gp41-mediated virus entry. *Nat. Med.* **1988**, *4*, 1302–1307.

[35] Yu, K.-L., et al. Fundamental structure–activity relationships associated with a new structural class of respiratory syncytial virus inhibitor. *Bioorg. Med. Chem. Lett.* **2003**, *13*, 2141–2144.

[36] Meanwell, N. A., et al. The regiospecific functionalization of 1,3-dihydro-2*H*-benzimidazol-2-one and structurally related cyclic urea derivatives. *J. Org. Chem.* **1995**, *60*, 1565–1582.

[37] Yu, K.-L., et al. Respiratory syncytial virus fusion inhibitors: 2. Benzimidazol-2-one derivatives. *Bioorg. Med. Chem. Lett.* **2004**, *14*, 1133–1137.

[38] Byrd L. G.; Prince, G. A. Animal models of respiratory syncytial virus infection. *Clin. Infect. Dis.* **1997**, *25*, 1363–1368.

[39] Domachowske, J. B.; Bonville, C. A.; Rosenberg, H. F. Animal models for studying respiratory syncytial virus infection and its long term effects on lung function. *Pediatr. Infect. Dis. J.* **2004**, *23*, S228–S234.

[40] Prince, G. A., et al. Respiratory syncytial virus infection in inbred mice. *Infect. Immun.* **1979**, *26*, 764–766.

[41] Sudo, K., et al. Mouse model of respiratory syncytial virus infection to evaluate antiviral activity in vivo. *Antiviral Chem. Chemother.* **1999**, *10*, 135–139.

[42] Kong, X., et al. An immunocompromised BALB/c mouse model for respiratory syncytial virus infection. *Virol. J.* **2005**, *2*, 3–11.

[43] Prince, G. A., et al. The pathogenesis of respiratory syncytial virus infection in cotton rats. *Am. J. Pathol.* **1978**, *93*, 771–791.

[44] Prince, G. A., et al. Immunoprophylaxis and immunotherapy of respiratory syncytial virus infection in the cotton rat. *Virus Res.* **1985**, *3*, 193–206.

[45] Prince, G. A.; Horswood, R. L.; Chanock, R. M. Quantitative aspects of passive immunity to respiratory syncytial virus infection in infant cotton rats. *J. Virol.* **1985**, *55*, 517–520.

[46] Grubbs, S. T.; Kania, S. A.; Potgieter, L. N. Prevalence of ovine and bovine respiratory syncytial virus infections in cattle determined with a synthetic peptide-based immunoassay. *J. Vet. Diagn. Invest.* **2001**, *13*, 128–132.

[47] Huntley, C. C., et al. RFI-641, a potent respiratory syncytial virus inhibitor. *Antimicrob. Agents Chemother.* **2002**, *46*, 841–847.

[48] Graham, B. S.; Rutigliano, J. A.; Johnson, T. R. Respiratory syncytial virus immunobiology and pathogenesis. *Virology* **2002**, *297*, 1–7.

[49] Wyde, P. R.; Wilson, S. Z.; Petrella, R.; Gilbert, B. E. Efficacy of high dose-short duration ribavirin aerosol in the treatment of respiratory syncytial virus infected cotton rats and influenza B virus infected mice. *Antiviral Res.* **1987**, *7*, 211–220.

[50] Wilson, S. Z., et al. Amantadine and ribavirin aerosol treatment of influenza A and B infection in mice. *Antimicrob. Agents Chemother.* **1980**, *17*, 642–648.

[51] Yu, K.-L., et al. Respiratory syncytial virus fusion inhibitors: 3. Water-soluble benzimidazol-2-one derivatives with antiviral activity in vivo. *Bioorg. Med. Chem. Lett.* **2006**, *16*, 1115–1122.

[52] Yu, K.-L., et al. Respiratory syncytial virus fusion inhibitors. 4. Optimization for orally bioavailability. *Bioorg. Med. Chem. Lett.* **2007**, *17*, 895–901.

[53] Cianci, C., et al. Oral efficacy of a respiratory syncytial virus inhibitor in rodent models of infection. *Antimicrob. Agents Chemother.* **2004**, *48*, 2448–2454.

[54] Wyde, P. R. Respiratory syncytial virus (RSV) disease and prospects for its control. *Antiviral Res.* **1998**, *39*, 63–79.

[55] Dischino, D. D., et al. Development of a photoaffinity label for respiratory syncytial inhibitors. *J. Radiolabelled Cpd. Radiopharm.* **2003**, *46*, 1105–1116.

[56] Cianci, C., et al. Targeting a binding pocket within the trimer-of-hairpins: small-molecule inhibition of viral fusion. *Proc. Natl. Acad. Sci. USA* **2004**, *101*, 15046–15051.

[57] Earp, L. J., et al. The many mechanisms of viral membrane fusion proteins. *Curr. Top. Microbiol. Immunol.* **2005**, *285*, 25–66.

[58] Matthews, J. M., et al. The core of the respiratory syncytial virus fusion protein is a trimeric coiled coil. *J. Virol.* **2000**, *74*, 5911–5920.

[59] Zhao, X., et al. Structural characterization of the human respiratory syncytial virus fusion protein core. *Proc. Natl. Acad. Sci. USA* **2000**, *97*, 14172–14177.

[60] Provencal, D. P., et al. Development of an efficient and scalable process of a respiratory syncytial virus inhibitor. *Org. Process Res. Dev.* **2004**, *8*, 903–908.

[61] Wang, X. A., et al. Respiratory syncytial virus fusion inhibitors: 5. Optimization of benzimidazole substitution patterns towards derivatives with improved activity. *Bioorg. Med. Chem. Lett.* **2007**, *17*, 4592–4598.

[62] Combrink, K. D., et al. Respiratory syncytial virus fusion inhibitors: 6. An examination of the effect of structural variation of the benzimidazol-2-one heterocycle moiety. *Bioorg. Med. Chem. Lett.* **2007**, *17*, 4784–4790.

[63] Sin, N., et al. Respiratory syncytial virus fusion inhibitors: 7. Structure–activity relationships associated with a series of isatin oximes that demonstrate antiviral activity in vivo. *Bioorg. Med. Chem. Lett.* **2009**, *19*, 4857–4862.

[64] Tidwell, R. R.; Geratz, J. D.; Dubovi, E. J. Aromatic amidines. Comparison of their ability to block respiratory syncytial virus induced cell fusion and to inhibit plasmin, urokinase, thrombin, and trypsin. *J. Med. Chem.* **1983**, *26*, 294–298.

[65] Tidwell, R. R.; Geratz, J. D.; Dubovi, E. J. Inhibition of respiratory syncytial virus by bis(5-amidino-2-benzimidazolyl)methane. *Virology* **1980**, *103*, 502–504.

[66] Dubovi, E. J., et al. Inhibition of respiratory syncytial virus–host cell interactions by mono- and diamidines. *Antimicrob. Agents Chemother.* **1981**, *19*, 649–656.

[67] Dubovi, E. J.; Geratz, J. D.; Tidwell, R. R. Enhancement of respiratory syncytial virus-induced cytopathology by trypsin, thrombin, and plasmin. *Infect. Immun.* **1983**, *40*, 351–358.

[68] Tidwell, R. R., et al. Suppression of respiratory syncytial virus infection in cotton rats by bis(5-amidino-2-benzimidazolyl)methane. *Antimicrob. Agents Chemother.* **1984**, *26*, 591–593.

[69] Douglas, J. L., et al. Small molecules VP-14637 and JNJ-2408068 inhibit respiratory syncytial virus fusion by similar mechanisms. *Antimicrob. Agents Chemother.* **2005**, *49*, 2460–2466.

[70] Douglas, J. L., et al. Inhibition of respiratory syncytial virus fusion by the small molecule VP-14637 via specific interactions with F protein. *J. Virol.* **2003**, *77*, 5054–5064.

[71] Andries, K., et al. Substituted benzimidazoles with nanomolar activity against respiratory syncytial virus. *Antiviral Res.* **2003**, *60*, 209–219.

[72] Bonfanti, J.-F., et al. Selection of a respiratory syncytial virus fusion inhibitor clinical candidate: improving the pharmacokinetic profile using the structure–property relationship. *J. Med. Chem.* **2007**, *50*, 4572–4584.

[73] Bonfanti, J.-F., et al. Selection of a respiratory syncytial virus fusion inhibitor clinical candidate: 2. Discovery of a morpholinopropylaminobenzimidazole derivative (TMC353121). *J. Med. Chem.* **2008**, *51*, 875–896.

[74] Bonfanti, J.-F. et al. Discovery of TMC-353121, a novel RSV fusion inhibitor with potent in vitro and in vivo activity. 47th Interscience Conference on Antimicrobial Agents and Chemotherapy, Chicago, Sept. 17–20, 2007. Poster F1-950.

[75] Wyde, P. R., et al. Antiviral efficacy of VP14637 against respiratory syncytial virus in vitro and in cotton rats following delivery by small droplet aerosol. *Antiviral Res.* **2005**, *68*, 18–26.

[76] Wyde, P. R., et al. Short duration aerosols of JNJ 2408068 (R170591) administered prophylactically or therapeutically protect cotton rats from experimental respiratory syncytial virus infection. *Antiviral Res.* **2003**, *60*, 221–231.

26

DISCOVERY AND DEVELOPMENT OF RSV604

JOANNA CHAPMAN AND G. STUART COCKERILL
Arrow Therapeutics, Ltd., London, UK

INTRODUCTION

Human respiratory syncytial virus (RSV) is a negative-strand RNA virus and is the most important respiratory pathogen that causes lower respiratory tract infections worldwide. Historically, it has been considered to be solely an infection of children. However, with the ever-increasing awareness of elderly and immunocompromised patient populations, this perception is changing. The medical literature is awash with studies reviewing the clinical and financial burden of RSV infections year after year, and yet the amount of research into antivirals against this virus remains small. A recent study investigated the total burden of RSV infection among young children in the United States [1]. They concluded that RSV infection was associated with considerable morbidity in children under 5 years of age and that control strategies that target only those considered high-risk had a limited effect on the total disease burden. Other studies going back over the past five years have reached the same conclusions [2–4]. These reports also found that RSV was responsible for more infant hospitalizations than were influenza, parainfluenza, or human metapneumovirus. The World Health Organisation (WHO) estimates that RSV causes 64 million infections and 160,000 deaths globally each year. They also state that children who experience a severe lower respiratory tract RSV infection have an increased risk of developing childhood asthma.

In the elderly population in 2003 it was found that 78% of RSV-associated deaths occurred in those aged 65 years or older [5]. Falsey et al. concluded that over four years RSV resulted in 177,500 hospital admissions and 14,000 deaths in the aged community in the United States [6]. They estimated that the hospitalization costs alone were more than $1 billion. Studies have shown that RSV is a serious cause of morbidity and mortality in immunocompromised adults. In their 2005 study, Ebbert and Limper found that 55% of patients died from RSV-associated complications [7]. RSV persistence has been demonstrated in some animals, such as guinea pigs [8] and cows [9]. Persistence is a major concern for some patients, such as those suffering from chronic obstructive pulmonary disease (COPD) or chronic heart problems.

The success of the passive immunization with the monoclonal antibody palivizumab (Synagis) given as a prophylactic treatment to high-risk groups, such as premature babies, demonstrates that there is a market for new RSV therapies. However, this treatment regimen is prohibitively expensive and its use is thus limited to the treatment of preterm infants in the United States. The effectiveness of ribavirin [10], the only licensed small-molecule antiviral against RSV, is questionable [11]. Its clinical benefits are small and not all patients respond. There is also possible deterioration of respiratory function and teratogenicity associated with its use.

It was recognized in 1969 that there was a medical need for a RSV vaccine [12], but progress in this field has been extremely slow. The National Institutes of Health (NIH) in the United States did develop a formalin-inactivated vaccine and conducted clinical trials in 1969, but the results were disastrous. It not only failed to provide immunity to RSV, but immunized children experienced a more severe disease when naturally infected with wild-type virus [13]. Other issues have hindered vaccine discovery. The age groups affected are neonates, with their immature immune systems, and the elderly, with deteriorating immunity, and the testing of vaccines in these age groups has inherent safety issues.

Antiviral Drugs: From Basic Discovery Through Clinical Trials, First Edition. Edited by Wieslaw M. Kazmierski.

An effective candidate would also be required to provide protection to both subtypes of RSV, which can be circulating at the same time. Currently, there are no vaccine candidates available for wide-scale testing.

RSV can be divided into two strains, A and B. They can be distinguished antigenically and have divergent nucleotide sequences [14–16]. The most variable protein is the attachment (G) protein, which shows only 53% amino acid identity between the two strains [14]. Both strains exhibit variation within the group, and phylogenetic analysis of the G-nucleotide sequence has resulted in the identification of multiple lineages for both A and B strains [17–19]. RSV infection is a global annual winter epidemic in temperate climates. Numerous studies have shown that both strains may coexist within an epidemic, but their relative incidence can vary. The predominant epidemic strain causing the epidemic can change from year to year, and both strains have been detected worldwide. For example, in Birmingham, UK they have identified a triennial cycle where RSV A was dominant except in every third year, when B was responsible for the outbreak [20]. In Finland the dominance was found to alternate every two years [21].

Drug discovery can utilize a range of live virus assays at the in vitro evaluation stage. At Arrow we employed a colorimetric readout utilizing XTT [2,3-bis(2-methoxy-4-nitro-5-sulfophenyl)-2*H*-tetrazolium-5-carboxanilide, disodium salt] to measure compound-mediated cell survival in the presence of the virus and performed secondary testing in cell ELISA and plaque [22] reduction assays. In vivo evaluation of compound effectiveness against RSV has several problems, however. The various disease models available have been reviewed [23] and include small-animal models such as the BALB/c mouse and cotton rat and larger-animal models such as primate and bovine. Each of these has its own set of problems. RSV does not replicate very well in rodent cells in vitro, and this is reflected by the large inoculum required and the small amount of virus recovered from the lungs of the animals. Primates can be infected with RSV, but these models are notoriously impractical and expensive. Bovine RSV has a clinical need of its own and manifests itself in a manner similar to human RSV. Studies in the calf are, however, hampered by the large amounts of test compound required. The end result is that no animal model of RSV infection demonstrates the human disease in its entirety and can be considered ideal.

The 15.2-kb genome of RSV contains 10 mRNA species encoding 11 distinct proteins. There are three transmembrane surface proteins (F, G, SH) important for attachment and entry, a matrix protein (M), a nucleocapsid protein (N) which wraps around the RNA genome, a phosphoprotein (P), a RNA polymerase (L), M2-1 and M2-2 proteins, and two nonstructural proteins (NS1, NS2). A transcriptase complex is formed between N, L, P, and M2-1, which transcribes the RSV genome once it has entered the cytoplasm of the host cell. This complex switches from transcription to replication by an unknown mechanism.

When Arrow Therapeutics began its RSV research program in 2001, there were a few companies investigating the inhibition of viral attachment and entry, but investigation of replication had proven fruitless. A number of compounds have been synthesized from various chemical classes that target either attachment or fusion of RSV. These have been summarized in a review by Sidwell and Bernard [24]. Subsequently, however, there has been slow progress with these fusion inhibitors in the clinic.

A ViroPharma compound, VP-14637, was described as a potent inhibitor of RSV fusion at concentrations in the low-nanomolar range [25]. It progressed to phase I trials but was not developed further. RFI-641 from Wyeth was first described in 2001 as an inhibitor of RSV [26]. They claim activity in three animal models of RSV infection, including African green monkeys [27]. In this study they showed that the compound was effective when dosed 24 h postinfection. It was reported that this compound entered clinical trials in 2001 [24], but no data are available from this trial and Wyeth has discontinued its development.

Other fusion inhibitors of note are JNJ-2408068 [28] and BMS-433771 [29]. JNJ-2408068 has potent anti-RSV activity in vitro. It is effective against both strains A and B [28]. A cotton rat study demonstrated antiviral activity in vivo with high lung concentration levels [30]. Johnson and Johnson identified the suboptimal pharmacokinetic properties of JNJ-2408068 and proceeded to identify TMC353121 as a clinical candidate [31,32]. BMS-433771 is thought to act by disrupting the hairpin structure of the RSV fusion protein. Similar to other fusion inhibitors, it had a low-nanomolar EC_{50} value vs. RSV in vitro. It was orally active in the mouse model but was not pursued for strategic reasons. There has been some research into small peptide fusion inhibitors [33], polymerase inhibitors (YM-53403) [34], and Alnylam Pharmaceuticals is developing siRNA treatment of RSV with ALN-RSV01. ALN-RSV01 had an EC_{50} of 0.7 nM against RSV in vitro [35]. Recently, Alnylam announced that its human proof-of-concept GEMINI trial with ALN-RSV01 showed statistically significant antiviral efficacy.

DISCOVERY

The first stage of the screening campaign at Arrow was the selection of a 20,000-member diverse component of the in-house collection. This component was screened against RSV virus in a whole-cell XTT cell survival assay. The process was laborious and resulted in a relatively high hit rate, but several distinct series were identified. Secondary plaque reduction and cell ELISA assays allowed us to eliminate certain compound classes of hit from our investigation, due to lack of consistent activity across the assay types. Further, to identify

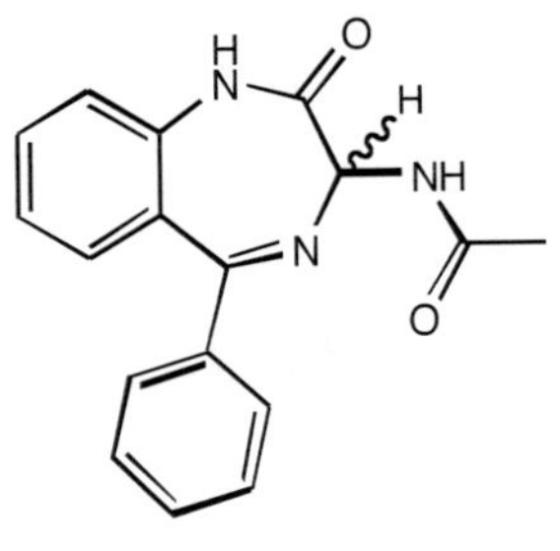

FIGURE 1 Lead representative of benzodiazepine hit series.

compounds that acted after the fusion event, time-of-addition studies were incorporated into our screening cascade. Compound was added to cells after RSV infection and compounds showing a significant drop in activity when dosed at 6 h postinfection were discarded for the purposes of this project. This process allowed identification of a series of racemic 1,4-benzodiazepines, exemplified by A-33903 (**1**) as nonfusion inhibitors (Fig. 1).

The lead acetamido-1,4-benzodiazepine analog (**1**) A-33903 exhibited EC_{50} values in the range 10 to 20 μM over all three assays. An EC_{50} of 9.7 ± 5.5 μM for RSV RSS strain was observed in the plaque reduction assay [36]. This molecule also demonstrated excellent pharmacokinetic properties in the rat, with a half-life of approximately 6 h and an oral bioavailability of 76%. This suggested that the core benzodiazepine was relatively stable to metabolism, with good absorption properties. Calculated physicochemical properties (molecular weight, 293; *c* log *P*, 1.55; tPSA 70.56) supported this series as a good starting point for lead optimization, with ample room for structural modifications.

Structural modifications to A-33903 (**1**) (see Fig. 2) showed that the unsubstituted benzodiazepine template was optimal for antiviral activity but that potency could be improved markedly by modification of the amide moiety. Increasing the size of the alkyl chain or branching in the chain gave a modest decrease in potency, as did incorporation of a cyclic substituent. Noticeable increases in potency were seen, however, when aromatic amides were tested, especially those containing electron-donating substituents. The *o*-methoxybenzamide (**3**) was the most potent analog of this type. However, it showed a very poor pharmacokinetic profile with low bioavailability (4%) and extremely high clearance (71 mL·min/kg) when dosed in the rat (Table 2). Addition of a second methoxy group retained activity (**4**), whereas chain lengthening (**5** and **6**) reduced activity. Other electron-donating substituents (e.g., dimethylamino) also led to reasonably potent molecules (**7**). Incorporation of a lipophilic electronically neutral substituent (cyclohexyl, **8**) resulted in a loss in potency. Other substitutions tended to lower activity.

Heteroaromatic compounds (e.g., **9**) also demonstrated excellent activity; however, the heteroaromatic and electron-rich aromatic amides suffered from poor pharmacokinetics (Fig. 2, examples **3** to **5**). Addition of halogens as groups blocking potential aromatic hydroxylation of electron-withdrawing substituents led to very potent molecules (**10** to **13**) with a wide range of metabolic vulnerability. The 5-fluoro analog (**13**) was virtually undetectable after oral dosing to rats, whereas incorporation of a 4-nitro substituent (**10**) gave a potent molecule that demonstrated good exposure combined with a low clearance and a 5.8-h half-life when orally dosed to rats at 25 mg/kg. Incorporation of a 4-trifluoromethyl group gave a compound that although having potent antiviral activity, was shown to be highly cell-toxic (data not shown). Generally, the series exhibited good half-lives and volumes of distribution in conjunction with low-to-moderate clearances, suggesting that these molecules would be well distributed in tissues relevant to RSV infection.

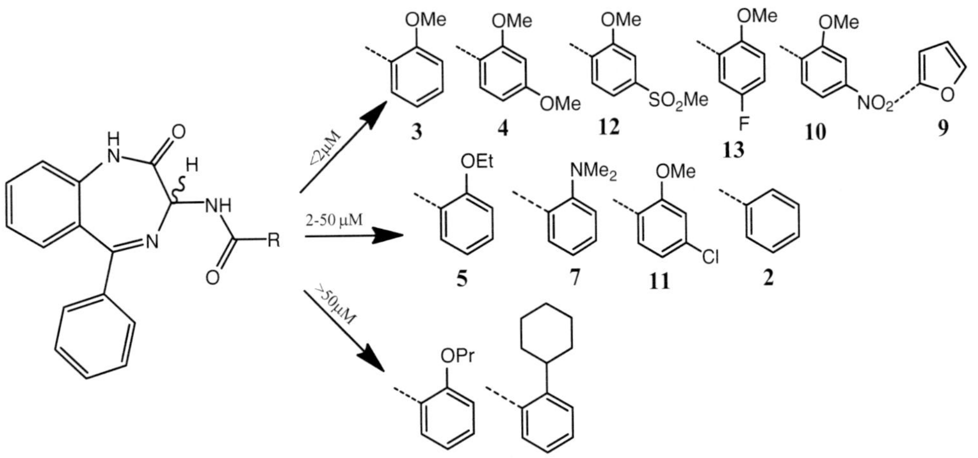

FIGURE 2 SAR expansion of the amide substituent in A-33903.

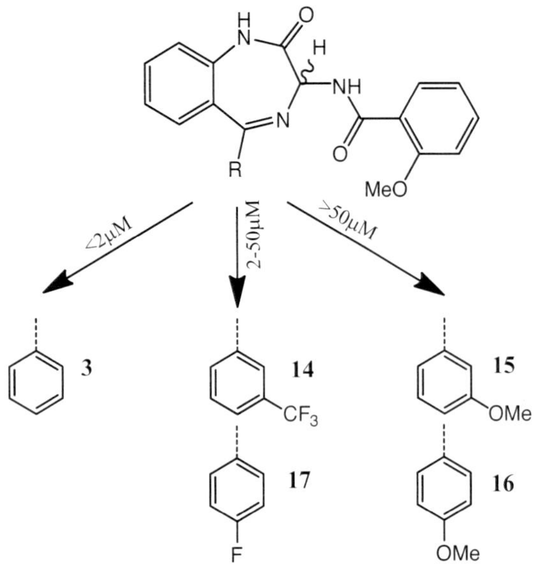

FIGURE 3 Pendant phenyl modifications.

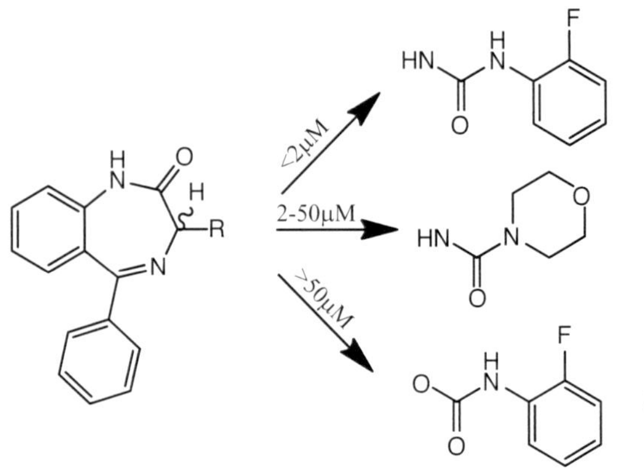

FIGURE 5 Urea and carbamate modifications.

Unless stated otherwise, all molecules exhibited no cell toxicity at 50 μM.

Replacement of the pendant phenyl ring with a methyl group led to poor activity, and an identical result was seen when the phenyl ring was replaced by cyclohexyl. Inactivity was also observed when the phenyl was modified to benzyl system or a pyridine ring (data not shown). Substitution on the pendant phenyl ring generally led to a lowering of potency. Only substitution at the *meta* position with electron-withdrawing groups (e.g., **14**), or at the *para* position with groups as small as fluorine (**17**) maintained any measurable antiviral activity, as shown in Figure 3. Substitution on the fused phenyl ring has also been investigated both with and without substitution on the pendant phenyl. Substitution at the 7 position with chlorine gave a slight loss in activity (**18**). All other substituents investigated to date at either the 7 or 8 position have led to reduction of antiviral activity (Fig. 4).

The importance of the NH groups in both the ring and substituent amide (or urea) was well demonstrated by the reduction in activity when either of these moieties was methylated (Fig. 4, example **19**). Replacement of the amide linking group by urea retained activity (Fig. 5, example **20**) and some modification of the terminal lipophilic group was possible. Modification of carbamate (**22**) was also possible with some drop in activity. Replacement of the amide moiety with a sulfonamide led to loss of activity (data not shown) and to a general increase in cell toxicity. A similar lack of activity was observed in benzylamine analogs when the amide carbonyl was removed.

In general, the structure–activity relationship (SAR) from the XTT assay was consistent with both other assays (plaque and ELISA), with good antiviral activity demonstrated. These compounds also showed excellent activity against a range of RSV strains (Long, B, and A2 strains; see Table 1) and also against a number of both A and B strain clinical isolates (data not shown).

Historically, the benzodiazepine skeleton is well documented as having high promiscuity in terms of pharmacological activity, we tested a number of our lead molecules

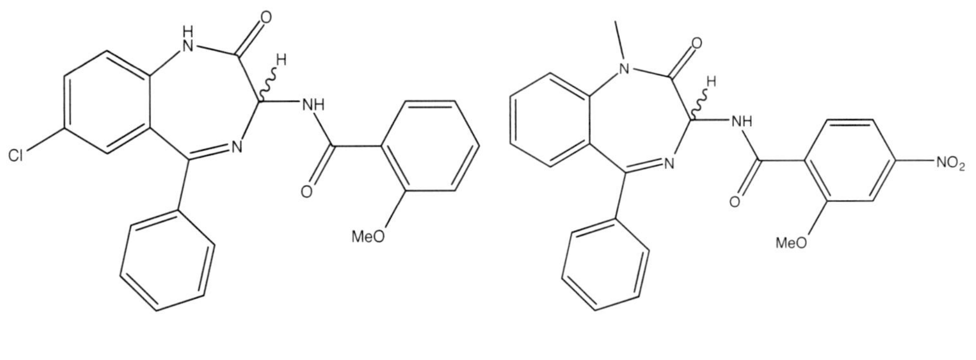

(18) EC_{50} 6.1 μM **(19)** EC_{50} >50 μM

FIGURE 4 Benzodiazepine core modifications.

TABLE 1 RSV Strain Data for Selected Compounds[a]

	ELISA				Plaque			
Compound	XTT	RSS	Long	B	A2	RSS	Long	B
1	8.6	9.3	17.6	17.8	N.T.	7.1	7.2	3.6
20	3.3	2.7	2.5	1.9	2.8	3.0	2.2	0.75
10	2.0	2.5	1.2	1.3	N.T.	1.8	0.9	<0.3

[a]All figures are EC_{50} values (μM). N.T., not tested.

in a Cerep diversity profile screen. This protocol involved testing molecules at a concentration of 10 μM against 68 receptors and 17 enzyme targets. The affinity for each target was measured by displacement of a radiolabeled ligand specific for each particular receptor or enzyme. The results are expressed in terms of the percentage of ligand displaced, and results of 50% or less are considered to be insignificant. The overall profile was very clean, and a notable lack of affinity for the central benzodiazepine receptor was demonstrated.

Representative pharmacokinetic data in vivo are shown in Table 2. As has been described, compounds are characterized by low clearance and good absorption and distribution properties. A series of compounds that showed a range of activities in addition to structural differences in the side chain and linker were chosen to be synthesized as chirally pure enantiomers to quickly examine any enantiomeric preference and trends. The results of two of these enantiomeric pairs are presented in Table 3. It was observed that in all cases the relative potency across the chiral and achiral forms remained the same, but the *S*-isomer showed greater activity than the racemate, and the *R*-isomer was consistently less potent.

With this initial indication of enantiospecific anti-RSV activity, the strategy within the chiral series was to optimize utilizing SARs gleaned from the racemic optimization process [37]. Particular attention was paid to substituents that would potentially modify physical properties and maintain or improve the PK profile of the series. Similarly, the unsubstituted 5-phenyl-1,3-dihydrobenzo[*e*][1,4]diazepin-2-one was used as the core structure for this optimization. A range of compounds were prepared as part of this strategy, with SAR trends entirely as observed in the racemic program. A summary of leading compounds is shown in Table 4, alongside their antiviral and comparative pharmacokinetic data. All compounds shown were orally bioavailable in the rat with low clearances and reasonable volumes of distribution. Compound 23, designated RSV604 upon licensing to Novartis, was chosen for progression, as it was the best overall of its peers. Compound 25 appeared a few months later as part of the lead optimization program and was designated as a backup to RSV604 [37]. A summary of SAR is shown in Figure 6. RSV604 inhibited viral replication but its mechanism was unknown. A series of experiments ensued to try and understand how this series of compounds exerted their antiviral effect.

Time-of-addition studies confirmed that this compound acted late in the replication cycle. Drug-resistant mutants to RSV604 were generated by performing multiple passages of virus with increasing concentrations of compound. A 10-fold increase in EC_{50} observed for RSV604 after eight passages increased to > 40-fold after three rounds of plaque picking in the presence of 25 μM compound where its EC_{50} value was 30.4 μM. The plaque-picked mutant was cross-resistant to other compounds from within the same chemical series but showed no resistance to ribavirin or a fusion inhibitor [38].

The complete genome of the plaque-picked RSV604-resistant virus was sequenced and mutations were identified in the conserved N-terminal region of the nucleocapsid gene only. These resulted in the amino acid changes I129L and L139I. An alignment of RSV strains revealed these residues to be conserved across A and B strains of the virus (Fig. 7). To confirm that these mutations were important for the resistance phenotype, reverse genetic experiments were carried

TABLE 2 Rat Pharmacokinetic Data for Selected Compounds[a]

Compound	C_{max} (ng/mL)	T_{max} (h)	$t_{1/2}$ (h)	*Cl* (mL·min/kg)	*Vd* (L/kg)	*F* (%)
1 (p.o.)	616	2.6	5.9	4.9	4.2	77
1 (i.v.)	2400	0.08	5.0	5.3	2.2	
3 (p.o.)	19.3	0.8	N.D.	N.D.	N.D.	4
3 (i.v.)	798	0.08	0.4	71.2	2.4	
20 (p.o.)	386	2.6	8.1	9.5	7.5	76
20 (i.v.)	1533	0.08	3.7	7.8	2.5	

[a]All compounds dosed at 2 mg/kg. N.D., not determined. Oral dose a suspension in 1% carboxymethylcellulose, i.v. dose by dilution of 100% DMSO solution into 10% w/v solution of hydroxypropyl β-cyclodextrin in phosphate-buffered saline to a total volume of 5 mL.

TABLE 3 Activity vs. RSV in XTT Assay of Racemates and Pure Enantiomers (μM)

	Racemate		*S*-Isomer		*R*-Isomer	
Compound	EC_{50}	TD_{50}	EC_{50}	TD_{50}	EC_{50}	TD_{50}
10	2.0	>50	0.9	>50	21.2	>50
20	3.5	>50	0.9	>50	27.8	>50

TABLE 4 Activity vs. RSV and Pharmacokinetics of Leading Chiral Benzodiazepines

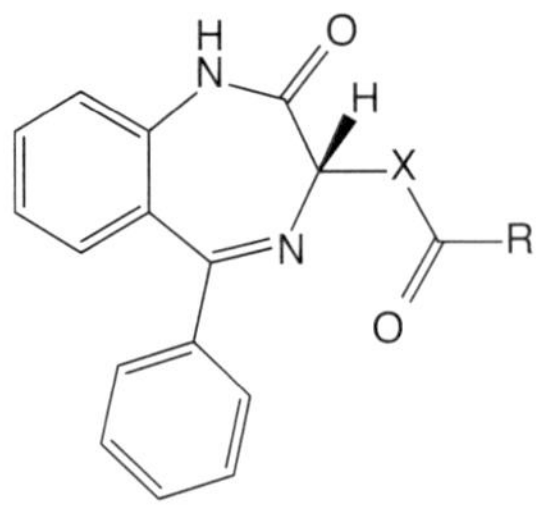

Compound	X	R	XTT (μM)		ELISA (μM)		Plaque (μM)		$C \log P$	Aqueous Solution pH7 (μg/mL)	Plasma Levels[a] (ng/mL)
			EC_{50}	TD_{50}	EC_{50}	TD_{50}	EC_{50}	TD_{50}			
23 (RSV604)	N	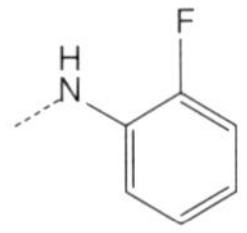	0.9	>50	1.4	>50	0.7	>50	3.02	4.1	C_{max} 1023 T_{max} 4 h
24	N	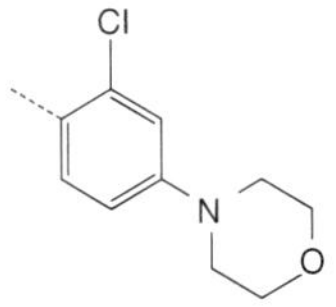	1.4	>50	1.5	>50	0.8	>50	2.67	0.9	C_{max} 204 T_{max} 6 h
25	N	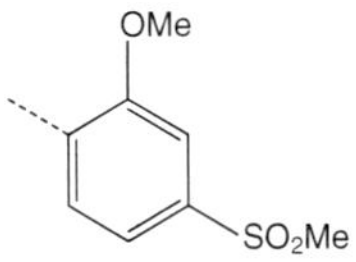	0.6	>50	0.6	>50	0.5	>50	1.88	22	C_{max} 2197 T_{max} 8 h

[a]20 mg/kg dosed orally as a suspension in 5% PEG-400 with 1% CMC in the rat.

out using a RSV antigenome plasmid. Recombinant mutant viruses were generated, fully sequenced, and analyzed. An I129L mutant was sixfold resistant to RSV604, L139I was sevenfold resistant, but a double mutant (I129L and L139I) was > 20-fold resistant. There was no significant difference in the replication capacities of these mutant viruses. This was a completely novel mechanism of action for a small molecule against RSV. The N protein is a highly conserved major structural protein that is involved in encapsidation of the RNA genome and is essential for replication and

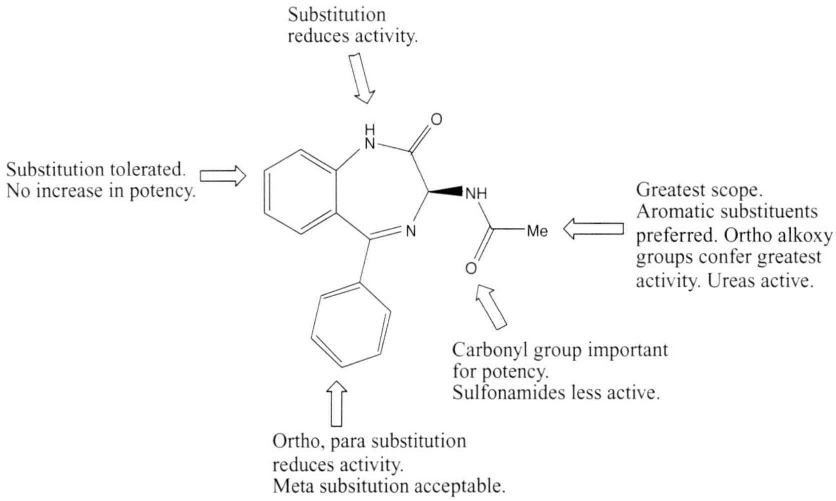

FIGURE 6 Summary of SAR.

```
A2  MALSKVKLNDTLNKDQLLSSSKYTIQRSTGDSIDTPNYDVQKHINKLCGMLLITEDANHK 60
RSS MALSKVKLNDTLNKDQLLSSSKYTIQRSTGDSIDTPNYDVQKHINKLCGMLLITEDANHK 60
B   MALSKVKLNDTLNKDQLLSSSKYTIQRSTGDNIDTPNYDVQKHLNKLCGMLLITEDANHK 60
    *******************************.***********:****************

A2  FTGLIGMLYAMSRLGREDTIKILRDAGYHVKANGVDVTTHRQDINGKEMKFEVLTLASLT 120
RSS FTGLIGMLYAMSRLGREDTIKILRDAGYHVKANGVDVTTHRQDINGKEMKFEVLTLSSLT 120
B   FTGLIGMLYAMSRLGREDTIKILKDAGYHVKANGVDITTYRQDINGKEMKFEVLTLSSLT 120
    ***********************:************:**:****************:***

            ↓         ↓
A2  TEIQINIEIESRKSYKKMLKEMGEVAPEYRHDSPDCGMIILCIAALVITKLAAGDRSGLT 180
RSS TEIQINIEIESRKSYKKMLKEMGEVAPEYRHDSPDCGMIILCIAALVITKLAAGDRSGLT 180
B   SEIQVNIEIESRKSYKKLLKEMGEVAPEYRHDSPDCGMIILCIAALVITKLAAGDRSGLT 180
    :***:************:******************************************

A2  AVIRRANNVLKNEMKRYKGLLPKDIANSFYEVFEKHPHFIDVFVHFGIAQSSTRGGSRVE 240
RSS AVIRRANNVLKNEMKRYKGLLPKDIANSFYEVFEKYPHFIDVFVHFGIAQSSTRGGSRVE 240
B   AVIRRANNVLKNEIKRYKGLIPKDIANSFYEVFEKHPHLIDVFVHFGIAQSSTRGGSRVE 240
    *************:******:**************:**:*********************
```

FIGURE 7 Mapping of resistance to RSV604 to the nucleocapsid protein. The partial sequence alignment (from amino acid 1 to 240) for the N protein from the human RSV strains A2 (protein ID AAB59852.1), RSS (protein ID NP044591.1), and subgroup B (protein ID AAB82431.1) is given. The highly conserved nature of this protein between different strains of RSV is denoted by asterisks. The position of amino acid changes observed for the resisting mutants derived vs. RSV604 are boldface and denoted by ↓. The substitutions are **I**129**L** and **L**139**I** (**I**, isoleucine; **L**, leucine).

transcription [39]. Crystallography studies with RSV N protein have been pursued and have revealed variable crystal morphology [40], but a high-resolution structure has not been published at this time. This makes it difficult to predict the effects of the mutations observed on the protein. However, with such a pivotal role in replication and transcription, it is highly likely that any effect on the N structure or function would be detrimental to the virus. This made the N protein an excellent antiviral target.

As discussed previously, no mechanistically relevant animal model was available for assessing the inhibition of replication of RSV in vivo. To gain an understanding of the efficacy of the compound in a model with relevance to human disease, we studied RSV604 in a human airway epithelial (HAE) model [41]. These differentiated human primary epithelial cell cultures recapitulate the morphology and physiology of the HAE. By infecting these cultures with GFP-expressing RSV, the progress of infection can be monitored. GFP-expressing RSV was added to the apical surface of the cells and RSV604 was concomitantly added to the medium on the basolateral surface. A dose of 1 μM inhibited virus replication by approximately 50%, and concentrations of 10 μM completely abolished infection. RSV604 was at least 20-fold more active than ribavirin in this model. Adding RSV604 as late as 24 h postinfection resulted in an inhibition of viral spread (Fig. 8).

RSV604 was tested against a panel of 40 RSV clinical isolates which covered both A and B strains, a 15-year span of infections, and both the northern and southern hemispheres. RSV604 was found to be equipotent, with an average EC_{50} of 0.8 ± 0.2 μM [38]. As a final point, resistant mutant studies on RSV604 showed amino acid changes in the same region of the N protein as other compounds in this series, such as A33903 (1), indicating the same mode of action [38]. Progression into preclinical evaluation was the next logical step for this compound.

SYNTHESIS

The synthetic sequence employed within the medicinal chemistry group at Arrow permitted synthesis of the requisite amounts for preclinical and early clinical trials. Following a precedented route [42], the racemic precursor **26** was produced from **27** in a satisfactory overall yield of 64% after some optimization (Scheme 1). Resolution of the enantiomers of **27** (Scheme 2) was originally achieved by forming a diastereomeric amide with (*S*)-Boc-phenylalanine. Subsequent deprotection and resolution by chromatographic separation was used to provide almost a kilogram of (*S*)-**27**. An attempt to utilize a diastereoisomeric crystallization approach was attempted but found to be capricious upon scale-up. This sequence, although sufficient to produce 2 kg in total in the time demanded for preclinical and clinical trials, had its limitations. Efforts were therefore made to circumvent the use of chromatography and the inherently low yielding resolution stage to provide a practical approach that would lend itself to the needs of the manufacturing process.

Reider and co-workers had previously described the resolution of the 1-methyl analog of **26** (**28**, R = Me, Scheme 3) via a crystallization-induced dynamic resolution (CIDR) [43]. In this process, the salt of one enantiomer, **29**, crystallized when the racemic amine was stirred with 1 equivalent of (*S*)-CSA in a suitable solvent. Epimerization of the

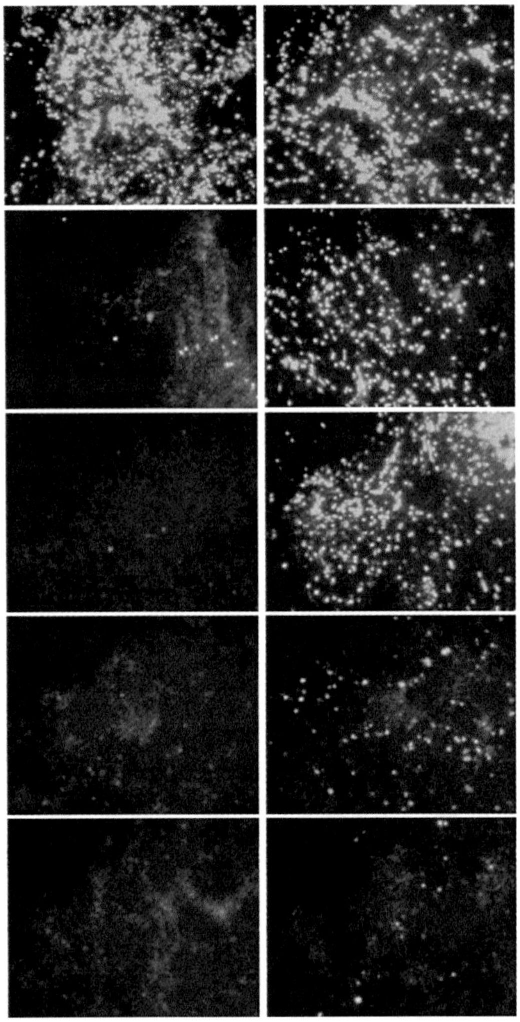

FIGURE 8 Dose-dependent inhibition of RSV replication in an in vitro model of human ciliated epithelium. RSV replication was measured visually by the expression of fluorescent green protein from the virus genome [41]. The top two panels show control cultures in the absence of drug. Compound (RSV604, ribavirin) was added to the basolateral media concomitantly with the virus at the concentrations indicated. (*See insert for color representation of the figure.*)

chiral center (effecting dynamic resolution) was achieved by reversibly condensing the amine with a catalytic amount of aromatic aldehyde. The α-proton within imine **30** thus formed was sufficiently acidic at ambient temperature and basicity for racemization to occur via the enol tautomer.

Encouraged by the precedent, a detailed analysis of whether CIDR could be applied successfully to unsubstituted amine **26** was undertaken. This involved attempted crystallizations of the resulting amine salts of a range of chiral organic acids [(*S*)-tartaric acid, (*S*)-CSA, *N*-Boc-(*S*)-phenylalanine, (*S*)-3-phenyllactic acid, (*S*)-mandelic acid, (*S*)-lactic acid, (*R*)-2,2-dimethyl-5-oxo-1,3-dioxolane-4-acetic acid] employing a variety of solvents (toluene, Et_2O, DCM, EtOH, EtOAc, *i*-Pr_2O, *i*-PrOAc). Varying amounts of water were also added (0.05 to 1 eq.), as this has been shown to aid the crystallization process [43]. All attempts to crystallize salts in this manner failed, with only crystals of racemic amine being isolated. These initial studies suggested that the physicochemical characteristics of amine **26** and its salts precluded this direct approach. A possible solution lay in the modification of the solubility of this ring system by substitution with lipophilic protecting groups, N1 substitution appeared the most reasonable position to start.

A range of protecting groups were investigated (R = Benzyl, *p*-methoxybenzyl, 2,4,6-trimethoxybenzyl, 2,4-dimethoxybenzyl, pivaloyloxymethyl, acetyl, methoxymethyl, and Boc. These were typically synthesized from **26** by treating with sodium hydride and quenching with the corresponding halide. All these derivatives exhibited much improved solubility in organic solvents, confirming the importance of this site on the physical properties.

The *p*-methoxybenzyl derivative **31** was investigated further, as it provided the most tractable synthesis (Scheme 4). Salts of **31** were treated with the same range of chiral organic acids as used previously with amine **26**. Initially, 0.5 equiv. of acid was used to assess if kinetic resolution could be achieved. A variety of solvents initially produced no crystal growth. However, addition of a small quantity of water (5%) to the *N*-boc-(*S*)-phenylalanine salt in toluene or diisopropyl ether followed by a brief exposure to ultrasound caused a dense crop of crystals to form immediately. The isolated crystals proved to have an enantiomeric purity of 95% in 45% yield. The experiment was then repeated with a catalytic amount (5%) of 3,5-dichlorosalicaldehyde, 0.1 equiv. of water in toluene, with the addition of seed crystals. After stirring overnight, the crystals formed were then isolated. Analysis showed them to have an enantiomeric excess of over 99%, with a chemical yield of 95%. Chiral high-performance liquid chromatography confirmed that the *S*-enantiomer required had been isolated. This experiment was repeated on scales ranging from 100 mg to 50 g, with reproducible results.

Deprotection of **32** to **33** proved unsuccessful by a number of methods. Synthesis of RSV604 (**23**) could still be achieved, however, by introduction of the urea moiety prior to deprotection. This deprotection was then achieved using thioanisole for 5 h. Yields for this reaction were excellent (> 95%), with chiral purity exceeding 99.5% e.e. An alternative route to functionalized amine **31** is now viable, as the reaction of **34** (R = PMB) with base and amyl nitrite under basic conditions provides a good yield of oxime **35**, whereas the analogous reaction of **26** (R = H) had earlier proved unsuccessful. This observation enabled us to pursue the route described by Bock et al. (Scheme 5, R = Me) [44]. The yields in Scheme 5 are at present unoptimized; however, the synthesis of RSV604 following this route has a combined yield

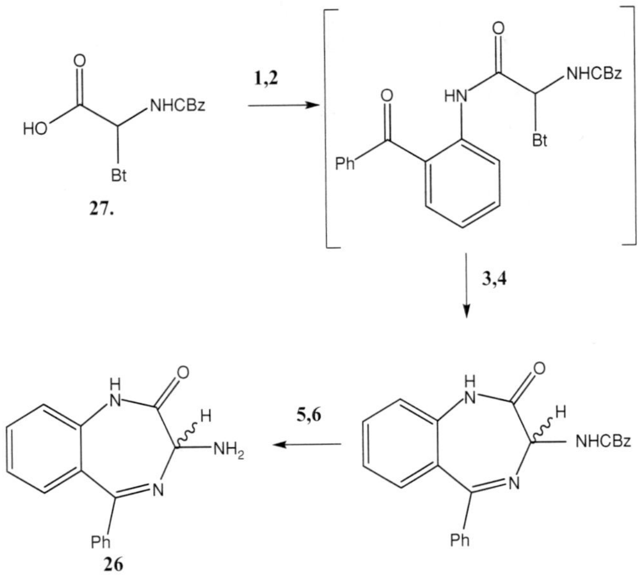

SCHEME 1 Synthesis of racemic benzodiazepine core. Reagents: (1) $COCl_2$, NMP, DCM, 5°C, 5 h; (2) 2-aminobenzophenone, 5°C, 5 h; (3) NH_3, MeOH, 5°C, 24 h; (4) NH_4OAc, AcOH, 5°C, 24 h; (5) HBr, AcOH, room temperature, 2 h, 73%; (6) K_2CO_3, 88%.

of 48% compared to 32% via the original route outlined in Schemes 1 and 2.

Initial stereochemical assignments were made in this series on the basis of the preparation of N-methylated Boc-D-phenylanaline diastereoisomers **36** and **37** and comparison with published data [44]. Preparation of a heavy atom containing urea derivative **38** allowed an unequivocal confirmation of structure via x-ray analysis. Compound **38** had the expected *S*-configuration at C3 (shown as C11 in the Ortep representation of **38** in Fig. 9) [37].

PRECLINICAL PHARMACOKINETIC AND TOXICOLOGY

As part of the preclinical process, an assessment of the absorption, distribution, metabolism, and excretion (ADME)

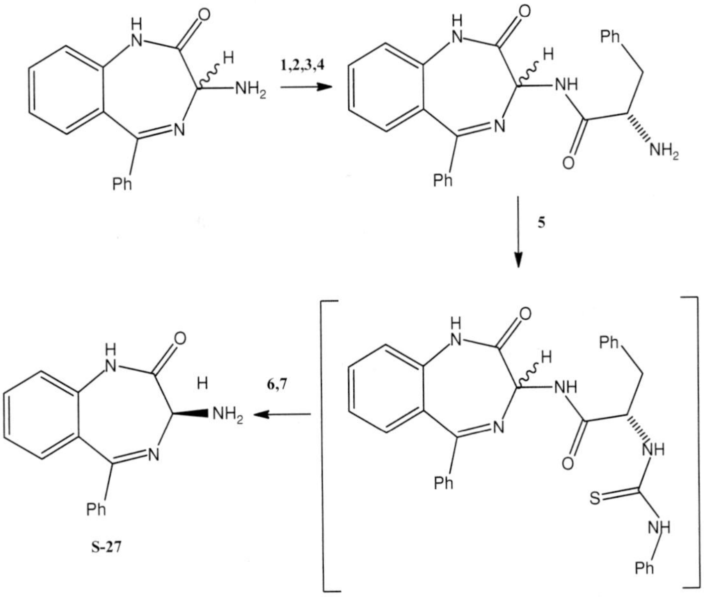

SCHEME 2 Resolution via separation of diasteroisomers. Reagents. (1) EDAC, Et_3N, N-Boc-Phe-OH, room temperature, 20 h; (2) HCl, EtOAc, 5°C, 3 h; (3) K_2CO_3; (4) separation 40%; (5) 95% PHNCS, room temperature, 18 h, 95%; (6) HBr, AcOH; (7) K_2CO_3, 90%.

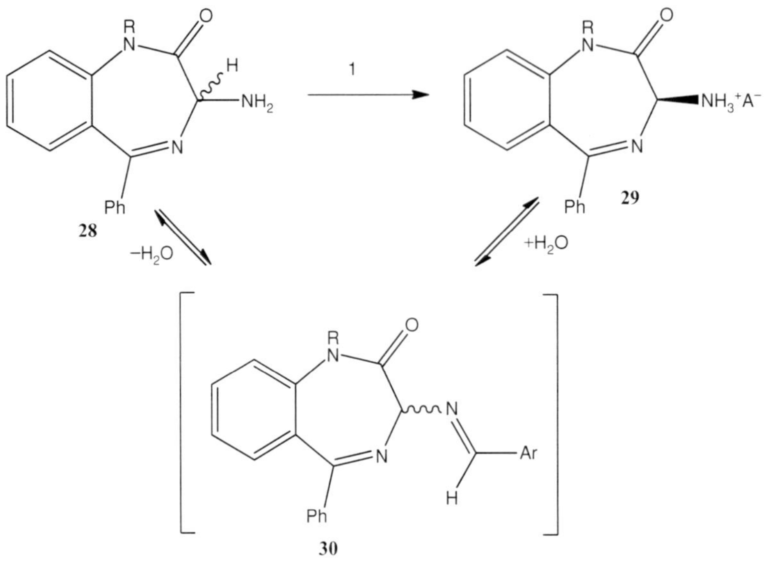

SCHEME 3 Crystallization-induced dynamic resolution (CIDR). Reagents: (1) AH, ARCHO, 5% H_2O, room temperature, 24 h.

characteristics of RSV604 was undertaken. In a focused selection of in vivo and in vitro experiments, the suitability for progression into safety assessment studies and, ultimately, clinical evaluation was determined. When a high-throughput equilibrium dialysis approach with LC-MS/MS detection was used, RSV604 showed high binding to serum proteins; $fu = 0.05$ (95% protein bound), with equivalence observed in rat, dog, and human sera. Rat and human microsomes were used to determine the susceptibility of RSV604 for oxidative metabolism. Both species displayed slow turnover with the apparent intrinsic clearance of 23.5 ± 2.8 and 4.5 ± 2.4 μL·min/mg of rat and human microsomal protein, respectively. This was supported by in vivo data described previously.

Rat in vivo pharmacokinetic (PK) characterization was carried out using both oral and intravenous routes of administration (Table 5). The plasma clearance was found to be low in the rat (7.2 mL·min/kg), which complemented the turnover results seen with the rat microsomes. The data also suggested that RSV604 would not be restricted to the systemic

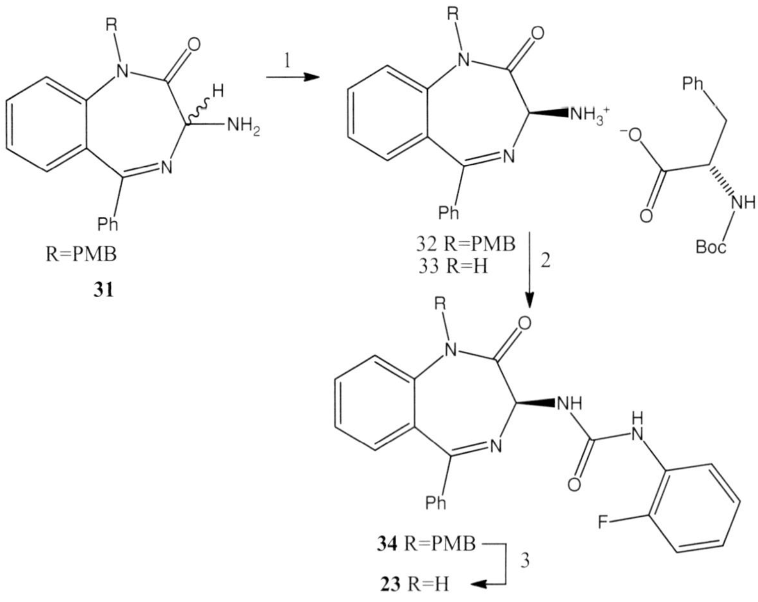

SCHEME 4 Synthesis of RSV604 via CIDR. Reagents: (1) 0.1 equiv. ARCHO, BocPheOH, 95%; (2) 2-fluorophenyl-NCO, DCM, Et3N, 90%; (3) 1 equiv. $AlCl_3$, PhSMe, 95%.

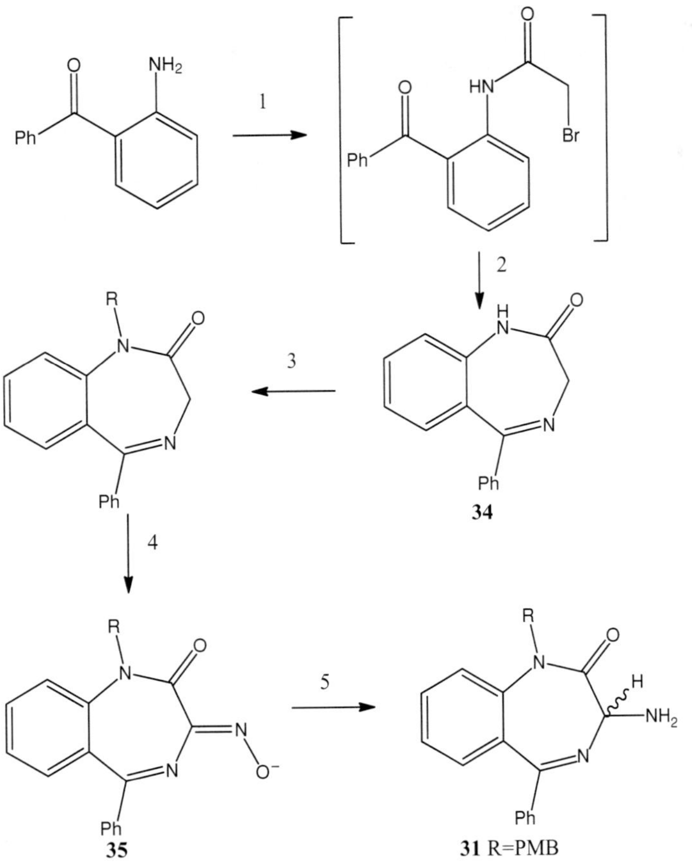

SCHEME 5 Alternative synthesis of advanced racemic amine **31**. Reagents: (1) Bromoacetyl bromide, H_2O, DCM, 0°C, 18 h; (2) NH_3, MeOH, 95% over two steps; (3) KOtBu, RCl, DMF, 0°C, room temperature, 1 h, 87%; (4) KOtBu, amyl nitrate, toluene, −5°C, 30 min, 76%; (5) H_2, 5% Ru/C, MeOH, 40 to 130 psi, 81%.

circulation and could have significant tissue distribution, since its high volume of distribution (2.2 L/kg) was much greater than the total body water. The rat PK data showed a prolonged exposure over the dosing interval and a half-life of 3 to 4 h. Rising doses of RSV604 up to 50 mg/kg in the rat showed a dose-related but less than proportional increase in AUC and C_{max}. Repeat-dose studies showed evidence of some accumulation over the dosing period.

Marmosets and dogs were evaluated as second species to assess nonrodent pharmacokinetics and support preclinical toxicological evaluation. Single- and multiple-dose studies in the marmoset showed a dose-related but subproportional increase in C_{max} and AUC. No accumulation was observed upon a repeat dose over 14 days. Initial dog studies showed poor and a variable absorption profile. Later studies showed a significant improvement with formulation.

In oral PK studies in colostrum-deprived calves [45], nasal mucosa showed significant levels of parent compound at trough. These data suggested that the compound was capable of reaching the target site of RSV infection at concentrations that exceed the bovine EC_{50} (123 ng/mL) at 24 h post-dose. These data provided confidence that efficacious target tissue concentrations could readily be achieved using an appropriate dosing regimen, thus providing an opportunity

TABLE 5 PK Properties of RSV604 Following Oral and Intravenous Administration to the Rat[a]

Route	Dose (mg/kg)	$AUC_{0\text{-inf}}$ (μg·h/mL)	C_{max} (μg/mL)	*Cip* (mL·min/kg)	V_{ss} (L/kg)	$t_{1/2}$ (h)
p.o.	5	10.9 (± 1.5)	0.91 (±0.1)	N.D.	N.D.	2.6 (± 0.2)
i.v.	5	11.7 (± 1.4)	3.3 (± 0.48)	7.2 (± 0.87)	2.2 (± 0.12)	3.8 (± 0.9)

[a]N.D., not determinable following oral administration.

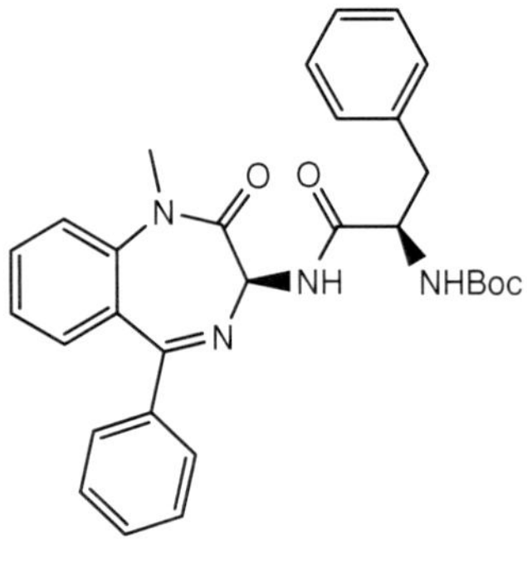

36

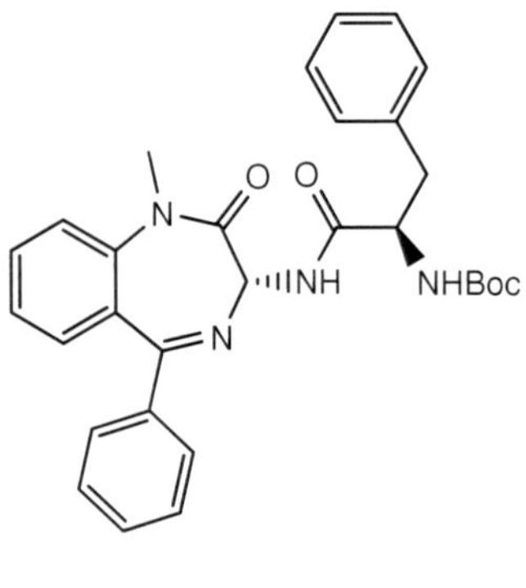

37

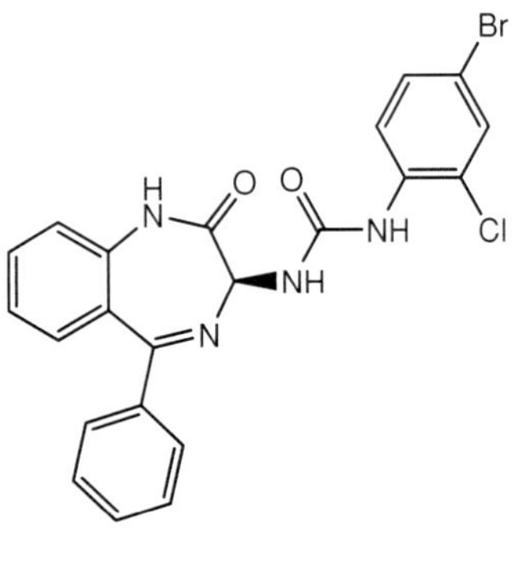

38

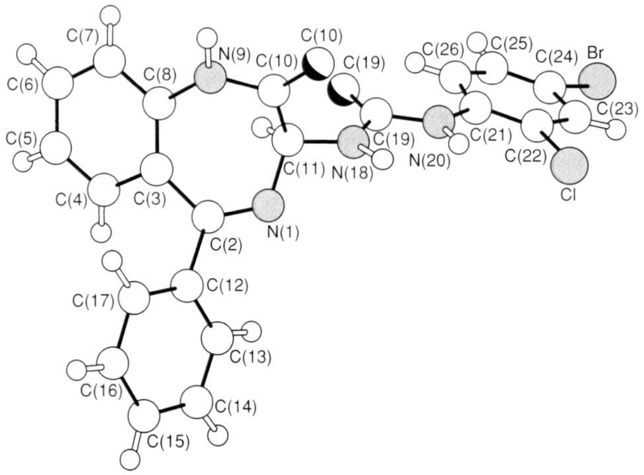

FIGURE 9 Key compounds associated with absolute stereochemistry assignment.

to demonstrate in vivo potency, assuming that these observations would extrapolate to humans.

In the species studied so far, oral doses were generally given in a lipid-based formulation to enhance bioavailability (*F*) and maximize exposure and circulating plasma levels of RSV604. The compound showed good absorption, with $F > 90\%$ at 5 mg/kg. When RSV604 was administered as a suspension in 1% carboxymethylcellulose (CMC), bioavailability was reduced to <40% at an equivalent dose, but dose proportionality in this formulation was demonstrated from 2 to 20 mg/kg. The apparent high bioavailability in the solubilized form correlated well with the low clearance and the in vitro experimentally determined apparent permeability coefficient (P_{app}) using a MDCK cell line of 13×10^{-6} cm/s, indicating that RSV604 had moderate to high passive permeability characteristics.

Although RSV604 has low plasma clearance, it has been shown to be a substrate for cytochrome P450 (CYP450) metabolism using the Bactosome recombinant isoform expression system. CYP450 3A4 was established to be the major contributor to the metabolism of the compound, with both 2C19 and 2D6 also implicated in metabolic turnover in vitro. To further assess the potential for RSV604 to undergo drug interaction when dosed in combination with other CYP450-metabolized therapeutics, CYP inhibition and induction were assessed. It was found to be a moderate inducer of CYP3A4 and CYP1A in a concentration-dependent manner but was demonstrated to have no inhibitory effect on the metabolism of specific probe substrates for CYPs 3A4, 1A2, 2D6, 2C9, or 2C19.

In vitro cell toxicity was investigated using three different cell lines (gastric, epithelial, and liver), and no significant toxicity was observed with growth inhibition figures in excess of 50 μM in all three lines. Ames bacterial mutagenicity, chromosomal aberration, and mouse micronucleus assays were also clean. No significant effects were observed in either hERG and Purkinje fiber assays. Minor action potential duration and tail current amplitude effects were followed up in a dog telemetry study, where no effects were observed.

Specifically, RSV604 was screened against a wide range of receptors in a CEREP screen [46]. Marginal activity was observed at CCKa and CCKb receptors at 10 μM, although no demonstratable clinical effect was expected from this activity. No significant effect was observed on the benzodiazepine

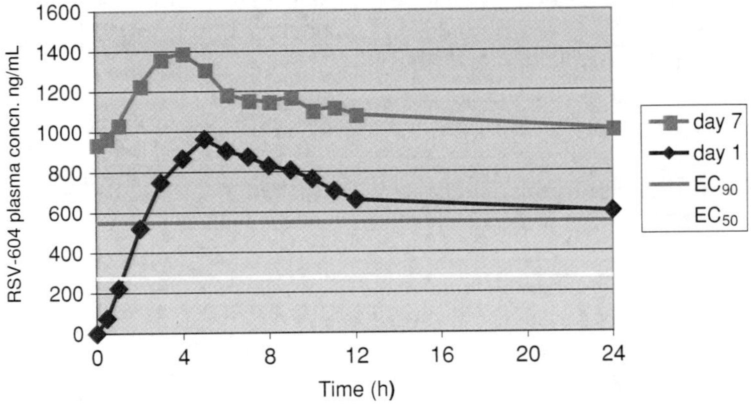

FIGURE 10 RSV604 human PK data, where volunteers received 600 mg on day 1 followed by 450 mg on days 2 to 7. (*See insert for color representation of the figure.*)

receptor. RSV604 progressed through escalating-dose studies (up to 500 mg/kg per day in rats and marmosets) and 14-day repeat-dose studies in these species (500 mg/kg per day in rats, 250 mg/kg per day in marmosets). No drug-related results were found at these doses in terms of either clinical pathology or histopathology. This profile allowed RSV604 to progress into phase 1 clinical studies with monitoring of cardiac function in healthy volunteers, as the dog telemetry study was viewed as limited by exposure.

PHASE I–III SAFETY AND EFFICACY

Single and multiple ascending-dose studies in healthy volunteers of up to 600 mg/day showed that RSV604 was well tolerated. No serious or severe adverse events were observed, and all adverse events were mild and not considered drug related. No clinically significant changes were observed in vital signs, ECGs, or from telemetry. Dosing after a high-fat meal improved bioavailability significantly. A further study looked at the safety, tolerability, and pharmacokinetic profile of 7 days' dosing of RSV604 in healthy male subjects. RSV604 was administered as an oral syrup suspension 30 min after completion of a high-fat meal. Plasma concentrations of RSV604 above the in vitro EC_{90} values were achieved (Fig. 10). Subjects given a loading dose of 600 mg RSV604 followed by 6 days of 450 mg exhibited trough concentrations above the in vitro EC_{90} at the end of day 1 and were $\geq 4 \times EC_{50}$ and $\geq 2 \times EC_{90}$ for the following 6 days.

Orally administered RSV604 was absorbed from the gastrointestinal tract and exhibited dose-dependent pharmacokinetics with biexponential elimination. The half-life of RSV604 was long, ranging from 30 to 76 h indicating suitability for once-daily administration. Over 7 days dosing there was a moderate increase in RSV604 exposure and a small decrease in half-life, indicating time-dependent elimination due to either drug metabolism autoinduction or an increase in renal clearance or a combination of both. No subjects were withdrawn from the study due to safety or tolerability concerns [47]. As a result, RSV604 was advanced into studies in patients.

The original proof-of-concept (POC) trial for RSV604 was designed to be a healthy volunteer challenge study, but a suitable high-titer virus stock proved difficult to manufacture at that time. As already discussed, the high-risk populations for RSV are the young, the elderly, and the immunocompromised. It was decided to conduct the RSV604 POC trial in adult hematopoietic stem cell transplant (HSCT) patients. RSV causes bronchiolitis, pneumonia, and long-term airflow obstruction problems in these patients. As a consequence, they are tested routinely for RSV once infected viral titers are high and RSV shedding is prolonged. At this time, there is no approved antiviral treatment for these patients. The disadvantage of using this patient group are the limited number of treatment centers and having patients clear of other infections. An RSV trial has its own problems with the seasonality of the virus and the narrow window of infection. The RSV604 POC trial was an extremely difficult one to set up and involved 10 centers in the United States, the U.K., Australia, and Spain. Many potential patients were excluded due to the severity of their underlying condition. It was the largest double-blind placebo-controlled study in HSCT recipients with RSV infection carried out at that time.

A pilot phase of the study was designed to determine the safety of RSV604 in HSCT patients and the PK of the compound with relation to the concurrent medications being taken by the individual patients. The objectives of the main phase were to identify an in vivo antiviral effect of RSV604 and a 2 log decrease in RSV viral load as determined by nasopharyngeal swabs and subsequent real-time polymerase chain reaction analysis. Secondary endpoints included safety and PK, RSV viral load during and after treatment, relationship between RSV exposure and antiviral activity, and the effect of RSV604 on symptoms and signs. The treatment regime was 600 mg on day 1 followed by 450 mg on days 2 to 5. RSV604 was taken after a high-calorie meal, and nasopharyngeal swabs were taken daily up to day 6 and again on day 12 post-treatment. The trial was double blind and placebo controlled. Recruitment for the trial proved difficult for the reasons mentioned.

Patients who achieved RSV604 levels greater than the in vitro EC_{90} had a bigger drop in RSV viral load than that of those who did not. Symptom improvement was also greater among patients who experienced higher RSV604 exposure. However, most patients on RSV604 had lower drug exposures than were predicted from the PK studies, and the RSV viral load difference at 72 h after start of treatment was not significantly different from that with placebo. The mean RSV604 trough levels did not exceed the EC_{90} value until day 3, there was large individual variation, and steady state was not achieved until the end of treatment. There were no serious adverse events, so overall, RSV604 was safe and well tolerated [48]. With its potent antiviral efficacy, unique mechanism of action, and oral bioavailability, RSV604 has great potential, and Novartis is continuing clinical studies.

FUTURE DIRECTIONS

A subsequent program at Arrow Therapeutics identified (*S*)-4-methanesulfonyl-2-methoxy-*N*-(2-oxo-5-phenyl-2,3-dihydro-1*H*-benzo[*e*][1,4]diazepin-3-yl)benzamide, **25** (A-315), as a backup molecule to RSV604. Compound **25** showed potent anti-RSV activity across the primary and secondary assays, with a different PK profile and improved aqueous solubility over RSV604. The exciting potential of the N-protein target as shown by RSV604 is tempered by the tractability of the target from a drug discovery point of view. A high-resolution crystal structure of the protein is needed but is proving very difficult to attain. The search for new inhibitors of RSV N-protein, or indeed any replication-targeted approach, is restricted to the use of whole virus infectious assays. Future drug discovery efforts may be aided by the use of RSV subgenomic replicon systems, in much the same way that HCV research has progressed over the last 10 years.

Work has continued on the identification of inhibitors of the RSV fusion protein, both at Arrow and elsewhere, with some success. Fusion is an essential process for RSV infection, so the fusion protein as a target remains worthy of further investigation. There is a clear unmet medical need for the treatment of RSV, and the financial burden of RSV infection year after year is huge. The development of new small-molecule antivirals is essential to protect vulnerable patient groups, as vaccine production continues to face major problems.

REFERENCES

[1] Hall, C. B.; Weinberg, G. A.; Iwane, M. K.; Blumkin, A. K.; Edwards, K. M.; Staat, M. A.; Auinger, P.; Griffin, M. R.; Poehling, K. A.; Erdman, D.; et al. The burden of respiratory syncytial virus infection in young children. *N. Engl. J. Med.* **2009**, *360*, 588–598.

[2] Iwane, M. K.; Edwards, K. M.; Szilagyi, P. G.; Walker, F. J.; Griffin, M. R.; Weinberg, G. A.; Coulen, C.; Poehling, K. A.; Shone, L. P.; Balter, S.; et al. Population-based surveillance for hospitalizations associated with respiratory syncytial virus, influenza virus and parainfluenza viruses among young children. *Pediatrics* **2004**, *113*, 1758–1764.

[3] Schanzer, D. L.; Langley, J. M.; Tam, T. W. S. Hospitalization attributable to influenza and other viral respiratory illnesses in Canadian children. *Pediatr. Infect. Dis. J.* **2006**, *25*, 795–800.

[4] Nicholson, K. G.; McNally, T.; Silverman, M.; Simons, P.; Stockton, J. D.; Zambon, M. C. Rates of hospitalisation for influenza, respiratory syncytial virus and human metapneumovirus among infants and young children. *Vaccine* **2006**, *24*, 102–108.

[5] Thompson, W. W.; Shay, D. K.; Weintraub, E.; Brammer, L.; Cox, N.; Anderson, L. J.; Fukuda, K. Mortality associated with influenza and respiratory syncytial virus in the United States. *JAMA* **2003**, *289*, 179–186.

[6] Falsey, A. R.; Hennessey, P. A.; Formica, M. A.; Cox, C.; Walsh, E. E. Respiratory syncytial virus infection in elderly and high-risk adults. *N. Engl. J. Med.* **2005**, *352*, 1749–1759.

[7] Ebbert, J. O.; Limper, A. H. Respiratory syncytial virus pneumonitis in immunocompromised adults: clinical features and outcome. *Respiration* **2005**, *72*, 263–269.

[8] Hegele, R. G.; Hayashi, S.; Bramley, A. M.; Hogg, J. C. Persistence of respiratory syncytial virus genome and protein after acute bronchiolitis in guinea pigs. *Chest* **1994**, *105*, 1848–1852.

[9] Valarcher, J. F.; Bourhy, H.; Lavenu, A.; Bourges-Abella, N.; Roth, M.; Andreoletti, O.; Ave, P.; Schelcher, F. Persistent infection of B lymphocytes by bovine respiratory syncytial virus. *Virology* **2001**, *291*, 55–67.

[10] Hruska, J. F.; Bernstein, J. M.; Douglas, R. G., Jr.; Hall, C. B. Effects of ribavirin on respiratory syncytial virus in vitro. *Antimicrob. Agents Chemother.* **1980**, *17*, 770–775.

[11] Ventre, K.; Randolph, A.G. Ribavirin for respiratory syncytial virus infection of the lower respiratory tract in infants and young children. *Cochrane Database Syst. Rev.* **2004**, CD000181.

[12] Englund, J. In search of a vaccine for respiratory syncytial virus: the saga continues. *J. Infect. Dis.* **2005**, *191*, 1036–1039.

[13] Kim, H. W.; Canchola, J. G.; Brandt, B. D.; Pyles, G.; Chanock, R. M.; Jensen, K.; Parrott, R. H. Respiratory syncytial disease in infants despite prior administration of antigenic inactivated vaccine. *Am. J. Epidemiol.* **1969**, *89*, 422–434.

[14] Johnson, P. R.; Spriggs, M. K.; Olmsted, R.A.; Collins, P. L. The G glycoprotein of human respiratory syncytial viruses of subgroups A and B: extensive divergence between antigenically related proteins. *Proc. Natl. Acad. Sci. USA* **1987**, *84*, 5625–5629.

[15] Johnson, P. R.; Collins, P. L. The fusion glycoproteins of human respiratory syncytial virus of subgroups A and B: sequence conservation provides a structural basis for antigenic relatedness. *J. Gen. Virol.* **1988**, *69*, 2623–2628.

[16] Johnson, P. R.; Collins, P. L. The 1B (NS2), 1C (NS1) and N proteins of human respiratory syncytial virus (RSV) of antigenic subgroups A and B: sequence conservation and divergence within RSV genomic RNA. *J. Gen. Virol.* **1989**, *70*, 1539–1547.

[17] Cane, P. A.; Matthews, D. A.; Pringle, C. R. Analysis of relatedness of subgroup A respiratory syncytial viruses isolated worldwide. *Virus Res.* **1992**, *25*, 15–22.

[18] Cane, P. A.; Matthews, D. A.; Pringle, C. R. Analysis of respiratory syncytial virus strain variation in successive epidemics in one city. *J. Clin. Microbiol.* **1994**, *32*, 1–4.

[19] Peret, T. C.; Hall, C. B.; Schnabel, K. C.; Golub, J. A.; Anderson, L. J. Circulation patterns of genetically distinct group A and B strains of human respiratory syncytial virus in a community. *J. Gen. Virol.* **1998**, *79*, 2221–2229.

[20] Cane, P. A. Molecular epidemiology of respiratory syncytial virus. *Rev. Med. Virol.* **2001**, *11*, 103–116.

[21] Waris, M. Pattern of respiratory syncytial virus epidemics in Finland: two-year cycles with alternating prevalence of groups A and B. *J. Infect. Dis.* **1991**, *163*, 464–469.

[22] McKimm-Breschkin, J. L. A simplified plaque assay for respiratory syncytial virus: direct visualisation of plaques without immunostaining. *J. Virol. Methods* **2004**, *120*, 113–117.

[23] Domachowske, J. B.; Bonville, C. A.; Rosenberg, H. F. Animal models for studying respiratory syncytial virus infection and its long term effects on lung function. *Pediatr. Infect. Dis. J.* **2004**, *23*, S228–S234.

[24] Sidwell, R. W.; Barnard, D. L. Respiratory syncytial virus infections: recent prospects for control. *Antiviral Res.* **2006**, *71*, 379–390.

[25] Douglas, J. L.; Panis, M. L.; Ho, E.; Lin, K.-Y.; Krawczyk, S. H.; Grant, D. M.; Cai, R.; Swaminathan, S.; Chen, X.; Cihlar, T. Small molecules VP-14637 and JNJ-2408068 inhibit respiratory syncytial virus fusion by similar mechanisms. *Antimicrob. Agents Chemother.* **2005**, *49*, 2460–2466.

[26] Nikitenko, A. A.; Raifeld, Y. E.; Wang, T. Z. The discovery of RFI-641 as a potent and selective inhibitor of the respiratory syncytial virus. *Bioorg. Med. Chem. Lett.* **2001**, *11*, 1041–1044.

[27] Weiss, W. J.; Murphy, T.; Lynch, M. E.; Frye, J.; Buklan, A.; Gray, B.; Lenoy, E.; Mitelman, S.; O'Connell, J.; Quartuccio, S.; Huntley, C. Inhalation efficacy of RFI-641 in an African green monkey model of RSV infection. *J. Med. Primatol.* **2003**, *32*, 82–88.

[28] Andries, K.; Moeremans, M.; Geyers, T.; Willebrords, R.; Sommen, C.; Lacrampe, J.; Janssens, F.; Wyde, P. R. Substituted benzimidazoles with nanomolar activity against respiratory syncytial virus. *Antiviral Res.* **2003**, *60*, 209–219.

[29] Cianci, C.; Yu, K.-L.; Combrink, K.; Sin, N.; Pearce, B.; Wang, A.; Civiello, R.; Voss, S.; Luo, G.; Kadow, K.; et al. Orally active fusion inhibitor of respiratory syncytial virus. *Antimicrob. Agents Chemother.* **2004**, *48*, 413–422.

[30] Wyde, P. R.; Chetty, S. N.; Timmerman, P.; Gilbert, B. E.; Andries, K. Short duration aerosols of JNJ 2408068 (R170591) administered prophylactically or therapeutically protect cotton rats from experimental respiratory syncytial virus infection. *Antiviral Res.* **2003**, *60*, 209–219.

[31] Bonfanti, J. F.; Doublet, F.; Fortin, J.; Lacrampe, J.; Guillemont, J.; Muller, P.; Queguiner, L.; Arnoult, E.; Gevers, T.; Janssens, P.; et al. Selection of a respiratory syncytial virus fusion inhibitor clinical candidate: 1. improving the pharmacokinetic profile using the structure–property relationship. *J. Med. Chem.* **2007**, *50*, 4572–4584.

[32] Bonfanti, J. F.; Meyer, C.; Doublet, F.; Fortin, J.; Muller, P.; Queguiner, L.; Gevers, T.; Janssens, P.; Szel, H.; Willebrords, R.; et al. Selection of a respiratory syncytial virus fusion inhibitor clinical candidate: 2. Discovery of a morpholinopropylaminobenzimidazole derivative (TMC353121). *J. Med. Chem.* **2008**, *51*, 875–896.

[33] Ni, L.; Zhao, L.; Qian, Y.; Zhu, J.; Jin, Z.; Chen, Y. W.; Tien, P.; Gao, G. F. Design and characterization of human respiratory syncytial virus entry inhibitors. *Antiviral Ther.* **2005**, *10*, 833–840.

[34] Sudo, K.; Miyazaki, Y.; Kojima, N.; Kobayashi, M.; Suzuki, H.; Shintani, M.; Shimizu, Y. YM-53403, a unique anti-respiratory syncytial virus agent with a novel mechanism of action. *Antiviral Res.* **2005**, *65*, 125–131.

[35] Alvarez, R.; Elbashir, S.; Borland, T.; Toudjarska, I.; Hadwiger, P.; John, M.; Roehl, I.; Shulga Morskyaya, S.; Martinello, R.; Kahn, J.; et al. RNAi-mediated silencing of the respiratory syncytial virus nucleocapsid defines a potent antiviral strategy. *Antimicrob. Agents Chemother.* **2009**, Jun 8. EPub.

[36] Carter, M. C.; Alber, D. G.; Baxter, R. C.; Bithell, S. K.; Budworth, J.; Chubb, A.; Cockerill, G. S.; Dowdell, V. C. L.; Henderson, E. A.; Keegan, S. J.; et al. 1,4-Benzodiazepines as inhibitors of respiratory syncytial virus. *J. Med. Chem.* **2006**, *49*, 2311–2319.

[37] Henderson, E. A.; Alber, D. G.; Baxter, R. C.; Bithell, S. K.; Budworth, J.; Carter, M. C.; Chubb, A.; Cockerill, G. S.; Dowdell, V. C. L.; Fraser, I. J.; et al. 1,4-Benzodiazepines as inhibitors of respiratory syncytial virus. the identification of a clinical candidate. *J. Med. Chem.* **2007**, *50*, 1685–1692.

[38] Chapman, J.; Abbott, E.; Alber, D. G.; Baxter, R. C.; Bithell, S. K.; Henderson, E. A.; Carter, M. C.; Chambers, P.; Chubb, A.; Cockerill, G. S.; et al. RSV604, a novel inhibitor of respiratory syncytial virus replication. *Antimicrob. Agents Chemother.* **2007**, *51*, 3346–3353.

[39] Collins, P. L.; Chanock, R. M.; Murphy, B. R. Respiratory syncytial virus. In *Fields Virology*, 4th ed., Knipe, D. M., Howley, P. M., Griffin, D. E., Lamb, R. A., Martin, M. A., Roizman, B.,

Straus, S. E., Eds.; Lippincott Williams & Wilkins, Philadelphia, 2001, pp. 1443–1485.

[40] Omari, K. E.; Scott, K.; Dhaliwal, B.; Ren, J.; Abrescia, N. G. A.; Budworth, J.; Lockyer, M.; Powell, K. L.; Hawkins, A. R.; Stammers, D. K. Crystallization and preliminary x-ray analysis of the human respiratory syncytial virus nucleocapsid protein. *Acta Crystallogr.* **2008**, *64*, 1019–1023.

[41] Zhang, L.; Peeples, M. E.; Boucher, R. C.; Collins, P. L.; Pickles, R. J. Respiratory syncytial virus infection of human airway epithelial cells is polarized, specific to ciliated cells and without obvious cytopathology. *J. Virol.* **2002**, *76*, 5654–5666.

[42] Sherrill, R. G.; Sugg, E. E. An improved synthesis and resolution of 3-amino-1,3-dihydro-5-phenyl-2H-1,4-benzodiazepin-2-ones. *J. Org. Chem.* **1995**, *60*, 730–734.

[43] Reider, P. J.; Davis, P.; Hughes, D. L.; Grabowski, E. J. J. *J. Org. Chem.* **1987**, *52*, 957–958.

[44] Bock, M. G.; DiPardo, R. M.; Evans, B. E.; Rittle, K. E.; Veber, D. F.; Freidinger, R. M.; Hirshfield, J.; Springer, J. P. *J. Org. Chem.* **1987**, *52*, 3232–3239.

[45] Gershwin, L. J.; Schelegle, E. S.; Gunther, R. A.; Anderson, M. L.; Woolums, A. R.; Larochelle, D. R.; Boyle, G. A.; Friebertshauser, K. E.; Singer, R. S. A bovine model of vaccine enhanced respiratory syncytial virus pathophysiology. *Vaccine* **1998**, *16*, 1225–1236.

[46] CEREP screen. See http://www.cerep.fr for details of screen and protocols.

[47] Dent, J.; Grieve, S.; Harland, R.; Alber, D.; Sanderson, B.; Lonsdale, F.; Thomson, E.; Smith, G.; Allan, G.; Powell, K. Multiple-dose safety and pharmacokinetics of A-60444, a novel compound active against respiratory syncytial virus (RSV). Poster F-483. 45th Annual Interscience Conference on Antimicrobial Agents and Chemotherapy, Washington, DC, Dec. 16–19, 2005.

[48] Marty, F. A double-blind, randomized, placebo-controlled study to evaluate the safety and efficacy of RSV604 in adults with respiratory syncytial virus infection following stem cell transplantation. IXth International Symposium on Respiratory Viral Infections, Causeway Bay, Hong Kong, Mar. 3–6, 2007.

PART IV

INFLUENZA, HEPATITIS B, AND CYTOMEGALOVIRUS INHIBITORS

27

DISCOVERY AND DEVELOPMENT OF INFLUENZA VIRUS SIALIDASE INHIBITOR RELENZA

ROBIN THOMSON AND MARK VON ITZSTEIN
Institute for Glycomics, Griffith University, Queensland, Australia

INTRODUCTION

Influenza has a significant impact on human health: Annual influenza epidemics exact a high toll in morbidity, estimated to be in the range of 3 to 5 million cases of severe illness, and mortality, with up to half a million deaths worldwide [1]. In addition, it has been estimated that a human-to-human-transmissible, highly pathogenic pandemic influenza virus could lead to about 62 million deaths worldwide [2]. In March 2009, an outbreak of infection with a novel influenza A virus (swine-origin H1N1 2009) began in Mexico and spread rapidly across the globe, and by the end of the year at least 12,000 deaths had been attributed to infection with the virus [3]. While the highly transmissible 2009 pandemic (H1N1) virus has, to date, caused a predominantly mild disease in patients with no underlying disease [4], human infection with the highly pathogenic avian-origin H5N1 influenza A virus, commonly referred to as "bird flu", has been significantly more severe and associated with a very high mortality rate [5]. However, although the H5N1 virus transmits zoonotically from infected poultry to humans, often with fatal consequences, such transmission remains inefficient, as does subsequent human-to-human transmission [6]. The situation of concurrently circulating highly transmissible pandemic A/H1N1 virus, and extremely aggressive avian A/H5N1 virus, brought into sharp focus the need for the global availability of effective influenza virus-specific antiviral agents to provide a first line of defense against an emerging pandemic virus.

Influenza Virus

Influenza virus belongs to the orthomyxoviridae family and has a single-stranded segmented RNA genome. The virus is subdivided into three serologically distinct types, A, B, and C, of which type C does not seem to cause significant disease. Influenza A viruses, which cause the most significant disease in humans [7], are further classified based on the antigenic properties of the two envelope-associated surface glycoproteins (Fig. 1A), hemagglutinin (HA: H1-16) and sialidase (neuraminidase, NA: N1-9) [7]. Viruses of all HA and NA subtypes have been recovered from aquatic birds (the biological reservoir of all influenza viruses), but only three HA subtypes (H1, H2, and H3) and two NA subtypes (N1 and N2) have established stable lineages in the human population since 1918 [7].

The replication cycle of influenza A virus (Figure 1B) presents a number of potential virus-specific drug targets (reviewed in [10–12]), including inhibition of the essential functions of the three viral surface glycoproteins: the lectin hemagglutinin, involved in cell entry and fusion; the M2 ion channel protein, involved in virus uncoating; and the glycohydrolase sialidase, which facilitates the release of new virus particles. The first influenza virus-specific drugs, developed in the mid-1960s, were the adamantane-based M2 ion channel inhibitors rimantadine and amantadine [13,14]. However, these drugs are effective only against influenza virus A infection (influenza B virus strains do not have an M2 ion channel), and both drugs have been reported

Antiviral Drugs: From Basic Discovery Through Clinical Trials, First Edition. Edited by Wieslaw M. Kazmierski.

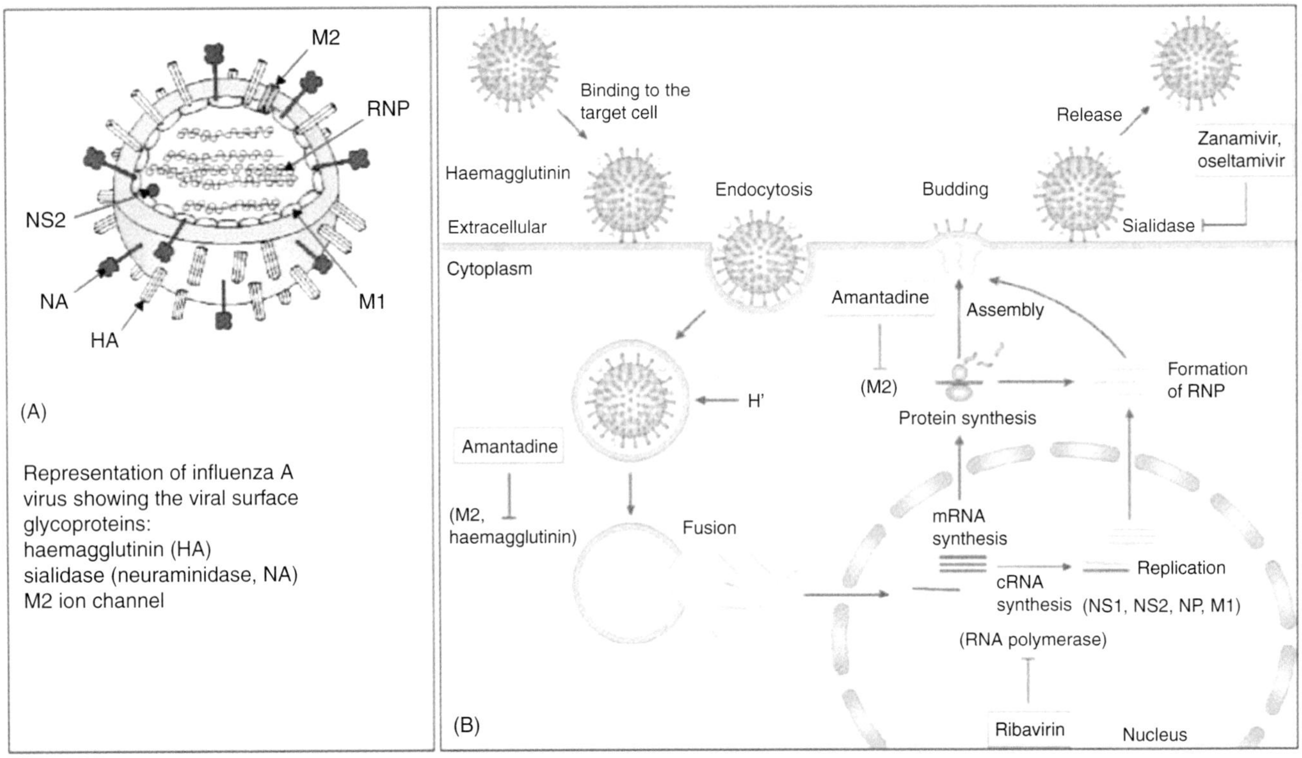

FIGURE 1 Schematic representations of (A) influenza A virus, and (B) its replication cycle, indicating the therapeutic intervention points targeted by current drugs. [(A) from [8], copyright © 2000, with permission from Elsevier; (B) from [9], with permission.]

not only to have significant side effects, but also lead to the rapid emergence of drug resistant influenza virus strains [7,10,14].

Both the viral hemagglutinin and sialidase have been considered as drug discovery targets, due to their roles in virus replication and propagation. The hemagglutinin mediates both the initial attachment of the virus to the target respiratory epithelium of host cells, via *N*-acetylneuraminic acid terminated cell-surface sialoglycoconjugates, and subsequent internalization of the virus and fusion of the viral envelope with the host-cell membrane [15]. A major role of the sialidase in the infective cycle is to facilitate release of virus progeny from the infected cell by cleaving the *N*-acetylneuraminic acid residues from cell surface and virus particle–associated sialoglycoconjugates (see **1**, Scheme 1) that would otherwise be bound by the HA of the new virus particles, keeping the particles aggregated at the cell surface [16,17]. The interplay between the receptor-binding (HA) and receptor-destroying (NA) functions is of major importance in the efficiency of viral replication [17].

A number of drug discovery approaches targeting the viral HA have been explored (reviewed in [12]) but to date have not led to a therapeutically active agent. The most significant recent advances in anti-influenza drug development have arisen from targeting the sialidase function. In this chapter we review the discovery and development of the first potent sialidase inhibitor–based anti-influenza drug zanamivir [18].

Influenza Virus Sialidase: Structure and Mechanism

Influenza virus sialidase (EC 3.2.1.18) is a tetrameric glycoprotein consisting of four identical subunits [19]. It has a box-shaped head attached to a long slender stalk [20]. The protein was first purified in the 1960s, the A/N2 sialidase was crystallized successfully in the late 1970s, and its x-ray crystal structure was solved soon thereafter [21,22] (reviewed in [19,20]). The x-ray crystal structures of influenza B and A/N9 sialidases were solved in the early 1990s, and a number of NA-complex structures since, but it was not until 2006 that structures of the clinically important A/N1 subtype were solved [23].

While the sequence homology between sialidases from influenza A and B viruses is around 30% and between influenza A virus subtypes is less than 50%, a number of amino acid residues are highly conserved between virtually all A and B virus subtypes [24]. With the resolution of the A/N2 structure, the relationship between these highly conserved residues spaced along the sialidase polypeptide "crystallized" when they were found to line the walls of the

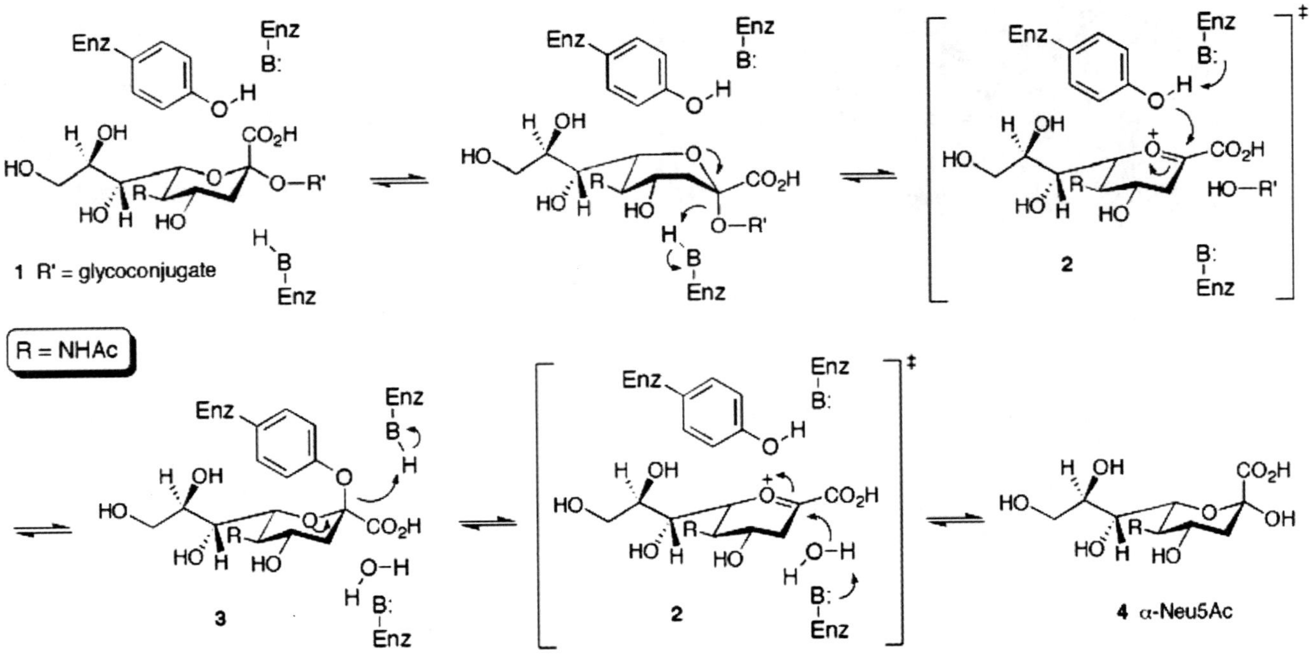

SCHEME 1 Proposed enzyme reaction mechanism of influenza virus sialidase showing the putative sialosyl-cation (**2**) and covalent sialosyl-enzyme (**3**) intermediates. The α-anomer of the product *N*-acetylneuraminic acid (α-Neu5Ac, **4**) formed initially undergoes rapid equilibration with the β-anomer.

enzyme active site [19,20]. The active site consists of a number of distinct adjoining pockets that are lined by eight highly conserved amino acid residues that make direct contact with a bound α-*N*-acetylneuraminic acid residue (α-Neu5Ac; see **4**, Scheme 1), as in the terminal residue of a sialoglycoconjugate substrate or the product of enzyme hydrolysis [25]. In addition, there are another 10 amino acid residues invariant in all strains of influenza virus within the vicinity of the active site that appear to be important primarily in the stabilization of the architecture of the active site [19].

Upon binding, an α-Neu5Ac residue is oriented within the active site through charge–charge interactions between the C1 carboxylate group and a cluster of three conserved arginine residues [25] (Fig. 2). Also important are the interactions of the C5 acetamido group, which is embedded in a pocket of the active site through hydrogen bonding of the carbonyl oxygen and the N—H to residue Arg152 and a buried water molecule, respectively. (Note: The numbering used throughout reflects that reported for influenza A virus N2 sialidase.) Favorable hydrophobic contacts to residues Trp178 and Ile222 are also made by the methyl of the C5 acetamido group. Additional hydrogen-bond networks are formed by the C8 and C9 hydroxyl groups of the glycerol side chain to the carboxylate oxygens of residue Glu276, while the C4 hydroxyl group associates with the carboxylate oxygen of Glu119. All of the amino acid residues mentioned above are fully conserved across the natural strains of influenza virus known to date [19].

Extensive biochemical studies of influenza virus and other sialidases have led to the proposed catalytic mechanism shown in Scheme 1. On binding of the terminal *N*-acetylneuraminic acid (Neu5Ac) residue of the substrate sialoglycoconjugate (**1** in Scheme 1), the Neu5Ac residue adopts a distorted boatlike conformation (seen in the x-ray structure of the A/N2:α-Neu5Ac complex [25]), facilitated in part by formation of a salt bridge between the Neu5Ac carboxylate and the triarginyl cluster (Arg118, Arg371, Arg292) [25]. Cleavage of the aglycon unit then appears to proceed via the formation of an enzyme-stabilized sialosyl cation intermediate (**2**) [26–28]. This may be trapped transiently as a covalent sialosyl-enzyme intermediate (**3**), as proposed for other sialidases [29], by nucleophilic attack of a strain-independent, highly conserved tyrosine residue positioned directly below the anomeric carbon (C2) of the *N*-acetylneuraminic acid moiety. Subsequent stereoselective reaction of the sialosyl cation, or covalent intermediate, with water affords initially α-Neu5Ac (**4**), which then mutarotates to the more thermodynamically stable anomer β-anomer.

SIALIDASE AS A DRUG DISCOVERY TARGET

Key for drug design against influenza virus sialidase was the finding from x-ray crystal structures [19] that despite high antigenic variability of the viral sialidase, a significant number of active-site residues are conserved in sialidases

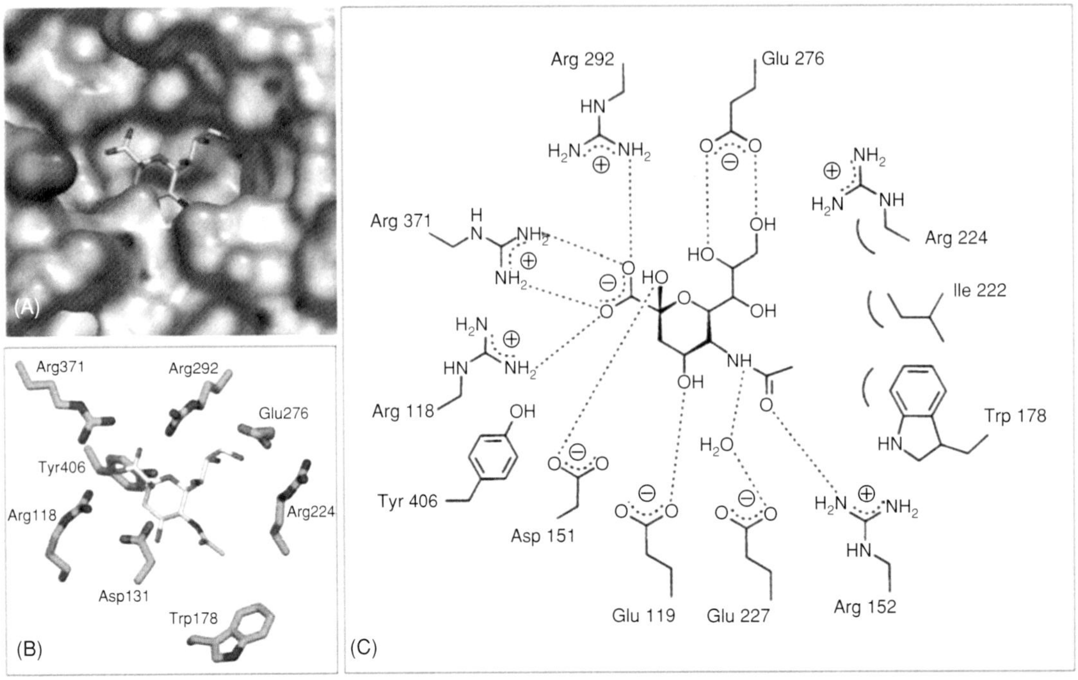

FIGURE 2 Representations of the A/N2:α-Neu5Ac (**4**) complex (pdb 2BAT). (A) View of active site with protein surface colored by electrostatic potential (blue, positive; red, negative). α-Neu5Ac carbons in yellow. (B) Key active-site residues surrounding α-Neu5Ac. (C) Schematic representation of the A/N2 active site showing some key interactions of α-Neu5Ac with conserved residues. Conserved interacting active site residues include Arg118, Arg371, Arg292, Glu276, Arg152, and Glu227. Hydrophobic interactions are made between the C5 acetamido methyl group and Ile222 and Trp178. Tyr406 and Asp151 are involved in enzyme catalysis [25]. (*See insert for color representation of the figure.*)

across all strains of influenza A and B viruses. This not only meant that sialidase was a good drug target against the highly mutating virus, but the conservation of key active-site residues across both A and B viruses provided an exciting opportunity for the development of compounds that could target all influenza A and B viruses. In addition, by targeting inhibitor interactions to conserved residues, it was hoped that the generation of viable mutants would not be facile.

Past work with inhibitors of influenza virus [30] and other [31] sialidases had identified the unsaturated *N*-acetylneuraminic acid derivative Neu5Ac2en **5** (Fig. 3) as a general micromolar inhibitor of viral and bacterial sialidases. It was postulated to be a mimic of the putative sialosyl cation intermediate (**2**) of the sialidase transition state, by virtue of its half-chair conformation [31]. The C5 trifluoroacetamido analog of Neu5Ac2en (**6**) was the most active inhibitor of influenza virus sialidase known to date ($K_i = 8 \times 10^{-7}$ M A/N1) [30] and showed effective inhibition of virus replication in tissue culture and inhibition of the elution of influenza virus from erythrocytes [32]. Neu5Ac2en itself inhibits both viral and mammalian sialidases, with K_i values in the micromolar range [33]; therefore, a drug design program based on the Neu5Ac2en template was aimed at both increasing the inhibitory potency against influenza virus sialidases, from A and B viruses, and installing functionality that would confer high inhibitory specificity for the viral enzyme.

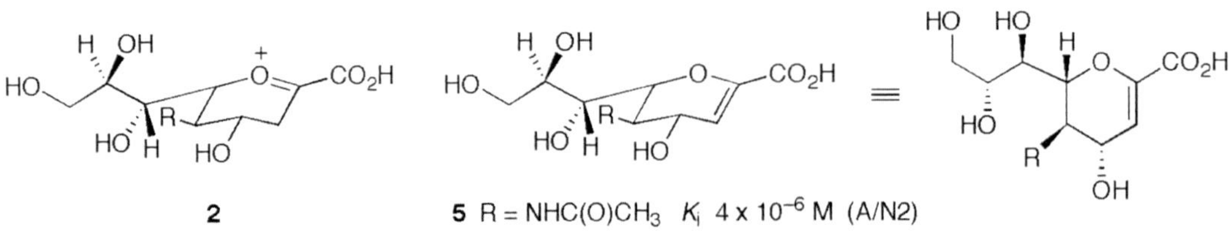

2

5 R = NHC(O)CH$_3$ K_i 4 x 10^{-6} M (A/N2)

6 R = NHC(O)CF$_3$ K_i 8 x 10^{-7} M (A/N1)

FIGURE 3

Structure-Based Drug Design on the Neu5Ac2en Template: The Discovery of Zanamivir (Relenza)

With detailed knowledge of the interactions between the highly conserved active-site residues and α-Neu5Ac (**4**) [25] (Fig. 2C) and Neu5Ac2en (**5**), the structure-based drug design effort was begun. Using the software program GRID [34], energetically favorable interactions between various functional group probes (such as carboxylate, amine, methyl group, and phosphate) and residues within the A/N2 NA active site were explored [35]. Overlaying the functional group "hot spots" with the known position of Neu5Ac2en (**5**) in the A/N2:Neu5Ac2en complex identified potential substitutions on the Neu5Ac2en template that would be predicted to increase binding affinity. From this study it became clear that replacement of the C4 hydroxyl group of Neu5Ac2en (**5**) by a more basic amine group (e.g., 4-amino-4-deoxy-Neu5Ac2en **7**) should enhance binding affinity as a result of salt bridge formation with conserved amino acid Glu119. Importantly, with further analysis it was evident that the C-4 hydroxyl binding pocket may also accommodate larger, more basic functional groups than the amine. This analysis, together with chemical intuition, led to the conclusion that a guanidino group incorporated at C4 of Neu5Ac2en (**8**) (Fig. 4), engaging most of the C4 binding pocket, could form substantial interactions with two highly conserved acidic amino acid residues (Glu119 and Glu227) via its terminal nitrogens.

The two target Neu5Ac2en derivatives, 4-amino-4-deoxy-Neu5Ac2en (**7**) and 4-deoxy-4-guanidino-Neu5Ac2en (**8**), were readily synthesized (see the following section) and evaluated as inhibitors of sialidases from both influenza A and B viruses [18,33]. Both derivatives were found to be potent competitive inhibitors of influenza virus sialidase in vitro, with K_i values 100- to 10,000-fold lower than the parent Neu5Ac2en [**7**: $K_i = 5 \times 10^{-8}$ M (A/N2); **8**: $K_i = 2 \times 10^{-10}$ M (A/N2), 7×10^{-10} M (B)] [18]. The 4-guanidino derivative **8** exhibited slow binding kinetics that further decreased the apparent K_i value against A/N2 sialidase to 3×10^{-11} M [18]. Both compounds also efficiently prevented in vitro and in vivo replication of both influenza A and B viruses [18] (reviewed in [36,37]).

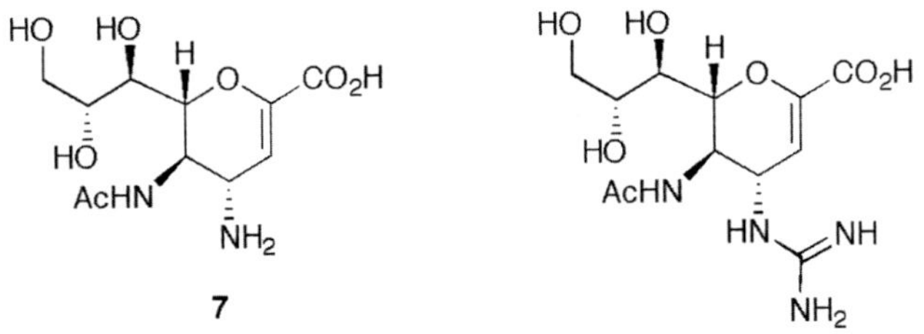

7

K_i 5×10^{-8} M (A/N2)

8 (zanamivir)

K_i 2×10^{-10} M (A/N2)

K_i 7×10^{-10} M (B)

FIGURE 4

Through x-ray crystal structure determination, both **7** [18] and **8** [18,38] were found to orient, in general, within the active site of influenza A/N2 sialidase in the manner predicted: most importantly, with neither compound causing any rearrangement of amino acids within the catalytic domain [18]. For 4-deoxy-4-guanidino-Neu5Ac2en (**8**), the predicted lateral binding between the terminal nitrogens of the guanidino group and Glu227 does occur, although Glu119 was found to be slightly further removed than predicted and stacked parallel to the guanidinyl group, but still within a distance close enough for electrostatic interactions [18,38]. The bulkier guanidino substituent of **8** was found to displace a water molecule from the C4 binding domain, accounting for some entropic gain as well as providing a logical reason for the slow binding properties reported for the compound [18]. Importantly, installation of the basic functionalities at the C4 position resulted in $\geq$ 10,000-fold selectivity for the inhibition of influenza virus sialidase compared with sialidases from mammalian origin [18,33].

The more potent compound, 4-deoxy-4-guanidino-Neu5Ac2en (**8**), was licensed by Glaxo in 1990 as a lead drug candidate under the generic name zanamivir. Zanamivir progressed successfully through the significant clinical studies required to evaluate a first-in-class drug. It gained regulatory approval as the first sialidase-targeting anti-influenza drug in 1999 under the trade name Relenza.

SYNTHESIS OF ZANAMIVIR AND BEYOND

Synthesis of 4-deoxy-4-guanidino-Neu5Ac2en (Zanamivir)

The original syntheses in the development of zanamivir began with an *in-house* chemoenzymatic synthesis of *N*-acetylneuraminic acid (Neu5Ac, **9**) (Scheme 2), which in the mid-1980s was predominantly isolated from natural sources, making it prohibitively expensive for a drug discovery pipeline. Today, driven in part by the requirement for synthesis of zanamivir, Neu5Ac is prepared commercially using either a chemoenzymatic or fully enzymatic conversion of GlcNAc to Neu5Ac, on a multiton scale.

Introduction of the amino substituent at C4 on the Neu5Ac2en template utilized the previously reported [39] unsaturated 4,5-oxazoline derivative **10**, prepared as shown in Scheme 3. Oxazoline (**10**) was originally synthesized by Lewis acid–catalyzed reaction of peracetylated Neu5Ac2en1Me (**11**) [40]. Subsequently [41], oxazoline (**10**) was synthesized directly from the peracetylated methyl ester of Neu5Ac (**12**) [42], thereby avoiding the chlorination step in the synthesis of **11**. Oxazoline (**10**) is readily hydrolyzed to the 4-*epi*-hydroxy derivative **13** (Scheme 4). Compounds

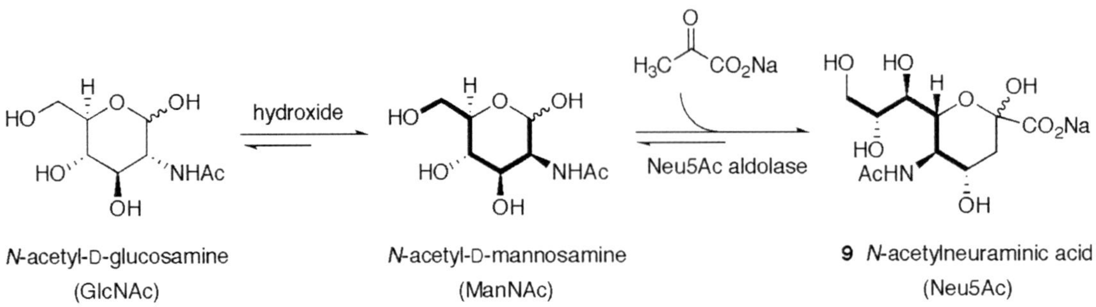

SCHEME 2 Synthesis of *N*-acetylneuraminic acid (Neu5Ac, **9**) from *N*-acetyl-D-glucosamine (GlcNAc).

10 and **13** both offered access to the desired 4-*N*-substituted Neu5Ac2en derivatives via stereoselective nucleophilic displacement at C4 with azide ion (Scheme 4).

The original strategy for the introduction of azide at C4 proceeded through activation of the C4-*epi*-hydroxyl group of **13** as a triflate (**14**), followed by displacement with sodium azide to give the key intermediate 4-azido derivative **15** in relatively low (24%) yield [43]. Subsequently, a direct opening of the oxazoline ring of **10** was utilized to introduce azide at C4 with high stereoselectivity for the C4 equatorial product (< 2% of C4 epimer **16** [40]) and significantly improved yield. Initial reaction conditions using lithium azide with acidic catalysis in DMF [40] were replaced by reaction with trimethylsilyl azide in *tert*-butanol on scale-up of the process [40,41]. Two alternative approaches to 4-azido derivative **15** from the 4-*epi*-OH derivative **13** have employed either Mitsunobu conditions (PPh_3, HN_3), which led to an epimeric mixture of **15** and **16** [42], or reaction of **13** with (less hazardous) diphenylphosphoryl azide [44].

Generation of the amino group at C4 encompassed the challenges of chemoselective reduction of the azide group in the presence of the 2,3-double bond and preservation of the free amino group in a compound prone to acetate migration. Chemoselective reduction of the azido group was first addressed by treating the fully protected azide **15** with hydrogen sulfide in pyridine, leading to the *O*-acetylated product **17** in moderate yield [43] (Scheme 5). Subsequently it was shown that chemoselective hydrogenation of the azido group could be accomplished on the fully protected azide using palladium on carbon at atmospheric pressure, with addition of acetic acid to form the salt of the amine in situ to prevent acetate migration (**15** → **17**, 72% yield [45]). Similarly, chemoselective hydrogenation of the fully deprotected azide derivative **18** [41] (or protected analogs [46]) could be accomplished using Lindlar catalyst. During structure–activity relationship (SAR) studies on zanamivir (e.g., investigating C5 substitution [47]), azide reduction was also carried out via phosphinimine formation with triphenylphosphine [42], giving the corresponding 4-amino derivatives in moderate (~45%) yields.

A number of reagents have been used for guanidinylation of the 4-amino group. The original syntheses used *S*-methylthiourea (**17** → **8**, 25% yield [43]) or AIMSA (aminoiminomethanesulfonic acid) (**7** → **8**, 57%

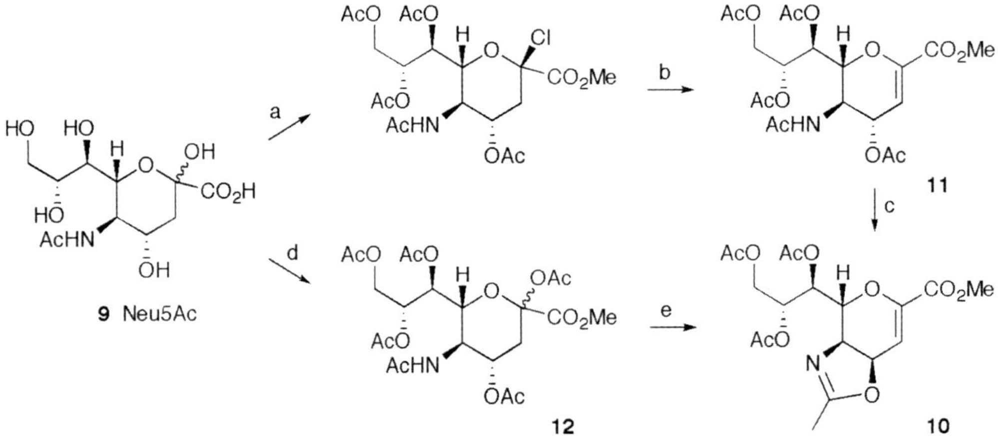

SCHEME 3 Reagents and conditions: (a) (i) MeOH, H^+; (ii) AcCl; b) DBU; (c) $BF_3{\cdot}OEt_2$, DCM/MeOH, 25 to 30°C, 16 h (96%) [40]; (d) (i) MeOH, H^+; (ii) Ac_2O, pyridine, DMAP; (e) TMSOTf, EtOAc, 52°C, 2.5 h [41].

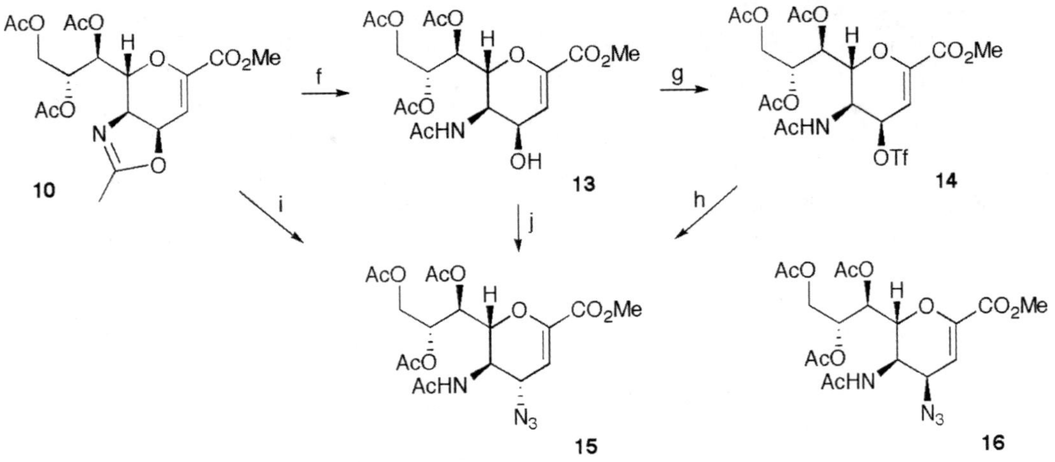

SCHEME 4 Reagents and conditions: (f) aqueous AcOH/EtOAc, room temperature (rt), 2 days [43]; (g) Tf_2O, DCM/pyridine, −30°C, 5 h; (h) NaN_3, Bu_4NHSO_4, DMF, rt, 16 h [24% for (g) and (h)] [43]; (i) LiN_3, Dowex (H^+), DMF, 80°C, 16 h (73% **15**, < 2% **16**) [40]; or $TMSN_3$, *t*-BuOH, 80°C, 4 h (83% [40,41]); (j) PPh_3, DEAD, HN_3, toluene, 0°C, 14 h (67% **15**, 17% **16**) [42]; or $(PhO)_2PON_3$, DBU, C_6H_6, rt, 5 h (87%) [44].

yield [41,45]). Subsequent syntheses during SAR studies (e.g., [46]) have used the more readily handled Boc-protected 1-guanylpyrazole [*N*,*N*′-bis(*tert*-butoxycarbonyl)-[1]-*H*-pyrazol-[1]-carboxyamidine].

Although *N*-acetylneuraminic acid is considered a relatively expensive starting material, the synthesis of zanamivir from this carbohydrate is straightforward and has been adapted to industrial-scale production [48]. Alternative syntheses of zanamivir and analogs beginning from cheaper carbohydrates such as gluconolactone [49] require significantly more steps.

Further Developments on the Neu5Ac2en Template: Toward Next-Generation Zanamivir

In the search for potent and selective sialidase inhibitors, significant research has been dedicated to the manipulation of every position on the Neu5Ac2en template. In particular, extensive SAR studies were carried out on this template during, and after, the development of zanamivir (**8**) (reviewed in [50,51]). These studies found that for the Neu5Ac2en template there appears to be a requirement to conserve the important interactions of the C1 carboxylate, a C5 acylamino

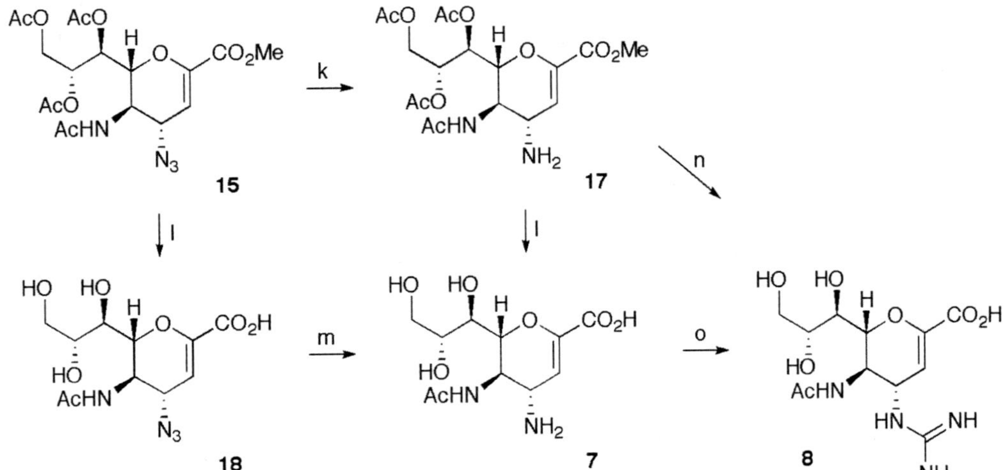

SCHEME 5 Reagents and conditions: (k) H_2S, pyridine, room temperature (rt), 16 h (56%) [43]; or H_2, Pd/C, MeOH/toluene/AcOH, rt, 1 h (72%) [45]; (l) (i) NaOMe, MeOH, rt, 2.5 h; (ii) aqueous NaOH, rt, 2 h [43]) or Et_3N, H_2O, rt, 7 h [41]; (m) H_2, Lindlar catalyst, H_2O, rt, 21 h [41]; (n) (i) $CH_3SC(NH)NH_2$, H_2O, 5°C, 7 days; (ii) NH_4OH, H_2O (25%) [43]; (o) $HO_3SC(NH)NH_2$, H_2O, K_2CO_3, 30 to 40°C to rt, 24 h (57%) [41,45].

group, and an amine or guanidino group at C4, for potent inhibition of influenza virus sialidase.

Further developments on the 4-deoxy-4-guanidino-Neu5Ac2en (zanamivir) template have been directed principally toward producing derivatives with improved pharmacokinetic properties. In this context, an alkoxyalkyl ester (prodrug) form of zanamivir, with a long alkyl chain [ester = $-(CH_2)_2O(CH_2)_{17}CH_3$] chosen to counteract the high hydrophilicity of the molecule, was reported to show significant protective effects against influenza (H1N1) infection in mice upon oral or intraperitoneal administration [52].

Functionalization Through the C7 Position of Zanamivir: The Development of Long-Acting Sialidase Inhibitors In complexes of influenza virus sialidase with Neu5Ac [25] and derivatives, including zanamivir [38], the C8 and C9 hydroxyl groups of the glycerol side chain form important interactions with sialidase active-site residue Glu276; however, the C7 hydroxyl group makes no direct interactions with the protein and is exposed to bulk solvent. This fact has been exploited in the development of C7 functionalized zanamivir derivatives with increased lipophilicity, but which also retain the important contributions of the C8 and C9 hydroxyl groups to the overall binding to influenza virus sialidase. This research has generated compounds that have improved pharmacokinetic properties over zanamivir and show promise as next-generation influenza virus sialidase inhibitors. The most notable of these compounds are the "simple" 7-*O*-methyl ether derivative of zanamivir (**19**) [46], and its C9 ester prodrug **20** [53,54], and divalent zanamivir linked through C7 (e.g., Fig. 5 **21**, [55]). Both exhibit the characteristic of long residence times in the lungs and are currently being forwarded in a joint venture between Daiichi Sankyo (Japan) and Biota (Australia) as long-acting influenza sialidase inhibitors for treatment of influenza.

The 7-*O*-methyl ether derivative of zanamivir (**19**) (R-125489, laninamivir) shows inhibitory potency similar to zanamivir in sialidase enzyme assay and in cell culture [46,53,54]. Significantly, the more lipophilic C9 acylated prodrug form of **20** (R-118958, CS8958, laninamivir octanoate) showed a strong protective effect in mice when administered intranasally 4 days prior to infection (with some efficacy also shown with dosage 7 days prior to infection), which is more effective than zanamivir in the same situation [53,54]. The prolonged efficacy seen in mice is potentially related to an observed increased residence time in the lungs. Prolonged retention of drug in humans has also been observed, with the active compound detected in the urine of healthy human subjects for more than 6 days after a single inhalation of **20** [53]. This is in contrast to zanamivir itself, which was not detected beyond 18 h after inhalation [53]. At the end of 2009, R-118958 (**20**) was progressing through phase III clinical trials as a long-acting, inhaled influenza virus sialidase inhibitor for once-only treatment and once-weekly prophylactic protection against influenza.

Concurrent with the development of laninamivir (**19**) has been the development of di- and polyvalent structures carrying zanamivir [55,56] (reviewed in [57]). For dimeric constructs, a distance between the two zanamivir residues of approximately 18 to 23 Å (a linker length of 14 to 18 atoms) (e.g., **21**) was found to give optimal inhibitory potency. Contributing to the inhibitory potency of the dimeric constructs may be their demonstrated ability to cause aggregation of (isolated) sialidase tetramers and whole virus [55]. The constructs inhibit virus replication in vitro and in vivo with approximately 100-fold more potency than that of monomeric zanamivir, after valency correction, and provide outstanding, long-lasting protective effects in a mouse model of influenza infection using a single intranasal dose at a significantly lower drug level than that of zanamivir [55]. They also showed extremely long residence times in the lungs of rats, with 100-fold greater concentration than zanamivir at 168 h. These characteristics have led to constructs such as **21** being forwarded into preclinical trials (Biota/Daiichi Sankyo) as once-weekly, low-dose therapeutic agents for the prevention or treatment of influenza virus infection [55].

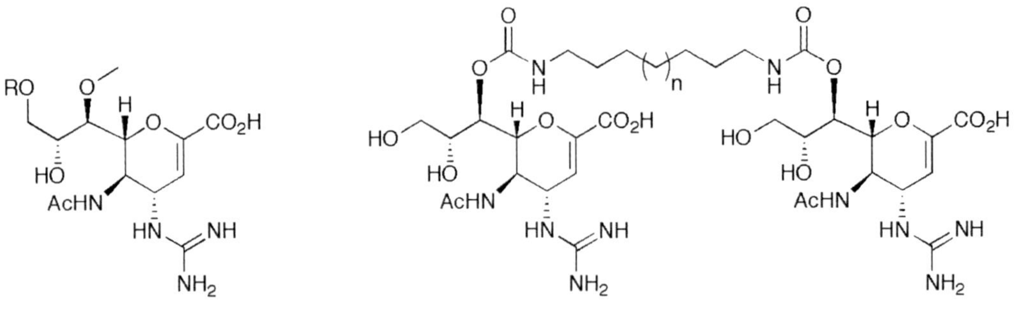

19 R = H (R-125489)

20 R = -C(O)C_7H_{15} (R-118958, CS8958)

21 n = 6, 8

FIGURE 5

Inhibitors Based on Noncarbohydrate Templates

The discovery of zanamivir, and the increasing availability of x-ray structural data for influenza virus sialidases in the 1990s provided a platform for further drug discovery targeting the sialidase. In particular, substantial effort has been employed in the development of inhibitors based on noncarbohydrate templates, with potent and selective inhibitors of influenza virus sialidase, and of influenza virus infection in vivo, being developed on the cyclohexene (**22**, **23**), cyclopentane (**24**), and pyrrolidine (**25**) templates (reviewed in [58]). Of these, oseltamivir carboxylate (**22**), in its prodrug form (**23**), is now used to treat and prevent influenza, and peramivir (**24**) is an investigational drug (see below). A full discussion of the development of these inhibitors is outside the scope of this chapter; the reader is directed to the review cited for further details beyond the brief overviews provided in the following sections.

Inhibitor Design Based on the Cyclohexene Template: Development of Oseltamivir (Tamiflu) Most noteworthy in the work using noncarbohydrate templates has been the development of the cyclohexene-based inhibitor **22** (GS 4071, oseltamivir carboxylate) and its orally bioavailable prodrug form (**23**) (GS 4104, oseltamivir) [60,61] (Gilead Sciences). Derived from natural shikimic acid, this template incorporates significant variations from the Neu5Ac2en-based inhibitors. These variations include replacement of the dihydropyran ring with a cyclohexene ring in which the double bond is placed to more closely mimic the putative sialosyl cation **2** of the enzyme transition state (Scheme 1) and replacement of the glycerol side chain with a hydrophobic aliphatic ether. Substantial SAR studies (reviewed in [61]) led to the development of the optimized structure **22** with a 3-pentyl ether side chain, and the carboxylate, amino, and acetamido groups mimicking 4-amino-4-deoxy-Neu5Ac2en (**7**).

Oseltamivir carboxylate (**22**) is a potent (K_i nM) and selective inhibitor of influenza virus sialidases [61] (Fig. 6), and an inhibitor of influenza A and B virus replication in vitro and in vivo, with potency similar to that of zanamivir [61,62]. Despite the more lipophilic side chain of **22**, compared to the glycerol side chain of zanamivir (**8**), the ethyl ester prodrug form (**23**) (oseltamivir) was necessary to achieve sufficient oral bioavailability [61]. Post absorption, oseltamivir is converted to the active form (**22**) by endogenous esterases [62]. Oseltamivir (**23**) was approved for the treatment of influenza in 1999 and is marketed by Roche under the trade name Tamiflu as an orally administered drug for treatment and prevention of influenza virus infection (reviewed in [62–64]).

Structural studies showed that the interactions of the carboxylate, amino, and acetamido substituents of **22** with the sialidase active-site residues are similar to those of the Neu5Ac2en-based inhibitors such as **7** [61]. However, to fully accommodate the hydrophobic 3-pentyl side chain, a previously unanticipated reorganization of the active site in the glycerol side-chain binding pocket takes place; the side-chain of conserved Glu276 (which interacts with the C8 and C9 hydroxyls of Neu5Ac2en-based inhibitors) reorientates outward from the glycerol side-chain binding domain to form a salt-bridge with Arg224 [61]. This rearrangement generates a substantial hydrophobic patch within this region that enables accommodation of one arm of the hydrophobic 3-pentyl side chain. Importantly, the necessity for this rearrangement for effective sialidase binding of, and inhibition by, **22** has been found to have implications for the development of clinically significant oseltamivir resistant virus strains. In certain A/H1N1 viruses, a mutation of His274 to Tyr prevents the reorientation of Glu276 and diminishes the binding affinity of **22**, leading to viable oseltamivir resistant viruses [65,66].

Inhibitor Design Using Five-Membered Ring Templates The underlying templates of the potent influenza sialidase inhibitors zanamivir (**8**; 5,6-dihydro-4*H*-pyran) and oseltamivir (**22**; cyclohexene) were chosen in part to provide a central ring that mimicked the half-chair conformation of

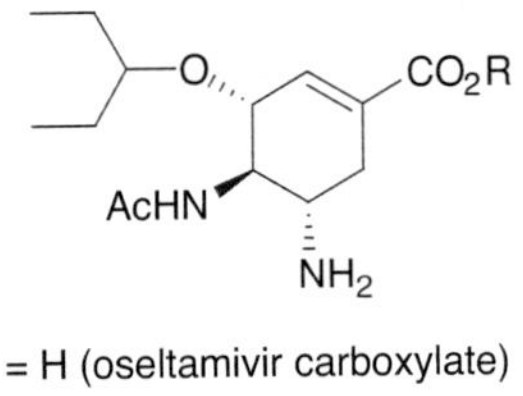

22 R = H (oseltamivir carboxylate)

IC_{50} 1.3 ± 0.2 nM (A/N2)

IC_{50} 1.1 ± 0.05 nM (B)

23 R = Et (oseltamivir)

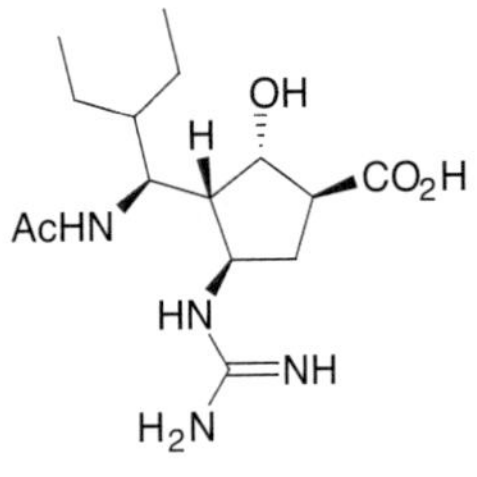

24 (peramivir)

IC_{50} 1.1 ± 0.02 nM (A/N2)

IC_{50} 0.21 ± 0.01 nM (B)

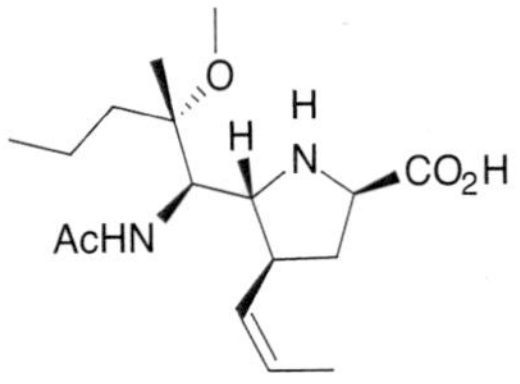

25 (A-315675)

IC_{50} 0.19 ± 0.01 nM (A/N2)

IC_{50} 0.14 ± 0.01 nM (B)

FIGURE 6 Potent influenza virus sialidase inhibitors developed on noncarbohydrate templates. Inhibition data against A/Tokyo/3/67 (H3N2) and B/Memphis/3/89 [cf. zanamivir (**8**): 0.086 ± 0.003 nM (A/N2) and 0.08 ± 0.01 nM (B)] is shown [59].

the putative sialosyl cation transition state **2** of the enzyme reaction (Scheme 1). A number of intensive research efforts have also been directed toward developing potent sialidase inhibitors based on alternative cyclic templates (reviewed in [58]). Two drug discovery programs in particular, using the five-membered ring cyclopentane and pyrrolidine templates, have produced the potent influenza virus sialidase inhibitors **24** [67] and **25** [59], respectively (Fig. 6). Extensive SAR studies were used to optimize substituent binding within the pockets of the sialidase active site.

The cyclopentane-based inhibitor **24** (BCX-1812, RWJ-270201, peramivir) (BioCryst Pharmaceuticals) [67], a selective influenza virus sialidase inhibitor with potency similar to that of zanamivir and oseltamivir, has progressed through a number of clinical trials. Although peramivir is still an investigational drug undergoing human clinical trials of both intravenous (BioCryst) and intramuscular [68] formulations, in early 2006 the U.S. Food and Drug Administration granted a fast-track designation of peramivir in an injectable formulation. In 2009 an Emergency Use Authorization was granted for intravenous administration of peramivir in seriously ill hospitalized patients with H1N1 2009 infection [69].

BIOLOGICAL EVALUATION OF ZANAMIVIR

In Vitro Enzyme Assay and Tissue Culture

Measurement of in vitro sialidase inhibitory activity against isolated influenza virus sialidase [33,59,70] and whole virus [70,71] has routinely been undertaken using a fluorimetric assay with the substrate 4-methylumbelliferyl *N*-acetyl-α-neuraminide, although other assay systems are also used [72,73]. Because of its slow-binding kinetics [18], zanamivir is routinely preincubated with the enzyme or virus before addition of substrate. It has been noted [73] that direct measurement of enzyme inhibition may have advantages when monitoring viruses for inhibitor susceptibility and may be more predictive of in vivo susceptibility than cell-based (plaque reduction) assays.

Zanamivir is a potent broad-spectrum (competitive) inhibitor of the sialidase activity of medically relevant human influenza A (H1N1, H2N2, and H3N2) and B viruses [18,59,70], with inhibition values in the low- to subnanomolar range. Zanamivir has also been shown to inhibit the sialidase activity of all nine NA subtypes, with IC_{50} values in the nanomolar range [71].

In tissue culture (plaque reduction assay in Madin–Darby canine kidney (MDCK) cells [73]), zanamivir effectively inhibited virus replication of laboratory-passaged human influenza A ($IC_{50} = 0.004$ to 0.014 μM) and B ($IC_{50} = 0.005$ μM) viruses [18,74]. In all cases, zanamivir inhibited virus replication at lower concentrations than did the M2 ion channel inhibitors amantadine and rimantadine, and ribavirin [74].

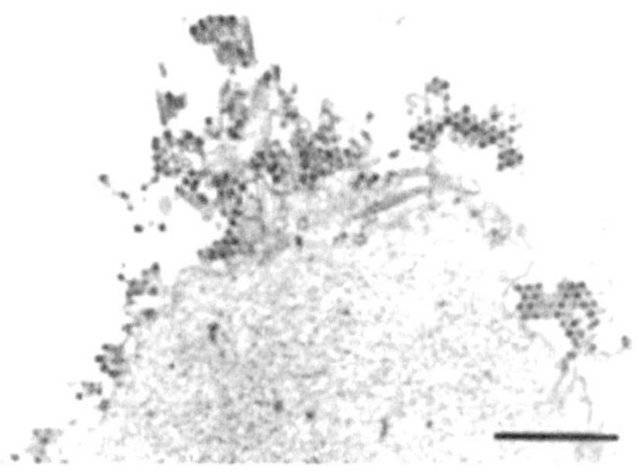

FIGURE 7 Electron micrograph of MDCK cell infected with influenza A virus in the presence of NA inhibitor, showing cell-surface aggregation of virus. Bar = 1 μM. (Image from K. Gopal Murti, St. Jude Children's Research Hospital, Memphis, TN. Reprinted from [8], copyright © 2000, with permission from Elsevier.)

It also reduced virus yields in human epithelial cells [37]. No cytotoxicity was observed at concentrations up to 10 mmol/L, where cytotoxicity was observed for the other anti-influenza drugs [74]. Zanamivir inhibited tissue culture growth of avian influenza A viruses (representing all NA subtypes [71]) at concentrations that were effective against human A/N1 and A/N2 viruses [36]. As anticipated, the sialidase inhibitors have been found to inhibit the release of virion progeny from infected cells, with cell-associated virus particles found in the presence of drug (Fig. 7).

Selectivity

Of concern is the possibility that the influenza virus sialidase inhibitors may inhibit the endogenous human sialidases. Zanamivir was shown to exhibit selective in vitro inhibition of influenza virus sialidase over mammalian [human lysosomal (Neu1) and sheep] sialidases, with inhibition of the mammalian sialidases being more than 100,000 times weaker than that of the viral sialidases [18,33]. A more recent evaluation of zanamivir inhibition of recombinant versions of the four human sialidases characterized to date reported micromolar inhibition of Neu3 (plasma membrane) and Neu2 (cytosolic) sialidases (K_i values of 4 and 14 μM, respectively) [75]. However, this inhibition is still substantially weaker than the low-nanomolar concentrations at which zanamivir blocks the activity of influenza virus sialidase. In addition, and significant with regard to potential inhibition of the human sialidases, radiolabeled zanamivir does not enter either uninfected or influenza infected MDCK cells [76].

Efficacy in Animal Models of Influenza Infection

Both mouse and ferret models of influenza infection have been used in the evaluation of zanamivir's in vivo efficacy. Ferrets are a preferred animal model for influenza infection, as they exhibit many of the typical signs of influenza infection, including fever [72]. They also have a similar receptor profile for the viral hemagglutinin on respiratory tract epithelial cells to that in humans and so can be used as a model of virus transmissibility [6].

In a mouse model of influenza infection (influenza A/N2 or B), intranasally administered zanamivir effectively reduced mortality, lung consolidation, and virus titers in the lung, with no virus growing back following the cessation of treatment [37]. In both mouse and ferret models, intranasally administered zanamivir was found to be 100 to 1000 times more active than amantadine or ribavirin, and retained efficacy when treatments were delayed until 24 h post-infection [36,37]. Zanamivir was found to have poor oral bioavailability in mice, and was inactive against influenza viruses when delivered by this route [37]. This was not unexpected given the known rapid excretion of orally administered sialic acid derivatives, including the zanamivir parent template Neu5Ac2en (**5**) [77].

Clinical Experience: Efficacy, Toxicity, and Resistance Development

In clinical trials, and subsequently in the clinical environment, zanamivir has been found to be effective in both the treatment and prophylaxis of influenza A and B virus infections. Although being approved in 1999 for the treatment of influenza virus infection, there is only limited clinical experience to date with zanamivir in nonexperimental human influenza. The outcomes of clinical trials undertaken during the development of zanamivir, and of its clinical use since approval, have been reported in a number of comprehensive reviews [36,37,64], from which some of the following discussion is drawn and to which the reader is directed for a more detailed discussion and primary references.

As anticipated from mouse studies [37], zanamivir was found to have poor oral bioavailability during human trials (mean oral bioavailability 2%; 500-mg dose; healthy adults) [37,78]. Upon oral inhaled (10-mg dose via Diskhaler; healthy adults) or intranasal (16-mg dose; healthy adults) administration, a "moderate" median of 10 to 20% of the dose was systemically absorbed, with maximum serum concentrations generally reached within 1 to 2 h [78]. Intravenously administered zanamivir (600-mg; healthy adults) had a half-life of approximately 2 h, with approximately 90% of the drug excreted unchanged in the urine [78]. Independent of the mode of administration, zanamivir was excreted unchanged [78].

After delivery of the drug by oral inhalation (Diskhaler), the mean disposition of the drug was 13% in the lungs and 78% in the oropharynx [36,37], indicating that the majority of the drug is being delivered directly to the major sites of influenza infection and replication [37]. Also important was the finding that after oral inhalation (1×10-mg dose, healthy adults), drug concentrations found in sputum and nasal washings at 12 h postdosing were significantly higher than the median IC_{50} for inhibition of the viral sialidase, indicating long retention of antiviral activity [37]. Intravenous delivery of zanamivir (600-mg dose) also showed distribution of drug to the respiratory mucosa [79].

Because of its limited oral bioavailability and the logic of delivery of the drug to the site of infection, zanamivir was formulated as a dry powder aerosol for delivery by oral inhalation using Glaxo's established Diskhaler technology. The drug is coadministered with lactose as vehicle (20 mg of lactose per 5 mg of zanamivir) [8]. The recommended dose for treatment is 10 mg twice daily for 5 days, beginning within 48 h after the onset of symptoms for adults, and within 36 h after onset of symptoms for children [64]. For prevention of influenza following exposure to an infected person, prophylactic treatment of 10 mg once daily for 10 days is recommended, while for prevention of influenza during a community outbreak (seasonal prophylaxis), the recommended treatment is 10 mg once daily for up to 28 days. Zanamivir is indicted for treatment of uncomplicated acute illness due to influenza A and B virus in adults and pediatric patients greater than 5 years of age who have been symptomatic for no more than 2 days. Zanamivir is also indicated for prophylaxis of influenza in adults and paediatric patients 5 years of age and older.

In the clinical setting, zanamivir is found to be effective for the treatment of both influenza A and B virus infections. For treatment, the primary clinical endpoint was set as the length of time to alleviation of major symptoms (fever, myalgia, headache, sore throat, cough) for at least 24 h. For zanamivir this was found to be a median of 1 to 1.5 days earlier relief of symptoms than for placebo when treatment was started within 36 to 48 h of infection [37,64,80]. Treatment appears to be of most benefit in those with preexisting disease and those with severe influenza symptoms [81]. Importantly, the effects of drug treatment are a reduction in the severity of illness [36,37] and in the incidence of secondary complications [64]. A significant reduction in the use of antibiotics was also seen in some clinical settings [80,82]. Zanamivir has also been shown to reduce the likelihood of influenza infection in a number of trials of prophylactic efficacy [37,64,83].

The availability of an intramuscular or intravenous formulation of an influenza sialidase inhibitor may be important in treating patients hospitalized with severe and potentially life-threatening influenza where inhaled dosing, or oral dosing in the case of Tamiflu, is not applicable. The more systemic forms of dosing may also provide greater protection against potential systemic infection by H5N1 viruses [5]. Intravenously administered zanamivir, which is still in the investigational phase, is distributed to the respiratory mucosa and is protective against infection and illness in experimental human influenza A infection [79]. Its clinical efficacy has recently been demonstrated in the successful treatment of two separate cases of H1N1 2009 influenza where the patients had compromised airway function [84,85].

Toxicity and Adverse Effects Zanamivir is generally well tolerated [64]. Concerns that inhaled zanamivir could reduce lung function and induce bronchospasm in asthmatic patients have not been borne out in clinical studies, where zanamivir was found not to affect pulmonary function adversely in high-risk subjects [37,64]. However, as a precaution, patients with underlying airway disease require careful monitoring and are advised to have a fast-acting bronchodilator at hand [64]. The potential for clinically relevant drug–drug interactions with zanamivir is considered to be low [37].

Resistance Development The generation of resistant viruses during clinical use of the influenza virus sialidase inhibitors zanamivir and oseltamivir is an obvious and significant concern. Virus growth in the presence of the sialidase inhibitors generally gives rise, in the first instance, to variants with changes in the hemagglutinin glycoprotein, and later to changes in the sialidase [73,86]. Owing to the fundamental interconnection between receptor-binding and receptor-destroying activities of the viral hemagglutinin and sialidase, respectively, in virus replication [17], viruses with a hemagglutinin with reduced affinity for the cell surface receptors may also have reduced reliance on sialidase activity for release of virion progeny from cells, and consequently, an altered sensitivity to the sialidase inhibitors [87]. This has been observed in surveys of neuraminidase inhibitor–resistant viruses.

As zanamivir and oseltamivir came to the market, a Global Neuraminidase Inhibitor Susceptibility Network was established to monitor the development of viruses resistant to these drugs [86]. To the end of 2009, no influenza viruses with a change in the sialidase causing resistance to zanamivir had been isolated from patients treated with the drug who have a competent immune system [65,88]. One variant influenza B virus (with Arg152Lys in the sialidase), however, was isolated from an immunocompromised patient [65].

Seasonal influenza viruses (A/H1N1, A/H3N2, and B) collected worldwide between October 2004 and March 2008 were found to be sensitive to inhibition by zanamivir, with IC_{50} values in the low-to subnanomolar range [89], in line with the findings from drug susceptibility surveillance of previous years. Although a mutation of the conserved Asp151 in a number of A/H3N2 viruses that has moderately reduced susceptibility to zanamivir (IC_{50} ~10 nM) was observed in the most recent survey [89], this variant has not (yet) been identified in clinically isolated viruses. An A/H1N1 sialidase variant with the mutation Q137K that confers reduced (36 [90] to 300 [88] fold) susceptibility to zanamivir has also recently been identified [88,90] after passaging a small number of clinical isolates in MDCK cells. This mutation did not compromise viral infectivity or transmissibility in a ferret model of influenza infection [88]. However, the mutation was not found in the original isolates, and its clinical relevance is unclear at this stage.

A number of sialidase variants (predominantly with changes at Glu119) arise in vitro during passage in the presence of zanamivir and oseltamivir (reviewed in [65,87]). Variations at Glu119 (A/N2, A/N9, B) that appear in the presence of zanamivir (Glu119 Gly, Ala, Asp) adversely affect the stability and activity of the enzyme [87,91] and virus replication in vitro [91]. However, the clinically relevant [65] oseltamivir-selected Glu119Val A/H3N2 variant showed less significant loss of sialidase activity, grew well in cell culture [91], and was transmissible in ferrets [92]. Importantly, this variant is sensitive to zanamivir as well as to peramivir (**24**) [93].

Resistance to oseltamivir (Tamiflu **23**), to date the more widely used influenza virus sialidase inhibitor, has been observed not only in the clinical setting (2% drug resistance in adults and up to 18% resistance in children [65]) but also in some circulating seasonal viruses [66,89]. In particular, since mid-2007 [89] there has been a significant increase in the frequency of oseltamivir-resistant seasonal A/H1N1 viruses with a His274Tyr mutation in the sialidase [66]. These variants can no longer accommodate the hydrophobic 3-pentyl side chain of oseltamivir. Importantly, the oseltamivir-resistant A/N1 His274Tyr variants are still sensitive to zanamivir and peramivir [66].

FUTURE OUTLOOK

Antiviral drug development including anti-influenza therapy discovery and development is a considerable challenge. The variable antigenic nature of the surface glycoproteins presents not only challenges for the discovery of new vaccines in a timely manner [94], but also appeares to hinder effective targeting of these proteins for drug discovery [10,11]. The discovery of zanamivir not only provided proof of concept for structure-based drug design but also delivered the first specific anti-influenza drug that targeted the virus's surface glycoprotein, sialidase. This inhibitor has the capacity to halt the spread of all strains of both influenza A and B virus, including the currently circulating seasonal and pandemic H1N1 as well as the much-publicized avian H5N1 virus.

While zanamivir was the first designer drug approved for the treatment of influenza infection, it has not been used widely in the treatment of nonexperimental human influenza infection. However, in clinical cases of influenza infection where zanamivir has been used, the outcomes have mirrored its successful clinical trial efficacy. Moreover, zanamivir was found to be well tolerated with a very limited side-effect profile.

What has been recognized in recent years is that there is a need for alternative drug administration methods, particularly for treatment in the circumstance where oral or inhaled dosing is not appropriate. This is now being addressed with the development of intravenous and intramuscular injection formulations of sialidase inhibitors [68,79]. In this context, and most interestingly, intravenous injection of zanamivir was found to provide positive outcomes in patients severely compromised by influenza infection [84,85]. Furthermore, and of significant interest, a "second-generation" zanamivir-based inhibitor is currently undergoing clinical trials as a long-acting sialidase inhibitor (LANI). These inhibitors require only a once-a-week dosing [54] and would offer an exciting alternative to existing drugs, which require twice-daily dosing.

The development of substantial resistance to the sialidase inhibitors is a fundamental issue of great concern. Significant resistance development to the most commonly used anti-influenza drug oseltamivir has confirmed the capacity of the virus to respond to drugs. Importantly, at present there is no significant resistance development in the clinical setting to zanamivir, although close monitoring of drug resistance development is essential. The threat of continuing resistance development demands a continued discovery and development of next-generation sialidase inhibitors, as well as other influenza virus inhibitors that target other essential viral proteins.

The arrival of the 2009–2010 influenza virus pandemic reinforced the importance of influenza virus sialidase–targeting inhibitors as anti-influenza drugs. These drugs have provided a first line of defense to treat and protect the human population in the event of a serious pandemic and, importantly, to buy time for vaccine development.

REFERENCES

[1] World Health Organisation. Fact Sheet 211: Influenza. Apr. 2009. Available at http://www.who.int/mediacentre/factsheets/fs211/en/.

[2] Murray, C. J. L., et al. Estimation of potential global pandemic influenza mortality on the basis of vital registry data from the 1918–20 pandemic: a quantitative analysis. *Lancet* **2006**, *368*, 2211–2218.

[3] World Health Organisation. Pandemic (H1N1) 2009: Update 81. Dec. 30, 2009. Available at http://www.who.int/csr/don/2009_12_30/en/index.html.

[4] Itoh, Y., et al. In vitro and in vivo characterization of new swine-origin H1N1 influenza viruses. *Nature* **2009**, *460*, 1021–1025.

[5] Beigel, J. H., et al. Avian influenza A (H5N1) infection in humans. *N. Engl. J. Med.* **2005**, *353*, 1374–1385.

[6] Maines, T. R., et al. Lack of transmission of H5N1 avian–human reassortant influenza viruses in a ferret model. *Proc. Natl Acad. Sci. USA* **2006**, *103*, 12121–12126.

[7] Nicholson, K. G.; Wood, J. M.; Zambon, M. Influenza. *Lancet* **2003**, *362*, 1733–1745.

[8] Gubareva, L. V.; Kaiser, L.; Hayden, F. G. Influenza virus neuraminidase inhibitors. *Lancet* **2000**, *355*, 827–835.

[9] von Itzstein, M. The war against influenza: discovery and development of sialidase inhibitors. *Nat. Rev. Drug Discov.* **2007**, *6*, 967–974.

[10] Meanwell, N. A.; Krystal, M. Taking aim at a moving target—inhibitors of influenza virus: 1. Virus adsorption, entry and uncoating. *Drug Discov. Today* **1996**, *1*, 316–324.

[11] Meanwell, N. A.; Krystal, M. Taking aim at a moving target—inhibitors of influenza virus: 2. Viral replication, packaging and release. *Drug Discov. Today* **1996**, *1*, 388–397.

[12] Lagoja, I. M.; De Clercq, E. Anti-influenza agents: synthesis and mode of action. *Med. Res. Rev.* **2008**, *28*, 1–38.

[13] Hay, A. J. The action of adamantanamines against influenza A viruses: inhibition of the M2 ion channel protein. *Semin. Virol.* **1992**, *3*, 21–30.

[14] Wintermeyer, S. M.; Nahata, M. C. Rimantidine: a clinical perspective. *Ann. Pharmacother.* **1995**, *29*, 299–310.

[15] Skehel, J. J.; Wiley, D. C. Receptor binding and membrane fusion in virus entry: the influenza hemagglutinin. *Annu. Rev. Biochem.* **2000**, *69*, 531–569.

[16] Palese, P., et al. Characterization of temperature sensitive influenza virus mutants defective in neuraminidase. *Virology* **1974**, *61*, 397–410.

[17] Wagner, R.; Matrosovich, M.; Klenk, H.-D. Functional balance between haemagglutinin and neuraminidase in influenza virus infections. *Rev. Med. Virol.* **2002**, *12*, 159–166.

[18] von Itzstein, M., et al. Rational design of potent sialidase-based inhibitors of influenza virus replication. *Nature* **1993**, *363*, 418–423.

[19] Colman, P. M. Influenza virus neuraminidase: structure, antibodies, and inhibitors. *Protein Sci.* **1994**, *3*, 1687–1696.

[20] Laver, G.; Garman, E. Pandemic influenza: its origin and control. *Microbes Infect.* **2002**, *4*, 1309–1316.

[21] Colman, P. M.; Varghese, J. N.; Laver, W. G. Structure of the catalytic and antigenic sites in influenza virus neuraminidase. *Nature* **1983**, *303*, 41–44.

[22] Varghese, J. N.; Laver, W. G.; Colman, P. M. Structure of the influenza virus glycoprotein antigen neuraminidase at 2.9 Å resolution. *Nature* **1983**, *303*, 35–40.

[23] Russell, R. J., et al. The structure of H5N1 avian influenza neuraminidase suggests new opportunities for drug design. *Nature* **2006**, *443*, 45–49.

[24] Smith, F. I.; Palese, P. Variation in the influenza virus genes: epidemiological, pathogenic and evolutionary consequences. In *The Influenza Viruses*, Krug, R. M., Ed., Plenum Press, New York, **1989**, pp. 319–350.

[25] Varghese, J. N., et al. The structure of the complex between influenza virus neuraminidase and sialic acid, the viral receptor. *Proteins* **1992**, *14*, 327–332.

[26] Chong, A. K., et al. Evidence for a sialosyl cation transition-state complex in the reaction of sialidase from influenza virus. *Eur. J. Biochem.* **1992**, *207*, 335–343.

[27] Taylor, N. R.; von Itzstein, M. Molecular modeling studies on ligand binding to sialidase from influenza virus and the mechanism of catalysis. *J. Med. Chem.* **1994**, *37*, 616–624.

[28] Thomas, A., et al. Is there a covalent intermediate in the viral neuraminidase reaction? A hybrid potential free-energy study. *J. Am. Chem. Soc.* **1999**, *121*, 9693–9702.

[29] Watts, A. G., et al. Structural and kinetic analysis of two covalent sialosyl-enzyme intermediates on *Trypanosoma rangeli* sialidase. *J. Biol. Chem.* **2006**, *281*, 4149–4155.

[30] Meindl, P., et al. Inhibition of neuraminidase activity by derivatives of 2-deoxy-2,3-dehydro-*N*-acetylneuraminic acid. *Virology* **1974**, *58*, 457–463.

[31] Miller, C. A.; Wang, P.; Flashner, M. Mechanism of *Arthrobacter sialophilus* neuraminidase: the binding of substrates and transition-state analogs. *Biochem. Biophys. Res. Commun.* **1978**, *83*, 1479–1487.

[32] Palese, P.; Compans, R. W. Inhibition of influenza virus replication in tissue culture by 2-deoxy-2,3-dehydro-*N*-trifluoroacetylneuraminic acid (FANA): mechanism of action. *J. Gen. Virol.* **1976**, *33*, 159–163.

[33] Holzer, C. T., et al. Inhibition of sialidases from viral, bacterial and mammalian sources by analogues of 2-deoxy-2,3-didehydro-*N*-acetylneuraminic acid modified at the C-4 position. *Glycoconj. J.* **1993**, *10*, 40–44.

[34] Goodford, P. J. A computational procedure for determining energetically favorable binding sites on biologically important macromolecules. *J. Med. Chem.* **1985**, *28*, 849–857.

[35] von Itzstein, M., et al. A study of the active site of influenza virus sialidase: an approach to the rational design of novel anti-influenza drugs. *J. Med. Chem.* **1996**, *39*, 388–391.

[36] Waghorn, S. L.; Goa, K. L. *Zanamivir.* Drugs **1998**, *55*, 721–725.

[37] Elliott, M. Zanamivir: from drug design to the clinic. *Philos. Trans. R. Soc. Lond. B.* **2001**, *356*, 1885–1893.

[38] Varghese, J. N.; Epa, V. C.; Colman, P. M. Three-dimensional structure of the complex of 4-guanidino-Neu5Ac2en and influenza virus neuraminidase. *Protein Sci.* **1995**, *4*, 1081–1087.

[39] Kumar, V.; Tanenbaum, S. W.; Flashner, M. Characterization of lewis-acid transformation-products from 2,3-unsaturated relatives of methyl *N*-acetylneuraminate during attempted glycoside synthesis. *Carbohydr. Res.* **1982**, *101*, 155–159.

[40] von Itzstein, M., et al. A convenient method for the introduction of nitrogen and sulfur at C-4 on a sialic acid analog. *Carbohydr. Res.* **1993**, *244*, 181–185.

[41] Chandler, M., et al. Synthesis of the potent influenza neuraminidase inhibitor 4-guanidino-Neu5Ac2en: x-ray molecular structure of 5-acetamido-4-amino-2,6-anhydro-3,4,5-trideoxy-D-*erythro*-L-*gluco*-nononic acid. *J. Chem. Soc. Perkin Trans.1* **1995**, 1173–1180.

[42] Schreiner, E., et al. Structural variations on *N*-acetylneuraminic acid: 20. Synthesis of some 2,3-didehydro-2-deoxysialic acids structurally varied at C-4 and their behavior towards sialidase from *Vibrio cholerae*. *Liebigs Ann. Chem.* **1991**, 129–134.

[43] von Itzstein, L. M., et al. (Biota Scientific Management Pty. Ltd., Australia). Preparation of derivatives and analogs of 2-deoxy-2,3-didehydro-*N*-acetylneuraminic acid as antiviral agents. WO 9116320, 1991.

[44] Scheigetz, J., et al. A Synthesis of 4-alpha-guanidino-2-deoxy-2,3-didehydro-*N*-acetylneuraminic Acid. *Org. Prep. Proc. Int.* **1995**, *27*, 637–644.

[45] von Itzstein, M.; Wu, W.-Y.; Jin, B. The synthesis of 2,3-didehydro-2,4-dideoxy-4-guanidinyl-*N*-acetylneuraminic acid: a potent influenza virus sialidase inhibitor. *Carbohydr. Res.* **1994**, *259*, 301–305.

[46] Honda, T., et al. Synthesis and anti-influenza virus activity of 7-O-alkylated derivatives related to zanamivir. *Bioorg. Med. Chem. Lett.* **2002**, *12*, 1925–1928.

[47] Smith, P. W., et al. Synthesis and influenza virus sialidase inhibitory activity of analogues of 4-guanidino-Neu5Ac2en (GG167) with modified 5-substituents. *Eur. J. Med. Chem.* **1996**, *31*, 143–150.

[48] Magano, J. Synthetic approaches to the neuraminidase inhibitors zanamivir (Relenza) and oseltamivir phosphate (Tamiflu) for the treatment of influenza. *Chem. Rev.* **2009**, *109*, 4398–4438.

[49] Liu, K.-G., et al. Synthesis of 4-azido-4-deoxy-Neu5,7,8,9Ac$_4$2en1Me: a key intermediate for the synthesis of GG167 from D-glucono-delta-lactone. *Org. Lett.* **2004**, *6*, 2269–2272.

[50] Bamford, M. J. Neuraminidase inhibitors as potential anti-influenza drugs. *J. Enzyme Inhib.* **1995**, *10*, 1–16.

[51] Rich, J. R.; Gehle, D.; von Itzstein, M. Design and synthesis of sialidase inhibitors for influenza virus infections. In *Comprehensive Glycoscience*, Kamerling, J. P., Boons, G.-J., Lee, Y., Suzuki, A., Tanigichi, N., Voragen, A. G. J., Eds., Elsevier, Oxford, UK, 2007, pp. 885–922.

[52] Liu, Z.-Y., et al. Synthesis and anti-influenza activities of carboxyl alkoxyalkyl esters of 4-guanidino-Neu5Ac2en (zanamivir). *Bioorg. Med. Chem. Lett.* **2007**, *17*, 4851–4854.

[53] Yamashita, M. R-118958, a unique anti-influenza agent showing high efficacy for both prophylaxis and treatment after a single administration: from the in vitro stage to phase I study. *Int. Congr. Ser.* **2004**, *1263*, 38–42.

[54] Yamashita, M., et al. CS-8958, a prodrug of the new neuraminidase inhibitor R-125489 shows long-acting anti-influenza virus activity. *Antimicrob. Agents Chemother.* **2009**, *53*, 186–192.

[55] Macdonald, S. J., et al. Potent and long-acting dimeric inhibitors of influenza virus neuraminidase are effective at a once-weekly dosing regimen. *Antimicrob. Agents Chemother.* **2004**, *48*, 4542–4549.

[56] Honda, T., et al. Synthesis and anti-influenza evaluation of polyvalent sialidase inhibitors bearing 4-guanidino-Neu5Ac2en derivatives. *Bioorg. Med. Chem. Lett.* **2002**, *12*, 1929–1932.

[57] Sun, X.-L. Recent anti-influenza strategies in multivalent sialyloligosaccharides and sialylmimetics approaches. *Curr. Med. Chem.* **2007**, *14*, 2304–2313.

[58] Chand, P. Recent advances in the discovery and synthesis of neuraminidase inhibitors. *Expert Opin. Ther. Patents* **2005**, *15*, 1009–1025.

[59] Kati, W. M., et al. In vitro characterization of A-315675, a highly potent inhibitor of A and B strain influenza virus neuraminidases and influenza virus replication. *Antimicrob. Agents Chemother.* **2002**, *46*, 1014–1021.

[60] Kim, C. U., et al. Influenza neuraminidase inhibitors possessing a novel hydrophobic interaction in the enzyme active site: design, synthesis, and structural analysis of carbocyclic sialic acid analogues with potent anti-influenza activity. *J. Am. Chem. Soc.* **1997**, *119*, 681–690.

[61] Lew, W.; Chen, X.; Kim, C. U. Discovery and development of GS 4104 (Oseltamivir): an orally active influenza neuraminidase inhibitor. *Curr. Med. Chem.* **2000**, *7*, 663–672.

[62] Doucette, K. E.; Aoki, F. Y. Oseltamivir: a clinical and pharmacological perspective. *Expert Opin. Pharmacother.* **2001**, *2*, 1671–1683.

[63] Oxford, J. Oseltamivir in the management of influenza. *Expert Opin. Pharmacother.* **2005**, *6*, 2493–2500.

[64] Moscona, A. Neuraminidase inhibitors for influenza. *N. Engl. J. Med.* **2005**, *353*, 1363–1373.

[65] Reece, P. A. Neuraminidase inhibitor resistance in influenza viruses. *J. Med. Virol.* **2007**, *79*, 1577–1586.

[66] Hurt, A. C., et al. Emergence and spread of oseltamivir-resistant A(H1N1) influenza viruses in Oceania, South East Asia and South Africa. *Antiviral Res.* **2009**, *83*, 90–93.

[67] Babu, Y. S., et al. BCX-1812 (RWJ-270201): Discovery of a novel, highly potent, orally active, and selective influenza neuraminidase inhibitor through structure-based drug design. *J. Med. Chem.* **2000**, *43*, 3482–3486.

[68] Bantia, S., et al. Anti-influenza virus activity of peramivir in mice with single intramuscular injection. *Antiviral Res.* **2006**, *69*, 39–45.

[69] Birnkrant, D.; Cox, E. The emergency use authorization of peramivir for treatment of 2009 H1N1 influenza. *N. Engl. J. Med.* **2009**, *361*, 2204–2207.

[70] Bantia, S., et al. Comparison of the anti-influenza virus activity of RWJ-270201 with those of oseltamivir and zanamivir. *Antimicrob. Agents Chemother.* **2001**, *45*, 1162–1167.

[71] Govorkova, E. A., et al. Comparison of efficacies of RWJ-270201, zanamivir, and oseltamivir against H5N1, H9N2, and other avian influenza viruses. *Antimicrob. Agents Chemother.* **2001**, *45*, 2723–2732.

[72] Sidwell, R. W.; Smee, D. F. In vitro and in vivo assay systems for study of influenza virus inhibitors. *Antiviral Res.* **2000**, *48*, 1–16.

[73] Tisdale, M. Monitoring of viral susceptibility: new challenges with the development of influenza NA inhibitors. *Rev. Med. Virol.* **2000**, *10*, 45–55.

[74] Woods, J. M., et al. 4-Guanidino-2,4-dideoxy-2,3-dehydro-*N*-acetylneuraminic acid is a highly effective inhibitor both of the sialidase (neuraminidase) and of growth of a wide range of influenza-A and influenza-B viruses in vitro. *Antimicrob. Agents Chemother.* **1993**, *37*, 1473–1479.

[75] Hata, K., et al. Limited inhibitory effects of oseltamivir and zanamivir on human sialidases. *Antimicrob. Agents Chemother.* **2008**, *52*, 3484–3491.

[76] Morris, S. J., et al. Role of neuraminidase in influenza virus–induced apoptosis. *J. Gen. Virol.* **1999**, *80*, 137–146.

[77] Nöhle, U.; Beau, J. M.; Schauer, R. Uptake, metabolism and excretion of orally and intravenously administered, double-labeled *N*-glycoloylneuraminic acid and single-labeled 2-deoxy-2,3-dehydro-*N*-acetylneuraminic acid in mouse and rat. *Eur. J. Biochem.* **1982**, *126*, 543–548.

[78] Cass, L. M. R.; Efthymiopoulos, C.; Bye, A. Pharmacokinetics of zanamivir after intravenous, oral, inhaled or intranasal administration to healthy volunteers. *Clin. Pharmacokinet.* **1999**, *36*(Suppl. 1), 1–11.

[79] Calfee, D. P., et al. Safety and efficacy of intravenous zanamivir in preventing experimental human influenza A virus infection. *Antimicrob. Agents Chemother.* **1999**, *43*, 1616–1620.

[80] Burch, J., et al. Antiviral drugs for the treatment of influenza: a systematic review and economic evaluation. *Health Technol. Assess.* **2009**, *13*, 1–265.

[81] Wutzler, P.; Vogel, G. Neuraminidase inhibitors in the treatment of influenza A and B: overview and case reports. *Infection (Munich, Ger.)* **2000**, *28*, 261–266.

[82] Vogel, G. E. Neuraminidase inhibitors in the management of influenza: experience of an outpatient practice. *Med. Microbiol. Immunol.* **2002**, *191*, 161–163.

[83] Khazeni, N., et al. Systematic review: safety and efficacy of extended-duration antiviral chemoprophylaxis against pandemic and seasonal influenza. *Ann. Intern. Med.* **2009**, *151*, 464–473.

[84] Kidd, I. M., et al. H1N1 Pneumonitis treated with intravenous zanamivir. *Lancet* **2009**, *374*, 1036.

[85] Gaur, A. H., et al. Intravenous zanamivir for oseltamivir-resistant 2009 H1N1 influenza. *N. Engl. J. Med.* **2010**, *362*, 88–89.

[86] Zambon, M.; Hayden, F. G. Position statement: global neuraminidase inhibitor susceptibility network. *Antiviral Res.* **2001**, *49*, 147–156.

[87] McKimm-Breschkin, J. L. Resistance of influenza viruses to neuraminidase inhibitors: a review. *Antiviral Res.* **2000**, *47*, 1–17.

[88] Hurt, A. C., et al. Zanamivir-resistant influenza viruses with a novel neuraminidase mutation. *J. Virol.* **2009**, *83*, 10366–10373.

[89] Sheu, T. G., et al. Surveillance for neuraminidase inhibitor resistance among human influenza A and B viruses circulating worldwide from 2004 to 2008. *Antimicrob. Agents Chemother.* **2008**, *52*, 3284–3292.

[90] Okomo-Adhiambo, M., et al. Host cell selection of influenza neuraminidase variants: implications for drug resistance monitoring in A(H1N1) viruses. *Antiviral Res.* **2010**, *85*, 381–388.

[91] Zürcher, T., et al. Mutations conferring zanamivir resistance in human influenza virus N2 neuraminidases compromise virus fitness and are not stably maintained in vitro. *J. Antimicrob. Chemother.* **2006**, *58*, 723–732.

[92] Yen, H.-L., et al. Neuraminidase inhibitor–resistant influenza viruses may differ substantially in fitness and transmissibility. *Antimicrob. Agents Chemother.* **2005**, *49*, 4075–4084.

[93] Mishin, V. P.; Hayden, F. G.; Gubareva, L. V. Susceptibilities of antiviral-resistant influenza viruses to novel neuraminidase inhibitors. *Antimicrob. Agents Chemother.* **2005**, *49*, 4515–4520.

[94] Cinatl, J., Jr.; Michaelis, M.; Doerr, H. W. The threat of avian influenza A (H5N1): IV. Development of vaccines. *Med. Microbiol. Immunol.* **2007**, *196*, 213–225.

28

DISCOVERY AND DEVELOPMENT OF ENTECAVIR

RICHARD WILBER, BRUCE KRETER, MARC BIFANO, STEPHANIE DANETZ, LOIS LEHMAN-MCKEEMAN, DANIEL J. TENNEY, NICHOLAS MEANWELL, ROBERT ZAHLER, AND HELENA BRETT-SMITH

Bristol-Myers Squibb Company Research and Development, Wallingford, Connecticut

INTRODUCTION

Hepatitis B infection represents a major global public health problem. Worldwide, it is estimated that over 2 billion people have been infected with hepatitis B virus (HBV), and over 350 million people are chronically infected [1]. The prevalence of chronic hepatitis B (CHB) infection varies by region, with the highest prevalence rates ($\geq 8\%$) observed in China, Southeast Asia, and sub-Saharan Africa [2]. In these high-prevalence areas, HBV infection is acquired mainly in early childhood, commonly by perinatal (vertical) transmission. In areas of lower prevalence, HBV infection is more often acquired during adulthood as a consequence of unprotected sexual intercourse or intravenous drug use.

The clinical course of CHB infection can be variable, with the activity of disease fluctuating over time. Four patterns of CHB infection have been identified [3,4]. People infected with HBV during early childhood typically enter an asymptomatic immune tolerance phase, which may last for up to four decades. Hepatitis B e antigen (HBeAg)-positive CHB (the immune clearance phase) is characterized by elevated alanine aminotransferase (ALT) levels and inflammation in the liver. Patients who develop HBeAg seroconversion typically enter an inactive carrier state, wherein HBV DNA falls to a low level and the disease is quiescent despite the continued presence of hepatitis B surface antigen (HBsAg) in the serum. However, in some individuals, the loss of HBeAg represents the spontaneous emergence of mutant HBV variants incapable of synthesizing HBeAg. This clinical presentation, termed HBeAg-negative CHB, is characterized by detectable viral replication in the absence of HBeAg antigen. Fluctuating levels of both HBV DNA and ALT are typically observed in HBeAg-negative CHB and are associated with a poor long-term prognosis.

Longitudinal studies on the natural history of HBV infection demonstrated that CHB was a significant risk factor for the development of cirrhosis [3]. In addition, HBV became one of the first viruses to be causally linked to a human cancer when Beasley et al. demonstrated the link between CHB and hepatocellular carcinoma (HCC) in 1981 [5]. As a result, there has been a focus on vaccination to prevent the spread of HBV and on drug therapy to minimize disease progression to cirrhosis and HCC in patients with CHB infection.

HBV vaccines targeted against the small envelope protein of HBV (principally HBsAg) are highly antigenic and effective in preventing HBV infection [6,7]. The vaccines used most commonly consist of HBsAg-viruslike particles expressed in recombinant yeast. Large-scale studies following universal vaccination of infants in Taiwan have demonstrated that vaccination (with or without hepatitis B immune globulin) can significantly reduce the incidence of both CHB infection and HCC in children [8–10].

Few options for treatment of CHB were approved when entecavir was first studied in human clinical trials in 1997. The first treatment to be approved for CHB was interferon α-2b. Significant numbers of patients achieved HBeAg loss after a 16-week course of subcutaneous injections [11]. However, treatment with interferon was associated with a wide range of adverse events, such as influenza-like symptoms, fatigue, anorexia, and weight loss. In 1998, lamivudine became the first nucleoside analog approved for the treatment of CHB after it was shown to be superior to placebo in terms

Antiviral Drugs: From Basic Discovery Through Clinical Trials, First Edition. Edited by Wieslaw M. Kazmierski.

of histologic improvement, HBV DNAsuppression, ALT normalization, and HBeAg seroconversion [12,13]. Resistance to lamivudine was rapidly recognized, and this develops in up to 70% of patients through five years of therapy [14]. Adefovir dipivoxil was subsequently shown to offer benefit for HBeAg-positive and HBeAg-negative CHB patients compared with placebo and was approved in 2002 [15,16]. Resistance to adefovir occurs at a slower rate than resistance to lamivudine, but still develops in up to 29% of patients through five years of therapy in HBeAg-negative patients [17]. Entecavir received approval for the treatment of CHB in 2005, followed by telbivudine in 2006 and tenofovir disoproxil fumarate in 2008.

Several recent advances in the field of CHB have led to a greater understanding of the natural history of this condition. The introduction of sensitive polymerase chain reaction (PCR)-based assays for the detection of HBV DNA has shown that many patients previously thought to have inactive CHB infection actually have detectable levels of HBV replication [18]. Findings from the R.E.V.E.A.L.-HBV cohort study demonstrated further that elevated HBV DNA levels are associated with an increasing risk of liver-related mortality, cirrhosis, and HCC [19–21]. Thus, recent CHB treatment guidelines state that suppression of HBV DNA to the lowest possible level is the primary goal of antiviral therapy [22,23].

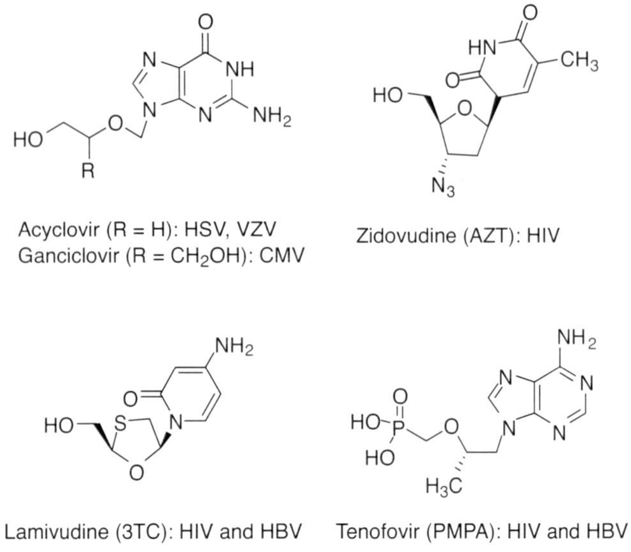

FIGURE 1 Antiviral activities of exemplary nucleoside and nucleotide analogs.

DISCOVERY

The discovery of entecavir stemmed from a research program at Bristol-Myers Squibb (BMS) targeting nucleoside analogs that would selectively inhibit viral polymerases while minimally interacting with host polymerases. The initial focus of the BMS nucleoside analog medicinal chemistry program was the herpes family viruses, in particular herpes simplex virus-1 and virus-2 (HSV-1 and HSV-2), varicella-zoster virus (VZV), and cytomegalovirus (CMV). It was recognized from the outset that nucleoside analogs have the potential to inhibit a wide range of pathogenic viruses. At the time the project was initiated, nucleoside analogs were being used or investigated for the treatment of a variety of viruses, including herpesviruses, human immunodeficiency virus (HIV), and HBV (Fig. 1) [24–29]. More recently, promising nucleoside analogs are also being developed for the treatment of hepatitis C virus (HCV) [25,27]. Consequently, as the project evolved, nucleoside analogs were not only screened against herpesviruses, but also against HBV, HCV, and HIV.

Nucleoside analogs are prodrugs (Fig. 2) which must first be converted to their corresponding triphosphate by cellular (and sometimes viral) kinases. The resulting triphosphates then serve as inhibitors of the viral polymerase, blocking viral replication. The primary screens in the vast majority of nucleoside analog drug discovery programs rely on measuring the ability of nucleoside analogs to inhibit viral replication in cell-based assays. Gaining a fuller understanding of the underlying phosphorylation and polymerase

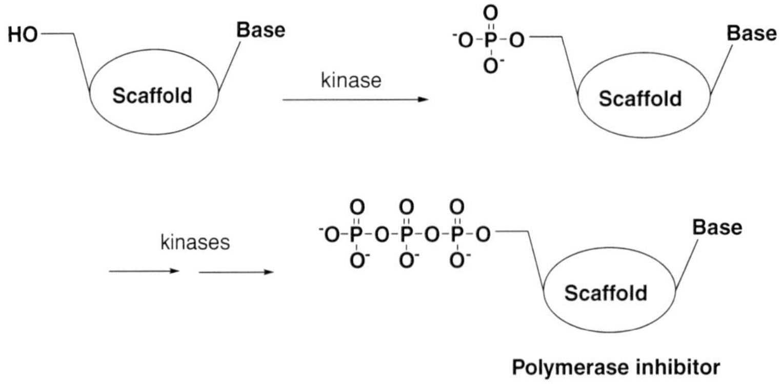

FIGURE 2 Nucleoside analog activation.

inhibition mechanisms is generally limited to select compounds that demonstrate activity of particular interest. Because of the multiple steps and enzymes involved in these cell-based assays, the structure–activity relationships (SARs) of nucleoside analogs are unpredictable, and small modifications may lead to dramatic differences in antiviral potency and selectivity.

When BMS initiated its nucleoside analog discovery program, the field was already mature, with much of the prior art in the field having focused on nucleobase analogs and acyclic ribose mimetics. A central hypothesis and theme behind the BMS nucleoside analog medicinal chemistry program was that the 2′-deoxyribose portion of the natural nucleosides serves as a scaffold that positions the hydroxyl and nucleobase moieties in certain bioactive position(s) in space. The pursuit of this hypothesis ultimately permitted a more focused exploration of the SARs of these agents.

The design of alternatives to the ribose scaffold is particularly challenging because the natural 2′-deoxynucleosides can adopt multiple "pseudorotational" conformations, several of which represent local minima of comparable energy, and little is understood about the bioactive conformation(s) of the natural nucleosides. As a result, the vast majority of scaffold designs ultimately result in inactive compounds. This challenge is further complicated by the fact that the activity of nucleoside analogs is dependent on the species of virus being tested and, to some extent, the cellular background. A corollary to this is the observation that the antiviral activity of a given nucleoside analog can sometimes encompass more than one viral species: for example, inhibition of HIV and HBV by lamivudine and tenofovir. A key breakthrough in the BMS nucleoside analog program was the discovery of oxetanocin (Nippon Kayaku) and, subsequently, lobucavir (BMS). Oxetanocin was reported to possess activity against the herpesviruses and HIV [30,31] and lobucavir against the herpesviruses, HIV, and HBV [32–35].

Unlike the conformationally flexible tetrahydrofuran ring found in the natural nucleosides, the oxetane and cyclobutane of oxetanocin and lobucavir, respectively, are conformationally rigid, adopting a single puckered conformation, as depicted in Figure 3. The activity of oxetanocin and lobucavir against herpesviruses, HBV, and HIV suggested that scaffold conformational flexibility is not essential for antiviral activity and that a rigid scaffold can be compatible with the inhibition of viral replication. Importantly, the rigid four-membered ring offered an opportunity to greatly simplify molecular modeling. Molecular mechanics (MM2) calculations were used to determine the local minima of proposed novel scaffolds, and the ability of such scaffolds to place the nucleobase (in particular guanine) and pseudo-4′-CH_2OH in positions similar to those found in lobucavir was a key criterion for establishing priorities. This paradigm led to the discovery of novel nucleoside analogs such as **1**, **2** [36,37], and entecavir [32,38], as depicted in Figure 4.

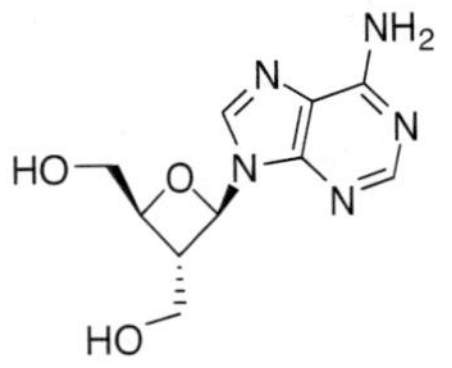

Oxetanocin: HSV and HIV

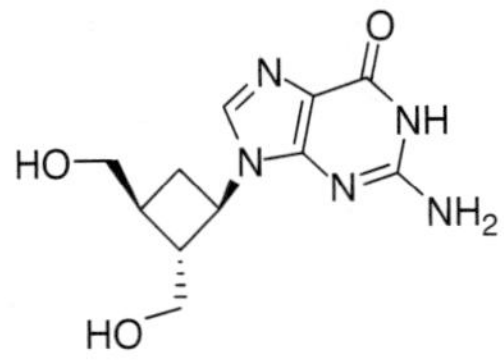

Lobucavir: HSV, VZV, CMV, HIV, HBV

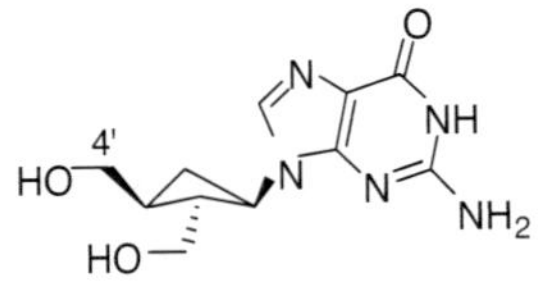

Lobucavir: Rigid Scaffold

FIGURE 3 Structures of oxetanocin and lobucavir.

The SARs surrounding entecavir are summarized in Table 1 and provide a stark illustration of the capricious nature of nucleoside mimetic SARs [32,38,39]. The only nucleoside analog conferring moderately potent HBV inhibitory activity was the adenine analog **2**, and this compound displayed an effective concentration 50 (EC_{50}) of 0.13 μM, which is 40-fold weaker than that of entecavir. The corresponding thymine (**3**) and 5-iodouracil (**4**) analogs displayed EC_{50} values of 100 and 10 μM, respectively. In addition, the activity of entecavir is critically dependent on the presence of the 3′-α-hydroxyl group. Inversion of the hydroxyl (**5**), replacement of the hydroxyl with an α- or β-azide (**6**, **7**) or fluorine (**8**, **9**), or formal elimination of the hydroxyl (**10**) results in a > 10,000-fold loss of activity. The failure of these analogs to express anti-HBV activity is difficult to interpret given the complex dependence of antiviral activity on sequential metabolic activation and subsequent recognition of the triphosphate as an HBV polymerase substrate.

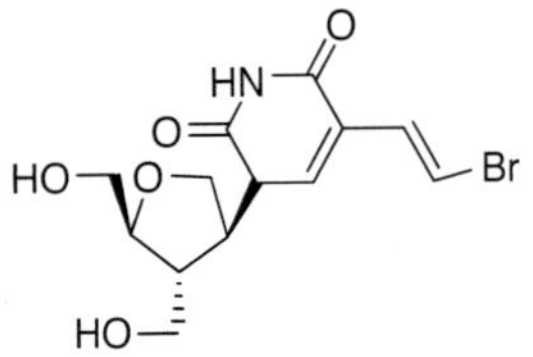

1: VZV and HSV

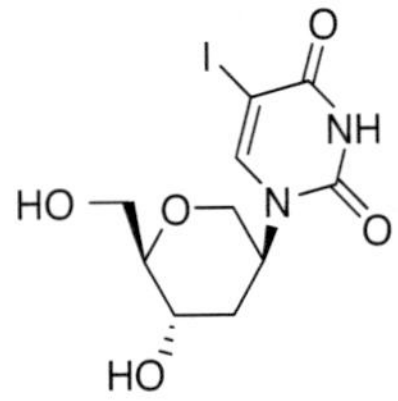

2: HSV

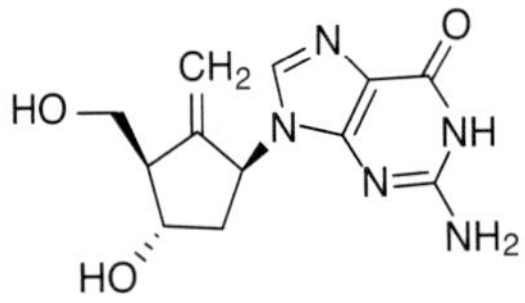

Entecavir: HBV

FIGURE 4 Novel nucleoside analogs discovered at BMS, including entecavir.

TABLE 1 Anti-HBV Activity of Nucleoside Analogs in HepG2.2.15 Cells

Compound	Structure	EC_{50} (μM)
1	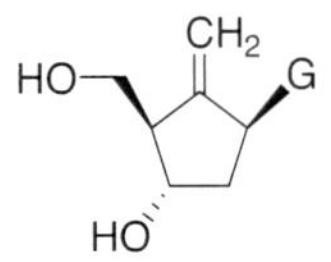 entecavir	0.003
2	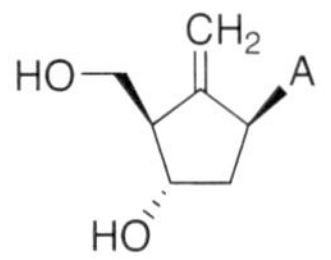	0.13
3	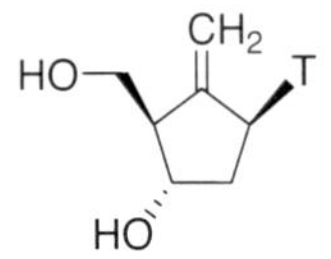	>100
4	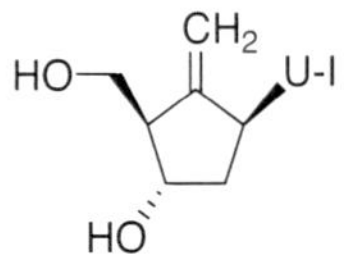	10
5	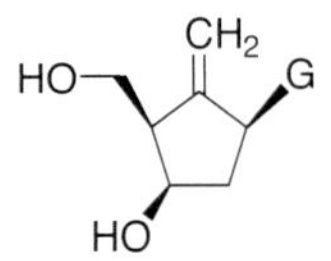	40
6	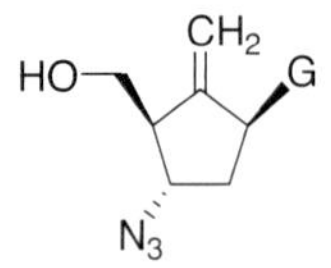	>100
7	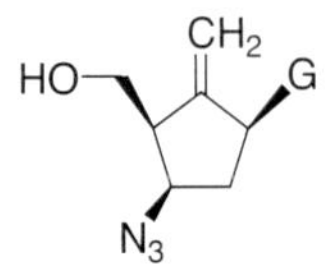	60
8	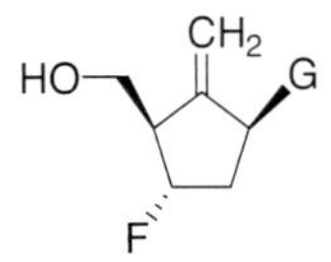	50
9	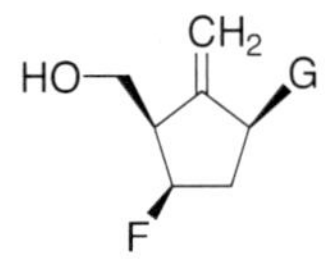	>100
10	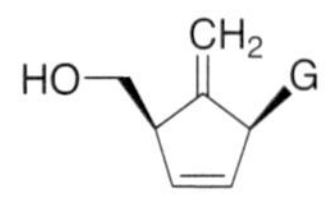	70

SYNTHESIS

The synthesis of entecavir is challenging, requiring the introduction of three stereocenters and an exocyclic methylene onto a cyclopentane ring [38]. Treatment of a cyclopentadienyl anion with benzyl chloromethyl ether followed by treatment with diisopinocampheyl borane and oxidation with hydrogen peroxide (Scheme 1) provided the alcohol **4** in 75% yield and 98% enantiomeric excess (e.e.). Hydroxyl-directed epoxidation using $VO(acac)_2$ provided the desired epoxide, and protection of the secondary alcohol gave **5** in 83% yield. The epoxide could then be regioselectively opened with *O*-benzylguanine/LiH, and the guanine NH_2 protected with a *p*-methoxytrityl group (**6**, 50% yield).

Oxidation of the secondary alcohol using Dess–Martin reagent and treatment of the resulting ketone with Nysted reagent gave the exocyclic olefin **7** in 75% yield. Deprotection of the *p*-methoxytrityl group with HCl and removal of the benzyl ether with BCl_3 provided entecavir in 82% yield.

Although the discovery synthesis above was sufficient to supply the drug substance needed for preclinical and early clinical development, the synthesis was unsuitable for later-stage development. For example, the formation of compound **4** from cyclopentadienyl anion and the formation of olefin **7** from the corresponding ketone both occurred with variable yields. As a result, alternative synthetic routes were devised for later-stage clinical development and manufacture.

PRECLINICAL TOXICOLOGY

Like other members of the nucleoside analog class, entecavir has potential toxic effects based on a common mode of action. Nucleoside analogs are activated by intracellular phosphorylation and compete with naturally occurring nucleotides for utilization by the viral polymerase. By substituting for the natural analog, these compounds halt the synthesis of viral DNA. Such a mechanism of action confers the potential to interfere with human genomic or nongenomic (mitochondrial) DNA replication. The preclinical program to investigate the potential toxic effects of entecavir included extensive in vitro and in vivo testing.

Potential effects on mitochondrial functioning were investigated using primer extension assays and studies in proliferating HepG2 cells. Results of primer extension assays showed that entecavir does not inhibit mitochondrial DNA polymerase γ and that the polymerase exhibits a strong preference for the natural substrate deoxyguanosine triphosphate, even in the presence of high concentrations of entecavir. Studies in proliferating HepG2 cells showed that exposures to entecavir many times (10- to 2500-fold) the maximal clinical exposure resulted in no demonstrated effect on mitochondrial

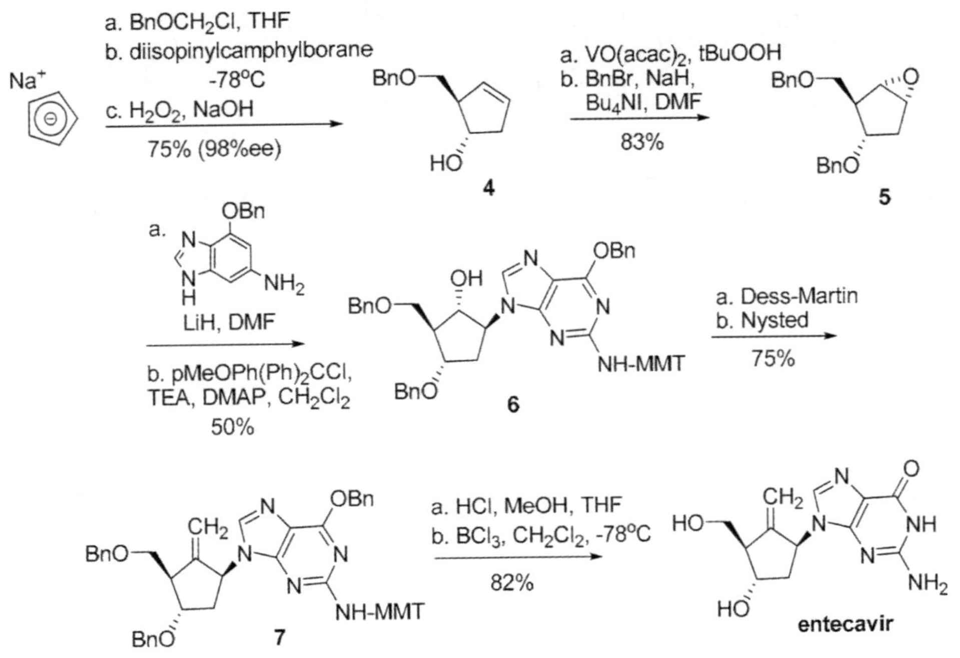

SCHEME 1 Discovery synthetic process for entecavir.

DNA levels or on the production of key mitochondrial proteins [32,40]. Levels of extracellular lactate also remained essentially unchanged in these studies, suggesting that entecavir has no effect on oxidative metabolism. Collectively, these results suggest that entecavir has little or no potential for mitochondrial toxicity.

Extensive in vivo toxicology evaluations were performed in (among others) mice, rats, dogs, and monkeys. Most nucleoside analogs are intended for long-term administration and as such must be evaluated in lifetime rodent assessments for tumorigenicity. Studies of entecavir were conducted in rats and mice at maximum tolerated doses over the life of the animal and compared with untreated control groups. Mice were administered entecavir, resulting in exposures of up to 75 times (for the 0.5-mg dose) and 42 times (for the 1.0-mg dose) human clinical exposures. Male rats were exposed to entecavir at levels of up to 62 times (0.5-mg dose) and 35 times (1.0-mg dose) human clinical exposures; female rats were exposed to levels up to 43 times (0.5 mg) and 24 times (1.0 mg) human clinical exposures. Complete histopathologic studies were performed on all animals at the time of death or at the end of the study.

Results showed increased incidences of tumors that presented in two major distinct patterns: lung tumors that were limited to mice and high-dose tumors in both mice and rats. The increased incidence of lung tumors in mice was observed at low exposure multiples (five times and three times the human exposure for the 0.5- and 1.0-mg dose, respectively) and resulted from early preneoplastic changes in the lung that were not observed in any other species. In contrast to the lung tumors in mice, all other tumors in rodents were seen only at higher exposure multiples; in mice at approximately 70 and 40 times the human exposures at the 0.5- mg and 1.0-mg doses, respectively, and in rats at ≥ 43 and ≥ 24 times the human exposures at the 0.5- and 1.0-mg doses, respectively. For these high-dose tumors, there were no preneoplastic or other relevant histopathologic changes observed in the affected tissues.

Genetic toxicology tests showed that as expected for a nucleoside analog, entecavir was clastogenic in human lymphocytes at high cytotoxic concentrations (10,000 times higher than the EC_{50} for HBV in human liver HepG2 cells). However, it did not induce micronuclei formation in an in vivo micronucleus study in rats, even at toxic doses. In other in vitro and in vivo genetic toxicology assays, including the Ames assay and the SHE-cell transformation assay, entecavir was negative. Collectively, these data suggest that the tumor findings in rodents following lifetime exposure to entecavir does not result from direct DNA damage.

The basis for the increased incidence of lung tumors in mice was investigated and the findings showed that the tumors arise from sustained proliferation of type II pneumocytes. Of note, the strain of mice used in the studies (CD-1) has a genetic predisposition to the spontaneous development of lung tumors that are thought to arise primarily from type II pneumocytes. Experiments showed that the stimulus for the entecavir-induced hyperplasia of type II pneumocytes is neither direct cytotoxicity to lung cells nor unique metabolism of entecavir in the mouse lung, and it was also shown that entecavir does not directly stimulate proliferation of type II pneumocytes. Rather, entecavir causes recruitment of alveolar macrophages into the mouse lung—a chemotactic effect on mouse monocytes mediated by chemokine receptor 2 (CCR2)—and this increased number of macrophages is required for proliferation of type II pneumocytes. Exposure to entecavir in the absence of macrophages was shown not to cause proliferation of type II pneumocytes. In summary, the investigations demonstrated that entecavir causes lung tumors in mice through increased cell replication in a tissue genetically predisposed to tumor development. The specific mechanism is entecavir-induced recruitment of macrophages whose presence is required to stimulate and sustain the proliferation of type II pneumocytes.

Evidence strongly suggests that the entecavir-induced changes observed in the mouse lung are species-specific. No histopathologic changes were noted in the lung of any other species evaluated, including rats, dogs, and monkeys. No lung tumors were noted in the rat carcinogenicity studies and, consistent with this finding, entecavir was shown not to be a potent chemoattractant for macrophages in rats. Monkeys administered entecavir at doses $\geq$ 100 times the human exposure at the 1.0-mg dose daily for one year showed no histopathologic changes in the lung. Most importantly, studies showed that entecavir is not chemotactic for human monocytes, even at concentrations as high as 6000 nM. Collectively, these results indicate that the recruitment of macrophages into the mouse lung elicited by entecavir and required for tumor development is specific to mice and not predictive of a similar effect in other species, including humans. Interspecies differences in CCR2 receptors may account for the differences in entecavir chemotactic activity in mice vs. other species.

Tumors at sites other than the mouse lung were observed only at the highest evaluated doses of entecavir and were not associated with histopathologic changes in the tissues affected. The possible mechanism(s) giving rise to these tumors were investigated. As noted above, results of genetic toxicology tests demonstrated that entecavir is not directly DNA-reactive; in addition, no evidence suggested that the tumors resulted from immunosuppression. It was proposed that the high-dose tumors might be caused by perturbations in intracellular deoxynucleotide triphosphate (dNTP) pools; since entecavir is a nucleoside analog requiring phosphorylation for antiviral activity, extremely high concentrations might result in imbalances in dNTP pools. It is generally recognized that balanced pools of dNTPs (dATP, dGTP, dCTP, and dTTP) are essential for DNA synthesis and repair, and that pathways for synthesis or salvage of dNTPs are therefore tightly regulated. In addition, perturbations in dNTP pools have previously been associated with various adverse effects, including tumor-promoting effects.

Experiments with entecavir in mouse lymphoma cell lines showed a dose–response effect with a threshold entecavir concentration associated with generalized imbalances in dNTPs. At concentrations below 10 μM, dNTP pools were not affected, whereas at concentrations between 10 and 100 μM, dCTP concentrations were decreased while other dNTPs remained unchanged. Exposure to entecavir at concentrations of 100 μM resulted in more generalized dNTP pool disruptions and, importantly, this was also the concentration above which entecavir was observed to be clastogenic. These results suggested both a threshold effect for dNTP imbalances and that the clastogenicity of entecavir at high doses is mediated by dNTP pool perturbations. Other nucleoside analogs (including penciclovir and ganciclovir) were similarly shown to cause dNTP pool imbalances and to exhibit mutagenicity at threshold levels.

In vivo studies supported the findings from mouse lymphoma cell lines. It was found that mice and rats administered entecavir at dosages at which liver tumors were observed (4 mg/kg for mice, 2.6 mg/kg for rats) also demonstrated severe dNTP pool imbalances in hepatocytes. These imbalances included a decrease in dGTP together with an increase in dATP levels. In contrast, when entecavir was administered at doses observed to be noncarcinogenic, no generalized imbalances in dNTP pools in hepatocytes were observed, but rather, only isolated decreases in dGTP concentrations. Such results are consistent with those of previous studies in cell cultures linking a generalized imbalance in purine pools (including increased dATP levels) to inhibition of DNA repair mechanisms. Further studies with entecavir showed that the carcinogenic doses in rodents were associated with entecavir triphosphate concentrations in hepatocytes exceeding 300 nM. These data support the conclusion that when a critical level of entecavir triphosphate is reached, dNTP pools are disrupted, thus impairing the fidelity of DNA replication and repair and increasing the likelihood of tumor development. The requirement of a threshold level for dNTP pool perturbation helps to explain why, with the exception of the mouse lung tumors (for which a specific mechanism has been identified), all entecavir-induced tumors were observed only at the highest dosages tested.

In summary, the investigations into the rodent tumor findings from preclinical carcinogenicity testing of entecavir demonstrate that the observed tumors in rodents are unlikely to be relevant to human safety. Only lung tumors in mice occurred at relatively low exposure levels, and these tumors were shown to arise from a species-specific mechanism. All other tumors occurred at extremely high exposures to entecavir and appear to result from perturbations of intracellular dNTP pools that arise only when threshold entecavir concentration is exceeded. For these high-dose tumors the difference between doses that increase tumor incidence in rodents and those that are used in humans suggest that the occurrence of entecavir-associated tumors in humans is unlikely. Indeed, to date, no increase in human malignancies associated with entecavir (or any nucleoside) has been observed in clinical trials or postmarketing studies.

ANIMAL MODELS

Entecavir has exhibited potent antiviral efficacy in woodchuck, duck, and transgenic mouse models of hepadnavirus infection. Eastern woodchucks (*Marmota monax*) chronically infected with woodchuck hepatitis virus (WHV) are an accepted model used to study the host response, pathogenesis, and efficacy of antiviral agents for CHB [41]. Importantly, these animals develop chronic hepatitis and HCC that is similar to that of humans, and oral administration of entecavir results in potent suppression of WHV replication. In an initial 4-week dose-ranging study in chronically infected woodchucks, 0.5 and 0.1 mg/kg per day of entecavir reduced serum WHV DNA by 3 $\log_{10}$ at week 4 [42]. In a subsequent 12-week dosing study, evaluated with a more sensitive PCR method, 0.1 mg/kg per day of entecavir resulted in a 7 $\log_{10}$ reduction in circulating WHV DNA to undetectable levels within 4 weeks in all animals. The majority of animals treated with 0.02 mg/kg entecavir also achieved undetectable viral DNA by 4 weeks. Treatment discontinuation resulted in a rebound of circulating WHV DNA in all animals, although some animals showed prolonged posttreatment suppression for up to 10 weeks. Importantly, assessment of liver WHV DNA replicative intermediates and covalently closed circular DNA (cccDNA) showed marked reductions as early as week 4 of treatment, reaching undetectable levels in several animals over the course of treatment. cccDNA suppression was maintained for up to 12 weeks beyond treatment discontinuation. In contrast, lamivudine (5 mg/kg per day) resulted in only modest reductions in circulating WHV DNA and no significant reductions in liver-replicative DNA intermediates or cccDNA. No evidence of toxicity was associated with entecavir treatment [42].

These dramatic results prompted a novel long-term study in which 8 weeks of daily treatment was followed by long-term weekly maintenance therapy [43]. Woodchucks were administered 0.5 mg/kg per day of oral entecavir for 8 weeks and were then taken off treatment or administered a weekly dosage of 0.5 mg/kg entecavir for 12 months (14 months total treatment) or for 34 months (36 months total treatment). The initial 8 weeks of daily therapy resulted in a reduction in circulating WHV DNA levels in all animals of 5 to 8 $\log_{10}$ pg/mL. For those animals with detectable virus after 8 weeks, the maintenance therapy resulted in further reductions in WHV DNA, with reductions of up to 8 $\log_{10}$ pg/mL by study end. All nine animals examined at the end of the maintenance phase had at least 4 $\log_{10}$ reductions in liver WHV DNA and cccDNA, with eight of the nine being below detectable limits (0.007 copy/cell for WHV DNA and 0.07 copy/cell for cccDNA). These results contrast with those for lamivudine and adefovir, where cccDNA levels were not reduced.

Whereas animals that were withdrawn from therapy after 8 weeks of dosing exhibited viral rebounds within 1 to 8 weeks of treatment discontinuation, nearly all animals withdrawn after 36 months achieved sustained suppression through the end of the study (5 months off treatment). These results emphasize that longer-term treatment results in more durable suppression off treatment. Importantly, the high incidence of HCC typically seen in these animals was reduced significantly by entecavir therapy, which also extended the survival time for the animals relative to historic controls. Although lamivudine and clevudine resistance can be observed as early as 6 months in the WHV model [44,45], entecavir resistance was not observed during this study.

The duck hepatitis B virus (DHBV)–infected Pekin duck (*Anas platyrhynchos*) model has provided antiviral assessments that correlate with clinical antiviral activity [46]. Entecavir showed efficacy in the DHBV model as a postexposure HBV therapy [47]. DHBV-infected ducklings treated with entecavir for 21 days showed dose-dependent reductions in serum and liver DHBV, as well as hepatic DHBV DNA and the stable cccDNA reservoir.

To model treatment of chronically infected patients, treatment of persistently infected ducks with 0.1 mg/kg/day of entecavir for 244 days yielded a 4 $\log_{10}$ reduction in serum DHBV DNA, up to a 3 $\log_{10}$ drop in serum DHBV surface antigen and reductions in liver DHBV and cccDNA [48]. Entecavir treatment, initiated 24 h prior to an inoculation with DHBV, restricted the spread of infection by about 1000-fold and ultimately led to the clearance of persistent virus in about 50% of persistently infected ducks [49]. These results probably arose from the development of an effective immune response under a reduced magnitude of DHBV infection.

Highly effective postexposure therapy of DHBV included entecavir with an effective vaccination strategy using a DNA vaccine expressing viral nucleocapsid and envelope protein antigens, followed by a second vaccination with recombinant fowlpox viruses expressing DHBV antigens [50]. Animals treated with entecavir only suppressed the spread of virus, but widespread viremia occurred in 60% of animals following cessation of entecavir therapy. However, the combination of entecavir and vaccination resulted in 100% of animals showing no DHBV infection in serum or liver at days 14 and 67. Thus, entecavir can be combined with effective vaccination to prevent postexposure persistent DHBV infection.

In the transgenic mouse model of HBV, 10-day oral administration of various dosages of entecavir, from 0.0032 to 3.2 mg/kg, displayed reductions in liver HBV DNA. As expected, expression of HBV proteins from the transgene was not affected [51].

PHASE I–III SAFETY AND EFFICACY

Phase I

The pharmacokinetics of entecavir have been assessed in a number of phase I studies, including single and multiple dose-ranging studies both in healthy subjects and in subjects with CHB, and in studies of subjects with hepatic and renal impairment. Entecavir was rapidly absorbed following oral administration of doses ranging from 0.1 to 1.0 mg, with the peak plasma concentration (C_{max}) generally occurring within 1 h of dosing [52]. Steady state was achieved after 6 to 10 days of once-daily administration. At steady state, C_{max} and area under the curve (AUC) increased in proportion to dose. For a 0.5-mg oral dose, C_{max} at steady state was 4.2 ng/mL and trough plasma concentration (C_{trough}) was 0.3 ng/mL [52–54]. For a 1.0-mg oral dose, C_{max} was 8.2 ng/mL and C_{trough} was 0.5 ng/mL. Food delayed the absorption of entecavir (1.0 to 1.5 h fed vs. 0.75 h fasted) and decreased C_{max} (by 44 to 46%) and AUC (by 18 to 20%) values. The apparent volume of distribution estimated (4000 to 8000 L) is in excess of the total body water, suggesting that entecavir is distributed extensively in the tissues [53,54]. Binding to human plasma proteins in vitro was approximately 13%.

Entecavir is eliminated predominately by the kidneys. In healthy volunteers, 62 to 73% of the dose administered was recovered unchanged from urine [52]. Renal clearance was independent of dose and ranged from 360 to 471 mL/min, suggesting that entecavir undergoes both glomerular filtration and net tubular secretion [53,54]. Entecavir has a long terminal elimination half-life of approximately 128 to 149 h, allowing for once-daily administration of the approved doses [52].

Entecavir is not a substrate, inhibitor, or inducer of the cytochrome P450 enzyme system [54]. Thus, the pharmacokinetics of entecavir are unlikely to be altered by coadministration of agents that are either metabolized by, inhibit, or induce the cytochrome P450 enzyme system. The steady-state pharmacokinetics of entecavir coadministered with lamivudine, adefovir, or tenofovir were not altered in interaction studies [55]. The pharmacokinetics of entecavir were also unaltered in patients with HIV–HBV coinfection who received entecavir in addition to highly active antiretroviral therapy [56].

The pharmacokinetics of entecavir have also been studied in special populations. A single 1.0-mg dose was studied in subjects with varying degrees of renal impairment, without CHB infection. The study demonstrated that reduced renal function leads to the accumulation of entecavir (increased C_{max} and AUC) and therefore dose adjustment is recommended for all patients with creatinine clearance < 50 mL/min. No dose adjustment is required in patients with hepatic impairment [57]. Entecavir AUC was increased by 29% in elderly subjects (aged ≥ 65 years) compared with younger subjects (aged 18 to 40 years), which was attributed to differences in renal function [58]. Therefore, entecavir dose should be adjusted according to renal function rather than age [53,54].

No significant differences in entecavir pharmacokinetics were observed according to gender or race [53,54]. Single- and multiple-dose pharmacokinetics of entecavir were studied in healthy subjects from the United States, China, and Japan. Steady-state exposure vs. dose (mg/kg) demonstrated a linear relationship in all three populations. The pharmacokinetics of entecavir in Japanese patients with CHB infection enrolled in two phase IIb clinical trials were compared with the pharmacokinetics of non-Japanese patients enrolled in three global phase II trials. A model-based analysis indicated that the pharmacokinetics of entecavir are similar in Japanese and global CHB patients, and that apparent differences in entecavir exposure were attributable to differences in the distributions of creatinine clearance in these patient populations.

Phase II–III

The efficacy and safety of once-daily oral entecavir for the treatment of CHB infection was assessed in several worldwide randomized double-blind phase II and III trials in both treatment-naive and lamivudine-refractory patients. In addition, entecavir was evaluated in separate registration studies in China and Japan. An initial placebo-controlled dose-ranging study examined four doses of entecavir administered once daily in nucleoside-naive CHB patients for 28 days [59]. This study demonstrated substantial HBV DNA reductions of 2.5 to 2.8 $\log_{10}$ copies/mL at the 0.5- and 1.0-mg dose levels. Based on these results, phase II dose-ranging studies were initiated in both naive and lamivudine-refractory patients to further evaluate the safety and antiviral efficacy of entecavir in comparison with lamivudine for a 24-week period. In naive CHB patients, daily treatment with entecavir at 0.1- and 0.5-mg doses was shown to be superior to treatment with lamivudine 100 mg in reducing HBV DNA as measured by PCR at week 22 ($p < 0.001$) [60]. Lamivudine-refractory CHB patients were defined as those who remained viremic after at least 24 weeks of lamivudine therapy or had documented lamivudine resistance–associated substitutions. The phase II dose-ranging study showed that significantly more patients receiving either entecavir 0.5 or 1.0 mg achieved the primary endpoint of undetectable HBV DNA by branched-chain DNA assay at week 24 compared with lamivudine-treated patients ($p < 0.001$) [61]. The entecavir 1.0-mg dose was also shown to provide superior HBV DNA reduction compared with the 0.5-mg dose.

Entecavir was approved for the treatment of CHB virus infection in adults with evidence of active viral replication and of either persistent elevations in serum aminotransferases (ALT or aspartate aminotransferase) or histologically active disease based on the results of three phase III double-blind double-dummy randomized controlled trials. These trials compared entecavir 0.5 mg daily with lamivudine 100 mg daily in HBeAg-positive and HBeAg-negative nucleoside-naive patients, and entecavir 1.0 mg daily vs continued lamivudine in HBeAg-positive lamivudine-refractory patients [62–64].

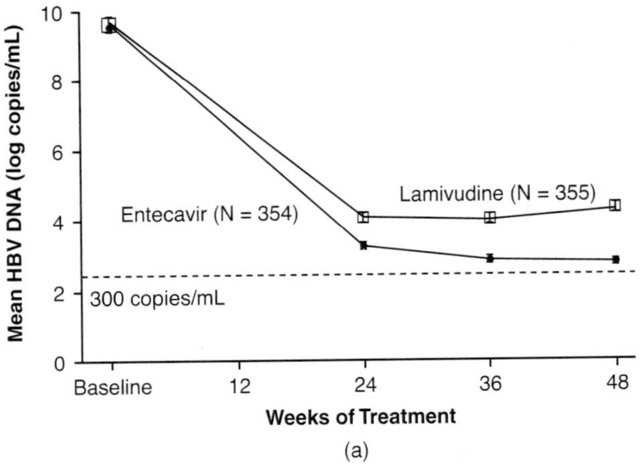

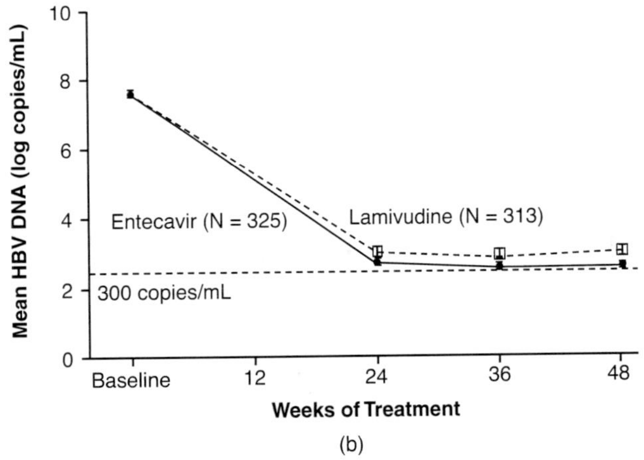

FIGURE 5 Mean HBV DNA levels through week 48 among (a) HBeAg-positive and (b) HBeAg-negative patients. (Reprinted with permission from *NEJM*.)

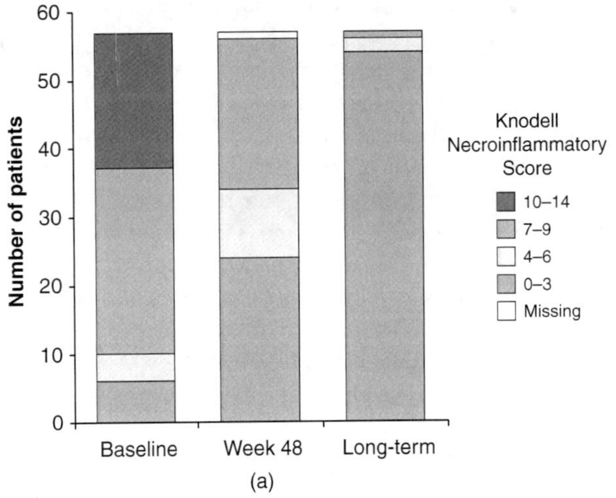

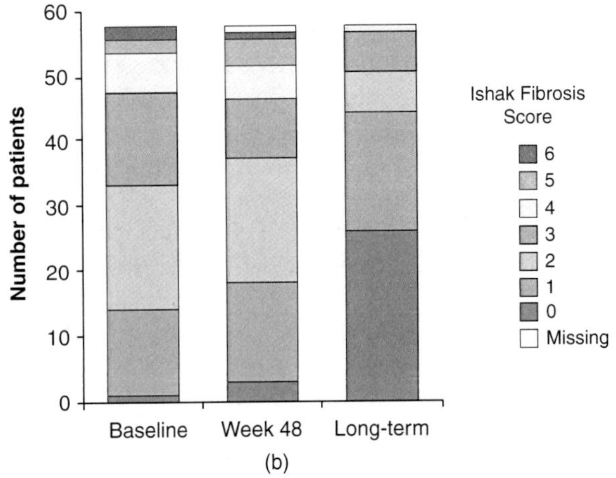

FIGURE 6 Distribution of (a) Knodell necroinflammatory and (b) Ishak fibrosis scores at phase III baseline after 48 weeks of entecavir treatment and at the time of long-term biopsy [median 6 years of entecavir treatment (range 3 to 7 years)]. (Reprinted with permission from *Hepatology*.) (*See insert for color representation of the figure.*)

In 709 nucleoside-naive HBeAg-positive CHB patients with high-baseline HBV DNA and elevated ALT, 48 weeks of entecavir treatment was shown to be superior to lamivudine for the primary endpoint of histologic improvement ($p < 0.001$) [62]. Entecavir was also superior to lamivudine for mean reduction in HBV DNA (–6.9 vs. –5.4 $\log_{10}$ copies/mL; $p < 0.001$; Fig. 5a), HBV DNA < 300 copies/mL by PCR assay (67% vs. 36%; $p < 0.001$) and ALT normalization (68% vs. 60%; $p < 0.001$). HBeAg seroconversion occurred in 21% of entecavir-treated patients compared with 18% of those treated with lamivudine. The safety profiles of entecavir and lamivudine were comparable. Among patients treated in year 2, a higher proportion of entecavir- vs. lamivudine-treated patients achieved HBV DNA < 300 copies/mL (74% vs. 37%) and ALT normalization (79% vs. 68%).

In 638 nucleoside-naive HBeAg-negative CHB patients who received either entecavir or lamivudine, histologic improvement after 48 weeks of treatment occurred in 70% of entecavir-treated patients compared with 60% of lamivudine-treated patients ($p = 0.01$) [63]. Mean reduction in HBV DNA was also higher with entecavir, as shown in Fig. 6b (–5.0 vs. –4.5 $\log_{10}$ copies/mL; $p < 0.001$), and higher proportions of entecavir-treated patients achieved HBV DNA < 300 copies/mL (90% vs. 72%; $p < 0.001$) and ALT normalization (78% vs. 71%; $p = 0.045$) compared with lamivudine-treated patients. Safety profiles were similar for the two study arms. Due to the study design, only a small number of patients continued blinded treatment in the second year.

A randomized comparative study of entecavir 1.0 mg or continued lamivudine 100 mg daily in lamivudine-refractory patients demonstrated superior histologic improvement in entecavir-treated patients at week 48 ($p < 0.0001$) [64]. Mean change in HBV DNA from baseline was –5.11 $\log_{10}$ copies/mL among entecavir-treated patients compared with

–0.48 $\log_{10}$ copies/mL in lamivudine-treated patients ($p < 0.0001$). Higher proportions of entecavir- vs. lamivudine-treated patients also achieved HBV DNA < 300 copies/mL ($p < 0.0001$) and ALT normalization ($p < 0.0001$). HBeAg seroconversion occurred in 11% of entecavir-treated patients compared with 4% of those who continued lamivudine therapy. The safety profile of entecavir was comparable to lamivudine, with fewer ALT flares in patients receiving entecavir. Among the 77 entecavir-treated patients who continued treatment in the second year, the proportion of patients with HBV DNA < 300 copies/mL increased from 21% to 40% and ALT normalization increased from 65% to 81%.

All patients enrolled in the entecavir phase III studies were eligible to enroll in a long-term rollover study and receive open-label entecavir 1.0 mg once daily for up to seven years. The long-term HBeAg-positive naive cohort included 146 patients with a treatment gap of ≤ 35 days between phase III and the rollover study. After five years of treatment, 94% of patients achieved HBV DNA < 300 copies/mL by PCR assay and 80% had normalized ALT levels [65]. The safety profile of entecavir in this long-term cohort was consistent with the phase III trials. The effect of long-term entecavir therapy on liver histology was examined in patients who underwent a repeat liver biopsy. Following a median of six years on therapy, histologic improvement was observed in 96% of naive HBeAg-positive or HBeAg-negative patients and improvement in fibrosis was observed in 88% of patients, including all 10 patients with advanced fibrosis or cirrhosis (Ishak fibrosis score 4 to 6) [66]. The distribution of Knodell necroinflammatory and Ishak fibrosis scores at baseline, week 48, and after long-term treatment are shown in Figure 6.

The antiviral efficacy and viral kinetics of entecavir 0.5 mg or adefovir dipivoxil 10 mg were compared in 66 HBeAg-positive patients treated for at least 52 weeks in an open-label phase IIIb study [67]. Entecavir was superior to adefovir in mean HBV DNA reduction at week 12 (–6.23 vs. –4.42 $\log_{10}$ copies/mL, respectively; $p < 0.0001$) and at weeks 24 and 48 (Fig. 7). Eighteen adefovir-treated patients in this study either failed to achieve HBV DNA < 300 copies/mL on adefovir therapy ($n = 14$) or relapsed off treatment ($n = 4$) and received treatment with entecavir 1.0 mg once daily [68]. All 18 patients experienced a rapid reduction in HBV DNA and increased rates of virologic suppression.

The efficacy and safety of entecavir 1.0 mg or adefovir 10 mg have also been compared in 195 HBeAg-positive and HBeAg-negative patients with decompensated cirrhosis (Child–Pugh score ≥ 7) [104]. Entecavir demonstrated superior antiviral activity to adefovir in this population. Mean change in HBV DNA at week 24 was –4.48 $\log_{10}$ copies/mL among entecavir-treated patients compared with –3.40 $\log_{10}$ copies/mL among adefovir-treated patients (treatment difference –1.40; $p < 0.0001$). Significantly higher proportions of entecavir-treated patients also achieved HBV DNA < 300 copies/mL and ALT normalization. Entecavir was well tolerated and the safety results were comparable between the treatment groups.

Separate registration programs of entecavir were conducted in China and Japan. In China, large phase III studies demonstrated results similar to those obtained in the global studies for both nucleoside-naive and lamivudine-refractory patients. In 519 nucleoside-naive patients, entecavir 0.5 mg was superior to lamivudine 100 mg daily for the primary endpoint, a composite of HBV DNA reduction to < 0.7 MEq/mL by branched-chain DNA assay and ALT < 1.25 × the upper limit of normal (ULN) ($p < 0.0001$), while the safety profiles of the treatment groups were comparable [69]. Among patients treated during year 2, higher proportions of entecavir-treated than lamivudine-treated patients achieved HBV DNA < 300 copies/mL by PCR assay (74% vs. 41%) and ALT ≤ 1 × ULN (96% vs. 82%) [70]. Entecavir therapy for lamivudine-refractory patients was also shown to be superior to placebo and resulted in a change in HBV DNA of –5.08 $\log_{10}$ copies/mL after 48 weeks [71].

Eligible patients from the phase III studies in China entered a long-term rollover study and, among 160 nucleoside-naive patients, three years of entecavir resulted in 89% of patients with HBV DNA < 300 copies/mL (increased from 74% at year 2) and 86% with ALT ≤ 1 × ULN [72]. Among 138 lamivudine-refractory patients, after three years of entecavir therapy, 55% had HBV DNA < 300 copies/mL and 65% had ALT ≤ 1 × ULN [73]. The safety profile of entecavir during long-term treatment remained consistent with the safety profiles observed during the earlier studies.

In Japan, three phase II bridging studies in nucleoside-naive and lamivudine-refractory patients demonstrated efficacy and safety results similar to those obtained in global registration studies [74–76]. Japanese patients who completed the phase II studies could enroll in a long-term rollover study and receive entecavir 0.5 or 1.0 mg daily (depending on whether they entered from nucleoside-naive or lamivudine-refractory studies). Among 167 nucleoside-naive patients who received a total of three years of entecavir, 88% had HBV DNA < 400 copies/mL, 90% had ALT ≤ 1 × ULN, and 26% achieved HBe seroconversion [77]. For a subset of 21 patients with evaluable long-term biopsies, 100% demonstrated histologic improvement and 57% showed improvement in fibrosis at year 3. Among 82 lamivudine-refractory patients treated for a total of three years with entecavir, 55% had HBV DNA < 400 copies/mL, 85% had ALT ≤ 1 × ULN, and 15% achieved HBeAg seroconversion [78]. For a subset of 16 patients with evaluable biopsies, 81% showed histologic improvement and 38% showed improvement in fibrosis at year 3. The safety profile of entecavir during long-term treatment remained consistent with the safety profile observed during the phase II studies.

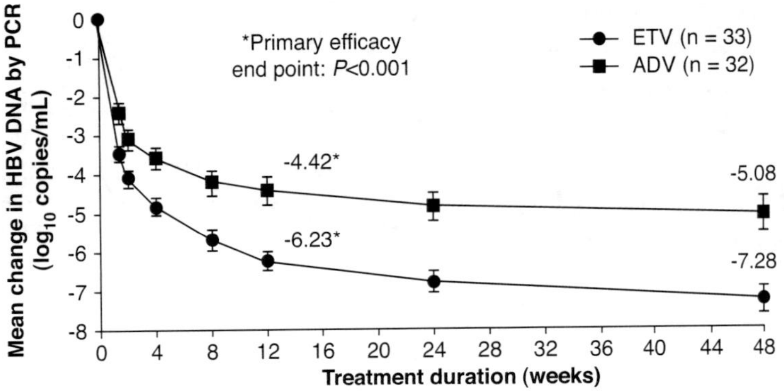

FIGURE 7 Mean HBV DNA reduction (log_{10} copies/mL) from baseline during treatment in study ETV-079.

IN VITRO ACTIVITY AND RESISTANCE

Cell culture studies have shown that entecavir possesses more potent activity against HBV replication than other approved anti-HBV nucleos(t)ides. In cell culture, entecavir is 550- to 675-fold more potent than adefovir [79–81] and 17- to 533-fold more potent than lamivudine [32,79,80,82]. Entecavir is phosphorylated efficiently to the active triphosphate in hepatic cells [82,83]. Entecavir triphosphate targets the HBV polymerase, where it competes for deoxyguanosine triphosphate and effectively inhibits three distinct phases of HBV DNA replication: priming, reverse transcription (minus-strand DNA), and synthesis of the positive-strand DNA [84]. Entecavir triphosphate is a potent (~ 50 nM) inhibitor of the HBV reverse transcriptase (RT) enzyme in vitro [80,82,84,85]. Entecavir displays modest (8-fold) cross-resistance to lamivudine-resistant HBV with tyrosine–methionine–aspartate–aspartate (YMDD) substitutions, but retains intrinsic potency (nM) in cell culture [80,82,85]. Kinetic and molecular modeling studies have shown that the entecavir triphosphate binding pocket is retained in the YMDD-mutant HBV RT [85].

HBV resistance to nucleos(t)ide therapies arises through changes in the "Palm" subdomain of the RT, the active site for nucleotide addition to the growing DNA chain. Clinical resistance to lamivudine arises through changes to the YMDD motif, with a change of RT residue methionine (M) 204 to isoleucine (I), valine (V), or rarely, serine (S). The M204V change is always found accompanied by a leucine (L) 180 change to M, and the L180M change can also accompany the other YMDD changes [86]. The L180 change increases the activity of impaired RT activity. Lamivudine-resistant HBV is fully cross-resistant to telbivudine and emtricitabine [86,87].

Resistance to adefovir, and cross-resistance to the related tenofovir, arises through the RT changes alanine (A) 181 to threonine (T) or V and/or an asparagine (N) 236 to T change (reviewed by Delaney [88] and Locarnini [87]). The A181 changes are unique in that they also emerge during lamivudine therapy and cause resistance to lamivudine [89]. Virologic resistance emerging in HBV isolates during entecavir therapy requires multiple substitutions in the viral RT. These include the primary lamivudine resistance substitutions (rtM204V/I ± rtL180M) plus an additional entecavir-specific change at rtT184, rtS202, or rtM250 [80,90]. This is in contrast with clinical resistance to the other approved HBV nucleos(t)ides, as discussed above, that emerge after selection of as few as a single substitution in the HBV RT. The multiple changes required for entecavir resistance indicate a uniquely high genetic barrier to resistance. In addition, the potent suppression of HBV replication observed with entecavir [62,63], combined with a requirement for multiple substitutions for resistance, and the impaired fitness of entecavir-resistant viruses, creates a high barrier to entecavir resistance in nucleoside-naive patients [91].

In the worldwide entecavir phase II and III clinical trials, genotypic resistance was assessed in patients with detectable HBV DNA at the end of each year of therapy. The RT domain of the HBV polymerase was amplified by PCR from patient serum and the products were sequenced directly [80]. Amino acid substitutions in conserved residues of the RT, emerging during entecavir treatment, were tested for phenotypic resistance to entecavir in culture. Phenotypic assays also included paired baseline and breakthrough isolates for patients experiencing virologic breakthrough on treatment.

The entecavir resistance program provided six years of follow-up on patients from six phase II and III clinical studies [92]. Serum samples were obtained from nucleoside-naive HBeAg-positive and HBeAg-negative patients enrolled in ETV-022 and ETV-027, respectively, and from lamivudine-refractory patients enrolled in studies ETV-026, ETV-014, and ETV-015 (orthotopic liver transplant patients with recurrent viremia).

In nucleoside-naive patients through six years of entecavir therapy, the cumulative probability of genotypic entecavir

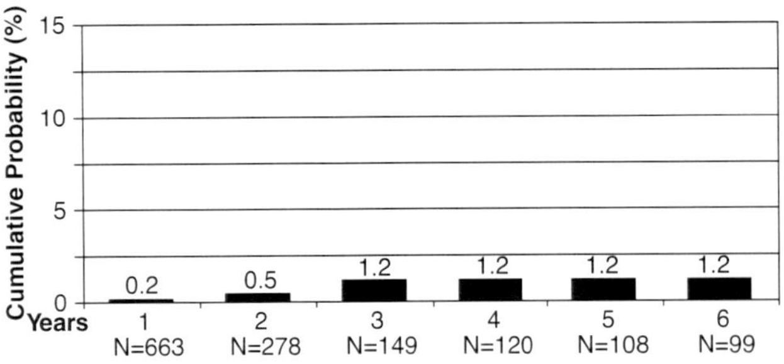

FIGURE 8 Cumulative probability of entecavir resistance (M204V ± L180M + T184, S202, and/or M250 substitutions) among nucleoside-naive HBeAg-positive and HBeAg-negative patients through six years of treatment.

resistance was 1.2% (Fig. 8) [92]. A reduced barrier to resistance was observed among lamivudine-refractory patients, as the lamivudine resistance mutations, a subset of changes required for entecavir resistance, preexist in this population. The cumulative probabilities of genotypic entecavir resistance and virologic breakthrough due to entecavir resistance among lamivudine-refractory patients were 57 and 50%, respectively, through six years of therapy [92].

Results from separate registration studies conducted in Japan support observations from the worldwide resistance cohort. Nucleoside-naive patients in these studies received three different doses of entecavir (0.01, 0.1, or 0.5 mg once daily) in the phase II studies (ETV-047 and ETV-053) and 0.5 mg in the rollover study ETV-060. Among the subset of patients ($n = 66$) who received the approved 0.5-mg dose of entecavir continuously for three years from phase II baseline through to the end of dosing in ETV-060, one patient developed entecavir resistance [93]. The cumulative probability of entecavir resistance in this population was 1.7% through three years. Among lamivudine-refractory patients treated with the recommended dose of entecavir (1.0 mg once daily) for three years in ETV-052 and ETV-060, the cumulative probabilities of genotypic entecavir resistance and virologic breakthrough due to entecavir resistance were 33% and 24%, respectively [78].

Kinetic and modeling studies of entecavir-resistant HBV RT revealed that resistance arises through reduced recognition of entecavir triphosphate by HBV RT—the "exclusion" model, well established for HIV nucleoside resistance (reviewed by Sarafianos et al. [94]). The rtT184 and rtS202 substitutions are modeled to further reduce the size of the entecavir triphosphate-binding pocket in the lamivudine-resistant enzyme by repositioning of the YMDD loop. In contrast, the rtM250 substitutions in HBV RT with lamivudine resistance reduce the binding pocket by repositioning of the HBV DNA template [95].

It is becoming increasingly recognized that combination therapy will probably aid the therapy of HBV patients with resistance to prior treatments [96]. The most useful combinations will include agents with nonoverlapping resistance profiles. Entecavir displays a unique resistance profile; it is active against viruses with adefovir and tenofovir resistance, as well as those with lamivudine resistance (reviewed by Locarnini [87]), including those with A181 substitutions [89]. The high barrier to resistance, along with the potency of entecavir, suggests that it could be an important component of combination therapy for treatment-experienced patients.

FUTURE DIRECTIONS

With the development of entecavir and more recently tenofovir for the treatment of CHB, physicians currently have the choice of two potent antiviral agents with apparently low resistance rates. The availability of potent antiviral agents is an important step forward in addressing the challenges of treating CHB, such as adequately controlling viral replication, assessing treatment duration and discontinuation, and the role of interferons and combination therapies.

The first challenge facing the CHB-treating physician is to adequately suppress viral replication. The importance of suppressing viral replication has been demonstrated in a number of clinical studies. First, the R.E.V.E.A.L.-HBV study, which was a natural history study in which patients did not receive treatment, demonstrated that elevated viral load was associated with an increased incidence of both cirrhosis and HCC [19,20]. Second, treatment with lamivudine has been shown to significantly reduce the rates of disease progression among CHB patients, including those with advanced liver disease [97,98]. Notably, increased rates of disease progression were observed among patients who developed lamivudine resistance in both studies, compared with those who remained sensitive to lamivudine. Thus, current treatment goals are to achieve sustained suppression of HBV replication to the lowest possible level, preventing the progression of HBV-related liver disease and minimizing the risk of resistance [22,23]. Therefore, it is recommended that treatment is initiated with a potent agent that has a high genetic barrier to resistance, which should allow the majority of patients to achieve suppression of viral replication to below the limit of detection of current HBV DNA assays.

A second challenge facing the physician is to determine the optimal duration of treatment and if or when treatment can be discontinued. Of the current agents licensed for the treatment of CHB, only the interferons have a defined duration of treatment, primarily as a result of their poor tolerability profile. Over a 48-week treatment period, pegylated interferon α-2a appears to offer an enhanced or accelerated immune response compared with treatment with nucleos(t)ide analogs, with higher rates of HBeAg seroconversion observed, although relatively few patients achieve HBsAg seroconversion [99]. However, long-term therapy with potent nucleos(t)ide analogs can result in comparable levels of serologic response, potentially reducing the role of interferons. Regimens combining potent antivirals with pegylated interferon α-2a could capitalize on the advantages of both agents and produce enhanced treatment responses. Results from the combination of pegylated interferon α-2a and lamivudine in phase III trials did not demonstrate any benefit over interferon monotherapy, although lamivudine treatment was discontinued after only 48 weeks [99,100]. Studies examining the combination of other antivirals, including entecavir, with pegylated interferon α-2a are currently ongoing. Limited data on finite treatment with nucleos(t)ide analogs is available. Hadziyannis et al. have demonstrated that among HBeAg-negative patients who received adefovir dipivoxil for five years before discontinuing therapy, the majority (67%) of patients sustained biochemical remission through a 22-month follow-up period [17].

The nature of the hepatitis B viral life cycle, which results in the formation of intracellular cccDNA, means that in the majority of cases the current CHB therapies are not able to fully eradicate the virus [101,102]. This represents a further challenge for treating physicians, particularly as more patients undergo immunosuppressive therapy for comorbidities. Immune suppression can result in the reactivation of CHB infection, highlighting the requirement for new regimens or strategies that can eradicate HBV (cccDNA) from hepatocytes.

Finally, combination regimens are likely to evolve to play an increasingly important role in the future of CHB treatment. As discussed previously, this may comprise the combination of an interferon with a nucleos(t)ide analog or the combination of two nucleos(t)ide analogs. At present, there is clear evidence demonstrating the efficacy of combination therapy in the treatment of patients with lamivudine-resistant CHB. However, the potential role of de novo combination therapy in nucleoside-naive patients is less certain. De novo combinations are likely to offer a clear advantage in terms of preventing the development of resistance, but this benefit needs to be weighed against the associated increased cost of treatment and increased risks of toxicity [103]. Trials examining the combination of entecavir and tenofovir in both naive and lamivudine-resistant patients are also currently ongoing.

REFERENCES

[1] World Health Organization. Hepatitis B. Fact Sheet 204, Mar. 6, 2009.

[2] Lavanchy, D. Hepatitis B virus epidemiology, disease burden, treatment, and current and emerging prevention and control measures. *J. Viral Hepatitis* **2004**, *11*, 97–107.

[3] Fattovich, G., et al. Natural history of chronic hepatitis B: special emphasis on disease progression and prognostic factors. *J. Hepatol.* **2008**, *48*, 335–352.

[4] Yim, H. J.; Lok, A. S. Natural history of chronic hepatitis B virus infection: what we knew in 1981 and what we know in 2005. *Hepatology* **2006**, *43*, S173–S181.

[5] Beasley, R. P., et al. Hepatocellular carcinoma and hepatitis B virus: a prospective study of 22, 707 men in Taiwan. *Lancet* **1981**, *2*, 1129–1133.

[6] Scolnick, E. M., et al. Clinical evaluation in healthy adults of a hepatitis B vaccine made by recombinant DNA. *JAMA* **1984**, *251*, 2812–2815.

[7] McAleer, W. J., et al. Human hepatitis B vaccine from recombinant yeast. *Nature* **1984**, *307*, 178–180.

[8] Hsu, H. M., et al. Efficacy of a mass hepatitis B vaccination program in Taiwan: studies on 3464 infants of hepatitis B surface antigen-carrier mothers. *JAMA* **1988**, *260*, 2231–2235.

[9] Chen, D. S., et al. A mass vaccination program in Taiwan against hepatitis B virus infection in infants of hepatitis B surface antigen-carrier mothers. *JAMA* **1987**, *257*, 2597–2603.

[10] Chang, M. H., et al. Universal hepatitis B vaccination in Taiwan and the incidence of hepatocellular carcinoma in children: Taiwan Childhood Hepatoma Study Group. *N. Engl. J. Med.* **1997**, *336*, 1855–1859.

[11] Hoofnagle, J. H., et al. Randomized, controlled trial of recombinant human alpha-interferon in patients with chronic hepatitis B. *Gastroenterology* **1988**, *95*, 1318–1325.

[12] Dienstag, J. L., et al. Lamivudine as initial treatment for chronic hepatitis B in the United States. *N. Engl. J. Med.* **1999**, *341*, 1256–1263.

[13] Lai, C. L., et al. A one-year trial of lamivudine for chronic hepatitis B: Asia Hepatitis Lamivudine Study Group. *N. Engl. J. Med.* **1998**, *339*, 61–68.

[14] Lok, A. S., et al. Long-term safety of lamivudine treatment in patients with chronic hepatitis B. *Gastroenterology* **2003**, *125*, 1714–1722.

[15] Hadziyannis, S. J., et al. Adefovir dipivoxil for the treatment of hepatitis B e antigen-negative chronic hepatitis B. *N. Engl. J. Med.* **2003**, *348*, 800–807.

[16] Marcellin, P., et al. Adefovir dipivoxil for the treatment of hepatitis B e antigen-positive chronic hepatitis B. *N. Engl. J. Med.* **2003**, *348*, 808–816.

[17] Hadziyannis, S. J., et al. Long-term therapy with adefovir dipivoxil for HBeAg-negative chronic hepatitis B for up to 5 years. *Gastroenterology* **2006**, *131*, 1743–1751.

[18] Pawlotsky, J. M. Molecular diagnosis of viral hepatitis. *Gastroenterology* **2002**, *122*, 1554–1568.

[19] Chen, C. J., et al. Risk of hepatocellular carcinoma across a biological gradient of serum hepatitis B virus DNA level. *JAMA* **2006**, *295*, 65–73.

[20] Iloeje, U. H., et al. Predicting cirrhosis risk based on the level of circulating hepatitis B viral load. *Gastroenterology* **2006**, *130*, 678–686.

[21] Iloeje, U. H., et al. Baseline HBV viral load and excess mortality associated with chronic hepatitis B infection: the REVEAL-HBV study. *Hepatology* **2007**, *44*(Suppl. 1), 540A.

[22] European Association for the Study of the Liver. EASL Clinical practice guidelines: management of chronic hepatitis B. *J. Hepatol.* **2009**, *50*, 227–242.

[23] Lok, A. S.; McMahon, B. J. Chronic hepatitis B. *Hepatology* **2007**, *45*, 507–539.

[24] De Clercq, E.; Field, H. J. Antiviral chemistry and chemotherapy's current antiviral agents FactFile (2nd edition): retroviruses and hepadnaviruses. *Antiviral Chem. Chemother.* **2008**, *19*, 75–105.

[25] De Clercq, E.; Field, H. J. Antiviral chemistry and chemotherapy's current antiviral agents FactFile 2008 (2nd edition): RNA viruses. *Antiviral Chem. Chemother.* **2008**, *19*, 63–74.

[26] Field, H. J.; De Clercq, E. Antiviral chemistry and chemotherapy's current antiviral agents FactFile (2nd edition): DNA viruses. *Antiviral Chem. Chemother.* **2008**, *19*, 51–62.

[27] De Clercq, E. The design of drugs for HIV and HCV. *Nat. Rev. Drug Discov.* **2007**, *6*, 1001–1018.

[28] Villarreal, E. C. Current and potential therapies for the treatment of herpes-virus infections. *Prog. Drug Res.* **2003**, *60*, 263–307.

[29] Papatheodoridis, G. V., et al. Therapeutic strategies in the management of patients with chronic hepatitis B virus infection. *Lancet Infect. Dis.* **2008**, *8*, 167–178.

[30] Shimada, N., et al. Oxetanocin, a novel nucleoside from bacteria. *J. Antibiot. (Tokyo).* **1986**, *39*, 1623–1625.

[31] Hoshino, H., et al. Inhibition of infectivity of human immunodeficiency virus by oxetanocin. *J. Antibiot. (Tokyo).* **1987**, *40*, 1077–1078.

[32] Innaimo, S. F., et al. Identification of BMS-200475 as a potent and selective inhibitor of hepatitis B virus. *Antimicrob. Agents Chemother.* **1997**, *41*, 1444–1448.

[33] Slusarchyk, W. A., et al. Synthesis of SQ-33,054, a novel cyclobutane nucleoside with potent antiviral activity. *Tetrahedron Lett.* **2009**, *30*, 6453–6456.

[34] Bisacchi, G. S., et al. Synthesis and antiviral activity of enantiomeric forms of cyclobutyl nucleoside analogues. *J. Med. Chem.* **1991**, *34*, 1415–1421.

[35] Hayashi, S., et al. Cyclobut-A and cyclobut-G, carbocyclic oxetanocin analogs that inhibit the replication of human immunodeficiency virus in T cells and monocytes and macrophages in vitro. *Antimicrob. Agents Chemother.* **1990**, *34*, 287–294.

[36] Tino, J. A., et al. Synthesis and antiviral activity of novel isonucleoside analogs. *J. Med. Chem.* **1993**, *36*, 1221–1229.

[37] Tino, J. A., et al. Antiviral tetrahydropyrans. U.S. Patent 5,314,893, **1994**.

[38] Bisacchi, G. S., et al. BMS-200475, a novel carbocyclic 2′-deoxyguanosine analog with potent and selective anti-hepatitis B virus activity in vitro. *Bioorg. Med. Chem. Lett.* **1997**, *7*, 127–132.

[39] Rudediger, E., et al. Novel 3′-deoxy analogs of the anti-HBV agent entecavir: synthesis of enantiomers from a single chiral epoxide. *Tetrahedron Lett.* **2009**, *45*, 739–742.

[40] Mazzucco, C. E., et al. Entecavir for treatment of hepatitis B virus displays no in vitro mitochondrial toxicity or DNA polymerase gamma inhibition. *Antimicrob. Agents Chemother.* **2008**, *52*, 598–605.

[41] Menne, S.; Cote, P. J. The woodchuck as an animal model for pathogenesis and therapy of chronic hepatitis B virus infection. *World J. Gastroenterol.* **2007**, *13*, 104–124.

[42] Genovesi, E. V., et al. Efficacy of the carbocyclic 2′-deoxyguanosine nucleoside BMS-200475 in the woodchuck model of hepatitis B virus infection. *Antimicrob. Agents Chemother.* **1998**, *42*, 3209–3217.

[43] Colonno, R. J., et al. Long-term entecavir treatment results in sustained antiviral efficacy and prolonged life span in the woodchuck model of chronic hepatitis infection. *J. Infect. Dis.* **2001**, *184*, 1236–1245.

[44] Zhou, T., et al. Emergence of drug-resistant populations of woodchuck hepatitis virus in woodchucks treated with the antiviral nucleoside lamivudine. *Antimicrob. Agents Chemother.* **1999**, *43*, 1947–1954.

[45] Zhu, Y., et al. Kinetics of hepadnavirus loss from the liver during inhibition of viral DNA synthesis. *J. Virol.* **2001**, *75*, 311–322.

[46] Jilbert, A. R., et al. Characterization of age- and dose-related outcomes of duck hepatitis B virus infection. *Virology* **1998**, *244*, 273–282.

[47] Marion, P. L., et al. Potent efficacy of entecavir (BMS-200475) in a duck model of hepatitis B virus replication. *Antimicrob. Agents Chemother.* **2002**, *46*, 82–88.

[48] Foster, W. K., et al. Entecavir therapy combined with DNA vaccination for persistent duck hepatitis B virus infection. *Antimicrob. Agents Chemother.* **2003**, *47*, 2624–2635.

[49] Foster, W. K., et al. Effect of antiviral treatment with entecavir on age- and dose-related outcomes of duck hepatitis B virus infection. *J. Virol.* **2005**, *79*, 5819–5832.

[50] Miller, D. S., et al. Antiviral therapy with entecavir combined with post-exposure "prime-boost" vaccination eliminates duck hepatitis B virus-infected hepatocytes and prevents the development of persistent infection. *Virology* **2008**, *373*, 329–341.

[51] Julander, J. G., et al. Characterization of antiviral activity of entecavir in transgenic mice expressing hepatitis B virus. *Antiviral Res.* **2003**, *59*, 155–161.

[52] Yan, J. H., et al. Entecavir pharmacokinetics, safety, and tolerability after multiple ascending doses in healthy subjects. *J. Clin. Pharmacol.* **2006**, *46*, 1250–1258.

[53] Baraclude® (entecavir) European Summary of Product Characteristics. Bristol-Myers Squibb Pharma EEIG, Apr. 2009.

[54] Baraclude® (entecavir) US Prescribing Information. Bristol-Myers Squibb Company, Jan. 2009.

[55] Bifano, M., et al. Lack of a pharmacokinetic interaction when entecavir is co-administered with lamivudine, adefovir, or tenofovir. *J. Hepatol* **2005**, *42*(Suppl. 2), 171.

[56] Zhu, M., et al. Lack of an effect of human immunodeficiency virus coinfection on the pharmacokinetics of entecavir

in hepatitis B virus-infected patients. *Antimicrob. Agents Chemother.* **2008**, *52*, 2836–2841.

[57] Bifano, M., et al. Hepatic impairment does not alter single-dose pharmacokinetics and safety of entecavir. *Hepatology* **2004**, *40* (Suppl. 1), 663A.

[58] Yan, J. H., et al. Effect of age and gender on single-dose pharmacokinetics of entecavir in healthy subjects. *Antiviral Ther.* **2004**, *9*, H23.

[59] de Man, R. A., et al. Safety and efficacy of oral entecavir given for 28 days in patients with chronic hepatitis B virus infection. *Hepatology* **2001**, *34*, 578–582.

[60] Lai, C. L., et al. Entecavir is superior to lamivudine in reducing hepatitis B virus DNA in patients with chronic hepatitis B infection. *Gastroenterology* **2002**, *123*, 1831–1838.

[61] Chang, T. T., et al. A dose-ranging study of the efficacy and tolerability of entecavir in lamivudine-refractory chronic hepatitis B patients. *Gastroenterology* **2005**, *129*, 1198–1209.

[62] Chang T. T., et al. A comparison of entecavir and lamivudine for HBeAg-positive chronic hepatitis B. *N. Engl. J. Med.* **2006**, *354*, 1001–1010.

[63] Lai, C. L., et al. Entecavir versus lamivudine for patients with HBeAg-negative chronic hepatitis B. *N. Engl. J. Med.* **2006**, *354*, 1011–1020.

[64] Sherman, M., et al. Entecavir for treatment of lamivudine-refractory, HBeAg-positive chronic hepatitis B. *Gastroenterology* **2006**, *130*, 2039–2049.

[65] Chang, T. T., et al. Entecavir treatment for up to 5 years in patients with hepatitis B e antigen-positive chronic hepatitis B.. *Hepatology* **2008**, *48* (Suppl. 1), 705A–706A.

[66] Chang, T. T., et al. Long-term entecavir therapy results in the reversal of fibrosis/cirrhosis and continued histologic improvement in patients with chronic hepatitis B. *Hepatology* **2010**, *52*, 886–893.

[67] Leung, N., et al. Early hepatitis B virus DNA reduction in hepatitis B e antigen-positive patients with chronic hepatitis B: a randomized international study of entecavir versus adefovir. *Hepatology* **2009**, *49*, 72–79.

[68] Leung, N., et al. Entecavir therapy in chronic hepatitis B patients previously treated with adefovir with incomplete response on-treatment or relapse off-treatment. *J. Hepatol.* **2009**, *50* (Suppl 1), S334.

[69] Yao, G., et al. Efficacy and safety of entecavir compared with lamivudine in nucleoside-naive patients with chronic hepatitis B: a randomized double-blind trial in China. *Hepatol. Int.* **2007**, *1*, 365–372.

[70] Yao, G., et al. Two-year results from a phase 3 study in nucleoside-naive patients in China (ETV-023). *Hepatol. Int.* **2007**, *1*, 124.

[71] Yao, G., et al. Entecavir for the treatment of lamivudine-refractory chronic hepatitis B patients in China. *Hepatol. Int.* **2007**, *1*, 373–381.

[72] Yao, G., et al. Three years of continuous treatment with entecavir results in high proportions of Chinese nucleoside-naive patients with undetectable HBV DNA: results from studies ETV-023 and -050. *Hepatol. Int.* **2008**, *2*, A162.

[73] Yao, G., et al. Three-year continuous entecavir treatment in Chinese patients who had previously failed lamivudine: results from studies ETV-056 and -50. *Hepatol. Int.* **2008**, *2*, A98.

[74] Suzuki, F., et al. Efficacy and safety of entecavir in lamivudine-refractory patients with chronic hepatitis B: randomized controlled trial in Japanese patients. *J. Gastroenterol. Hepatol.* **2008**, *23*, 1320–1326.

[75] Kobashi, H., et al. Efficacy and safety of entecavir in nucleoside-naive, chronic hepatitis B patients: phase II clinical study in Japan. *J. Gastroenterol. Hepatol.* **2009**, *24*, 255–261.

[76] Shindo, M., et al. Investigation of the antiviral activity, dose-response relationship and safety of entecavir following 24-week oral dosing in nucleoside-naive adult patients with chronic hepatitis B: a randomized double-blind phase II clinical trial in Japanese patients. *Hepatol. Int.* **2009**, *3*, 445–452.

[77] Takehara, T., et al. Efficacy and safety of 3 years treatment with entecavir in Japanese nucleoside-naive patients with chronic hepatitis B. *Hepatol. Int.* **2008**, *2*, A97–A98.

[78] Izumi, N., et al. Efficacy and safety of 3 years treatment with entecavir in lamivudine-refractory Japanese chronic hepatitis B patients. *Hepatol. Int.* **2008**, *2*, A186.

[79] Ono, S. K., et al. The polymerase L528M mutation cooperates with nucleotide binding-site mutations, increasing hepatitis B virus replication and drug resistance. *J. Clin. Invest.* **2001**, *107*, 449–455.

[80] Tenney, D. J., et al. Clinical emergence of entecavir-resistant hepatitis B virus requires additional substitutions in virus already resistant to lamivudine. *Antimicrob. Agents Chemother.* **2004**, *48*, 3498–3507.

[81] Yang, H., et al. Cross-resistance testing of next-generation nucleoside and nucleotide analogues against lamivudine-resistant HBV. *Antiviral Ther.* **2005**, *10*, 625–633.

[82] Levine, S., et al. Efficacies of entecavir against lamivudine-resistant hepatitis B virus replication and recombinant polymerases in vitro. *Antimicrob. Agents Chemother.* **2002**, *46*, 2525–2532.

[83] Yamanaka, G., et al. Metabolic studies on BMS-200475, a new antiviral compound active against hepatitis B virus. *Antimicrob. Agents Chemother.* **1999**, *43*, 190–193.

[84] Seifer, M., et al. In vitro inhibition of hepadnavirus polymerases by the triphosphates of BMS-200475 and lobucavir. *Antimicrob. Agents Chemother.* **1998**, *42*, 3200–3208.

[85] Langley, D. R., et al. Inhibition of hepatitis B virus polymerase by entecavir. *J. Virol.* **2007**, *81*, 3992–4001.

[86] Das, K., et al. Molecular modeling and biochemical characterization reveal the mechanism of hepatitis B virus polymerase resistance to lamivudine (3TC) and emtricitabine (FTC). *J. Virol.* **2001**, *75*, 4771–4779.

[87] Locarnini, S. Primary resistance, multidrug resistance, and cross-resistance pathways in HBV as a consequence of treatment failure. *Hepatol. Int.* **2008**, *2*, 147–151.

[88] Delaney, W. E. Progress in the treatment of chronic hepatitis B: long-term experience with adefovir dipivoxil. *J. Antimicrob. Chemother.* **2007**, *59*, 827–832.

[89] Villet, S., et al. Impact of hepatitis B virus rtA181V/T mutants on hepatitis B treatment failure. *J. Hepatol.* **2008**, *48*, 747–755.

[90] Tenney, D. J., et al. Two-year assessment of entecavir resistance in lamivudine-refractory hepatitis B virus patients reveals different clinical outcomes depending on the resistance substitutions present. *Antimicrob. Agents Chemother.* **2007**, *51*, 902–911.

[91] Tenney, D. J., et al. Long-term monitoring shows hepatitis B virus resistance to entecavir in nucleoside-naive patients is rare through 5 years of therapy. *Hepatology* **2009**, *49*, 1503–1514.

[92] Tenney, D. J., et al. Entecavir maintains a high genetic barrier to HBV resistance through 6 years in naive patients. *J. Hepatol.* **2009**, *50* (Suppl. 1), S10.

[93] Yokosuka, O., et al. Three-year assessment of entecavir resistance in nucleoside-naive and lamivudine-refractory Japanese patients with chronic hepatitis B. *Hepatol. Int.* **2008**, *2*, A161.

[94] Sarafianos, S. G., et al. Structure and function of HIV-1 reverse transcriptase: molecular mechanisms of polymerization and inhibition. *J. Mol. Biol.* **2009**, *385*, 693–713.

[95] Walsh, A., et al. Mechanistic characterization of entecavir resistance in lamivudine resistant hepatitis B virus. *Antiviral Res.* **2006**, *70*, A36.

[96] Zoulim, F., et al. Antiviral-resistant hepatitis B virus: Can we prevent this monster from growing? *J. Viral Hepatol.* **2007**, *14*(Suppl. 1), 29–36.

[97] Liaw, Y. F., et al. Lamivudine for patients with chronic hepatitis B and advanced liver disease. *N. Engl. J. Med.* **2004**, *351*, 1521–1531.

[98] Yuen, M. F., et al. Long-term lamivudine therapy reduces the risk of long-term complications of chronic hepatitis B infection even in patients without advanced disease. *Antiviral Ther.* **2007**, *12*, 1295–1303.

[99] Lau, G. K., et al. Peginterferon alfa-2a, lamivudine, and the combination for HBeAg-positive chronic hepatitis B. *N. Engl. J. Med.* **2005**, *352*, 2682–2695.

[100] Marcellin, P., et al. Peginterferon alfa-2a alone, lamivudine alone, and the two in combination in patients with HBeAg-negative chronic hepatitis B. *N. Engl. J. Med.* **2004**, *351*, 1206–1217.

[101] Werle-Lapostolle, B., et al. Persistence of cccDNA during the natural history of chronic hepatitis B and decline during adefovir dipivoxil therapy. *Gastroenterology* **2004**, *126*, 1750–1758.

[102] Wong, D. K., et al. One-year entecavir or lamivudine therapy results in reduction of hepatitis B virus intrahepatic covalently closed circular DNA levels. *Antiviral Ther.* **2006**, *11*, 909–916.

[103] Terrault, N. A. Benefits and risks of combination therapy for hepatitis B. *Hepatology* **2009**, *49*, S122–S128.

[104] Liaw, Y. F., et al. Efficacy and safety of entecavir vs adefovir in chronic hepatitis B patients with evidence of hepatic decompensation. *Hepatology* **2009**, *50* (Suppl. 4). 505A.

29

BENZIMIDAZOLE RIBONUCLEOSIDES: NOVEL DRUG CANDIDATES FOR THE PREVENTION AND TREATMENT OF CYTOMEGALOVIRUS DISEASES

KAREN K. BIRON
Pathfinder Pharmaceuticals, Inc., Durham, North Carolina

KRISTJAN S. GUDMUNDSSON
University of Iceland, Reykjavik, Iceland

JOHN C. DRACH
School of Dentistry, University of Michigan, Ann Arbor, Michigan

INTRODUCTION: CLINICAL NEED AND CHEMISTRY INSIGHTS

Human cytomegalovirus (HCMV) is one of eight viruses belonging to the Herpesviridae family; all of which are significant human pathogens. One characteristic of herpesviruses is their ability to establish lifelong latency in their hosts and to reactivate well after the initial infection. Consequently, reactivation during immunosuppression can lead to recurrent disease episodes. Although initial infection with HCMV in immunocompetent individuals usually is mild and transitory, reactivation can lead to sight- and life-threatening "opportunistic" infections in immunocompromised persons such as AIDS patients, allogeneic bone marrow recipients, and organ transplant patients [1,2]. HCMV also is among the leading causes of birth defects in the United States [3,4] and has implicated links to atherosclerosis [5] and glioblastoma [6].

In the early to mid-1980s, the growing epidemic of HIV infection spurred the search for new antiviral drugs. In addition to the urgent need for antiretroviral treatments, one of the late-stage opportunistic infections of AIDS, CMV retinitis, prompted drug discovery efforts in both academic and pharmaceutical laboratories. The approval of the first truly selective anti-herpes drug, the nucleoside analog acyclovir [9-(2-hydroxyethoxymethyl)guanine; Zovirax] in 1982 provided a major advancement in the prevention and treatment of diseases caused by herpes simplex and, subsequently, varicella-zoster viruses [7]. Unfortunately, this drug was not potent enough for the treatment of established CMV diseases, and its more bioavailable prodrug valacyclovir (L-valyl ester of acyclovir; Valtrex, GlaxoSmithKline) showed a limited benefit in the prophylaxis of CMV disease in bone marrow and solid organ transplant recipients [8–10]. The closely related purine nucleoside analog ganciclovir [GCV, 9-(2-hydroxy-1-(hydroxymethyl)ethoxy)methylguanine, Hoffman–La Roche] [11] subsequently provided the necessary potency for the treatment of established CMV diseases and it quickly became the treatment of choice. The analogous L-valine ester prodrug valGCV generated plasma levels and clinical efficacy comparable to intravenous GCV, and it remains the gold standard to date [12]. However, the hematopoetic and renal toxicities of GCV and valGCV compromise patient safety, and resistance arises with prolonged treatment of immunocompromised transplant patients [13,14].

The mechanism of action of GCV involves two viral gene products: the pUL97 protein kinase, which catalyzes the initial phosphorylation of GCV [15], and pUL54, the viral

Antiviral Drugs: From Basic Discovery Through Clinical Trials, First Edition. Edited by Wieslaw M. Kazmierski.

DNA polymerase, which is the ultimate target of this viral DNA synthesis inhibitor [16]. Two other broad-spectrum anti-herpes drugs also inhibit CMV DNA synthesis and are approved for CMV treatment. Due to safety concerns and their intravenous routes of administration, the use of foscarnet (a pyrophosphate analog, Astra Zeneca [17]) and cidofovir (a nucleotide analog, Gilead Sciences, Inc. [18]) is limited. Since all three drugs target the viral DNA polymerase, cross-resistance can occur [19]. Consequently, there was a need for a safer, orally bioavailable drug with a different mode of action.

EARLY BENZIMIDAZOLE LEAD COMPOUNDS: TCRB AND BDCRB

It was in this environment that the University of Michigan team of Leroy Townsend and John Drach under the sponsorship of the National Institute for Allergy and Infectious Diseases began to investigate anticancer compounds synthesized in Townsend's laboratory for antiviral activities. Initially directed at examining the activity of pyrrolo [2,3-*d*]pyrimidine nucleosides [20], the research was broadened to other classes of heterocycles and nucleoside analogs synthesized by Townsend's group. One fruitful starting point involved the study of 2,5,6-trichloro-1-(β-D-ribofuranosyl)benzimidazole (TCRB, **2**), a compound originally synthesized as a potential anticancer drug [21]. Although TCRB was inactive as an anticancer compound, it was highly selective against HCMV at noncytotoxic concentrations in both plaque and yield reduction assays [22]. This was a surprising result because it is closely related to the broad-spectrum transcription inhibitor DRB [23] (see Fig. 1), which is not selective against HCMV. The addition of chlorine to the 2-position of DRB to give TCRB not only made the molecule active against HCMV but also greatly reduced cytotoxicity. Many analogs then were synthesized and evaluated, leading to the conclusion that TCRB, its 2-bromo homolog (BDCRB; **3**, Fig. 1), and their 5′-deoxy analogs were among the most active compounds [24].

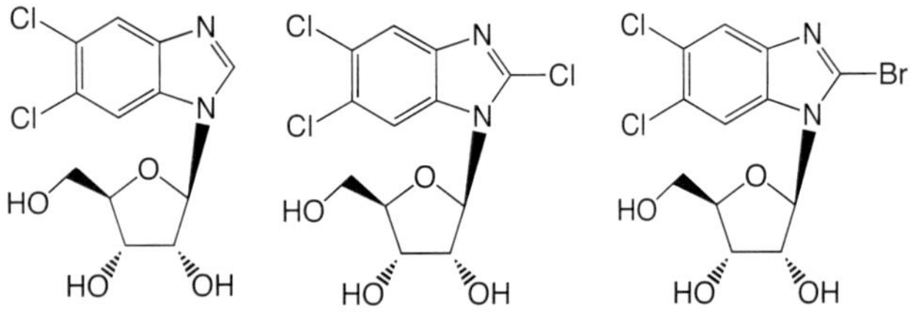

1 DRB **2** TCRB **3** BDCRB

FIGURE 1 Structures of halogenated benzimidazole-D-ribonucleosides.

The spectrum of antiviral activity of TCRB (**2**) and BDCRB (**3**) is very specific and is limited to cytomegaloviruses (CMVs). The compounds are equally active against human and rhesus CMV [25]), less active against guinea pig CMV [26], and weakly active or inactive against rodent CMVs. Surprisingly, neither compound has significant activity against other herpesviruses, including herpes simplex virus types 1 and 2, varicella zoster virus, and human herpes virus 6. Similarly, the compounds are inactive against respiratory viruses, including influenza A, influenza B, respiratory syncytial virus, and adenovirus strains 5 and 7. They are also inactive against measles virus; enteroviruses such as coxsackie A9, coxsackie B1, ECHO viruses 7 and 9, and polio virus; human immunodeficiency virus; and human papiloma virus.

Activity (IC_{50} or IC_{90} values) against laboratory strains of HCMV, such as Towne and AD169, ranged from 0.1 μM to approximately 3 μM in various plaque and yield reduction assays. This is two- to fivefold more active than GCV and is at least 100-fold lower than concentrations cytotoxic to cultured cells or human progenitor cells [22,27]. Activity against clinical isolates was similar to that seen against laboratory strains. TCRB and BDCRB also were active against strains of HCMV carrying clinically significant GCV resistance mutations in the UL97 gene, and against HCMV strains bearing mutations in DNA polymerase associated with GCV or cidofovir resistance.

Mechanism-of-action studies with TCRB and BDCRB in our laboratories provided several surprises. First, unlike other nucleoside analogs with antiviral activity (which typically are converted to corresponding triphosphates that inhibit nucleic acid polymerases), BDCRD is not anabolized to its mono-, di-, or triphosphate nor incorporated into DNA or RNA [24]. Furthermore, as mentioned above, these 5′-deoxy analogs cannot be phosphorylated and are more active than TCRB and BDCRB. Thus, the compounds appear to act as such, without metabolism to nucleotides.

Also surprising and again unlike other nucleoside antivirals, TCRB and BDCRB did not inhibit DNA, RNA, or protein synthesis. Apparently at odds with lack of inhibition of viral DNA synthesis, HCMV-infected cells treated with TCRB contained many viral particles, but few had encapsidated DNA. Because herpes DNA replication proceeds with the generation of high-molecular-weight concatemers or branched-chain molecules that must be cleaved to genome length at packaging into viral capsids, this led us to hypothesize and prove that TCRB and BDCRB inhibited viral DNA processing (maturation), not DNA synthesis [28] (see Fig. 2). McVoy and Nixon [29] refined this hypothesis and showed that some DNA of approximate genome length is formed in the presence of BDCRB. They proposed a more detailed model in which genome maturation is not totally inhibited by BDCRB. Concatemer packaging can occur at a low frequency by continuing beyond the cleavage point appropriate

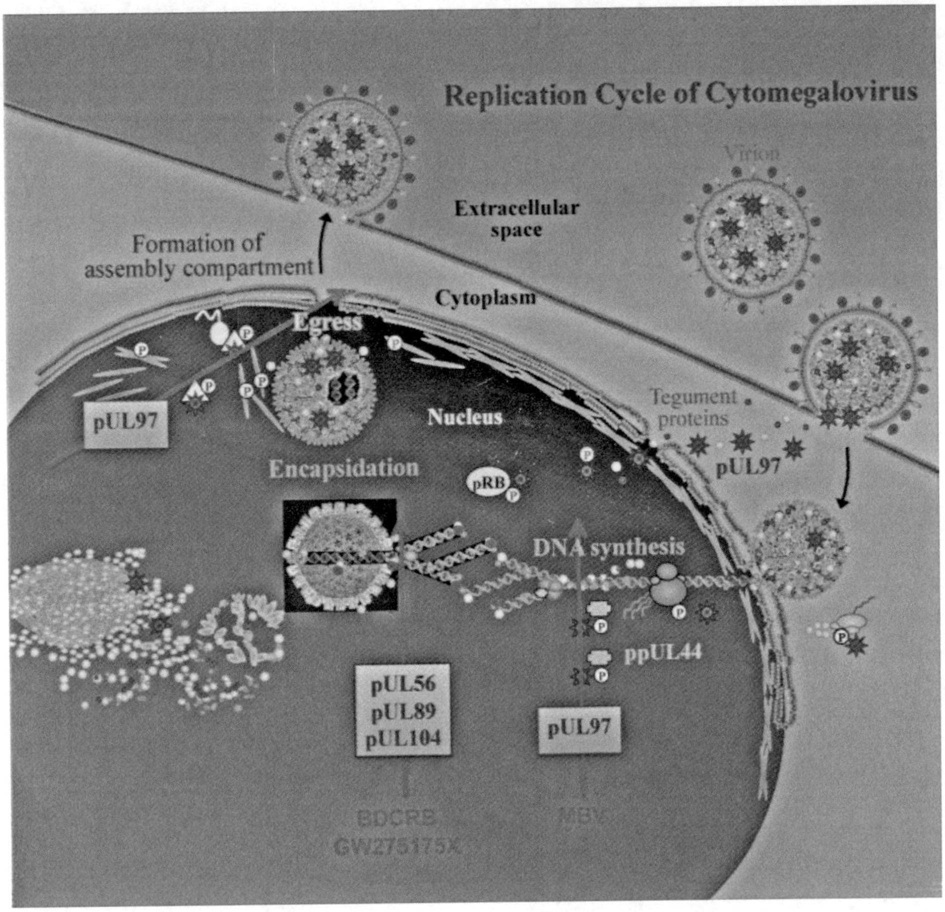

FIGURE 2 Inhibition of human cytomegalovirus replication by benzimidazole nucleosides. Inhibition of key aspects of the replication cycle by maribavir (MBV), BDCRB, and GW275175X are illustrated by red arrows. HCMV proteins inhibited by or involved in the action of the compounds are shown in boxes attached to the arrows. (*See insert for color representation of the figure.*)

for normal genome formation. This gives rise to a nonfunctional structure that we also observed and termed "monomer plus" DNA [28].

Genetic approaches were also used in our laboratories to explore the mechanism of action of TCRB and BDCRB. Selection of HCMV resistant to TCRB or BDCRB and marker transfer studies established that resistance mapped to amino acids 344 and 355 of gene UL89. This indicated that its gene product (pUL89) was the target for the compounds and that pUL89 is involved in HCMV DNA processing [28]. Studies with a different HCMV isolate selected for greater resistance to TCRB established that the product of another gene, UL56, was also involved in the action of TCRB and BDCRB [30]. These data first suggested to us that the gene products of UL89 and UL56 act as part of a maturation complex similar to the two-subunit "terminase" found in bacteriophage [31]. In fact, the mechanism in HCMV may be more complex. We have identified a L21F mutation in gene UL104 (which encodes the viral portal protein) of an HCMV strain resistant to TCRB and BDCRB [32]. An association between the portal protein of HCMV and the terminase has been found by Bogner and co-workers [33].

Terminases are enzymes responsible for the packaging of unit-length genomes into procapsids. Typically, these are multifunctional heteroligomers wherein one protein catalyzes the ATP-dependent translocation into preformed capsids while the other cleaves DNA concatemers into genome length. They are highly conserved in many double-stranded DNA viruses, including bacteriophages [31] and herpesviruses [34]. The HCMV terminase consists of the large subunit pUL56 and the small pUL89 [34,35], whose interaction domains have been identified [36]. pUL56 mediates sequence-specific DNA binding and ATP hydrolysis [37,38]; pUL89 is required for duplex nicking [35,36]. As shown by the genetic studies of benzimidazole-resistant HCMV described above, terminase subunits pUL89 and pUL56 are involved in the action of BDCRB. Biochemically, Scheffczik et al. demonstrated that BDCRB inhibits the nicking activity of pUL89 and therefore leads to inhibition of viral DNA cleavage [35]. Sequence analysis and modelling studies by Champier et al. supported these biochemical results by showing the TCRB/BDCRB resistance mutations D344E and A355T are close to a putative ATPase motor motif [39]. Interestingly, BDCRB inhibits the pUL56-associated ATPase activity as well [40]. In addition, Champier et al. [41] identified two putative leucine zippers that might be involved in pUL56 dimerization and/or pUL56 protein–protein interactions. Based on their modeling and our observation that the BDCRB-resistance mutation in pUL56 is in a zinc finger [30], they postulated that BDCRB could block the recognition site formed by two zinc fingers of a pUL56 dimer [41].

DNA packaging also requires the involvement of a portal protein, pUL104. Portal proteins are oligomers that form a channel at one vertex of the capsid enabling the insertion of DNA into the capsid [42]. Since DNA packaging is ATP dependent and the portal protein has no enzymatic activity, the interaction of these two proteins is essential. Such interaction with the large terminase subunit pUL56 was blocked by a BDCRB homolog [33], thereby strongly suggesting that BDCRB action is complex, involving both inhibition of enzymatic activities and interaction among at least three proteins. Nonetheless, it is conceivable that a single underlying mechanism exists, such as inhibition of ATP hydrolysis by the benzimidazole-D-ribonucleosides.

EXPANDED BENZIMIDAZOLE STRUCTURE–ACTIVITY RELATIONSHIPS

Despite the excellent in vitro activity of TCRB (**2**) and BDCRB (**3**) against HCMV, pharmacokinetic and drug metabolism studies in rats and monkeys showed that TCRB and BDCRB were metabolized too rapidly by glycosidic bond cleavage to be good clinical drug candidates [43]. Subsequent studies showed that *N*-methylpurine DNA glycosylase and 8-oxoguanine DNA glycosylase could cleave the glycosidic bond in BDCRB [44]. As the pharmacokinetic lability of the lead compounds BRCRD and TCRB became apparent, chemical exploration of the series was expanded greatly. Through the partnership of chemists and biologists at the University of Michigan and the Burroughs Wellcome company, several hundred compounds were synthesized and evaluated in one or both laboratories. Many of these had potent in vitro antiviral activity, and it was necessary to carefully examine the SAR using chemical and biological criteria to guide optimization.

Initially, compound rankings were based on antiviral potency and selectivity. The program consisted of a primary high-throughput 96-well viral DNA hybrid capture assay; confirmatory plaque reduction or yield reduction assays, both with concurrent cytotoxicity controls; followed by cytotoxicity assessments in human B and T and progenitor cells. Promising hits were evaluated in a rodent pharmacokinetic screen for bioavailability, and if reasonably bioavailable and stable, compounds were then evaluated in monkeys. Early toxicological evaluations consisted of acute rodent single-dose and 14-day toxicology screens, safety pharmacology screens, and in vitro liver microsomal assays. Ultimately, select lead compounds proceeded into 30-day dose-ranging studies in rats or monkeys.

A major advantage of this discovery program was the fact that the cell-based viral replication screen for biological activity enabled the discovery of compounds with novel and distinct mechanisms of action, whose targets were not yet functionally defined. This primary screen approach preselected for soluble compounds that would enter cells and exert antiviral inhibition at $< 10\ \mu M$ with a therapeutic index (ratio of IC_{50} for cell/EC_{50} antiviral activity) > 10. The goal was to increase both the antiviral potency and therapeutic window with analog synthesis.

Many chemical modifications were made on the benzimidazole base and the sugar moieties. Soon after the discovery of the anti-HCMV activity of TCRB, additional 2-substituted analogs were prepared, including 2-alkylthio, 2-benzylthio [45], 2-amino, 2-bromo, and 2-iodo analogs [22]. As mentioned previously, the 2-bromo derivative (**3**, BDCRB) was even more potent against HCMV than was TCRB. Later, the 2-isopropyl- (**4**) and the 2-cyclopropylamines (**5**) were shown to be potential replacements for the 2-chlorine or 2-bromine in TCRB/BDCRB, which had the additional benefit of reducing the overall number of halogens in the molecule (Fig. 3).

Although much of the initial SAR work was focused on the 5,6-dichloro substituents on the benzimidazole moiety, significant effort was devoted to exploring if other substitution patterns would improve anti-HCMV activity or selectivity (Fig. 3). Thus, 2,5-dichloro- (**6**), 2,6-dichloro- (**7**) [46], 2,4,6-trichloro- (**8**), and 2,4,5-trichlorobenzimidazole ribonucleosides (**9**) [47] were prepared. The dichloro analogs showed little anti-HCMV activity, but the 2,4,6- and 2,4,5-trichloro analogs **8** and **9** were three- to fivefold less active than the 2,5,6-trichlorosubstituted TCRB (**2**).

Having shown the 2,5,6-substitution pattern to be optimal, the nature of the 5- and 6-substituents was explored. Thus, 2-chloro-5,6-difluoro- (**10**), 2-chloro-5,6-dibromo- (**11**), and 2-chloro-5,6-diiodo-(**12**) benzimidazole ribosides were prepared. The 5,6-difluoro derivative **10** was inactive and nontoxic, whereas both the dibromo **11** and diiodo **12** were almost as active against HCMV as was TCRB. However, compounds **11** and **12** were significantly more cytotoxic than TCRB, thus offering no net improvement [48]. Several additional multisubstituted benzimidazole ribonucleosides were prepared, including tetrahalo-substituted analogs. Several of these were more potent against HCMV than BDCRB [49], but given their generally greater cytotoxicity along with higher molecular weight, these did not offer improvement over TCRB and BDCRB.

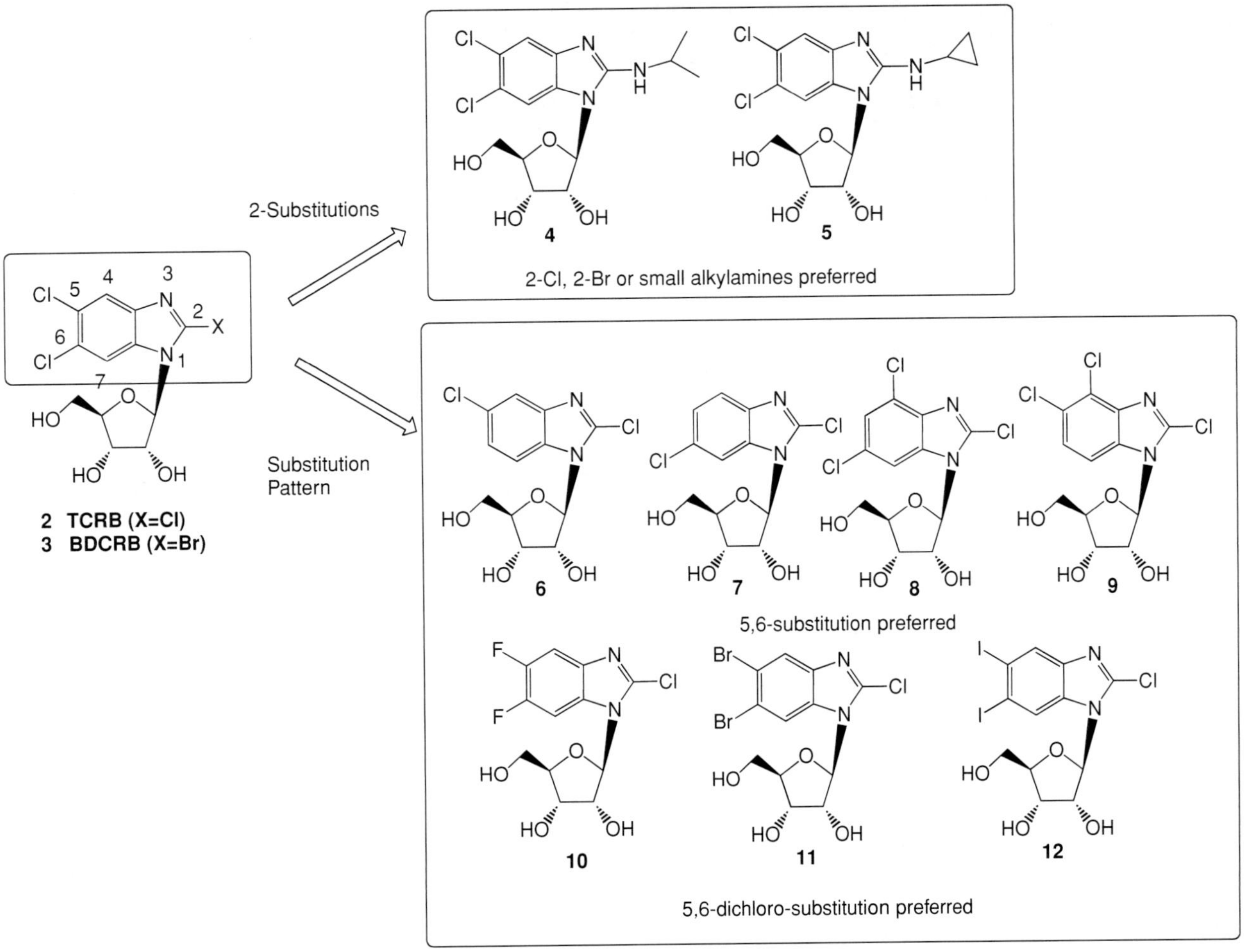

FIGURE 3 Changes to the substitution pattern of the heterocycle in benzimidazole-D-ribonucleosides TCRB and BDCRB (**2**, **3**) that affected antiviral activity.

To investigate if the benzimidazole could be replaced with a smaller heterocycle, a series of polyhalogenated imidazole nucleosides, such as 2,4,5-trichloroimidazole ribonucleoside (**13**, Fig. 4), were prepared. These polyhalogenated imidazole nucleosides were inactive (and noncytotoxic) and therefore not pursued further [50].

A series of TCRB analogs in which the benzimidazole was extended dimensionally were also prepared. These included 2,6,7-trichloro-1-(β-D-ribofuranosyl)naptho[2,3-*d*] imidazole (**14**) [51], 2,6,7-trichloro-1-(β-D-ribofuranosyl) imidazo[4,5-*b*]quinoline (**15**), and 2,6,7-trichloro-3-(β-D-ribofuranosyl)imidazo[4,5-*b*]quinoline (**16**) [52]. These extended analogs showed similar or less activity than TCRB but were more cytotoxic, resulting in a smaller selectivity window. These efforts indicated that a bicyclic heterocycle such as the benzimidazole was preferred for optimal activity and selectivity.

Many changes were also made to the carbohydrate portion (ribofuranosyl) of TCRB/BDCRB; some of which were prompted by the pharmacokinetic liability of the glycosidic bond [43], as discussed above. Carbocyclic analogs (Fig. 5) received considerable attention for their close structural similarity to the ribose series and stability of the glycosidic bond. The carbocyclic analog of BDCRB, **17**, was prepared, initially as a mixture of D- and L-like isomers. This carbocyclic analog (**17**) had promising anti-HCMV activity, being only slightly less active than BDCRB (**3**). Separation of the D- and L-like isomers then revealed that the L-carbocyclic (**19**) was at least 20-fold more potent than the corresponding D-like analog (**18**), and that the L-like carbocyclic BDCRB derivative **19** had activity similar to that of BDCRB [53]. Several additional carbocyclic analogs, such as the 2-isopropylamine-substituted carbocyclic derivatives **20** (D) and **21** (L), were prepared and, surprisingly, the L-like isomer was the most active against HCMV at noncytotoxic concentrations [53].

In general, several of the carbocyclic benzimidazole nucleosides showed excellent potency but often were somewhat more cytotoxic than the ribofuranose derivatives, resulting in somewhat lower selectivity. Importantly, the fact that the carbocyclic L-like analogs (such as **19** and **21**, Fig. 5) were

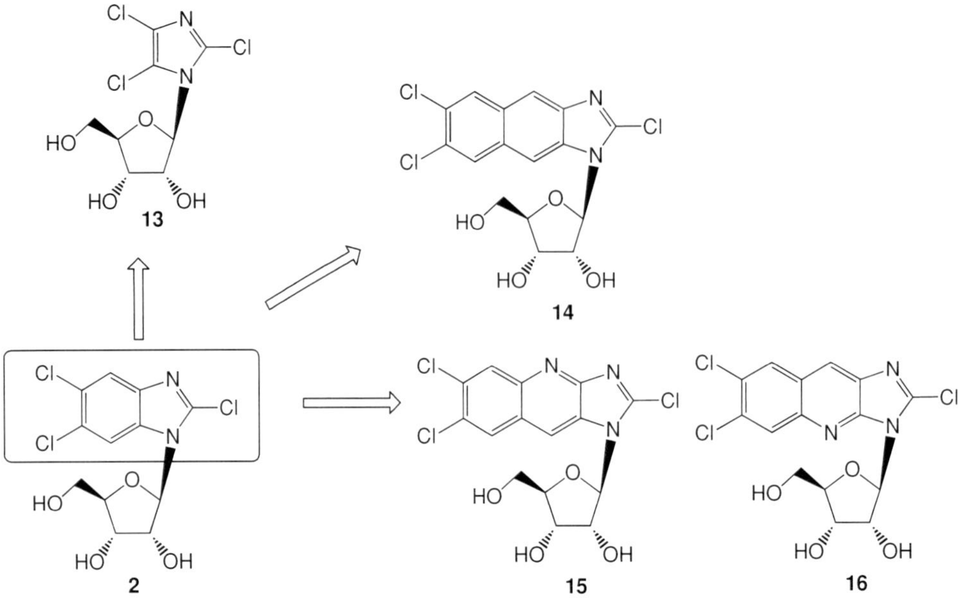

FIGURE 4 Imidazole (**13**) or linearly extended nucleoside analogs (**14** to **16**) that were inactive or less active than TCRB (**2**) against human cytomegalovirus.

found to be more active than the corresponding D-like analogs prompted increased emphasis on synthesizing both D- and L-analogs for carbohydrate modification.

In parallel with the carbocyclic synthetic effort, a large number of L-ribofuranosyl benzimidazoles, wherein the benzimidazole substitution pattern was changed, were prepared [54–58]. Again the 5,6-dichloro-substitution pattern was preferred for the L-isomers. However, for the L-analogs, a small alkylamine (e.g., isopropylamine) was an alternative substituent in the 2-position, whereas for the D-analogs the preferred 2-substituent was a halogen (chlorine or bromine). In retrospect, these differences in structure–activity trends are not surprising in view of the fact that the L-benzimidazole nucleosides have been shown to have a different mode of action

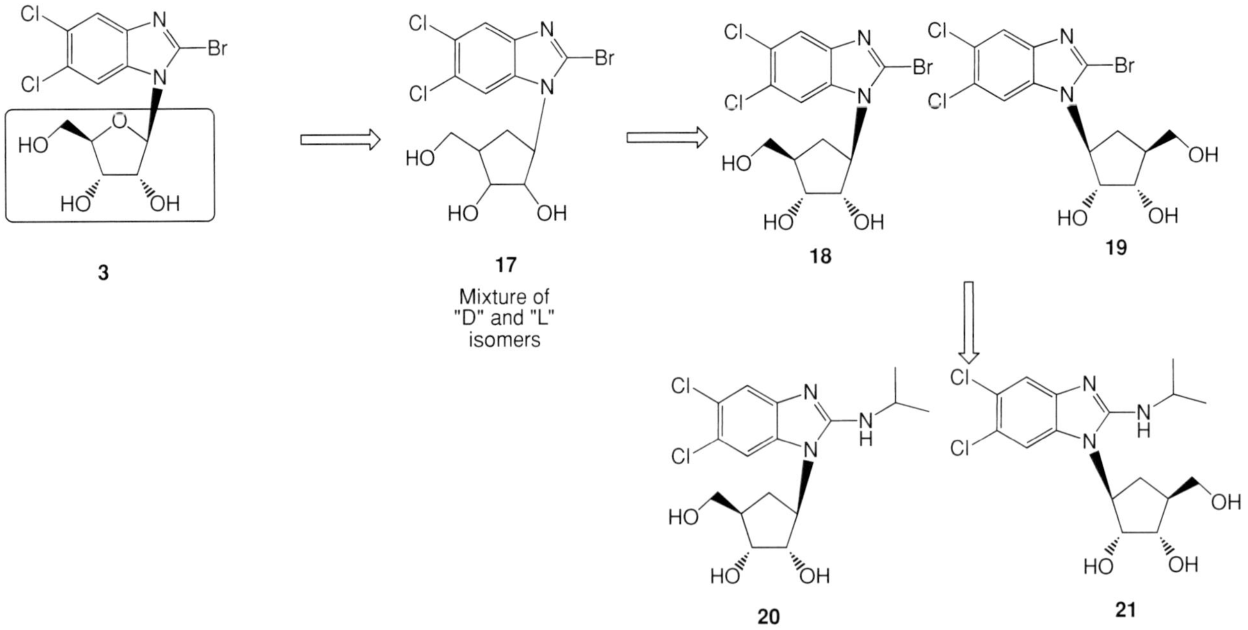

FIGURE 5 Carbocyclic benzimidazoles (**17** to **21**) related to BDCRB (**3**) that were active against human cytomegalovirus.

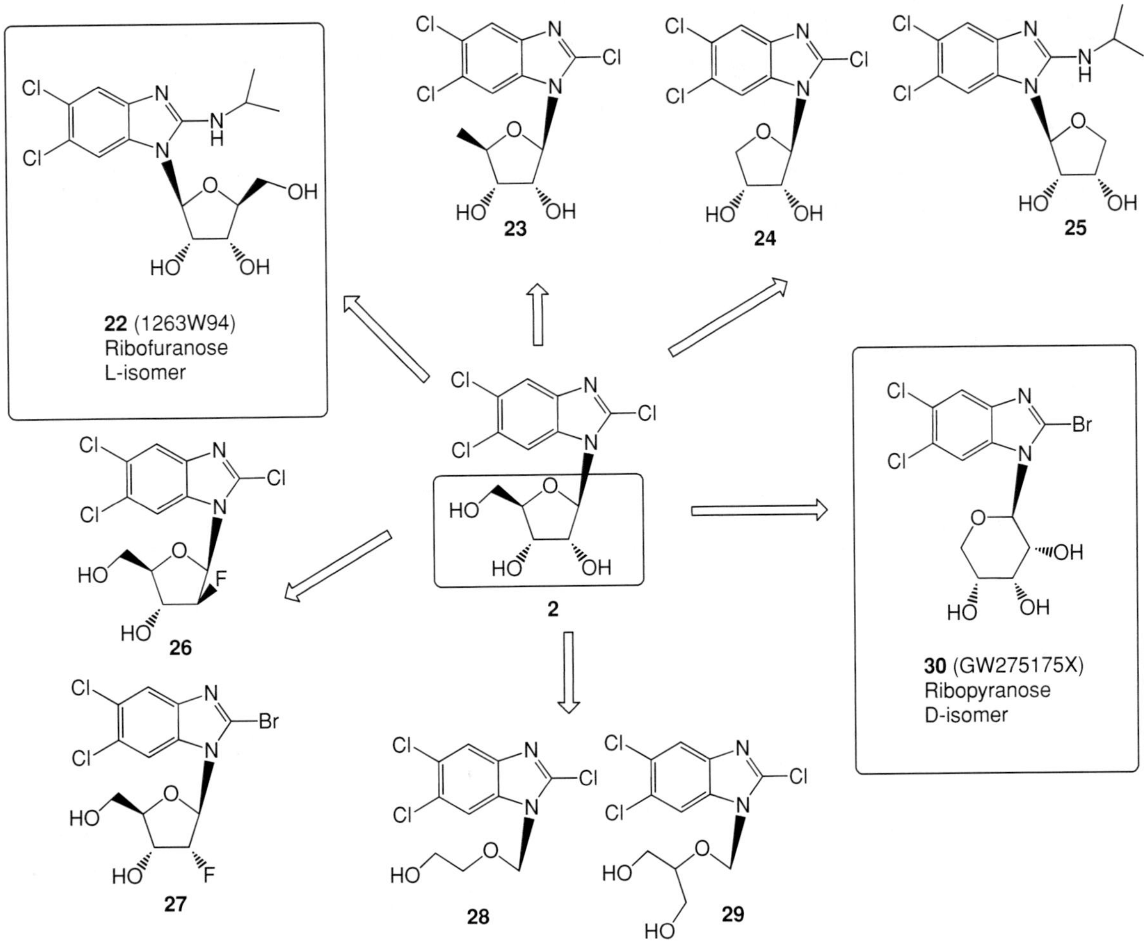

FIGURE 6 Other changes to the carbohydrate moiety of benzimidazole nucleosides that affected antiviral activity.

than the D-benzimidazole nucleosides (see Fig. 2 and below). From a large number of L-benzimidazole nucleosides prepared, compound **22** (1263W94, maribavir) [54,57] showed good in vitro antiviral activity and selectivity [59]. Moreover, in vivo pharmacokinetic, pharmacological, and toxicological profiles were sufficient for clinical evaluation [60].

Early structure–activity relationship (SAR) work focusing on the ribofuranosyl portion of TCRB and BDCRB had established that the 5′-hydroxyl group was not required for activity. Indeed, the D-5′-deoxy-TCRB analog **23** was about fivefold more potent than TCRB (**2**) against HCMV [24].

Further work showed that the entire 5′-hydroxymethyl group could be removed to yield D-benzimidazole erythrofuranosyl derivatives (**24**, Fig. 6) that were about five- to 10-fold more potent than the corresponding ribofuranosyl derivative, TCRB (**2**) [61]. Benzimidazole L-erythrofuranosyl nucleosides were also prepared (e.g., **25**) but were less active (five- to 10-fold) than their corresponding D-ribofuranosyl analogs as well as less active than maribavir (**22**). Thus, even though the D-erythrofuranosyl derivatives were more active than the corresponding D-ribose derivatives, this was not the case for the L-erythrofuranosyl derivatives [61].

Additional studies on the D-ribofuranosyl benzimidazoles, aimed at improving stability of the glycosidic bond, by replacing the 2′-OH group with fluorine gave the 2-fluoroarabinose derivative **26** and the 2-fluororibose derivative **27** [62]. The 2-fluoroarabinose analog of TCRB (**26**) was about two- to threefold less active than TCRB, whereas the 2-fluororibose analog of BDCRB (**27**) was about 20-fold less active than BDCRB. Furthermore, the fluorinated derivatives were more cytotoxic than the ribosyl analogs, resulting in fluorinated carbohydrate derivatives not being pursued further.

More dramatic changes of the carbohydrate portion, such as replacement of the ribofuranosyl portion with the acyclic (hydroxyethoxy)methyl group (**28**) or the (dihydroxypropoxy)methyl group (**29**) resulted in almost complete loss of activity [63]. A number of other carbohydrate derivatives, including 2′-deoxyribose [64,65], lyxose [66], xylopyranoside, and ribopyranoside derivatives, were prepared. Among these the ribopyranosides [67] were especially

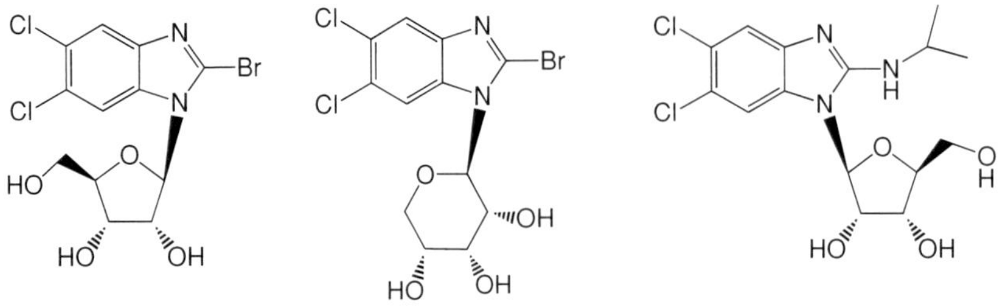

FIGURE 7 Comparison of the structure of BDCRB to the two benzimidazole nucleosides (GW275175X and maribavir) that progressed into clinical trials.

interesting, with the D-ribopyranoside 2-bromo-5,6-dichlorobenzimidazole (**30**) showing anti-HCMV activity similar to the ribofuranosyl analog BDCRB (**3**), Fig. 7. Moreover, it had good selectivity and an in vivo pharmacokinetic, pharmacological, and toxicological profile suitable for progression into clinical trials [68].

This effort demonstrated that a carbohydrate (ribofuranosyl or ribopyranosyl) or carbocyclic group was required for good antiviral activity, whereas acyclic derivatives showed much reduced potency against HCMV. In general, SAR for the carbohydrate was not as clear as for the benzimidazole heterocycle, with several differences emerging between the D and L series, due to their different mode of action (see below).

Finally, effort was focused on attempts to replace the benzimidazole with a different bicyclic heterocycle, such as imidazo[1,2-*a*]pyridine or indole. Both of these heterocycles would allow the benzimidazole halogene to be placed in desirable positions on the heterocycle. Replacement of the benzimidazole with an imidazopyridine was accomplished by synthesis of the 2,6,7-trichloro-3-(β-D-ribofuranosyl)imidazo[1,2-*a*]pyridine C-nucleoside analog of TCRB [69]. Surprisingly despite very striking similarity to TCRB, this imidazopyridine derivative was totally inactive against HCMV. Subsequently, indole N-nucleoside analogs of TCRB [70] were also prepared, again showing limited anti-HCMV activity. Further exploration into replacing the benzimidazole system was curtailed because benzimidazole nucleosides, such as **22** (1263W94) and **30** (GW275175X), showed excellent preclinical properties and were synthetically highly tractable.

GW275175X: PRECLINICAL AND CLINICAL STUDIES

The in vitro antiviral spectrum of GW275175X was similar to that of BDCRB and TCRB: active against HCMV only. As predicted, GW275175X was effective against clinical wild-type strains and against strains resistant to the clinically available CMV drugs, and was cross-resistant to BDCRB-resistant mutants that encoded alterations in the terminase components pUL89 and pUL56 [68]. The relative potency of GW275175X and GCV for the laboratory strain AD169 was comparable in standard plaque-reduction and DNA hybridization assays [68]. Significantly, GW275175X was three- to fivefold less inhibitory to the growth of human marrow progenitor cells than was GCV. Theoretically, this would provide a therapeutic advantage in the marrow and stem cell transplant populations. Biochemical studies of CMV DNA synthesis and maturation in the presence of GW275175X confirmed a block to the maturational cleavage of the high-molecular viral DNA, analogous to the inhibition mechanism of BDCRB and TCRB [30].

Pharmacokinetic evaluation of GW275175X in both mouse and monkey established that the instability problem of the parent BDCRB had been solved. In those two species, GW275175X was readily orally bioavailable (~90%) and showed a moderate-to-high volume of distribution, a low-to-moderate clearance rate, and a relatively long plasma half-life. There was no evidence of significant metabolism or glycosidic cleavage. Metabolic stability was also seen in a series of in vitro human liver microsomal extract studies. GW275175X exhibited good brain penetration in the mouse after oral dosing. Human serum protein binding was approximately 92%, which predicted adequate free drug levels for antiviral efficacy. Toxicological evaluations supported the advancement of this compound into human trials [71].

A phase I randomized double-blind placebo-controlled trial in healthy subjects was conducted, and results established that the drug was well tolerated at all doses without serious adverse events or clinical laboratory abnormalities (GlaxoSmithKline, internal data). The encouraging phase I PK and early safety profile of GW275175X would have enabled its continued development, but its developmental status was considered against the more advanced stage of the L-benzimidazole analog maribavir (MBV) and the declining CMV retinitis market following the introduction of HAART (highly active antiretroviral therapy) for HIV-infected

TABLE 1 Comparison of Properties and Preclinical Studies with BDCRB and Maribavir

Parameter or Study	BDCRB	Maribavir
Sugar portion of molecule	D-ribose	L-ribose
Phosphorylation at the 5′ position not necessary for antiviral activity	True	True
Potent inhibition of HCMV	Yes	Yes
Active vs. HCMV resistant to GCV, CDV, and PFA	Yes	Yes
Noncytotoxic to human diploid and bone marrow progenitor cells at concentrations well in excess of antiviral activity	Yes	Yes
Inhibits cellular metabolism in antiviral dose range	No	No
Inhibits viral protein synthesis	No	No
Inhibits viral RNA synthesis	No	No
Inhibits viral DNA synthesis	No	Yes
Inhibits viral DNA polymerase	No	No
Inhibits viral DNA processing	Yes	No
Inhibits viral nucleocapsid egress from infected cell nucleus	No	Yes
Oral bioavailability	Partial	Good
Half-life and pharmacokinetics in vivo	Poor	Good
Progressed into clinical trials	No	Yes

patients. Thus, this promising compound was shelved as a backup to MBV in the late 1990s.

MARIBAVIR: ANTIVIRAL ACTIVITY AND MECHANISM OF ACTION

The precedent strategy of converting a nucleoside carbohydrate moiety from the D-sugar to the unnatural L analog in this benzimidazole series achieved the expected reductions in metabolic instability and cytotoxicity, as described above, resulting in the clinical candidate maribavir (MBV). In addition, this strategy increased the potency, and for MBV, completely changed the mechanism of action and slightly altered the spectrum of antiviral activity. MBV not only showed potent inhibition of HCMV, but also inhibited the in vitro lytic replication of Epstein–Barr virus [72]. Weak activity against HHV-6 [73] has also been reported. No other herpesviruses were reported susceptible, nor were HIV, HBV, HCV, influenza A, and HPV 59,74].

Interestingly, the L-sugar benzimidazole analogs did not inhibit the CMV pUL56 and pUL89 "terminase"-mediated processing of viral DNA, based on gel analyses of viral DNA size following MBV treatment. Instead, we initially observed a strong concentration and time-dependent reduction in viral DNA synthesis in growth-arrested human MRC-5 lung fibroblasts [59]. Other investigators, however, saw only a modest reduction in viral DNA synthesis in active MRC-5 cells or in human foreskin fibroblasts, yet they observed potent but highly variable reductions in viral yields or plaque formation. Our culture conditions had been optimized to provide reproducible EC_{50} values during compound series screening and for selection of resistant virus. Subsequent studies in several laboratories demonstrated that MBV interfered with capsid egress from the nucleus [73]. Thus, the mechanism of action was clearly different from that of the β-D benzimidazole riboside analogs (see Table 1 and Fig. 2). The structural similarities of MBV to a nucleoside analog prompted studies that ruled out any direct effect on the viral DNA polymerase function during viral DNA synthesis. MBV was not anabolized to phosphate forms in CMV-infected or uninfected cells. Furthermore, the chemically synthesized mono-, di-, and triphosphates of MBV did not inhibit viral DNA polymerase in vitro or the mammalian cellular polymerase α [59].

The activity profile, chemical, and preclinical properties supported the advancement of MBV toward clinical development. Mechanism-of-action studies of this interesting 1994 lead actually progressed at a slower pace than the critical activities required for an IND, and all were disrupted by a corporate merger. The drug candidate moved into phase 1 clinical studies in 1996 without knowledge of the viral target or exact mechanism of action, based solely on in vitro antiviral potency, preclinical safety, and pharmacokinetic properties. There was a level of confidence that the target was viral in nature, based on the successful laboratory selection of drug-resistant viral strains in vitro.

We ultimately identified the CMV-encoded protein kinase pUL97 as the primary target by using traditional marker transfer techniques to map the resistance of a laboratory-derived mutant strain (BW2916R) of AD169 [59]. Independent confirmation of the pUL97 as a major target of MBV emerged from a protein kinase screen in which the phosphorylation of a histone substrate by pUL97 was strongly inhibited by MBV (IC_{50} = 3 nM). The selectivity of maribavir for this CMV kinase was suggested by the lack of inhibitory activity against a panel of 70 mammalian kinases [75]. These screens included cell cycle kinases known to be upregulated by viral infection [76]. A second genetic site associated with

MBV resistance was mapped to the UL27 ORF in maribavir-resistant laboratory strains of Towne and AD169 [77,78]. The pUL27 encodes nuclear localization signals and motifs for protein kinase phosphorylation, but its function remains under study as of 2011 [78a].

At the time of the identification of MBV's primary target in 1999, little was known about the role of the pUL97 in the CMV replication cycle beyond its identification as the viral kinase responsible for the intracellular monophosphorylation of GCV [79]. Subsequently, a laboratory deletion mutant provided important clues to the various steps affected by loss of pUL97 function [80]. These included reduced phosphorylation of the viral polymerase processivity factor pUL44 [81,82], reduced viral DNA synthesis [59,83], altered intracellular distribution of the pp65 tegument protein [84,85], and a strong inhibition of capsid egress from the cell nucleus [83–87]. The UL97 deletion strain provided a unique tool to define the roles of the HCMV pUL97 in the virus life cycle, and maribavir served as a confirmatory biochemical knockout/ modulator of function in the infected treated cells.

The CMV pUL97 protein kinase not only regulates several viral replication functions, but it also affects host cell activities [88–91]. Two key examples of pUL97's modulation of the host-cell cycle are the exciting discovery of the hyperphosphorylation of the Rb oncoprotein, thus relaxing the brakes on cell cycle progression [73,85,92], and the demonstration that pUL97 mimics the regulatory functions of cdc2 and can phosphorylate the eukaryotic elongation factor 1delta [90]. These host cell functions presumably adjust the cell's metabolic state to better support viral growth, but such a mechanism calls into question the validity of pUL97 as a drug target. Will the drug be active in the diverse tissues and organs infected by CMV? Indeed, maribavir has shown an unusual variability in laboratory potency and mechanism of action according to the physiologic state of the cells and even cell type [59,93]. However, in vitro selectivity and mechanism studies and preclinical safety studies are consistent with the overall good safety profile observed so far in the clinic. Mechanism studies support the possibility that maribavir's antiviral action could affect multiple events across the life cycle of the virus, thus providing many opportunities to reduce viral replication and disease production.

There are no good animal models of infection with human CMV to confirm drug efficacy studies with this new drug target and thus confirm target validity. However, CMV growth in human tissues implanted in SCID-hu mice was reduced after oral dosing [94], suggesting antiviral action of the drug. Perhaps the importance of pUL97 to viral pathogenesis can be inferred by consideration of the pUL97 kinase homologs across the herpesviruses, where some animal models of virus infection exist. These protein kinase homologs are highly conserved in catalytic and regulatory regions, with some divergence from mammalian protein kinases [95–97]. The HSV1 and the VZV homologs (pUL13 and gene 47 protein kinases, respectively) have been shown to be required for tissue tropism and disease pathogenesis [98,99]. These findings are supportive of pUL97 as a valid target, but the real proof is in successful demonstration of efficacy with a selective pUL97 inhibitor in the clinic. Maribavir offers the opportunity for proof of principle.

MARIBAVIR: PRECLINICAL STUDIES

Maribavir progressed through a series of preclinical tests to evaluate pharmacokinetics and safety on its journey toward the clinic. The overall profile for a safer, orally bioavailable drug was achieved. The key pharmacokinetic parameters determined in rats and monkeys were 50 to 90% oral bioavailability, dose-proportional plasma levels, reasonable volume of distribution and half-life, and clearance mediated mainly by biliary secretion with some enterohepatic recirculation [60,100]. The major metabolite in animals and in human liver microsomal extract studies was the N-dealkylated derivative BW4469W94, and this was also the major metabolite recovered in vivo.

Toxicology studies indicated a safety profile acceptable for further drug development. The studies included acute oral and intravenous studies, chronic 1-month studies with oral dosing in rats and mice, and chronic 6-month treatments in rats and monkeys [60]. The minimum no-effect dose in the 1-month rat study was 100 mg/kg per day, and in the 1-month monkey study was 180 mg/kg per day (plasma C_{max} = 8 μg/mL). Adverse effects noted included increases in liver weights, neutrophils, and monocytes at the higher doses in the female rats. In monkeys, 1-month treatments resulted in mild reversible decreases in erythroid populations and increases in reticulocytes. Chronic exposures of rats at 25, 100, and 400 mg/ kg per day, and monkeys at 100, 200, and 500 mg/kg per day for 6 months and one year (monkey study only) resulted in mild but reversible treatment-related effects, such as elevations of white blood cells, anemias, and liver enzyme functions. Both rat and monkey experienced a mild-to-moderate mucosal hyperplasia of the intestinal tract, which presented as altered stools or diarrhea at the higher doses. This hyperplasia was partially reversed in the 1-month recovery period. The long-term significance of this hyperplasia is unknown.

Genetic toxicology studies showed improvements over the marketed CMV drugs including the in vitro Ames assay (up to 650 μg/plate), and in vivo micronucleus assays (up to 1200 mg/kg single oral doses) were negative. In the in vitro mouse lymphoma assay, maribavir was mutagenic in the absence of metabolic activation, at concentrations cytotoxic to cultured cells, whereas results were equivocal in the presence of liver microsomal S9 extracts [60,100]. Reproductive toxicology studies in standard rabbit and murine systems also suggested that maribavir was a safer alternative then existing anti-HCMV agents (GlaxoSmithKline; internal data). Other safety studies conducted but not published included the in-life carcinogenicity study (ViroPharma, Inc.; internal data).

MARIBAVIR: PHASE I–III CLINICAL STUDIES

Maribavir now has advanced through several phase I and II studies and into the first phase III trials. The published results for the early phase I and II clinical studies were promising and are summarized here.

Two phase I trials of MBV investigated the safety and tolerability of single oral escalating doses; one was conducted in healthy volunteers ($n = 13$, doses of 50 to 1600 mg) and one in HIV-infected subjects ($n = 17$, doses of 100 to 1600 mg) [101]. The key PK parameters for humans were defined in these studies: rapid absorption of oral doses, peak concentrations (C_{max}) observed 1 to 3 h post-dose, and dose-proportional increases in area under the concentration curve ($AUC_{0\text{-}\infty}$). Elimination was rapid, with a plasma half-life of 3 to 5 h at all doses. In contrast to the animal ADME results, MBV was excreted in the urine after extensive metabolism, with < 2% of the dose recovered as unchanged MBV and 20 to 40% of the dose recovered as the N-dealkylated metabolite 4469W94. Human liver microsomal studies suggested that the liver cytochrome P450 isozyme Cyp3A4 was predominantly responsible for metabolic clearance. The major metabolite 4469W94 showed a 2-h delay in T_{max} and a slower clearance rate. No anti-HCMV activity in vitro has been noted for 4469W94 (GlaxoSmithKline; internal data). The consumption of a high-fat meal somewhat delayed the T_{max} of MBV and decreased $AUC_{0\text{-}\infty}$ and C_{max} by approximately 30% [101].

Both MBV and its key metabolite were highly protein bound: > 97% and 92%, respectively. The high degree of protein binding of MBV is a concern for bioavailability of active free drug, although it reportedly binds primarily to serum albumin and exhibits relatively low affinity binding in kinetic studies in vitro [59,100].

The first clinical trial to explore the antiviral action of MBV provided exciting data to validate the drug mechanism of action, and it exhibited activity which suggested that the protein binding did not abrogate drug action at the lower doses [102]. The study was a placebo-controlled dose-escalating trial of oral MBV in HIV-infected subjects, a subset of whom shed CMV in semen (5000 genome copies/mL or greater) Subjects were treated for 28 days with one of six dose regimens: 100, 200, or 400 mg t.i.d., or 600, 900, or 1200 mg b.i.d. or with placebo. Viral load reduction was assessed in samples from patients receiving the four lower doses by titration of infectious virus in semen by plaque assay or by quantitation of total CMV DNA using a developmental quantitative PCR method (Roche Diagnostics). MBV reduced viral load across the four doses in the range 2.9 to 3.7 $\log_{10}$ pfu/mL (Table 2) in a dose-dependent manner. Interestingly, the viral genome reductions as measured by the quantitative PCR showed only a modest drop (range of 1.1 to 1.5 log 10 genome copies) in this same time frame. This result may be consistent with a mechanism of action of a UL97 protein kinase inhibitor, in which noninfectious virus is formed via the block to capsid egress but scores positive in the DNA assay until cleared biologically.

TABLE 2 Reduction of CMV by MBV in a Phase I Study in HIV-Infected Men

	Change in Semen CMV Viral Load ($\log_{10}$)		
	Infectious Titers		PCR
MBV Dose (mg)	Day 14	Day 28	Day 28
100 t.i.d.	−1.1	−2.9	−1.11
200 t.i.d.	−1.6	−3.7	−1.27
400 t.i.d.	−2.5	−3.7	−1.28
600 b.i.d.	−2.7	−3.4	−1.25

Source: [102].

In this phase I study, viral load reductions were also observed in urine, in blood ($n = 1$, 4.81 $\log_{10}$ reduction to the lower limits of assay quantitation), and in saliva of one subject with measurable load before therapy. Thus, MBV was active in viral load reduction in several tissue compartments, although the number of subjects in the analyses was small.

Similar positive results were reported for a subsequent study in CMV retinitis patients who received oral doses of 800 mg t.i.d., or 1200 mg b.i.d. daily for 7 days to establish steady-state concentrations in the ocular fluids, as a measure of its potential to treat retinitis [103]. Reductions of CMV DNA in blood by polymerase chain reaction of 0.26, 1.1, and 1.9 log 10 were observed in the three subjects who had CMV detectable at baseline. The intravitreal levels achieved with these doses exceeded MBV EC_{50} values reported by several assay methods. These results suggest that MBV should be seriously considered for the congenital CMV indication. The basic pharmacokinetic and safety features of MBV characterized in these early GSK-sponsored phase I studies were consistent with those observed in subsequent phase I and II studies.

The clinical safety record for MBV reported as of July 2009 is promising, and results have been relatively consistent across all the phase I and II studies published. MBV was generally well tolerated; taste disturbance was the most frequently reported adverse event (> 80% of treated subjects and 20% of placebo recipients). This dose-related taste disturbance was described as a transient bitter or metallic taste. Other reported adverse events that were deemed related to MBV administration included nausea, diarrhea, and headache [101–103]; there were no noteworthy clinical laboratory abnormalities or issues related to vital signs. In the HIV-infected population of the POC trial, five subjects discontinued the drug because of a diffuse macropapular rash (grade 2) that resolved off the drug; four of these patients had a history of allergic reactions [102]. No such rash has been reported in subsequent studies in other patient populations, including transplant recipients. Overall, MBV exhibits a safety profile superior to current treatments.

In 2003, MBV was licensed by GSK to ViroPharma, Inc., to continue development for the prophylaxis and treatment of CMV diseases [104]. ViroPharma expanded the phase I and II studies to explore the safety and pharmacokinetics of MBV in specialized patient populations, such as the renally impaired and those receiving concomitant medications that were known to interact with liver enzymes. A phase I drug–drug interaction study was conducted as a double-blind placebo-controlled trial in 20 healthy volunteers administered 400 mg b.i.d. oral MBV along with a modified five-drug phenotyping cocktail [105]. Results indicated no effect of MBV on the metabolic activities of P450 CYP1A2, CYP2C9, CYP3A, NAT-2 (*N*-acetyltransferase-2), or xanthine oxidase, whereas decreased activity was noted for CYP2C19 and CYP2D6 [105].

In 2006, ViroPharma announced promising preliminary data from a phase II clinical trial in allogeneic stem cell transplant (SCT) recipients that demonstrated successful prophylaxis of CMV reactivation [106]. The trial was a randomized double-blind placebo-controlled study of three oral doses of MBV (100 mg b.i.d., 400 mg q.d., and 400 mg b.i.d., or placebo for up to 12 weeks ($n = 111$ subjects). Patients were regularly monitored for CMV reactivation using standard quantitative assays for CMV pp65 antigenemia or plasma CMV DNA by PCR methods. If the threshold for CMV reactivation was reached, study medication was discontinued and patients were treated with institutional standard of care (generally, preemptive CMV drug treatment). ViroPharma reported a statistically significant reduction in the numbers of subjects who required preemptive intervention: 57% for placebo, vs. 15, 30, and 15% for MBV at 100 mg b.i.d., 400 mg q.d., and 400 mg b.i.d., respectively. There were no cases of CMV disease in the MBV-treated arms of the study, whereas three cases were reported in the placebo group. These exciting results are notable in two respects: (1) The antiviral activity of MBV translated into clinical benefit, which is the most relevant POC endpoint, and (2) there was no dose-response apparent within this trial between 100 and 400 mg b.i.d. This is in contrast to the antiviral activity results of the first POC trial in HIV-infected subjects [102].

The positive results encouraged ViroPharma to move forward in 2006 with a phase III pivotal study in the allogeneic SCT recipients, in which they were treated prophylactically with the 100-mg b.i.d. dose in a monitoring design similar to that used in the pilot study. However, preliminary results announced in early 2009 indicated that in the trial as designed, MBV failed to reach the primary endpoints for the study [107]. Consequently, an NDA for MBV has not yet been submitted to the FDA.

There are many reasons why an antiviral agent that is active in vitro could fail in the context of a clinical study. One plausible explanation in this case of the failed phase III SCT study is inadequate drug exposure at the MBV 100 mg b.i.d. dose. Ultimately, a dose-range pilot POC trial is designed to explore the dose-antiviral response relationship in order to select the optimal safe and effective dose for the registrational studies. As a general rule, for the expanded clinical populations in the registrational phase III trial, one aims for the highest dose supported by safety studies, and certainly that shown in POC to provide clear antiviral effect. The possibility that the SCT trial dose of 100 mg b.i.d was suboptimal is supported by the subsequent report of successful CMV viremia reductions by higher-dose MBV treatment of six transplant recipients who were failing conventional therapy due to drug resistance and/or refractory invasive disease [108]. All responded with $> 1 \log_{10}$ decrease in blood CMV DNA by PCR within 6 weeks of administration of oral MBV, starting at a 400-mg b.i.d. dose, and four of the six became CMV DNA undetectable between days 10 and 41. This small and uncontrolled study provides optimism that MBV could be a useful therapeutic tool in the transplant setting.

The potential for MBV therapy to select for drug resistance in the clinical setting is yet to be determined, with its implications for treatment durability and class positioning. GCV treatment failures are associated with the emergence of drug-resistant strains under conditions of prolonged therapy in highly immunocompromised patients [10,13]. MBV resistance has been modeled in the laboratory by the use of an engineered laboratory strain deficient in the CMV exonuclease repair function of the polymerase (T2294; see ref. 109). Viral strains of T2294 passaged under MBV have generated both single and double mutants in an accelerated fashion, encoding changes in the UL97 ORF at the following codons: H411L/N/Y, T409M, and V355A. Another at L397R is analogous to the original AD169-resistant strain selected with the carbocyclic analog of MBV [59]. These resistant strains showed a wide range of resistance to MBV; however, all remained susceptible to GCV in vitro [109]. Interestingly, one of the five SOT patients with the highest baseline viremia and who was rescued with MBV treatment developed virus with the H411Y and T409M mutations at rebound of viremia after 3 months [108], thus recapitulating one of the laboratory mutations [109]. The encouraging lack of cross-resistance of the MBV-resistant strains to GCV and PFA, and vice versa, suggests that MBV will be a useful addition to the current treatments for CMV disease in the transplant population.

THE BENZIMIDAZOLE DISCOVERY PROGRAM: A LOOK BACK

The development program for the benzimidazole ribosides for CMV diseases is notable in several respects.

1. It is an outstanding example of a successful collaborative partnership of academia, pharmaceutical industry and government entities where scientists worked persistently across institutional barriers.

2. The approach used to discover the large series of active benzimidazole nucleosides and their highly specific activity against CMV was based on lead-directed synthesis followed by testing that depended on virological endpoints in cultured cells, and not upon inhibition of a preselected target by the high-throughput screening methods then coming into vogue at large pharmaceutical companies. Not only did the approach succeed in putting drugs into the clinic but it also identified five new antiviral targets! Thus, the discovery approach was very successful.

3. In another break from the traditional approach to viral target-based drug discovery, MBV progressed into clinical trials without knowledge of the ultimate drug target and mechanism of action. It also progressed without POC in an animal model because the drug is not active against nonprimate CMVs used in such models. Nonetheless, the criteria for advancement were very rational, stringent, and included antiviral potency by the most relevant assays, in vitro selectivity, animal safety, satisfactory pharmacokinetics, and so on.

4. This program evolved during an unstable time of corporate consolidations; the disruptive effects of two major mergers resulted in developmental delays beyond the first POC study in 1997. Maribavir was caught in this unfortunate series of events, and is still not available to patients in 2011, 17 years after original discovery and 14 years after the first successful POC.

The benzimidazole CMV discovery program began in University of Michigan laboratories and the Burroughs Wellcome company (privately funded by the Wellcome Trust) with their combined emphasis on both basic science and medical need in drug discovery. It exemplified a scientifically based effort that provided the opportunity for true innovation in target discovery. This successful collaboration ultimately succeeded in placing into clinical trials two drugs from a novel series of benzimidazole ribosides. Overall development results to date indicate that MBV will provide a safe alternative to conventional anti-HCMV therapies for treatment and rescue options in the transplant setting.

Acknowledgments

We thank Mark N. Prichard for providing his figure on the functions of UL97 kinase [73], which we modified to produce Figure 2. We gratefully acknowledge the seminal and indispensable contributions of our colleague, mentor, and friend, Leroy B. Townsend. Without his interests in benzimidazole nucleosides that go back to the 1960s, the exceptional productivity of his laboratory, and his enthusiasm and encouragement, there would have been no discovery of benzimidazoles as drugs to treat CMV disease.

REFERENCES

[1] Mocarski, E. S., Jr.; Shenk, T.; Pass, R. F. Cytomegaloviruses: In *Fields Virology*, 5th ed., Knipe, D. M., Howley, P. M., Eds., Lippincott Williams & Wilkins, Philadelphia, **2006**, pp. 2701, 2772.

[2] Lischka, P.; Zimmermann, H. Current antiviral strategies to combat cytomegalovirus infections in transplant recipients. *Opin. Pharmacol.* **2008**, *8*, 541–548.

[3] Alford, C. A.; Britt, W. J. Cytomegalovirus. In *The Human Herpesviruses*, Roizman, B., Whitley, R. J., Lopez, C., Eds., Raven Press, New York, 1993, pp. 227–255.

[4] Nassetta, L.; Kimberlin, D.; Whitley, R. Treatment of congenital cytomegalovirus infection: implications for future therapeutic strategies. *J. Antimicrob. Chemother.* **2009**, *63*, 862–867.

[5] Gravel, S.-P.; Servant, M. J. Roles of an IkB kinase-related pathway in human cytomegalovirus-infected vascular smooth muscle cells: a molecular link in pathogen-induced proatherosclerotic conditions. *J. Biol. Chem.* **2005**, *280*, 7477–7486.

[6] Miller, G. A viral link to glioblastoma? *Science* **2009**, *323*, 30–31.

[7] Elion, G. B.; Furman, P. A.; Fyfe, J. A.; de Miranda, P.; Beauchamp, L.; Schaeffer, H. J. Selectivity of action of an antiherpetic agent, 9-(2-hydroxyethoxymethyl)guanine. *Proc. Nat. Acad. Sci. USA* **1977**, *74*, 5716–5720.

[8] Lowance, D.; Neumayer, H. H.; Legendre, C. M.; Squifflet, J. P.; Kovarik, J.; Brennan, P. J.; Norman, D.; Mendez, R.; Keating, M. R.; Coggon, G. L.; et al. Valacyclovir for the prevention of cytomegalovirus disease after renal transplantation. International Valacyclovir Cytomegalovirus Prophylaxis Transplantation Study Group. *N. Engl. J. Med.* **1999**, *340*, 1462–1470.

[9] Hodson, E. M.; Jones, C. A.; Webster, A. C.; Strippoli, G. F.; Barclay, P. G.; Kable, K.; Vimalachandra, D.; Craig, J. C. Antiviral medications to prevent cytomegalovirus disease and early death in recipients of solid-organ transplants: a systematic review of randomised controlled trials. *Lancet* **2005**, *365*, 2105–2115.

[10] Biron, K. K. Antiviral drugs for cytomegalovirus diseases. *Antiviral Res.* **2006**, *71*, 154–163.

[11] Cytovene-IV (ganciclovir sodium for intravenous infusion only) and Cytovene (ganciclovir capsules for oral administration only). Package insert. Roche Laboratories, Inc., **2009**.

[12] Cvetkovic, R. S.; Wellington, K. Valganciclovir: a review of its use in the management of CMV infection and disease in immunocompromised patients. *Drugs* **2005**, *65*, 859–878.

[13] Erice, A. Resistance of human cytomegalovirus to antiviral drugs. *Clin. Microbiol. Rev.* **1999**, *12*, 286–297.

[14] Gilbert, C.; Boivin, G. Human cytomegalovirus resistance to antiviral drugs. *Antimicrob. Agents Chemother.* **2005**, *49*, 873–883.

[15] Biron, K. K.; Fyfe, J. A.; Stanat, S. C.; Leslie, L. K.; Sorrell, J. B.; Lambe, C. U.; Coen, D. M. A human cytomegalovirus mutant resistant to the nucleoside analog 9-([2-hydroxy-1-(hydroxymethyl)ethoxy]methyl)guanine (BW B759U) induces reduced levels of BW B759U triphosphate. *Proc. Nat. Acad. Sci. USA* **1986**, *83*, 8769–8773.

[16] Chou, S.; Lurain, N. S.; Thompson, K. D.; Miner, R. C.; Drew, W. L. Viral DNA polymerase mutations associated with drug resistance in human cytomegalovirus. *J. Infect. Dis.* **2003**, *188*, 32–39.

[17] Foscavir (foscarnet injection). Package insert. AstraZeneca, Inc., **2000**.

[18] Vistide (cidofovir injection). Package insert. Gilead Sciences, Inc., **1996**.

[19] Field, A. K.; Biron, K. K. "The end of innocence" revisited: resistance of herpesviruses to antiviral drugs. *Clin. Microbiol. Rev.* **1994**, *7*, 1–13.

[20] Townsend, L. B.; Drach, J. C.; Wotring, L. L.; Vittori, S.; Pudlo, J. S.; Swayze, E. E.; Gupta, P.; Maruyama, T.; Saxena, N.; Coleman, L. A.; et al. Design, synthesis and studies on the structure activity relationships of certain pyrrolo[2,3-*d*]pyrimidine nucleosides and structurally related analogs as potential antineoplastic and antiviral agents. *Farmaco* **1991**, *46*, 113–139.

[21] Townsend, L. B.; Revankar, G. R. Benzimidazole nucleosides, nucleotides, and related derivatives. *Chem. Rev.* **1970**, *70*, 389–438.

[22] Townsend, L. B.; Devivar, R. V.; Turk, S. R.; Nassiri, M. R.; Drach, J. C. Design, synthesis, and antiviral activity of certain 2,5,6-trihalo-1-(β-D-ribofuranosyl)benzimidazoles. *J. Med. Chem.* **1995**, *38*, 4098–4105.

[23] Tamm, I.; Sehgal, P. B. Halobenzimidazole ribosides and RNA synthesis of cells and viruses. *Adv. Virus Res.* **1978**, *22*, 187–258.

[24] Krosky, P. M.; Borysko, K. Z.; Nassiri, M. R.; Devivar, R. V.; Ptak, R. G.; Davis, M. G.; Biron, K. K.; Townsend, L. B.; Drach, J. C. Phosphorylation of β-D-ribosyl-benzimidazoles is not required for activity against human cytomegalovirus. *Antimicrob. Agents Chemother.* **2002**, *46*, 478–486.

[25] North, T. W.; Sequar, G.; Townsend, L. B.; Drach, J. C.; Barry, P. A. Rhesus cytomegalovirus is similar to human cytomegalovirus in susceptibility to benzimidazole nucleosides. *Antimicrob. Agents Chemother.* **2004**, *48*, 2760–2765.

[26] Nixon, D. E.; McVoy, M. A. Dramatic effects of 2-bromo-5,6-dichloro-1-β-D-ribofuranosyl benzimidazole riboside on the genome structure, packaging, and egress of guinea pig cytomegalovirus. *J. Virol.* **2004**, *78*, 1623–1635.

[27] Nassiri, M. R.; Emerson, S. G.; Devivar, R. V.; Townsend, L. B.; Drach, J. C.; Taichman, R. S. Comparison of benzimidazole nucleosides and ganciclovir on the in vitro proliferation and colony formation of human bone marrow progenitor cells. *Br. J. Haematol.* **1996**, *93*, 273–279.

[28] Underwood, M. R.; Harvey, R. J.; Stanat, S. C.; Hemphill, M. L.; Miller, T.; Drach, J. C.; Townsend, L. B.; Biron, K. K. Inhibition of HCMV DNA maturation by a benzimidazole ribonucleoside is mediated through the UL89 gene product. *J. Virol.* **1998**, *72*, 717–725.

[29] McVoy, M. A.; Nixon, D. E. Impact of 2-bromo-5,6-dichloro-1-β-D-ribofuranosyl benzimidazole riboside and inhibitors of DNA, RNA, and protein synthesis on human cytomegalovirus genome maturation. *J. Virol.* **2005**, *79*, 11115–11127.

[30] Krosky, P. M.; Underwood, M. R.; Turk, S. R.; Feng, K. W.-H.; Jain, R. K.; Ptak, R. G.; Westerman, A. C.; Biron, K. K.; Townsend, L. B.; Drach, J. C. Resistance of human cytomegalovirus to benzimidazole ribonucleosides maps to two open reading frames: UL89 and UL56. *J. Virol.* **1998**, *72*, 4721–4728.

[31] Catalano, C. E. The terminase enzyme from bacteriophage lambda: a DNA-packaging machine. *Cell Mol. Life Sci.* **2000**, *57*, 128–148.

[32] Komazin, G.; Townsend, L. B.; Drach, J. C. Role of a mutation in human cytomegalovirus gene UL104 in resistance to benzimidazole ribonucleosides. *J. Virol.* **2004**, *78*, 710–715.

[33] Dittmer, A.; Drach, J. C.; Townsend, L. B.; Fischer, A.; Bogner, E. Interaction of the putative HCMV portal protein pUL104 with the large terminase subunit pUL56 and its inhibition by benzimidazole-D-ribonucleosides. *J. Virol.* **2005**, *79*, 14,660–14,667.

[34] Bogner, E. Human cytomegalovirus terminase as a target for antiviral chemotherapy. *Rev. Med. Virol.* **2002**, *12*, 115–127.

[35] Scheffczik, H.; Savva, C. G. W.; Holzenburg, A.; Kolesnikova, L.; Bogner, E. The terminase subunits pUL56 and pUL89 of human cytomegalovirus are DNA-metabolizing proteins with toroidal structure. *Nucleic Acids Res.* **2002**, *30*, 1695–1703.

[36] Thoma, C.; Borst, E.; Messerle, M.; Rieger, M.; Hwang, J.-S.; Bogner, E. Identification of the interaction domain of the small terminase subunit pUL89 with the large subunit pUL56 of human cytomegalovirus. *Biochemistry* **2006**, *45*, 8855–8863.

[37] Hwang, J.-S.; Bogner, E. ATPase activity of the terminase subunit pUL56 of human cytomegalovirus. *J. Biol. Chem.* **2002**, *277*, 6943–6948.

[38] Scholz, B.; Rechter, S.; Drach, J. C.; Townsend, L. B. Bogner, E. Identification of the ATP-binding site in the terminase subunit pUL56 of human cytomegalovirus. *Nucleic Acids Res.* **2003**, *31*, 1426–1433.

[39] Champier, G.; Hantz, S.; Couvreux, A.; Stuppfler, S.; Mazeron, M. C.; Bouaziz, S.; Denis, F.; Alain, S. New functional domains of human cytomegalovirus pUL89 predicted by

sequence analysis and three-dimensional modeling of the catalytic site. *Antiviral Ther.* **2007**, *12*, 217–232.

[40] Savva, C. G. W.; Holzenburg, A.; Bogner, E. Insights into the structure of human cytomegalovirus large terminase subunit pUL56. *FEBS Lett.* **2004**, *563*, 135–140.

[41] Champier, G.; Couvreux, A.; Hantz, S.; Rametti, A., Mazeron, M. C.; Bouaziz, S.; Denis, F.; Alain, S. Putative functional domains of human cytomegalovirus pUL56 involved in dimerization and benzimidazole D-ribonucleoside activity. *Antiviral Ther.* **2008**, *13*, 643–654.

[42] Holzenburg, H.; Dittmer, A.; Bogner, E. Assembly of monomeric human cytomegalovirus pUL104 into portal structures. *J. Gen. Virol.* **2009**, *90*, 2381–2385.

[43] Good, S. S.; Owens, B. S.; Townsend, L. B.; Drach, J. C. The disposition in rats and monkeys of 2-bromo-5,6-dichloro-1-(β-D-ribofuranosyl)-benzimidazole (BDCRB) and its 2,5,6-trichloro congener (TCRB). *Antiviral Res.* **1994**, *23*(S1), 103.

[44] Lorenzi, P. L.; Landowski, C. P.; Brancale, A.; Song, X.; Townsend, L. B.; Drach, J. C.; Amidon, G. L. *N*-Methylpurine DNA glycosylase and 8-oxoguanine DNA glycosylase metabolize the antiviral nucleoside 2-bromo-5,6-dichloro-1-(β-D-ribofuranosyl)benzimidazole. *Drug Metab. Dispos.* **2006**, *34*, 1070–1077.

[45] Devivar, R.; Kawashima, E.; Revenkar, G.; Breitenbach, J. M.; Kreske, E. D.; Drach, J. C.; Townsend, L. B. Benzimidazole ribonucleosides: design, synthesis, and antiviral activity of certain 2-(alkylthio-) and 2-(benzylthio)-5,6-dichloro-1-(β-D-ribofuranosyl)benzimidazoles. *J. Med. Chem.* **1994**, *37*, 2942–2949.

[46] Zou, R.; Ayres, K. R.; Drach, J. C.; Townsend, L. B. Synthesis and antiviral evaluation of certain disubstituted benzimidazole ribonucleosides. *J. Med. Chem.* **1996**, *39*, 3477–3482.

[47] Zou, R.; Drach, J. C.; Townsend, L. B. (**1997**). Design, synthesis, and antiviral evaluation of 2-substituted 4,5-dichloro- and 4,6-dichloro-1-β-D-ribofuranosylbenzimidazoles as potential agents for human cytomegalovirus infections. *J. Med. Chem.* **1997**, *40*, 802–810.

[48] Zou, R.; Drach, J. C.; Townsend, L. B. Design, synthesis, and antiviral evaluation of 2-chloro-5,6-dihalo-1-β-D-ribofuranosylbenzimidazoles as potential agents for human cytomegalovirus infections. *J. Med. Chem.* **1997**, *40*, 811–818.

[49] Hwang, J.-S. Kregler, O. Schilf, R.; Bannert, N.; Drach, J. C.; Townsend, L. B.; Bogner, E. Identification of acetylated, tetrahalogenated benzimidazole D-ribonucleosides with enhanced activity against human cytomegalovirus. *J. Virol.* **2007**, *81*, 11604–11611.

[50] Chien, T.-C.; Saluja, S. S.; Drach, J. C.; Townsend, L. B. Synthesis and antiviral evaluation of polyhalogenated imidazole nucleosides: dimensional analogues of 2,5,6-trihalo-1-(β-D-ribofuranosyl)benzimidazoles. *J. Med. Chem.* **2004**, *47*, 5743–5752.

[51] Zhu, Z.; Drach, J. C.; Townsend, L. B. Synthesis of 2,6,7-trichloro-1-(β-D-ribofuranosyl)naptho[2,3-*d*]imidazole: a linear dimensional analogue of the antiviral agent TCRB. *J. Org. Chem.* **1998**, *63*, 977–983.

[52] Zhu, Z.; Lippa, B.; Drach, J. C.; Townsend, L. B. Design, synthesis, and antiviral evaluation of tricyclic nucleosides (dimensional probes) as analogues of certain antiviral polyhalogenated benzimidazole ribonucleosides. *J. Med. Chem.* **2000**, *43*, 2430–2437.

[53] Townsend, L. B.; Drach, J. C.; Good, S. S.; DaLuge, S. M.; Martin, M. C. Therapeutic nucleosides. U.S. Patent 5,534,535, July 9, 1996.

[54] Chamberlain, S. D.; Daluge, S. M., Koszalka, G. W. Antiviral benzimidazole nucleoside analogues and methods for their preparation. U.S. Patent 5,998,605, Dec. 7, 1999.

[55] Chamberlain, S. D.; Daluge, S. M.; Koszalka, G. W.; Tidwell, J. H.; Drach, J. C.; Townsend, L. B. Antiviral benzimidazole nucleoside analogues and a method for their preparation. U.S. Patent 6,077,832, June 20, 2000.

[56] Chamberlain, S. D.; Koszalka, G. W.; Tidwell, J. H.; van Draanen, N. L-Benzimidazole nucleosides. U.S. Patent 6,204,249, Mar. 20, 2001.

[57] Chamberlain, S. D.; Tidwell, J. H. Benzimidazole and its ribonucleoside. U.S. Patent 6,307,043, Oct. 23, 2001.

[58] Tidwell, J. H.; Chamberlain, S. D.; Freeman, G. A.; Chan, J. H.; Koszalka, G. W.; Townsend, L. B.; Drach, J. C. Benzimidazole derivatives for the treatment of viral infections. U.S. Patent 6,413,938, July 2, 2002.

[59] Biron, K. K.; Harvey, R. J.; Chamberlain, S. C.; Good, S. S.; Smith, A. A., III; Davis, M. G.; Talarico, C. L.; Miller, W. H.; Ferris, R.; Dornsife, R. E.; et al. Potent and selective inhibition of human cytomegalovirus replication by 1263W94: a benzimidazole L-riboside with a unique mode of action. *Antimicrob. Agents Chemother.* **2002**, *46*, 2365–2372.

[60] Koszalka, G. W.; Johnson, N. W.; Good, S. S.; Boyd, L.; Chamberlain, S. C.; Townsend, L. B.; Drach, J. C.; Biron, K. K. Preclinical and toxicology studies of 1263W94, a potent and selective inhibitor of human cytomegalovirus replication. *Antimicrob. Agents Chemother.* **2002**, *46*, 2373–2380.

[61] Gudmundsson, K. S.; Tidwell, J.; Lippa, N.; Koszalka, G. W.; van Draanen, N.; Ptak, R. G.; Drach, J. C.; Townsend, L. B. Synthesis and antiviral evaluation of halogenated β-D- and L-erythrofuranosylbenzimidazoles. *J. Med. Chem.* **2000**, *43*, 2464–2472.

[62] Gudmundsson, K. S.; Freeman, G. A.; Drach, J. C.; Townsend, L. B. Synthesis of fluorosugar analogues of 2,5,6-trihalo-1-(β-D-ribofuranosyl)benzimidazoles. *J. Med. Chem.* **2000**, *43*, 2473–2478.

[63] Saluja, S.; Zou, R.; Drach, J. C.; Townsend, L. B. Structure–activity relationships among 2-substituted 5,6-dichloro-, 4,6-dichloro-, and 4,5-dichloro-1[(2-hydroxyethoxy)methyl]- and 1[(1,3-dihydroxy-2-propoxy) methyl]-benzimidazoles. *J. Med. Chem.* **1996**, *39*, 881–891.

[64] Chan, J. H.; Chamberlain, S. D.; Biron, K. K.; Davis, M. G.; Harvey, R. J.; Selleseth, D. W.; Dornsife, R. E.; Dark, E. H.; Frick. L. W.; Townsend, L. B.; et al. Synthesis and evaluation of a series of 2′-deoxy analogues

of the antiviral agent 5,6-dichloro-2-isopropylamnio-1-(L-ribofuranosyl)-1*H*-benzimidazole (1263W94). *Nucleosides Nucleotides Nucleic Acids* **2000**, *19*, 101–123.

[65] Zou, R.; Kawashima, E.; Freeman, G. A.; Koszalka, G. W.; Drach, J. C.; Townsend, L. B. Design, synthesis and antiviral evaluation of 2-deoxy-D-ribosides of substituted benzimidazoles as potential agents for human cytomegalovirus infections. *Nucleosides Nucleotides* **2000**, *19*, 125–153.

[66] Migawa, M. T.; Girardet, J.-L.; Walker, J. A.; Koszalka, G. A. Chamberlain, S. D.; Drach, J. C.; Townsend, L. B. Design, synthesis, and antiviral activity of α-nucleosides: D- and L-isomers of lyxofuranosyl- and (5-deoxylyxofuranosyl) benzimidazoles. *J. Med. Chem.* **1998**, *41*, 1242–1251.

[67] Drach, J. C.; Townsend, L. B.; Boyd, F. L.; Chamberlain, S. D.; Daluge, S. M.; Deaton, D. N.; Andersen, M. W.; Freeman, G. A. Benzimidazole derivatives. U.S. Patent 6,455,507, Sept. 24, 2002.

[68] Underwood, M. R.; Ferris, R. G.; Selleseth, D. W.; Davis, M. G.; Drach, J. C.; Townsend, L. B.; Biron, K. K.; Boyd, F. L. Mechanism of action of the ribopyranoside benzimidazole GW275175X against human cytomegalovirus. *Antimicrob. Agents Chemother.* **2004**, *48*, 1647–1651.

[69] Gudmundsson, K. S.; Drach, J. C.; Townsend, L. B. Synthesis of the first C3 ribosylated imidazo[1,2-*a*]pyridine C-nucleoside by enantioselective construction of the ribose moiety. *J. Org. Chem.* **1998**, *63*, 984–989.

[70] Chen, J. J.; Wei, Y.; Drach. J. C.; Townsend, L. B. Synthesis and antiviral evaluation of trisubstituted indole *N*-nucleosides as analogues of 2,5,6-trihalo-1-(β-D-ribofuranosyl)benzimidazoles. *J. Med. Chem.* **2000**, *43*, 2449–2456.

[71] Biron, K. K. Following acyclovir: the quest for a more potent anti-CMV drug. Gertrude B Elion Memorial Award Lecture. *Antiviral Res.* **2009**, *82*, 2009. Abstract 15.

[72] Zacny, V. L.; Gershburg, E.; Davis, M. G.; Biron, K. K.; Pagano, J. S. Inhibition of Epstein–Barr virus replication by a benzimidazole L-riboside: novel antiviral mechanism of 5,6-dichloro-2-(isopropylamino)-1-beta-L-ribofuranosyl-1*H*-benzimidazole. *J. Virol.* **1999**, *73*, 7271–7277.

[73] Prichard, M. N. Function of human cytomegalovirus UL97 kinase in viral infection and its inhibition by maribavir. *Rev. Med. Virol.* **2009**, *19*, 215–229.

[74] Williams, S. L.; Hartline, C. B.; Kushner, N. L.; Harden, E. A.; Bidanset, D. J.; Drach, J. C.; Townsend, L. B.; Underwood, M. R.; Biron, K. K.; Kern, E. R. In vitro activities of benzimidazole D- and L-ribonucleosides against herpesviruses. *Antimicrob. Agents Chemother.* **2003**, *47*, 2186–2192.

[75] Truesdale, A. T.; Biron, K. K.; Ellis, B. P.; Miller, W. H.; Wood, E. R. Mode of inhibition studies with MBV and the CMV kinase UL97. 32nd International Herpesvirus Workshop, Asheville, NC, 2007. Abstract 10.27.

[76] Jault, F. M.; Jault, J. M.; Ruchti, F.; Fortunato, E. A.; Clark, C.; Corbeil, J.; Richman, D. D.; Spector, D. H. Cytomegalovirus infection induces high levels of cyclins, phosphorylated Rb, and p53, leading to cell cycle arrest. *J. Virol.* **1995**, *69*, 6697–6704.

[77] Komazin, G.; Ptak, R. G.; Emmer, B. T.; Townsend, L. B.; Drach, J. C. Resistance of human cytomegalovirus to the benzimidazole L-ribonucleoside maribavir maps to UL27. *J. Virol.* **2003**, *77*, 11499–11506.

[78] Chou, S.; Marousek, G. I.; Senters, A. E.; Davis, M. G.; Biron, K. K. Mutations in the human cytomegalovirus UL27 gene that confer resistance to maribavir. *J. Virol.* **2004**, *78*, 7124–7130.

[78a] Reitsma, J.M.; Savaryn, J.P.; Faust, K.; Sato, H.; Halligan, B.D.; Terkune, S.S. Antiviral inhibition targeting the HCMV kinase pUL97 requires pUL27-dependent degradation of Tip60 acetyltransferase and cell-cycle arrest. *Cell Host Microbe* **2011**, *9*, 103–114.

[79] Sullivan, V.; Talarico, C. L.; Stanat, S. C.; Davis, M.; Coen, D. M.; Biron, K. K. A protein kinase homologue controls phosphorylation of ganciclovir in human cytomegalovirus-infected cells. *Nature* **1992**, *359*, 85.

[80] Prichard, M. N.; Gao, N.; Jairath, S.; Mulamba, G.; Krosky, P.; Coen, D. M.; Parker, B. O.; Pari, G. S. A recombinant human cytomegalovirus with a large deletion in UL97 has a severe replication deficiency. *J. Virol.* **1999**, *73*, 5663–5670.

[81] Krosky, P. M.; Baek, M. C.; Jahng, W. J.; Barrera, I.; Harvey, R. J.; Biron, K. K.; Coen, D. M.; Sethna, P. B. The human cytomegalovirus UL44 protein is a substrate for the UL97 protein kinase. *J. Virol.* **2003**, *77*, 7720–7727.

[82] Marschall, M.; Freitag, M.; Suchy, P.; Romaker, D.; Kupfer, R.; Hanke, M.; Stamminger, T. The protein kinase pUL97 of human cytomegalovirus interacts with and phosphorylates the DNA polymerase processivity factor pUL44. *Virology* **2003**, *311*, 60–71.

[83] Wolf, D. G.; Courcelle, C. T.; Prichard, M. N.; Mocarski, E. S. Distinct and separate roles for herpesvirus-conserved UL97 kinase in cytomegalovirus DNA synthesis and encapsidation. *Proc. Nat. Acad. Sci. USA* **2001**, *98*, 1895–1900.

[84] Kamil, J. P.; Coen, D. M. Human cytomegalovirus protein kinase UL97 forms a complex with the tegument phosphoprotein pp65. *J. Virol.* **2007**, *81*, 10659–10668.

[85] Prichard, M. N.; Sztul, E.; Daily, S. L.; Perry, A. L.; Frederick, S. L.; Gill, R. B.; Hartline, C. B.; Streblow, D. N.; Varnum, S. M.; Smith, R. D.; Kern, E. R. Human cytomegalovirus UL97 kinase activity is required for the hyperphosphorylation of retinoblastoma protein and inhibits the formation of nuclear aggresomes. *J. Virol.* **2008**, *82*, 5054–5067.

[86] Krosky, P. M.; Baek, M. C.; Coen, D. M. The human cytomegalovirus UL97 protein kinase, an antiviral drug target, is required at the stage of nuclear egress. *J. Virol.* **2003**, *77*, 905–914.

[87] Marschall, M.; Marzi, A.; aus dem Siepen P.; Jochmann, R.; Kalmer, M.; Auerochs, S.; Lischka, P.; Leis, M.; Stamminger, T. Cellular p32 recruits cytomegalovirus kinase pUL97 to redistribute the nuclear lamina. *J. Biol. Chem.* **2005**, *280*, 33357–33367.

[88] Baek, M. C.; Krosky, P. M.; Pearson, A.; Coen, D. M. Phosphorylation of the RNA polymerase II carboxyl-terminal domain in human cytomegalovirus-infected cells and in vitro by the viral UL97 protein kinase. *Virology* **2004**, *324*, 184–193.

[89] Kawaguchi, Y.; Matsumura, T.; Roizman, B.; Hirai, K. Cellular elongation factor 1delta is modified in cells infected with representative alpha-, beta-, or gammaherpesviruses. *J. Virol.* **1999**, *73*, 4456–4460.

[90] Kawaguchi, Y.; Kato, K. Protein kinases conserved in herpesviruses potentially share a function mimicking the cellular protein kinase cdc2. *Rev. Med. Virol.* **2003**, *13*, 331–340.

[91] Michel, D.; Mertens, T. The UL97 protein kinase of human cytomegalovirus and homologues in other herpesviruses: impact on virus and host. *Acta Biochim. t Biophys.* **2004**, *1697*, 169–180.

[92] Hume, A. J.; Finkel, J. S.; Kamil, J. P.; Coen, D. M.; Culbertson, M. R.; Kalejta, R. F. Phosphorylation of retinoblastoma protein by viral protein with cyclin-dependent kinase function. *Science* **2008**, *320*, 797–799.

[93] Chou, S.; Van Wechel, L. C.; Marousek, G. I. Effect of cell culture conditions on the anticytomegalovirus activity of maribavir. *Antimicrob. Agents Chemother.* **2006**, *50*, 2557–2559.

[94] Kern, E. R.; Hartline, C. B.; Rybak, R. J.; Drach, J. C.; Townsend, L. B.; Biron, K. K.; Bidanset, D. J. Activities of benzimidazole D- and L-ribonucleosides in animal models of cytomegalovirus infections. *Antimicrob. Agents Chemother.* **2004**, *48*, 1749–1755.

[95] Chee, M. S.; Lawrence, G. L.; Barrell, B. G. Alpha-, beta-, and gammaherpesviruses encode a putative phosphotransferase. *J. Gen. Virol.* **1989**, *70*(Pt. 5), 1151–1160.

[96] Hanks, S. K.; Quinn, A. M.; Hunter, T. The protein kinase family: conserved features and deduced phylogeny of the catalytic domains. *Science* **1988**, *241*, 42–52.

[97] Smith, R. F.; Smith, T. F. Identification of new protein kinase-related genes in three herpesviruses, herpes simplex virus, varicella-zoster virus, and Epstein–Barr virus. *J. Virol.* **1989**, *63*, 450–455.

[98] Coulter, L. J.; Moss, H. W.; Lang, J.; McGeoch, D. J. A mutant of herpes simplex virus type 1 in which the UL13 protein kinase gene is disrupted. *J. Gen. Virol.* **1993**, *74*(Pt. 3), 387–395.

[99] Moffat, J. F.; Zerboni, L.; Sommer, M. H.; Heineman, T. C.; Cohen, J. I.; Kaneshima, H.; Arvin, A. M. The ORF47 and ORF66 putative protein kinases of varicella-zoster virus determine tropism for human T cells and skin in the SCID-hu mouse. *Proc. Nat. Acad. Sci. USA* **1998**, *95*, 11969–11974.

[100] Biron, K.; Maribavir: a promising new antiherpes therapeutic agent. In *New Concepts of Antiviral Therapy*, Bogner, E., Holzenburg, A., Eds., Springer-Verlag, New York, 2006.

[101] Wang, L. H.; Peck, R. W.; Yin, Y.; Allanson, J.; Wiggs, R.; Wire, M. B. Phase I safety and pharmacokinetic trials of 1263W94, a novel oral anti-human cytomegalovirus agent, in healthy and human immunodeficiency virus-infected subjects. *Antimicrob. Agents Chemother.* **2003**, *47*, 1334–1342.

[102] Lalezari, J. P.; Aberg, J. A.; Wang, L. H.; Wire, M. B.; Miner, R.; Snowden, W.; Talarico, C. L.; Shaw, S.; Jacobson, M. A.; Drew, W. L. Phase I dose escalation trial evaluating the pharmacokinetics, anti-human cytomegalovirus (HCMV) activity, and safety of 1263W94 in human immunodeficiency virus-infected men with asymptomatic HCMV shedding. *Antimicrob. Agents Chemother.* **2002**, *46*, 2969–2976.

[103] Hendrix, C.; Kuppermann, B. D.; Dunn, J. P.; Wang, L. H.; Starns, E.; Snowden, B. W.; Hamzeh, F.; Wire, M. B. A phase I trial to evaluate the ocular (intravitreal) penetration of 1263W94 after multiple dose, oral administration in AIDS patients with CMV retinitis. Interscience Conference on Antimicrobial Agents and Chemotherapy, Toronto, Ontario, Canada, 2000.

[104] Lu, H.; Thomas, S. Maribavir (ViroPharma). *Curr. Opin. Invest. Drugs* **2004**, *5*, 898–906.

[105] Ma, J. D.; Nafziger, A. N.; Villano, S. A.; Victory, J.; Bertino, J. S. Single and multiple dose pharmacokinetics (PK) of maribavir (MB) in healthy adults. American Society for Clinical Pharmacology and Therapeutics (ASCPT) Annual Meeting, Orlando, Florida, FL, 2005.

[106] ViroPharma, Inc. Press release, Mar. 29, 2006. Viro Pharma announces positive Phase 2 results demonstrating that Maribavir significantly reduces CMV reactivation. Available at http://www2.prnewswire.com/cgi-bin/stories.pl?ACCT=104&STORY=/www/story/03-29-2006/0004329626&EDATE=. Accessed Oct. 6, 2009.

[107] ViroPharma, Inc. Press release, Feb. 13, 2009. ViroPharma announces discontinuation of Maribavir Phase 3 Study in liver transplant patients. Available at http://phx.corporate-ir.net/phoenix.zhtml?c=92320&p=irol-newsArticle&ID=1256496&highlight=. Accessed Oct. 6, 2009.

[108] Avery, R.; Marty, F.; Strasfeld, L.; Lee, I.; Arrieta, A.; Chou, S.; Villano, S. Oral maribavir (MBV) for treatment of resistant or refractory cytomegalovirus (CMV) infections in transplant recipients. 49th Interscience Conference on Antimicrobial Agents and Chemotherapy, San Francisco, 2009.

[109] Chou, S.; Marousek, G. I. Accelerated evolution of maribavir resistance in a cytomegalovirus exonuclease domain II mutant. *J. Virol.* **2008**, *82*, 246–253.

INDEX

(*S*)-9-(2,3-dihydroxypropyl)adenine [(*S*)-DHPA], 85
1263W94, 423
3TC (lamivudine), 64, 88, 96, 103, 108, 113, 191, 415
4-hydroxycoumarins, 48, 49
9-(2-phosphonylmethoxyethyl)adenine (PMEA), 99

A-33903, 369
Abacavir, 64, 69, 87, 88, 97, 98, 103
ABC (abacavir), 64, 69, 87, 88, 97, 98, 103
α-ketoamide, 159, 162, 212, 213, 240, 245, 250, 251, 252, 274, 330
Anti-influenza drug, 386, 389, 394, 396
Antiviral therapy, 169, 220, 254, 317, 322, 402
ARTEMIS, 37, 39, 40, 41
Aspartyl protease, 20, 24, 30, 42, 47, 49, 50
Asymmetric synthesis, 50, 51
Atazanavir, 3
Atripla, 88
Atropisomer, 140, 147, 178
Attachment, 118, 146, 150, 151, 152, 155, 156, 158, 159, 160, 329, 336, 341, 350, 368
Azapeptide, 3
Azt (zidovudine), 52, 64, 87, 90, 97, 103, 109, 115, 149

Balapiravir, 287
BALB/c mouse model, 347, 348, 356
Banana streak virus (BSV), 85
Baraclude, 414
BDCRB, 418
Benzimidazol-2-one, 355–362
Benzimidazole ribosides, 420, 429
Benzodiazepine, 369, 370, 375, 379
Benzotriazole, 280, 355, 363
BI 201335, 225, 234
BILN 2061, 225, 227, 230, 234, 273, 274, 276, 277, 291
bis-(5-amidino-2-benzimidazolyl)methane (BABIM), 361, 363
bis(isopropyloxycarbonyloxymethyl)-[(*R*)-9-(2-phosphonylpropyl)adenine], 88
bis(POC)-PMPA, 88
BMS 262362, 3
BMS-378806, 118, 152–155, 159–161
BMS-433771, 358–363, 368
BMS-488043, 152
BMS-663749, 155
Boceprevir, 229, 239, 249–252, 263, 274

Caco-2, 119, 121, 152, 154, 158, 276, 292, 296
CASTLE, 13, 14, 16, 17
CCR5, 15, 50, 117, 137, 181
CD4, 13, 36, 118, 124, 127, 128, 130, 134, 137, 145, 149, 151, 159, 160, 161, 191, 192, 193
CD81, 329, 331, 336
Celsentri, 181
Chronic hepatitis B, 88, 92, 99
Chronic hepatitis C, 257, 305, 313
Cidofovir [(*S*)-HPMPC], 85
Clinical isolate, 11, 33, 52, 63, 76, 81, 88, 109, 154, 159, 163, 262, 321, 358, 370, 373, 396
Combination therapy, 14, 42, 52, 59, 67, 93, 149, 190, 234, 235, 257, 267, 282, 284, 300, 321, 329, 334, 336, 412
Concatemer, 418
Cotton rat, 346–349, 352, 355–357, 361, 368, 381
Covalent inhibitor, 225, 257
Cyclooctylpyranones, 49
Cyclophilin, 317–324
Cyclosporin, 318–324
CYP3A4, 3, 7, 12, 25, 69, 108, 121, 133, 144, 155, 185, 189, 332, 379, 427
Cytochrome P450 3A, 12, 53

Antiviral Drugs: From Basic Discovery Through Clinical Trials, First Edition. Edited by Wieslaw M. Kazmierski.

d4T (stavudine), 103, 394
Darunavir, 19, 22, 31, 41, 56, 64, 89, 94, 192, 270
ddC (zalcitabine), 103
DDE motif, 198
ddI (didanosine), 13, 87, 88, 90, 92, 94
Diazirine, 359, 360, 362
Didanosine (ddI), 13, 87, 88, 90, 92, 94
Dihydropyrone, 49
Dihydroxypyrimidines, 185
Diketo acid, 163, 169, 170, 180, 182, 194, 197, 199
DIONE, 41
Direct antiviral, 216, 257, 264, 284, 318
DMPK, 50, 184, 296
D-ribo, 418, 420, 421, 423, 424
Drug resistance, 19, 22, 23, 29, 31, 268, 319, 396, 397, 428
Drug-drug interactions, 185, 189
DUET, 37, 77

Efavirenz, 12, 13, 14, 74, 92, 148, 195
Efficacy (antiviral), 67, 89, 145, 202, 233, 263, 287, 299, 317, 321, 325, 378, 366, 380, 407, 410
Elvitegravir, 15, 77, 89, 170, 197, 202
Emtricitabine (FTC), 65, 87, 89, 90, 93, 94, 97, 100, 103, 149, 160, 411, 415
Enfuvirtide Fuzeon, 54, 55, 77, 94, 118, 181, 192, 194, 202
Entecavir, 92, 401
Entry inhibitor, 56, 149, 151, 161, 329, 330, 333, 336
Etravirine, 37, 71, 94

FTC (emtricitabine), 65, 87, 89, 90, 93, 94, 97, 100, 103, 149, 160, 411, 415
Fusion inhibitor, 59, 94, 117, 129, 181, 202, 342, 345, 347, 349, 353, 356, 361–365, 368, 369, 371
Fusion protein (F protein), 216, 341, 343, 359, 380

Genetic barrier, 82, 186, 193, 264, 270, 289, 317, 322, 323, 325, 363, 411, 416
gp120, 118, 124, 128, 149, 151
GS-9137, 89, 170, 197
GW275175X, 419, 424

HAART, 29, 31, 424
HCV polymerase, 182, 185, 222, 291, 300
HCV protease inhibitor, 210, 220, 273, 288, 331
HCV replicon, 216, 221, 263, 264, 265, 287, 289, 290, 298, 300, 308, 321, 322, 323
HDP (hexadecyloxypropyl)-cidofovir, 88
HEP-2 cells, 358
Hepatitis B, 55, 85, 92, 95, 191, 383, 401, 407, 413
Hepatitis B virus (HBV), 55, 85, 88, 92, 401, 405, 413
Hepatitis C, 55, 79, 194, 207, 209, 220, 222, 225, 236, 239, 250, 254, 273, 282, 287, 305, 317, 325, 329, 402
Hepatitis C virus, 209, 220, 225, 250, 254, 287, 305, 313, 317, 329
Hepatocyte, 11, 25, 63, 108, 156, 171, 177, 180, 189, 209, 239, 262, 278, 326, 330, 333, 406, 413
hERG, 109, 119, 122, 125, 140, 250, 379
Herpesvirus, 88, 289, 402, 403, 417–419, 425, 430
High genetic barrier, 163, 263, 412
Highly active antiretroviral therapy, 16, 19, 29, 59, 88, 98, 103, 114, 117, 149, 408
HIV integrase mutants, 187, 193
HIV protease inhibitor, 13, 15, 47, 48, 49, 56, 110, 149, 170
HIV-1 protease inhibitor, 3, 4, 15, 19, 29, 42, 48, 56, 262, 267
Host cell, 104, 181, 273, 305, 329, 335, 336, 341
Host factor, 317–325
Human airway epithelial (HAE) model, 373
Human cytomegalovirus, 149, 417, 419, 422, 429
Human immunodeficiency virus, 1, 15, 19, 30, 31, 42, 56, 71, 85, 114, 197, 203, 254, 358, 402
Human rhinovirus, 358
Hydroxyethylene isostere, 3

Influenza virus, 381, 385
Integrase, 15, 56, 59, 94, 151, 163, 181, 197
Integrase inhibitor, 15, 56, 94, 163, 177, 181, 182, 186, 193, 197, 199, 201
Integration, 182, 195, 198, 203, 321
INTELENCE, 35, 71
InterMune, 257, 269
Isentress, 181, 187, 190, 193
ITMN-191, 239, 257, 258, 262

JNJ-2408068, 342, 343–345, 368
JTK-303, 197

Ketoamide, 159, 212, 213, 240, 245, 247, 250, 251, 252, 330
Keto-enol acid, 197

Lamivudine (3TC), 64, 88, 96, 103, 108, 113, 191, 415
Lamivudine-refractory, 408, 409, 412
Lipophilicity, 119, 142, 184, 293, 296, 392
Log P, 55, 75, 119, 169, 184, 292, 296, 333, 369
L-ribo, 314, 422

Macrocyclic inhibitor, 226, 227, 242, 243, 245, 253, 263, 266, 276
Maraviroc, 15, 56, 77, 83, 94, 117, 145, 181
Maribavir, 419, 423
MBV, 419, 424–429
MK-0536, 163
MMMF, 167, 169, 178
Monoketo acid, 197
Monotherapy, 13, 15, 17, 31, 41, 65, 83, 88, 92, 111, 127, 140, 144, 155, 190, 202, 234, 257, 263–269, 299, 334, 413
Motaviizumab (Numax), 353
Murine (Moloney) sarcoma virus, 85

N protein, 380
Neuraminidase, 385, 396, 397
NIM811, 318–323
N-methylpyrimidones, 185
NNRTI, 35, 52, 59, 72, 78, 81, 103, 149
NNRTI-resistant HIV-1, 77, 78, 81
Noncovalent, 225, 262, 273
Non-nucleoside reverse transcriptase inhibitor, 59, 184,
NRTI, 19, 29, 35, 69, 71, 89, 92, 103, 109, 113, 149

NS3 protease, 209, 210, 214, 221, 225, 226, 230, 235, 241, 244, 251, 287, 322, 323
NS3 protease inhibitor, 220, 323
NS3/4A inhibitor, 259, 263, 273
NS5B, 182, 257, 264, 268, 282, 286, 291, 305, 309, 312, 317, 319, 324
NtRTI, 87, 89, 94, 103
Nucleoside, 14, 35, 44, 59, 71, 85, 93, 94, 103, 109, 117, 149, 181, 264, 279, 287, 287, 289, 305, 323, 401, 421, 425

ODE (octadecyloxyethyl)-cidofovir, 88
Oral bioavailability, 3, 7, 12, 15, 24, 48, 50, 75, 88, 119, 139, 153, 183, 189, 231, 264, 276, 293, 297, 303, 310, 313, 333, 361, 369, 380, 393
Otitis media, 353
Oxadiazole, 158, 187, 189

Palivizumab (Synagis), 353, 354, 367
Parainfluenza-3 virus, 354, 358, 367, 381
Peginterferon, 209, 220, 221, 264, 268, 334
Pegylated interferon, 209, 257, 273, 299, 305, 317, 325, 329, 412
Peptidomimetic, 24, 47, 226
Permeability, 75, 121, 150, 153, 156, 158, 160, 169, 183, 225, 259, 276, 292, 296, 357
PF-232798, 117
Pharmacophore, 48, 139
Pharmasset, 269, 305
Photoaffinity reagent, 359
PL-100, 19
PMPApp, 87
PMPDAPpp, 88
Pneumovirus, 367
Polymerase, 88, 90, 95, 104, 109, 182, 185, 216, 222, 257, 264, 273, 287, 289, 291, 300, 305, 309, 317, 322, 368, 380, 402, 411
POWER, 35
PPL-100, 19, 24, 25
Predicted human clearance, 171, 177
Pre-exposure prophylaxis (PrEP), 100
Prezista, 31
Prodrug, 19, 24, 88, 94, 155, 156, 159, 292, 294–297, 302, 310, 312, 392, 402, 417
Protease inhibitor, 3, 11, 13, 19, 31, 42, 47, 52, 54, 77, 92, 98, 103, 110, 117, 143, 145, 149, 170, 181, 192, 197, 210, 212, 216, 220, 234, 237, 257, 273, 279, 284, 291, 302, 323, 331, 363
Protein binding, 7, 13, 27, 34, 40, 52, 123, 143, 153, 159, 169, 183, 190, 265, 278, 333, 361, 424, 427
PSI-6130, 291, 305, 306–314
Pyranoside, 423, 424

QT_c prolongation, 140

R1479, 289, 291–299, 306, 307
R1626, 287, 292, 297, 299, 301
R7227, 257, 268, 426
Raltegravir, 15, 42, 45, 56, 77, 83, 94, 163, 181, 187, 199
Replicon, 213–216, 220–221, 230, 244, 247, 252–3, 259–260, 263–266, 276, 288, 289, 291–292, 298, 300, 307, 310, 312, 318, 321
Resistance selection assay, 344
Respiratory syncytial virus (RSV), 341, 353,, 355, 360, 367, 380
Reversible inhibitor, 182, 211
RG7128, 305, 310, 312, 313
Ribavirin, 220, 22, 230, 239, 252, 257, 267, 273, 282, 284, 287, 292, 300, 305, 312, 313, 317, 325, 329, 341, 352, 354, 367, 371, 374, 381, 394, 395
Ribonucleoside, 114, 292, 306, 417, 420
Rilpivirine, 59
Ritonavir, 9, 11, 14, 29, 47, 54, 55, 89, 147
Ritonavir boosting, 29, 53, 55
RNA-dependent RNA polymerase, 182, 273, 288, 305, 306, 322
Roche, 21, 118, 132, 269, 287, 289, 299, 301, 393, 417, 427
RSV long A strain, 363
RSV604, 371

Scavenger receptor B-1, 330
SCH 417690, 137
Sch 503034, 249
Sch-6, 244, 249
SCH-D, 137
Sendai virus, 354, 358
Serine protease, 211, 212, 225, 231, 236, 239, 257, 261, 273, 317, 363
Serine trap, 240, 252
Serine-139, 239, 251
Sialic acid, 395
Sialidase, 385
STAT-C, 220, 222, 238, 302, 314
Stavudine (d4T), 103, 394
Strand transfer, 163, 169, 182, 195, 197, 201
Structure-based drug design, 210, 240, 255, 389, 396

TCRB, 418
Telaprevir, 209, 210, 213, 257, 263, 266, 274
Tenofovir disoproxil fumarate (TDF), 88
Terminase, 419
Tetrahydronaphthyridine, 163
Time-of-addition experiment, 149, 343, 345, 347, 349, 358
Tipranavir, 19, 22, 33, 38, 47, 77, 94, 110, 111
Tissue retention, 342, 344, 345
TITAN, 33, 36, 37
TMC114, 31, 32, 34, 36, 37, 39, 42
TMC278, 59
TMC278-C201, 65
TMC278-C204, 65
TMC278-C209 (ECHO), 66
TMC278-C215 (THRIVE), 66
TMC353121, 344
TMC-353121, 364
TMC435, 239, 273
Tropism, 127, 130, 132, 426
Truvada, 88
TVR, 221

UGT1A1, 12, 108, 189, 332
UL104, 419
UL27, 426

UL56, 419
UL89, 419
UL97, 425
Unboosted atazanavir, 12
Unconjugated bilirubin, 236

Vicriviroc, 15, 119, 132, 137
Viral load, 31, 36, 38, 41, 53, 65, 78, 90, 111–113, 118, 121, 145, 155, 191, 193, 202, 221, 231–236, 257, 264, 268, 282, 289, 299, 300, 325, 333, 349, 380, 427
Viral resistance, 19, 47, 79, 114, 192, 266, 313
VP-14637, 368

X-ray crystal structure, 24, 48, 55, 252, 258, 386
XTT assay, 368, 370, 371

Zalcitabine (ddC), 103
Zidovudine (AZT), 52, 64, 87, 90, 97, 103, 109, 115, 149

Printed in the USA/Agawam, MA
September 21, 2026

910661.040